Yearbook of Intensive Care and Emergency Medicine

Edited by J.-L. Vincent

Yearbook of Intensive Care and Emergency Medicine 2009

Edited by J.-L. Vincent

With 172 Figures and 96 Tables

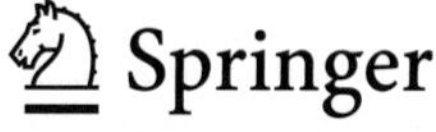

Prof. Jean-Louis Vincent
Head, Department of Intensive Care
Erasme Hospital, Université libre de Bruxelles
Route de Lennik 808, B-1070 Brussels, Belgium

ISBN 978-3-540-92275-9 Springer-Verlag Berlin Heidelberg New York

ISSN 0942-5381

Springer is a part of Springer Science+Business Media
springer.com

Typesetting: FotoSatz Pfeifer GmbH, D-82166 Gräfelfing
Printing: Stürtz GmbH, D-97080 Würzburg

21/3150 – 5 4 3 2 1 0 – Printed on acid-free paper

Table of Contents

IV Proposed Targets for New Therapies

V Septic Shock

VI Intravenous Fluids

VII Hemodynamic Support

VIII Airway Management

IX Mechanical Ventilation

X Respiratory Monitoring

XI Perioperative Management

XVI Nutrition

XVII Glucose Control

XVIII Adrenal Function

XIX Coagulation

XX Neurological Aspects

XXI Malignancies

XXII Drug Dosing

XXIII Sedation and Analgesia

XXIV ICU Management

XXV End-of-Life Issues

List of Contributors

Abdel-Razeq SS
Section of Trauma, Surgical Critical Care, and Surgical Emergencies
Yale University School of Medicine
330 Cedar Street, BB-310
New Haven, CT 06520
USA

Abraham E
Department of Medicine
University of Alabama at Birmingham
BDB 420, 1530 3rd Avenue S
Birmingham, AL 35294–0012
USA

Ackland GL
Department of Anesthesia
Stanford University Medical Center
300 Pasteur Drive
Stanford, CA 94305
USA

Adams F
Department of Intensive Care
Princess Alexandra Hospital
Ipswich Road
Brisbane, QLD 4102
Australia

Aguilar G
Department of Anesthesiology and Critical Care
Hospital Clinico Universitario de Valencia
Avenida Blasco Ibanez 17
46010 Valencia
Spain

Ali FSM
Department of Emergency Medicine
King Fahad Specialist Hospital
PO Box 15215
Dammam 31444
Saudi Arabia

Ali NA
Division of Pulmonary, Allergy, Critical Care, and Sleep Medicine
Department of Internal Medicine
201G DHLRI
Columbus, OH 43210
USA

Amato MBP
Respiratory Intensive Care Unit
University of Sao Paulo School of Medicine
Av Dr Arnaldo 455
01246–903 Sao Paulo, SP
Brazil

Araujo DV
Department of Internal Medicine
Medical Sciences School
Universidade do Estado do Rio de Janeiro
Rio de Janeiro
Brazil

Asfar P
Department of Intensive Care and Hyperbaric Medicine
Centre Hospitalo-Universitaire
Rue Dominique Larrrey
49933 Angers
France

Azoulay E
Department of Intensive Care
Hôpital Saint-Louis
1 Avenue Claude Vellefaux
75010 Paris
France

Baessler B
Department of Anesthesiology
and Intensive Care
University of Bonn
Sigmund-Freud-Str. 25
53105 Bonn
Germany

Baudouin S
Department of Anesthesia
Royal Victoria Infirmary
Queen Victoria Road
Newcastle upon Tyne, NE2 4HH
United Kingdom

Beale R
Department of Adult Critical Care
Guy's and St Thomas' NHS Foundation
Trust
St Thomas' Hospital, 1st Floor East Wing
Westminster Bridge Road
London, SE1 7EH
United Kingdom

Beck J
Department of Pediatrics
St Michael's Hospital
30 Bond Street
Toronto, ON M5B 1W8
Canada

Belda FJ
Department of Anesthesiology
and Critical Care
Hospital Clinico Universitario de
Valencia
Avenida Blasco Ibanez 17
46010 Valencia
Spain

Benoit DD
Department of Intensive Care
Ghent University Hospital
De Pintelaan 185
9000 Ghent
Belgium

Berg A
Department of Anesthesia and
Intensive Care
Karolinska Institute
Huddinge University
14186 Stockholm
Sweden

Berg RA
Department of Anesthesiology
and Critical Care
The Children's Hospital of Philadelphia
34th Street and Civic Center Boulevard
Philadelphia, PA 19104
USA

Berger MM
Department of Adult Intensive Care
and Burns
Centre Hospitalier Universitaire
Vaudois
Rue du Bugnon 47
1011 Lausanne
Switzerland

Boer W
Department of Nephrology
Atrium Medical Center
6410 CX Heerlen
Netherlands

Böhm SH
CSEM Nanomedicine Division
Research Centre for Nanomedicine
Schulstrasse 1
7302 Landquart
Switzerland

Brady W
Department of Emergency Medicine
University of Virginia Health System
1215 Lee Street
Charlottesville, VA 22908-0699
USA

Brander L
Department of Intensive Care
University Hospital Inselspital
30110 Bern
Switzerland

Breukers RMBGE
Department of Intensive Care
VU University Medical Center
De Boelelaan 1117
1081 HV Amsterdam
Netherlands

Brunkhorst FM
Department of Anesthesiology
and Intensive Care
Friedrich-Schiller University
Erlanger Allee 101
07743 Jena
Germany

Camporota L
Department of Adult Critical Care
Guy's and St Thomas' NHS Foundation
Trust
St Thomas' Hospital, 1st Floor East Wing
Westminster Bridge Road
London, SE1 7EH
United Kingdom

Chanques G
Intensive Care Unit, Department of
Anesthesiology (DAR B)
CHU, Hôpital Saint Eloi
80 avenue Augustin Fiche
34295 Montpellier Cedex 5
France

Chen J
The Simpson Center for Health Systems
Research
Liverpool Hospital
Locked Bag 7103
Liverpool BC, NSW 1871
Australia

Chinnery P
Mitochondrial Research Group
Institute of Ageing and Health
Newcastle University
Newcastle upon Tyne, NE2 4HH
United Kingdom

Chiolero RL
Department of Adult Intensive Care
and Burns
Centre Hospitalier Universitaire
Vaudois
Rue du Bugnon 47
1011 Lausanne
Switzerland

Cinel I
Department of Critical Care
Cooper University Hospital
One Cooper Plaza
Dorrance Building, Suite 393
Camden, NJ 08103
USA

Cohen J
General Intensive Care Unit
Rabin Medical Center
Campus Beilinson
Petah Tikva 49100
Israel

Cook D
Department of Anesthesia, Critical
Care and Pain
Birmingham Heartlands Hospital
Bordesley Green East
Birmingham, B9 5SS
United Kingdom

Corrêa F
Department of Anesthesiology
and Intensive Care
Friedrich-Schiller University
Erlanger Allee 103
07743 Jena
Germany

Costa ELV
Respiratory Intensive Care Unit
University of Sao Paulo School
of Medicine
Av Dr Arnaldo 455
01246–903 Sao Paulo, SP
Brazil

Costa MG
Department of Anesthesia and Intensive Care
Azienda Ospedaliero-Universitaria S.M. della Misericordia
P.le S. M. Misericordia 15
33100 Udine
Italy

Creagh-Brown BC
Department of Critical Care
Royal Brompton Hospital
Sydney Street
London, SW3 6NP
United Kingdom

Darmon M
Department of Intensive Care
Hôpital Saint-Louis
1 Avenue Claude Vellefaux
75010 Paris
France

Davies SJ
Department of Anesthetics
York Hospital
Wigginton Road
York, YO31 8HE
United Kingdom

Decruyenaere JM
Department of Intensive Care
Ghent University Hospital
De Pintelaan 185
9000 Ghent
Belgium

De laet IE
Department of Intensive Care
ZNA Stuivenberg
Lange Beeldekensstraat 267
2060 Antwerp
Belgium

Della Rocca G
Department of Anesthesia and Intensive Care
Azienda Ospedaliero-Universitaria S.M. della Misericordia
P.le S. M. Misericordia 15
33100 Udine
Italy

Dellinger RP
Department of Critical Care Medicine
Cooper University Hospital
One Cooper Plaza
Dorrance Building, Suite 393
Camden, NJ 08103
USA

DeMichele SJ
Strategic and International R & D
Abbott Nutrition
3300 Stelzer Road
Columbus, OH 43219
USA

Depuydt PO
Department of Intensive Care
Ghent University Hospital
De Pintelaan 185
9000 Ghent
Belgium

Devarajan P
Department of Nephrology and Hypertension
Cincinnati Children's Hospital Medical Center
University of Cincinnati
3333 Burnet Avenue
Cincinnati, OH 45229-3039
USA

De Waele JJ
Surgical Intensive Care Unit
Ghent University Hospital
De Pintelaan 185
9000 Ghent
Belgium

Draisma A
Department of Intensive Care
Radboud University Nijmegen Medical Center
PO Box 9101
6500 HB Nijmegen
Netherlands

Dubin A
Unit of Applied Pharmacology
Faculty of Medical Science
La Plata National University
1900 La Plata, Buenos Aires
Argentina

Dupont H
Department of Anesthesiology
and Intensive Care
Centre Hospitalier Universitaire
d'Amiens
Place Victor Pauchet
80054 Amiens Cedex
France

Duranteau J
Department of Anesthesiology
and Surgical Intensive Care
CHU de Bicêtre
78 rue du Général Leclerc
94275 Le Kremlin Bicêtre Cedex
France

Edul VSK
Unit of Applied Pharmacology
Faculty of Medical Science
La Plata National University
1900 La Plata, Buenos Aires
Argentina

Enkhbaatar P
Investigational Intensive Care Unit
Department of Anesthesiology
The University of Texas Medical Branch
301 University Blvd
Galveston, TX 77555-0833
USA

Ertmer C
Department of Anesthesiology
and Intensive Care
University Hosptial of Münster
Albert-Schweitzer-Str. 33
48149 Münster
Germany

Esen F
Department of Anesthesiology
and Intensive Care
Medical Faculty of Istanbul
University of Istanbul
Capa Klinikleri
34093 Istanbul
Turkey

Evans TW
Department of Critical Care
Royal Brompton Hospital
Sydney Street
London, SW3 6NP
United Kingdom

Ferguson ND
Toronto Western Hospital
399 Bathurst Street, 2MCL-411M
Toronto, ON M5T 2S8
Canada

Ferrando C
Department of Anesthesiology
and Critical Care
Hospital Clinico Universitario de
Valencia
Avenida Blasco Ibanez 17
46010 Valencia
Spain

Gabriella C
Department of Anesthesia and
Intensive Care
Azienda Ospedaliero-Universitaria S.M.
della Misericordia
P.le S. M. Misericordia 15
33100 Udine
Italy

Gallo D
Department of Emergency Medicine
University of Virginia Health System
1215 Lee Street
Charlottesville, VA 22908-0699
USA

Gama de Abreu M
Department of Anesthesiology
and Intensive Care
University Hospital Carl Gustav Carus
Fetscherstr. 74
01307 Dresden
Germany

Gao-Smith F
Department of Anesthesia, Critical
Care and Pain
Birmingham Heartlands Hospital
Bordesley Green East
Birmingham, B9 5SS
United Kingdom

GAUGLITZ GG
Department of Dermatology
and Allergology
Ludwig Maximilians University
Frauenlobstrasse 9–11
80337 Munich
Germany

GIAMARELLOS-BOURBOULIS EJ
4th Department of Internal Medicine
Attikon University Hospital
1 Rimini Street
Athens, 124 62
Greece

GONZALEZ LIMA R
Department of Mechanical Engineering
Escola Politecnica
University of Sao Paulo
Av Prof Melo Moraes 2231
05508–030 Sao Paulo, SP
Brazil

GOODMAN S
General Intensive Care Unit
Department of Anesthesiology
and Critical Care
Hadassah Hebrew University Medical
Center
PO Box 12000
Jerusalem, 91120
Israel

GREEN DW
Department of Anesthesiology
King's College Hospital
Denmark Hill
London, SE5 9RS
United Kingdom

GRIFFITHS RD
Pathophysiology Unit
School of Clinical Sciences
University of Liverpool
Liverpool, L69 3GA
United Kingdom

GROENEVELD ABJ
Department of Intensive Care
VU University Medical Center
De Boelelaan 1117
1081 HV Amsterdam
Netherlands

GROUNDS RM
Department of Anesthesiology
and Intensive Care
Friedrich-Schiller-University
Erlanger Allee 101
07743 Jena
Germany

HANSEN K
Cancer Center Proteomics Core
University of Colorado Denver
UCD Anschutz Medical Campus, RC-1
South, L18–1303
PO Box 6511, Campus Box 8119
Aurora, CO 80045
USA

HARROIS A
Department of Anesthesia and Surgical
Intensive Care
CHU de Bicêtre
78 rue du Général Leclerc
94275 Le Kremlin Bicêtre Cedex
France

HARTOG C
Department of Anesthesiology
and Intensive Care
Friedrich-Schiller University
Erlanger Allee 101
07743 Jena
Germany

HEYMANN A
Department of Anesthesiology and
Intensive Care
Campus Charité Mitte und Campus
Virchow-Klinikum
Charité-Universitätsmedizin Berlin
Augustenburger Platz 1
13353 Berlin
Germany

HILLMAN K
The Simpson Center for Health Systems
Research
Liverpool Hospital
Locked Bag 7103
Liverpool BC, NSW 1871
Australia

Hommes TJ
Academic Medical Center
University of Amsterdam
Meibergdreef 9, G2–129
1105 AZ Amsterdam
Netherlands

Honoré PM
Department of Intensive Care
St-Pierre Para-Universitary Hospital
Avenue Reine Fabiola 9
1340 Louvain-la-Neuve
Belgium

Huang SJ
Department of Intensive Care
Nepean Clinical School
University of Sydney
Sydney, NSW 2750
Australia

Huet O
Department of Anesthesia and Surgical Intensive Care
CHU de Bicêtre
78 rue du Général Leclerc
94275 Le Kremlin Bicêtre Cedex
France

Hüter L
Department of Anesthesiology and Intensive Care
Friedrich Schiller University
Erlanger Allee 101
07740 Jena
Germany

Ince C
Department of Translational Physiology
Academic Medical Center
University of Amsterdam
Meibergdreef 9
1105 AZ Amsterdam
Netherlands

Jaber S
Intensive Care Unit, Department of Anesthesiology
CHU, Hôpital Saint Eloi
80 avenue Augustin Fiche
34295 Montpellier Cedex 5
France

Jeschke MG
Galveston Burns Unit
Shriners Hospitals for Children
815 Market Street
Galveston, TX 77550
USA

Joannes-Boyau O
Department of Anesthesia and Intensive Care II
University of Bordeaux II
33600 Pessac
France

Jolliet P
Department of Intensive Care
University Hospital
1211 Geneva 14
Switzerland

Jones AT
Department of Intensive Care Medicine
St Thomas Hospital
Westminster Bridge Road
London, SE17 EH
United Kingdom

Jung B
Intensive Care Unit, Department of Anesthesiology
CHU, Hôpital Saint Eloi
80 avenue Augustin Fiche
34295 Montpellier Cedex 5
France

Kaplan LJ
Section of Trauma, Surgical Critical Care, and Surgical Emergencies
Yale University School of Medicine
330 Cedar Street, BB-310
New Haven, CT 06520
USA

Kipnis E
Department of Surgical Intensive Care
Hôpital Huriez
Centre Hospitalier Régional Universitaire de Lille
1 rue Michel Polonovski
59037 Lille
France

Kopp R
Department of Surgical Intensive Care
RWTH Aachen University
52074 Aachen
Germany

Kowalewski S
Chair of Computer Science 11
RWTH Aachen University
52074 Aachen
Germany

Krinsley JS
Department of Critical Care
Stamford Hospital
Columbia University College
of Physicians and Surgeons
190 W Broad St.
Stamford, CT 06902
USA

Kruger P
Intensive Care Unit
Princess Alexandra Hospital
Ipswich Road
Woolloongabba, Brisbane
Australia

Kuiper MA
Department of Intensive Care
Medical Center Leeuwarden
PO Box 888
8901 BR Leeuwarden
Netherlands

Laureys S
Coma Science Group
Cyclotron Research Centre
University of Liège
Sart-Tilman-B30
4000 Liège
Belgium

Lautrette A
Department of Nephrology
and Intensive Care
CHU Gabriel Montpied
58 rue Montalembert
63000 Clermont-Ferrand
France

Legriel S
Department of Intensive Care
Hôpital André Mignot
177 rue de Versaille
78150 Le Chesnay
France

Leonhardt S
Philips Chair of Medical Information
Technology
RWTH Aachen University
52074 Aachen
Germany

Lepape A
Intensive Care Unit
Centre Hospitalier Lyon-Sud
Chemin du Grand Revoyet
69495 Pierre-Benite
France

Levesque E
Department of Intensive Care
Hôpital Paul Brousse
12, Av Paul Vaillant Couturier
94800 Villejuif
France

Levi M
Department of Medicine (F-4)
Academic Medical Center
University of Amsterdam
Meibergdreef 9
1105 AZ Amsterdam
Netherlands

Lewin III JJ
The Johns Hopkins Medical Institutions
600 N. Wolfe Street
Carnegie 180
Baltimore, MD 21287-6180
USA

Liu X
Therapeutics Research Unit
Princess Alexandra Hospital
Ipswich Road
Woolloongabba, Brisbane, QLD 4102
Australia

Loh NHW
Pathophysiology Unit
School of Clinical Sciences
University of Liverpool
Liverpool, L69 3GA
United Kingdom

Lorne E
INSERM ERI-12
Université Jules Verne de Picardie
Centre Hospitalier Universitaire
d4amiens
Place Victor Pauchet
80054 Amiens Cedex
France

Luepschen H
Department of Anesthesiology
and Intensive Care
University of Bonn
Sigmund Freud Strasse 25
53105 Bonn
Germany

Malbrain MMLG
Department of Intensive Care
ZNA Stuivenberg
Lange Beeldekensstraat 267
2060 Antwerp
Belgium

Marx G
Department of Intensive Care
University Hospital
RWTH Aachen
Pauwelsstr. 30
52074 Aachen
Germany

McLean AS
Department of Intensive Care
Nepean Clinical School
University of Sydney
Sydney NSW 2750
Australia

Meersseman W
Medical Intensive Care Unit
University Hospital
Herestraat 49
3000 Leuven
Belgium

Menon DK
Division of Anesthesia
University of Cambridge
Addenbrooke's Hospital
Cambridge, CB2 2QQ
United Kingdom

Metzger A
Department of Critical Care
Cooper University Hospital
One Cooper Plaza
Dorrance Building, Suite 393
Camden, NJ 08103
USA

Mirski MA
Department of Anesthesiology
and Critical Care
Division of Neuroanesthesia/
Neurosciences Critical Care
The Johns Hopkins Hospital
600 N. Wolfe Street, Meyer 8–140
Baltimore, MD 21287
USA

Monneret G
Flow Cytometry Unit
Immunology Laboratory
Hôpital E. Herriot 5
Place d'Arsonval
69437 Lyon cedex 03
France

Monnet X
Department of Medical Intensive Care
Hôpital de Bicêtre
78 rue du Général Leclerc
94270 Le Kremlin-Bicêtre
France

Morelli A
Department of Anesthesiology and
Intensive Care
University of Rome „La Sapienza"
Viale del Policlinico 155
00161 Rome
Italy

Muders T
Department of Anesthesiology and Intensive Care
University of Bonn
Sigmund Freud Strasse 25
53105 Bonn
Germany

Mueller C
Department of Medicine
University Hospital
Petersgraben 4
4031 Basel
Switzerland

Müller-Werdan U
Department of Medicine III
Universitätsklinikum Halle
Martin-Luther-University
Halle-Wittenberg
Ernst-Grube Str. 40
06097 Halle/Saale
Germany

Nacul FE
Department of Anesthesiology and Intensive Care
Friedrich-Schiller University
Erlanger Allee 103
07743 Jena
Germany

Nadkarni VM
Department of Anesthesiology and Critical Care
The Children's Hospital of Philadelphia
34th Street and Civic Center Boulevard
Philadelphia, PA 19104
USA

Neumar RW
Department of Emergency Medicine
University of Pennsylvania School of Medicine
Hospital of the University of Pennsylvania
3400 Spruce Street
Philadelphia, PA 19104–4283
USA

Nishisaki A
Department of Anesthesiology and Critical Care
The Children's Hospital of Philadelphia
34th Street and Civic Center boulevard
Philadelphia, PA 19104
USA

Nolan JP
Department of Anesthesiology and Intensive Care
Royal United Hospital
Combe Park
Bath, BA1 3NG
United Kingdom

Noveanu M
Department of Medicine
University Hospital
Petersgraben 4
4031 Basel
Switzerland

Ochola J
Department of Intensive Care
Princess Alexandra Hospital
199 Ipswich Road
Brisbane, QLD 4102
Australia

Oelke A
Department of Medicine III
Universitätsklinikum Halle
Martin-Luther-University
Halle-Wittenberg
Ernst-Grube-Str. 40
06097 Halle/Saale
Germany

Patterson AJ
Department of Anesthesia
Stanford University Medical Center
300 Pasteur Drive
Stanford, CA 94305
USA

Pelosi P
Department of Ambient Health and Safety
Service of Anesthesia B
Ospedale di Circolo
University of Insubria
Viale Borri 57
21100 Varese
Italy

Perkins GD
Warwick Medical School Clinical Trials Unit
University of Warwick
Warwick, CV4 7AL
United Kingdom

Pickkers P
Department of Intensive Care
Radboud University Nijmegen Medical Center
PO Box 9101
6500 HB Nijmegen
Netherlands

Pines JM
Department of Emergency Medicine
University of Philadelphia
Pennsylvania School of Medicine
Philadelphia, PA 19104-4283
USA

Pinsky MR
Department of Critical Care Medicine
606 Scaife Hall
3550 Terrace Street
Pittsburgh, PA 15261
USA

Poelaert J
Department of Anesthesiology and Perioperative Medicine
UZ Brussel
Laarbeeklaan 101
1090 Brussels
Belgium

Polito A
General Intensive Care Unit
Raymond Poincaré Teaching Hospital (AP-HP)
104 boulevard Raymond Poincaré
92380 Garches
France

Pontes-Arruda A
Intensive Care Nutrition Department
Fernandes Tavora Hospital
Rua Ildefonso Albano 777/403
Fortaleza, Ceara 60115-000
Brazil

Powell E
Department of Anesthesia, Critical Care and Pain
Birmingham Heartlands Hospital
Bordesley Green East
Birmingham, B9 5SS
United Kingdom

Preiser JC
Department of Intensive Care
Centre Hospitalier Universitaire de Liège
Domaine Universitaire Sart Tilman B35
4000 Liège 1
Belgium

Pustavoitau A
Departments of Anesthesiology and Critical Care
Johns Hopkins Hospital
Meyer 8-140, 600 N. Wolfe St
Baltimore, MD 21287
USA

Putensen C
Department of Anesthesiology and Intensive Care
University of Bonn
Sigmund Freud Strasse 25
53105 Bonn
Germany

Pyle A
Mitochondrial Research Group
Institute of Ageing and Health
Newcastle University
Newcastle upon Tyne, NE2 4HH
United Kingdom

Quiroz Martinez H
Interdepartmental Division of Critical Care
Toronto Western Hospital
399 Bathurst Street, 2MCL-411M
Toronto, ON M5T 2S8
Canada

Radermacher P
Sektion Anästhesiologische
Pathophysiologie und
Verfahrensentwicklung
Universitätsklinikum
Parkstrasse 11
89073 Ulm
Germany

Rahman West R
Department of Intensive Care
St George's Hospital
Blackshaw Road
London, SW17 0QT
United Kingdom

Rehberg S
Investigational Intensive Care Unit
Department of Anesthesiology
The University of Texas Medical Branch
301 University Blvd
Galveston, TX 77555-0833
USA

Reichlin T
Department of Medicine
University Hospital
Petersgraben 4
4031 Basel
Switzerland

Reinhart K
Department of Anesthesiology
and Intensive Care
Friedrich-Schiller University
Erlanger Allee 101
07743 Jena
Germany

Rhodes A
Department of Intensive Care
St George's Hospital
Blackshaw Road
London, SW17 0QT
UK

Ristagno G
Weil Institute of Critical Care Medicine
35100 Bob Hope Drive
Rancho Mirage, CA 92270
USA

Roberts MS
Intensive Care Unit
Princess Alexandra Hospital
Ipswich Road
Woolloongabba, Brisbane, QLD 4102
Australia

Robin E
Department of Surgical intensive Care
Hôpital Huriez
Centre Hospitalier Régional
Universitaire de Lille
1 rue Michel Polonovski
59037 Lille
France

Rooyackers O
Department of Anesthesia and
Intensive Care
Karolinska Institute
Huddinge University
14186 Stockholm
Sweden

Roumier M
Department of Medical Intensive Care
Hôpital Saint-Louis
1 Avenue Claude Vellefaux
75010 Paris
France

Sakr Y
Department of Anesthesiology
and Intensive Care
Friedrich-Schiller University
Erlanger Allee 103
07743 Jena
Germany

Saliba F
Hepatobiliary Center
Hôpital Paul Brousse
12, Av Paul Vaillant Couturier
94800 Villejuif
France

Samama CM
Department of Anesthesiology
and Intensive Care
Hotel-Dieu University Hospital
1 Place du Parvis de Notre-Dame
75181 Paris Cedex 04
France

Scales DC
Department of Critical Care
Sunnybrook Health Sciences Centre
2075 Bayview Avenue, Room D108
Toronto, ON M4N 3M5
Canada

Schroeder S
Department of Anesthesiology
and Intensive Care
Westküstenklinikum Heide
Esmarchstrasse 50
25746 Heide
Germany

Schuerholz T
Department of Intensive Care
University Hospital
RWTH Aachen
Pauwelsstr. 30
52074 Aachen
Germany

Schultz MJ
Department of Intensive Care and
Laboratory of Experimental Intensive
Care and Anesthesiology
Academic Medical Center at the
University of Amsterdam
Meibergdreef 9
1105 AZ Amsterdam
Netherlands

Seeling M
Department of Anesthesiology
and Intensive Care
Campus Charité Mitte und Campus
Virchow-Klinikum
Charité-Universitätsmedizin Berlin
Augustenburger Platz 1
13353 Berlin
Germany

Shapiro M
General Intensive Care Unit
Rabin Medical Center
Campus Beilinson
Petah Tikva 49100
Israel

Sharshar T
General Intensive Care Unit
Raymond Poincaré Teaching Hospital
(AP-HP)
104 boulevard Raymond Poincaré
92380 Garches
France

Shaw A
Department of Anesthesiology
Duke University Medical Center
Durham, NC 27710
USA

Shawcross D
Department of Hepatology
King's College Hospital
Denmark Hill
London, SE5 9RS
United Kingdom

Shukri K
Department of Critical Care
King Fahad Specialist Hospital
PO Box 15215
Dammam 31444
Saudi Arabia

Siami S
General Intensive Care Unit
Raymond Poincaré Teaching Hospital
(AP-HP)
104 Boulevard Raymond Poincaré
92380 Garches
France

Silva E
Intensive Care Unit
Hospital Albert Einstein
Sao Paulo, SP 05651–901
Brazil

Sinderby C
Department of Critical Care
St Michael's Hospital
30 Bond Street
Room 4–072, Queen Wing
Toronto, ON M5B 1W8
Canada

Singer P
General Intensive Care Unit
Rabin Medical Center
Campus Beilinson
Petah Tikva 49100
Israel

Smith J
Department of Adult Critical Care
Guy's and St Thomas' NHS Foundation Trust
St Thomas' Hospital, 1st Floor East Wing
Westminster Bridge Road
London, SE1 7EH
United Kingdom

Smith M
Department of Neuroanesthesia and Neuroscience Critical Care
The National Hospital for Neurology and Neurosurgery
University College London Hospitals
Queen Square
London, WC1N 3BG
United Kingdom

Soar J
Department of Anesthetics
and Intensive Care
Southmead Hospital
North Bristol NHS Trust
Bristol, BS10 5NB
United Kingdom

Souweine B
Department of Nephrology
and Medical Intensive Care
CHU Gabriel Montpied
58 rue Montalembert
63000 Clermont-Ferrand
France

Spagnesi L
Department of Anesthesia
and Intensive Care
Azienda Ospedaliero-Universitaria S.M. della Misericordia
P.le S. M. Misericordia 15
33100 Udine
Italy

Spies C
Department of Anesthesiology and Intensive Care
Campus Charité Mitte und Campus Virchow-Klinikum
Charité-Universitätsmedizin Berlin
Augustenburger Platz 1
13353 Berlin
Germany

Spieth PM
Department of Anesthesiology and Intensive Care
University Hospital Carl Gustav Carus
Fetscherstrasse 74
01307 Dresden
Germany

Spriet I
Pharmacy Department
University Hospital
Herestraat 49
3000 Leuven
Belgium

Spronk PE
Department of Intensive Care
Gelre Hospitals (Lukas site),
PO Box 9014
7300 DS Apeldoorn
Netherlands

Sprung CL
General Intensive Care Unit
Department of Anesthesiology and Critical Care
Hadassah Hebrew University Medical Center
PO Box 12000
Jerusalem, 91120
Israel

Stafford-Smith M
Department of Anesthesiology
Duke University Medical Center
Erwin Road
Durham, NC 27710
USA

Stevens RD
Division of Neurosciences Critical Care
Departments of Anesthesiology,
Critical Care Medicine, Neurology
and Neurosurgery
Johns Hopkins Hospital
Meyer 8–140, 600 N. Wolfe St
Baltimore, MD 21287
USA

Suarez Sipmann F
Department of Critical Care
Fundacion Jimenez Diaz-UTE
Avda de los Reyes Catolicos 2
28010 Madrid
Spain

Swaminathan M
Department of Anesthesiology
Duke University Medical Center
Erwin Road
Durham, NC 27710
USA

Szabó C
Department of Anesthesiology
The University of Texas Medical Branch
610 Texas Avenue
Galveston, TX 775553
USA

Tang BM
Department of Intensive Care
Nepean Clinical School
University of Sydney
Sydney NSW 2750
Australia

Tang W
Weil Institute of Critical Care
35100 Bob Hope Drive
Rancho Mirage, CA 92270
USA

Tassaux D
Department of Intensive Care
University Hospital
1211 Geneva 14
Switzerland

Teboul JL
Department of Intensive Care
Hôpital de Bicêtre
78 rue du Général Leclerc
94270 Le Kremlin-Bicêtre
France

Thonnard M
Coma Science Group
Cyclotron Research Centre
University of Liège
Sart-Tilman-B30
4000 Liège
Belgium

Traber DL
Investigational Intensive Care Unit
Department of Anesthesiology
The University of Texas Medical Branch
301 University Blvd
Galveston, TX 77555–0833
USA

Trof RJ
Department of Intensive Care
VU University Medical Center
De Boelelaan 1117
1081 HV Amsterdam
Netherlands

Tugrul S
Department of Anesthesiology and
Intensive Care
Medical Faculty of Istanbul
University of Istanbul
Capa Klinikleri
34093 Istanbul
Turkey

Tusman G
Department of Anesthesiology
Hospital Privado de Comunidad
Cordoba 4545
7600 Mar del Plata
Argentina

Vallet B
Department of Surgical Intensive Care
Hôpital Huriez
Centre Hospitalier Régional
Universitaire de Lille
1 rue Michel Polonovski
59037 Lille
France

van der Hoeven JG
Department of Intensive Care Medicine
Radboud University Nijmegen
Medical Center
PO Box 9101
6500 HB Nijmegen
Netherlands

Van der Poll T
Academic Medical Center
University of Amsterdam
Meibergdreef 9, G2–129
1105 AZ Amsterdam
Netherlands

Vanhaudenhuyse A
Coma Science Group
Cyclotron Research Centre
University of Liège
Sart-Tilman-B30
4000 Liège
Belgium

van Zijl P
Department of Radiology
John Hopkins Hospital
Baltimore, MD 21205
USA

Venet F
Immunology Laboratory
Hôpital E. Herriot 5
Place d'Arsonval
69437 Lyon cedex 03
France

Venkatesh B
Department of Intensive Care
Princess Alexandra & Wesley Hospitals
Brisbane, QLD 4102
Australia

Vignaux L
Department of Intensive Care
University Hospital
1211 Geneva 14
Switzerland

Weber S
Department of Anesthesiology and
Intensive Care
University of Bonn
Sigmund-Freud-Strasse 25
53105 Bonn
Germany

Weiss YG
General Intensive Care Unit
Department of Anesthesiology
and Critical Care
Hadassah Hebrew University
Medical Center
PO Box 12000
Jerusalem, 91120
Israel

Wendon J
Liver Intensive Care Unit and Institute
of Liver Studies
King's College Hospital
Denmark Hill
London, SE5 9RS
United Kingdom

Werdan K
Department of Medicine III
Universitätsklinikum Halle
Martin-Luther-University
Halle-Wittenberg
Ernst-Grube-Str. 40
06097 Halle/Saale
Germany

Wernerman J
Department of Anesthesia
and Intensive Care K32
Karolinska Institute
Huddinge University
14186 Stockholm
Sweden

Westphal M
Department of Anesthesiology
and Intensive Care
University Hosptial of Münster
Albert-Schweitzer-Str. 33
48149 Münster
Germany

WIERSINGA WJ
Academic Medical Center
University of Amsterdam
Meibergdreef 9, G2–129
1105 AZ Amsterdam
Netherlands

WILLIAMS M
Division of Anesthesia
University of Cambridge
Addenbrooke's Hospital
Cambridge, CB2 2QQ
United Kingdom

WILSON RJT
Department of Anesthetics
York Hospital
Wigginton Road
York, YO31 8HE
United Kingdom

WUNSCH H
Department of Anesthesiology
Columbia Presbyterian Medical Center
622 W 168th St, PH5–505
New York, NY 10032
USA

YEUNG J
Academic Department of Anesthesia,
Critical Care and Pain
Heart of England NHS Foundation
Trust
Bordesley Green East
Birmingham, B9 5SS
United Kingdom

Common Abbreviations

AKI	Acute kidney injury
ALI	Acute lung injury
APACHE	Acute physiology and chronic health evaluation
ARDS	Acute respiratory distress syndrome
CABG	Coronary artery bypass graft
COPD	Chronic obstructive pulmonary disease
CPB	Cardiopulmonary bypass
CPP	Cerebral perfusion pressure
CPR	Cardiopulmonary resuscitation
CRP	C-reactive protein
CT	Computed tomography
CVP	Central venous pressure
DIC	Disseminated intravascular coagulopathy
EEG	Electroencephalogram
EKG	Electrocardiogram
EVLW	Extravascular lung water
FiO_2	Inspired fraction of oxygen
FRC	Functional residual capacity
HES	Hydroxyethyl starch
HSP	Heat shock protein
ICG	Indocyanine green
ICP	Intracranial pressure
ICU	Intensive care unit
IL	Interleukin
LPS	Lipopolysaccharide
MAP	Mean arterial pressure
MAPK	Mitogen-activated protein kinase
MRI	Magnetic resonance imaging
NF-κB	Nuclear factor-kappa B
NO	Nitric oxide
NOS	Nitric oxide synthase
PAC	Pulmonary artery catheter
PAOP	Pulmonary artery occlusion pressure
PEEP	Positive end-expiratory pressure
ROS	Reactive oxygen species
$ScvO_2$	Central venous oxygen saturation
SIRS	Systemic inflammatory response syndrome
SOFA	Sequential organ failure assessment
SvO_2	Mixed venous oxygen saturation
TLR	Toll-like receptor
TNF	Tumor necrosis factor

I Genomics and Proteomics

Rethinking Sepsis: New Insights from Gene Expression Profiling Studies

B.M. Tang, S.J. Huang, and A.S. McLean

Introduction

Critically ill patients encompass an enormously heterogeneous population and, as such, therapeutic interventions, including drug therapy, can produce multiple outcomes in different patient subgroups. For example, researchers not only look for an 'average effect' of a drug on a typical patient, but also seek to understand individual variability. The presence of variability impacts significantly on the success of clinical trials and failure to identify this variability can result in the clinical trial being under-powdered to detect a treatment effect. For clinicians, failure to recognize variability can result in unintended toxicity or excessive harm in certain patients. Hence, understanding variability is critically important in both research and clinical practice.

Nowhere is the relevance of patient variability more evident than in sepsis. Over the last two decades, numerous clinical trials have been conducted, all producing mixed results. It has been commonly observed that various patient populations responded differently to the same drug, ranging from marginal beneficial effect in some subgroups, to nil effect or increased toxicity in others.

Investigators have attempted to address the heterogeneity issue by stratifying patients into groups who have different baseline mortality risk. Theoretically, identifying those patients who are most likely to respond to treatment will ensure maximal benefits and minimal harms. In the case of recombinant activated protein C (drotecogin alfa (activated)), such subgroups have been identified [1, 2]. For many other drugs, no particular subgroups were found, although investigators have long suspected patient heterogeneity was the reason for failure in these trials [3].

There is now an increased recognition that our failure to give the right treatment to the right patient reflects our current limitations in identifying and measuring heterogeneity in critically ill patients [4, 5]. In this chapter, we will redefine heterogeneity in sepsis patients using a simple conceptual model. We then review findings from recent studies that provide new insights into the sources of heterogeneity in these patients.

How to Identify and Measure Heterogeneity

Current methods to define patient heterogeneity in sepsis are grossly inadequate. Traditional criteria such as age, clinical settings or disease severity are commonly used to enlist patients into clinical trials. However, these are crude measures of the inherent heterogeneity of a very complex syndrome in a diverse patient population.

Although simple physiological parameters (e.g., systemic inflammatory response syndrome [SIRS] criteria), organ level indices (e.g., circulatory failure), or a combination of both (e.g., APACHE score) have been proved to be helpful in epidemiological studies, they are too non-specific as criteria to stratify patients in clinical trials. With the exception of recombinant activated protein C and anti-tumor necrosis factor (TNF) therapy, attempts to select patients based on disease severity or baseline mortality risk have consistently failed, as evidenced from analyses of clinical trials on anti-coagulant therapy, anti-inflammatory drugs, or low-dose corticosteroids [11, 12]. Investigators can also measure a vast array of physiological parameters and serum cytokines in sepsis patients. However, we do not know how these measurements relate to the observed heterogeneity, nor do we know how they can be used to predict a patient's possible response to a new drug. Consequently, there is currently no agreed upon method to identify and measure heterogeneity in sepsis patients.

Sources of Heterogeneity in Sepsis Patients

The sources of heterogeneity are multiple and manifest at different levels. Study and patient level variables (e.g., trial design, disease severity) are easy to discern, as this information is readily available from published reports of clinical trials. Our current understanding of heterogeneity derives mainly from these variables [8]. While the data from these variables is useful, they represent only the tip of an iceberg (**Fig. 1**).

The iceberg model provides a qualitative overview of the sources of heterogeneity. The complexity of the data increases progressively downwards in this model (**Fig. 1**). Data on organ and cellular level variables demonstrate a diverse range of complex behavior exhibited by different organs (e.g., liver vs. kidney) [9] and different cells

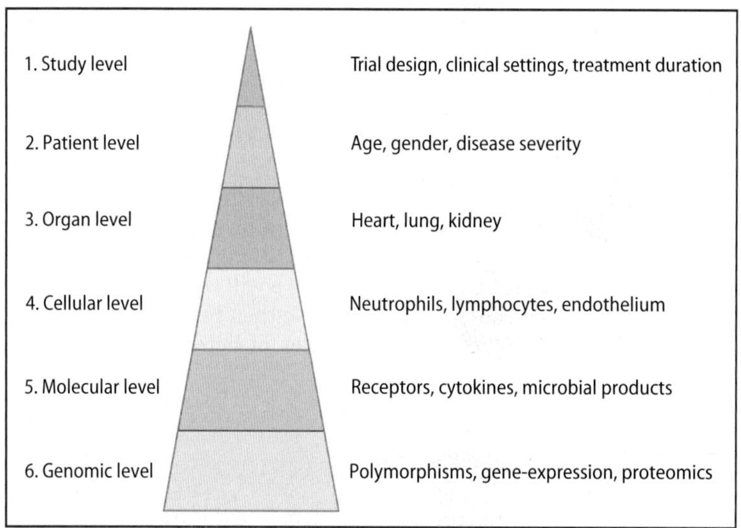

Fig. 1. The iceberg model to conceptualize the sources of heterogeneity in sepsis trials. Variables on the upper levels of the model are easier to discern and study. Complexity of the data increases towards the lower levels, with most variables yet to be discovered or understood at the genomic level.

(e.g., leukocytes vs. endothelium) [10]. Data from molecular level studies are even more complex, with over 50 mediators found to be involved at multiple points during the host response to sepsis [11].

The highest level of complexity, however, lies at the genomic level. Here, a vast myriad of data is accessible to only a handful of researchers in a few highly specialized research institutions. Yet, these data are potentially the richest source of information and may help us identify and measure the observed clinical heterogeneity in sepsis patients. Here, we will highlight some important findings from this rapidly expanding area of research.

New Insights from Gene-expression Studies

The field of genomic science includes the study of genetic polymorphism, proteomics, and gene-expression profiling (see **Table 1** for more details). The emerging fields of proteomics and genetic polymorphism have been reviewed elsewhere [12, 13]. This chapter will focus on insights obtained from studies of gene-expression profiling, a field with the most promising potential to assist us understand the sources of heterogeneity in sepsis.

Over the last 5 years, we have undertaken a large scale, systematic interrogation of the host response in sepsis at a transcriptional level [14–16]. The microarray technique is a powerful tool that allows us to sift through a massive amount of the

Table 1. Glossary

Proteomics: A new technology that involves large-scale study of protein composition and function. Typically, it involves cataloguing all the expressed proteins in a particular cell or tissue type, using techniques such as two-dimensional gel electrophoresis or mass spectrometry. A single mass spectrometry experiment can identify over 2,000 proteins.

Gene-expression profiling: A high-throughput technology that measures the activity of thousands of genes at once, to create a global picture of cellular function. Cells respond changes in their environment by making messenger RNA (i.e., gene-expression), which in turn encodes for various proteins that carry out the appropriate cellular function. A single experiment can measure an entire genome simultaneously, in some cases over 25,000 genes. This technology therefore provides a more global picture than proteomics.

Polymorphism: A common biological phenomenon in which phenotype variations arise due to difference in DNA sequence among individuals. The most frequent type of polymorphism is the single-nucleotide polymorphism (SNP), which can be a substitution, a deletion, or an insertion of a single nucleotide. It is thought to be one of the causes of the individual variability in the susceptibility to infectious disease.

Microarray: The commonest platform used in gene-expression profiling experiments. It is a two-dimensional grid of DNA genes or gene fragment spots, usually arranged on a glass slide or silicone wafer. A typical microarray contains 10,000–200,000 microscopic probes. The probes on the microarray are either a short oligonucleotide or a cDNA. Probe-target hybridization is usually detected and quantified by fluorescence-based detection. This allows the determination of relative abundance of nucleic acid sequences in the sample.

Network Analysis: An analysis method that seeks to study the relationships and interactions between various parts of a cell signaling system (metabolic pathways, organelles, cells, and organisms) and to integrate this information to understand how biological systems function.

genetic information contained within the human genome (see **Table 1** for more details). We examined the gene-expression profiles of 164 critically ill patients admitted to the intensive care unit (ICU) of a university-affiliated teaching hospital. The patient cohort consists of a full range of sepsis syndromes (from sepsis to septic shock) in a wide variety of clinical settings (medical, surgical and obstetric). Our findings reveal some interesting insights with regard to transcriptional heterogeneity.

Limitation of Current Risk Stratification Methods

Our data shows that there is no difference in the host response between sepsis, severe sepsis, and septic shock at a transcriptional level. Classification of septic patients into sepsis, severe sepsis, and septic shock is one of the commonest ways to stratify patient into different risk groups and is supported by a large amount of data from epidemiological studies [17]. However, the use of these criteria has failed to identify treatment-responsive groups in most clinical trials. Fundamental questions have therefore been raised on the effectiveness of such criteria to define the complex range of heterogeneity found in septic patients [18]. Our data provide the first genomic evidence that the grouping of patients based on such criteria is too limited to represent the full spectrum of heterogeneity in sepsis patients. A more precise definition of the subgroups in sepsis is needed, perhaps by using not just simple clinical variables (e.g., heart rate or creatine values), but also more sophisticated methods such as genomic studies.

Host Response in Sepsis is More Complex Than Previously Thought

Investigators have delivered a huge amount of molecular information on sepsis at an unprecedented level of complexity. This is well demonstrated by a seminal study by Calvano et al., in which volunteers were given endotoxin and their gene-expression profiles measured [19]. A total of 3,714 genes were found to have their expression intensity altered by the endotoxin challenge. This is an impressively large number because it represents over 14 % of the protein-coding genes. When these genes were followed at 2, 4, 6, 9 and 24 hours, more complex changes were exhibited. In addition, the authors performed network analysis (see **Table 1** for more details) and reported a further discovery of a vast interconnecting network of cellular activities. For example, by honing in on just one gene alone (i.e., nuclear factor kappa B), the authors unveiled a total of 619 interactions between 150 genes. With over three thousand genes showing simultaneous changes, the number of potential interactions is immeasurable. The immense complexity of these data provides an exciting opportunity to develop a potentially more powerful method to classify sepsis patients into clinically relevant and molecularly precise subgroups.

There Is Strong Evidence of Heterogeneity at the Genomic Level

Patient subgroups can be identified using gene-expression studies, but first there is a need to explore all the genomic variability within any defined population of sepsis patients. To this end, we recently undertook a review of all the gene-expression studies that had identified genomic markers of sepsis [14–16, 20–22]. We performed a pair-wise comparison of all the signature genes between each study. Our analysis of these studies reveals two important findings (**Fig. 2**).

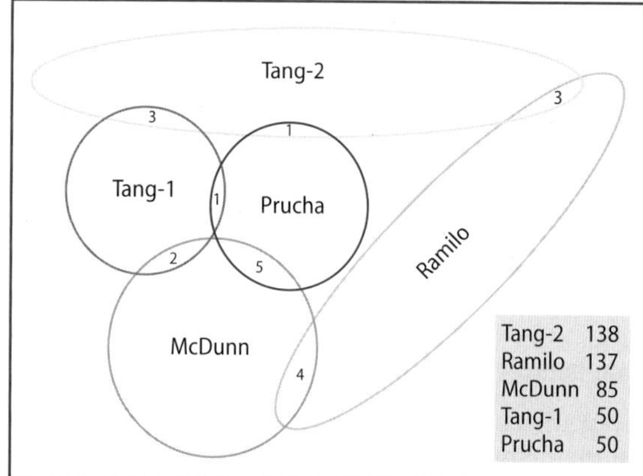

Fig. 2. List of putative genes in sepsis. Total number of genes in each data set is shown in the insert. References for included studies: Tang-2 [14], Ramilo [20], McDunn [21], Tang-1 [15], Prucha [22]

First, there are over 400 signature genes that were identified as putative genomic markers of human sepsis. The vast majority of these genes have never been studied in the past. These data sets contain valuable sources of information and could potentially lead to the discovery of novel pathways which may help researchers explain heterogeneity. In fact, many of these genes are subsequently identified to be those involved in nucleosome assembly, signal transduction, transcription/translation regulation, and control of protein complex assembly.

The second finding is that there is minimal overlapping in the lists of signature genes among studies. The genomic markers of sepsis seem to vary from one patient population to another. This finding persists even after the analysis is restricted to studies that had comparable study design, disease spectrum, or clinical settings. This finding indicates that the spectrum of heterogeneity at a transcriptional level is large. It is likely that the current studies revealed only a very small portion of this enormous variability.

Genomic Heterogeneity

To explore genomic heterogeneity further in the context of biological pathways, we recently conducted network analysis (see **Table 1** for more details) using our microarray datasets. We examined all the relevant biological pathways implicated in sepsis, including those involved in immunity and inflammatory responses. We then compared our findings to other gene-expression studies that used similar analysis techniques [19, 23, 24]. These analyses addressed two important questions: 1) what give rise to genomic heterogeneity; 2) where are the main sources of variability?

What Gives Rise To Genomic Heterogeneity?

Our analyses suggest that the vast connectivity of the molecular signaling system gives rise to heterogeneity. Traditionally, cellular function is conceptualized as individual components working in a linear fashion to produce a series of predictable biological effect. However, network analysis data suggest a far more complex picture. It shows that cellular functions are governed by vast gene regulatory networks. While there are main hubs in these networks, there are also extensive collateral sub-networks that will provide alternative routes. This is akin to the airline network, where travelers can arrive at the same destination via complex re-routing or the use of alternative airlines. Consequently, there is a large amount of redundancy in its signaling system. To complicate matters further, there are conflicting feedback loops acting on each hub. For any given biological signal, multiple outcomes are possible depending on a variety of factors, such as the temporal pattern of each feedback loop and summation of individual stimuli. Cellular function is therefore a result of an integrative process. Such a system gives rise to a huge potential for variability and, hence, heterogeneity.

Main Sources of Genomic Variability

Given the enormity and the complexity of the data, investigators need to hone into the main sources of the variability. Our data, along with those from other studies [19, 23, 24], allow us to narrow our focus down to four gene regulatory networks (**Fig. 3**).

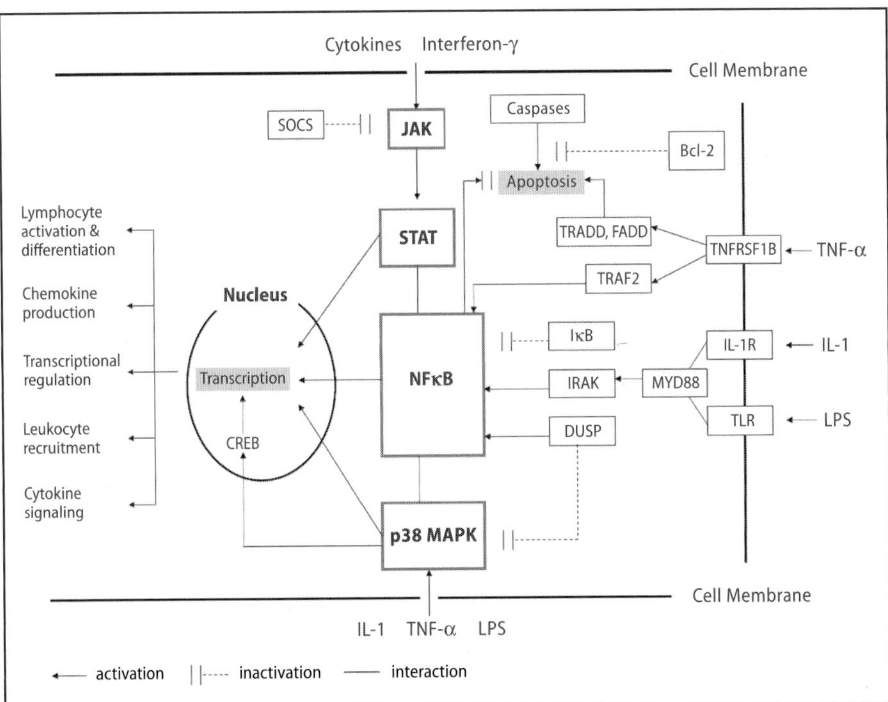

Fig. 3. Four gene regulatory networks (JAK, STAT, NF-κß and p38 MAPK). BCL2: B-cell CLL/lymphoma 2; CREB: cAMP responsive element binding protein; DUSP: dual specificity phosphatase; FADD: Fas-associated death domain protein; IFNGR: interferon gamma receptor; IκB: inhibitor of kappa-B; IL-R: interleukin-1 receptor; IRAK: interleukin-1 receptor-associated kinase; JAK: Janus kinase; LPS: lipopolysaccharide; MAPK: mitogen activated protein kinase; MyD88: myeloid differentiation primary response gene 88; NF-κB: nuclear factor kappa-B; SOCS: suppressor of cytokine signaling; STAT: transducer and activator of transcription protein; TLR: Toll-like receptor; TNF: tumor necrosis factor; TNFRSF1B: TNF receptor superfamily, member 1B; TRADD: TNF receptor-associated death domain protein; TRAF2: TNF receptor-associated factor-2.

All four networks have been implicated in the immune response to sepsis. Although other molecular networks have also been implicated, these four networks are the most consistent findings reported by the gene-expression studies we surveyed. While each network has been extensively studied in the past, the gene-expression studies provide a global overview of all these networks and their individual components. They reflect a growing body of data that will help researchers explain heterogeneity. However, these data represent only a glimpse of the vast genomic landscape. We still do not fully understand the complex inter-relationship between these networks and the dynamic interaction between components of each pathway. More in-depth studies focusing on gene regulatory networks are therefore needed in the future.

Further Questions on an Existing Sepsis Model

Our analysis of the gene-expression studies also revealed two unexpected findings with regard to the role of the immune response. First, there is a noticeable absence of the activation of pro-inflammatory genes. According to the currently accepted model of sepsis, the host response is a biphasic process in which an initial hyper-inflammatory phase is followed by a later, anti-inflammatory phase that manifests as functional immune suppression [25]. This has not been supported by data from the gene-expression studies we surveyed, where investigators rarely reported the activation of well-known inflammatory genes, such as TNF, interleukin (IL)-1, IL-2, IL-6, or IL-10. Second, the gene-expression studies suggest that immune suppression is present in both the early and late phases of sepsis. Again, this is in contrast to the established model of sepsis where immune suppression is thought to occur later. In fact, it is now well established that the simplistic strategy of treating early sepsis as a pro-inflammatory phenomenon has been proven ineffective.

Put together, these data suggest that the established model of sepsis is too simplistic to account for the wide range of immune abnormalities observed in sepsis patients. The insight that both hyper-immune and hypo-immune status can occur early in sepsis further reinforces our notion that the pathogenesis of sepsis is much more complex and heterogeneous than we previously thought.

There are important therapeutic implications of the above findings. First, sepsis has long been defined as a pro-inflammatory or hypo-inflammatory syndrome. Such a dichotomization ignores the complexity of sepsis and leads to simplistic strategies such as neutralizing elevated cytokines or replacing a compound when its serum level is low. Second, septic patients have been treated as an immunologically homogeneous group. However, there are likely to be many heterogeneous immune phenotypes. Giving drugs without sufficient information about the patient's underlying immunological status can result in benefit in some phenotypes but harm in others.

With an increased recognition of immunological heterogeneity, some authors are now advocating that the immune status needs to be accurately assessed before patients are recruited into clinical trials [26]. However, currently available biomarker assays capture only a fraction of all known immune abberations in sepsis. For example, serum measurements of inflammatory cytokines (e.g. IL-1, IL-6, or TNF-α) are widely used. But a far greater number of molecules have been observed to be abnormally elevated in septic patients. Functional testing of immune cells (e.g., cell proliferation or human-leukocyte antigen [HLA]-DR expression) has also been used, but it measures only a few pathways and hence provides only a partial view of the over-

I

all immunological status. Here, we propose that a gene-expression profiling technique is better suited to assess global immune dysfunction in sepsis.

Functional Mapping of Sepsis Genome to Monitor Immune Function

Gene-expression profiling can be used to characterize the immunological status of septic patients on a genome-wide scale. This is because there are advantages of this technique over conventional biomarker assays. First, gene-expression profiling can handle much larger volumes of data, often measuring thousands of genes simultaneously. This capability is unmatched by conventional assays. Second, many cellular dysfunctions are often unmeasurable by normal assays, because their expression is downregulated or their expressed proteins are below the dynamic range of detection. These dysfunctions can be easily detected by gene-expression profiling.

We undertook gene-expression analysis of thirty-five critically ill patients (sepsis = 25, control = 10). Circulating mononuclear cells were used because these cells play a major role in the immune response in sepsis. We then compared the gene-expression profile of the sepsis and control patients. The analysis was performed on over 130 biological pathways, including those known to be involved in immunological functions. Some of the important findings are presented in **Table 2**.

Table 2. Biological pathways implicated in sepsis

	BioCarta Pathway	Pathway description	Number of genes	p-value
1	h_crebPathway	Transcription factor CREB and its extracellular signals	9	1e-05
2	h_egfr_smrtePathway	MAPK inactivation of SMRT co-repressor	8	1e-05
3	h_hcmvPathway	Human cytomegalovirus and MAPK pathways	8	1e-05
4	h_hdacPathway	Control of skeletal myogenesis by HDAC & calcium/calmodulin-dependent kinase (CaMK)	12	1e-05
5	h_mapkPathway	MAPK signaling pathway	28	1e-05
6	h_p38mapkPathway	p38 MAPK signaling pathway	23	1e-05
7	h_tollPathway	Toll-like receptor pathway	13	1e-05
8	h_dspPathway	Regulation of MAPK pathways through dual specificity phosphatases	6	9.11e-05
9	h_SARSpathway	SARS coronavirus protease	7	9.63e-05
10	h_stressPathway	TNF/stress related signaling	7	9.67e-05
11	h_tall1Pathway	TACI and BCMA stimulation of B cell immune responses.	7	9.84e-05
12	h_fMLPpathway	fMLP induced chemokine gene expression in HMC-1 cells	11	0.0001511
13	h_biopeptidesPathway	Bioactive peptide induced signaling pathway	13	0.0001688
14	h_41bbPathway	The 4–1BB-dependent immune response	7	0.000176

Table 2. *(cont.)*

	BioCarta Pathway	Pathway description	Number of genes	p-value
15	h_pyk2Pathway	Links between Pyk2 and MAPKs	9	0.0003106
16	h_nfatPathway	NFAT and hypertrophy of the heart (Transcription in the broken heart)	12	0.0003726
17	h_eif4Pathway	Regulation of eIF4e and p70 S6 kinase	15	0.0006778
18	h_Ccr5Pathway	Pertussis toxin-insensitive CCR5 signaling in macrophage	9	0.001729
19	h_keratinocytePathway	Keratinocyte differentiation	15	0.0021693
20	h_arenrf2Pathway	Oxidative stress induced gene expression Via Nrf2	11	0.0022934
21	h_GATA3pathway	GATA3 participate in activating the Th2 cytokine gene expression	10	0.0026139
22	h_ranklPathway	Bone remodeling	5	0.0040675
23	h_IL12Pathway	IL12 and Stat4 dependent signaling pathway in Th1 development	17	0.0041499
24	h_ifnaPathway	IFN alpha signaling pathway	8	0.0043606
25	h_egfPathway	EGF signaling pathway	8	0.0179649
26	h_gleevecpathway	Inhibition of cellular proliferation by gleevec	7	0.0537086
27	h_ifngPathway	IFN gamma signaling pathway	6	0.0820155
28	h_tcraPathway	Lck and Fyn tyrosine kinases in initiation of TCR activation	23	0.1777127
29	h_asbcellPathway	Antigen dependent B cell activation	9	0.2645085
30	h_bbcellPathway	Bystander B cell activation	9	0.2645085

As expected, well known pathways such as Toll-like receptor (TLR) or TNF signaling are confirmed to be involved in sepsis. However, our analysis also discovered a large number of pathways, many of which have not been studied previously with regard to their involvement in sepsis. This analysis demonstrates that it is feasible to assay immunological dysfunction on a global scale and to yield highly valuable biological information regarding the roles of both established and unknown pathways. Based on the data above, we hypothesize that a comprehensive architecture of the gene regulatory network of immune response in sepsis can be constructed using gene-expression data. Such a database should include transcriptional information on: 1) all functional pathways; 2) all possible interactions between genes and molecules; 3) how the system functions as a whole in response to perturbations (e.g., to trauma, ischemia, or infectious stimuli); 4) mathematical modeling which will help investigators predict the existence of hidden interactions or feedback loops.

I

Conclusion

Based on the review above, we would argue for a greater appreciation of the complexity of the immune status in sepsis. Current models of sepsis are limited in their ability to account for the huge range of heterogeneity in sepsis patients. New data show that immunological dysfunction gives rise to much of the observed variability. We, therefore, propose that functional mapping of immunological aberrations by gene-expression studies holds the key to the understanding, measuring, and monitoring of heterogeneity in sepsis patients. Such a database will allow future researchers to better understand the variability of drug response. In the long term, it will help clinicians design drug treatment based on individual variability; this is the ultimate goal of individualized medicine.

References

1. Laterre PF (2007) Clinical trials in severe sepsis with drotrecogin alfa (activated). Crit Care 11 (Suppl 5):S5
2. Ely EW, Laterre P-F, Angus D, et al (2003) Drotrecogin alfa (activated) administration across clinically important subgroups of patients with severe sepsis. Crit Care Med 31: 12–19
3. Carlet J, Cohen J, Calandra T, Opal S, Masur H (2008) Sepsis: Time to reconsider the concept. Crit Care Med 36: 1–3
4. Levy M, Fink M, Marshall J, et al (2003) 2001 SCCM/ESICM/ACCP/ATS/SIS International Sepsis Definitions Conference. Crit Care Med 31: 1250–1256
5. Marshall J, Vincent J-L, Fink MP, et al (2003) Measures, markers, and mediators: towards a staging system for clinical sepsis. Crit Care Med 31: 1560–1567
6. Macias WL, Nelson D, Williams M, Garg R, Janes J, Sashegyi A (2005) Lack of evidence for qualitative treatment by disease severity interactions in clinical studies of severe sepsis. Crit Care 9: R607–622
7. Minneci PC, Deans KJ, Banks SM, Eichacker PQ, Natanson C (2004) Meta-analysis: The effect of steroids on survival and shock during sepsis depends on the dose. Ann Intern Med 141: 47–56
8. Macias W, Vallet B, Bernard GR, et al (2004) Sources of variability on the estimate of treatment effect in the PROWESS trial: implications for the design and conduct of future studies in severe sepsis. Crit Care Med 32: 2385–2391
9. Dear J, Yasuda H, Hu X, et al (2006) Sepsis-induced organ failure is mediated by different pathways in the kidney and liver: acute renal failure is dependent on MyD88 but not renal cell apoptosis. Kidney Int 69: 832–836
10. Annane D, Bellissant E, Cavaillon J (2005) Septic shock. Lancet 365: 63–78
11. Marshall J (2003) Such stuff as dreams are made on: mediator-directed therapy in sepsis. Nat Rev Drug Discov 2: 391–405
12. Holmes CL, Russell JA, Walley KR (2003) Genetic polymorphisms in sepsis and septic shock: role in prognosis and potential for therapy. Chest 124: 1103–1115
13. Nguyen A, Yaffe M (2003) Proteomics and systems biology approaches to signal transduction in sepsis. Crit Care Med 31: S1-S6
14. Tang B, McLean A, Dawes I, Huang S, Lin R (2008) Gene-expression profiling of peripheral blood mononuclear cells in sepsis. Crit Care Med (in press)
15. Tang B, McLean A, Dawes I, Huang S, Lin R (2007) The use of gene-expression profiling to identify candidate genes in human sepsis. Am J Respir Crit Care Med 176: 676–684
16. Tang B, McLean A, Dawes I, Huang S, Cowley M, Lin R (2008) Gene-expression profiling of gram-positive and gram-negative sepsis in critically ill patients. Crit Care Med 36: 1125–1128
17. Calandra T, Cohen J (2005) The international sepsis forum consensus conference on definitions of infection in the intensive care unit. Crit Care Med 33: 1538–15 48
18. Abraham E, Matthay M, Dinarello C, et al (2000) Consensus conference definitions for sepsis, septic shock, acute lung injury, and acute respiratory distress syndrome: Time for a reevaluation. Critical Care Medicine 28: 232–235

19. Calvano SE, Xiao W, Richards DR, et al (2005) A network-based analysis of systemic inflammation in humans. Nature 437: 1032–1037
20. Ramilo O, Allman W, Chung W, et al (2007) Gene expression patterns in blood leukocytes discriminate patients with acute infections. Blood 109: 2066–2077
21. McDunn J, Husain K, Polpitiya A, et al (2008) Plasticity of the systemic inflammatory response to actue infection during critical illness: development of the riboleukogram. PlosOne 3: e1564
22. Prucha M, Ruryk A, Boriss H, Moller E, Zazula R, Russwurm S (2004) Expression profiling: toward an application in sepsis diagnostics. Shock 22: 29–33
23. Shanley TP, Cvijanovich N, Lin R, et al (2007) Genome-level longitudinal expression of signaling pathways and gene networks in pediatric septic shock. Mol Med 13: 495–508
24. Johnson S, Lissauer M, Bochicchio G, Moore R, Cross A, Scalea T (2007) Gene expression profiles differentiate between sterile SIRS and early sepsis. Ann Surg 245: 611–621
25. Hotchkiss R, Karl I (2003) The pathophysiology and treatment of sepsis. N Engl J Med 348: 138–150
26. Monneret G, Venet F, Pachot A, Lepape A (2008) Monitoring immune dysfunction in the septic patient: a new skin for the old ceremony. Mol Med 14: 64–78

I

Mitochondrial Genetics and Sepsis

A. Pyle, P. Chinnery, and S. Baudouin

Introduction

Mitochondria are intracellular organelles that generate the principal source of cellular energy in the form of adenosine triphosphate (ATP). In a highly efficient process, mitochondria convert both carbohydrate and fat into high-energy phosphate compounds by a series of intermediate steps involving electron transfer. Emerging data implicate mitochondrial damage and dysfunction as critical factors in the pathogenesis of sepsis.

Oxidative Phosphorylation and ATP Generation

Mitochondria are present in all nucleated cells. They possess a smooth outer membrane and a convoluted inner membrane, the folds of which are termed cristae. Together the two membranes create an intermembrane space.

The primary role of mitochondria is to produce cellular energy, in the form of ATP, by a process called oxidative phosphorylation. The five multi-subunit enzyme complexes (I-V) of the oxidative phosphorylation system are located within the mitochondrial inner membrane (**Fig. 1**). Each complex itself is composed of multiple subunits; complex I is the largest with over 40 subunits. During oxidative phosphor-

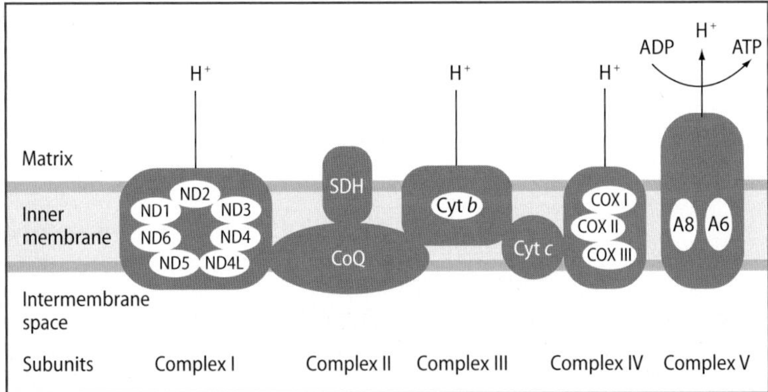

Fig. 1. Diagrammatic representation of the mitochondrial respiratory chain showing the major components: complexes I (NADH dehydrogenase), II (succinate dehydrogenase and coenzyme Q10), III (cytochrome c reductase), IV (cytochrome c oxidase) and V (ATP synthase) and the genes encoded by each complex.

ylation, electrons are transferred down these redox enzyme complexes, known as the electron transport chain. Through this process, energy is released and is used to transport protons out through the inner mitochondrial membrane into the intermembranous space. This produces an electrochemical gradient that is utilized by complex V as a source of energy to condense adenosine diphosphate (ADP) to make ATP.

An efficient oxidative phosphorylation system producing ATP is said to be tightly coupled. Alternatively, if the mitochondria are less efficient at generating ATP they are partially uncoupled and generate heat. Therefore, the mitochondrial oxidative phosphorylation system must be tightly regulated to generate a balance between ATP generation for energy and heat to maintain body temperature. Uncoupling proteins (UCP) are members of the mitochondrial transport carrier family [1]. UCP1 promotes the leakage of protons through the mitochondrial inner membrane. This uncouples ATP production from substrate oxidation, leading to increased oxygen consumption and ultimately heat production.

Reactive Oxygen Species

The mitochondrial electron transport chain is one of the pathways that produces oxidants and free radicals in the body. Reactive oxygen species (ROS), such as superoxide and hydrogen peroxide, are toxic by-products of cellular metabolism. At complex I and III of the mitochondrial electron transport chain, electrons may leak to molecular oxygen, causing the production of superoxide. Approximately 1–2 % of the oxygen consumed by mitochondria is converted to ROS. As ROS function as cellular messengers, they can broadly influence gene expression, cell proliferation, energy metabolism and mitochondrial biogenesis.

Mitochondria are the major intracellular source of ROS. It is known that ROS production from mitochondria increases with age [2]. Excessive ROS production can impair mitochondrial function and influence cell viability. Production of ROS is associated with damage to DNA, lipids and proteins, cellular proliferation, the expression of UCP, and the maintenance of mitochondrial membrane potential [3]. Mitochondria can increase the synthesis of ROS during hypoxia which triggers an increase in oxygen delivery to the cell and glycolytic metabolism [4].

Oxidative stress and damage by ROS can cause damage to bases and sugar phosphates in addition to single- or double-strand breaks in mitochondrial DNA (mtDNA). This ultimately leads to the occurrence of somatic mtDNA mutations. The accumulation of these mutations can result in dysfunction of the respiratory chain. In theory, this can lead to increased ROS production and further mtDNA mutations [5].

Apoptosis

Mitochondria are critical for cellular homeostasis. However, they also play an important role in regulating programmed cell death, or apoptosis (as opposed to death by necrosis which is not programmed). Apoptosis is triggered by both intrinsic and extrinsic pathways. Oxidative stress can induce the intrinsic pathway of apoptosis. The mitochondrial regulation of apoptosis occurs during the initiation and regulation of the intrinsic pathway. Lethal agents cause the mitochondria to release cytochrome c and other pro-apoptotic proteins into the cytosol. Here they induce or amplify the activation of apoptotic caspases [6]. Mitochondrial oxidative stress has been implicated in cell death. As cellular metabolism relies on ATP production from mitochondria, any damage e.g., from ROS, affecting respiratory chain function may influence cell viability.

Mitochondria and Sepsis

A considerable body of evidence has accumulated implicating mitochondrial dysfunction in sepsis (reviewed in [7]). The multiple organ dysfunction that characterizes sepsis is poorly understood but is accompanied by impaired cellular oxygen uptake despite adequate tissue perfusion. It is thought that cellular oxygen consumption is impaired primarily at the level of the mitochondrion, ultimately leading to a decrease in energy production.

Several of the inflammatory mediators released during sepsis have been shown to inhibit oxidative phosphorylation [8]. Ultra-structural changes in mitochondria have also been observed in animals with sepsis [9] and in patients who died in critical care with multiple organ failure (MOF) [10]. Subtle defects of complex I and ATP depletion have been observed in the skeletal muscle of septic patients who subsequently die [11].

It is possible that mitochondrial damage in critical illness leads to increased electron leakage and ROS generation. The intense inflammatory response during sepsis also results in increased inducible nitric oxide (NO) synthase (iNOS) activity and reactive nitrogen species production. NO is thought to play an important role in sepsis patients as it has an inhibitory effect on electron transport chain complexes, thus leading to the generation of electrons through relative blockade of the respiratory chain [12]. However, depending upon the concentration and release time of NO, studies have demonstrated that low levels of NO stimulate mitochondrial proliferation during sepsis [13].

Mitochondrial Genetics

Mitochondria probably originated as free-living bacteria-like organisms. At some point in evolution they were engulfed by primitive, nucleated, anaerobic cells and became symbiotic [14]. They contain their own DNA (mtDNA) which is present in high copy number in human cells. mtDNA is a small circular double stranded molecule, 16.5 kb in length (**Fig. 2**). It consists of a heavy (purine rich) and light chain (pyrimidine rich). The 37 genes of the mitochondrial genome encode 13 essential components of the oxidative phosphorylation system, as well as two ribosomal RNAs and 22 transfer RNAs [15]. Nuclear genes code for the remaining and majority of the mitochondrial respiratory chain proteins. They are translated by cytosolic ribosomes with a mitochondrial targeting sequence that directs them into the mitochondrion.

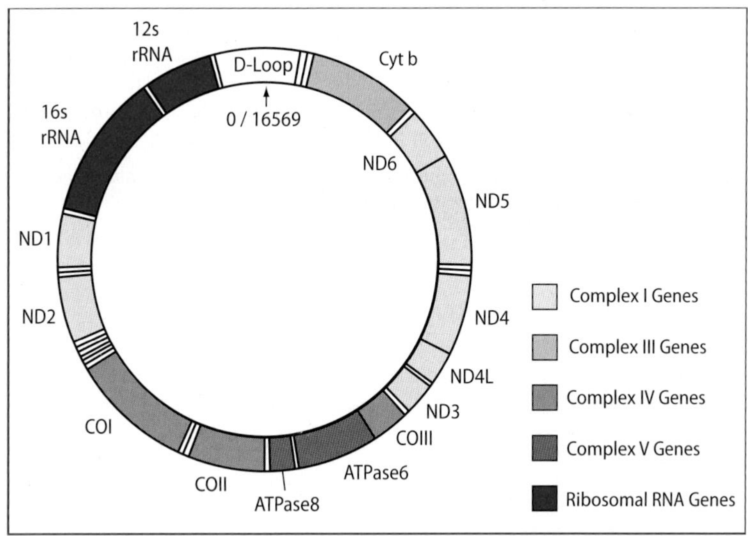

Fig. 2. The human mitochondrial DNA (mtDNA) genome demonstrating the location of the complex genes

Mitochondrial Haplogroups

mtDNA is inherited almost exclusively through the maternal lineage, and does not undergo significant recombination. The high mutation rate of mtDNA is due to its lack of protective histones, inefficient DNA repair mechanisms, and exposure to the mutagenic effects of oxygen radicals generated by oxidative phosphorylation [16]. These mutations are completely random and can affect any base in the mitochondrial genome in either the coding or non-coding regions. Therefore, the rate of mtDNA sequence evolution is much higher than that of the average nuclear gene [17]. Consequently a substantial number of mtDNA single nucleotide polymorphisms (SNPs) have accumulated, sequentially along radiating maternal lineages. In turn, these have diverged as human populations, colonizing different geographical regions of the world. These specific SNPs are known as mtDNA haplogroups [18]. Different mtDNA haplogroups are associated with major global ethnic groups [19]. The majority of Europeans belong to one of nine haplogroups: H, J, T, U, K, V, W, I, X, with haplogroup H being the most common (44 %) [20].

The geographical variation observed in mtDNA haplogroups could reflect selection acting on specific lineages. Ruiz-Pesini and colleagues hypothesized that certain mtDNA haplogroups cause a decrease in coupling efficiency, leading to lower ATP generation and increased heat production. These particular haplogroups are thought to have been positively selected for during radiation of modern humans into colder climates [21]. However this hypothesis was later tested using a bioenergetic test on the specific mtDNA variants. The authors found that mitochondria from Arctic haplogroups had similar or increased coupling efficiency when compared to tropical haplogroups [22]. Moreover, a further study observed no evidence for climate-induced geographical varied selection [23].

Table 1. Definitions of common genetic terms

Genetic term	Definition
Adaptive selection	Selection favoring advantageous alleles/traits. This allows advantageous alleles to become prevalent in the natural population
Cybrid	A hybrid cell produced by fusing a cell nucleus with a cell of the same or a different species whose nucleus has been removed
Genetic drift	The process by which gene frequencies are changed by the process of random sampling in a small population
Non-synonymous	A substitution that replaces one codon with another that encodes a different amino acid
Purifying selection	Selection acting against deleterious alleles. This prevents harmful alleles becoming prevalent in the natural population
Recombination	The exchange and rearrangement of DNA
Single nucleotide polymorphism	A change in which a single base in the DNA differs from the usual base at that position
Synonymous	A substitution that replaces one codon with another that encodes the same amino acid

The various influences of random genetic drift, positive selection, or purifying selection that eliminate non-synonymous changes in mtDNA sequence variation remain uncertain (**Table 1**). Kivisild and co-workers produced further evidence for non-random processes affecting the evolution of the human mtDNA encoded proteins [24]. Although functional studies have failed to identify a biochemical consequence of mtDNA haplogroups [25], these effects could be subtle and only be manifest on an evolutionary scale.

A recent study investigated the historical genetic diversity of ancient human mtDNA genotypes and compared them to modern mtDNA genotypes from England, Europe, and the Middle East. The investigators found a higher genetic diversity in the ancient samples. This could be the result of genetic drift, selection, or stochastic processes. Examples include the Black Death in 1347 which led to a loss of 50 % of the European population and the Great Plague of 1665 in which 20 % of the London population died [26]. This work provides circumstantial evidence that major environmental insults, including pandemic infections, have influenced mtDNA evolution.

Haplogroups and Human Disease

Multiple associations have been documented between clinical conditions and mtDNA haplogroups. These include some neurodegenerative diseases, ageing, and, more recently, survival in human sepsis. Analysis of patients with Parkinson's disease demonstrated a 22 % reduction in the risk of development of Parkinson's disease in patients in the UKJT haplogroup cluster [27]. Another study found that European individuals with haplogroup J or K were significantly less likely to develop Parkinson's disease compared to those with haplogroup H [28]. De Benedictis and co-workers found that in a group of healthy centenarians, haplogroup J was significantly overrepresented, therefore linking haplogroup J with longevity [29].

A longitudinal clinical and genetic study of 150 patients with severe sepsis demonstrated that on admission to intensive care, the haplogroup distribution was similar to a large age-matched control group from the same region. However, survival in the haplogroup H patients was significantly better than other patients at 28 days, hospital discharge and six month follow-up [30]. Examination of mtDNA haplogroups in severe sepsis in the Chinese Han population revealed that haplogroup R, one of the three main haplogroups of the Han population, predicts a survival advantage [31].

Haplogroups and Mitochondrial Function

Evidence has emerged, over recent years, to link different mtDNA haplogroups with alterations in the phenotypic expression of mitochondrial activity. Leber hereditary optic neuropathy (LHON) is a rare cause of inherited blindness primarily due to three pathogenic mtDNA mutations (11778G>A, 14484T>C and 3460G>A). The penetrance of the 11778G>A and 14484T>C mutations is markedly influenced by the background mtDNA haplogroup [32]. Sperm motility is strongly dependent upon ATP supplied by oxidative phosphorylation activity. Haplogroup H has been associated with increased sperm motility and the T haplogroup with reduced motility [33]. A further study illustrates that several sublineages of haplogroup U were associated with differences in sperm motility and vitality [34]. However, the mechanism by which the haplogroup exerts its functional effect upon mitochondria in sperm function is unclear. Differences in haplogroup distributions have been revealed between long distance runners and sprinters in a study of elite Finnish athletes [35], but the number of subjects was small, and this result must be confirmed before firm conclusions can be drawn.

The haplotypes associated with decreased survival in sepsis [30] could have a direct effect on ATP levels, leading to reversible cellular dysfunction, reduced respiratory chain function with increased levels of ROS, and ultimately cellular apoptosis; uncoupling of mitochondria could result in increased heat generation. mtDNA SNPs could also influence phenotypic variation in humans. However, a study using a cybrid cellular model did not reveal any significant respiratory defect in haplogroups J or T cybrids [36]. A more recent investigation studied the bioenergetic capacities and coupling efficiencies of mitochondria in transmitochondrial cybrids [25]. These cybrids harbored mitochondria with either haplogroup H or haplogroup T, with identical nuclear backgrounds. At the mitochondrial and cellular level, the results demonstrated no significant bioenergetic differences in these mitochondria. Therefore, the mtDNA haplogroup could affect mitochondrial proliferation or signaling but it does not appear to affect coupling efficiency in cells [25]. However, the effect could be too subtle to be detected by conventional techniques, only becoming manifest at times of extreme stress. An investigation into oxidative phosphorylation performance and ROS production in mouse cells with different mtDNA variants demonstrated that mtDNA haplotypes produce different levels of ROS and their growth in galactose is affected [37]. Further work is needed in this area.

Mitochondrial Biogenesis

Mitochondrial biogenesis involves multiple transcriptional regulation pathways that require the expression of nuclear and mitochondrial genes. The number of mtDNA molecules doubles in every cell cycle, under normal physiological conditions. When

I

conditions change, the mtDNA copy number can be altered according to the energy need of the cell. Animal models of sepsis have demonstrated depletion in the number of heart [38] and liver [39] mitochondria. Mitochondrial dysfunction in sepsis is associated with a decrease in mitochondrial number. This depletion could be associated with a decrease in oxidative phosphorylation activity and impaired oxygen use or hypoxia which is associated with sepsis. In a recent short term survival study, it was found that mtDNA copy number was low when compared to controls. In recovering patients, the copy number increased over time compared to those that did not survive [40].

Data suggest a role for mitochondrial biogenesis in the response to inflammatory conditions. A recent study found that mitochondrial biogenesis can restore both mitochondrial number and oxidative metabolism, after selective damage to the organelles [41].

Conclusion

There is strong evidence that changes in mitochondrial function occur in human sepsis. The underlying cause/s of these changes remains uncertain but a failure of adequate energy production is plausible. mtDNA is a small, plasmid-like structure which is inherited almost exclusively down the maternal line. The mitochondrial genome contains a number of common single base variations which together define a set of inherited haplogroups. These haplogroups may influence mitochondrial function, particularly at times of intense cellular stress. The frequency of these haplogroups may have been influenced by natural selection due to infectious disease. Their diversity may, therefore, explain some of the variation in outcome from severe infection.

References

1. Echtay KS (2007) Mitochondrial uncoupling proteins--what is their physiological role? Free Radic Biol Med 43: 1351–1371
2. Sohal RS, Ku HH, Agarwal S, Forster MJ, Lal H (1994) Oxidative damage, mitochondrial oxidant generation and antioxidant defenses during aging and in response to food restriction in the mouse. Mech Ageing Dev 74: 121–133
3. Echtay KS, Roussel D, St-Pierre J, et al (2002) Superoxide activates mitochondrial uncoupling proteins. Nature 415: 96–99
4. Chandel NS, Maltepe E, Goldwasser E, Mathieu CE, Simon MC, Schumacker PT (1998) Mitochondrial reactive oxygen species trigger hypoxia-induced transcription. Proc Natl Acad Sci USA 95: 11715–11720
5. Lee HC and Wei YH (2007) Oxidative stress, mitochondrial DNA mutation, and apoptosis in aging. Exp Biol Med (Maywood) 232: 592–606
6. Kroemer G, Dallaporta B, Resche-Rigon M (1998) The mitochondrial death/life regulator in apoptosis and necrosis. Annu Rev Physiol 60: 619–642
7. Bayir H, Kagan VE (2008) Bench-to-bedside review: Mitochondrial injury, oxidative stress and apoptosis--there is nothing more practical than a good theory. Crit Care 12: 206
8. Geng Y, Hansson GK, Holme E (1992) Interferon-gamma and tumor necrosis factor synergize to induce nitric oxide production and inhibit mitochondrial respiration in vascular smooth muscle cells. Circ Res 71: 1268–1276
9. Simonson SG, Welty-Wolf K, Huang YT, et al (1994) Altered mitochondrial redox responses in gram negative septic shock in primates. Circ Shock 43: 34–43
10. Vanhorebeek I, De Vos R, Mesotten D, Wouters PJ, De Wolf-Peeters C, Van den Berghe G (2005) Protection of hepatocyte mitochondrial ultrastructure and function by strict blood glucose control with insulin in critically ill patients. Lancet 365: 53–59

11. Brealey D, Brand M, Hargreaves I, et al (2002) Association between mitochondrial dysfunction and severity and outcome of septic shock. Lancet 360: 219–223
12. Protti A, Singer M (2006) Bench-to-bedside review: potential strategies to protect or reverse mitochondrial dysfunction in sepsis-induced organ failure. Crit Care 10: 228
13. Nisoli E, Clementi E, Paolucci C, et al (2003) Mitochondrial biogenesis in mammals: the role of endogenous nitric oxide. Science 299: 896–899
14. Margulis L (1971) Symbiosis and evolution. Sci Am 225: 48–57
15. Anderson S, Bankier AT, Barrell BG, et al (1981) Sequence and organization of the human mitochondrial genome. Nature 290: 457–465
16. Wallace DC (1994) Mitochondrial DNA sequence variation in human evolution and disease. Proc Natl Acad Sci USA 91: 8739–8746
17. Miyata T, Hayashida H, Kikuno R, Hasegawa M, Kobayashi M, Koike K (1982) Molecular clock of silent substitution: at least six-fold preponderance of silent changes in mitochondrial genes over those in nuclear genes. J Mol Evol 19: 28–35
18. Torroni A, Schurr TG, Cabell MF, et al (1993) Asian affinities and continental radiation of the four founding Native American mtDNAs. Am J Hum Genet 53: 563–590
19. Quintana-Murci L, Semino O, Bandelt HJ, Passarino G, McElreavey K, Santachiara-Benerecetti AS (1999) Genetic evidence of an early exit of Homo sapiens sapiens from Africa through eastern Africa. Nat Genet 23: 437–441
20. Torroni A, Huoponen K, Francalacci P, et al (1996) Classification of European mtDNAs from an analysis of three European populations. Genetics 144: 1835–1850
21. Ruiz-Pesini E, Mishmar D, Brandon M, Procaccio V, Wallace DC (2004) Effects of purifying and adaptive selection on regional variation in human mtDNA. Science 303: 223–226
22. Amo T, Brand MD (2007) Were inefficient mitochondrial haplogroups selected during migrations of modern humans? A test using modular kinetic analysis of coupling in mitochondria from cybrid cell lines. Biochem J 404: 345–351
23. Elson JL, Turnbull DM, Howell N (2004) Comparative genomics and the evolution of human mitochondrial DNA: assessing the effects of selection. Am J Hum Genet 74: 229–238
24. Kivisild T, Shen P, Wall DP, et al (2006) The role of selection in the evolution of human mitochondrial genomes. Genetics 172: 373–387
25. Amo T, Yadava N, Oh R, Nicholls DG, Brand MD (2008) Experimental assessment of bioenergetic differences caused by the common European mitochondrial DNA haplogroups H and T. Gene 411: 69–76
26. Topf AL, Gilbert MT, Fleischer RC, Hoelzel AR (2007) Ancient human mtDNA genotypes from England reveal lost variation over the last millennium. Biol Lett 3: 550–553
27. Pyle A, Foltynie T, Tiangyou W, et al (2005) Mitochondrial DNA haplogroup cluster UKJT reduces the risk of PD. Ann Neurol 57: 564–567
28. van der Walt JM, Nicodemus KK, Martin ER, et al (2003) Mitochondrial polymorphisms significantly reduce the risk of Parkinson disease. Am J Hum Genet 72: 804–811
29. De Benedictis G, Rose G, Carrieri G, et al (1999) Mitochondrial DNA inherited variants are associated with successful aging and longevity in humans. Faseb J 13: 1532–1536
30. Baudouin SV, Saunders D, Tiangyou W, et al (2005) Mitochondrial DNA and survival after sepsis: a prospective study. Lancet 366: 2118–2121
31. Yang Y, Shou Z, Zhang P, et al (2008) Mitochondrial DNA haplogroup R predicts survival advantage in severe sepsis in the Han population. Genet Med 10: 187–192
32. Torroni A, Petrozzi M, D'Urbano L, et al (1997) Haplotype and phylogenetic analyses suggest that one European-specific mtDNA background plays a role in the expression of Leber hereditary optic neuropathy by increasing the penetrance of the primary mutations 11778 and 14484. Am J Hum Genet 60: 1107–1121
33. Ruiz-Pesini E, Lapena AC, Diez-Sanchez C, et al (2000) Human mtDNA haplogroups associated with high or reduced spermatozoa motility. Am J Hum Genet 67: 682–696
34. Montiel-Sosa F, Ruiz-Pesini E, Enriquez JA, et al (2006) Differences of sperm motility in mitochondrial DNA haplogroup U sublineages. Gene 368: 21–27
35. Niemi AK, Majamaa K (2005) Mitochondrial DNA and ACTN3 genotypes in Finnish elite endurance and sprint athletes. Eur J Hum Genet 13: 965–969
36. Baracca A, Solaini G, Sgarbi G, et al (2005) Severe impairment of complex I-driven adenosine triphosphate synthesis in leber hereditary optic neuropathy cybrids. Arch Neurol 62: 730–736

I

37. Moreno-Loshuertos R, Acin-Perez R, Fernandez-Silva P, et al (2006) Differences in reactive oxygen species production explain the phenotypes associated with common mouse mitochondrial DNA variants. Nat Genet 38: 1261 – 1268
38. Watts JA, Kline JA, Thornton LR, Grattan RM, Brar SS (2004) Metabolic dysfunction and depletion of mitochondria in hearts of septic rats. J Mol Cell Cardiol 36: 141 – 150
39. Crouser ED, Julian MW, Huff JE, Mandich DV, Green-Church KB (2006) A proteomic analysis of liver mitochondria during acute endotoxemia. Intensive Care Med 32: 1252 – 1262
40. Cote HC, Day AG, Heyland DK (2007) Longitudinal increases in mitochondrial DNA levels in blood cells are associated with survival in critically ill patients. Crit Care 11: R88
41. Haden DW, Suliman HB, Carraway MS, et al (2007) Mitochondrial biogenesis restores oxidative metabolism during Staphylococcus aureus sepsis. Am J Respir Crit Care Med 176: 768 – 777

Lung Proteomics in Intensive Care

E. Kipnis and K. Hansen

Introduction

The advent of routinely available genomics and sequencing of the human genome, among others, associated with advances in technology previously limited to biochemical research, and in bioinformatics has brought the new field of proteomics within the reach of the life sciences and even clinical research. Important hypotheses are increasingly being generated in lung disease by biomarker identification from screening of clinical samples. However, proteomics, ideally suited for biomarker discovery, is only just emerging as a field of research in intensive care and has, to date, mostly been applied to serum in studies of sepsis [1 – 5]. The purpose of this chapter is to overview the rationale, basics, methods, pitfalls, applications, and future directions for lung proteomics in intensive care.

The Search for Biomarkers

What is a Biomarker?

A biomarker is a clinically available biomolecule (most often the concentration of a protein in a biological sample such as serum) that should either be able to increase physiopathological knowledge about a disease process in order to ultimately develop new therapeutic prospects or be able to detect a pathological process in order to aid diagnosis and treatment. In order for a biomarker to be useful, it must be associated with a disease or a specific phase/stage of disease with high sensitivity and specificity. Ideally, variations in its concentration should predict the clinical evolution of the disease [6].

The classical paradigm of medical research has been to accumulate physiopathological knowledge of disease, from this knowledge to formulate hypothesis-driven research, from hypothesis-driven research to identify candidate biomolecules with a suspected relation to disease, and then to test their ability in disease prediction, diagnosis, staging or prognosis. However, with the advances in genomics and proteomics, this paradigm has been reversed (**Fig. 1**). Such techniques offer the possibility of screening samples for hundreds of biomarkers (or genes translated to biomarkers) and, therefore, allow direct identification of candidate biomarkers of disease. From these identifications, hypotheses as to their role are advanced, and research is designed to explore the possibilities. From this research, new pathophysiological insights to disease are sometimes revealed.

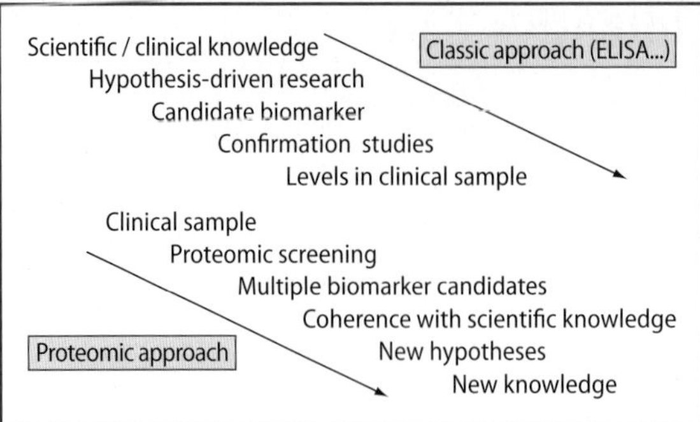

Fig. 1. Classic versus proteomic approach to biomarker discovery. The 'Classic' approach relies on hypothesis-driven basic research derived from scientific knowledge and focused on one or a few known proteins which seem good candidate biomarkers to be tested in confirmation studies of their levels in clinical samples. The proteomic approach starts from the clinical samples which are screened for the differential expression of any proteins, many of which will be candidate biomarkers from which new pathophysiological hypotheses may be made and eventually confirmed adding to scientific knowledge in addition to their diagnostic or prognostic use.

The Need for Proteomics in the Intensive Care Unit

The two major and often intricate diseases leading to critical illness are sepsis and acute lung injury (ALI) and their most severe forms, septic shock and acute respiratory distress syndrome (ARDS). The hallmarks of these diseases are that they are so heterogeneous that they barely qualify as diseases, rather they are clinical syndromes caused by a diversity of etiologies leading to organ injury and failure through a wide array of pathophysiological pathways. Their heterogeneity increases when taking into account the variety of underlying predisposing conditions as well as the timepoint at which a given patient is diagnosed and treated. Therefore, the diseases for which biomarkers are most needed in the ICU are so complex that it is very improbable that any lone biomarker identified from 'classical' approaches will be successful [7]. This is supported by the literature where potential biomarkers sometimes perform excessively well in the very 'pure' experimental models in which they are established only to become, if anything at all, gross biomarkers of severity in the intensive care unit (ICU). Procalcitonin, which is a biomarker of infection in non-severely ill patients in the emergency room, loses its discriminative power and becomes generically indicative of severity in the ICU [8]. Likewise, brain natriuretic peptide (BNP), which is a biomarker of increased ventricular filling pressures and left ventricular dysfunction, cannot discriminate these patients in a critical care cohort [9]. Therefore, it would be more coherent in complex and overly heterogeneous diseases such as sepsis and ALI/ARDS, to have a comprehensive system-wide approach in order to identify 'profiles' of protein expression that may vary according to disease state in order to truly identify the ongoing pathophysiological processes at any given timepoint rather than severity alone which most clinicians can assess clinically and with routine analyses.

Genomics versus Proteomics

It could be argued that genomics has already fulfilled this goal and provided the intensive care community with more potential biomarkers, genetic profiles, and transcriptomes than it can handle [10–12]. However, the use of genomics raises several issues. First, DNA or RNA extraction from clinical samples is often difficult. Second, one gene can lead to multiple messenger RNAs through splicing, RNA editing, and other mechanisms [13]. Third, protein expression does not correlate strictly with mRNA levels [14]. Finally, proteins undergo various posttranslational modifications (glycosylation, phosphorylation, ubiquitination, methylation...) which lead to further varying gene products [15]. Furthermore, the identification of an upregulated or downregulated gene in a disease process may be so far removed from the disease process itself through multiple and often redundant regulation processes, that it is difficult to gain any useful insight concerning the disease. Therefore, it is difficult to directly extrapolate pathophysiological significance from genomic or transcriptomic studies without identifying expressed proteins related to the genes. Proteomics, however, holds the promise of directly identifying relevant proteins that can subsequently be detected as biomarkers.

Lung Proteomics

Basics

Proteomics is the comprehensive study of the protein complement to a genome. Although the term is often misused and covers many definitions, the principle it conveys is the comprehensive identification of a full set of proteins in any given biological system (organism, tissue, biological fluid, cell, cell fraction, or organelle). In addition to large scale identification of proteins, it has come to designate the large scale study of protein post-translational modifications, interactions, localizations, activities, and functions, or any associations thereof. Proteomics can be used in several general ways. First, as was the case in genomics, the race is on to proteomically characterize all simple organisms such as yeast and pathogens as well as various normal human and animal cells, tissues, or fluids in order to develop reference libraries and maps of normally expressed proteins. Second, proteomics can simply be a tool, just as polymerase chain reaction (PCR) has become a routine benchtop tool, used to identify proteins in a sample as part of a step in a non-proteomic experiment. Even as a tool, the advantage of proteomic techniques such as mass-spectroscopy is that they do not rely on possessing specific antibodies as in enzyme-linked immunosorbent assays (ELISA) and, therefore, do not necessitate knowing exactly which protein is being searched for. Finally, proteomics can be the center of hypothesis-driven studies of proteins differentially expressed in different samples, different states, or at different timepoints in order to identify novel biomarkers.

What Intensivists Should Know About Proteomic Methods

This chapter does not aim to be a complete review of all proteomics and the lung, and the reader is encouraged to consult other detailed reviews on the topic [16, 17]. Rather, the following are basic principles and important caveats that intensivists should keep in mind when confronted with information from the emerging field of proteomics in intensive care.

As specified above, not all protein science qualifies as 'proteomics', which implies a scale in the screening or study of proteins. Thus, in-depth study of a protein, bioinformatic extrapolation of protein 'expression' from genomic data, and simultaneous or multiplex ELISA of several proteins do not qualify as proteomic studies. Protein arrays and microarrays are sometimes covered by the term but they lack any ability to detect non-predetermined proteins.

An increasing and constantly innovative array of techniques may be applied to the large-scale study of proteins in biological samples but major complete workflows involve the same basic steps: Protein extraction from the sample, protein denaturation, protein separation and degradation into polypeptidic fragments/peptides, ionization, further separation and fragmentation simultaneously to mass detection in a mass spectrometer, protein sequencing and identification from bio-informatic processing of mass spectrometer data searched against databases, and optional confirmation of some identifications through Western blot. An overview of the steps involved in a proteomic workflow leading to protein sequencing and identification is given in **Figure 2**.

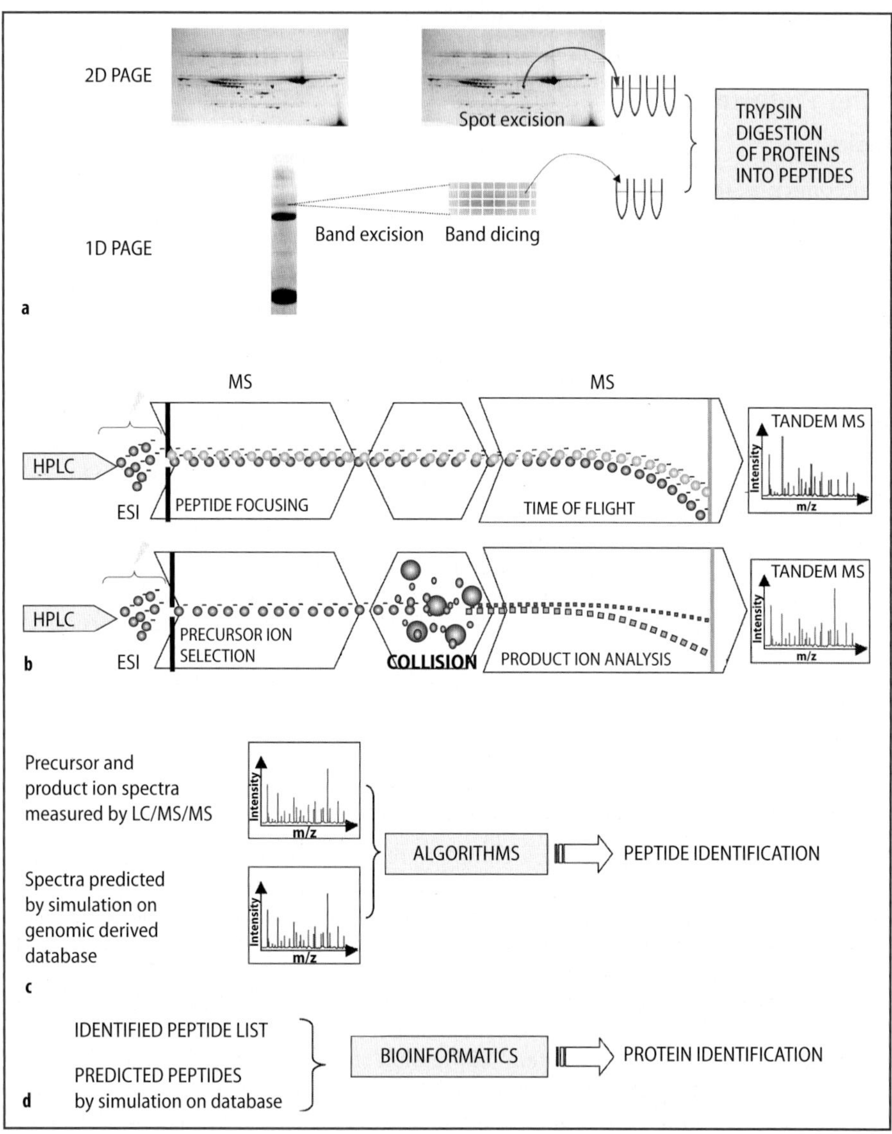

Fig. 2 (*legend see p. 27*)

Table 1 lists most of the steps, techniques, and principles involved in proteomics with a short description. It is important to understand that many combinations of different steps allow the design of different proteomic analysis workflows. Likewise, each technique involved is a field of expertise in itself with its own advantages, limitations and caveats which cannot be listed here.

Table 1. Tools, steps, techniques and principles involved in proteomics.

Methods	Principles
Protein separation	*Separation of proteins based on physical properties*
1D PAGE	Molecular weight (MW)-based separation on acrylamide gels
2D PAGE	Isoelectric point (pI) and MW-based separation on acrylamide gels
Capillary electrophoresis	MW-based separation in a conductive liquid medium
Liquid Chromatography	Proteins dissolved in a solvent passed through a stationary phase
Reversed Phase	Non-polar stationary phase; hydrophobicity-based separation
Ion Exchange	Charged stationary phase; charge-based separation
Affinity	Selective protein-binding-based separation
Protein digestion	*Enzymatic cleavage of proteins into peptides*
Trypsin	Carboxyl cleavage of peptide chains between lysine and arginine
Peptide ionization	*Modifying peptide charge to facilitate its detection by MS*
Electrospray	Ionization from the liquid phase pressured through an electric field
Laser desorption (LDI)	Laser energy ionization
Matrix assisted (MALDI)	Ionization from, and facilitated by, a solid phase chemical matrix
MALDI Imaging	In-situ ionization of analytes from frozen tissue
Surface-enhanced (SELDI)	Chemical or immunocapture surfaces for selective ionization

(*Cont. see p. 28*)

◁

Fig. 2. Proteomic workflow. **a** Protein separation by electrophoresis (1DPAGE, 2D PAGE) followed by the manual or automated excision of spots or bands which are diced and submitted to tryptic digestion of proteins into peptides best suited for mass spectrometric sequencing. **b** Peptide separation is achieved first by online liquid chromatography on a reversed phase microscale capillary high performance liquid chromatography (HPLC) column or ion-exchange column, which elutes peptides into an electrospray needle in which peptides are vaporized by pressure though a microscopic needle and ionized through application of a high electric potential. In tandem mass spectroscopy (Tandem LC/MS/MS), a first mass spectrometer, a mass analyzer, selectively filters ionized peptides of a focused mass/charge (m/z) range into the second mass spectrometer, which determines their precise m/z ratio. In a fraction of a second the whole apparatus switches modes, and for the same peptides being ionized, the first mass spectrometer selects peptides at a given m/z which it then sends into a collision chamber in which this ionized peptide or 'precursor ion' is fragmented by collision with inert gas molecules producing 'product ions'. The product ions are introduced into the second mass spectrometer which determines their m/z ratios. Therefore, for any given peptide in a sample, its m/z and the m/z of its fragments are determined leading to a specific precursor/product profile. **c** Peptide identification is either by complex *'de novo'* sequencing (not shown) and/or simpler matching of precursor and product ion m/z profiles with profiles extrapolated from the theoretical digestion of protein sequences from a genome-derived database. **d** Lists of identified peptides are used to interrogate databases through bioinformatics in order to match them with predicted lists of peptides from simulated tryptic digestion of proteins derived from genomic databases and identify proteins in the sample.

Table 1. *(cont.)*

Methods	Principles
Peptide mass/charge (m/z) determination: Mass Spectroscopy (MS)	*Separation of peptide ions according to their mass-to-charge ratio. All involve acceleration followed by detection of ions*
Time-of-flight MS (TOF)	Ions accelerated through an electrical field and measure of time they take to reach a detector (time-of-flight)
Ion trap (3D, IT)	Ions are trapped in an acceleration cell and sequentially detected upon ejection from the field
Linear ion trap	Ions trapped in a two dimensional quadrupole field
Ion cyclotron resonance (ICR)	Detecting of an image current produced by ions cyclotroning (rotating) ions in the presence of a magnetic field
Quadrupole (Q)	Oscillating electrical fields selectively stabilize or destabilize ions passing through a radio frequency (RF) quadrupole field
Peptide/protein identification	*Methods used in proteomics for protein identification*
Immunoblotting of 1D or 2D PAGE gels	Proteins are detected using specific antibodies
2D PAGE + staining vs. reference map	Matching spots on compared gels based on location and pattern
Mass fingerprinting	MS: peptide peak comparison w/ database (can successfully be used to identify purified proteins)
Mass tag search	Tandem MS/MS: peptide sequencing (can be used to identify proteins in complex mixtures)
Expression profile comparisons	*Methods to obtain relative or absolute protein abundances between two or more samples*
2D PAGE	Spot intensity comparisons between different sample/gels
DIGE	Differentially fluorescent-stained samples run on the same gel, each fluorescent wavelength is scanned to compare spot intensity
SELDI	Bio-informatic comparisons of spectral peak profiles (usually peptide and protein ions, without identification)
Label Free (spectral counting, spectral peak intensity/integration)	Samples are run separately and peptide identifications or peak intensities are compared to evaluate protein abundance
Stable isotope labeling (ICAT, O16/O18, SILAC)	Two or more samples are labeled with light and heavy forms of a modification reagent. Samples are mixed and relative quantification is determined from relative ion intensity measured by MS
Stable isotope isobaric labeling (iTRAQ)	Multiple peptide modifying reagents contain combinations of stable heavy isotopes to yield a "tag" of the same mass. Multiple samples each labeled with one of the tags are mixed. Relative quantification from peptide fragmentation spectra which yield tagged reporter ions

Information can also be obtained at various intermediate steps. Indeed, proteins separated first through electrophoresis according to their charge and then according to their molecular weight on a polyacrylamide gel, a separation technique known as 2D PAGE, can be visualized by staining and sometimes identified through comparisons with known migration profiles. Bands from 1D gels or spots from 2D gels can be excised and digested for mass spectoscopic analysis. Further separation through high-pressure liquid chromatography (HPLC) is a mandatory step for some mass spectrometric workflows [18], such as tandem mass spectroscopy, but matrix assisted laser desorption/ionization (MALDI) can be performed directly on digested proteins or even on a frozen tissue sample in imaging mass spectroscopy (MALDI-IMS). Likewise, macropeptide fragments and even some entire proteins can be directly ionized and analyzed through mass spectroscopy in techniques such as MALDI or surface-enhanced laser desorption/ionization (SELDI), which can generate proteomic profiles or 'peptide mass fingerprints' without going all the way to full protein sequencing. However, definitive identification through peptide sequencing requires full fractionation and mass spectroscopy analysis in a tandem mass spectroscopy approach.

Caveats

Proteomics is an emerging field which is far from having reached the technical maturity of genomics and the technology ranges from the deceptively simple, such as gel electrophoresis which is available in any research laboratory but is operator dependent and necessitates expertise, to the extremely sophisticated, such as mass spectroscopic techniques which require an entire infrastructure, technical maintenance, and bio-informatic expertise. These technical issues in themselves lead to many sources of error which cannot be reviewed here, but it must be remembered when taking into account results from proteomic experiments that we are not dealing with routine benchtop analyses. For the non-proteomics expert, the most important caveats are: Protein abundance, clinical sample complexity, interindividual variability, necessity of genome-derived databases for protein identification, non-constant ionization of peptides, and bio-informatic complexity.

Protein abundance is a major problem in proteomics. Indeed, be it robust techniques such as 2D PAGE or highly sensitive ones such as mass spectroscopy, the extreme dynamic range of protein expression [18] leads to the 'masking' of low abundance proteins [19], which may be the most interesting biological signals, by high abundance proteins such as acute phase reactants which are often well-known and non-specific signals. Indeed, in the seminal studies of protein expression in bronchoalveolar lavage (BAL) fluid, several overabundant *serum* proteins such as serum albumin, hemoglobin and immmunoglobulin chains, and acute phase reactants represent many of the proteins identified in lung proteomics [20]. This is probably due in part to moderate alveolar capillary barrier permeability disorders induced by the BAL procedure itself [21]. While increases in serum proteins in BAL fluid during ALI due to increased alveolar capillary barrier permeability are pertinent, they are well documented and do not represent novel findings. Serum albumin identified in BAL fluid is a typical example. Several strategies addressing this problem are possible. First, abundant proteins of little interest, such as albumin, can be removed from the sample by immunocapture purification and various ultracentrifugation methods [22]. Second, and this leads to the problem of sample complexity, one can study a sample that does not normally contain as many proteins or is not as easily contaminated by serum as BAL fluid. This explains why some of the best results using SELDI, which does not identify proteins as such but rather an expression profile or 'fingerprint', have been obtained in amniotic fluid, a simple sample containing several orders of magnitude less proteins than serum allowing the prediction of amniotic fluid inflammation, infection, and neonatal sepsis [1]. The other problem posed by overly complex samples is interindividual variability. In highly complex samples such as serum, there are so many expressed proteins from myriad pathways involved in simultaneous processes that it is almost impossible to discriminate whether an expression signal detected by differential expression proteomic studies is due to the studied disease or a confounding factor such as interindividual variability. This has also been termed the "hamburger effect" by Diamandis [23] who doubted that SELDI cancer studies in which protein profiles did not even detect cancer-specific proteins could discriminate between profiles due to cancer itself and profiles due to the subjects having eaten a hamburger prior to the test, or any other source of interinvidual variability [23, 24]. When taking into account the heterogeneity of ALI/ARDS cases, this leads to a serious plea for 'simple' samples in ICU lung proteomics.

Proteomics, as any other high-tech field, is not an end in itself and is only as valuable as what it is used on and in which context. The principle of 'garbage-in, garbage-out' holds as well as in any other biological research field. In proteomics, this phenomenon is even increased by the sensitivity of the methods used in proteomics leading to 'garbage-in, *more* garbage-out' [25]. Any flaw in study design, sample processing, sample handling, sample contamination, equipment maintenance and handling, and bioinformatic/biostatistical processing will lead to flawed results [23–25]. The bioinformatics involved in protein identification are highly complex and often rely on various commercial or in-house developed software which differ in their treatment of data as well as in the biostatistical algorithms they are based upon [26, 27]. Furthermore, protein identification relies on information derived from genome databases in the form of protein databases which vary in design, completeness according to organism, available information, and data curation [27]. It must also be remembered that many of the genes from which protein identification is derived code for proteins which are still unknown or poorly studied or whose function is not yet determined, thus limiting the yield of information [27].

Finally, one of the most subtle caveats is that, regardless of the increasing sensitivity of mass spectroscopic equipment, it is not because a peptide/protein is not detected, that it is not there. Indeed, limits to the equipment sensitivity, 'masking' by other more abundant proteins, and the unpredictable ionization of peptide/proteins lead to many proteins being undetected even in thorough, well design proteomic workflows. The opposite is also true, i.e., it is not because a protein is detected that it is necessarily there. When tandem mass spectroscopy is applied directly to peptide mixtures, protein sequences are inferred from peptide sequences, and while some large peptide sequences definitely point to certain proteins, other peptide sequences can point to several proteins. This leads to the possible over-identification of certain proteins without the certainty of their presence which is why protein identifications in such experiments are reported with confidence scores [27].

Applications in ALI/ARDS

In vitro

Proteomic analysis of airway surface liquid in a cytokine-stimulated human bronchial epithelial cell monolayer model yielded many candidate biomarkers among which gelsolin was considered the most promising [28].

In vivo Animal Models

In a 2D-PAGE followed by mass spectrometric identifications, Signor et al. identified proteins which were differentially expressed in rats challenged with lipopolysaccharide (LPS) compared to controls [29]. Acute phase reactants, such as T-kininogen I and II, alpha-1-antitrypsin, and haptoglobin, increased whereas lung-specific proteins, such as Clara cell 10 kDa secretory protein (CC10), and pulmonary surfactant-associated protein B (SP-B), decreased in the LPS-challenge. In isolated alveolar type II cells from rats submitted to hepatic ischemia-reperfusion, Hirsch et al. [30] found, using quantitative proteomics through isobaric sample labeling, that hepatic ischemia-reperfusion increased the expression of metabolism and oxidative-stress related proteins.

Clinical Studies

In a landmark clinical study comparing plasma and pulmonary edema fluid from 16 ALI patients and BAL fluid from 12 normal subjects, Bowler et al. [20], in one of the first applications of clinical lung proteomics to ALI, using 2D PAGE and MALDI, identified several protein modifications which seemed specific to ALI. A study which perfectly illustrates the new dynamics of biomarker discovery that stem from proteomics is the study by Schnapp et al. [31]. Following the steps we described in our introduction, the authors went from the proteomic screening of clinical BAL samples from ARDS patients, to the identification of known biomarkers of lung injury and proteins previously unreported in ARDS from which they then formulated a hypothesis which they tested at the bench leading to the findings of a novel insulin-like growth factor-binding protein-3 (IGFBP-3) pathway in ARDS pathogenesis [31].

In a study of infectious exacerbation of inflammatory lung diseases but not ALI per se, Gray et al. using SELDI-time-of-flight (TOF), studied the relative quantitative profile of peptides in the fluid phase of sputum from patients with cystic fibrosis before and after antibiotic treatment for an infective exacerbation [32]. The authors found that calgranulin A and calgranulin B, which were increased in sputum from infected cystic fibrosis patients, subsequently decreased upon treatment of infection.

In another human study of BAL fluid, de Torre et al. [33] compared the quantitative protein profiles from healthy volunteers with a respiratory challenge of LPS or saline using SELDI. LPS challenge led to an increase over time of several proteins which were then identified through 2D PAGE as apolipoprotein A1, and calcium-binding proteins, S100A8 and S100A9. Furthermore, they found the same protein expression profile in BAL fluid from ARDS patients. Lung proteomics can also be applied to the study of the therapeutic modulation of disease states. In an original proteomic experiment, Bozinovski et al. identified six proteins that were induced by respiratory LPS challenge and were resistant to dexamethasone treatment, among which S100A8 which was abundantly expressed in BAL fluid [34]. In a more recent work, Chang et al. in a differential gel-electrophoresis (DIGE) experiment followed by MALDI/TOF/TOF, compared BAL fluid from ARDS patients at different time-points and BAL fluid from healthy volunteers [35]. In addition to observing that differentially expressed proteins were mostly in the ARDS day 1 versus normal comparison, they also performed a bioinformatic analysis of protein interactions from which they concluded that S100A8 and S100A9 could be key proteins in ARDS pathophysiology. A picture is, therefore, slowly emerging in which certain proteins such as gelsolin or the S100 protein family seem poised to be key proteins in ARDS and deserve further research as to their role.

Future Directions

Epithelial Lining Fluid

Concerning protein abundance and sample complexity in lung proteomics, looking for relevant samples less complex than BAL fluid may be a valuable approach. Indeed, an alternative sample, directly sampled epithelial lining fluid, rather than indirectly recovered and diluted under the form of BAL fluid, has recently been obtained by bronchoscopic use of a specially designed apparatus, the bronchoscopic microsampling probe, or BMS probe [36]. In a preliminary study, we successfully retrieved undiluted epithelial lining fluid from the BMS probe tip and submitted it to proteomic characterization [37]. We found that, although we used an experimental animal (rabbit) that has incomplete databases for protein identification and low protein loads, we identified more (43 versus 30) non-redundant proteins than Bow-

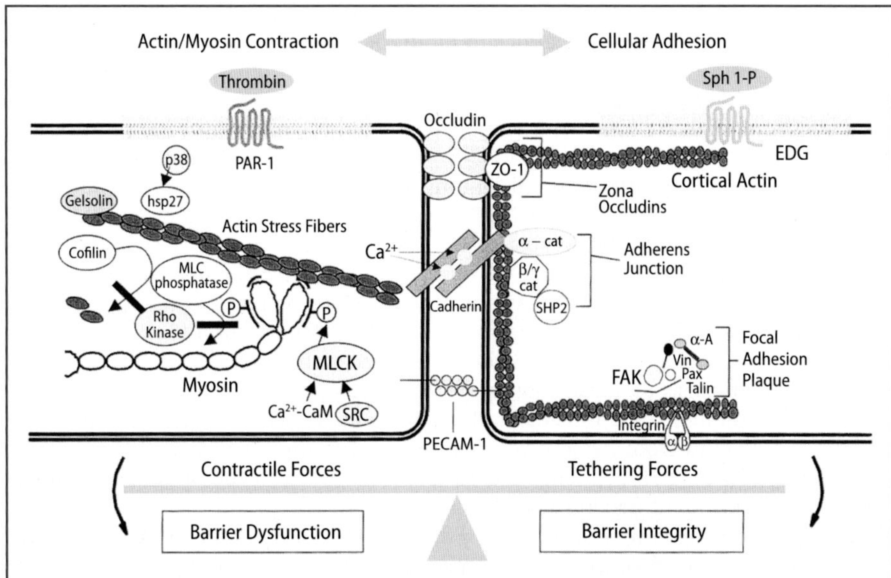

Fig. 3. Proteins involved in lung endothelial integrity detected in epithelial lining fluid. An overview of the proteins involved in either the cytoskeletal tethering or contractile forces of lung endothelial cells either maintaining endothelial integrity or leading to alveolar capillary barrier dysfunction (from [38] with permission). Proteomic analysis of undiluted epithelial lining fluid simultaneously identified several proteins from the pathway leading to barrier dysfunction: Gelsolin, cofilin, HSP27, and actin.

ler et al. [20] who used high protein loads and complete human genome derived databases. Furthermore, most of the non-redundant proteins we identified in epithelial lining fluid (86 %) were distinct from the usual high abundance proteins previously identified in serum or BAL fluid studies. Data-mining the Medline database further demonstrated that the proteins identified were relevant to lung disease in general and to ALI/ARDS in particular. To illustrate the relevance of the proteins identified in epithelial lining fluid to the study of ALI pathophysiology, **Figure 3** shows two opposing pathways driving the forces in balance in lung endothelial permeability [38]. We simultaneously identified in epithelial lining fluid, several proteins involved in the pathway – gelsolin, cofilin, heat shock protein (HSP)27, and actin. Additionally to its low protein complexity, epithelial lining fluid as recovered through the BMS probe, is not as salt-laden as BAL fluid obtained through lavage with saline which hampers proteomic analysis and necessitates preparative processing steps [22]. Furthermore, the BMS probe can be used non-bronchoscopically through a Combicath® which should allow more routine use in the intensive care setting.

Exhaled Breath Condensates

Another sample of interest could be exhaled breath condensates. Exhaled breath condensates have already been collected from ventilated patients allowing assessment of oxidative stress [39], multiplex cytokine measurement [40], and pH [41]. Exhaled breath condensate from healthy volunteers has been subjected to proteomic analysis showing it was a valid candidate sample for exploration of lung disease [42]. Most interestingly, a recent study collected exhaled breath condensates from 24 ventilated patients with ALI/ARDS and from 10 healthy volunteers which were all submitted to proteomic analysis through 1D PAGE followed by MALDI-TOF [43]. The authors identified three proteins, cytokeratins 2, 9, and 10, which were only expressed in ventilated ALI/ARDS patients and whose detection was correlated to peak inspiratory pressure, positive end-expiratory pressure (PEEP) and ARDS score, but not to serum inflammatory markers, such as C-reactive protein (CRP) and procalcitonin, nor to pro-inflammatory cytokines, such as interleukin (IL)-6 or IL-8 in either serum or exhaled breath condensates. Since exhaled breath condensate may be continuously collected in ventilated patients [41], this opens the perspective that once pertinent biomarkers of ALI/ARDS have been discovered through exhaled breath condensates proteomics, they could be monitored continuously on-line.

Decreasing the Noise to Discover the Signal

The concept of studying biomarkers over time is crucial. Indeed, as previously explained, general protein expression levels, especially in complex biological fluid samples, generate 'noise' which may vary interindividually unrelated to the studied processes and either mask signals or, even worse, induce false signals [23, 24]. Thus, searching for answers in heterogeneous diseases, such as sepsis or ALI/ARDS, occurring in such an inhomogeneous group as critically ill patients by comparing the expression of potential biomarkers between individuals may be an ill-suited approach. Indeed, the potential 'noise' due to the various host responses occurring in critically ill patients may drown out the signal. Likewise, it is exceedingly difficult to determine which phase of a pathophysiological process a critically ill patient is in, leading to the study of patients which are undoubtedly in different stages of disease, again drowning biological signals in noise. One strategy to cancel out this 'noise' may be to use subjects as their own controls, comparing the expression of potential biomarkers *intra*individually rather than *inter*individually over time. Indeed, a profile of variations may emerge when following biological processes over time in a given patient. Rather than a single biomarker at one timepoint being the signal, the evolution over time of one or more biomarkers with a certain profile may become the signal. It may even emerge that this profile could characterize the evolution of disease allowing 'calibration' of studied patients according to their disease stage. This, in turn, would allow greater homogeneity in intensive care studies and further facilitate studies. This paradigm shift is starting in critical care and has been addressed in a recent editorial raising the issue of new statistical and modeling methods relevant to this approach [44].

Another approach is to cancel out the noise by comparing protein expression in an organ area involved in a process to that in an uninvolved organ area. This strategy was used in a non-proteomic study of LPS-induced lung inflammation in which LPS was administered in healthy volunteers selectively to one lung allowing the comparison of BAL fluid from the involved lung to BAL fluid recovered from the 'control' lung in the same subject [45]. The BMS probe allows such 'internal' controls by selective sampling, which we have used in proteomic studies of exhaled breath condensates proximal to suspected peripheral lung cancer showing differential expression of proteins compared to the controlateral lung (unpublished data).

Proteomic studies relevant to intensive care are not limited to the sole areas of sepsis or ALI/ARDS. Indeed, proteomic screening for biomarkers has identified many potential biomarkers or expression profiles for ICU-related diseases, such as pulmonary embolism [46], lung infection [47], lung allograft rejection [48], and severe acute respiratory syndrome (SARS) [49].

As a highly technology-dependent field, constant technological advances will lead to increases in proteomic sensitivity, reliability, and reproducibility. These advances concern every aspect of proteomics, including sample preparation and separation methods, such as microfluidics and capillary electrophoresis, protein labeling techniques for comparative or quantitative proteomics, mass spectrometer performance, and data analysis solutions [50].

Conclusion

While proteomics should not be considered as an end in itself, to avoid an upcoming deluge of studies using proteomics as a publication 'gimmick', it is an emerging field of research which, used appropriately, has the capacity to yield a great deal of new pertinent information in the study of the pathophysiology of complex diseases, such as ALI/ARDS, which has, until recently, dwelled on either well-known non-specific inflammatory biomarkers or genomic information too far removed from the physiological processes involved. As such, we believe the intensive care community should familiarize itself with the methods, inherent limitations, and perspectives involved and embrace proteomics. Future research in ALI/ARDS should incorporate proteomics into the design of major projects and intensive care researchers should seek collaboration with proteomic scientists.

References

1. Buhimschi CS, Bhandari V, Hamar BD, et al (2007) Proteomic profiling of the amniotic fluid to detect inflammation, infection, and neonatal sepsis. PLoS Med 4:e18
2. Crouser ED, Julian MW, Huff JE, Mandich DV, Green-Church KB (2006) A proteomic analysis of liver mitochondria during acute endotoxemia. Intensive Care Med 32: 1252–1262
3. Holly MK, Dear JW, Hu X, et al (2006) Biomarker and drug-target discovery using proteomics in a new rat model of sepsis-induced acute renal failure. Kidney Int 70: 496–506
4. Kalenka A, Feldmann RE Jr, Otero K, Maurer MH, Waschke KF, Fiedler F (2006) Changes in the serum proteome of patients with sepsis and septic shock. Anesth Analg 103: 1522–1526
5. Ren Y, Wang J, Xia J, et al (2007) The alterations of mouse plasma proteins during septic development. J Proteome Res 6: 2812–2821
6. Manolio T (2003) Novel risk markers and clinical practice. N Engl J Med 349: 1587–1589
7. Ackland GL, Mythen MG (2007) Novel biomarkers in critical care: utility or futility? Crit Care 11:175
8. Becker KL, Snider R, Nylen ES (2008) Procalcitonin assay in systemic inflammation, infection, and sepsis: clinical utility and limitations. Crit Care Med 36: 941–952
9. McLean AS, Huang SJ, Hyams S, et al (2007) Prognostic values of B-type natriuretic peptide in severe sepsis and septic shock. Crit Care Med 35: 1019–1026
10. Garcia JG, Moreno Vinasco L (2006) Genomic insights into acute inflammatory lung injury. Am J Physiol Lung Cell Mol Physiol 291:L1113–1117
11. Meyer NJ, Garcia JG (2007) Wading into the genomic pool to unravel acute lung injury genetics. Proc Am Thorac Soc 4: 69–76
12. Nonas SA, Finigan JH, Gao L, Garcia JG (2005) Functional genomic insights into acute lung injury: role of ventilators and mechanical stress. Proc Am Thorac Soc 2: 188–194
13. Poly WJ (1997) Nongenetic variation, genetic-environmental interactions and altered gene expression. III. Posttranslational modifications. Comp Biochem Physiol A Physiol 118: 551–572
14. Gygi SP, Rochon Y, Franza BR, Aebersold R (1999) Correlation between protein and mRNA abundance in yeast. Mol Cell Biol 19: 1720–1730
15. Witze ES, Old WM, Resing KA, Ahn NG (2007) Mapping protein post-translational modifications with mass spectrometry. Nat Methods 4: 798–806
16. Bowler RP, Ellison MC, Reisdorph N (2006) Proteomics in pulmonary medicine. Chest 130: 567–574
17. Hirsch J, Hansen KC, Burlingame AL, Matthay MA (2004) Proteomics: current techniques and potential applications to lung disease. Am J Physiol Lung Cell Mol Physiol 287:L1–23
18. Sandra K, Moshir M, D'Hondt F, Verleysen K, Kas K, Sandra P (2008) Highly efficient peptide separations in proteomics Part 1. Unidimensional high performance liquid chromatography. J Chromatogr B Analyt Technol Biomed Life Sci 866: 48–63
19. Jiang X, Ye M, Zou H (2008) Technologies and methods for sample pretreatment in efficient proteome and peptidome analysis. Proteomics 8: 686–705
20. Bowler RP, Duda B, Chan ED, et al (2004) Proteomic analysis of pulmonary edema fluid and plasma in patients with acute lung injury. Am J Physiol Lung Cell Mol Physiol 286: L1095–1104
21. Feng NH, Hacker A, Effros RM (1992) Solute exchange between the plasma and epithelial lining fluid of rat lungs. J Appl Physiol 72: 1081–1089
22. Plymoth A, Lofdahl CG, Ekberg-Jansson A, et al (2003) Human bronchoalveolar lavage: biofluid analysis with special emphasis on sample preparation. Proteomics 3: 962–972
23. Diamandis EP (2004) Analysis of serum proteomic patterns for early cancer diagnosis: drawing attention to potential problems. J Natl Cancer Inst 96: 353–356
24. Garber K (2004) Debate rages over proteomic patterns. J Natl Cancer Inst 96: 816–818
25. Zhang Z, Chan DW (2005) Cancer proteomics: in pursuit of "true" biomarker discovery. Cancer Epidemiol Biomarkers Prev 14: 2283–2286
26. Domon B, Aebersold R (2006) Challenges and opportunities in proteomics data analysis. Mol Cell Proteomics 5: 1921–1926
27. Nesvizhskii AI, Aebersold R (2005) Interpretation of shotgun proteomic data: the protein inference problem. Mol Cell Proteomics 4: 1419–1440
28. Candiano G, Bruschi M, Pedemonte N, et al. (2007) Proteomic analysis of the airway surface

I

liquid: modulation by proinflammatory cytokines. Am J Physiol Lung Cell Mol Physiol 292:L185–198
29. Signor L, Tigani B, Beckmann N, Falchetto R, Stoeckli M (2004) Two-dimensional electrophoresis protein profiling and identification in rat bronchoalveolar lavage fluid following allergen and endotoxin challenge. Proteomics 4: 2101–2110
30. Hirsch J, Niemann CU, Hansen KC, et al (2008) Alterations in the proteome of pulmonary alveolar type II cells in the rat after hepatic ischemia-reperfusion. Crit Care Med 36: 1846–1854
31. Schnapp LM, Donohoe S, Chen J, et al (2006) Mining the acute respiratory distress syndrome proteome: identification of the insulin-like growth factor (IGF)/IGF-binding protein-3 pathway in acute lung injury. Am J Pathol 169: 86–95
32. Gray RD, MacGregor G, Noble D, et al (2008) Sputum proteomics in inflammatory and suppurative respiratory diseases. Am J Respir Crit Care Med 178: 444–452
33. de Torre C, Ying SX, Munson PJ, Meduri GU, Suffredini AF (2006) Proteomic analysis of inflammatory biomarkers in bronchoalveolar lavage. Proteomics 6: 3949–3957
34. Bozinovski S, Cross M, Vlahos R, et al (2005) S100A8 chemotactic protein is abundantly increased, but only a minor contributor to LPS-induced, steroid resistant neutrophilic lung inflammation in vivo. J Proteome Res 4: 136–145
35. Chang DW, Hayashi S, Gharib SA, et al (2008) Proteomic and computational analysis of bronchoalveolar proteins during the course of the acute respiratory distress syndrome. Am J Respir Crit Care Med 178: 701–709
36. Ishizaka A, Watanabe M, Yamashita T, et al (2001) New bronchoscopic microsample probe to measure the biochemical constituents in epithelial lining fluid of patients with acute respiratory distress syndrome. Crit Care Med 29: 896–898
37. Kipnis E, Hansen K, Sawa T, et al (2008) Proteomic analysis of undiluted lung epithelial lining fluid. Chest 134: 338–345
38. Dudek SM, Garcia JG (2001) Cytoskeletal regulation of pulmonary vascular permeability. J Appl Physiol 91: 1487–1500
39. Gessner C, Hammerschmidt S, Kuhn H, et al (2003) Exhaled breath condensate nitrite and its relation to tidal volume in acute lung injury. Chest 124: 1046–1052
40. Sack U, Scheibe R, Wotzel M, et al (2006) Multiplex analysis of cytokines in exhaled breath condensate. Cytometry A 69: 169–172
41. Walsh BK, Mackey DJ, Pajewski T, Yu Y, Gaston BM, Hunt JF (2006) Exhaled-breath condensate pH can be safely and continuously monitored in mechanically ventilated patients. Respir Care 51: 1125–1131
42. Griese M, Noss J, von Bredow C (2002) Protein pattern of exhaled breath condensate and saliva. Proteomics 2: 690–696
43. Gessner C, Dihazi H, Brettschneider S, et al (2008) Presence of cytokeratins in exhaled breath condensate of mechanical ventilated patients. Respir Med 102: 299–306
44. Clermont G (2007) Modeling longitudinal data in acute illness. Crit Care 11:152
45. Nick JA, Coldren CD, Geraci MW, et al (2004) Recombinant human activated protein C reduces human endotoxin-induced pulmonary inflammation via inhibition of neutrophil chemotaxis. Blood 104: 3878–3885
46. Li SQ, Qi HW, Wu CG, et al (2007) Comparative proteomic study of acute pulmonary embolism in a rat model. Proteomics 7: 2287–2299
47. Ventura CL, Higdon R, Kolker E, Skerrett SJ, Rubens CE (2008) Host airway proteins interact with Staphylococcus aureus during early pneumonia. Infect Immun 76: 888–898
48. Nelsestuen GL, Martinez MB, Hertz MI, Savik K, Wendt CH (2005) Proteomic identification of human neutrophil alpha-defensins in chronic lung allograft rejection. Proteomics 5: 1705–1713
49. Yip TT, Cho WC, Cheng WW, et al (2007) Application of ProteinChip array profiling in serum biomarker discovery for patients suffering from severe acute respiratory syndrome. Methods Mol Biol 382: 313–331
50. Malmstrom J, Lee H, Aebersold R (2007) Advances in proteomic workflows for systems biology. Curr Opin Biotechnol 18: 378–384

II Inflammatory Response

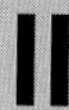

The Host Response to Sepsis

T.J. Hommes, W.J. Wiersinga, and T. van der Poll

Introduction

Sir William Osler, probably the most influential physician in the English-speaking world at the turn of the century more than a hundred years ago, wrote the following about sepsis in his famous text book, The Evolution of Modern Medicine (1904): "Except on few occasions, the patient appears to die from the body's response to infection rather than from it". The assumption that sepsis is the consequence of an overwhelming inflammatory reaction of the patient to microorganisms was widely accepted for many years. Current knowledge indicates that this paradigm is oversimplified and only partially true. The original theory that sepsis mortality is caused by an overstimulated immune system was based on studies in animals that were infused with large doses of bacteria or bacterial products, in particular lipopolysaccharide (LPS), the toxic component of the Gram-negative bacterial cell wall. Such infusions result in a brisk systemic release of an array of pro-inflammatory mediators of which many have been found to be directly responsible for the death of the host. In a hallmark manuscript published in 1985, Beutler and colleagues reported that elimination of the early activity of the pro-inflammatory cytokine, tumor necrosis factor (TNF)-α, after intravenous injection of LPS prevented death in mice [1]. Two years later, these results were confirmed by Tracey and colleagues, who showed that a monoclonal anti-TNF-α antibody protected baboons against lethal Gram-negative sepsis [2]. Since then, anti-TNF-α therapies have been found to be protective in a number of sepsis models in which bacteria or bacterial products were administered systemically as a bolus or a brief infusion [3]. In addition, neutralization of another pro-inflammatory cytokine, interleukin (IL)-1, also reduced lethality induced by LPS or living bacteria in animals [4, 5]. These landmark findings revolutionized thinking about sepsis pathogenesis and treatment and made researchers and physicians believe that finally sepsis mortality, which had remained unacceptably high, could be reduced by 'magic bullets' targeting TNF-α and/or IL-1. We know now that virtually all clinical sepsis trials with anti-TNF-α strategies and recombinant IL-1 receptor antagonist (IL-1ra) failed. Moreover, many other anti-inflammatory therapies failed to alter the outcome of patients with sepsis. Clearly, the hypothesis that excessive inflammation is the main underlying cause for an adverse outcome of a septic patient is not correct, at least not generally speaking. In this chapter, we will describe new insights into components of the integral reaction of the host to sepsis. Important pathways activated during the host response to sepsis are depicted in **Figure 1**.

II

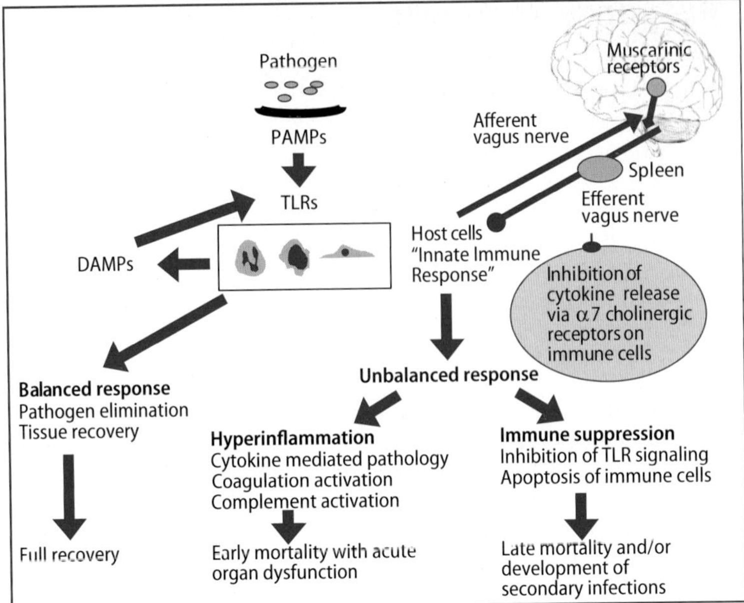

Fig. 1. The host response to sepsis. The interaction between pathogens and the host is mediated initially via an interaction between PAMPs (pathogen-associated molecular pathogens) and TLRs (Toll-like receptors). This interaction can result in the release of alarmins or DAMPs (danger-associated molecular patterns) that have the ability to further amplify the inflammatory response at least in part via TLRs. The initial inflammation activates afferent signals that are relayed to the nucleus tractus solitarius; subsequent activation of vagus efferent activity, mediated by central muscarinic receptors in the brain, inhibits cytokine synthesis via pathways dependent on the $\alpha7$ subunit of acetylcholine receptors on macrophages and other cells through the so-called cholinergic anti-inflammatory pathway (the inflammatory reflex). The resulting innate response of immune cells can result in a balanced reaction leading to pathogen elimination and tissue recovery or an unbalanced reaction that on the one hand can lead to exaggerated inflammation and tissue injury and on the other hand to immune suppression caused by immune cell apoptosis and enhanced expression of negative regulators of TLR signaling.

Epidemiology and Genetic Variability

Sepsis is the second leading cause of death in non-coronary intensive care units (ICUs) and the 10th leading cause of death overall. During the last two decades the incidence of sepsis increased from 83 per 100,000 population in 1979 to 240 per 100,000 population in 2000, representing an annual increase of 9 % [6]. In this period, the average age of patients with sepsis increased from 57 to 61 years. Although mortality rates during the last two decades have declined, the concurrently rising incidence of sepsis resulted in a tripling of the number of deaths related to sepsis to 44 per 100,000 population in 2000 [6]. Organ failure has a cumulative effect on mortality: Whereas mortality due to sepsis without organ failure is approximately 15 %, patients with three or more failing organs die in 70 % of cases [6]. Septic shock, defined as sepsis plus refractory hypotension, has a crude mortality of 45–60 %.

The response to infection varies between individuals. This variability, at least in part, is related to a number of external determinants, including the virulence and the load of the etiologic pathogen and the interval between onset of disease and initiation of treatment. In addition, comorbidity is of major importance: Patients with underlying disease are more likely to develop sepsis, in particular those with cancer, immunodeficiency, and chronic organ failure [6]. It is likely, however, that internal determinants, i.e., the genetic makeup of the host, also play an important role in the susceptibility to sepsis. This hypothesis is supported by the fact that sepsis occurs more frequently in men than in women (annual relative risk 1.28) and in non-white persons than in white persons (annual relative risk 1.90) [6]. Recent evidence indicates that more subtle genetic variations, resulting from so-called single nucleotide polymorphisms (SNPs), may also impact on the development and outcome of sepsis. It is unlikely that one SNP will have a major impact on the susceptibility and/or outcome of sepsis, but when several predisposing SNPs are present, a certain phenotype may become apparent. Several sepsis-gene association studies have been conducted seeking to determine the influence of genetic variation on the host response to infection [7]. Although associations between individual SNPs and outcome have been identified, published data are not consistent most likely due to small sample sizes [7]. It is without doubt that our knowledge of the impact of genetic variation of the host will increase tremendously in the years to come. High throughput assays that can genotype hundreds of thousands of SNPs in a single experiment will be of great value here.

Pathogen Recognition Systems

The innate immune system is able to detect pathogens via a limited number of pattern-recognition receptors (PRRs) [8]. PRRs recognize conserved motifs that are expressed by pathogens but absent in higher eukaryotes; these microbial components are known as pathogen-associated molecular patterns (PAMPs). PRRs activate distinct cellular responses aimed at killing the invading microorganism. The best studied PAMP is LPS, which is a component of the outer membrane of Gram-negative bacteria. Other major bacterial PAMPs with likely relevance for the pathogenesis of sepsis include lipoteichoic acid, peptidoglycan, lipopeptides, flagellin and bacterial DNA; important fungal PAMPs are zymosan and (phospholipo)mannan [8]. Additionally, PRRs may warn the host of imminent danger through their ability to recognize endogenous mediators released upon injury. Such endogenous danger signals have been named 'alarmins' or 'danger-associated molecular patterns' (DAMPs).

The Toll-like family of receptors (TLR) plays a central role as PRRs in the initiation of cellular innate immune responses (**Fig. 2**). TLRs are the first to detect host invasion by pathogens and initiate immune responses [8]. Thirteen mammalian homologs of *Drosophila* Toll (TLRs 1 to 13) have been identified. Of these, humans (but not mice) express TLR10, whereas mice (but not humans) express TLR11, -12 and -13. All TLRs are single-spanning transmembrane proteins with leucine-rich extracellular domains and with a cytoplasmic part largely composed of a so-called TIR (Toll/interleukin [IL]-1 receptor/Resistance) domain. Ligands for most TLRs have been described; Table 1 summarizes TLR specificity for several bacterial and fungal PAMPs with likely relevance for sepsis. TLRs can be expressed on the cell surface (TLR1, -2, -4, -5 and -6) or in intracellular compartments, in particular within the endosomes (TLR3, -7, -8 and -9).

It should be noted that each pathogen expresses multiple PAMPs and thus triggers multiple TLRs. *Escherichia coli* for example harbors LPS (a TLR4 ligand), pepti-

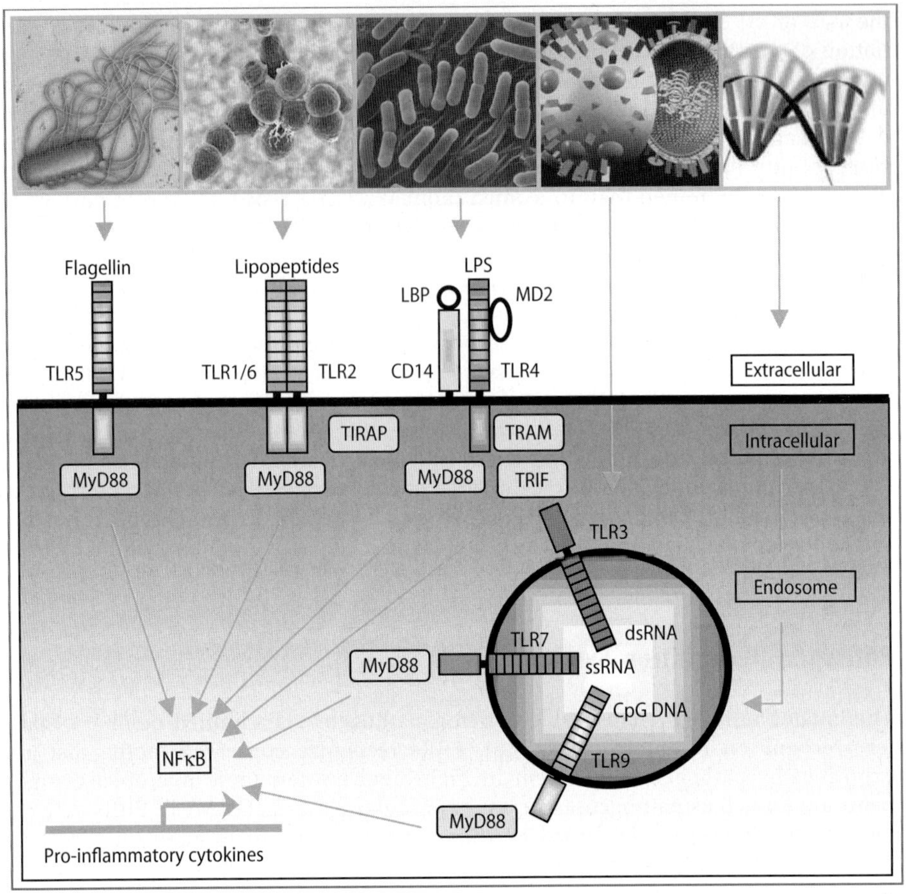

Fig. 2. Toll-like receptors (TLR) and pathogen recognition. The TLR family discriminates between specific patterns of microbial components. TLR2, which can associate with TLR1 and TLR6, is essential for the recognition of microbial lipopeptides. TLR4 recognizes lipopolysaccharide (LPS). LPS first binds to LPS-binding-protein (LBP), which transfers LPS to CD14. Binding of LPS to CD14 leads to the association of CD14 with MD-2 and TLR4. TLR5 is a receptor for flagellin. TLR9 is the CpG DNA receptor, whereas TLR3 and TLR7 are implicated in the recognition of viral double-stranded RNA (dsRNA) and single-stranded RNA (ssRNA), respectively. After TLR stimulation, the adaptor molecule myeloid differentiation primary-response protein 88 (MyD88) is recruited. This will lead to the release of nuclear-factor-κB (NF-κB) which will result in the transcription of a whole range of inflammatory genes. Next to MyD88, the adaptor molecules, Toll/interleukin-1 receptor (TIR)-domain-containing-adaptor-protein (TIRAP), TIR-domain-containing-adaptor-protein-inducing-interferon-β (TRIF) and TRIF-related-adaptor-molecule (TRAM) have been identified. TIRAP is essential for MyD88-dependent signaling through TLR2 and TLR4. TRIF is essential for the TLR3 and TLR4-mediated activation of the MyD88-independent pathway. TRAM is involved in TLR4 mediated MyD88-independent/TRIF-dependent signaling pathways.

doglycan, lipoproteins (both TLR2 ligands), flagellin (a TLR5 ligand) and CpG DNA (a TLR9 ligand). The complexity of the interaction between innate immune receptors and fungi was recently illustrated by an elegant investigation showing that three distinct components of the cell wall of *Candida albicans* are recognized by four different host receptors: N-linked mannosyl residues are detected by the mannose

II

Table 1. Pathogen and danger associated molecular patterns and their recognition by Toll-like receptors (TLR)

	Species	TLR
Pathogen-associated molecular patterns (PAMPs)		
Bacteria		
Lipopolysaccharide	Gram-negative bacteria	TLR4
Lipoteichoic acid	Gram-positive bacteria	TLR2*
Peptidoglycan	Most bacteria	TLR2
Triacyl lipopeptides	Most bacteria	TLR1/TLR2
Diacyl lipopeptides	*Mycoplasma* spp	TLR2/ TLR6
Porins	Neisseria	TLR2
Flagellin	Flagellated bacteria	TLR5
CpG DNA	Bacteria	TLR9
Unknown	Uropathogenic bacteria	TLR11[ü]
Fungus		
Zymosan	*Saccharomyces cerevisiae*	TLR2/TLR6
Phospholipomannan	*Candida albicans*	TLR2
Mannan	*Candida albicans*	TLR4
O-linked mannosyl residues	*Candida albicans*	TLR4
β-glucans	*Candida albicans*	TLR2[§]
Danger-associated molecular patterns (DAMPs)**		
Heat shock proteins	Host	TLR4
Fibrinogen, fibronectin	Host	TLR4
Hyaluronan	Host	TLR4
Biglycans	Host	TLR4
HMGB1	Host	TLR4, TLR2

The table shows PAMPs and DAMPs with likely relevance for sepsis (PAMPs expressed by viruses and parasites are not shown). *For detection of lipoteichoic acid from some pathogens, TLR6 functions as a coreceptor for TLR2; [ü]TLR11 is not functional in humans; [§]in collaboration with dectin-1; **recent studies describe a role for TLRs in acute injury using rodent models of hemorrhagic shock, ischemia and reperfusion, tissue trauma and wound repair, and various toxic exposures: these studies have implicated TLR4 as a major factor in the initial injury response. The table shows endogenous mediators identified as TLR4 ligands.

receptor, O-linked mannosyl residues are sensed by TLR4, and β-glucans are recognized by the dectin/TLR2 complex [9].

Although at first sight, the TLR signaling pathway seems overwhelming in complexity, it is fascinating to see that the innate immune response signals through a channel of relatively low complexity: The entire TLR family signals via four adapter proteins (myeloid differentiation primary-response protein 88 [MyD88], TIR-domain-containing-adaptor-protein [TIRAP], TIR-domain-containing-adaptor-protein-inducing-IFN-β [TRIF], and TRIF-related-adaptor-molecule [TRAM]), which together with a number of protein kinases take care of the recognition and response to microbial molecules. Importantly, TLR signaling is tightly regulated in order to avoid detrimental inflammatory responses; as such, several negative regulators of TLRs have been identified, including MyD88 short, IL-1R-associated kinase [IRAK]-M, ST2, single-immunoglobulin-IL-1R-related-molecule [SIGIRR] and Toll-interacting protein [TOLLIP] [10]. It is beyond the scope of this review to discuss the signaling cascade elicited by TLR triggering in detail. It is sufficient to state here that given their central role in the recognition of microbes, TLRs likely play a central role in sepsis pathogenicity. In this respect, one has to remember that TLRs are, on the one hand, essential for the early detection of pathogens, but on the other hand may also cause excessive inflammation after uncontrolled stimulation. Thus, whereas TLR4 deficient mice are totally protected against the toxic effects of LPS, these animals are more susceptible to several Gram-negative infections [11]. Similarly, TLR2 deficient mice are protected against lethal shock induced by heat killed *Bacillus subtilis* [12], but are more susceptible to some infections with viable Gram-positive bacteria, including *Staphylococcus aureus* [13].

Triggering receptor expressed on myeloid cells-1 (TREM-1) amplifies the TLR-mediated inflammatory response to microbial products [14]. TREM-1, which signals through the adaptor protein, DAP12, is strongly and specifically expressed on monocytes and neutrophils from patients with sepsis. Of diagnostic importance, high concentrations of plasma soluble TREM-1 can indicate infection in patients with systemic inflammatory response syndrome (SIRS). Blockade of TREM-1 protected mice against LPS-induced shock, as well as microbial sepsis caused by live *E. coli* or cecal ligation and puncture. In addition, a synthetic peptide mimicking a short, highly conserved domain of soluble TREM-1 protected septic animals from hyper-responsiveness and death [14].

TLRs detect pathogens at either the cell surface or in lysosomes/endosomes. Pathogens that invade the cytosol are recognized by various cytoplasmic PRRs. Nucleotide-binding oligodimerization domain proteins, NOD1 and NOD2, contribute to the detection of peptidoglycan in the cytosol [8]. In addition, bacterial infection leads to activation of caspase-1 in a protein complex that has been termed the "NALP3-inflammasome" [15]. NALP3, also known as cryopyrin or CIAS, regulates the activity of caspase-1, an enzyme responsible for the secretion of three IL-1 family members implicated in host defense against infection: IL-1β, IL-18 and IL-33. Caspase-1 plays a detrimental role in overwhelming inflammation, such as induced by bolus injection of high dose LPS, as indicated by the fact that caspase-1 deficient mice are resistant against LPS-induced lethality. In murine infection models, however, caspase-1 has a positive impact on host defense. In this respect the dual role of caspase-1 resembles the bimodal roles of TLR2 and -4 in severe infection.

The exponentially increasing knowledge of the pathways that activate the innate immune system will lead to novel interventions seeking to improve the outcome of sepsis. At present, several therapeutic agents are under investigation in clinical trials involving patients with sepsis. Strategies aiming to interfere with TLR signaling include two TLR4 antagonists (E5564, Eisai, and TAK-242, Takeda). It can be expected that other compounds influencing pathogen recognition systems will be developed for clinical testing in the future.

Coagulation and Anticoagulation

Patients with sepsis almost invariably show evidence of activation of the coagulation system [16]. Although the majority of sepsis patients do not have clinical signs of disseminated intravascular coagulation (DIC), patients with a laboratory diagnosis of this syndrome are known to have a worse outcome than patients with normal coagulation parameters. In addition, several clinical studies have suggested that sepsis-related DIC is associated with not only a high mortality but also organ dysfunction, and that attenuation of coagulation may ameliorate organ failure in this condition [16, 17].

Tissue factor is regarded as the primary initiator of coagulation in sepsis [16]. Interaction of tissue factor with factor VIIa results in the activation of factor X either directly or indirectly through the activation of factor IX. Activated factor X converts prothrombin to thrombin, which finally induces the conversion of fibrin to fibrinogen, thereby inducing the formation of a blood clot. Of note, in addition to its traditional cell-associated form, tissue factor antigen and procoagulant activity have also been detected in cell-free plasma. Circulating tissue factor resides in microparticles that can be shed from leukocytes, endothelial cells, vascular smooth muscle cells, and platelets [16].

The pivotal role of tissue factor in the activation of coagulation during a systemic inflammatory response syndrome, such as produced by endotoxemia or severe sepsis, has been established by many different experiments. In particular, a number of different strategies that prevent the activation of the VIIa-tissue factor pathway in endotoxemic humans and chimpanzees, and in bacteremic baboons abrogated the activation of the common pathway of coagulation [16]. In accordance, mice with an almost complete absence of tissue factor had reduced coagulation, inflammation and mortality relative to control mice upon administration of high dose LPS [18]. Similarly, a deficiency of tissue factor expression by hematopoietic cells reduced LPS-induced coagulation, inflammation, and mortality, suggesting that hematopoietic cells are the major pathologic site of tissue factor expression during endotoxemia [18].

Blood clotting is controlled by three major anticoagulant proteins: tissue factor pathway inhibitor (TFPI), antithrombin, and activated protein C (APC) [16]. During severe sepsis the activities of TFPI, antithrombin and the protein C-APC system are impaired, which together with enhanced tissue factor-dependent coagulation results in a shift toward a net procoagulant state. In septic primates, the administration of either TFPI, antithrombin, or APC attenuated consumptive coagulopathy [16] and large clinical trials in sepsis patients have been completed [19–22]. Only APC was found to reduce 28-day mortality in patients with severe sepsis [19]; importantly, APC was not effective in patients with severe sepsis and a low risk of death [22]. Recently, the European licensing authority has requested Eli Lilly to perform another placebo-controlled trial with APC in adult patients with severe sepsis; this trial (PROWESS-SHOCK) was recently initiated.

In recent years, much attention has been given to the role of protease-activated cell receptors (PARs) in linking coagulation and inflammation [23]. The PAR family consists of four members, PAR-1 to PAR-4, which are localized in the vasculature on endothelial cells, mononuclear cells, platelets, fibroblasts, and smooth muscle cells [23]. Low concentrations of thrombin activate PAR-1, whereas high concentrations are required to activate PAR-3 and PAR-4. In primary endothelial cells, APC signaling is mediated through PAR-1, which induces a number of genes that are known to downregulate pro-inflammatory signaling pathways and that inhibit apoptosis, thereby providing molecular evidence for anti-inflammatory effects of APC [24].

Kaneider et al. [25] utilized cell penetrating peptides (so-called pepducins) to delineate the roles of PAR-1 and PAR-2 in LPS shock and sepsis induced by cecal ligation and puncture. Using either agonistic or antagonistic pepducins targeted at PARs, they provided evidence that activation of PAR-1 is harmful during the early phases of endotoxemia and sepsis, facilitating pulmonary leak and DIC, but becomes beneficial at later stages in a PAR-2 dependent way by a mechanism that involved a time-dependent switch in the inflammatory functions of endothelial PAR-1, dependent on the ability of PAR1 to transactivate PAR-2 [25]. This intriguing time dependent switch of PAR-1 from an exacerbating receptor to a protective receptor is consistent with studies showing that PAR-1 deficiency conferred no net survival benefit in models of endotoxemia or sepsis [18, 25]. Remarkably, PAR-1 deficiency was reported to protect mice against LPS induced lethality in an LD80 model of endotoxemia [26]. While PAR-1 deficient mice initially developed levels of inflammatory markers indistinguishable from wild type mice, they showed reduced late-stage inflammation. In a series of elegant experiments, support was provided for the hypothesis that beyond the very early host response to a severe infection a tight interaction exists between coagulation and inflammation, driven by the interaction between thrombin and PAR-1 [26]. Clearly, the studies on the role of PAR-1 and PAR-2 in endotoxic shock and sepsis discussed here [18, 25, 26] are not fully consistent, although differences can at least in part be explained by differences in the severity of the insults.

Immune Suppression and Apoptosis

Although severe infection is still considered to result in an early phase of hyperinflammation by most investigators, the extent and duration of this period likely varies considerably due to differences in comorbidity, nutritional status, age, and genetic background of the patient on the one hand and the initial source of the infection, the virulence of the causative organism, and the size of the infectious inoculum on the other hand [27]. In most if not all patients who survive the acute phase of sepsis, a prolonged state of immune suppression evolves, a condition referred to as immunoparalysis. The majority of patients who are enrolled in sepsis trials display evidence for this state of reduced immune responsiveness: Their blood leukocytes are less capable of releasing pro-inflammatory cytokines upon stimulation with bacteria or bacterial products. Some investigators have challenged the concept that sepsis results in sequential hyperinflammatory and anti-inflammatory phases; it has been suggested that these different responses may occur simultaneously or that the anti-inflammatory reaction may predominate from the start [28].

Although immunoparalysis has been regarded beneficial in the sense that it counteracts a potentially devastating pro-inflammatory response, it can also lead to an inability to clear infection and a subsequent predisposition to nosocomial infection. Recent work has provided insight into the mechanisms of immune suppression in sepsis. Hotchkiss and Nicholson have shown that large numbers of lymphocytes and gastrointestinal epithelial cells die by apoptosis during sepsis [29]. Apoptosis is a physiological process by which cells are eliminated in a controlled manner ('programmed suicide') in order to limit damage to surrounding tissue. Apoptotic cells produce anti-inflammatory cytokines and elicit anergy, which impairs the response to pathogens; necrotic cells cause immune stimulation and enhance defense against microbials. Experimental data have provided firm evidence for a causal role of enhanced apoptosis in the pathogenesis of sepsis, i.e., prevention of apoptosis of lymphocytes on the intestinal epithelium improved survival in experimental sepsis [29].

HMGB1 and RAGE

High-mobility group box 1 protein (HMGB1) is a nuclear protein present in almost all eukaryotic cells, where it functions to stabilize nucleosome formation, regulating the expression of several genes [30]. HMGB1 has been implicated as a late acting pro-inflammatory cytokine in the pathogenesis of sepsis. Mice challenged with a bolus dose of LPS started to release HMGB1 into their circulation with a delay of approximately 10 hours, and an anti-HMGB1 antibody protected against LPS-induced lethality even when the administration was postponed until after the peak levels of TNF-α and IL-1 had been reached [31]. Even more impressively, anti-HMGB1 treatment was found to increase survival in a model of abdominal sepsis caused by cecal ligation and puncture; anti-HMGB1 was protective when given 24 hours after the surgical procedure, at a time when most animals had already developed signs of lethargy and sickness behavior [32]. Also, delayed administration of A box, a DNA binding domain within HMGB1 that acts as an inhibitor of HMGB1 activity, rescued mice from death after cecal perforation [32]. Considering that the therapeutic window for anti-HMGB1 therapies is much wider than for TNF neutralizing strategies, inhibitors of HMGB1 may be valuable as an adjunctive therapy for severe sepsis.

It is uncertain whether highly purified HMGB1 can directly activate cells. It has been suggested that other molecules bound by HMGB1 are at least in part responsible. Nonetheless, several receptors have been implicated in mediating the cellular effects of HMGB1, including TLR2 and -4, and the receptor for advanced glycation end products (RAGE) [30, 33]. RAGE is a promiscuous receptor that interacts with diverse ligands such as advanced glycation end products, S100/calgranulins, amyloid A, leukocyte adhesion receptors, *E. coli* curli operons, and HMGB1; activation of RAGE leads to the activation of nuclear factor-kappa B (NF-κB) and mitogen-activated protein kinase (MAPK) pathways [34]. The potential role of RAGE signaling in sepsis pathophysiology has been documented in mice exposed to cecal ligation and puncture: both RAGE deficient mice and wild-type mice treated with soluble RAGE were partially protected against lethality in this model of severe sepsis [35, 36]. Further research is warranted to address the therapeutic potential of RAGE (ligand) inhibitors in sepsis.

The Cholinergic Anti-inflammatory Pathway

The cholinergic nervous system, and in particular the vagus nerve, plays an important role in limiting inflammatory responses [37]. In the so-called cholinergic anti-inflammatory pathway, enhanced efferent activity of parasympathetic nerve endings results in the release of acetylcholine, which by a specific action on α7 cholinergic receptors on macrophages suppresses pro-inflammatory cytokine production. Disruption of this neural-based system by vagotomy renders animals more vulnerable to LPS toxicity. Conversely, electrical stimulation of the efferent vagus nerve prevented the development of shock and attenuated the release of TNF-α, whereas stimulation of α7 cholinergic receptors by specific agonists, such as nicotine, attenuated systemic inflammation and improved the outcome of mice with polymicrobial abdominal sepsis [37]. Recent evidence indicates that, within the brain, central muscarinic receptors play a role in activating the cholinergic anti-inflammatory pathway [38] and that the spleen is an essential peripheral part of the cholinergic anti-inflammatory reflex [39]. Together, these preclinical data suggest that stimulation of the vagus nerve and/or pharmacologic α7 cholinergic receptor agonists may be a useful strategy in the treatment of the severe inflammation accompanying sepsis.

Macrophage Migration Inhibitory Factor

Macrophage migration inhibitory factor (MIF) is a cytokine that can be produced by many different cell types. Serum MIF levels are elevated in patients with sepsis, and even higher levels occur in patients with septic shock [40]. MIF regulates innate immune responses through modulation of TLR4: When MIF-deficient mice were challenged with LPS they showed a defective response as a direct result of decreased TLR4 expression [41]. MIF-directed therapies might offer a new treatment opportunity for sepsis. Inhibition of MIF activity with neutralizing anti-MIF antibodies protected mice from septic shock [40]. Furthermore, a specific small molecule inhibitor of MIF, named ISO-1, partially protected mice from sepsis induced by endotoxin or cecal ligation and puncture [42].

C5a and C5a Receptor

Although traditionally the complement system has been considered a central part of host defense against invading pathogens, complement activation may also contribute to an adverse outcome of sepsis [43]. The importance of C5a for the outcome of sepsis has been highlighted by several investigations using different animal models of sepsis wherein blockade of C5a proved beneficial. Infusion of anti-C5a antibodies improved hemodynamic parameters in pigs infused with LPS or live *E. coli* and reduced mortality in primates with *E. coli* sepsis and rats subjected to cecal ligation and puncture [43]. Interventions seeking to block C5a signaling represent promising targets for sepsis treatment. As with other anti-inflammatory strategies, an important goal of complement inhibition in patients with an infection would be to avoid disrupting the role of complement in host defense, while effectively preventing the pathological activities of complement activation products.

Conclusion

Sepsis has traditionally been regarded as the result of an exacerbated detrimental inflammatory response towards invading bacteria. However, recent insights have forced us to rethink this sepsis paradigm. Although some septic patients succumb from the initial exacerbated hyper-inflammatory response, most patients die during the following extended period of immunodepression. Bimodal interactions between inflammation and coagulation can give rise to a vicious cycle, eventually leading to dramatic events such as are manifested in severe sepsis and DIC. A careful balance between the inflammatory and anti-inflammatory response is vital for a successful host response to sepsis.

References

1. Beutler B, Milsark IW, Cerami AC (1985) Passive immunization against cachectin/tumor necrosis factor protects mice from lethal effect of endotoxin. Science 229: 869–871
2. Tracey KJ, Fong Y, Hesse DG, et al (1987) Anti-cachectin/TNF monoclonal antibodies prevent septic shock during lethal bacteraemia. Nature 330: 662–664
3. Lorente JA, Marshall JC (2005) Neutralization of tumor necrosis factor in preclinical models of sepsis. Shock 24 (Suppl 1): 107–119

4. Ohlsson K, Bjork P, Bergenfeldt M, Hageman R, Thompson RC (1990) Interleukin-1 receptor antagonist reduces mortality from endotoxin shock. Nature 348: 550–552
5. Fischer E, Marano MA, Van Zee KJ, et al (1992) Interleukin-1 receptor blockade improves survival and hemodynamic performance in Escherichia coli septic shock, but fails to alter host responses to sublethal endotoxemia. J Clin Invest 89: 1551–1557
6. Martin GS, Mannino DM, Eaton S, Moss M (2003) The epidemiology of sepsis in the United States from 1979 through 2000. N Engl J Med 348: 1546–1554
7. Arcaroli J, Fessler MB, Abraham E (2005) Genetic polymorphisms and sepsis. Shock 24: 300–312
8. Akira S, Uematsu S, Takeuchi O (2006) Pathogen recognition and innate immunity. Cell 124: 783–801
9. Netea MG, Gow NA, Munro CA, et al (2006) Immune sensing of Candida albicans requires cooperative recognition of mannans and glucans by lectin and Toll-like receptors. J Clin Invest 116: 1642–1650
10. Liew FY, Xu D, Brint EK, O'Neill LA (2005) Negative regulation of toll-like receptor-mediated immune responses. Nat Rev Immunol 5: 446–458
11. Beutler B, Rietschel ET (2003) Innate immune sensing and its roots: the story of endotoxin. Nat Rev Immunol 3: 169–176
12. Meng G, Rutz M, Schiemann M, et al (2004) Antagonistic antibody prevents toll-like receptor 2-driven lethal shock-like syndromes. J Clin Invest 113: 1473–1481
13. Takeuchi O, Hoshino K, Akira S (2000) Cutting edge: TLR2-deficient and MyD88-deficient mice are highly susceptible to Staphylococcus aureus infection. J Immunol 165: 5392–5396
14. Klesney-Tait J, Turnbull IR, Colonna M (2006) The TREM receptor family and signal integration. Nat Immunol 7: 1266–1273
15. Ogura Y, Sutterwala FS, Flavell RA (2006) The inflammasome: first line of the immune response to cell stress. Cell 126: 659–662
16. Schouten M, Wiersinga WJ, Levi M, van der Poll T (2008) Inflammation, endothelium, and coagulation in sepsis. J Leukoc Biol 83: 536–545
17. Dhainaut JF, Shorr AF, Macias WL, et al (2005) Dynamic evolution of coagulopathy in the first day of severe sepsis: relationship with mortality and organ failure. Crit Care Med 33: 341–348
18. Pawlinski R, Pedersen B, Schabbauer G, et al (2004) Role of tissue factor and protease-activated receptors in a mouse model of endotoxemia. Blood 103: 1342–1347
19. Bernard GR, Vincent JL, Laterre PF, et al (2001) Efficacy and safety of recombinant human activated protein C for severe sepsis. N Engl J Med 344: 699–709
20. Warren BL, Eid A, Singer P, et al (2001) Caring for the critically ill patient. High-dose antithrombin III in severe sepsis: a randomized controlled trial. JAMA 286: 1869–1878
21. Abraham E, Reinhart K, Opal S, et al (2003) Efficacy and safety of tifacogin (recombinant tissue factor pathway inhibitor) in severe sepsis: a randomized controlled trial. JAMA 290: 238–247
22. Abraham E, Laterre PF, Garg R, et al (2005) Drotrecogin alfa (activated) for adults with severe sepsis and a low risk of death. N Engl J Med 353: 1332–1341
23. Coughlin SR (2000) Thrombin signalling and protease-activated receptors. Nature 407: 258–264
24. Riewald M, Petrovan RJ, Donner A, Mueller BM, Ruf W (2002) Activation of endothelial cell protease activated receptor 1 by the protein C pathway. Science 296: 1880–1882
25. Kaneider NC, Leger AJ, Agarwal A, et al (2007) 'Role reversal' for the receptor PAR1 in sepsis-induced vascular damage. Nat Immunol 8: 1303–1312
26. Niessen F, Schaffner F, Furlan-Freguia C, et al (2008) Dendritic cell PAR1-S1P3 signalling couples coagulation and inflammation. Nature 452: 654–658
27. van der Poll T, Opal SM (2008) Host-pathogen interactions in sepsis. Lancet Infect Dis 8: 32–43
28. Munford RS, Pugin J (2001) Normal responses to injury prevent systemic inflammation and can be immunosuppressive. Am J Respir Crit Care Med 163: 316–321
29. Hotchkiss RS, Nicholson DW (2006) Apoptosis and caspases regulate death and inflammation in sepsis. Nat Rev Immunol 6: 813–822
30. Lotze MT, Tracey KJ (2005) High-mobility group box 1 protein (HMGB1): nuclear weapon in the immune arsenal. Nat Rev Immunol 5: 331–342

II

II

31. Wang H, Bloom O, Zhang M, et al (1999) HMG-1 as a late mediator of endotoxin lethality in mice. Science 285: 248–251
32. Yang H, Ochani M, Li J, et al (2004) Reversing established sepsis with antagonists of endogenous high-mobility group box 1. Proc Natl Acad Sci USA 101: 296–301
33. van Zoelen MA, Yang H, Florquin S, et al (2008) Role of Toll-like receptors 2 and 4, and the receptor for advanced glycation end products (RAGE) in HMGB1 induced inflammation in vivo. Shock (in press)
34. van Zoelen MA, van der Poll T (2008) Targeting RAGE in sepsis. Crit Care 12: 103
35. Liliensiek B, Weigand MA, Bierhaus A, et al (2004) Receptor for advanced glycation end products (RAGE) regulates sepsis but not the adaptive immune response. J Clin Invest 113: 1641–1650
36. Lutterloh EC, Opal SM, Pittman DD, et al (2007) Inhibition of the RAGE products increases survival in experimental models of severe sepsis and systemic infection. Crit Care 11: R122
37. Tracey KJ (2007) Physiology and immunology of the cholinergic antiinflammatory pathway. J Clin Invest 117: 289–296
38. Pavlov VA, Ochani M, Gallowitsch-Puerta M, et al (2006) Central muscarinic cholinergic regulation of the systemic inflammatory response during endotoxemia. Proc Natl Acad Sci USA 103: 5219–5223
39. Huston JM, Ochani M, Rosas-Ballina M, et al (2006) Splenectomy inactivates the cholinergic antiinflammatory pathway during lethal endotoxemia and polymicrobial sepsis. J Exp Med 203: 1623–1628
40. Calandra T, Echtenacher B, Roy DL, et al (2000). Protection from septic shock by neutralization of macrophage migration inhibitory factor. Nat Med 6: 164–170
41. Roger T, David J, Glauser MP, Calandra T (2001) MIF regulates innate immune responses through modulation of Toll-like receptor 4. Nature 414: 920–924
42. Al-Abed Y, Dabideen D, Aljabari B, et al (2005) ISO-1 binding to the tautomerase active site of MIF inhibits its pro-inflammatory activity and increases survival in severe sepsis. J Biol Chem 280: 36541–36544
43. Guo RF, Ward PA (2005) Role of C5a in inflammatory responses. Annu Rev Immunol 23: 821–852

Endotoxin Tolerance: Mechanisms and Clinical Applicability

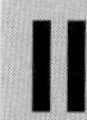

A. Draisma, J.G. van der Hoeven, and P. Pickkers

Introduction

Lipopolysaccharide (LPS) is a glycolipid that constitutes the major portion of the outermost membrane of Gram-negative bacteria. LPS is considered one of the most powerful microbial stimulants of immune and non-immune cells. The immune system responds to LPS with a systemic production of pro- and anti-inflammatory cytokines, such as tumor necrosis factor (TNF)-α, interleukin (IL)-6 and IL-10, primarily aimed to eliminate invading pathogens and subsequently curtail the immune response. Although pro-inflammatory cytokines are indispensable for the control of the growth and dissemination of the pathogen, excessive release of these cytokines, together with LPS-induced effects on endothelial cells, results in the clinical syndrome of septic shock and multiple organ failure.

Tolerance to repeated administration of endotoxin was first noticed when typhoid vaccine was administered as a pyrogen to induce fever to slow the progress of *Treponoma pallidum* infection within the central nervous system. With repeated administrations, the vaccine showed progressive loss of efficacy as a pyrogen, and an increase in dose was required to achieve the desired pyrogenic effect. In 1942, Favorite and Morgan administered purified LPS to humans for the first time and described the development of tolerance after repeated injections [1]. Furthermore, it was observed in the 1960s that animals receiving low dose LPS had a markedly reduced mortality when challenged with a subsequent 'lethal' injection of endotoxin. In the following years, endotoxin tolerance not only provided protection against a subsequent identical insult with LPS, but also against other insults, specifically against ischemia-reperfusion injury, a phenomenon called 'cross-tolerance'. This chapter will focus on the development of endotoxin tolerance and its effect on endothelial function in humans. Furthermore it explores the possible clinical applicability, as cross-tolerance could protect against ischemia-reperfusion injury in certain patient groups.

Mechanisms of Endotoxin Tolerance

Toll-like Receptors

Toll-like receptors (TLRs) recognize specific pathogen-associated molecular patterns. Ten members of the so called TLR family have so far been identified in humans. Various TLRs are involved in the recognition of different microbial products. Although TLRs do not exhibit specificity for a single microbial product, they are individually responsive to a limited group of molecules. Besides stimulation of

TLR4 by endotoxin, a wide variety of bacterial products, DNA and RNA viruses, fungi and protozoa play an important role through stimulation of other TLRs. For example, LPS and heat shock protein (HSP) signal via TLR4, Gram-positive peptidoglycan through TLR1 and 2, TLR3 is implicated in the recognition of viral double-stranded RNA, TLR5 recognizes bacterial flagellin, and single-stranded RNA viruses signal via TLR7. Since the discovery of the various TLRs it has become clear that they act in concert in the signaling cascade following ligand-specific stimulus. The resultant production and release of cytokines demonstrates a different spectrum per TLR. Also, the development of tolerance is not similar for each cytokine that is released, showing the complexity of this response. Interestingly, the development of tolerance after repeated exposure to LPS results not only in tolerance to subsequent TLR4 stimulation both *in vivo* as well as *in vitro*, but also results in a diminished cytokine response after subsequent stimulation of TLR2, 3 and 5 *ex vivo* [2–5]. In contrast, endotoxemia does not induce tolerance to subsequent stimulation with a TLR7 agonist [6], indicating that the development of tolerance is differentially regulated dependent on the specific TLR that is stimulated and the cytokine that is measured.

Anti-inflammatory Hypothesis and Leukocyte Reprogramming

The mechanisms by which endotoxin tolerance develops are still not completely clear and over the last decades several pathophysiological pathways have been proposed (**Table 1**). The 'anti-inflammatory hypothesis' is based on the finding that endotoxin tolerance does not attenuate the release of different cytokines similarly, resulting in attenuated levels of pro-inflammatory cytokines with concomitant increased levels of anti-inflammatory cytokines, leading to the observed tolerance. Indeed, *in vitro* experiments show that LPS tolerance is associated with an increased expression of the anti-inflammatory cytokines, IL-10 [7, 8], IL-1 receptor antagonist (Il-1ra) [9] or transforming growth factor (TGF)β [9, 10]. However, the role of IL-10 has become controversial as numerous studies do not show enhanced expression of IL-10 in whole blood or in animal *in vivo* studies. Finally, IL-10 knock-out mice show the dispensability of this anti-inflammatory cytokine in the development of endotoxin tolerance [11].

The anti-inflammatory cytokine, TGFβ, also appears to be involved in the development of LPS tolerance in *in vitro* and animal sepsis studies [9, 10], because after administration of TGFβ, animals become tolerant to LPS, whereas in animals that are infused with antibodies aimed to neutralize TGFβ, no tolerance to LPS develops [9]. In humans, repeated infusions of LPS result in a diminished release of both pro- and anti-inflammatory cytokines, such as TNF-α, IL-6, IL-1ra and IL-10, within 5 days, in contrast to LPS-induced circulating TGFβ levels, which increase to the same

Pathophysiological pathways	
1970	"Hyper-Inflammation"
1980	"LPS tolerance"
1990	"SIRS, CARS, MARS"
1996	"Immune paralysis"
1997	"Monocyte-deactivation"
1998	"Anti-inflammatory hypothesis"
2005	"Leukocyte reprogramming"

Table 1. An overview of terms used to describe the development of endotoxin tolerance with regard to pathophysiological pathways. Over time, investigation of endotoxin tolerance has moved from soluble, secreted factors to the signal transduction machinery that resides on and inside cells.

LPS: lipopolysaccharide; SIRS: systemic inflammatory response syndrome: CARS: compensatory anti-inflammatory response syndrome, MARS: mixed antagonist response syndrome

Table 2. Alterations in signaling pathways and chromatin remodeling with the induction of lipopolysaccharide (LPS) tolerance are referred to as "leukocyte reprogramming". An overview of proposed mechanisms is presented during the development of endotoxin tolerance with regard to intra/extracellular changes.

Proposed mechanisms for endotoxin tolerance	Effect
Extracellular/receptor level	
CD14	↕
TLR4	↓
Cytosolic level	
IRAK	↓
Iκ-Bα	↑
Erk 1/2	↓
MAP3K	↓
p50/p50	↑
p38	↓
p50/p65	↓
Nuclear level	
NF-κB	↓

TLR: Toll like receptor; IRAK: interleukin-1 receptor associated kinase; Iκ-Bα: inhibitory proteins; Erk: extracellular signal-related kinase; MAP3K: mitogen-activated protein kinase; NF-κB: Nuclear factor-kappa B

extent after administration of LPS on day 5 compared to day 1 [12]. These results indicate that TGFβ may play a role in the development of LPS tolerance and that during this development, production of TGFβ is not downregulated in contrast to other measured cytokines.

Partly in accordance with the above, the investigation of endotoxin tolerance has moved from soluble, secreted factors to the signal transduction machinery that resides on and inside cells. Alterations in signaling pathways and chromatin remodeling with the induction of LPS tolerance are referred to as "leukocyte reprogramming" [13, 14]. Experiments show a reduced capacity of leukocytes from septic patients to produce pro-inflammatory cytokines while other (intra)cellular signaling pathways are unaltered (**Table 2**). Selection of different subpopulations of leukocytes may also play a role in this phenomenon. Therefore, it is now clear that endotoxin tolerance is not synonymous with global downregulation of the immune response.

Endothelial Function and Microcirculation during LPS Tolerance

Whereas the endothelium was once regarded as the wallpaper of blood vessels, an inert cell layer, it is now clear that the complete opposite is true. During critical illness, e.g., sepsis, the endothelial cell can be viewed as both a victim and a perpetrator of the inflammatory response as it plays a central role in the (dys)regulation of vascular tone. Hemodynamic instability with inadequate vasodilation combined with simultaneous presence of inadequate vasoconstriction in different vascular beds represent typical characteristics of septic shock. This dysregulation of vascular tone in septic patients is the consequence of an attenuated vasoconstrictive response to catecholamines, while at the same time the endothelium-dependent vasodilatory response is also impaired. Production of inducible nitric oxide (NO) synthase (iNOS) with subsequent generated NO is thought to be responsible as it has been observed that endothelial cells of blood vessel walls upregulate iNOS and subsequent huge amounts of NO cause systemic vasodilation [15–17]. In septic models, this excessive NO production also accounts for downregulation of physiologically essential endothelial NO-synthase (eNOS) leading to the observed attenuated endothelium-dependent vasodilatory response [18–20].

The precise mechanism between inflammation and endothelial dysfunction is not completely understood. It is unclear whether LPS exerts a direct effect on endothelial function through activation of TLR4 receptors that are present on endothelial cells [19], or whether the LPS-induced cytokines or other inflammatory mediators are primarily responsible for endothelial dysfunction. The latter suggestion is supported by the fact that in humans *Salmonella typhi* vaccination is associated with short-term impairment of endothelium-dependent dilation in conduit and resistance vessels that parallels the inflammatory response [22]. Experimental human endotoxemia studies combined with forearm blood flow measurements demonstrate the presence of endothelial dysfunction during endotoxemia as the acetylcholine-induced vasodilatory response in the human forearm is attenuated during endotoxemia, whereas the vasodilatory response to sodium nitroprusside is unaffected [19, 23]. Repeated LPS infusions for 5 consecutive days resulted in a marked attenuation of the acetylcholine-induced vasodilatory response on day 1, whereas this effect was not present on day 5, associated with the diminished release of cytokines (Draisma et al. unpublished data). This suggests that LPS-induced cytokine production mediates the observed endothelial dysfunction, although downregulation of the TLR4 receptor or altered intracellular signaling in the endothelial cell cannot be ruled out.

Endothelial cell activation can also be measured by the release of von Willebrand factor (vWF), as this is one of the first factors to be released after administration of endotoxin [24]. Repeated LPS administrations cause peak levels of vWF 6 hours after LPS administration on day 1, but not on day 5, which is another indication for the presence of endothelial dysfunction during endotoxemia which does not occur once LPS tolerance develops [12]. Hence, LPS-induced cytokine release results in activation of iNOS, leading to downregulation of eNOS and endothelial dysfunction, whereas these processes do not occur during LPS tolerance.

The complex interplay between NO and LPS tolerance is also illustrated by the fact that selective iNOS inhibition abolishes the development of tolerance to stimulation with a TLR5 agonist, but does not influence development of tolerance to either TLR2 or 4 agonist stimulation [6].

In the last decade, the role of the microcirculation during systemic inflammation has been increasingly investigated. Near infrared spectroscopy (NIRS) and sidestream dark field imaging (SDF) are non-invasive bedside techniques for continuous, real time monitoring of the microcirculation, and one of the most striking findings has been the heterogeneity of microcirculatory flow during different disease states. More importantly, microvascular blood flow is more severely altered in non-survivors than in survivors of sepsis. Indeed, microcirculatory alterations improve rapidly in septic shock survivors but not in patients dying of multiple organ failure regardless of whether the shock resolves or not. Different patterns of microvascular alterations in septic shock patients could, therefore, characterize their outcome [25]. Interestingly, the increase in tissue oxygenation after local ischemia measured by NIRS is also related to the severity of the septic state and patient outcome [7]. It has been observed that during experimental acute endotoxemia, microvascular flow is decreased (SDF imaging) in addition to an attenuated endothelium-dependent ischemia-mediated increase in tissue oxygenation (NIRS) and an attenuated pharmacologically-induced endothelium-dependent vasodilatory response to acetylcholine (venous occlusion plethysmography). In addition, these microvascular changes are no longer present after repeated LPS administration, related to the development of LPS tolerance (Draisma et al., unpublished data).

Clinical Applicability and Therapeutic Possibilities

Cross-tolerance

Although endotoxin has been used to induce tolerance against a subsequent identical stimulus, it has also been demonstrated that endotoxin provokes tolerance against other forms of injury, a phenomenon called 'cross tolerance'. A vast number of animal experiments demonstrate that pre-treatment with endotoxin results in protection against hepatic [27–30], pancreatic [31], lung [23, 33] and renal ischemia-reperfusion injury [34, 35]. In patients undergoing an elective intervention during which there is a high risk of ischemia-reperfusion injury, pre-treatment with LPS to induce tolerance may improve their outcome. Major vascular surgery and elective organ transplantation are examples of patient groups which may benefit. However, whether this LPS tolerance-mediated protection against ischemia-reperfusion injury also exists in humans *in vivo* is unknown.

It is possible to detect ischemia-reperfusion injury in humans *in vivo* with use of ^{99m}Tc annexin A5 scintigraphy as annexin A5 binds to negatively charged phosphatidylserine [36]. In general, the ischemia-induced injury results in a flip-flop of the phosphatidylserine molecules in the ischemic cell membranes allowing radiolabeled annexin A5 to bind this molecule and visualize this ischemia-induced injury through 99mTc annexin A5 scintigraphy. As such, targeting of radiolabeled annexin A5 can be used to detect early and reversible ischemia-reperfusion injury in humans *in vivo* [37, 38]. Nevertheless, using this method, LPS tolerance does not provide protection against ischemia-induced injury (Draisma et al., unpublished work). This negative finding is associated with the lack of complement activation observed directly following reperfusion, suggesting that this ischemia-reperfusion model is too mild to induce an ischemia-induced inflammatory response that could be down-regulated by the presence of LPS tolerance. More severe ischemia, e.g., following myocardial infarction does result in an inflammatory response in humans [39] suggesting that during these circumstances LPS tolerance may exert a protective effect. For this reason, it cannot be excluded that LPS tolerance may provide protection against ischemia-reperfusion injury in humans *in vivo*, but apparently the ischemia-reperfusion injury must be severe enough to elicit an ischemia-induced inflammatory response.

The previously described induction of LPS tolerance in humans *in vivo* was brought about by repeated injections of 2 ng/kg LPS for 5 consecutive days. As a consequence, volunteers experienced flu-like symptoms and fever during the first few days, which subsided during the development of LPS tolerance. For cardiovascular compromised patients this would limit the clinical applicability. Of clinical importance, an incremental LPS dose protocol starting at 0.2 ng/kg LPS and increasing to 2.0 ng/kg on day 4 and 5, results in an equal degree of LPS tolerance, but the subjects remain almost completely free of symptoms and no fever or relevant cardiovascular changes are observed. Therefore, this incremental LPS dose schedule would be easier to apply in clinical practice (**Table 3**).

II

Table 3. Clinical, hemodynamic and inflammatory parameters comparing two different lipopolysaccharide (LPS) administration protocols to develop LPS tolerance. In one group, 2 ng/kg LPS was administered daily for 5 consecutive days. In the other group, an incremental dose protocol was used with 0.2 ng/kg LPS on the first day, followed by 0.5 ng/kg on day 2; 1 ng/kg LPS on day 3; 2 ng/kg LPS on day 4 and 5. The symptom score consisted of backache, shivering, nausea, headache and muscle ache. The volunteers were asked to score each of these complaints every 30 minutes after LPS administration from day 1 until 5 ranging from "not present" (score 0) up to "most severe ever" (score 5). The maximum score of each subject was used to calculate a group mean. Temperature levels were obtained every 30 minutes after LPS administration from day 1 until day 5 using a tympanic thermometer (°C). Heart rate and mean arterial pressure data were obtained by use of an arterial cannula and therefore monitored continuously. Both groups developed LPS tolerance indicated by the attenuated levels of pro-inflammatory cytokine, tumor necrosis factor (TNF)-α on day 5. After the first LPS administration, all displayed parameters are significantly more pronounced in the one daily dose group compared to the incremental group, whereas the development of LPS tolerance on day 5 was not different between the two groups, indicating that a similar degree of LPS tolerance was obtained associated with less symptoms in the incremental dose group, making this schedule easier to apply in clinical practice.

	Daily 2 ng/kg LPS group		Incremental LPS dose group	
	Day 1: 2 ng/kg	Day 5: 2 ng/kg	Day 1: 0.2 ng/kg	Day 5: 2 ng/kg
Symptom score	6.1±0.8	0.3±0.2	0.6+0.3	1.6±0.6
Δ Temperature (°C)	1.810.2	1.010.1	0.5±0.1	1.0+0.2
Δ Heart rate (/min)	35±7	13±1	12±6	11±6
Δ Mean arterial pressure (mmHg)	−20+2	−14±4	−5±3	−13±5
max. TNFα (pg/ml)	927±182	31±9	15±0	27±5
max. IL-6 (pg/ml)	1785±230	201+38	30±5	222±38
max. IL-10 (pg/ml)	155±28	20±3	12±1	18±1

Conclusions

It is possible to induce endotoxin tolerance in humans *in vivo* by repeated LPS administration associated with attenuated levels of most pro- and anti-inflammatory cytokines, with the exception of TGFβ. In addition, LPS tolerance is associated with less endotoxemia-induced endothelial dysfunction in humans *in vivo*. Whether or not LPS tolerance provides protection against ischemia-reperfusion injury in humans remains to be elucidated. In view of the fact that LPS tolerance can be easily and safely induced in humans, and with regards its putative beneficial effects in certain patient groups, further research is warranted.

References

1. Favorite GO, Morgan HR (1942) Effects produced by the intravenous injection in man of a toxic antigenic material derived from eberhtella typhosa: clinical, hematological, chemical and serological studies. J Clin Invest 21: 589–599
2. Sato S, Nomura F, Kawai T, et al (2000) Synergy and cross-tolerance between toll-like receptor (TLR) 2- and TLR4-mediated signaling pathways. J Immunol 165: 7096–7101
3. Lehner MD, Morath S, Michelsen KS, Schumann RR, Hartung T (2001) Induction of cross-tolerance by lipopolysaccharide and highly purified lipoteichoic acid via different Toll-like receptors independent of paracrine mediators. J Immunol 166: 5161–5167
4. Jiang W, Sun R, Wei H, Tian Z (2005) Toll-like receptor 3 ligand attenuates LPS-induced liver injury by down-regulation of toll-like receptor 4 expression on macrophages. Proc Natl Acad Sci U S A 102: 17077–17082

5. Mizel SB, Snipes JA (2002) Gram-negative flagellin-induced self-tolerance is associated with a block in interleukin-1 receptor-associated kinase release from toll-like receptor 5. J Biol Chem 277: 22414–22420
6. Draisma A, Dorresteijn M, Pickkers P, van der Hoeven JG (2008) The effect of systemic iNOS inhibition during human endotoxemia on the development of tolerance to different TLR-stimuli. Innate Immun 14: 153–159
7. Shimauchi H, Ogawa T, Okuda K, Kusumoto Y, Okada H (1999) Autoregulatory effect of interleukin-10 on proinflammatory cytokine production by Porphyromonas gingivalis lipopolysaccharide-tolerant human monocytes. Infect Immun 67: 2153–2159
8. Frankenberger M, Pechumer H, Ziegler-Heitbrock HW (1995) Interleukin-10 is upregulated in LPS tolerance. J Inflamm 45: 56–63
9. Randow F, Syrbe U, Meisel C, et al (1995) Mechanism of endotoxin desensitization: involvement of interleukin 10 and transforming growth factor beta. J Exp Med 181: 1887–1892
10. Sly LM, Rauh MJ, Kalesnikoff J, Song CH, Krystal G (2004) LPS-induced upregulation of SHIP is essential for endotoxin tolerance. Immunity 21: 227–239
11. Berg DJ, Kuhn R, Rajewsky K, et al (1995) Interleukin-10 is a central regulator of the response to LPS in murine models of endotoxic shock and the Shwartzman reaction but not endotoxin tolerance. J Clin Invest 96: 2339–2347
12. Draisma A, Pickkers P, Bouw M, van der Hoeven J (2008) Development of endotoxin tolerance in humans in vivo. Crit Care Med (in press)
13. Zhang X, Morrison DC (1993) Lipopolysaccharide structure-function relationship in activation versus reprogramming of mouse peritoneal macrophages. J Leukoc Biol 54: 444–450
14. Cavaillon JM, Adib-Conquy M (2006) Bench-to-bedside review: endotoxin tolerance as a model of leukocyte reprogramming in sepsis. Crit Care 10: 233–240
15. Wang P, Ba ZF, Chaudry IH (1994) Administration of tumor necrosis factor-alpha in vivo depresses endothelium-dependent relaxation. Am J Physiol 266: H2535-H2541
16. Clapp BR, Hingorani AD, Kharbanda RK, et al (2004) Inflammation-induced endothelial dysfunction involves reduced nitric oxide bioavailability and increased oxidant stress. Cardiovasc Res 64: 172–178
17. Bhagat K, Vallance P (1997) Inflammatory cytokines impair endothelium-dependent dilatation in human veins in vivo. Circulation 96: 3042–3047
18. Wang P, Ba ZF, Chaudry IH (1995) Endothelium-dependent relaxation is depressed at the macro- and microcirculatory levels during sepsis. Am J Physiol 269: R988-R994
19. Pleiner J, Mittermayer F, Schaller G, MacAllister RJ, Wolzt M (2002) High doses of vitamin C reverse Escherichia coli endotoxin-induced hyporeactivity to acetylcholine in the human forearm. Circulation 106: 1460–1464
20. Heitzer T, Schlinzig T, Krohn K, Meinertz T, Munzel T (2001) Endothelial dysfunction, oxidative stress, and risk of cardiovascular events in patients with coronary artery disease. Circulation 104: 2673–2678
21. Faure E, Thomas L, Xu H, Medvedev A, Equils O, Arditi M (2001) Bacterial lipopolysaccharide and IFN-gamma induce Toll-like receptor 2 and Toll-like receptor 4 expression in human endothelial cells: role of NF-kappa B activation. J Immunol 166: 2018–2024
22. Hingorani AD, Cross J, Kharbanda RK, et al (2000) Acute systemic inflammation impairs endothelium-dependent dilatation in humans. Circulation 102: 994–999
23. Pickkers P, Dorresteijn MJ, Bouw MP, van der Hoeven JG, Smits P (2006) In vivo evidence for nitric oxide-mediated calcium-activated potassium-channel activation during human endotoxemia. Circulation 114: 414–421
24. van Deventer SJ, Buller HR, ten Cate JW, Aarden LA, Hack CE, Sturk A (1990) Experimental endotoxemia in humans: analysis of cytokine release and coagulation, fibrinolytic, and complement pathways. Blood 76: 2520–2526
25. Sakr Y, Dubois MJ, De Backer D, Creteur J, Vincent JL (2004) Persistent microcirculatory alterations are associated with organ failure and death in patients with septic shock. Crit Care Med 32: 1825–1831
26. Creteur J, Carollo T, Soldati G, Buchele G, De Backer D, Vincent JL (2007) The prognostic value of muscle StO2 in septic patients. Intensive Care Med 33: 1549–1556
27. Colletti LM, Remick DG, Campbell DA Jr (1994) LPS pretreatment protects from hepatic ischemia/reperfusion. J Surg Res 57: 337–343

28. Dominguez FE, Siemers F, Flohe S, Nau M, Schade FU (2002) Effects of endotoxin tolerance on liver function after hepatic ischemia/reperfusion injury in the rat. Crit Care Med 30: 165–170
29. Fernandez ED, Flohe S, Siemers F, et al (2000) Endotoxin tolerance protects against local hepatic ischemia/reperfusion injury in the rat. J Endotoxin Res 6: 321–328
30. Yoshidome H, Kato A, Edwards MJ, Lentsch AB (1999) Interleukin-10 suppresses hepatic ischemia/reperfusion injury in mice: implications of a central role for nuclear factor kappaB. Hepatology 30: 203–208
31. Obermaier R, Drognitz O, Grub A, et al (2003) Endotoxin preconditioning in pancreatic ischemia/reperfusion injury. Pancreas 27: e51-e56
32. Friedrich I, Spillner J, Lu EX, et al (2003) Induction of endotoxin tolerance improves lung function after warm ischemia in dogs. Am J Physiol Lung Cell Mol Physiol 284: L224-L231
33. Markart P, Schmidt R, Ruppert C, et al (2005) Ischemic and endotoxin pre-conditioning reduce lung reperfusion injury-induced surfactant alterations. J Heart Lung Transplant 24: 1680–1689
34. Godet C, Goujon JM, Petit I, et al (2006) Endotoxin tolerance enhances interleukin-10 renal expression and decreases ischemia-reperfusion renal injury in rats. Shock 25: 384–388
35. Heemann U, Szabo A, Hamar P, et al (2000) Lipopolysaccharide pretreatment protects from renal ischemia/reperfusion injury : possible connection to an interleukin-6-dependent pathway. Am J Pathol 156: 287–293
36. Rongen GA, Oyen WJ, Ramakers BP, et al (2005) Annexin A5 scintigraphy of forearm as a novel in vivo model of skeletal muscle preconditioning in humans. Circulation 111: 173–178
37. Riksen NP, Zhou Z, Oyen WJ, et al (2006) Caffeine prevents protection in two human models of ischemic preconditioning. J Am Coll Cardiol 48: 700–707
38. Riksen NP, Oyen WJ, Ramakers BP, et al (2005) Oral therapy with dipyridamole limits ischemia-reperfusion injury in humans. Clin Pharmacol Ther 78: 52–59
39. Yellon DM, Hausenloy DJ (2007) Myocardial reperfusion injury. N Engl J Med 357: 1121–1135

Oxidative Stress and Endothelial Dysfunction during Sepsis

O. Huet, A. Harrois, and J. Duranteau

Introduction

The endothelium is an active tissue that plays a pivotal role in maintaining cardiovascular homeostasis. The endothelium ensures the quality of both the global and microcirculation. It forms an interface between blood and tissues. The human body contains approximately 10^{13} endothelial cells, an area of 4000 to 7000 m^2. This size is one of the reasons why endothelium must be considered an organ. Physiological functions of endothelial cells are: 1) to control vascular tone and blood flow by a local balance between vasodilators (paracrine release of diffusible vasodilator mediators, such as nitric oxide [NO], prostacyclin) and vasopressors (endothelin-1 [ET-1]); 2) to keep blood in a fluid state by preventing thrombosis; 3) to control the exchange of fluid and macromolecules between the blood and the tissues; and 4) to control the local balance between pro- and anti-inflammatory mediators.

Reactive oxygen species (ROS) and reactive nitrogen species (RNS) have several potentially important effects on endothelial function and are implicated both in physiological regulation and in disease pathophysiology [1–3]. The effects of ROS on endothelial cells are dependent on the amount and the sites of production of ROS, but also on the processes that degrade or scavenge ROS. The imbalance between the production of ROS and their effective removal by non-enzymatic and enzymatic antioxidant systems could induce endothelial dysfunction with alteration of vascular tone, increase in cell adhesion properties (leukocyte and platelet adhesion), increase in vascular wall permeability and a pro-coagulant state.

Endothelial dysfunction appears to be critical during septic shock, and its activation is involved in microcirculatory impairment and organ dysfunction. During sepsis, the endothelium becomes both a target and a source of ROS and RNS. Exogenous sources of ROS and RNS are mainly phagocytes; however, endothelial cells can also generate ROS and RNS which may help to initiate and perpetuate the development of a systemic inflammatory response and subsequently cause organ dysfunction.

Sources and Actions of ROS and RNS in the Endothelium during Sepsis

The endothelium represents both a source and a target for ROS released in the vasculature in sepsis, although other cells in the vessel wall as well as the inflammatory cells also play important roles. During sepsis, stimulated inflammatory cells, such as neutrophils and macrophages, produce large amounts of ROS and RNS [4, 5]. This production of ROS and RNS is a crucial mechanism for neutrophils and macrophages to damage or kill microorganisms and contributes to part of the host defense against bacterial spread. Oxygen burst can also cause cell damage, and the endothelium is one of the first targets of ROS.

During sepsis, a large number of components (e.g., pro- and anti-inflammatory cytokine balance, degree of leukocyte activation, oscillatory shear stress) and conditions (hypoxia, reperfusion injury) are responsible for endothelial superoxide ($O_2\cdot^-$) production. Endothelial sources of $O_2\cdot^-$ that are implicated in endothelial dysfunction include mitochondria, xanthine oxidase (XO), uncoupled NO synthases (NOS), cytochrome P450 enzymes, and NADPH oxidases. In addition, enzymes such as lipoxygenases may also generate $O_2\cdot^-$. Increasing evidence supports the idea that ROS generated from mitochondria contribute significantly to endothelial cell dysfunction. The mitochondrial respiratory chain can be a major source of $O_2\cdot^-$ [6, 7]. During oxidative phosphorylation, 1–4 % of oxygen may be incompletely reduced in the mitochondrial respiratory chain, resulting in $O_2\cdot^-$ formation, mainly at complex I (NADH coenzyme Q reductase) and complex III (ubiquinol Cyt c reductase) of the mitochondrial respiratory chain. Increased mitochondrial $O_2\cdot^-$ generation appears to be particularly prominent in situations of metabolic perturbation. For example, hyperglycemia, hypoxia, and ischemia/reperfusion induce $O_2\cdot^-$ production. Moreover, pro-inflammatory cytokines (tumor necrosis factor [TNF]-α) may directly induce mitochondrial $O_2\cdot^-$ production [8] .

Our group has tested the capacity of the plasma of patients in septic shock as a whole to induce ROS production in naïve human umbilical vein endothelial cells (HUVEC) [9]. For this purpose, we used a fluorescence technique which has been widely used by our group and others to quantify ROS production in HUVEC. We found that plasma from patients treated for septic shock induced ROS formation in naive HUVEC, and that the extent of ROS production was higher in non-survivors than in survivors and was correlated with mortality and with criteria of the severity of septic shock as assessed by the sequential organ failure assessment (SOFA) score and simplified acute physiology score (SAPS) II (**Fig. 1**) [9]. This experiment therefore demonstrated the ability of the plasma to induce ROS production independent of any direct effect of sepsis mediated by circulating cells on the endothelial cells. This observation may be of clinical relevance because during septic shock, infection and

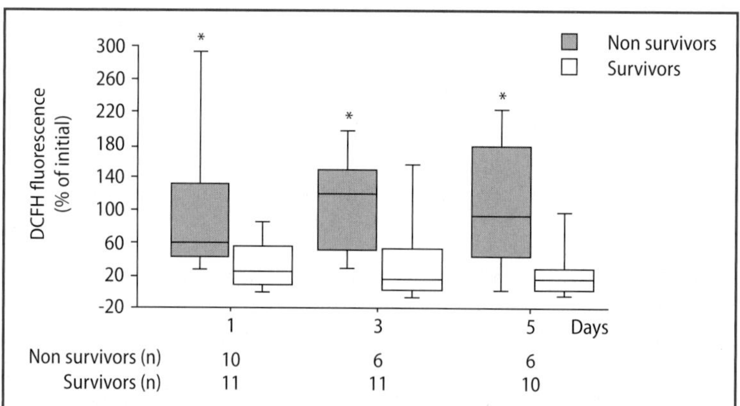

Fig. 1. Patients in septic shock. Changes in reactive oxygen species (2′-7′DCFH levels) are significantly higher at Day 1, Day 3, and Day 5 in non-survivors than in survivors (ANOVA, p = .0015). Values are means ± SD. From [9] with permission.

II

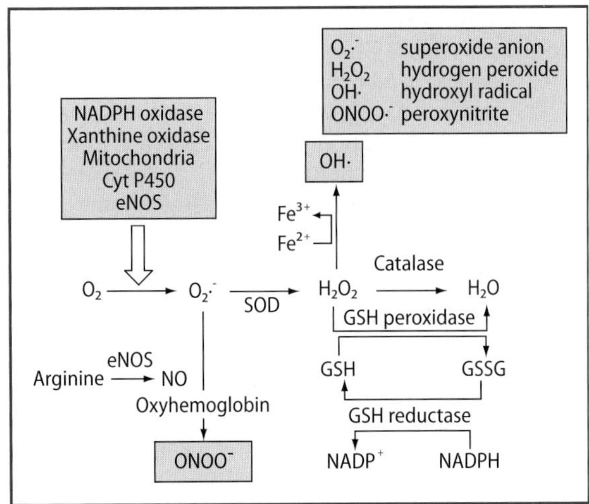

Fig. 2. Enzymatic and non-enzymatic antioxidant systems. NOS: nitric oxide synthase; SOD: superoxide dismutase; GSH: glutathione

the inflammatory response are initially spatially limited. Subsequently however, a systemic inflammatory response and organ dysfunction at a distance from the initial infection site can occur, events for which endothelial cell activation is a key factor.

The effects of $O_2\cdot^-$ generated within the endothelial cell are dependent on the amount of $O_2\cdot^-$ generated and on the ability of antioxidant systems to control this $O_2\cdot^-$ production. The deleterious effects of ROS can be modulated by enzymatic and non-enzymatic antioxidant systems that can either specifically inhibit ROS formation or facilitate ROS conversion into inactive components. Antioxidant systems comprise non-enzymatic molecules and specific antioxidant enzymes. Non-enzymatic antioxidants in endothelial cells include uric acid, ascorbic acid (vitamin C), α-tocopherol (vitamin E), and glutathione (GSH). GSH is the major thiol antioxidant in endothelial cells, serving as a substrate for glutathione peroxidase to eliminate lipid hydroperoxides and hydrogen peroxide (H_2O_2), whereby it becomes converted to GSH disulfide (GSSG). Normally, GSSG is maintained at levels $< 1\%$ of total GSH. Enzymatic antioxidants in endothelial cells include superoxide dismutases (SOD), catalase, the thioredoxin system, glutathione peroxidase, and heme oxygenase (HO) (**Fig. 2**). SODs convert $O_2\cdot^-$ to H_2O_2. H_2O_2 is then degraded to water by catalase or glutathione peroxidase. Copper/zinc SOD (CuZnSOD) is suggested to be the predominant SOD isoform in endothelium. An interesting point is that CuZnSOD expression is upregulated by shear stress and is related to cellular redox state. Under physiological conditions, endothelial cell antioxidant defenses are able to control $O_2\cdot^-$ production and to prevent production of two powerful oxidants: The hydroxyl radical (OH·) and peroxynitrite ($ONOO^-$) (**Fig. 2**).

Mechanisms of Endothelial Dysfunction during Sepsis

Increasing evidence supports the idea that the principal cause of endothelial cell dysfunction during sepsis is cell injury [3, 10, 11]. It is essential to understand the difference between endothelial cell dysfunction and endothelial cell activation. An activated endothelial cell responds by the acquisition of a new endothelial function which is going to be beneficial for the host. Dysfunction is the failure to adequately perform a homeostatic function. Significant injury leads to endothelial cell desquamation and release of membrane vesicles known as exosomes or microparticles with an increased thrombotic propensity.

ROS cytotoxicity is always due to the association of two phenomena, i.e., an increase in ROS production and a decrease in antioxidants. Huet et al. [12] reported that the ROS cytotoxicity induced by plasma from septic shock patients seems mainly to be due to a rapid decrease (4 hours) of intracellular GSH concentrations in HUVEC. GSH concentration is one of the critical determinants of endothelial cell damage during septic shock.

Neither $O_2\cdot^-$ nor NO is particularly toxic *in vivo* because $O_2\cdot^-$ is rapidly removed by SODs and NO is rapidly removed by its rapid diffusion into red blood cells where it is converted to nitrate by reaction with oxyhemoglobin. However, when NO is in the high nanomolar range, NO may outcompete SOD and react with $O_2\cdot^-$ to generate $ONOO^-$ ($O_2\cdot$- reacts with NO at a significantly faster rate than with SOD, $k = 6.7 \times 10^9$ $mol.l^{-1}.s^{-1}$). Under pro-inflammatory conditions, simultaneous production of $O_2\cdot^-$ and NO can occur to increase production 1,000-fold, which will increase the formation of $ONOO^-$ by 1,000,000-fold [17]. Thus, even modest increases in the production of $O_2\cdot^-$ and NO will greatly stimulate the formation of $ONOO^-$. This reaction is associated with a decrease in NO availability. Excess H_2O_2 might induce OH· formation by the Fenton reaction ($H_2O_2 + Fe^{++} \Rightarrow OH\cdot + OH\cdot + Fe^{III}$) or Haber-Weiss cycle ($H_2O_2 + O_2\cdot^- \Rightarrow OH\cdot + OH\cdot + O_2$) when in the presence of transition metals like copper or iron.

A large body of evidence supports a key role of $ONOO^-$ in cell cytotoxicity [11, 13, 14]. The half-life of $ONOO^-$ is short (10–20 ms), but sufficient to cross biological membranes. Thus, $ONOO^-$ diffuses and reacts within one to two cell diameters. In comparison, OH· is so reactive that it will react within a very short diffusion distance (≈ less than the diameter of a protein). Once formed, $ONOO^-$ causes cell injury by oxidizing biological molecules. In addition, it can yield hydroxyl radical and nitrogen dioxide (NO_2^-). Through these reactions, $ONOO^-$ in activated macrophages and in endothelial cells damages protein, lipid, and DNA (**Fig. 3**). Moreover, $ONOO^-$ can react with most of the components of the electron transport chain including complexes I and III [13, 14 (**Fig. 3**). $ONOO^-$ may reach mitochondria either from extramitochondrial compartments or may be directly produced within the mit-

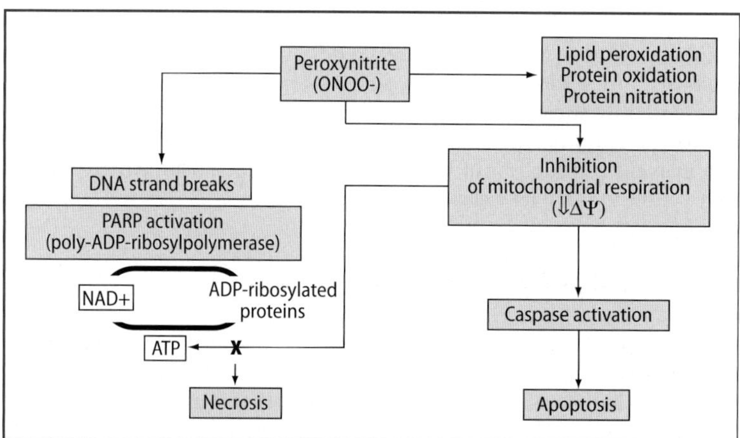

Fig. 3. Mechanisms of peroxynitrite-mediated cell death. PARP: poly-ADP ribose polymerase

ochondria. Indeed, mitochondria can produce both NO, by the activity of a Ca^{2+}-sensitive mitochondrial NOS (mtNOS) and $O_2^{\cdot-}$, due to the natural leak of electrons from the mitochondrial respiratory chain. $ONOO^-$ may mediate apoptosis by permeabilization of the mitochondrial outer membrane. Mitochondrial outer membrane permeabilization allows the efflux of various pro-apoptotic signaling molecules, which promote cell death or by a phenomenon termed mitochondrial permeability transition. Mitochondrial permeability transition describes the permeabilization of the inner mitochondrial membrane. The permeability transition pore results in the dissipation of mitochondrial membrane potential, resulting in cessation of electron transfer and ATP production. Futhermore, $ONOO^-$ nitrates and inhibits manganese (Mn)SOD preventing the breakdown of locally produced superoxide, which further fuels the formation of $ONOO^-$. $ONOO^-$ may induce DNA damage with activation of the DNA repair enzyme, poly-ADP ribose polymerase (PARP-1) (**Fig. 3**). Upon severe DNA injury, overactivation of PARP-1 depletes the cellular stores of NAD^+, an essential cofactor of the glycolytic pathway, the tricarboxylic acid cycle, and the mitochondrial electron transport chain. As a result, the loss of NAD^+ leads to a marked decrease in the cellular pools of ATP, resulting in cellular dysfunction and cell death ('suicide hypothesis' after irreversible DNA injury). Whereas apoptosis is a typical consequence of low to moderate concentrations of $OHOO^-$, exposure of cells to higher concentrations has been associated with necrosis.

$OHOO^-$ may also oxidize the essential NOS cofactor, tetrahydrobiopterin (BH_4), and induce endothelial NOS (eNOS) uncoupling. NOS is composed of a homodimeric complex that includes an enzymatic site with reductase activity along with a site with oxidase activity. NO formation is the result of two successive reactions. The first consists of molecular oxygen formation that hydroxylates guanidino-nitrogenated L-arginine to form N^G-hydroxyl-L-arginine. The second reaction consists of N^G-hydroxyl-L-arginine oxidation and leads to NO and L-citrullin formation. The cofactor, BH_4, is necessary for both reactions. When BH_4 is missing, NOS can become 'uncoupled', leading to the generation of $O_2^{\cdot-}$. Uncoupled NOS is responsible for $O_2^{\cdot-}$ production and thereby an increase in oxidative stress [15–17]. In addition to increased catabolism or degradation, another reason for BH_4 depletion may be its reduced synthesis. NOS uncoupling results in loss of endothelial vasodilation properties due to the decrease in NO availability and an increase in oxidative stress. ROS therefore play a pivotal role in the vasomotor disturbances seen in septic shock.

Conclusion

Endothelial activation and dysfunction play a role in the pathogenesis of sepsis [18, 19]. The endothelium is one of the first targets of systemic inflammation due to sepsis. Vasomotor tone modification, leukocyte and platelet adhesion, capillary leak, and a pro-coagulant state lead to a global decrease and heterogeneity in capillary perfusion as well as a decrease in tissue oxygen extraction capacities. Endothelial dysfunction is involved in microcirculatory impairment and organ dysfunction. ROS and RNS have several potentially important effects on endothelial function and are implicated both in physiological regulation and in disease pathophysiology [19]. During sepsis, the endothelium becomes both a target and a source of ROS and RNS. Exogenous sources of ROS and RNS are mainly phagocytes. A large body of evidence supports a key role of $ONOO^-$ in cell cytotoxicity [1, 10, 20]. $ONOO^-$ contributes to mitochondrial dysfunction by a range of mechanisms and induces both necrotic and apoptotic cell death [11, 21]. Understanding the mechanisms underlying the generation of ROS and RNS in endothelial cells and the causes of endothelial dysfunction in sepsis may help in the development of therapeutic strategies to tackle endothelial dysfunction and microcirculatory failure in sepsis. However, even though some studies have shown encouraging results by antagonizing ROS, none has clearly demonstrated an absolute benefit for antioxidant strategies; this is one of the most important therapeutic challenges to be investigated in the near future.

References

1. Halliwell B, Zhao K, Whiteman M (1999) Nitric oxide and peroxynitrite. The ugly, the uglier and the not so good: a personal view of recent controversies. Free Radic Res 31: 651–669
2. Budinger GR, Duranteau J, Chandel NS, Schumacker PT (1998) Hibernation during hypoxia in cardiomyocytes. Role of mitochondria as the O2 sensor. J Biol Chem 273: 3320–3326
3. Cerwinka WH, Cooper D, Krieglstein CF, Ross CR, McCord JM, Granger DN (2003) Superoxide mediates endotoxin-induced platelet-endothelial cell adhesion in intestinal venules. Am J Physiol Heart Circ Physiol 284:H535–541
4. Sikora JP (2002) Immunotherapy in the management of sepsis. Arch Immunol Ther Exp (Warsz) 50: 317–324
5. Fialkow L, Wang Y, Downey GP (2007) Reactive oxygen and nitrogen species as signaling molecules regulating neutrophil function. Free Radic Biol Med 42: 153–164
6. Therade-Matharan S, Laemmel E, Carpentier S, et al (2005) Reactive oxygen species production by mitochondria in endothelial cells exposed to reoxygenation after hypoxia and glucose depletion is mediated by ceramide. Am J Physiol Regul Integr Comp Physiol 289:R1756–1762
7. Duranteau J, Chandel NS, Kulisz A, Shao Z, Schumacker PT (1998) Intracellular signaling by reactive oxygen species during hypoxia in cardiomyocytes. J Biol Chem 273: 11619–11624
8. Corda S, Laplace C, Vicaut E, Duranteau J (2001) Rapid reactive oxygen species production by mitochondria in endothelial cells exposed to tumor necrosis factor-alpha is mediated by ceramide. Am J Respir Cell Mol Biol 24: 762–768
9. Huet O, Obata R, Aubron C, et al (2007) Plasma-induced endothelial oxidative stress is related to the severity of septic shock. Crit Care Med 35: 821–826
10. Chung HY, Yokozawa T, Kim MS, et al (2000) The mechanism of nitric oxide and/or superoxide cytotoxicity in endothelial cells. Exp Toxicol Pathol 52: 227–233
11. Brown GC, Borutaite V (1999) Nitric oxide, cytochrome c and mitochondria. Biochem Soc Symp 66: 17–25
12. Huet O, Cherreau C, Nicco C, et al (2008) Pivotal role of glutathione depletion in plasma-induced endothelial oxidative stress during sepsis. Crit Care Med 36: 2328–2334
13. Li H, Forstermann U (2000) Nitric oxide in the pathogenesis of vascular disease. J Pathol 190: 244–254
14. Radi R, Cassina A, Hodara R (2002) Nitric oxide and peroxynitrite interactions with mitochondria. Biol Chem 383: 401–409
15. Thum T, Fraccarollo D, Schultheiss M, et al (2007) Endothelial nitric oxide synthase uncoupling impairs endothelial progenitor cell mobilization and function in diabetes. Diabetes 56: 666–674
16. Gao YT, Roman LJ, Martasek P, Panda SP, Ishimura Y, Masters BS (2007) Oxygen metabolism by endothelial nitric-oxide synthase. J Biol Chem 282: 28557–28565
17. Sullivan JC, Pollock JS (2006) Coupled and uncoupled NOS: separate but equal? Uncoupled NOS in endothelial cells is a critical pathway for intracellular signaling. Circ Res 98: 717–719
18. Ince C (2004) Microcirculation in distress: a new resuscitation end point? Crit Care Med 32: 1963–1964
19. Li JM, Shah AM (2004) Endothelial cell superoxide generation: regulation and relevance for cardiovascular pathophysiology. Am J Physiol Regul Integr Comp Physiol 287:R1014–1030
20. Rada BK, Geiszt M, Kaldi K, Timar C, Ligeti E (2004) Dual role of phagocytic NADPH oxidase in bacterial killing. Blood 104: 2947–2953
21. Cadenas E (2004) Mitochondrial free radical production and cell signaling. Mol Aspects Med 25: 17–26

Measurement of Carbon Monoxide: From Bench to Bedside

F. Corrêa, F.E. Nacul, and Y. Sakr

Introduction

Carbon monoxide is produced endogenously by the class of enzymes known collectively as heme oxygenase (HO) [1]. The inducible form of HO, HO-1, has been reported to have cytoprotective and anti-oxidant activities [1]. In addition, other studies have suggested that endogenously generated carbon monoxide has protective and beneficial effects on a vast array of responses against multiple organ injury, inflammation, apoptosis, cell proliferation, vasoconstriction and systemic and pulmonary hypertension [2–5]. The initial evidence supporting a beneficial action of carbon monoxide originated from studies on lung injury in animals [6] and was reproduced later in other tissues, including the heart, liver, kidney, intestine and the reticulo-endothelial system [2, 7].

Although still limited in number, several human studies have reported carbon monoxide concentrations in various diseases, such as asthma, chronic obstructive pulmonary disease (COPD), cystic fibrosis, and hemolytic anemia, and in critically ill patients. The results of these studies have raised important questions concerning the association between carbon monoxide concentrations and disease activity and the potential prognostic value of carbon monoxide concentrations.

Carbon Monoxide Measurement

Approximately 80 % of the carbon monoxide produced in the body is exhaled [8], which makes breath measurement a potentially viable way to monitor changes in HO-enzyme activity. Carbon monoxide can be measured in real time or in collected

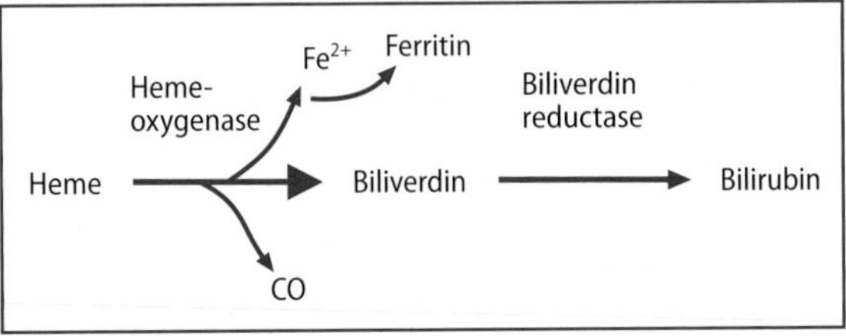

Fig. 1. Schematic representation of the production of carbon monoxide (CO), biliverdin, bilirubin, and iron from heme. Most endogenous CO production originates from active heme metabolism although a portion may arise from lipid peroxidation and drug metabolism reactions. Hemoxygenase cleaves the tetrapyrrolic ring of cellular heme moieties liberating CO and equimolar amounts of free iron and biliverdin with reduction of NADPH. Biliverdin is in turn converted into bilirubin by the cytosolic enzyme biliverdin reductase.

breath, and there is some debate as to which procedure is most accurate and reproducible [9]. However, monitoring exhaled carbon monoxide (CO_{ex}) has some limitations. Ambient carbon monoxide concentrations and tobacco smoking may alter the bronchial carbon monoxide value [10]. Furthermore, variations in ventilation may result in transient changes in the concentrations of CO_{ex} [11], which can also limit the accuracy of measurements. In addition, estimation of carboxyhemoglobin from CO_{ex} measurements is considered to be inaccurate in patients with severe airflow obstruction [12]. Another limitation is the fact that measuring end-tidal carbon monoxide is not possible in patients requiring high-frequency oscillatory ventilation or nasal continuous positive airway pressure (CPAP). Finally, CO_{ex} concentrations appear to be elevated in healthy subjects with viral upper respiratory tract infection [13].

Alternatively, carbon monoxide concentrations can be measured by assessing arterial carboxyhemoglobin, since there is a significant correlation between the arterial carboxyhemoglobin concentration and CO_{ex} [14]. However, some old blood gas analyzers may not be sensitive enough and have been shown to significantly underestimate the arterial carboxyhemoglobin [15]. The calibration of the wavelength specific for carboxyhemoglobin is also important for accurate determination of carboxyhemoglobin concentrations [16].

Carbon Monoxide Concentrations in Critically Ill Patients

Patients requiring intensive care demonstrate perturbations of the immune system and upregulation of potentially protective systems, including HO-1 expression and the products of its enzymatic activity, i.e., carbon monoxide, biliverdin, and iron (**Fig. 1**) [17]. Sepsis, severe sepsis, and septic shock, with their associated systemic inflammatory response, represent the most common cause of death in patients admitted to intensive care units (ICUs), with an associated mortality of 20 to 60 % [18]. These syndromes are associated with dysregulation of the homeostatic mechanisms that act to minimize intracellular and systemic oxidative stress [19]. Ample evidence has been provided that carbon monoxide acts as a potent anti-inflammatory molecule, both *in vitro* and *in vivo* [4]. Exposure of macrophages to low concentrations of carbon monoxide selectively inhibited the expression of lipopolysaccharide (LPS)-induced pro-inflammatory cytokines (tumor necrosis factor [TNF]-α, interleukin [IL]-1β and macrophage inflammatory protein [MIP]-1β), while increasing the LPS expression of anti-inflammatory cytokines (IL-10) [4]. In addition, it was also demonstrated that HO-1 was induced in the lung as well as in the kidney, the liver, the intestine, and the brain in a rat model of sepsis [20], suggesting that HO-1 may be inducible in various organs in massive inflammation such as sepsis [21]. Widespread overexpression of HO-1 has been described in a mouse model of sepsis [22]. This anti-inflammatory effect of carbon monoxide has been shown to affect several intracellular signaling pathways, including guanylyl-cyclase which generates cGMP and the mitogen-activated protein kinase (MAPK) system [23]. Other possible signaling mechanisms would entail interaction with Ca2+ modulated K+ channels [24, 25].

Several studies have demonstrated that CO_{ex} concentrations [11, 21, 26–28] or the carboxyhemoglobin concentration in the blood [21, 29–33] are increased in medical and surgical critically ill patients (**Table 1**). The correlation between CO_{ex} and arterial carboxyhemoglobin concentrations was studied by Scharte et al. [27], who reported that although CO_{ex} was increased in critically ill patients, it did not correlate with arterial or venous carboxyhemoglobin. These findings are in contrast to

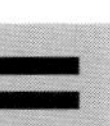

Table 1. Carbon monoxide levels in critically ill patients

First author/Year	Setting	Design	Sample	CO measurement	Main results
Melley 2007 [33]	Cardiothoracic ICU	Prospective	All patients admitted to ICU in a 15 month period (n = 1,267)	aHbCO	Low minimum and high maximum aHbCO were associated with increased mortality. After adjustment for age, gender, illness severity, and other relevant variables, a lower minimum aHbCO was associated with an increased risk of death from all causes. aHbCO correlated with markers of the inflammatory response
Scharte 2006 [26]	Critically ill	Prospective	Mechanically ventilated, critically ill patients (n = 95)	CO_{ex}	CO production correlated weakly with the multiple organ dysfunction score. Patients suffering from cardiac disease produced significantly higher amounts of CO_{ex} compared to critically ill controls
Morimatsu 2006 [21]	Mixed ICU	Prospective	Consecutive critically ill patients (n = 29) vs. healthy control subjects (n = 8)	CO_{ex}	Median CO_{ex} concentration was significantly higher in critically ill patients compared with control. No correlation among CO_{ex}, disease severity, and degree of inflammation. Strong trend for higher CO_{ex} concentration in survivors than in non-survivors
Mayr 2005 [60]	Experimental endotoxemia	Prospective	Healthy male non-smokers (n = 13)	vHbCO	LPS infusion transiently increased plasma concentrations of TNF-α, IL-6 and IL-8, as well as IL-1α and IL-1β mRNA levels. These LPS-induced changes were not influenced by CO inhalation
Sakamoto 2005 [61]	CABG surgery	Prospective	Patients undergoing CAGB (n = 45)	Serum HbCO	HbCO, TNF-α, and IL-1β significantly increased after surgery. There was a weak correlation between HbCO and inflammatory mediators
Eletr 2004 [36]	Surgical ICU	Prospective	Non-smoking, mechanically ventilated patients after gastrointestinal surgery (n = 30)	aHbCO and vHbCO	a-vHbCO was not correlated to any parameter, whereas aHbCO and central vHbCO concentrations were positively related with TNF-α, IL-6 and procalcitonin.
Shi 2003 [32]	Sepsis Septic shock	Prospective	Children with sepsis/ septic shock (n = 12) vs. control healthy children (n = 30)	Plasma CO	CO concentrations were increased in patients compared with controls. Patients with septic shock had higher plasma CO concentrations than those without shock
Zegdi 2002 [28]	Severe sepsis	Prospective	Severe sepsis patients (n = 24) vs. control subjects (n = 5). All mechanically ventilated.	CO_{ex}	Endogenous CO production was higher in the sepsis group during the first 3 days of treatment in comparison to the control group. Survivors of sepsis had a significantly higher endogenous CO production on day 1 compared to non-survivors

Table 1. *(cont.)*

First author/Year	Setting	Design	Sample	CO measurement	Main results
Zegdi 2000 [11]	Medical ICU	Prospective	Mechanically ventilated, critically ill patients (n = 9)	CO_{ex}	CO was easily detected in the exhaled breath of mechanically ventilated patients and CO lung excretion was markedly but transiently dependent on inspired oxygen fraction
Shi 2000 [31]	Neonatal sepsis	Prospective	Term septic newborn (n = 7) vs. healthy neonates control (n = 30)	Plasma CO	Plasma CO concentrations were significantly higher in the group with sepsis at the time of admission to the neonatal intensive care unit than in the healthy controls
Scharte 2000 [27]	Surgical ICU	Prospective	Critically ill patients (n = 30) vs. non-smokers healthy control (n = 6)	CO_{ex}	ICU patients showed significantly higher CO_{ex} as well as total CO production compared to controls. There were no correlations between CO_{ex}, arterial, and central venous blood HbCO
Moncure 1999 [30]	Trauma ICU	Prospective	Blood samples from patients admitted to ICU > 24h (n = 45)	Plasma HbCO	HbCO concentrations were higher in septic than in stressed and non-septic non-stressed patients. HbCO concentrations in samples obtained from patients in shock were higher than those from patients not in shock
Sedlacek 1999 [35]	Surgical ICU	Retrospective	Blood samples (n = 5569) of critically ill patients	HbCO	There was no correlation between lactate and HbCO concentrations.
Meyer 1998 [29]	Surgical ICU		Critically ill patients (n = 59) vs. healthy control (n = 29)	aHbCO and vHbCO	aHbCO and vHbCO, were significantly higher in the ICU patients. aHbCO was significantly higher than vHbCO.
Hunter 1994 [34]	Surgical ICU	Prospective	Consecutive admissions (n = 32)	aHbCO	There was a positive correlation between aHbCO and the APACHE II score. HbCO correlated with an increase in the white blood cell count.
Leikin 1986 [62]	Emergency department	Retrospective	Acute exacerbation of cardiopulmonary disease (n = 229)	aHbCO	Significant increases in HbCO were found in patients admitted to the ICU and with proven myocardial infarction over a control group.

ICU: intensive care unit; CO_{ex}: exhaled carbon monoxide; HbCO: carboxyhemoglobin concentration; a-vHbCO: arterio-venous carboxyhemoglobin concentration difference; CABG: coronary artery by-pass graft; aHbCO: arterial carboxyhemoglobin concentration; vHbCO: venous carboxyhemoglobin concentration; TNF: tumor necrosis factor; IL: interleukin those reported by Morimatsu et al. [21], who demonstrated a significant correlation between CO_{ex} and arterial carboxyhemoglobin concentrations. An important difference between these two studies was the sensitivity of the blood gas analyzer used. In the study by Morimatsu et al. [21], the authors used a more recent blood gas analyzer, 25 times more sensitive than the analyzer used by Scharte et al. and with calibration of the wavelength specific to carboxyhemoglobin, which allowed accurate determination of carboxyhemoglobin [16]. In addition, the analyzer used in the study by Scharte et al. [27] was shown to significantly underestimate the arterial carboxyhemoglobin concentrations [15]. Morimatsu et al. [21], also showed a significant correlation among CO_{ex}, carboxyhemoglobin concentrations in arterial blood, and total serum bilirubin in critically ill patients. Another important finding of this study [21], was that CO_{ex} concentrations were correlated with serum indirect bilirubin, but not with serum direct bilirubin in these patients. These findings led the authors to suggest that in critically ill patients there may be increased extracorpuscular heme catabolism, leading to the induction of HO-1 and resultant production of carbon monoxide and indirect bilirubin [21].

The first study to evaluate the relationship between carbon monoxide concentrations and sepsis was performed by Moncure et al. [30], who showed significantly elevated carboxyhemoglobin concentrations during stress, sepsis, and shock states in a group of patients admitted to a trauma ICU. However, these authors found an overlap between sepsis and stress carboxyhemoglobin sample values, limiting the clinical usefulness of the assays in predicting sepsis [30]. Shi et al. [31] investigated a small group of newborn infants with sepsis and reported that plasma carbon monoxide concentrations were significantly higher in the seven newborns with sepsis at the time of admission to the neonatal ICU than in the healthy controls. It was also found that the increased carbon monoxide concentrations were related to enhanced NO production during neonatal sepsis. Another study [32] evaluated 12 pediatric patients with sepsis syndrome and showed that plasma carbon monoxide concentrations were significantly increased in the group with sepsis syndrome, and that increased plasma carbon monoxide concentrations were higher in patients with septic shock than in those with sepsis but without shock. Zedgi et al. [28] also found that endogenous carbon monoxide production was higher in patients with severe sepsis during the first 3 days of treatment in comparison to the control group.

The clinical significance of the measurement of carbon monoxide concentration as a marker of inflammation in critical illness has been explored in some studies. Hunter et al. [34] analyzed data from 32 patients admitted to a surgical ICU and found a positive correlation between arterial carboxyhemoglobin concentrations and the APACHE II and white blood cell (WBC) count. Conversely, Sedlacek et al. [35] analyzed 5322 blood samples on which simultaneous lactate and carboxyhemoglobin determinations were performed and found no correlation between lactate and carboxyhemoglobin concentrations. However, the retrospective nature of this study [35], and the lack of information about the smoking status of patients and the presence of mechanical ventilation are some of the important limitations of this study. Moncure et al. [30], studied carbon monoxide concentrations in 45 trauma victims admitted to a trauma ICU, not mechanically ventilated, and could not demonstrate any relationship among carboxyhemoglobin concentrations, WBC count, APACHE III scores and Injury Severity Scores (ISS). In addition, in a group of 30 non-smoking, mechanically ventilated patients admitted to a surgical ICU after gastrointestinal surgery, no correlation was found between arteriovenous carboxyhemoglobin difference and IL-6, procalcitonin (PCT), or TNF-α [36]. However, arterial and central venous carboxyhemoglobin concentrations were positively correlated to plasma concentrations of TNF-α, IL-6 and PCT and not correlated with C-reactive protein (CRP) or leukocyte count [36]. Melley et al. [33] studied a cohort of 1267 patients admitted to a general ICU (82 % admitted after cardiac surgery) and found that carboxyhemoglobin concentration correlated significantly with CRP and serum bilirubin concentrations; there was no correlation between WBC count and carboxyhemoglobin concentration.

The role of carbon monoxide concentration as a mediator of critical illness and organ dysfunction has also been evaluated. A group of 29 non-smoking, mechanically ventilated patients (predominantly surgical) was studied by Morimatsu et al. [21]; no correlation was found between CO_{ex} and the sequential organ failure assessment (SOFA) score, WBC count or CRP. However, Scharte et al. [26] evaluated 95 mechanically ventilated, critically ill patients and found that CO_{ex} concentrations correlated weakly with the multiple organ dysfunction score.

The relationship between carbon monoxide concentrations and outcome in ICU patients has been evaluated also. Moncure et al. [30], studied carbon monoxide concentrations in a group of 45 patients admitted to a trauma ICU and found that carboxyhemoglobin concentrations in survivors did not differ significantly from those of patients who died. Zedgi et al. [28], studying carbon monoxide production in patients with severe sepsis, found that survivors of sepsis initially had higher endogenous carbon monoxide production. A limitation of this study, however, was that the sample size was not big enough to determine whether the level of endogenous carbon monoxide production was an independent predictor of survival in severe sepsis. Morimatsu et al. [21] also compared CO_{ex} concentrations in survivors and non-survivors in a group of critically ill patients (predominantly surgical patients), and found that survivors tended to have higher concentrations of CO_{ex} than non-survivors. Nonetheless, the difference did not reach statistical significance also because of a limited sample size. Melley et al. [33], reported that, after adjustment for age, gender, illness severity, and other relevant variables, a lower minimum arterial carboxyhemoglobin concentration was associated with an increased risk of death from all causes. These authors also showed that an elevated maximum arterial carboxyhemoglobin was also significantly associated with higher mortality rates. Since both low minimum and high maximum concentrations of arterial carboxyhemoglobin in patients were associated with increased intensive care mortality, the authors suggested that although HO-1 activity is protective, excessive induction may be deleterious, and that there may be an optimal range for HO activity and the liberation of its products.

In summary, CO_{ex} and carboxyhemoglobin concentrations are increased in various subgroups of critically ill patients including medical, surgical and post-traumatic ICU patients. CO_{ex} and carboxyhemoglobin are associated with the degree of inflammation and the extent of organ dysfunction especially in association with sepsis syndromes. In addition, carbon monoxide concentrations correlate well with outcome in critically ill patients.

Carbon Monoxide Concentrations and Lung Diseases

HO is present in the pulmonary vascular endothelium and alveolar macrophages and is upregulated by oxidative stress [37], inflammatory cytokines, and NO [38]. These findings imply a role of endogenous carbon monoxide in inflammatory airway diseases. There is enough evidence to support a role for inflammatory activity and the presence of oxidative stress in many lung disorders: Many cytokines are involved in asthmatic inflammation, including IL-1, IL-6, and TNF [39]; histological examination reveals neutrophil accumulation and infiltration in the lung in bacterial pneumonia [40]; increased levels of reactive oxygen species in neutrophils and bronchoalveolar lavage fluid have been found in inflammatory lung diseases such as cystic fibrosis and acute respiratory distress syndrome (ARDS) [41]; production of various inflammatory factors, including pro-inflammatory cytokines [42], reactive oxygen species [43], and NO [44], is observed in patients with idiopathic pulmonary fibrosis and active fibrosing alveolitis. These factors may upregulate HO-1 production directly [45] or via the synthesis of NO [46].

Carbon monoxide concentrations have been measured in a number of patients with different inflammatory lung conditions (**Table 2**). Increased carbon monoxide concentrations were a consistent finding in several studies in patients with different diseases, such as bronchial asthma [47–49], COPD [50], bronchiectasis [51], silicosis [52], idiopathic pulmonary fibrosis [14], acute pneumonia [14], cystic fibrosis [53] and bronchopulmonary dysplasia [54].

The first study to investigate carbon monoxide concentrations in asthma patients was performed in 1997 by Zayasu et al. [47], who reported higher CO_{ex} concentrations in adult asthma patients not receiving inhaled corticosteroids than in nonsmoking healthy control subjects. The potential use of carbon monoxide concentrations to monitor asthma activity in adults was studied by Yamaya et al. [49] who found that asthma exacerbations were associated with increased CO_{ex} concentrations. CO_{ex} was also reported to be higher in *unstable* severe asthmatics than in *stable* severe asthmatics [55]. Furthermore, a reduction in CO_{ex} was observed in adult asthmatic patients after treatment with inhaled or oral corticosteroids [14, 47–49]. However, Kong et al. [56] noted that even in asthma patients with acute exacerbation requiring hospitalization, CO_{ex} concentrations were not different from those measured in stable asthmatics and healthy controls. The results of this study [56] may be confounded by the fact that the majority (61 %) of the asthma patients with acute exacerbation had been treated with inhaled corticosteroids prior to hospitalization.

Carbon monoxide concentration as a potential marker of COPD activity was studied by Yasuda et al. [50] who reported significantly higher arterial blood carboxyhemoglobin concentrations in patients with COPD during exacerbations than those in stable condition before exacerbations. In addition, in the patients with COPD at stage II and stage III (but not at stage IV), CO_{ex} concentrations during the exacerbations were higher than those during stable conditions. Biernacki et al. [57] suggested that measurement of carbon monoxide in exhaled air can detect an increased inflammatory process within the airways, which has been caused by infection. In their study, these authors [57] showed an elevation of CO_{ex} in the majority of patients with lower respiratory tract infection, which subsequently decreased after treatment with antibiotics. A relation between CO_{ex} and the severity of pneumonia has also been demonstrated [58].

CO_{ex} concentrations as a non-invasive marker of cystic fibrosis was evaluated by Antuni et al. [59] who found increased CO_{ex} concentrations in patients with stable cystic fibrosis, and further increased concentrations in unstable patients. Likewise, Paredi et al. [44] reported that patients with cystic fibrosis not receiving steroid treatment had higher CO_{ex} concentrations than treated patients.

In summary, increased carbon monoxide concentrations are a consistent finding in several studies in patients with different diseases, such as bronchial asthma, COPD, bronchiectasis, silicosis, idiopathic pulmonary fibrosis, acute pneumonia,

Table 2. Carbon monoxide levels in patients with lung diseases

First author/Year	Disease	Design	Sample	CO measurement	Main results
May 2007 [54]	Bronchopulmonary dysplasia (BPD)	Prospective	Prematurely born with BPD (n = 14) vs. prematurely born without BPD (n = 36)	End-tidal CO (ETCO)	Infants who developed BPD had higher ETCO concentrations compared with the rest of the cohort on days 7, 14, 21, and 28.
Ohara 2006 [63]	Asthma	Prospective	Healthy (n = 188) vs. asthmatic stable (n = 29) vs. Asthmatic unstable (n = 22)	CO_{ex}	CO_{ex} concentrations were significantly elevated during acute asthma exacerbations, and partially recovered after treatment with β2-agonist and SCG in children with mild episodic asthma.
Yasuda 2005 [50]	COPD	Prospective	COPD pts (n = 58) vs. ex-smokers control subjects (n = 61)	CO_{ex}, aHbCO, vHbCO and a-vHbCO	aHbCO concentrations in stable patients were higher than those in control subjects. The HbCO concentrations in patients during exacerbations were higher than under stable conditions. a-vHbCO differences in patients during exacerbations did not differ from patients under stable conditions and from control subjects. aHbCO concentrations were higher in more severely ill patients.
Pearson 2005 [64]	Asthma	Prospective	Atopic asthma pts (n = 69)	CO_{ex}	At baseline there was no association between CO_{ex} and lung function or bronchial reactivity. In the longitudinal analysis, a rise in CO_{ex} was associated with improvement in bronchial reactivity
Yasuda 2004 [52]	Silicosis	Prospective	Elderly patients with silicosis (n = 48) vs. control group (n = 48). All were men and ex-smokers.	aHbCO and CO_{ex}	The aHbCO concentrations, CO_{ex} and serum CRP values were significantly higher in patients with silicosis than in controls. In patients with silicosis, aHbCO concentrations and CRP values during exacerbations were significantly higher than in patients with stable conditions.
Beck-Ripp 2004 [65]	Asthma, CF	Prospective	Healthy children (n = 20), stable CF-pts (n = 17), and steroid-naive asthmatics (n = 15)	CO_{ex}	CO_{ex} was not flow dependent in any of the three groups. Elevated CO_{ex} was found in asthmatics but not in CF-children
Yasuda 2004 [66]	Pulmonary and non-pulmonary inflammatory diseases	Prospective	Asthma (n = 18) and pneumonia (n = 33) vs. acute pyelonephritis (n = 28) and acute rheumathoid arthritis (n = 16) vs. control (n = 22)	aHbCO and vHbCO	Arterial and vHbCO was higher in patients with pulmonary and extra-pulmonary inflammation compared with those in control subjects. a-vHbCO differences in patients with inflammatory pulmonary diseases were higher than those with non-pulmonary inflammatory diseases and control subjects

Table 2. *(cont.)*

First author/Year	Disease	Design	Sample	CO measurement	Main results
Ramirez 2004 [10]	Asthma	Prospective	Adult with mild asthma without steroid treatment (n = 105)	CO_{ex}	CO_{ex} concentrations rose significantly after bronchial challenge with histamine. On stepwise multiple linear regression analysis, CO_{ex} only correlated significantly with continuous index of responsiveness.
Yasuda 2002 [14]	Asthma, pneumonia, IPF	Prospective	Control subjects (n = 34) vs. asthma pts (n = 24) vs. pneumonia (n = 52) vs. IPF (n = 21)	aHbCO and CO_{ex}	HbCO in patients with asthma during exacerbations, pneumonia at the onset of illness, and IPF was significantly higher than those in control subjects. In 20 patients with asthma the HbCO concentration decreased after 3 weeks of treatment with oral glucocorticoids
Kong 2002 [56]	Asthma	Prospective	Non-smoking "acute" asthmatics (hospitalized, n = 33); vs. "stable" asthmatics (n = 35); vs. healthy controls (n = 22)	CO_{ex}	CO_{ex} initial concentrations in acute asthmatics, stable asthmatics and controls were similar. In acute asthmatics, initial CO_{ex} did not correlate with duration of hospitalization, doses of intravenous corticosteroids, doses of nebulized salbutamol, PEF (% predicted) or FEV1 (% predicted)
Zanconato 2002 [48]	Asthma	Prospective	"Acute" exacerbation asthmatic children (n = 30) vs. control healthy children (n = 29)	CO_{ex}	Before therapy, CO_{ex} concentrations were higher in asthmatic children than in healthy controls. After prednisone therapy, there was a slight but non-significant decrease in CO_{ex}.
Zetterquist 2002 [67]	Asthma, CF	Prospective	Steroid-naïve asthmatics (n = 32) vs. steroid-treated asthmatics (n = 24, 16 allergic rhinitis; 9 CF) vs. non-smoking healthy control (n = 30)	CO_{ex}	No significant increase in FeCO in the groups of patients with inflammatory airway disorders compared to controls. FeNO was significantly elevated in steroid-naïve asthmatics and subjects with allergic rhinitis, but not in steroid-treated asthmatics and subjects with cystic fibrosis
Biernacki 2001 [57]	Lower respiratory tract infection	Prospective	Patients with symptoms of LRTI (n = 35)	CO_{ex}	Patients had elevated CO_{ex} concentrations at the moment of infection diagnosis and a decrease in CO_{ex} concentration after a course of antibiotics and clinical improvement
Khatri 2001 [68]	Asthma	Prospective	Atopic asthmatic (n = 8) vs. healthy control (n = 6)	CO_{ex}	CO_{ex} of asthmatics was not higher than that of control individuals at baseline, decreased immediately after allergen challenge, and returned to baseline levels during the late asthmatic response

Table 2. *(cont.)*

First author/Year	Disease	Design	Sample	CO measurement	Main results
Yamaya 2001 [55]	Asthma	Prospective	Mild asthmatics (n = 20) vs. moderate asthmatics treated with inhaled corticosteroids (n = 20) vs. stable asthmatics treated with high dose inhaled corticosteroids and oral corticosteroids once a month over 1 year (n = 15)	CO_{ex}	CO_{ex} concentrations in unstable severe asthmatics were significantly higher than those in stable severe asthmatics. CO_{ex} concentrations in mild and moderate asthmatics did not differ significantly from those in non-smoking control subjects. There was a significant relationship between the CO_{ex} concentrations and forced expiratory volume in one second in all asthmatic patients.
Antuni 2000 [59]	CF	Prospective	CF stable (n = 29) vs. CF unstable (n = 15) vs. non-smoking healthy control (n = 12)	CO_{ex}	CO_{ex} concentrations increased in the stable CF group, and further increased in the unstable group. A significant correlation was found between the deterioration in FEV1 and CO_{ex} concentrations
Paredi 1999 [44]	Asthma	Prospective	Atopic steroid-naive non-smoking asthmatics (n = 18) vs. non-smoking controls (n = 37)	CO_{ex}	CO_{ex} increased during early and late asthmatic reactions independent of the change in airway caliber
Paredi 1999 [53]	CF		CF steroid treated (n = 15) vs. CF steroid untreated (n = 14) vs. control (n = 15)	CO_{ex}	The concentration of CO_{ex} was significantly higher in patients with CF. Patients not receiving steroid treatment had higher CO concentrations than treated patients
Yamaya 1999 [49]	Asthma	Prospective	"Acute" exacerbation asthmatic pts (n = 20)	CO_{ex}	Asthma exacerbations caused a decrease in PEFR and a rise in CO_{ex} in all patients, and treatment with oral glucocorticoids reversed these changes in both parameters.
Uasuf 1999 [69]	Asthma		Asthmatic children (n = 29) vs. healthy control children (n = 40)	CO_{ex}	CO_{ex} concentrations were significantly higher in children with persistent asthma compared with those in children with infrequent episodic asthma and healthy children.

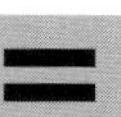

Table 2. *(cont.)*

First author/Year	Disease	Design	Sample	CO measurement	Main results
Yamaya 1998 [13]	URTIs	Prospective	Pts with URTIs (n = 20) vs. non- smoking control (n = 10) vs. smoking control (n = 10)	CO_{ex}	In subjects with URTI, CO_{ex} was significantly higher during the acute phase of URTIs than that in nonsmoking control subjects. CO_{ex} during the acute phase of URTIs decreased after 3 wk of recovery and CO_{ex} values in subjects who had recovered from URTIs did not differ significantly from those in non-smoking control subjects.
Horváth 1998 [9]	Asthma	Prospective	Non-steroid treated asthmatic (n = 37) vs. regular inhaled steroids treated asthmatic (n = 25) vs. healthy subjects (n = 37)	CO_{ex}	CO_{ex} was significantly increased in 37 non-steroid treated asthmatic patients compared with 37 healthy subjects, but was similar to normal in 25 patients who received corticosteroids.
Horváth 1998 [51]	Bronchiectasis	Prospective	Non-smoking pts with bronchiectasis (n = 42) vs. non-smoking healthy control (n = 37)	CO_{ex}	CO_{ex} was raised in patients with bronchiectasis, both treated and not treated, compared with normal subjects
Zayasu 1997 [47]	Asthma	Prospective	Treated asthmatic (n = 30) vs. untreated asthmatic (n = 30) vs. non-smoking control (n = 30) vs. smokers control (n = 20)	CO_{ex}	CO_{ex} was higher in asthmatic patients not receiving inhaled corticosteroids and similar in asthmatic patients receiving inhaled corticosteroids compared with those in non-smoking healthy control subjects. There was a decrease in CO_{ex} concentrations after corticosteroid therapy

CO_{ex}: exhaled carbon monoxide; HbCO: carboxyhemoglobin concentration; a-vHbCO: arterio-venous carboxyhemoglobin concentration difference; CF: cystic fibrosis; aHbCO: arterial carboxyhemoglobin concentration; vHbCO: venous carboxyhemoglobin concentration; FeCO: fractional concentration of CO in expired gas; FeNO: fractional exhaled nitric oxide; PEFR: peak expiratory flow rate; URTIs: upper respiratory tract infections; IPF: idiopathic pulmonary fibrosis; COPD: chronic obstructive pulmonary disease

Table 3. Carbon monoxide and other diseases

First author/Year	Disease	Design	Sample	CO measurement	Results
Hampson 2007 [70]	Hemolytic anemia	Case-report	61-yr-old non-smoking diabetic man	Serum HbCO	Case report of a patient with hemolytic anemia and elevation of serum HbCO
Sylvester 2005 [71]	Sickle-cell disease	Prospective	Children with sickle-cell anaemia (n = 87) vs. controls (n = 26)	$ETCO_{ex}$	Positive correlations were found between the ETCO and HbCO and bilirubin concentrations, and a significant negative correlation between the ETCO and hemoglobin concentrations. The mean and SD ETCO concentrations of the sickle-cell disease children were significantly higher than those of the controls
Ziemann-Gimmel 2004 [72]	Retroperitoneal hematoma	Case-report	41-yr-old man with large bilateral spontaneous adrenal hemorrhage and retroperitoneal hematoma	vHbCO	The vHbCO concentration was persistently elevated in a patient with retroperitoneal hematoma needing massive blood transfusion
Sears 2001 [73]	Sickle-cell disease	Cross-sectional	Patients with sickle-cell disease (n = 32)	Serum HbCO	Significant correlation between serum HbCO and hematocrit, reticulocyte count, unconjugated bilirubin concentration, and percentage of irreversibly sickled cells. There was no significant correlation between HBCO and measures of the vaso-occlusive severity of the disease
Paredi 1999 [74]	Diabetes	Cross-sectional	Patients with type 1 diabetes (n = 8) vs. type 2 (n = 16) vs. healthy control (n = 37)	CO_{ex}	CO_{ex} was higher in patients with diabetes compared to the controls. There was a positive correlation between CO_{ex} and the incidence of glycemia
Thunedborg 1995 [75]	Chronic hemodialysis	Prospective	Patients on chronic hemodialysis (n = 69)	Serum HbCO	In non-smokers treated with erythropoietin (EPO), there was a correlation between HbCO and the weekly EPO dose. In smoking patients not given EPO, HbCO correlated well with the number of cigarettes smoked.
Coburn 1966 [76]	Hemolytic anemia	Prospective	Patients with hemolytic anemia (n = 7)	vHbCO	The rate of CO production was elevated in patients with hemolytic anemia

CO_{ex}: exhaled carbon monoxide; ETCO: end-tidal carbon monoxide; HbCO: carboxyhemoglobin concentration; vHbCO: venous carboxyhemoglobin concentration.

cystic fibrosis and bronchopulmonary dysplasia. Carbon monoxide concentrations increase in acute exacerbations of pulmonary diseases and may be helpful in monitoring the effect of therapy in these patients.

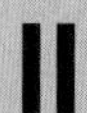

Carbon Monoxide Concentrations and Other Diseases

Hematological diseases characterized by hemolysis may also influence carbon monoxide concentrations. CO_{ex} concentrations have been shown to distinguish between children with hemolytic disorders, including beta-thalassemia and hereditary spherocytosis, and healthy controls (**Table 3**).

Conclusion

Increased carbon monoxide concentrations are a consistent finding in various diseases, including bronchial asthma, COPD, bronchiectasis, silicosis, idiopathic pulmonary fibrosis, acute pneumonia, cystic fibrosis and bronchopulmonary dysplasia. Carbon monoxide concentrations increase in acute exacerbations of pulmonary diseases and may be helpful in monitoring the effect of therapy in these patients. CO_{ex} and carboxyhemoglobin concentrations are also increased in various subgroups of critically ill patients, including medical, surgical and post-trauma ICU patients. CO_{ex} and carboxyhemoglobin concentrations are associated with the degree of inflammation and the extent of organ dysfunction especially in association with sepsis syndromes. In addition, carbon monoxide concentrations correlate well with outcome in critically ill patients. Measurement of CO_{ex} has some limitations including interference by tobacco smoking, variations in ventilation, the presence of severe airflow obstruction, and viral upper respiratory tract infection. Alternatively, carbon monoxide concentrations can be measured by assessing arterial carboxyhemoglobin concentrations. However, sensitive, well calibrated devices are required for accurate measurements.

References

1. Maines MD (1997) The heme oxygenase system: a regulator of second messenger gases. Annu Rev Pharmacol Toxicol 37: 517–554
2. Kim HP, Ryter SW, Choi AM (2006) CO as a cellular signaling molecule. Annu Rev Pharmacol Toxicol 46: 411–449
3. Ryter SW, Morse D, Choi AM (2004) Carbon monoxide: to boldly go where NO has gone before. Sci STKE 2004: RE6
4. Otterbein LE, Bach FH, Alam J, et al (2000) Carbon monoxide has anti-inflammatory effects involving the mitogen-activated protein kinase pathway. Nat Med 6: 422–428
5. Zuckerbraun BS, Chin BY, Wegiel B, et al (2006) Carbon monoxide reverses established pulmonary hypertension. J Exp Med 203: 2109–2119
6. Otterbein LE, Mantell LL, Choi AM (1999) Carbon monoxide provides protection against hyperoxic lung injury. Am J Physiol 276: L688-L694
7. Ryter SW, Alam J, Choi AM (2006) Heme oxygenase-1/carbon monoxide: from basic science to therapeutic applications. Physiol Rev 86: 583–650
8. Vreman HJ, Baxter LM, Stone RT, Stevenson DK (1996) Evaluation of a fully automated end-tidal carbon monoxide instrument for breath analysis. Clin Chem 42: 50–56
9. Horvath I, Donnelly LE, Kiss A, Paredi P, Kharitonov SA, Barnes PJ (1998) Raised levels of exhaled carbon monoxide are associated with an increased expression of heme oxygenase-1 in airway macrophages in asthma: a new marker of oxidative stress. Thorax 53: 668–672

10. Ramirez M, Garcia-Rio F, Vinas A, Prados C, Pino JM, Villamor J (2004) Relationship between exhaled carbon monoxide and airway hyperresponsiveness in asthmatic patients. J Asthma 41: 109–116
11. Zegdi R, Caid R, Van De Louw A, et al (2000) Exhaled carbon monoxide in mechanically ventilated critically ill patients: influence of inspired oxygen fraction. Intensive Care Med 26: 1228–1231
12. Togores B, Bosch M, Agusti AG (2000) The measurement of exhaled carbon monoxide is influenced by airflow obstruction. Eur Respir J 15: 177–180
13. Yamaya M, Sekizawa K, Ishizuka S, Monma M, Mizuta K, Sasaki H (1998) Increased carbon monoxide in exhaled air of subjects with upper respiratory tract infections. Am J Respir Crit Care Med 158: 311–314
14. Yasuda H, Yamaya M, Yanai M, Ohrui T, Sasaki H (2002) Increased blood carboxyhaemoglobin concentrations in inflammatory pulmonary diseases. Thorax 57: 779–783
15. Westphal M, Eletr D, Bone HG, et al (2002) Arteriovenous carboxyhemoglobin difference in critical illness: fiction or fact? Biochem Biophys Res Commun 299: 479–482
16. Singer P, Hansen H (1988) Suppression of fetal hemoglobin and bilirubin on oximetry measurement. Blood Gas News 8: 12–17
17. Maines MD, Gibbs PE (2005) 30 some years of heme oxygenase: from a "molecular wrecking ball" to a "mesmerizing" trigger of cellular events. Biochem Biophys Res Commun 338: 568–577
18. Vincent JL, Sakr Y, Sprung CL, et al (2006) Sepsis in European intensive care units: results of the SOAP study. Crit Care Med 34: 344–353
19. Salvemini D, Cuzzocrea S (2002) Oxidative stress in septic shock and disseminated intravascular coagulation. Free Radic Biol Med 33: 1173–1185
20. Fujii H, Takahashi T, Nakahira K, et al (2003) Protective role of heme oxygenase-1 in the intestinal tissue injury in an experimental model of sepsis. Crit Care Med 31: 893–902
21. Morimatsu H, Takahashi T, Maeshima K, et al (2006) Increased heme catabolism in critically ill patients: correlation among exhaled carbon monoxide, arterial carboxyhemoglobin, and serum bilirubin IXalpha concentrations. Am J Physiol Lung Cell Mol Physiol 290: L114-L119
22. Wiesel P, Patel AP, DiFonzo N, et al (2000) Endotoxin-induced mortality is related to increased oxidative stress and end-organ dysfunction, not refractory hypotension, in heme oxygenase-1-deficient mice. Circulation 102: 3015–3022
23. Ryter SW, Otterbein LE (2004) Carbon monoxide in biology and medicine. Bioessays 26: 270–280
24. Wu L, Cao K, Lu Y, Wang R (2002) Different mechanisms underlying the stimulation of K(Ca) channels by nitric oxide and carbon monoxide. J Clin Invest 110: 691–700
25. Dubuis E, Potier M, Wang R, Vandier C (2005) Continuous inhalation of carbon monoxide attenuates hypoxic pulmonary hypertension development presumably through activation of BKCa channels. Cardiovasc Res 65: 751–761
26. Scharte M, von Ostrowski TA, Daudel F, Freise H, Van Aken H, Bone HG (2006) Endogenous carbon monoxide production correlates weakly with severity of acute illness. Eur J Anaesthesiol 23: 117–122
27. Scharte M, Bone HG, Van Aken H, Meyer J (2000) Increased carbon monoxide in exhaled air of critically ill patients. Biochem Biophys Res Commun 267: 423–426
28. Zegdi R, Perrin D, Burdin M, Boiteau R, Tenaillon A (2002) Increased endogenous carbon monoxide production in severe sepsis. Intensive Care Med 28: 793–796
29. Meyer J, Prien T, Van Aken H, et al (1998) Arterio-venous carboxyhemoglobin difference suggests carbon monoxide production by human lungs. Biochem Biophys Res Commun 244: 230–232
30. Moncure M, Brathwaite CE, Samaha E, Marburger R, Ross SE (1999) Carboxyhemoglobin elevation in trauma victims. J Trauma 46: 424–427
31. Shi Y, Pan F, Li H, et al (2000) Plasma carbon monoxide levels in term newborn infants with sepsis. Biol Neonate 78: 230–232
32. Shi Y, Pan F, Li H, et al (2003) Carbon monoxide concentrations in paediatric sepsis syndrome. Arch Dis Child 88: 889–890
33. Melley DD, Finney SJ, Elia A, Lagan AL, Quinlan GJ, Evans TW (2007) Arterial carboxyhemoglobin level and outcome in critically ill patients. Crit Care Med 35: 1882–1887

34. Hunter K, Mascia M, Eudaric P, Simpkins C (1994) Evidence that carbon monoxide is a mediator of critical illness. Cell Mol Biol (Noisy-le-grand) 40: 507–510
35. Sedlacek M, Halpern NA, Uribarri J (1999) Carboxyhemoglobin and lactate levels do not correlate in critically ill patients. Am J Ther 6: 241–244
36. Eletr D, Reich A, Stubbe HD, et al (2004) Arteriovenous carboxyhemoglobin difference is not correlated to TNF-alpha, IL-6, PCT, CRP and leukocytes in critically ill patients. Clin Chim Acta 349: 75–80
37. Camhi SL, Alam J, Otterbein L, Sylvester SL, Choi AM (1995) Induction of heme oxygenase-1 gene expression by lipopolysaccharide is mediated by AP-1 activation. Am J Respir Cell Mol Biol 13: 387–398
38. Kim YM, Bergonia HA, Muller C, Pitt BR, Watkins WD, Lancaster JR, Jr. (1995) Loss and degradation of enzyme-bound heme induced by cellular nitric oxide synthesis. J Biol Chem 270: 5710–5713
39. Lavrovsky Y, Drummond GS, Abraham NG (1996) Downregulation of the human heme oxygenase gene by glucocorticoids and identification of 56b regulatory elements. Biochem Biophys Res Commun 218: 759–765
40. Stockley RA (1995) Role of inflammation in respiratory tract infections. Am J Med 99: 8S-13S
41. Chabot F, Mitchell JA, Gutteridge JM, Evans TW (1998) Reactive oxygen species in acute lung injury. Eur Respir J 11: 745–757
42. Kovacs EJ, DiPietro LA (1994) Fibrogenic cytokines and connective tissue production. FASEB J 8: 854–861
43. Goldstein RH, Fine A (1995) Potential therapeutic initiatives for fibrogenic lung diseases. Chest 108: 848–855
44. Paredi P, Kharitonov SA, Loukides S, Pantelidis P, du Bois RM, Barnes PJ (1999) Exhaled nitric oxide is increased in active fibrosing alveolitis. Chest 115: 1352–1356
45. Yamada N, Yamaya M, Okinaga S, et al (2000) Microsatellite polymorphism in the heme oxygenase-1 gene promoter is associated with susceptibility to emphysema. Am J Hum Genet 66: 187–195
46. Nathan C, Xie QW (1994) Regulation of biosynthesis of nitric oxide. J Biol Chem 269: 13725–13728
47. Zayasu K, Sekizawa K, Okinaga S, Yamaya M, Ohrui T, Sasaki H (1997) Increased carbon monoxide in exhaled air of asthmatic patients. Am J Respir Crit Care Med 156: 1140–1143
48. Zanconato S, Scollo M, Zaramella C, Landi L, Zacchello F, Baraldi E (2002) Exhaled carbon monoxide levels after a course of oral prednisone in children with asthma exacerbation. J Allergy Clin Immunol 109: 440–445
49. Yamaya M, Sekizawa K, Ishizuka S, Monma M, Sasaki H (1999) Exhaled carbon monoxide levels during treatment of acute asthma. Eur Respir J 13: 757–760
50. Yasuda H, Yamaya M, Nakayama K, et al (2005) Increased arterial carboxyhemoglobin concentrations in chronic obstructive pulmonary disease. Am J Respir Crit Care Med 171: 1246–1251
51. Horvath I, Loukides S, Wodehouse T, Kharitonov SA, Cole PJ, Barnes PJ (1998) Increased levels of exhaled carbon monoxide in bronchiectasis: a new marker of oxidative stress. Thorax 53: 867–870
52. Yasuda H, Ebihara S, Yamaya M, Mashito Y, Nakamura M, Sasaki H (2004) Increased arterial carboxyhemoglobin concentrations in elderly patients with silicosis. J Am Geriatr Soc 52: 1403–1404
53. Paredi P, Shah PL, Montuschi P, et al (1999) Increased carbon monoxide in exhaled air of patients with cystic fibrosis. Thorax 54: 917–920
54. May C, Patel S, Peacock J, Milner A, Rafferty GF, Greenough A (2007) End-tidal carbon monoxide levels in prematurely born infants developing bronchopulmonary dysplasia. Pediatr Res 61: 474–478
55. Yamaya M, Hosoda M, Ishizuka S, et al (2001) Relation between exhaled carbon monoxide levels and clinical severity of asthma. Clin Exp Allergy 31: 417–422
56. Kong PM, Chan CC, Lee P, Wang YT (2002) An assessment of the role of exhaled carbon monoxide in acute asthmatic exacerbations in hospitalised patients. Singapore Med J 43: 399–402
57. Biernacki WA, Kharitonov SA, Barnes PJ (2001) Exhaled carbon monoxide in patients with lower respiratory tract infection. Respir Med 95: 1003–1005

58. Bartlett JG, Mundy LM (1995) Community-acquired pneumonia. N Engl J Med 333: 1618–1624
59. Antuni JD, Kharitonov SA, Hughes D, Hodson ME, Barnes PJ (2000) Increase in exhaled carbon monoxide during exacerbations of cystic fibrosis. Thorax 55: 138–142
60. Mayr FB, Spiel A, Leitner J, et al (2005) Effects of carbon monoxide inhalation during experimental endotoxemia in humans. Am J Respir Crit Care Med 171: 354–360
61. Sakamoto A, Nakanishi K, Takeda S, Ogawa R (2005) Does carboxy-hemoglobin serve as a stress-induced inflammatory marker reflecting surgical insults? J Nippon Med Sch 72: 19–28
62. Leikin JB, Vogel S (1986) Carbon monoxide levels in cardiac patients in an urban emergency department. Am J Emerg Med 4: 126–128
63. Ohara Y, Ohrui T, Morikawa T, et al (2006) Exhaled carbon monoxide levels in school-age children with episodic asthma. Pediatr Pulmonol 41: 470–474
64. Pearson P, Lewis S, Britton J, Fogarty A (2005) Exhaled carbon monoxide levels in atopic asthma: a longitudinal study. Respir Med 99: 1292–1296
65. Beck-Ripp J, Latzin P, Griese M (2004) Exhaled carbon monoxide is not flow dependent in children with cystic fibrosis and asthma. Eur J Med Res 9: 518–522
66. Yasuda H, Sasaki T, Yamaya M, et al (2004) Increased arteriovenous carboxyhemoglobin differences in patients with inflammatory pulmonary diseases. Chest 125: 2160–2168
67. Zetterquist W, Marteus H, Johannesson M, et al (2002) Exhaled carbon monoxide is not elevated in patients with asthma or cystic fibrosis. Eur Respir J 20: 92–99
68. Khatri SB, Ozkan M, McCarthy K, et al (2001) Alterations in exhaled gas profile during allergen-induced asthmatic response. Am J Respir Crit Care Med 164: 1844–1848
69. Uasuf CG, Jatakanon A, James A, Kharitonov SA, Wilson NM, Barnes PJ (1999) Exhaled carbon monoxide in childhood asthma. J Pediatr 135: 569–574
70. Hampson NB (2007) Carboxyhemoglobin elevation due to hemolytic anemia. J Emerg Med 33: 17–19
71. Sylvester KP, Patey RA, Rafferty GF, Rees D, Thein SL, Greenough A (2005) Exhaled carbon monoxide levels in children with sickle cell disease. Eur J Pediatr 164: 162–165
72. Ziemann-Gimmel P, Schwartz DE (2004) Increased carboxyhemoglobin in a patient with a large retroperitoneal hematoma. Anesth Analg 99: 1800–2, table
73. Sears DA, Udden MM, Thomas LJ (2001) Carboxyhemoglobin levels in patients with sickle-cell anemia: relationship to hemolytic and vasoocclusive severity. Am J Med Sci 322: 345–348
74. Paredi P, Biernacki W, Invernizzi G, Kharitonov SA, Barnes PJ (1999) Exhaled carbon monoxide levels elevated in diabetes and correlated with glucose concentration in blood: a new test for monitoring the disease? Chest 116: 1007–1011
75. Thunedborg P, Nielsen AL, Brinkenfeldt H, Brahm J, Jensen HA (1995) Carbon monoxide in chronic uraemia related to erythropoietin treatment and smoking habits. Scand J Urol Nephrol 29: 21–25
76. Coburn RF, Williams WJ, Kahn SB (1966) Endogenous carbon monoxide production in patients with hemolytic anemia. J Clin Invest 45: 460–468

Monitoring Immune Dysfunction in Septic Patients: Toward Tailored Immunotherapy

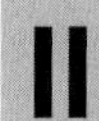

F. Venet, A. Lepape, and G. Monneret

Introduction

Septic syndromes represent a major although largely under-recognized healthcare problem worldwide accounting for thousands of deaths every year [1–3]. Mortality remains high ranging from 20 % for sepsis to over 50 % for septic shock despite almost 20 years of anti-inflammatory clinical trials [1–3]. The inability of these therapies to mitigate the devastating effects of this condition indicates that the initial hypotheses for sepsis pathophysiology may have been misconstrued or inadequately addressed. Two major explanations have been proposed: 1) Septic patients have mainly been treated as a group despite the extreme heterogeneity characterizing this population [1]; 2) The postulate that death after sepsis is solely due to an overwhelming pro-inflammatory immune response may actually be inaccurate [1, 3]. Indeed, several lines of evidence have now established that death from septic shock is probably due to the effect of distinct mechanisms over time [1–3]. Early in the course of the disease, a massive release of inflammatory mediators (normally designed to trigger an immune response against pathogens) is occurring that may be responsible for organ dysfunction and hypoperfusion [1, 3]. Concomitantly, the body develops compensatory mechanisms to prevent overwhelming inflammation and dampen an overzealous anti-infectious response [1–3]. These negative feedback mechanisms, although having protective effects during the first initial hours, may paradoxically become deleterious as they persist over time leading to immune paralysis (**Fig. 1**) [1, 3]. Indeed, considerable clinical and experimental evidence indicates that patients rapidly present with numerous compromised immune functions [1, 3]. As our capacity to treat patients during the very first hours of shock has improved (early and aggressive initial supportive therapy) [1], many patients now survive this critical step but eventually die later in a state of immunosuppression that is illustrated by difficulty fighting the primary bacterial infection and decreased resistance to secondary nosocomial infections [1, 3]. Consequently, immunostimulatory therapies are now considered as an innovative strategy for the treatment of sepsis [1, 3]. However, the first critical step is to be able to identify patients who would actually benefit from these therapies [2, 3]. Indeed, in the absence of specific clinical signs of immune status, it is critical to determine the best biological tools to stratify patients according to their immune status (a missing step in most previous clinical trials) [1–3]. This would define the right action (i.e., stimulating innate immunity and/or adaptive immunity, blocking apoptosis, restoring other altered functions) at the right time (early or delayed treatment) in the right patient (individualized/tailored therapy).

Although the mechanistic and molecular bases for sepsis-induced immunosuppression are not exhaustively established, several features of the condition have been

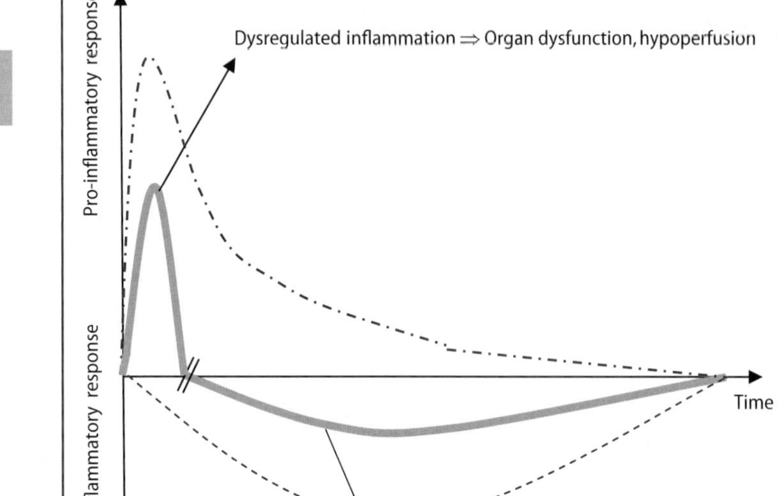

Fig. 1. Simplified description of systemic pro- and anti-inflammatory immune responses over time after septic shock. Dashed lines: pro- or anti-inflammatory responses; bold line: result at the systemic level. The shift from a pro-inflammatory to an anti-inflammatory immune response predominant at the systemic level likely occurs within 24 hours after the diagnosis of shock.

already described including enhanced leukocyte apoptosis, lymphocyte anergy, and deactivated monocyte functions [1, 3]. This review will focus on the immune dysfunctions described so far in septic patients regarding monocytes and T lymphocytes (as examples of innate and adaptive immune cells) and their potential use as biomarkers on a routine standardized basis for prediction of adverse outcome or occurrence of secondary nosocomial infections and for guidance of putative immunotherapy.

Monocyte Dysfunction

Monocytes from septic patients are mainly characterized by a decreased capacity to mount a pro-inflammatory reaction upon secondary bacterial challenge and by impairment in antigen presentation likely due to the lowered expression of major histocompatibility class II molecules (MHC class II).

Functional Testing

Since it directly measures *ex vivo* the capacity of a cell population to respond to an immune challenge, functional testing represents the gold standard method to establish immune alterations. Several groups have investigated the capacity of septic patients' monocytes to release pro-inflammatory cytokines in response to lipopolysaccharide (LPS), other Toll-like receptor (TLR) agonists, or whole bacteria *in vitro* (see recent review in [4]). These tests represent reliable methods to assess the phenomenon of endotoxin tolerance defined as a reduced responsiveness to a secondary LPS challenge following a first inflammatory response [4]. Monocytes from patients usually present with a diminished capacity to release tumor necrosis factor (TNF)-α, interleukin (IL)-1α, IL-6, IL-12, whereas the release of anti-inflammatory mediators (IL-1 receptor antagonist [IL-1ra], IL-10) is not affected or is even slightly increased [4]. This observation shows that LPS can still activate monocytes but that the intracellular signaling pathways have been turned to favor production of anti-inflammatory molecules, therefore supporting the concept of leukocyte reprogramming [4]. However, although this test is considered as a good method to assess monocyte hyporesponsiveness after sepsis, it is not suitable for routine analysis/diagnosis.

Cell Surface Marker Expression

In terms of molecules expressed on monocytes, which are readily measured by standardized flow cytometry protocols, numerous studies have been performed regarding the measurement of HLA-DR (human leukocyte antigen-DR). In septic patients, decreased cell-surface expression of HLA-DR has regularly been observed on circulating monocytes [3]. As opposed to assessment of circulating mediators, the major advantage of measuring a cell surface marker such as mHLA-DR is that its level of expression is the result of the sum of the effects of multiple mediators that may all be regulated during septic shock. For example, mHLA-DR expression has been shown to be positively and negatively regulated by cytokines such as interferon (IFN)-γ and IL-10 as well as by corticoids and catecholamines [3]. There is now a general consensus that a diminished mHLA-DR expression is a reliable marker for the development of immunosuppression in critically ill patients [3]. Indeed, the decrease in mHLA-DR expression has been assessed as a predictor for septic complications after trauma, surgery or pancreatitis. In these studies, low levels of mHLA-DR (< 40 % of positive monocytes, normal > 90 %) were observed in patients who subsequently developed nosocomial infections [3]. In contrast, in injured patients with uneventful recovery, mHLA-DR rapidly returned to normal values (in general in less than 1 week). Similar results in burn patients and after septic shock also indicate that a low mHLA-DR expression is associated with secondary septic/nosocomial events [3, 5]. Finally, decreased mHLA-DR has been shown to be predictive of adverse outcome in different groups of critically ill patients. This has recently been observed in burn patients [5] and after severe sepsis and septic shock [3].

Mechanisms Responsible for Monocyte Dysfunction

Among all the cytokines released by monocytes and increased after sepsis, IL-10 is the sole cytokine to consistently correlate with mHLA-DR values [6]. IL-10 production is increased after sepsis and has been shown to predict mortality [1, 3]. Given its properties in suppressing the synthesis of numerous pro-inflammatory cytokines [7], this continued release may contribute to the immune dysfunctions observed after septic shock and thus may augment susceptibility to secondary microbial invasion [7]. Gogos et al. showed that IL-10 and IL-10/TNF-α ratios, among a panel of various cytokines (IL-1, IL-6, soluble TNF receptor [sTNF-R] I and II), were the most powerful predictors of mortality in patients with severe sepsis both at admission and 48 hours later [8]. We extended these results in a group of 38 patients by illustrating that IL-10 levels remained higher in non-survivors until 15 days after the onset of septic shock [6]. In particular, high IL-10 concentrations at the beginning of shock were negatively correlated with the nadir of mHLA-DR measurements during the 2 weeks of monitoring [6]. Consequently, this initial value of IL-10 may reflect the severity of the forthcoming immunoparalysis.

Increased monocyte apoptosis has also been described after sepsis [9, 10]. Adrie et al. observed that septic patients exhibited an increased percentage of monocytes with depolarized mitochondria (as a marker of apoptosis) when compared with healthy individuals [11]. Furthermore, among septic patients, this percentage was significantly higher in non-survivors than in survivors. However, one limitation in assessing the incidence of monocyte/macrophage apoptosis is that some of these changes may represent an increased role in clearance of apoptotic cells, which may make these cells look overtly more apoptotic as a result of handling a greater amount of apoptotic material [10]. With that said, the down modulation of CD14 expression on monocytes after septic shock (a cell surface marker decreased during monocyte apoptosis) tends to confirm this increased apoptotic process especially because its downregulation was more pronounced in patients who were not going to survive [12].

Restoration of Monocyte Functions

Based on the above, several innovative immunotherapies may be proposed (**Table 1**).

AS101, with the capacity to inhibit IL-10, has been demonstrated to increase survival in septic mice [13]. Although it can be argued that blocking a single mediator in a context where many inhibitory pathways are involved/activated, may remain inefficient [2], this molecule has been shown to act through different mechanisms (inhibition of IL-10, activation of macrophage functions, inhibitor of IL-1beta converting enzyme) and, therefore, remains a valuable potential therapeutic strategy [3].

Table 1. Monocyte dysfunction in the septic patient: Potential biomarkers and therapies

	Biomarker	Technique	Targeted therapy
Functional testing	↓ *ex vivo* cytokine production after TLR agonist stimuli	ELISA or CBA	GM-CSF G-CSF IFN-γ
Cytokines	↑ plasma IL-10	ELISA or CBA	AS101
Cell surface marker expression	↓ mHLA-DR ↓ CD14, CD86, GM-CSF, CX3CR1 ...	FCM	GM-CSF G-CSF IFN-γ
Apoptosis	Depolarized mitochondria ↓ CD14	FCM	GM-CSF G-CSF IFN-γ

TLR: Toll-like receptor; ELISA: enzyme-linked immunosorbent assay; CBA: cytometric bead array; HLA-DR: human leukocyte antigen-DR; FCM: flow cytometry; IFN: interferon; G-CSF: granulocyte colony-stimulating factor; GM-CSF: granulocyte macrophage colony-stimulating factor; IL: interleukin

Several molecules have already been used (IFN-γ, granulocyte-colony stimulating factor [G-CSF], granulocyte/macrophage-colony stimulating factor [GM-CSF]) to stimulate monocyte functions with interesting preliminary results *ex vivo* (increased mHLA-DR expression, restoration of cytokine production) [1, 3]. Several prospective randomized multicenter clinical trials using IFN-γ have been conducted in trauma patients [1, 3]. However, despite interesting results regarding secondary endpoints in some subgroups of patients (decreased severity of nosocomial infections, decreased mortality in infected patients), the results were inconclusive in terms of overall mortality or infection rates [1, 14–15]. Presneill et al. [16] published preliminary data regarding the use of GM-CSF in 10 patients with sepsis-induced respiratory failure. These authors observed a modest improvement in gas exchange, resolution of acute respiratory distress syndrome (ARDS) and alveolar leukocyte phagocytic functions, but no enhanced survival rate. In a prospective, randomized, placebo-controlled trial, Rosenbloom and colleagues investigated whether GM-CSF treatment could improve leukocyte function and mortality in 40 septic patients [17]. These investigators observed a higher leukocyte count, increased mHLA-DR, and better resolution of infections in the treated group but again no difference in mortality. Nevertheless, it should be noted that these trials were designed without patient stratification and drug efficacy should be assessed only in patients with prior established impairment in monocyte function.

T Lymphocyte Dysfunction

Due to their ability to interact not only with cells of the innate immune system but also with other cells of the adaptive response, T lymphocytes play a central role in the anti-infectious immune response both as effectors and regulators of this response [1]. This role is illustrated by the description of increased mortality, decreased bacterial clearance, and an altered pro-inflammatory immune response after polymicrobial septic challenge in mice lacking both T and B cells [1, 18]. A growing body of evidence has now confirmed that the lymphocyte-mediated immune response may be dysfunctional after severe sepsis and may play a major role in the development of a state of immunosuppression in such patients [1, 18].

Functional Testing

Lymphocyte anergy is illustrated by the observation of the loss of the delayed-type hypersensitivity reaction to recall skin tests antigens in patients [1, 18]. This loss of hypersensitivity has been well described and is known to be associated with mortality and with the development of secondary infections [1, 18–19]. Indeed, a marked decrease in lymphocyte proliferation in response to antigens (tuberculin, tetanus toxin) or non-specific (phytohemagglutinin, concanavalin A, anti-CD3, anti-CD28 antibodies) stimulation has been described in patients after severe injuries (sepsis, major surgery, severe burn or trauma) [1, 19]. Most importantly, it has been observed that the severity of this state of anergy correlates with poor outcome [1, 18], increased occurrence of infectious complications, and subsequent multiorgan failure in patients [18, 19]. The measurement of cell proliferation *in vitro*, usually performed with peripheral blood mononuclear cells (i.e., lymphocytes and monocytes), investigates the capacity of lymphocytes to proliferate and of monocytes to present antigens (when performed with recall antigens) in a single test. Proliferation is usually assessed by ^{3}H-thymidine uptake or more recently by the use of fluorescent probes (like CFSE). However, as proliferation tests require long incubation times (2–3 days for mitogens, 5–7 days for recall antigens), they are not suitable for clinical decision-making and are not performed on a routine basis.

Cell Surface Marker Expression

T lymphocytes have been characterized by the overexpression of inhibitory co-receptors during immunoparalysis. It has recently been demonstrated in trauma patients that anergic T cells presented with increased programmed death-1 (PD-1), CD47 and cytotoxic T-lymphocyte-associated antigen-4 (CTLA4) expression that would facilitate preferential triggering of negative signaling pathways during T-cell stimulation [20] and, therefore, lead to lymphocyte anergy. Moreover, this increase in co-repressor receptors (in particular CTLA4) appears to be associated with a decrease in the expression of co-activator receptors such as CD28 or CD3, which could also play a role in the development of immunoparalysis [18, 21]. However, in contrast with mHLA-DR, only fragmental data are available regarding the correlation between these markers of lymphocyte suppression and mortality/morbidity and the development of nosocomial infections in patients.

Finally, one likely major characteristic of T lymphocyte dysfunction after severe injury is the increase among patients' circulating lymphocytes of a cell-population with known regulatory properties [18]. CD4$^+$CD25$^+$ regulatory T lymphocytes (Treg) have recently been reported as a potent regulatory T cell lineage playing an essential role in the control of both adaptive and innate immune responses [18]. An increase in the percentage of Treg has been described in septic shock patients [22]. Importantly, this increase was observed immediately after the diagnosis of sepsis; however, it persisted only in non-surviving patients in association with an augmented CTLA4 expression. A similar increase in Treg percentage has been observed in trauma patients and in mice after polymicrobial septic challenge and stroke [18]. We recently observed a strong correlation between the increased Treg/effector ratio measured in whole blood after septic shock and the decreased proliferative response of patients' lymphocytes after mitogenic stimulation. This suggests not only that the measurement of the Treg percentage may represent a reliable marker for the diagnosis of lymphocyte dysfunction in patients but also that these cells may play a central role in the development of immunoparalysis after sepsis.

Mechanism Responsible for Lymphocyte Dysfunction

It is generally agreed that apoptotic cell death represents the major mechanism triggering sepsis-induced lymphocyte anergy/dysfunction [1–2, 10]. After sepsis and severe trauma, this has been shown to be associated with a marked decrease in the number of circulating lymphocytes that is correlated with the development of nosocomial infections in these patients [1, 10, 18].

Pioneering autopsy studies by Hotchkiss et al. disclosed a profound, progressive, apoptosis-induced loss of cells of the adaptive immune system in the spleen, blood and gut-associated lymphoid tissue of adults who had died of sepsis [23–25]. Although no loss of CD8$^+$ T cells or natural killer cells occurred, sepsis markedly decreased the levels of B and CD4$^+$ T cells [25]. This loss was especially important because it occurred during life-threatening infectious process, while clonal expansion of these cells might have been expected [25]. Accordingly, Le Tulzo et al.

observed a marked increase in apoptosis of circulating lymphocytes from septic shock patients compared with critically ill patients without sepsis and healthy volunteers [26]. This induced a profound and persistent lymphopenia associated with poor outcome [26]. Bilbault et al. observed a severe downregulation in the expression of the anti-apoptotic gene, Bcl-2, in circulating mononuclear cells from patients with severe sepsis [27]. This was associated with a reduced T-cell count and an increase in annexin-V labeling. Most importantly, immediately after the onset of severe sepsis this decrease was higher in non-survivors than in survivors. A second study by this group confirmed these results by measuring Bax/Bcl-xl and Bax/Bcl-2 ratios in septic shock patients [28]. However, one major limitation to the use of apoptosis measurements as markers for immunoparalysis may be the drawbacks inherent to this type of experiment, such as the need for rapid processing of the samples (especially regarding annexin-V staining) which is hardly compatible with their use in ICUs [29]. Furthermore, as methods used for studying apoptosis may often have a significant rate of false positive results (especially the deoxyuridine triphosphate nick-end labeling assay), it is recommended that apoptosis be established on the basis of two or more methods of detection, including DNA-hypoploidy, morphology, DNA laddering, annexin-V staining, active caspase-3 or mitochondrial permeability measurements [2, 10].

Restoration of Lymphocyte Functions

Augmenting T cell function and fighting lymphopenia may, therefore, represent a valuable therapeutic strategy after sepsis (**Table 2**). IL-7 is an essential cytokine for T lymphocyte development, survival, expansion and maturation in humans [30]. Phase I clinical trials in cancer and in patients infected with human immunodeficiency virus (HIV) have shown that T cell expansion can be achieved at doses that are well tolerated [27]. In line with these findings, ligands of co-activator receptors for effector T lymphocytes may also possess beneficial effects. As an illustrative example, recent results by Scumpia et al. have shown that anti-glucocorticoid-induced TNF receptor family related gene (GITR) agonistic antibodies were

Table 2. Lymphocyte dysfunction in the septic patient: Potential biomarkers and therapies

	Biomarker	Technique	Targeted therapy
Functional testing	↓ proliferation after antigenic or non-specific stimulation	^{3}H-thymidine uptake or CFSE probes	IL-7 IVIG
Cell surface marker expression	↑ inhibitory receptors: PD1, CTLA4, CD47... ↓ co-activator receptors: CD28, CD3 ↑ % Treg	FCM	Anti-GITR agonistic abs IVIG
Apoptosis	↓ T cell count ↑ Annexin V staining ↓ Bcl2 expression protein/gene Bax/Bcl-xl or Bax/Bcl2 ratios	FCM RT-PCR/FCM RT-PCR/FCM	IL-7 Caspase-inhibitors Ritonavir

CFSE: carboxyfluorescein succinimidyl ester; IVIG: intravenous immunoglobulin; FCM: flow cytometry; GITR: glucocorticoid-induced tumor necrosis factor receptor; RT-PCR: Real time polymerase chain reaction; IL: interleukin; Treg: CD4$^+$CD25$^+$ regulatory T lymphocytes able to restore lymphocyte proliferation, prevent CD3 down-modulation, decrease bacteremia, and increase survival in a mice model of sepsis [31]. Intravenous use of immunoglobin has also been proposed as an adjuvant treatment for sepsis. However, to date, its benefits remain unclear [1]. The authors of recent meta-analyses recommend conducting larger clinical trials with patient stratification [32].

Finally, strategies designed at blocking apoptosis, including caspase-inhibitors, overexpression of Bcl-2, and inhibition of Fas/FasL signaling, have demonstrated survival improvement in animal models of sepsis [10]. That said, so far no therapeutic strategy has been developed sufficiently to reach clinical use. An alternative may be provided by HIV protease inhibitors, the activity of which is partly mediated through anti-apoptotic effects. Administration of ritonavir improved survival in a murine model of sepsis, even when given after the onset of the disease [33]. As these protease inhibitors are well tolerated in patients, we may expect exciting possibilities in sepsis. A phase I trial is currently underway investigating the effects of these drugs to boost the immune system in healthy volunteers (www.clinicaltrials.gov NCT00346619). Of note, drugs aimed at blocking apoptosis may be used as adjunctive agents in association with molecules targeting monocytes or leukocytes.

Conclusion

Our understanding of the pathogenesis of sepsis has been oversimplified during the past few decades and, as a result, many clinical trials have addressed the pro-inflammatory side when there was no evidence that hyper-inflammation was dominant in patients. Several issues require further definition before we can gain a complete picture of events leading to immunosuppression (e.g., Are the major sepsis-induced

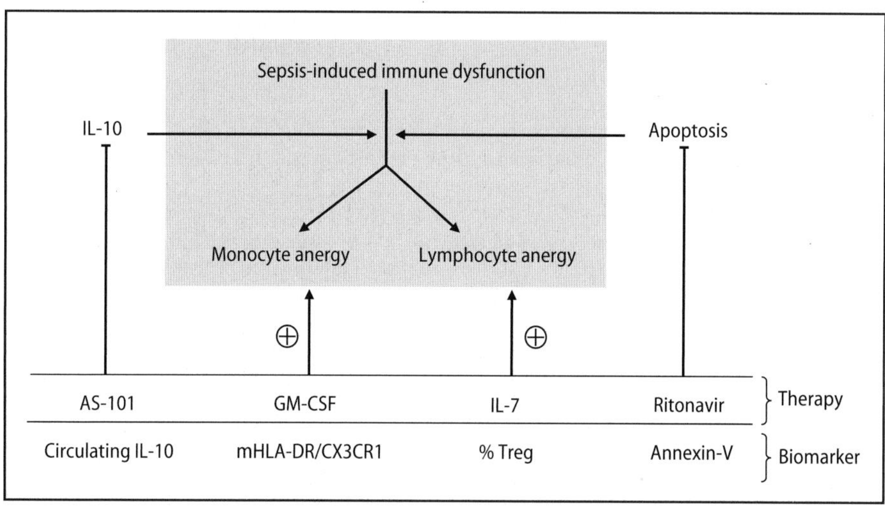

Fig. 2. Monitoring immune dysfunctions in septic patients: Toward tailored immunotherapy. Sepsis-induced immune dysfunction (lymphocyte and monocyte anergy) likely mediated by increased interleukin (IL)-10 and apoptosis might be treated by innovative and specific therapies administered based on measurements of selective biomarkers in patients before initiation of treatment. Treg: $CD4^{+}CD25^{+}$ regulatory T lymphocytes; GM-CSF: granulocyte macrophage colony-stimulating factor

inhibitory mechanisms fully elucidated? How large a part is played by physician-induced immunosuppression, as sedatives, catecholamines, and insulin are all immunsuppressive agents? Is the cellular energetic status crucial in maintaining immune functions? How important is the neuroendocrine-mediated part of immunosuppression? How preponderant is immune failure among other organ failures? Could immune dysfunction be just another organ failure?). Nevertheless, we can reasonably state that patients with sepsis have features consistent with immunosuppression. Consequently, stimulating the patient's immune system may be a promising therapeutic strategy. Although we cannot predict which of these therapies will be efficacious, they surely deserve to be fully and minutely investigated when considering the high mortality that characterizes septic syndromes. However, so as not to repeat the mistakes of the past, an absolute prerequisite for future clinical trials is to systematically assess patients' immune functions prior to inclusion so as to be able to define individualized immunotherapy (**Fig. 2**).

References

1. Hotchkiss RS, Karl IE (2003) The pathophysiology and treatment of sepsis. N Engl J Med 348: 138–150
2. Remick DG (2007) Pathophysiology of sepsis. Am J Pathol 170: 1435–1444
3. Monneret G, Venet F, Pachot A, Lepape A (2008) Monitoring immune dysfunctions in the septic patient: a new skin for the old ceremony. Mol Med 14: 64–78
4. Cavaillon JM, Adib-Conquy M (2007) Determining the degree of immunodysregulation in sepsis. Contrib Nephrol 156: 101–111
5. Venet F, Tissot S, Debard AL, et al (2007) Decreased monocyte human leukocyte antigen-DR expression after severe burn injury: Correlation with severity and secondary septic shock. Crit Care Med 35: 1910–1917
6. Monneret G, Finck ME, Venet F, et al (2004) The anti-inflammatory response dominates after septic shock: Association of low monocyte HLA-DR expression and high interleukin-10 concentration. Immunol Lett. 95: 193–198
7. Oberholzer A, Oberholzer C, Moldawer LL (2002) Interleukin-10: A complex role in the pathogenesis of sepsis syndromes and its potential as an anti-inflammatory drug. Crit Care Med 30: S58–S63
8. Gogos CA, Drosou E, Bassaris HP, Skoutelis A (2000) Pro- versus anti-inflammatory cytokine profile in patients with severe sepsis: A marker for prognosis and future therapeutic options. J Infect Dis 181: 176–180
9. Williams TE, Ayala A, Chaudry IH (1997) Inducible macrophage apoptosis following sepsis is mediated by cysteine protease activation and nitric oxide release. J Surg Res 70: 113–118
10. Wesche DE, Lomas-Neira JL, Perl M, Chung CS, Ayala A (2005) Leukocyte apoptosis and its significance in sepsis and shock. J Leukoc Biol 78: 325–337
11. Adrie C, Bachelet M, Vayssier-Taussat M, et al (2001) Mitochondrial membrane potential and apoptosis peripheral blood monocytes in severe human sepsis. Am J Respir Crit Care Med 164: 389–395
12. Venet F, Pachot A, Debard AL, et al (2006) Human CD4+CD25+ regulatory T lymphocytes inhibit lipopolysaccharide-induced monocyte survival through a Fas/Fas ligand-dependent. mechanism. J Immunol 177: 6540–6547
13. Kalechman Y, Gafter U, Gal R, et al (2002) Anti-IL-10 therapeutic strategy using the immunomodulator AS101 in protecting mice from sepsis-induced death: dependence on timing of immunomodulating intervention. J Immunol 169: 384–392
14. Polk HC Jr, Cheadle WG, Livingston DH, et al (1992) A randomized prospective clinical trial to determine the efficacy of interferon-gamma in severely injured patients. Am J Surg 163: 191–196
15. Dries DJ, Jurkovich GJ, Maier RV, et al (1994) Effect of interferon gamma on infection-related death in patients with severe injuries. A randomized, double-blind, placebo-controlled trial. Arch Surg 129: 1031–1041

16. Presneill JJ, Harris T, Stewart AG, Cade JF, Wilson JW (2002) A randomized phase II trial of granulocyte-macrophage colony-stimulating factor therapy in severe sepsis with respiratory dysfunction. Am J Respir Crit Care Med 166: 138–143
17. Rosenbloom AJ, Linden PK, Dorrance A, Penkosky N, Cohen-Melamed MH, Pinsky MR (2005) Effect of granulocyte-monocyte colony-stimulating factor therapy on leukocyte function and clearance of serious infection in nonneutropenic patients. Chest 127: 2139–2150.
18. Venet F, Chung CS, Monneret G, et al (2008) Regulatory T cell populations in sepsis and trauma. J Leukoc Biol 83: 523–535
19. Lederer JA, Rodrick ML, Mannick JA (1999) The effects of injury on the adaptive immune response. Shock 11: 153–159
20. Bandyopadhyay G, De A, Laudanski K, et al (2007) Negative signaling contributes to T-cell anergy in trauma patients. Crit Care Med 35: 794–801
21. Venet F, Bohe J, Debard AL, Bienvenu J, Lepape A, Monneret G (2005) Both percentage of gammadelta T lymphocytes and CD3 expression are reduced during septic shock. Crit Care Med 33: 2836–2840
22. Monneret G, Debard AL, Venet F, et al (2003) Marked elevation of human circulating CD4+CD25+ regulatory T cells in sepsis-induced immunoparalysis. Crit Care Med 31: 2068–2071
23. Hotchkiss RS, Tinsley KW, Swanson PE, et al (2002) Depletion of dendritic cells, but not macrophages, in patients with sepsis. J Immunol 168: 2493–2500
24. Hotchkiss RS, Swanson PE, Freeman BD, et al (1999) Apoptotic cell death in patients with sepsis, shock and multiple organ dysfunction. Crit Care Med 27: 1230–1251
25. Hotchkiss RS, Tinsley KW, Swanson PE, et al (2001) Sepsis-induced apoptosis causes progressive profound depletion of B and CD4+ T lymphocytes in humans. J Immunol 166: 6952–6963.
26. Le Tulzo Y, Pangault C, Gacouin A, et al (2002) Early circulating lymphocyte apoptosis in human septic shock is associated with poor outcome. Shock 18: 487–494
27. Bilbault P, Lavaux T, Lahlou A, et al (2004) Transient Bcl-2 gene down-expression in circulating mononuclear cells of severe sepsis patients who died despite appropriate intensive care. Intensive Care Med 30: 408–415
28. Bilbault P, Lavaux T, Launoy A, et al (2007) Influence of drotrecogin alpha (activated) infusion on the variation of Bax/Bcl-2 and Bax/Bcl-xl ratios in circulating mononuclear cells: a cohort study in septic shock patients. Crit Care Med 35: 69–75
29. Greineder CF, Nelson PW, Dressel AL, Erba HP, Younger JG (2007) In vitro and in silico analysis of annexin V binding to lymphocytes as a biomarker in emergency department sepsis studies. Acad Emerg Med 14: 763–771
30. Alpdogan O, van den Brink MR (2005) IL-7 and IL-15: therapeutic cytokines for immunodeficiency. Trends Immunol 26: 56–64
31. Scumpia PO, Delano MJ, Kelly-Scumpia KM, et al (2007) Treatment with GITR agonistic antibody corrects adaptive immune dysfunction in sepsis. Blood 110: 3673–3681
32. Turgeon AF, Hutton B, Fergusson DA, et al (2007) Meta-analysis: intravenous immunoglobulin in critically ill adult patients with sepsis. Ann Intern Med 146: 193–203
33. Weaver JG, Rouse MS, Steckelberg JM, Badley AD (2004) Improved survival in experimental sepsis with an orally administered inhibitor of apoptosis. FASEB J 18: 1185–1191

III Current and Future Management of Sepsis

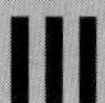

Source Control in the ICU

J.J. De Waele, M.M.L.G Malbrain, and I.E. De Laet

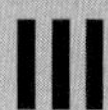

Introduction

Source control is generally considered one of the oldest, most important and most obvious strategies in the management of infections. 'Ubi pus ibi evacua' is a Latin aphorism that dates back to the early days of medicine, but is still widely used to stress the importance of source control. Although source control is generally considered to be the cornerstone of the management of several infections, it is also the least 'hyped' strategy, and therefore gets little overall attention in the literature.

In the Surviving Sepsis Campaign guidelines [1], the focus is mostly on resuscitation, antibiotic treatment, and ancillary strategies such as anti-inflammatory therapies, and source control may, therefore, appear underappreciated. A lot of questions remain unanswered regarding the necessity, timing, and methodology of source control, and how these factors impact the outcome of patients with sepsis. A possible explanation for the relative lack of apparent interest in source control may lie in the perception that the source control of infection is only a problem in surgical infections, and once, this was indeed true. The 'source control' concept originated in the management of complicated intra-abdominal infections, but over time, physicians treating various types of infection realized that this concept and the components it consists of, can be applied to other surgical and non surgical infections.

What is 'Source Control'?

In the context of complicated intra-abdominal infections, source control is often defined as the purely mechanical control of gastrointestinal content leaking into the peritoneal cavity. Surgeons often intuitively feel that source control equals surgery, rather than considering the surgical intervention to be part of a source control approach to the patient with intra-abdominal infections.

The concept 'source control' consists of 'all physical measures undertaken to eliminate a source of infection, to control ongoing contamination, and to restore premorbid anatomy and function' [2]. All the different aspects of this definition are important, but the elimination of the source and the control of ongoing contamination determine the early and long term success of the treatment. Restoration of anatomy and complete function can be performed in a delayed fashion when prolonging the surgical intervention may be harmful to the patient at the first operation (which is the basis of the 'damage control' concept).

Although this definition may seem straightforward, it describes the desired result instead of the proposed technique used to get there. Therefore, it is no surprise that source control can be interpreted in different ways, and that 'adequate source control' is not clearly defined. There are few data on the interobserver agreement of what adequate source control means when applied to a particular patient. In a recent study, Suding et al. studied 247 patients who failed treatment for complicated intra-abdominal infection. Interobserver agreement between two independent experts was (very) low, especially in patients with abscesses and in more severely ill patients [3]. It is not clear what impact this has on the management of the critically ill patient.

Elements of Source Control

Source control is based on four principles: Drainage, debridement, decompression and restoration of anatomy and function. All four principles are important as such, but in the individual patient, they can be applied independently, and at different moments; this is especially relevant in the critically ill patient, and obviates the need for involvement of intensivists regarding the timing and extent of the procedure in the critically ill patient.

Drainage

Drainage consists of evacuating the contents of an abscess, and by so-doing, creating a controlled fistula – if there is a connection to an epithelium lined lumen, such as an intestine – or creating a sinus if there is no such connection. The efficiency of the drain used is very important: It should be sized adequately to allow complete evacuation of the abscess. If the abscess cannot be drained completely, source control will fail. The use of additional drains can be considered, but it should be remembered that some abscesses or infections cannot be drained adequately. In these instances, debridement of necrotic tissues or removal of gastrointestinal contents may be necessary.

Drainage of an abscess can be performed surgically or percutaneously, often using ultrasound or computed tomography (CT) scan [4]. Percutaneous drainage is preferred for most situations, provided that adequate drainage is possible, and no debridement or repair of anatomical structures is necessary. Percutaneous drainage can also be used as a temporizing strategy even if debridement is indicated, or resection of part of the gastrointestinal tract is necessary. Especially in critically ill patients, where a surgical intervention can be difficult because of inflammation at the site of the infection and coagulopathy, this approach may be a valuable alternative.

Surgical drainage is indicated when percutaneous drainage fails, or when percutaneous drainage cannot be performed, for example when multiple abscesses are present, or when the presence of bowel loops between the abdominal wall and the abscess prevent passing a needle and guidewire to introduce the drain. It is often difficult to recognize failure of percutaneous drainage, but the clinical picture of ongoing sepsis a few days after percutaneous drainage should trigger a new search for a residual infection. In most cases, failure of percutaneous drainage is caused by ongoing contamination of the abscess due to a connection with an intestine, ineffective drains (too small for the content to be drained), or presence of tissues that need debridement. At this point, the aspect or volume of the drain effluent is notoriously unreliable and should not be used as a basis to guide therapy.

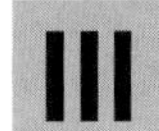

Decompression

Decompression may involve decompressing distended bowel in cases of (impending) obstruction or of intra-abdominal hypertension (IAH).

Debridement

Debridement should consist of removing dead tissue and foreign material from the abdominal cavity. This can only be accomplished surgically, and the extent to which this should be done remains a controversial topic. Some surgeons favor a minimalistic approach, which consists of removing dead tissue and using gauze to remove any pus present, whereas others promote an aggressive approach of high volume peritoneal lavage, and meticulous removal of all fibrin adherent to the intestines or abdominal wall. The latter carries a higher risk for iatrogenic bowel injuries, and has also been associated with a higher rate of postoperative abscesses. Therefore, a minimal aggressive approach should be preferred.

Restoration of Anatomy and Function

Restoration of anatomy and function is the final step in the management of complicated intra-abdominal infections, and as such often the goal of the surgical intervention. Examples are the perforation of the gastric ulcer that needs closure, or the inflamed appendix that needs resection. In most patients, restoration of anatomy and function can be established at the first operation, but in some patients, it needs to be delayed until the condition of the patient allows a sometimes lengthy procedure, and until tissue healing is adequate. This should be assessed on an individual basis but, generally, it is advised not to unnecessarily prolong surgical intervention in patients who are in shock, or who have severe organ dysfunction. In patients with severe acute pancreatitis who were treated surgically, we found that severity of disease at the moment of surgery was independently associated with increased mortality [5].

In some patients, this delay of a definitive procedure can take months, and the patient may even be discharged home before an attempt is made to restore anatomy and function, for example, restore continuity in a patient who underwent Hartmann's procedure for perforated diverticulitis.

Do we need to perform Source Control?

Although the application of source control in the treatment of infections seems only logical, a firm scientific basis for this is lacking. No controlled randomized trial has been performed, and the limited data available come from descriptive studies in which an increased mortality is reported in patients with intra-abdominal infections who were managed non-operatively [6, 7]. Koperna and Schulz described increased mortality when surgery was delayed for more than 48 hours in patients requiring relaparotomy for persistent abdominal sepsis; this effect was observed in all patients irrespective of the severity of disease, and was almost 100 % in patients with APACHE II scores of 20 or higher who were not operated on in time [8]. In another study in patients with complicated intra-abdominal infections, failure to clear the abdomen resulted in a much higher risk for dying, but also timing proved to be important, with increasing mortality when source control was delayed [9]. This has also been demonstrated in patients with necrotizing skin and soft tissue infections [10], but for most types of infection, data are lacking.

In infected pancreatic necrosis, it has been suggested that source control can or should be delayed until after the first 2 to 3 weeks [11, 12]. An increased mortality has been described in patients undergoing early surgery [13], but it should be considered that the majority of these patients did not have infected, but sterile, pancreatic necrosis. It is not clear if the increased mortality rate in a prospective study [14] of early versus late surgery was not caused by the surgical procedure and complications related to that surgical procedure. Other studies could not find a survival benefit of delaying surgery [15]. The decision to intervene in patients with infected pancreatic necrosis should be based on the clinical condition of the patient, the location and extent of the necrosis, but above all, should be individualized.

When to Perform Source Control?

Source control can and should be applied in the management of all patients presenting with sepsis, and not only in patients with surgical infections such as intra-abdominal infections or necrotizing skin and soft tissue infections, two conditions most often associated with source control. Although it may appear more important in the two above examples, removal of infected devices, drainage of abscesses and removal of necrosis is important in any kind of infection, irrespective of the focus.

The Role of the Intensivist

Patients with severe sepsis are often treated in an intensive care unit (ICU) from the moment the diagnosis is established, and the intensivist is routinely involved in the management of these patients. In parallel, the role of surgical and medical specialities on the ICU is decreasing, especially in closed units.

The role of the intensivist is crucial to determine the need for, timing and extent of source control measures that should be applied to the patient. Establishing a diagnosis is an essential first step in this process. This not only requires obtaining appropriate cultures, but also the identification of the focus of the infection. Thorough clinical examination, imaging techniques when necessary, and directed diagnostic studies should be performed in parallel with fluid resuscitation, empiric antibiotic administration, and supportive measures. Once a diagnosis has been obtained, the concept of source control should be applied to the patient and the search for a focus of infection that is amenable to one or more elements of the source control approach should be undertaken. **Table 1** lists a number of common infections with specific issues that should be considered in each case. When a patient has already undergone a source control procedure, it is even more challenging to recognize failed source control, and determine the need for a new intervention.

The next step is to determine the optimal intervention for the needs of the patient. It is obvious that adequate source control should aim at eliminating infection and controlling ongoing contamination. But adequate source control goes beyond that, acting to cause minimal damage to the patient and his/her physiology; this narrow balance between fully eradicating the infectious focus from the patient

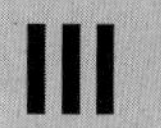

Table 1. Source control measures for specific infections

Clinical (suspected) diagnosis	Consider	Source control
Pneumonia	Empyema	Drainage of pleural effusion
Secondary peritonitis	Ongoing contamination due to perforation	Exteriorization of leaking GI tract, drainage of peritoneal fluids
Pancreatitis	Infected pancreatic necrosis	Debridement of necrotic tissue
Urinary tract infection	Catheter-related urinary tract infection	Remove catheter
Bacteremia	Catheter-related blood stream infection	Remove catheter
Skin and soft tissue infections	Necrotizing skin and soft tissue infections	Resection of necrotic tissue – explore when suspected on clinical grounds
Pyelonephritis	Urinary tract lithiasis	Debridement – lithiasis removal
Mediastinitis	Esophageal perforation	Surgical drainage
Sinusitis	Abscess formation	Aspiration and drainage – remove nasogastric/nasotracheal tube
Acalculous cholecystitis	Abscess, hydrops	Percutaneous drainage – cholecystectomy
Pericarditis		Drainage of pericardial fluid

Table 2. Indications for surgical versus percutaneous drainage

Percutaneous drainage preferable	Surgical drainage preferable
• One well defined abscess • Absence of ongoing contamination from gastrointestinal tract or other focus • Thin contents • No or minimal associated necrosis • 'Hostile' abdomen • Difficult to access visceral abscess	• Multiple abscesses • Ongoing contamination from gastrointestinal tract or other focus • Associated necrosis • Thick contents • Failed percutaneous drainage • Infected pancreatic necrosis • Abscess inaccessible to percutaneous drainage (e.g., inter-loop abscess)

and limiting harm to the patient, is crucial in the management of infections, especially in the critically ill, in whom additional intraoperative damage may have dramatic consequences. Drainage, as an example, can be accomplished by surgery or by percutaneous drainage. **Table 2** lists the conditions that may favor a surgical or percutaneous approach. When debridement is necessary in addition to drainage, a surgical approach may be preferred. The timing of surgery is also essential, yet often difficult to determine in individual cases.

What if Source Control is Impossible or Fails?

In some patients, source control is impossible to accomplish in one surgical intervention, because the disease process cannot be completely eradicated during the surgical procedure, e.g., in patients with retroperitoneal necrosis, diffuse peritonitis or intestinal ischemia. Although source control may fail in all infections, this is a typical problem in critically ill patients with complicated intra-abdominal infections. Those patients are candidates for more aggressive strategies like open abdomen treatment, or planned re-laparotomies. On-demand re-laparotomies are associated with reduced costs and use of hospital resources in this setting [16]; use of planned re-laparotomy as a routine strategy in the management of patients is no longer warranted. However, both options should be part of the armamentarium of the surgeon dealing with severe complicated intra-abdominal infections, rather than sticking unconditionally to either. Several techniques are available to temporarily close the abdomen without creating insurmountable nursing problems.

Failed source control often has a dramatic impact on postoperative morbidity and mortality, and is more important in determining outcome than antibiotic failure. Usually, it is the consequence of inadequate surgery – bad choice of type of operation, bad timing or bad technique – although patient factors with a 'hostile' abdomen and fragile intestines are also important. Severe sepsis and multiple organ dysfunction syndrome are systemic consequences of persistent infection, but local complications may also occur, such as IAH.

Diagnosis of failed source control is often difficult, and clinical examination is often unreliable. Imaging can be helpful, but in some patients explorative laparoscopy or -tomy must be used as a diagnostic tool as well [17], especially in patients in whom intestinal ischemia is suspected.

The therapy of complicated intra-abdominal infections can itself cause numerous complications, which further compromise the outcome. Intraoperative trauma to intestines is common, but erosion of drains into blood vessels or intestines is also possible. Surgical intervention can add to the trauma, and perforation during insertion of percutaneously placed drains can also occur.

In these patients, open abdomen techniques are often used to deal with the ongoing peritonitis, and planned or unplanned re-laparotomies may be necessary to deal with recurrent intraabdominal abscesses and collections. This clinical picture of persistent or recurrent peritonitis, nowadays referred to as tertiary peritonitis, has been associated with a high mortality rate [18]. Often infection with nosocomial organisms such as methicillin-resistant *Staphylococcus aureus* (MRSA), methicillin resistant coagulase-negative staphylococci, *Pseudomonas* or *Candida* species is found, although it is difficult to discriminate between infection and colonization. It is not clear if tertiary peritonitis is a cause rather than a consequence of disease severity [19], and a clear definition of the syndrome is lacking.

Special Considerations in Critically Ill Patients

Timing of Source Control

As a general rule, the source control procedure should be performed as soon as possible, and certainly within 6 hours after diagnosis. Stabilization of the patient is highly desirable before any source control procedures are started, but stabilization may not be feasible in some patients. Planning of the procedure and discussion with the surgeon and/or other specialities involved should take place before stabilization is accomplished.

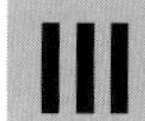

Definitive Therapy or Temporary Measures

As addressed before, collateral damage inflicted by the source control procedure should be minimal, and therefore, a minimally invasive procedure performed at the bedside is to be preferred, provided that it fulfils the requirements of an adequate source control procedure. Obviously, the risks of general anesthesia, or transportation to the interventional radiology suite should be weighed against the benefit of a more directed or definitive procedure. In patients with borderline coagulation parameters, surgical blood loss may add to the risk for postoperative bleeding and complications related to it.

The ongoing need for resuscitation should not be used as an argument against a source control procedure; fluid resuscitation should continue when a patient leaves the ICU, and full monitoring should be available at any location where this kind of patient is treated.

Damage control principles should be applied when physiology is unstable (impaired coagulation, metabolic disturbances with acidosis, hypothermia, and poor tissue perfusion among many). The patient should be returned to the ICU as soon as possible for correction of these disturbances; completion of the surgical procedure, including restoring gastrointestinal continuity or proper wound closure, can be deferred until circumstances are more favorable.

In case of rapidly progressive disease, with necrotizing fasciitis as a typical example, the same principles apply, but stabilization should not be pursued before surgery is performed. Bedside procedures are often recommended in these cases to gain time and to avoid transportation to the operating room.

How to Recognize Failed Source Control?

This is one of the most challenging issues, depending on the location of the infection. When there is ongoing necrosis in patients with necrotizing skin and soft tissue infections, or overt leakage of gastrointestinal contents from an open abdominal wound, the diagnosis of failed source control is obvious, and the need for re-intervention easily established. When there is failed source control in closed spaces such as the peritoneum or pleura, it is far more difficult to confirm the clinical suspicion. Currently, there is no diagnostic test available for failed source control; the use of simple inflammatory mediators such as fever, white blood cell count or C-reactive protein (CRP), may be limited by the occurrence of infections at other sites in ICU patients. Recently, Lepouse et al. retrospectively studied the role of procalcitonin as a predictor of the need for re-laparotomy; the authors found that persistent elevation of procalcitonin levels was associated with positive findings at re-laparotomy [20].

An important predictor seems to be the dynamics of organ dysfunction. When the patient further deteriorates, or deteriorates after initial improvement, this may be an indication that there is ongoing uncontrolled infection. This can be assessed by calculating daily sequential organ failure assessment (SOFA) scores. Recently, van Ruler et al. looked for parameters associated with positive findings at re-laparotomy after previous surgery for secondary peritonitis [21]. Age (OR 0.97, per 10 year), postoperative fever > 39 °C (OR 6.24), PaO_2/FiO_2 ratio (OR 0.99), heart rate (OR

1.02) and the postoperative hemoglobin level (OR 0.41) were all significantly associated with the need for re-laparotomy. Remarkably, none of the intraoperative findings, such as extent of peritonitis, etiology or focus of the intra-abdominal infection, played a role when the postoperative variables were entered in the model. Systemic bacteremia may also give a clue. In a study on blood stream infections of abdominal origin, the occurrence of a breakthrough blood stream infection (defined as an infection occurring after at least 48 hours of adequate antibiotic therapy) pointed to inadequate source control in 13/18 patients [22].

When failed source control is suspected based on any of the above parameters, the next step is to confirm this when there is no clear-cut indication for re-laparotomy; in some patients, obvious abdominal findings such as rebound tenderness or guarding with or without other signs or symptoms may be enough to advocate re-exploration. For obvious reasons, the role of clinical examination of the abdomen may be limited in the ICU; when findings are negative, few conclusions can be drawn from it, but when positive, they remain a very important tool. Consultation with the surgeon who performed the original surgical procedure is mandatory, as specific details of the surgical procedure may be helpful to guide further management of the patient. In some patients with a high probability of failed source control, for example a patient with gastrointestinal ischemia where borderline ischemic bowel was left *in situ*, a planned re-laparotomy should be considered. As a general tool, the use of planned re-laparotomy has not been demonstrated to be superior in the management of complicated intra-abdominal infections.

Conclusion

Source control is the cornerstone of the management of surgical infections, and antibiotics should be considered not more than an adjunct to source control. But source control also has an important role in non-surgical infections, and the need for source control should be evaluated early in the management of patients with severe sepsis. The critically ill patient is a unique challenge, as the physiology of the patient may make diagnosis more difficult and such patients may require specific interventions as a temporizing strategy. The role of the intensivist is essential in determining the specific needs of the patient, and in tailoring the therapeutic strategy to the individual patient. Adequate source control goes beyond source control *per se*, and includes optimal type and timing of the intervention and limited damage to the anatomy and physiology of the patient.

References

1. Dellinger RP, Levy MM, Carlet JM, et al (2008) Surviving Sepsis Campaign: international guidelines for management of severe sepsis and septic shock: 2008. Intensive Care Med 34: 17–60
2. Schein M, Marshall J (2002) Source Control. A Guide to the Management of Surgical Infections. Springer, Heidelberg
3. Suding PN, Orrico RP, Johnson SB, Wilson SE (2008) Concordance of interrater assessments of surgical methods to achieve source control of intra-abdominal infections. Am J Surg 196: 70–73
4. Montgomery RS, Wilson SE (1996) Intraabdominal abscesses: image-guided diagnosis and therapy. Clin Infect Dis 23: 28–36
5. De Waele J, Hoste E, Blot S, et al (2004) Perioperative factors determine outcome after surgery for severe acute pancreatitis. Crit Care 8: R504 – R511

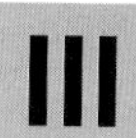

6. Wacha H, Hau T, Dittmer R, Ohmann C (1999) Risk factors associated with intraabdominal infections: a prospective multicenter study. Peritonitis Study Group. Langenbecks Arch Surg 384: 24–32
7. Grunau G, Heemken R, Hau T (1996) Predictors of outcome in patients with postoperative intra-abdominal infection. Eur J Surg 162: 619–625
8. Koperna T, Schulz F (2000) Relaparotomy in peritonitis: prognosis and treatment of patients with persisting intraabdominal infection. World J Surg 24: 32–37
9. Mulier S, Penninckx F, Verwaest C, et al (2003) Factors affecting mortality in generalized postoperative peritonitis: multivariate analysis in 96 patients. World J Surg 27: 379–384
10. Elliott DC, Kufera JA, Myers RA (1996) Necrotizing soft tissue infections. Risk factors for mortality and strategies for management. Ann Surg 224: 672–683
11. Muller CA, Vogeser M, Belyaev O, et al (2006) Role of endogenous glucocorticoid metabolism in human acute pancreatitis. Crit Care Med 34: 1060–1066
12. Nathens AB, Curtis JR, Beale RJ, et al (2004) Management of the critically ill patient with severe acute pancreatitis. Crit Care Med 32: 2524–2536
13. De Waele J, Vogelaers D, Decruyenaere J, et al (2004) Infectious complications of acute pancreatitis. Acta Clin Belg 59: 90–96
14. Mier J, Leon EL, Castillo A, et al (1997) Early versus late necrosectomy in severe necrotizing pancreatitis. Am J Surg 173: 71–75
15. De Waele JJ, Hoste E, Blot SI, et al (2004) Perioperative factors determine outcome after surgery for severe acute pancreatitis. Crit Care 8: R504–511
16. van Ruler O, Mahler CW, Boer KR, et al (2007) Comparison of on-demand vs planned relaparotomy strategy in patients with severe peritonitis: a randomized trial. JAMA 298: 865–872
17. Hutchins RR, Gunning MP, Lucas DN, et al (2004) Relaparotomy for suspected intraperitoneal sepsis after abdominal surgery. World J Surg 28: 137–141
18. Nathens AB, Rotstein OD, Marshall JC (1998) Tertiary peritonitis: clinical features of a complex nosocomial infection. World J Surg 22: 158–163
19. Evans HL, Raymond DP, Pelletier SJ, et al (2001) Tertiary peritonitis (recurrent diffuse or localized disease) is not an independent predictor of mortality in surgical patients with intraabdominal infection. Surg Infect (Larchmt) 2: 255–263
20. Lepouse C, Murat O, Nicolai F, et al (2008) Postoperative procalcitonin kinetics: An indicator for therapeutic strategy in peritonitis? Intensive Care Med 34 (Suppl 1):S123 (abst)
21. van Ruler O, Lamme B, Gouma DJ, et al (2007) Variables associated with positive findings at relaparotomy in patients with secondary peritonitis. Crit Care Med 35: 468–476
22. De Waele JJ, Hoste EA, Blot SI (2008) Blood stream infections of abdominal origin in the intensive care unit: characteristics and determinants of death. Surg Infect (Larchmt) 9: 171–177

IgM-enriched Immunoglobulins in Sepsis

F. Esen and S. Tugrul

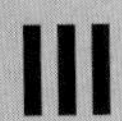

Introduction

The role of intravenous immunoglobulins (IVIGs) as an adjunctive treatment in sepsis has been a subject of debate for years. The main critique has been the lack of randomized trials of adequate size showing the effect of IVIGs on outcome. For that reason, many of the guidelines on sepsis have not addressed the use of IVIG treatment. Likewise, the Surviving Sepsis Guidelines [1] did not consider the use of immunoglobulins in adult patients with sepsis.

As an adjunctive therapy in adults with sepsis, the use of immunoglobulins was first reported in the early 1980s [2], and studies completed through the 1990s were reviewed by the Cochrane collaboration [3]; this began the series of meta-analyses on immunoglobins in sepsis. In the Cochrane review of IVIGs for the treatment of sepsis, IVIGs were reported to significantly reduce mortality in patients with sepsis [3]. However the authors concluded that due to the small size of the trials, the evidence was insufficient to support a definitive conclusion. The Cochrane review also included a retrospective subgroup analysis comparing IgM-enriched IVIG with standard polyclonal IgG IVIG. In this subgroup analysis of 11 trials, a *post hoc* sub-analysis according to the type of IVIG demonstrated a greater reduction in mortality among patients given IgM-enriched immunoglobulin compared with standard immunoglobulin. To date, five newer meta-analyses on the use of polyclonal immunoglobulins as adjunctive therapy for sepsis have been published [4–8]. Compared with the Cochrane statement, these meta-analysis included more trials and study patients, including the large Score-Based Immunoglobulin G Therapy of patients with Sepsis (SBITS) study [9] using a standard IgG preparation in patients with severe sepsis. The results of each meta-analysis were very similar to the results of the Cochrane meta-analysis, which showed a reduction in mortality with a standard IgG IVIG administration, and a greater risk reduction with an IgM-enriched preparation.

In the latest meta-analysis, Kreymann et al. [4] summarized the data for two groups of studies using IgM-enriched IVIG or IgG IVIG. The authors included 8 smaller trials with IgM-enriched immunoglobulins, including 560 adult patients in whom the estimate of the pooled effect on mortality showed a relative risk of 0.66 (a 34 % relative reduction in mortality) with no substantial heterogeneity. The results were even better in neonate trials with 352 patients in 5 studies with a 50 % relative reduction in mortality. The comparison of IgM-enriched IVIG and IgG IVIG showed a strong trend in favor of IgM-enriched treatment both in adults and in neonates. As already reported in the Cochrane meta-analysis [3], these data again confirmed that preparations enriched with IgA and IgM (IgGAM) yielded better results than IgG preparations. What is superior about IgM over IgG and why do IgM-enriched preparations seem to work better in patients with sepsis? To answer this question, the current review will address the mechanism by which IVIGs work in sepsis, and give brief information about the different nature of IVIGs and their effects on the treatment of sepsis. In addition to experimental evidence on the mechanism of action of immunoglobulins, we will mainly focus on the effects of IgM-enriched immunoglobulins and their clinical use in the management of sepsis.

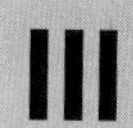

Mechanisms of Action of IVIG in Sepsis

IVIG is a therapeutic preparation of normal human polyclonal IgG obtained from a large number of healthy blood donors. The efficacy and tolerance of immunoglobulins from human plasma have been shown to be optimal since, compared with synthetic drugs, they have been shown to be highly specific. Initially introduced as a replacement therapy for patients with immune deficiencies, IVIG is now being used for the treatment of autoimmune and systemic inflammatory diseases. Besides these medical conditions, evidence suggests that many other conditions, such as inflammatory disorders with an imbalance in the cytokine network could benefit from IVIG treatment [10]. In sepsis, the use of IVIGs represents a therapeutic effort to positively modulate the immune response, thereby preventing organ dysfunction. Immunoglobulins might exert beneficial effects in sepsis by several mechanisms, like providing antibody against pathogen-specific lipopolysaccharides (LPS), enhancing phagocytic function, modulating cytokine responses, acting synergistically with antibiotics, and, most importantly, neutralizing endo- and exo-toxins [11].

Owing to their molecular structure, IVIGs react directly with viruses, bacteria, and toxins and also activate immunobiological activities in the body [10]. Studies have shown that IVIG preparations contain a broad spectrum of opsonic and neutralizing antibodies directed against a variety of antimicrobial agents. In addition to direct neutralization of these antigens, other modes of action contributing to the beneficial effect in systemic inflammatory diseases have been described for IVIG. These include blockade of Fc receptors on phagocytic cells, modulation of Fc receptor expression, interference with complement activation and the cytokine network, modulation of dendritic cell activity, and T and B cell activation. Thus, IVIGs have multiple modes of action which act synergistically [10].

Based on the differences in the amino acid sequences in the constant region of the heavy chains, immunoglobulins can be divided into five different classes (IgG, IgM, IgA, IgD, and IgE). Each class of immunoglobulin differs markedly in physical and biological properties from the other classes. IgM is the first class of antibody produced in the immune response. IgM is a larger molecule compared with IgG, and the concentration of IgM is 8–10 times lower than the concentration of IgG. Moreover, the half-life of the smaller IgG molecule is four times longer than that of the large IgM molecule [12].

Standard immunoglobulin preparations for intravenous administration contain class IgG immunoglobulin as the main component, while IgA and IgM immunoglobulins are present in small quantities. Although pure IgG preparations are known to be effective, IgM as well as IgG substitution appears desirable in cases like neonatal sepsis, which correlates with a physiologically-determined IgM deficiency in the newborn [13]. For IgM substitution, an intravenous IgM preparation (Pentaglobin, Biotest Pharma GmbH, Dreieich, Germany) was developed and introduced for clinical use in 1985, comprised of IgG (76 %), IgA (12 %), and IgM (12 %) (IgGAM). The efficacy of this preparation has been demonstrated in various ways [13]. The immunoglobulin concentration and antibody activity of this product was tested, demonstrating 99 % immunoglobulin purity, with very low anti-complement activity, which accounts for its tolerability to the same degree as standard intravenous IgG preparations.

Differences between IgG- and IgM-enriched Immunoglobulins

In vivo and *in vitro* studies have demonstrated that IgM is much more potent in general functions compared with IgG. The pentameric form of IgM has been suggested to contribute to superior efficacy in toxin neutralization and bacterial agglutination compared with IgG antibodies and has been shown to be very efficient at fixing complement and enhancing opsonization [14, 15].

A pre-eminent property of IgM is its capacity to produce pronounced activation of complement, which leads to irreversible damage of the bacterial membrane. More IgG molecules are required to damage the cell than IgM molecules. Moreover, the potency of IgM antibodies in the agglutination of large and complex structures, e.g., salmonella, is 10 times greater than that of IgG. In the same system, the killing of bacteria by IgM is more effective, since IgM activates 100–400 times more complement than IgG [12]. In the opsonization of bacteria, IgM has been shown to be 1000 times more active than IgG and IgM produces more antibody against endotoxin (LPS). The anti-LPS antibody content of commercial IVIGs was examined using LPS preparations from *Escherichia coli*, *Klebsiella*, and the *Pseudomonas aeruginosa* serotypes which occur most frequently in Gram-negative septicemia [16]. Three different IgG products and one IgM-enriched product were tested. The mean antibody levels were significantly higher in the IgM fraction of the IgM-enriched product compared with pure IgG products, which indicated that natural antibodies against bacterial LPS might belong primarily to the IgM class. The endotoxin neutralizing capacities of IgM and IgG were also assessed in an endotoxic shock model [17]. Maximal endotoxin inactivation was achieved after 15 min with the IgM-enriched preparation; however, the addition of two pure IgG preparations did not reveal a significant effect on endotoxin recovery. The inactivation was much lower with a standard IgG preparation than that obtained after the addition of the IgM-enriched immunoglobulin. Endotoxin-induced cytokine release from whole blood was not influenced by IgG; however, IgM administration significantly decreased the release of tumor necrosis factor (TNF)-α and interleukin (IL)-1 in a concentration-dependent manner. What about exotoxins? In an *in vitro* study [18], investigators compared the ability of different immunoglobulin preparations containing IgG, IgM, and IgA to neutralize the activity of streptococcal pyrogenic exotoxin (SpeA). All immunoglobulin preparations markedly inhibited the mitogenic and cytokine-inducing activity of SpeA. Moreover, the comparative neutralization effects of the IgM-enriched preparation on streptococcal exotoxin showed that both IgM and IgA are potent inhibitors of group A superantigens and pentaglobin containing IgGAM was significantly more potent on streptococcal exotoxin than the preparation containing only IgG.

The toxin inhibitory activity of intravenous IgGAM was studied in experimental endotoxemia induced by the intraperitoneal inoculation of a sublethal dose of *E. coli* and the subsequent intravenous administration of an antimicrobial agent [19]. The aim was to investigate whether a protective effect can be achieved in endotoxemia by application of IgM-enriched polyclonal immunoglobulin. The prophylactic administration of IgGAM significantly attenuated the antibiotic-induced increase in endotoxin activity as compared to the albumin control group. This decrease in endotoxemia was also shown to be associated with reduced levels of circulating IL-6. This synergistic effect occurring following the combined administration of pentaglobin with antibiotics was also confirmed in an experimental model of fecal peritonitis [20]. The effect of pentaglobin and piperacillin individually and in combination was investigated with particular emphasis on the role of intervention timings on survival rates in septic rats. The combined treatment with piperacillin plus pentaglobin provided better results as compared to the individual effects. The best results occurred with the earliest (4 h) administration, but the drugs showed no protection if the treatment was delayed 8 h following induction of peritonitis, indicating the effectiveness of early treatment with intravenous IgGAM [20].

Another potential difference in the mechanism of action of IgG and IgM is their effects on endotoxin-induced capillary perfusion failure and the resulting tissue integrity and organ function. Evidence suggests that the endotoxin-induced interaction of leukocytes with the endothelium at the microcirculatory level is a major cause of the microvascular injury responsible for perfusion failure and organ dysfunction. In an experimental study [21], the *in vivo* effects of clinically-used immunoglobulin preparations on microcirculatory mechanisms were analyzed in an endotoxemia model. Both intravenous IgM and IgG preparations markedly attenuated the endotoxin-induced leukocyte adherence in arterioles and venules at 8 h of endotoxemia. At 24 h, however, intravenous IgM was capable of further reducing venular leukocyte adherence, whereas IgG did not show a protective effect compared with controls. The protective effect of IgM was also evident with the measurement of functional capillary density (FCD). IgM application significantly ameliorated the LPS-induced decrease in FCD, whereas intravenous IgG did not provide protection against microvascular perfusion failure. Very recently, the protective effects of IgM on tissue integrity following secondary hyperinflammatory tissue damage caused by LPS were evaluated in an established model of endotoxemia [22]. The augmentation of host defense by IgM was not associated with collateral tissue damage, thus IgM substitution had an especially beneficial effect on LPS-induced pulmonary damage. The pulmonary protective effects of IgM substitution were demonstrated histologically and on a score-based evaluation. Significantly reduced alveolar damage, especially with respect to alveolar edema, interstitial edema, and hemorrhage was evident with the administration of IgM-enriched immunoglobulin. Similar pulmonary protective effects were shown in a rat acute respiratory distress model. Lachmann et al. [23] showed that translocation of *Klebsiella pneumonia* from the lung into the systemic circulation was reduced after IgM application, signifying a protective IgM effect on the alveolar-capillary barrier.

Clinical Significance of IgM-enriched IVIG

Clinical studies with IgM-enriched immunoglobulins in a mixed patient population of septic patients or more homogeneous groups for prophylactic use (primarily after cardiac surgery) showed a trend toward reduced morbidity and mortality; however, the lack of a significant difference in these studies was attributed, at least in part, to the small number of patients included in the studies (**Table 1**). After its introduction as an endotoxin-neutralizing technology, intravenous IgM-enriched immunoglobu-

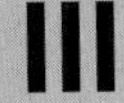

Table 1. Randomized control trials of IgM-enriched IVIG therapy in patients with sepsis

Reference	Population	No. of Patients	Mortality	p value
Schedel et al. [24]	Gram-negative sepsis patients with high endotoxin levels	69	IVIG: 1/27 Control: 9/28	0.012
Tugrul et al. [25]	Medical and surgical severe sepsis patients	42	IVIG: 5/21 Control: 7/21	0.73
Karatzas et al. [26]	Medical and surgical severe sepsis and septic shock patients	68	IVIG: 8/34 Control: 14/34	0.05
Rodriguez et al. [27]	Intra-abdominal sepsis patients	56	IVIG: 8/29 Control: 13/27	0.17
Hentrich et al. [28]	Neutropenic patients with hematologic disorders with sepsis	211	IVIG: 27/103 Control: 29/103	0.93

lin was assessed in a homogeneous septic patient population with high endotoxin levels [24]. Patients within 24 hours after the onset of septic shock with endotoxemia were randomized to receive IgM-enriched immunoglobulins with the hypothesis that eliminating endotoxin as early as possible might improve the clinical course of septic shock. The study was discontinued after the evaluation of the data from 55 patients, since the difference between the mortality rates (4 % vs. 32 %) was statistically significant in favor of the therapy. There was a statistically significant decrease in the APACHE II score beyond the 5th day after inclusion and the serum concentration of endotoxin was significantly reduced in IgM-treated patients within 24 hours after inclusion. In a mixed patient population with severe sepsis, our group evaluated the effects of IgM-enriched IVIG treatment on progression of organ failure and development of septic shock [25]. The patient population had severe sepsis and was obtained from the medical and surgical ICUs, regardless of the causative organism. Patients randomized to receive pentaglobin were treated for 3 consecutive days and followed up for 8 days in terms of inflammatory parameters and organ dysfunction. Mortality was not an endpoint in the study. A marked trend in favor of IgGAM treatment was demonstrated; however, the power of the study was not sufficient to make any clear conclusion. Procalcitonin (PCT) levels, as a marker of the severity of the inflammatory response, declined consistently in the treatment group, however this decline did not correspond with the clinical course, which was reflected by unchanged sequential organ failure assessment (SOFA) scores throughout the study, yet a trend in reduced incidence of septic shock and 28-day mortality was evident. In a similar protocol including 68 ICU patients with severe sepsis, Karatzas et al. [26] reported a significant reduction in mortality, especially in the IgM-enriched immunoglobulin-treated patients with an APACHE II score ranging between 20 and 29.

Most recently, the impact of high dose IgM-enriched immunoglobulin and antibiotic therapy was assessed in a more homogeneous group of critically ill patients with proven intra-abdominal sepsis [27]. The administration of intravenous IgM-enriched immunoglobulin in addition to antibiotic therapy produced a 20 % reduction in mortality, although this difference was not statistically significant. In the subset of patients with appropriate antibiotic therapy, a significant reduction in the mortality of IVIG treated patients was reported with reductions in the relative and absolute risk of death by 74 and 25 %, respectively.

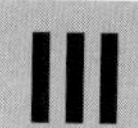

One of the largest studies on the use of IVIG in septic patients with chemotherapy-induced severe neutropenia has been recently published [28]. Two hundred eleven neutropenic patients with hematologic malignancies were randomized to receive intravenous IgGAM or albumin for 3 consecutive days. The study failed to document any benefit of IVIG therapy based on the 28-day mortality rate. Likewise, there was no significant difference in the duration of organ failure between the two arms; however, in all patients who survived with failing organs, there was a trend favoring intravenous IgGAM treatment. The choice of study population included in this trial [28] has been questioned with respect to representing the precise population of septic patients for IVIG treatment. These were low grade sepsis patients showing none or one organ failure with a relatively low mortality, and it has been suggested that these patients may not represent the target population for IVIG treatment to show any benefit on mortality.

Recently, the results of two large studies on the effects of standard G class IVIG treatment on a target group of sepsis patients (SBITS) [9] and post-cardiac surgery patients with severe systemic inflammatory response syndrome (SIRS) have been published [29]. The SBITS study revealed no reduction in mortality by administration of intravenous IgG in the entire study population, or in the subgroups. Given the statistical power, the study did not bolster the hope for IVIG therapy in septic patients. These results were further supported by a second large study in post-cardiac surgery patients with severe sepsis (the Early Supplemental Severe SIRS treatment with IVIG in score-identified high-risk patients after Cardiac Surgery study, ESSICS) [29]. The investigators of the SBITS and ESSICS studies have claimed that this failure with intravenous IgG does not necessarily exclude a survival benefit of IgM-enriched IVIG preparations, as suggested in previous meta-analyses [4–8].

The prophylactic use of IVIGs has been considered in surgical patients to reduce the incidence of infection and occurrence of sepsis and septic shock; however, results have been conflicting. In a clinical trial, Pilz et al. [30] showed that early supplemental IVIG treatment improved disease severity and may improve prognosis in prospectively APACHE II score-identified high-risk post-cardiac surgical patients. The same group [31] carried out a randomized prospective trial to compare the clinical course using a polyvalent IgG versus an IgGAM preparation in these high risk post-cardiac surgery patients. The study endpoints gave similar results for both immunoglobulin treatment regimens; however, with respect to serum IgM, only the IgGAM preparation led to significantly increased levels. Polyclonal IgM-enriched immunoglobulins did not significantly reduce the mortality rate in the overall study population; however, in the subgroup of patients with severe sepsis, they significantly improved the survival rate [32].

The prophylactic use of IgM-enriched solutions has been considered in high risk cardiosurgical patients to reduce the rate of infectious complications after open heart surgery. It has been suggested that the occurrence of postoperative infections is related to a pre-existing impairment of the immune system. Pre-operative anergic patients showing impaired cutaneous delayed type hypersensitivity responses were chosen as a high risk group for postoperative infection, and randomized to receive IgGAM 4 hours after surgery [33]. The infection rate was higher in the anergic patients compared to the normergic patients, and there was a significant reduction in infectious complications with IgM-enriched immunoglobulins in the anergic group compared with the control group [33]. Further studies compared two different IVIG preparations (IgG versus IgGAM), rather than two groups of patients treated with or without IVIGs [31, 34]. Two studies compared the efficacy of standard IgG and IgGAM in sepsis or in post-cardiac surgical patients at high risk for sepsis. No significant differences were noted between the two preparations in these patients. In the sepsis trial [34], patients treated with either IgG or IgGAM were compared with untreated controls, and there was a significant reduction in mortality with IgGAM when compared with controls, whereas no significant benefit was demonstrated for the standard IgG group.

An additional interesting finding is the beneficial effects of early treatment with IgM-enriched immunoglobulins on critical illness polyneuropathy (CIP) in patients with Gram-negative severe sepsis and septic shock, which has not yet been described for adjunctive intravenous IgG. In a retrospective study evaluating the incidence of CIP in patients with Gram-negative sepsis and organ dysfunction [35], investigators reported that patients who had been treated with IgGAM showed no signs of CIP during electrophysiologic examination. Similar results were also demonstrated in the SBITS trial [9], in which a shorter duration of mechanical ventilation was correlated with IVIG treatment. Amelioration in the motor response accounted for the effect on critical illness neuropathy, which might explain the shorter duration of mechanical ventilation in the treatment arm.

Conclusion

After more than 25 years of work examining IVIG therapy in sepsis, there are no recommendations for IVIG in the latest guidelines. A tangible explanation is that those studies with positive results were all small trials of low quality and the largest trial (SBITS) did not show the expected benefit with the standard IgG preparation. However, does this also apply to IgM-enriched immunoglobulins? There is enough *in vivo* and *in vitro* evidence showing the superiority of IgM-enriched IVIGs in experimental sepsis, and the clinical data are certainly not negligible and deserve to be considered. There may be some questions and concerns in terms of the power and the quality of the studies; however, no trial with IgM-enriched immunoglobulins demonstrated significantly different results, and tests of heterogeneity were not significant among the trials. Moreover, the latest meta-analyses, including 8 trials with nearly 600 patients, raised the possibility of a significant benefit with the use of IgM-enriched immunoglobulins in adult and neonatal septic patients [4].

It is clear that to better elucidate which patients would benefit from IgM-enriched immunoglobulin treatment, further trials are necessary. For the time being, the data suggest that the patients most likely to benefit from IgM-enriched IVIG are surgical ICU patients with Gram-negative septic shock. We believe that there is a need for larger clinical trials to confirm the effectiveness of this product in reducing mortality in sepsis. However, there is a question to be answered concerning the design of these trials: Will single-center, well-designed randomized controlled trials be adequate to obtain conclusive data concerning IgM-enriched IVIG therapy, or is it unavoidable that a large multicenter randomized controlled trial be called for in the next sepsis guidelines?

References

1. Dellinger RP, Carlet JM, Masur H, et al (2004) Surviving Sepsis Campaign Management Guidelines Committee. Surviving Sepsis Campaign guidelines for management of severe sepsis and septic shock. Crit Care Med 32: 858–873
2. Ziegler EJ, McCutchan JA, Fierer J, et al (1982) Treatment of Gram-negative bacteremia and shock with human antiserum to a mutant Escherichia coli. N Engl J Med 307: 1225–1230
3. Alejandria MM, Lansang MA, Dans LF, Mantaring JB (2002) Intravenous immunoglobulin for treating sepsis and septic shock. Cochrane Database Syst Rev CD0011090
4. Kreymann KG, de Heer G, Nierhaus A, Kluge S (2007) Use of polyclonal immunoglobulins as adjunctive therapy for sepsis or septic shock. Crit Care Med 35: 2677–2685
5. Norrby-Teglund A, Haque KN, Hammarström L (2006) Intravenous polyclonal IgM-enriched immunoglobulin therapy in sepsis: a review of clinical efficacy in relation to microbiological aetiology and severity of sepsis. J Intern Med 260: 509–516
6. Laupland KB, Kirkpatrick AW, Delaney A (2007) Polyclonal intravenous immunoglobulin for the treatment of severe sepsis and septic shock in critically ill adults: a systematic review and meta-analysis. Crit Care Med 35: 2686–2692
7. Pildal J, Gøtzsche PC(2004) Polyclonal immunoglobulin for treatment of bacterial sepsis: a systematic review. Clin Infect Dis 39: 38–46
8. Turgeon AF, Hutton B, Fergusson DA, et al (2007) Meta-analysis: intravenous immunoglobulin in critically ill adult patients with sepsis. Ann Intern Med 146: 193–203
9. Werdan K, Pilz G, Bujdoso O, et al (2007) Score-based immunoglobulin G therapy of patients with sepsis: the SBITS study. Crit Care Med 35: 2693–2701
10. Negi VS, Elluru S, Sibéril S, et al (2007) Intravenous immunoglobulin: an update on the clinical use and mechanisms of action. J Clin Immunol 27: 233–245
11. Werdan K (2001) Intravenous immunoglobulin for prophylaxis and therapy of sepsis. Curr Opin Crit Care 7: 354–361
12. Stephan W (1989) Investigations to demonstrate the antibacterial and antitoxic efficacy of an IgM-Enriched intravenous immunoglobulin preparation. In: Faist E, Ninnemann J, Green D (eds) Immune Consequences of Trauma; Shock and Sepsis. Springer-Verlag, Heidelberg, pp 501–507
13. Stephan W, Dichtelmüller H, Schedel I (1985) [Properties and efficacy of a human immunoglobulin M preparation for intravenous administration]. Arzneimittelforschung 35: 933–936
14. Garbett ND, Matharu GS, Cole PJ (1989) Defective opsonization of Haemophilus influenzae by sera of elderly patients. Clin Exp Immunol 76: 73–75
15. Rieben R, Roos A, Muizert Y, Tinguely C, Gerritsen AF, Daha MR (1999) Immunoglobulin M-enriched human intravenous immunoglobulin prevents complement activation in vitro an in vivo in a rat model of acute inflammation. Blood 93: 942–951
16. Trautmann M, Held TK, Susa M, et al (1998) Bacterial lipopolysaccharide (LPS)-specific antibodies in commercial human immunoglobulin preparations: superior antibody content of an IgM-enriched product. Clin Exp Immunol 111: 81–90
17. Berger D, Schleich S, Seidelmann M, Berger HG (1993) Antiendotoxic therapy with polyclonal and polyvalent immunoglobulins: in vitro an in vivo studies. In: Faist E Meakins JL, Schildberg FW (eds) Host Defense Dysfunction in Trauma, Shock and Sepsis. Springer-Verlag, Heidelberg, pp 1164–1174
18. Norrby-Teglund A, Ihendyane N, Kansal R, et al (2000) Relative neutralizing activity in polyspecific IgM, IgA, and IgG preparations against group A streptococcal superantigens. Clin Infect Dis 31: 1175–1182
19. Oesser S, Schulze C, Seifert J (1999) Protective capacity of an IgM/IgA-enriched polyclonal immunoglobulin-G preparation in endotoxemia. Res Exp Med 198: 325–339
20. Jacobs S, Sobki S, Morais C, Tariq M. (2000) Effect of pentaglobin and piperacillin on survival in a rat model of faecal peritonitis: importance of intervention timings. Acta Anaesthesiol Scand 44: 88–95
21. Hoffman JN, Fertmann JM, Vollmar B, Laschke MW, Jauch KW, Menger MD (2008) Immunoglobulin M-enriched human intravenous immunoglobulins reduce leukocyte-endothelial cell interactions and attenuate microvascular perfusion failure in normotensive endotoxemia. Shock 29: 133–139

III

22. Stehr SN, Knels L, Weissflog C, et al (2008) Effects of IGM-enriched solution on polymorphonuclear neutrophil function, bacterial clearance, and lung histology in endotoxemia. Shock 29: 167–172
23. Lachmann RA, van Kaam AH, Haitsma JJ, Verbrugge SJ, Delreu F, Lachmann B (2004) Immunoglobulin M-enriched intravenous polyclonal immunoglobulins reduce bacteremia following Klebsiella pneumoniae infection in an acute respiratory distress syndrome rat model. Exp Lung Res 30: 251–260
24. Schedel I, Dreikhausen U, Nentwig B, et al (1991) Treatment of gram-negative septic shock with an immunoglobulin preparation: A prospective, randomized clinical trial. Crit Care Med 19: 1104–1113
25. Tugrul S, Ozcan PE, Akinci O, et al (2002) The effects of IgM-enriched immunoglobulin preparations in patients with severe sepsis. Crit Care 6: 357–362
26. Karatzas S, Boutzouka E, Venetsanou K, Myrianthefs P, Fildisis G, Baltopoulos G (2002) The effects of IgM-enriched immunoglobulin preparations in patients with severe sepsis: another point of view. Crit Care 6: 543–544
27. Rodríguez A, Rello J, Neira J, et al (2005) Effects of high-dose of intravenous immunoglobulin and antibiotics on survival for severe sepsis undergoing surgery. Shock 23: 298–304
28. Hentrich M, Fehnle K, Ostermann H, et al (2006) IgMA-enriched immunoglobulin in neutropenic patients with sepsis syndrome and septic shock: a randomized, controlled, multiple-center trial. Crit Care Med 34: 1319–1325
29. Werdan K, Pilz G, Müller-Werdan U, et al (2008) Immunoglobulin G treatment of postcardiac surgery patients with score-identified severe systemic inflammatory response syndrome--the ESSICS study. Crit Care Med 36: 716–723
30. Pilz G, Kreuzer E, Kaab S, Appel R, Werdan K (1994) Early sepsis treatment with immunoglobulins after cardiac surgery in score-identified high-risk patients. Chest 105: 76–82
31. Pilz G, Appel R, Kreuzer E, Werdan K (1997) Comparison of early IgM-enriched immunoglobulin vs polyvalent IgG administration in score-identified postcardiac surgical patients at high risk for sepsis. Chest 111: 419–426
32. Buda S, Riefolo A, Biscione R, et al (2005) Clinical experience with polyclonal IgM-enriched Immunoglobulins in a group of patients affected by sepsis after cardiac surgery. J Cardiothorac Vasc Anesth 19: 440–445
33. Kress HG, Scheidewing C, Schmidt H, Silber R (1999) Reduced incidence of postoperative infection after intravenous administration of an immunoglobulin A- and immunoglobulin M-enriched preparation in anergic patients undergoing cardiac surgery. Crit Care Med 27: 1281–1287
34. Haque K, Remo C, Bahakim H (1995) Comparison of two types of intravenous immunoglobulins in the treatment of neonatal sepsis. Clin Exp Immunol 101: 328–333
35. Mohr M, Englisch L, Roth A, Burchardi H, Zielmann S (1997) Effects of early treatment with immunoglobulin on critical illness polyneuropathy following multiple organ failure and gram-negative sepsis. Intensive Care Med 23: 1144–1149

Clarithromycin: A Promising Immunomodulator in Sepsis

E.J. Giamarellos-Bourboulis

Introduction

Severe sepsis and septic shock are among the leading causes of death, representing the 10th most common cause of death in the United States of America [1]. The high mortality rates, ranging between 35 and 50 % despite adequate antimicrobial treatment [2], have encouraged intense research efforts to better understand the mechanisms underlying the pathogenesis of sepsis. As a consequence, sepsis syndrome is now recognized as a complex entity created by an intense inflammatory reaction that is generated in the host after stimulation of the innate and adaptive immune systems by bacterial components [3].

Understanding that sepsis is a hyper-inflammatory reaction of the host triggered by invading bacteria created the need for therapies aimed at modulating the exaggerated host response. Numerous experimental and clinical studies have been published in this field. Anti-endotoxin antibodies, anti-tumor necrosis factor (TNF)-α antibodies, soluble TNF-α receptors, recombinant human activated protein C (rhAPC), low dose hydrocortisone, and intensive insulin therapy are just some of the compounds that have been proposed. Clinical trials with most of these agents have failed to disclose any clinical benefit or have shown limited clinical efficacy. Published guidelines by the Surviving Sepsis Campaign [4] have restricted the application of immunotherapy to only three arms: a) Administration of rhAPC with a 2B grade of evidence in patients with an APACHE II> 25; b) low dose hydrocortisone with a 2C grade of evidence in patients with septic shock; and c) tight glucose monitoring to maintain glucose concentrations below 150 mg/dl with a 2C grade of evidence in patients with severe sepsis and septic shock. The above mentioned low grades of evidence, often resulting from the serious adverse effects of the suggested immunotherapies, underline the need for the evolution of new strategies of immuno-intervention with greater clinical efficacy and without serious adverse events.

The present chapter analyzes the evolution of intravenously administered clarithromycin as an immunomodulator in sepsis. The chapter is organized into three parts: a) Evidence from observational studies about promising anti-inflammatory effects of macrolides in pneumonia; b) presentation of the effect of clarithromycin in experimental studies of sepsis; and c) analysis of results from one recent randomized trial showing considerable clinical efficacy of clarithromycin in patients with ventilator-associated pneumonia (VAP) and sepsis.

Indirect Evidence for an Immunomodulatory effect of Macrolides in Pneumonia

Macrolides have been shown to be effective in chronic inflammatory disorders of the lower respiratory tract, namely diffuse panbronchiolitis and cystic fibrosis [5]. Diffuse panbronchiolitis is a chronic obstructive disease of the airways leading to early death due to respiratory failure and cor pulmonale. Survival has been considerably prolonged after introduction of erythromycin into the daily treatment of these patients in 1979. Daily oral administration of 500 mg of clarithromycin is the treatment of choice nowadays. Four randomized clinical trials have been published in patients with cystic fibrosis. In all these trials, enrolled patients were allocated to either placebo or azithromycin. Administration of azithromycin was accompanied by improvement of respiratory function, as shown by an increase in the forced expiratory volume in one second (FEV_1) and by a considerable reduction in exacerbations of the disease [6–9].

In all the above studies, the proposed mechanism of action of macrolides may involve either a direct effect on *Pseudomonas aeruginosa* colonizing the airways of the patients or an effect on the immune system of the host [5]. This mechanism of action is difficult to demonstrate in acute inflammation of the airways, namely in pneumonia, and no randomized trial has ever been conducted to provide such evidence. As a consequence, only indirect evidence is available, coming from retrospective observational studies. Results of these studies are summarized in **Table 1** [10–14]. A common denominator of these studies is the positive effect of the administration of a macrolide on patient outcome. Addition of a macrolide to a β-lactam was consistently accompanied by a considerable reduction in mortality. This was particularly pronounced when pneumonia was aggravated by bacteremia or severe sepsis. One probable explanation for the clinical benefit seen with macrolides could be their effect against atypical pathogens. However, even when the analysis included only patients infected by *Streptococcus pneumoniae*, the macrolide benefit was still apparent [10, 11]. The only evidence opposing a beneficial effect of macrolides in patients with pneumococcal pneumonia comes from analysis of a prospective cohort

Table 1. Summary of retrospective observational trials providing indirect evidence for an immunomodulatory effect of macrolides in pneumonia.

1st author [ref]	Number of patients	Effect of macrolide
Martinez [10]	409 patients with pneumococcal bacteremia	Addition of a macrolide to a β-lactam reduced the relative risk for death 2.5-fold
García Vázquez [11]	1391 patients with CAP	Therapy with β-lactam+ macrolide reduced mortality (6.9 %) compared to monotherapy with β-lactam (13.3 %)
Lodise [12]	2349 episodes of CAP and bacteremia	Independent factor connected with: ↓ in-hospital mortality, ↓ 30-day mortality
Metersky [13]	1560 patients with CAP	Therapy with β-lactam+ macrolide reduced mortality (18.4 %) than monotherapy with fluoroquinolone (36.6 %)
Restrepo [14]	237 patients with CAP and severe sepsis	Addition of a macrolide to antimicrobials decreased mortality in patients with macrolide-resistant pathogens

CAP: community-acquired pneumonia; ↓: reduction

of 638 Spanish patients. In these patients, addition of a macrolide to a β-lactam did not have any influence on mortality [15].

Lessons from Animal Studies

Clarithromycin was chosen as the most promising candidate among the macrolides for immunomodulation in sepsis. Selection was based on its *in vitro* efficacy and on its pharmacokinetics. *In vitro* studies showed that clarithromycin inhibited the production of interleukin (IL)-8 by both human monocytes and by monocytes of the THP-1 human leukemia cell line after stimulation with cell lysates of *P. aeruginosa* and of *Escherichia coli*. The effect of clarithromycin was dose-dependent and was greater at concentrations closer to 10 μg/ml in the growth medium; the effect was mediated through inhibition of nuclear factor-kappa B (NF-κB) [16]. Concentrations of clarithromycin in the epithelial lining fluid, which is the site of invading microorganisms in pneumonia, after oral administration range between 15 and 70 μg/ml [17]; those of azithromycin are equal to 1 μg/ml [18]. The need for concentrations close to 10 μg/ml to inhibit IL-8 production by monocytes, which are only achieved in the epithelial lining fluid by clarithromycin, led to its selection for further animal studies.

The efficacy of intravenously administered clarithromycin was tested in a series of animal studies [19–24]. Experimental sepsis was induced in rabbits by a model of complicated acute pyelonephritis closely resembling the human situation. In that model, the upper part of the ureter was ligated close to the renal pelvis and the offending pathogen was inoculated above the ligation inside the pelvis. Bacterial challenge was induced by bloodstream isolates from patients with severe sepsis. These isolates were antimicrobial-susceptible *E. coli*, multidrug-resistant *P. aeruginosa*, and pandrug-resistant *Klebsiella pneumoniae*. Clarithromycin did not affect *in vitro* bacterial growth of the selected isolates in time-kill assays. It was administered to animals either in parallel with bacterial inoculation or after bacterial challenge and upon presentation of signs of sepsis. These time windows for the administration of clarithromycin were selected in order to evaluate its efficacy in a model of late sepsis and to avoid past mistakes in which proposed immunomodulators were proven effective as pre-treatment but ineffective in clinical trials [25].

Clarithromycin was administered as either two consecutive intravenous doses for just one day or as one daily dose for three consecutive days. The rationale of dosing was to achieve serum levels close to 10 μg/ml. In all experiments, a single dose of amikacin was administered either alone or with clarithromycin. This was done in an attempt to simulate clinical practice where some antimicrobials are prescribed even for infections by multidrug-resistant pathogens. For infections by susceptible *E. coli* and multidrug-resistant *P. aeruginosa*, survival was the primary end-point. For infections by pandrug-resistant *K. pneumoniae*, animals were sacrificed at standard time intervals to assess tissue histopathology. Concentrations of endotoxins, TNF-α and malondialdehyde (MDA) were estimated in serum at serial time intervals. Blood monocytes were also isolated and assessed for their *ex vivo* release of TNF-α and for the intracellular activity of caspase-3.

Results from these animal studies [19–24] revealed that clarithromycin, either alone or in co-administration with amikacin, prolonged survival considerably. This was accompanied by improvement in oxygen saturation and heart rate. Although all animals had the same degree of endotoxemia and thus the same risk of developing

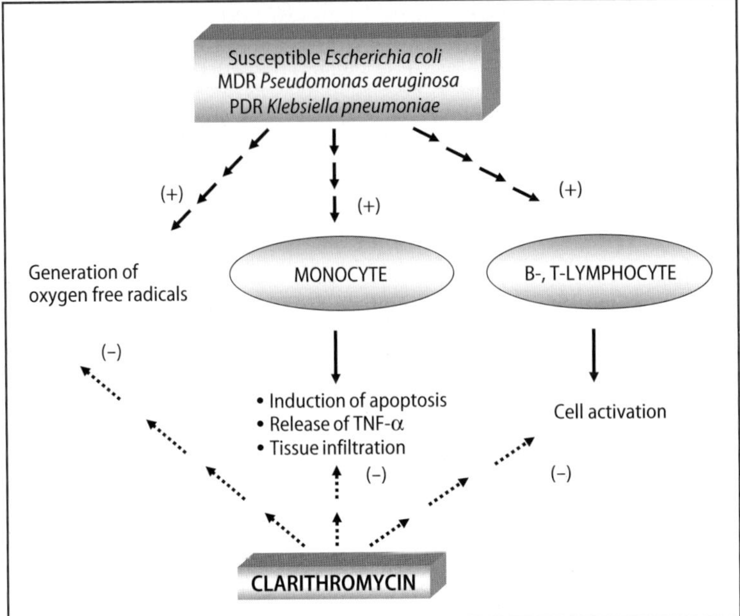

Fig. 1. Proposed mechanisms of action of clarithromycin based on experimental studies in sepsis. MDR: multidrug-resistant; PDR: pandrug-resistant; TNF: tumor necrosis factor; (+): activation; (–): inhibition

a septic reaction, those treated with clarithromycin had lower serum levels of TNF-α and MDA. This finding suggested attenuation of the systemic inflammatory response and of the generation of oxygen free radicals. Clarithromycin did not affect tissue growth of the test isolates. Pathology scores for the kidney, liver, lung and spleen were, however, lower among clarithromycin-treated animals than controls. More precisely, clarithromycin attenuated: a) peribronchial inflammation in the lung; b) mononuclear inflitration and necrosis in the liver and kidney; and c) activation of B- and T-cell rich areas in spleen. The effect of clarithromycin was most notable on the function of monocytes. Induction of apoptosis was attenuated as evidenced by a decrease in the intracellular activity of caspase-3; *ex vivo* release of TNF-α was also decreased.

The goal of the treatment regimen was achieved since serum levels of clarithromycin within two hours after the end of the infusion ranged between 5 and 10 μg/ml. The mode of action of clarithromycin, based on knowledge derived from animal studies, is summarized in **Figure 1**. Monocytes and lymphocytes appear to be the most likely cell targets of clarithromycin due to amelioration of the function of monocytes and to the reduction of tissue infiltration by mononuclear cells observed in animal studies.

Clinical Efficacy of Clarithromycin as an Immunomodulator in Sepsis

The promising results of experimental studies led us to design a randomized clinical trial of the immunomodulatory effect of clarithromycin in patients with sepsis. It is postulated that part of the failure of previous clinical trials with immunomodulators was due to the inclusion of heterogenous groups of patients, namely patients with sepsis caused by different types of infections [25]. In our trial, all patients had the same underlying infection causing sepsis, namely VAP. A total of 200 patients were enrolled in a prospective double-blind, placebo-controlled, randomized trial over the period June 2004-November 2005. Patients were allocated to either placebo or clarithromycin. One gram of clarithromycin diluted in 250 ml of 5 % glucose was infused within one hour through a central catheter once daily. This regimen was expected to provide serum levels of clarithromycin within those required to demonstrate its immunomodulatory properties, as assessed by preliminary pharmacokinetic studies [26]. The administered antimicrobials were selected by the attending physicians. Primary end-points were sepsis-related mortality, progression to multiple-organ dysfunction and resolution of VAP [27].

One hundred patients received placebo and another 100 patients received clarithromycin. There were no differences between groups in baseline characteristics, namely age, sex, APACHE II scores, and number of failing organs. All patients were screened for the underlying pathogen by quantitative cultures of tracheobronchial secretions. Cultures yielding a pathogen at a count $\geq 1 \times 10^6$ colony forming units (cfu)/ml were considered positive. There were no differences between the groups in the types of causative pathogens. Gram-negative bacteria alone were identified as underlying pathogens in 68 placebo-treated and 66 clarithromycin-treated patients. The most frequent pathogens were *Acinetobacter baumannii* in 43 and 36 patients, respectively, and *P. aeruginosa* in 12 and 17 patients, respectively. Based on the antibiograms of the pathogens, initial empirical antimicrobial coverage was active against 62.7 % of pathogens isolated from placebo-treated patients and against 75.4 % of pathogens isolated from clarithromycin-treated patients ($p = 0.44$ between groups). Tracheobronchial secretions were sampled again at follow-up. Eradication of the pathogen was achieved in 25.4 % and 33.8 % of cases, respectively, on day 5 ($p = 0.31$ between groups) and in 31.3 % and 29.2 % of cases, respectively, on day 10 ($p = 0.82$ between groups).

Sepsis-related mortality was 25 % in the placebo group and 23.3 % in the clarithromycin group. Odds ratio (OR) for death from septic shock and multiple organ failure was 19.00 (95 % confidence intervals: 5.64–64.03) in placebo-treated patients. It was reduced to 3.78 (95 % confidence intervals: 1.36–10.45) in clarithromycin-treated patients ($p = 0.043$ between groups). VAP resolved in 72.2 % of survivors treated with placebo and in 79.9 % of survivors treated with clarithromycin. Median time to resolution of VAP was 15.5 days in the placebo group and 10.0 days in the clarithromycin group. Comparative cumulative curves of the time to resolution of VAP for each treatment arm are shown in **Figure 2**. The mean clinical pulmonary infection scores (CPIS) for the placebo and the clarithromycin group on study enrolment were 7.92 and 7.62, respectively ($p = 0.29$). These decreased to 6.10 and 5.23, respectively, on day 5 of follow-up ($p = 0.016$) and to 5.88 and 5.09, respectively, on day 10 of follow-up ($p = 0.032$).

Weaning from mechanical ventilation was performed in 58.6 % of placebo-treated patients within a median period of 22.5 days, and in 72.5 % of clarithromycin-treated patients within a median period of 16.0 days. Comparative cumulative curves of the time to weaning for each treatment arm are shown in **Figure 3**. Eight and 14 patients of the placebo and clarithromycin groups, respectively, progressed to develop multiple organ failure. The mean time to progression to multiple organ failure was 3.38 and 5.78 days, respectively ($p = 0.047$ between groups). The two groups did not differ regarding the occurrence of serious adverse events.

III

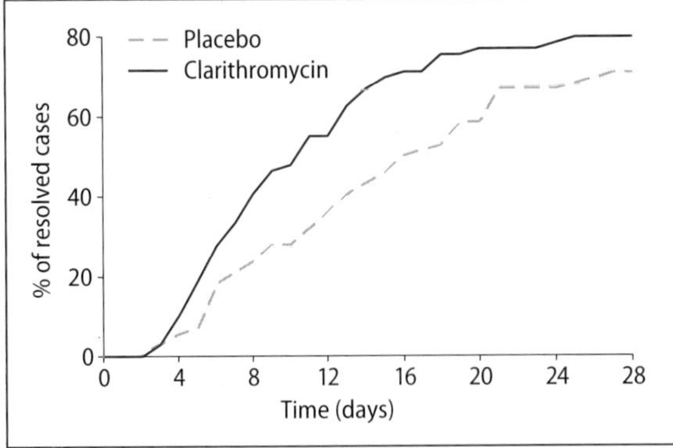

Fig. 2. Cumulative incidence of the resolution of ventilator-associated pneumonia (VAP) within the follow-up period of 28 days ($p = 0.011$ between groups). Analysis comprised survivors. From [27] with permission.

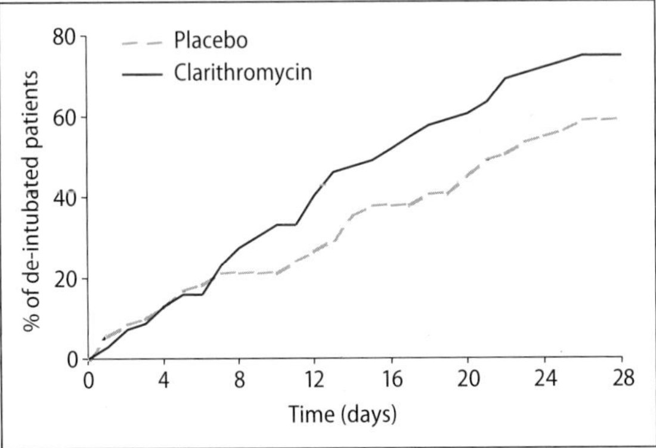

Fig. 3. Cumulative time to weaning from mechanical ventilation among placebo- and clarithromycin-treated patients ($p = 0.049$ between groups). Analysis comprised survivors. From [27] with permission.

The analysis of the randomized clinical trial [27] clearly showed that administration of clarithromycin was beneficial for the patients. This benefit was related to an improvement in the underlying infection and to an effect on the septic mechanism. The beneficial effect of clarithromycin in VAP was shown by: a) earlier resolution of VAP; and b) earlier weaning from mechanical ventilation. The effect of clarithromycin on the septic mechanism is supported by: a) the above mentioned similarities of both groups regarding disease severity and adequacy of antimicrobial therapy; b) the reduction in the relative risk of death due to septic shock and multiple organ dysfunction; and b) the prolongation of time to progression to multiple organ dysfunction.

Conclusion

Results of the trial discussed above [27] are very encouraging since statistical benefit was apparent with only 100 patients enrolled per treatment arm. However, to fully elucidate the future role of clarithromycin as an immunomodulator, further investigation is necessary. A second randomized trial in 600 patients with microbiologically or clinically documented sepsis by Gram-negative bacteria started in July 2007. This study is being conducted in six centers in Greece after approval by the National Ethics Committee (No 76306/13.06.2007) and the National Organization for Medicines (No 76305/15.02.2007). Enrolled patients have sepsis and primary or secondary Gram-negative bacteremia or intrabdominal infection or acute pyelonephritis. Clarithromycin seems a promising and safe new strategy for immunointervention in sepsis. The ongoing trial may verify its clinical efficacy.

References

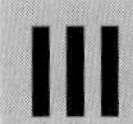

1. Heron M (2007) Deaths: leading causes for 2004. Natl Vital Stat Rep 56: 1–95
2. Engel C, Brunkhorst FM, Bone HG, et al (2007) Epidemiology of sepsis in Germany: results from a national prospective multicenter study. Intensive Care Med 33: 606–618
3. Hotchkiss RS, Karl IE (2003) The pathophysiology and treatment of sepsis. N Engl J Med 348: 138–150
4. Dellinger RP, Levy MM, Carlet JM, et al (2008) Surviving Sepsis Campaign: international guidelines for management of severe sepsis and septic shock: 2008. Crit Care Med 36: 296–327
5. Giamarellos-Bourboulis EJ (2008) Macrolides beyond the conventional antimicrobials: a class of potent immunomodulators. Int J Antimicrob Agents 31: 12–20
6. Wolter J, Seeney S, Bell S, Bowler S, Masel P, McCormack J (2002) Effect of long term treatment with azithromycin on disease parameters in cystic fibrosis: a randomized trial. Thorax 57: 212–216
7. Equi A, Balfour-Lynn IM, Bush A, Rosenthal M (2002) Long term azithromycin in children with cystic fibrosis: a randomized, placebo-controlled crossover trial. Lancet 360: 978–984
8. Saiman L, Marshall BC, Mayer-Hamblett N, et al (2003) Azithromycin in patients with cystic fibrosis chronically infected with *Pseudomonas aeruginosa*. A randomized controlled trial. JAMA 290: 1749–1756
9. Clement A, Tamalet A, Leroux E, Ravilly S, Fauroux B, Jais JP (2006) Long term effects of azithromycin in patients with cystic fibrosis: a double blind, placebo controlled trial. Thorax 61: 895–902
10. Martínez JA, Horcajada JP, Almela M, et al (2003) Addition of a macrolide to a beta-lactam-based empirical antibiotic regimen is associated with lower in-hospital mortality for patients with bacteremic pneumococcal pneumonia. Clin Infect Dis 36: 389–395
11. García Vázquez E, Mensa J, Martínez JA, et al (2005) Lower mortality among patients with community-acquired pneumonia treated with a macrolide plus a beta-lactam agent versus a beta-lactam agent alone. Eur J Clin Microbiol Infect Dis 24: 190–195
12. Lodise TP, Kwa A, Cosler L, Gupta R, Smith RP (2007) Comparison of β-lactam and macrolide combination therapy versus fluoroquinolone monotherapy in hospitalized veterans affairs patients with community-acquired pneumonia. Antimicrob Agents Chemother 51: 3977–3982
13. Metersky ML, Ma A, Houck PM, Bratzler DW (2007) Antibiotics for bacteremic pneumonia: improved outcomes with macrolides but not fluoroquinolones. Chest 131: 466–473
14. Restrepo MI, Mortensen EM, Waterer GW, Wunderink RG, Coalson JJ, Anzueto A (2009) Impact of macrolide therapy on mortality for patients with severe sepsis due to pneumonia. Eur Respir J (in press)
15. Aspa J, Rajas O, Rodriguez de Castro F, et al (2006) Impact of initial antibiotic choice on mortality from pneumococcal pneumonia. Eur Respir J 27: 1010–1019
16. Kikuchi T, Hagiwara K, Honda Y, et al (2002) Clarithromycin suppresses lipopolysaccharide-induced interleukin-8 production by human monocytes through AP-1 and NF-κB transcription factors. J Antimicrob Chemother 49: 745–755
17. Darkes MJ, Perry CM (2003) Clarithromycin extended-release tablet: a review of its use in the management of respiratory tract infections. Am J Respir Med 2: 175–201.
18. Danesi R, Lupetti A, Barbara C (2003) Comparative distribution of azithromycin in lung tissue of patients given oral daily doses of 500 and 1000 mg. J Antimicrob Chemother 51: 939–945
19. Giamarellos-Bourboulis EJ, Adamis T, Laoutaris G, et al (2004) Immunomodulatory clarithromycin treatment of experimental sepsis and acute pyelonephritis caused by multidrug-resistant *Pseudomonas aeruginosa*. Antimicrob Agents Chemother 48: 93–99

20. Giamarellos-Bourboulis EJ, Antonopoulou A, Raftogiannis M, et al (2006) Clarithromycin is an effective immunomodulator when administered late in experimental pyelonephritis by multidrug-resistant *Pseudomonas aeruginosa*. BMC Infect Dis 6: 31
21. Giamarellos-Bourboulis EJ, Baziaka F, Antonopoulou A, et al (2005) Clarithromycin co-administered with amikacin attenuates systemic inflammation in experimental sepsis by *Escherichia coli*. Int J Antimicrob Agents 25: 168–172
22. Giamarellos-Bourboulis EJ, Adamis T, Sabracos L, et al (2005) Clarithromycin: immunomodulatory therapy of experimental sepsis and acute pyelonephritis by *Escherichia coli*. Scand J Infect Dis 37: 48–54
23. Giamarellos-Bourboulis EJ, Tziortzioti V, Koutoukas P, et al (2006) Clarithromycin is an effective immunomodulator in experimental pyelonephritis caused by pan-resistant *Klebsiella pneumoniae*. J Antimicrob Chemother 57: 937–944.
24. Baziaka F, Giamarellos-Bourboulis EJ, Raftogiannis M, et al (2008) Immunomodulatory effect of three-day continuous administration of clarithromycin for experimental sepsis due to multidrug-resistant *Pseudomonas aeruginosa*. J Chemother 20: 63–68
25. Vincent JL, Sun Q, Dubois MJ (2003) Clinical trials of immunomodulatory therapies in severe sepsis and septic shock. Clin Infect Dis 34: 1084–1093
26. Giamarellos-Bourboulis EJ (2008) Immunomodulatory therapies for sepsis: unexpected effects with macrolides. Int J Antimicrob Agents (in press)
27. Giamarellos-Bourboulis EJ, Pechère JC, Routsi C, et al (2008) Effect of clarithromycin in patients with sepsis and ventilator-associated pneumonia. Clin Infect Dis 46: 1157–1164

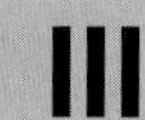

High-flow Hemofiltration as an Adjunctive Therapy in Sepsis

P.M. Honoré, O. Joannes-Boyau, and W. Boer

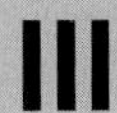

Introduction

Almost ten years ago, standard hemofiltration was often provided at 1 or 2 l/h of ultrafiltration and only in pre-dilution mode. However, practice began to change as results from new studies were published in the early 2000s demonstrating a beneficial effect on outcome of increasing the ultrafiltration rate to 35 ml/kg/h in patients with acute kidney injury (AKI). Two methods of high volume hemofiltration (HVHF), with different underlying concepts and results, became prevalent: Continuous high volume hemofiltration (CHVH) providing 50 to 70 ml/kg/h 24 hours a day, and intermittent high volume hemofiltration (IHVH) with brief, very high volume treatment at 100 to 120 ml/kg/h for 4 to 8 hours (previously called 'pulse' HVHF). Two recently published studies [1, 2] highlight the crucial role of adequate dosage of continuous venovenous hemofiltration (CVVH), demonstrating that, in critically ill patients with renal failure, a dose of 35 ml/kg/hour was associated with dramatic improvement in survival of nearly 20 %. The incorporation of the results from these studies into daily clinical practice can now be deemed to be urgent, although the results of other ongoing confirmatory (or not) studies are awaited. In a world increasingly guided by evidence based medicine, two level I studies lead to a Grade A recommendation, and this intervention should, therefore, be applied by every intensivist instigating continuous hemofiltration, while awaiting the results of the ongoing studies. Nevertheless, the implementation process is exposed to a number of potential difficulties. These encompass items such as blood flow requirements, vascular access problems, pre-and post-dilution policy, type of membranes used, as well as restitution fluid and the possible need for associated dialysis. Implementation of these findings will necessitate a collaborative network between medical staff members and the entire nursing staff.

Mechanism of Action: Hemofiltration as a New Shield against the 'Chaos Theory' and 'Complex Non-linear Systems' in Sepsis

Hemofiltration was first used in AKI, which is an independent factor for increased severity of illness and poor outcome in critically ill patients. Early studies had shown that the mortality rate of patients requiring renal replacement therapy (RRT) for AKI in the ICU was nearly twice as high compared to those without AKI (62.8 vs 38.5 %) [3, 4]. This suggests, therefore, that AKI is independently responsible for increased mortality, even if RRT is used. In fact, while standard RRT significantly reduced mortality in patients with AKI in comparison with mortality rates before

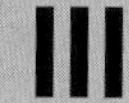

RRT was used, mortality rates were still not as low as in patients without AKI. The new concept of 'purification plasma challenge' was then developed to try to decrease mortality. Systemic inflammatory response syndrome (SIRS), sepsis and septic shock, and acute pancreatitis are known to be the leading causes of AKI in ICU patients, creating an immunologic disturbance with a cytokine storm. Sepsis and inflammatory pathologies disrupt homeostasis with a cellular and humoral response, generating secretion of cytokines such as interleukins and tumor necrosis factor (TNF)-α. Over the years, many attempts have been made to block some parts of the inflammatory cascade or to destroy specific components; some positive results were obtained in animal models but were not translated into clinical benefit [5]. It has been suggested that a large and non-specific reduction in cytokines in the blood compartment could in theory reduce mortality more than simply concentrating on removing or blocking one specific element [6]. However, this approach is complicated by the fact that neither the pharmacodynamics nor the pharmacokinetics of cytokines and other immune components are well known, not even their precise functions. Some of the leading theories in this field are provided by current experts in hemofiltration. First, the 'peak concentration hypothesis' of Ronco and Bellomo postulates that removing the peak cytokine concentration from the blood circulation during the early phase of sepsis could stop the inflammatory cascade and the accumulation of free cytokines, which are the leading cause of organ damage and homeostasis disruption [7, 8].

The second concept is called the 'threshold immunomodulation hypothesis', also called the 'Honore' concept [9, 10]. In this concept, the removal of cytokines does not only affect the cytokine concentration in the blood stream but also in the tissues. Indeed, when cytokine concentrations are reduced in the blood, blood and tissue concentrations may equilibrate to remove the immune components trapped in the organs. This could explain why no crucial reduction in cytokine concentration is observed in the blood stream during hemofiltration, because cytokines from the organs permanently replace those lost in the blood. The third theory, which has been proposed by Di Carlo, sheds new light on the mediator delivery hypothesis, in which the use of HVHF with a high volume of crystalloid fluids (3 to 5 l/hour) is able to increase the lymphatic flow by 20 to 40 fold [11, 12]. Indeed, this increase is correlated with the infusion of a high dose of fluids. Since cytokines and other immune components are transported by the lymphatic stream, this could explain their removal even though large amounts of cytokines were not found in ultrafiltration fluid [13]. Thus, the use of high volumes of exchange fluid might be the principal motor of cytokine removal.

To achieve a wider view of these theories, we need to explore the new paradigm of chaos and 'complex non-linear systems' in sepsis and SIRS [14]. The principal goal underlying these theories is not only removal of cytokines but also immunomodulation and control of the inflammatory response, which becomes deleterious when it surpasses its designed purpose. Indeed, the immune response of the host against septic aggression could be compared to a complex non-linear system which is defined by the infinite number of possible actions in response to a lone stimulus. In a complex non-linear system, e.g., the situation by which a flight of butterflies in China can change the weather in Boston three days later, a bacterial attack or cytokine secretion will have repercussions in the whole body. This explains why homeostasis is not a state of stability *per se* but rather the ability to stay stable while the status is permanently changing. Yet this incredible adaptability is halted when the system is drowned by an excess of information and when the 'endocrine effect' of cytokines and other immune messages are lost in the storm [15, 16]. The resources of the body system become depleted, and the complex non-linear system becomes a linear system, with only one course of action. This heralds the onset of multiple organ dysfunction syndrome. It may be that hemofiltration could play a role at this point by decreasing the cytokine storm and by allowing the efficacy of the immune messages to be recovered. Thus, the system's own resources increase, allowing a return of the complex non-linear system and homeostasis

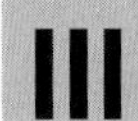

Recent Animal Trials and Clinical studies Highlighting the Crucial Roles of Dosing and Timing

Studies have shown benefits in terms of survival when 'early' and 'large' hemofiltration doses were applied in septic animals. Early use of hemofiltration has been thoroughly investigated in animal models [17, 18]. In most of the earlier studies, hemofiltration was used before or just after the injection of a bolus or even before the infusion of endotoxin. It was only in the late 1990s that investigators started to wait about 6 to 12 hours before using HVHF after a sepsis challenge, thereby 'allowing' the animals to become extremely ill, hemodynamically unstable, and to develop early multiple organ dysfunction before starting hemofiltration [19]. In this way, animal models were able to 'mimick' some aspects of the clinical situation. Only animal models in which HVHF was applied early proved to be very beneficial (some spectacularly), mainly due to the fact that in addition to early application, the investigators administered a much 'stronger' dose of HVHF. However, the differences between human and animal models do not allow these results to be extrapolated to humans. One of the greatest remaining problems with human studies (and especially the mechanistic studies) is the fact that the number of patients is very limited since the technique is so expensive. Moreover, clinical studies have fallen far short of the mean exchange obtained in animal models (only 40 ml/kg/h versus 100 ml/kg/h in animal studies) [20]. As a consequence, many effects seen in animal models can never be reproduced in human settings owing to the use of inadequate doses of HVHF. On the other hand, there is huge variability between clinical trials concerning the range of doses applied, ranging from 1 to 15 fold in the recent studies [20]. The foundations of the high volume technique were laid by Ronco and co-workers who showed that in their subgroup of sepsis patients, increasing the volume of treatment from 35 to 45 ml/kg/h could improve outcome [1]. That study effectively demonstrated that hemofiltration could be considered as a viable medication in the ICU. The volume of treatment not only has to be adapted to body weight but also to the severity of illness of ICU patients. If non-septic acute renal failure is being treated, then a lower dose may be optimal; however, a septic patient with AKI may need a higher dose close to 50 or 70 ml/kg/hour and perhaps even higher or with different modalities for catecholamine-resistant septic shock, refractory hypodynamic septic shock, or even acute severe pancreatitis. At the end of the 1990s, Journois et al. used HVHF (100 ml/kg/h) in 20 children during cardiac surgery and reported a reduction in postoperative blood loss, earlier extubation time, and reduced cytokine plasma levels [21]. The first large study using pulse HVHF, at about 100 ml/kg/hour for 4 consecutive hours (then 35 ml/kg/hour), was in 20 septic patients with refractory hypodynamic shock [22–24]. In this study, pulse HVHF-treated patients had a dramatically increased survival compared with classical treatment. The observed mortality (55 %) was significantly lower than that predicted by

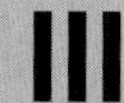

two severity scores (79 %). However, some patients were hemodynamic non-responders (9/20) with disastrous mortality rates. At the same time, a monocenter study by Oudemans Van Straaten and colleagues, with a prospective cohort design of mainly cardiac surgery patients with oliguria (306 patients), showed an observed mortality that was statistically lower in the group treated by intermittent HVHF with a mean volume of 3.8 l/h (nearly 50 ml/kg/h for a 70 kg patient) than the predicted mortality evaluated by three validated severity scores [25].

Studies in the early twentieth century concentrated on effects on hemodynamic response and cytokine removal; for example, Cole et al. showed interesting hemodynamic improvement in septic patients treated by HVHF [26]. Recently, a South American team headed by Cornejo did a study similar to that by Honoré et al. [22] and obtained comparable results [27]. They created an algorithm based on the international recommendations for sepsis treatment and incorporated intermittent HVHF (100 ml/kg/h for a single 12 hour period) as a salvage therapy for patients in refractory septic shock [27]. However, as in the study by Honoré et al. [22], although the observed mortality (40 %) was lower than the expected one (60 %), there was also a responder and a non-responder group. In contrast, Joannes-Boyau and colleagues studied the effect of HVHF at 50 ml/kg/h maintained for 96 hours in patients with septic shock with multiple organ dysfunction syndrome [28], and found that, although results in terms of mortality were comparable to those in previous studies (45 % observed vs 70 % predicted), all the patients were hemodynamic responders. A retrospective study by Piccinni et al. recently reported the same results with HVHF maintained at 45 ml/kg/h in 40 septic patients, in comparison with a historical group who were treated by standard CVVH [29]. Finally, a prospective study by Ratanarat et al. confirmed the earlier results of Honoré [22] and Cornejo [27], with a similar protocol of pulse HVHF (85 ml/kg/h for 6–8 hours) in 15 septic patients with multiple organ dysfunction syndrome [30]. All these studies were only single center, non-randomized and uncontrolled, but they all showed the same results and proved that HVHF can be delivered safely. The sole difference in results among the studies is in the occurrence of hemodynamic responders and non-responders in studies using intermittent hemofiltration which was not reported in studies using the continuous method.

A single study comparing HVHF with standard CVVH was conducted by Bouman et al.; 106 patients were randomized into three groups – early HVHF (within the first 12 hours of AKI), early standard CVVH, and late standard CVVH [31]. There were no differences in terms of 28-day mortality or recovery of renal function, but no statistical conclusions could be drawn owing to the lack of power, with only 35 patients in each group. Indeed, the very specific patient population, most coming from cardiac surgery, perhaps explains the low mortality rate, making the possibility of finding any statistical differences among the groups even more remote. Several studies, in particular in Asia, have also explored the effects of HVHF in severe acute pancreatitis. Wang et al. in animals [32] and humans [33] and Jiang et al. in humans [34] demonstrated the clinical benefit of HVHF in this context. They studied the effects of HVHF alone, or in comparison with standard CVVH, on mortality and organ function recovery and showed a clear benefit in using high volumes with early initiation.

While all these studies were promising, it is now time for larger studies and randomized controlled trials. The results from one such study, the so-called VA/NIH study were published in 2008 [35]. This was a very large and well conducted randomized study comparing two different doses of CRRT (20 vs 35 ml/kg/h) and two different intensities of intermittent RRT depending on the hemodynamic status of the patient; nevertheless several criticisms have been made [36, 37], including regarding the supposed 35 ml/kg dose of CVVH in the intensive treated group which was split into 18 ml/kg/h of dialysis (1500 ml/h) and 17 ml/kg/h of convection rate, giving an actual dose of roughly 15 ml/kg/h (when taking into account the pre-dilution modality instead of full post-dilution). Additionally, the patients were enrolled in the study after being a mean of roughly 7 days in the ICU and roughly 10 days in the hospital which represents a considerably longer delay in treatment than used in any other study. Of note also, more than 65 % of the patients received either intermittent hemodialysis or sustained low efficiency dialysis (SLED) treatment within 24 hours prior to the randomization. Needless to say, the results of the ANZICS clinical trials group renal study (clinicaltrials.gov number NCT00221013) comparing augmented with normal RRT in severe acute renal failure are eagerly awaited.

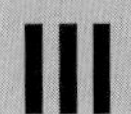

A recent animal study has also highlighted the direct action of hemofiltration on the cellular mitochondria of the septic myocardium [38]. Indeed, this study was able to demonstrate that hemofiltration could reverse the negative effects of sepsis on myocardial mitochondrial respiratory chain complex activity in porcine septic shock [38]. This study could be seen as the missing link between the hemodynamic effects of HVHF and its effects on outcome.

Practical Aspects for the Bedside Clinician

New treatment volumes imply changes in hemofiltration practice so as to guarantee the efficacy and safety of the technique. Indeed, to reach 60 or 100 ml/kg/h of treatment volume, important principles need to be respected. First, a high blood flow is necessary to maintain a filtration fraction below 25 %, a level above which 'protein cake' clogging in the membrane becomes a major concern. In our practice, in order to attain an exchange flow of 35 ml/kg/h even in very heavy patients (up to 120 kg), we have, for nearly 8 years, used a constant high blood flow of 300 ml/min which allows the clinician to run a hemofiltration device at 35 ml/kg/h with a filtration fraction below 25 % even in patients with a body weight of 120 kg as long as the blood flow is equal to 300 ml/min (**Table 1**). However, to attain such a blood flow, excellent vascular access is required, with a large catheter (13.5 or 14 French), using an adequate location (right jugular is the best followed by femoral approach, while the subclavian route should not to be used) [39] and good structure (coaxial with 360° arterial intake). Second, the best restitution fluid is probably buffered bicarbonate and should be administered 1/3 in pre-dilution and 2/3 in post-dilution, i.e., the best compromise between loss of treatment efficacy and optimization of blood rheology [40]; in patients with citrate anticoagulation, the proportions of pre-and post-dilution might be different [41]. The choice of membrane is also primordial and a highly biocompatible synthetic filter with a high exchange surface is recommended (1.7 to 2.1 m^2). Temperature control is not important with low fluid exchange volumes but becomes essential when the volume increases dramatically. Two systems are possible for temperature control: Heating the fluid before restitution or heating the blood directly. Empirically heating the replacement fluid seems preferable to heating the blood, owing to possible deleterious effects of high temperatures on the blood. However, to date no problems have been recorded and the two systems have demonstrated their safety and efficacy. The new machines specifically dedicated to high volumes have extremely sensitive and precise pressure control and volume bal-

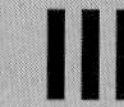

Table 1. How to reach an exchange flow of 35 ml/kg/h with a fixed blood flow of 300 ml/min

Weight/kg	Therapeutic dose 35 ml/kg/h	Pre-Dilution 1/3 therapeutic dose	Post-Dilution 2/3 therapeutic dose	
50	1800	600	1200	
55	1900	600	1300	
60	2100	700	1400	
65	2300	800	1500	FF.13 %
70	2400	800	1600	
75	2600	900	1700	
80	2700	900	1800	
85	3000	1000	2000	
90	3200	1100	2100	FF.17 %
95	3300	1100	2200	
100	3500	1200	2300	
105	3700	1200	2500	
110	3900	1300	2600	
115	4000	1300	2700	
120	4200	1400	2800	FF.23 %

FF: filtration fraction

ance functions. Furthermore, it is important to stay in the normal pressure range for optimal use of high flow hemofiltration. Indeed, staying below -120 mmHg of arterial pressure is indicative of a catheter problem and likely early machine failure. The same is true with a venous line, where high pressure indicates catheter or bubble trap clotting. The transmembrane pressure reflects the state of clogging in the filter while a high pressure indicates that many fibers are clogged. To alleviate the pressure problem, it is recommended that treatment is stopped when the patient is being nursed or moved, especially with high volumes. HVHF also requires adequate management and control of fluid exchange and small solutes. In fact, small molecules are largely removed during hemofiltration and strict monitoring of sodium, glucose, and acid-base balance is mandatory. Detection of infection during hemofiltration may be difficult as this technique can blunt hyperthermia but recent studies have showed interesting new tools for early detection of infection in these conditions [42]. Adaptation of antimicrobials during HVHF is also crucial in order to avoid underdosing [43]. Finally, on-line techniques may be crucial in the future [44]. Widespread application of fluid substitution in hemofiltration at 35 ml/kg/h remains surprisingly lacking; despite the evidence, recent unpublished surveys have shown that less than 50 % of units are applying this scientifically sound regimen.

Future Directions Regarding the Use of Hemofiltration in Sepsis

In terms of recommendations for clinical practice, patients with septic AKI should receive a renal replacement dose of at least 35 ml/kg/hour (level II evidence and grade C recommendation) [45] and probably a higher dose if they have septic shock. As discussed earlier, the VA/NIH study did not have enough power to change this recommendation in view of its shortcomings [36, 37]. Catecholamine-resistant septic

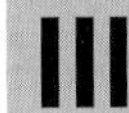

shock, either hypo- or hyperdynamic, could be seen as an indication for HVHF (level V evidence and grade E recommendation) for clinicians experienced in HVHF therapies [23, 24, 45]. However, HVHF should be integrated into practice algorithms for use as a salvage therapy in ICUs as no other treatment has proved its efficacy in these patients with a very high risk of mortality [27]. HVHF should be reserved for patients with AKI; although the benefit of early treatment has been shown, initiating RRT before renal injury is not yet recommended. In fact, the best time to start hemofiltration may be the renal injury state (creatinine × 2 from baseline or oliguria < 0.5 ml/kg over the preceding 12 hours) from the RIFLE (Risk, Injury, Failure, Loss, and End-stage Kidney) classification which could represent the best compromise between early initiation and renal impairment [46]. To evaluate HVHF, more, larger prospective randomized studies are needed which must respect certain conditions. First, the safest technique must be used, but this requirement is the easiest to meet as new hemofiltration machines are much safer and more efficient. Second, we need to define the exact time to start hemofiltration in relation to the start of sepsis and AKI. The best policy is to use a common classification for AKI, such as RIFLE, and to start in the first 24 hours following the onset of sepsis. Third, it is of primordial importance to define the volume of treatment according to body size in ml/kg/h. Finally, we should develop a greater understanding of the mechanisms of sepsis and SIRS in order to identify the targets for HVHF. In future trials, it would be interesting to detect any potential interference or possible synergy between HVHF and drotrecogin alfa (activated), for example. The best design for the use of hemofiltration still remains to be defined and the sequences and the duration of high volume 'rushes' need to be established [47]. Although prolonged HVHF seems more able to stop the initial inflammatory storm and late immunoparalysis, the efficiency and practicability of pulse high volume should be explored. While several large randomized trials are currently in progress investigating hemofiltration doses in AKI patients, only one is comparing HVHF with standard CVVH (The IVOIRE (hIgh VOlume in Intensive Care) study, clinicaltrials.gov ID NCT00241228). This study will try to expand the findings of the initial study by Ronco and colleagues [1] to septic patients. Indeed, this large randomized study will include patients with septic shock plus AKI, as defined by the RIFLE classification. After computerized randomization, patients will receive HVHF at either 35 or 70 ml/kg/h. This study will try to demonstrate that 'higher' doses (i.e., 70 ml/kg/hour) will further improve the survival rate from septic AKI in ICU patients at 28, 60, and 90 days. The first interim analysis will be performed when 150 patients have been included and this is expected to happen sometime in 2009.

Conclusion

The use of hemofiltration has steadily increased in the last decade, from a simple treatment for AKI to adjunctive therapy for sepsis or other acute episodes of SIRS, such as acute pancreatitis. The story is continuing to evolve and we can be sure that with the development of further technology and better understanding of the pathology, hemofiltration doses and the efficacy of the machines will be better defined. For the moment, 35 ml/kg/h should be the standard hemofiltration dose in ICUs for all patients with AKI, while in some situations, like sepsis, the dose should be increased as a salvage therapy in view of the high mortality rates in these patients. However, more trials are needed before HVHF can be recommended as routine treatment in

ICUs, in order to determine the best scheme of use and to obtain some form of consensus. In recent years, a number of techniques have been studied and developed in the field of RRT in the septic patient. Manipulation of ultrafiltrate dose, membrane porosity, mode of clearance, and combinations of techniques have yielded promising findings. However, at present, conclusive evidence based on well designed, randomized controlled trials remains scarce, limiting the practical implementation of many techniques in daily practice outside the context of a study. From the few well designed and documented studies that we have so far, it is safe to say that optimalization of delivered dose in RRT has a proven positive effect. An ultrafiltration rate between 35 and 45 ml/kg/h, with adjustment for predilution and down time, can be recommended for the septic patient until other data are available. The results of further dose outcome studies with higher ultrafiltration rates will likely be the stepping stone to further improvements in daily clinical practice. Hybrid techniques will also likely have a role in the expanding field of RRT in the septic patient in the near future [48, 49].

References

1. Ronco C, Bellomo R, Homel P, et al (2000) Effects of different doses in continuous veno-venous haemofiltration. Lancet 356: 26–30
2. Saudan P, Niederberger M, De Seigneux S, et al (2006) Adding a dialysis dose to continuous hemofiltration increases survival in patients with acute renal failure. Kidney Int 70: 1312–1317
3. Metnitz PG, Krenn CG, Steltzer H, et al (2002) Effects of acute renal failure requiring renal replacement therapy on outcome in critically ill patients. Crit Care Med 30: 2051–2058
4. Mehta RL, McDonald B, Gabbai FB, et al (2001) Collaborative Group for treatment of ARF in the ICU. A randomized clinical trial of continuous versus intermittent dialysis for acute renal failure. Kidney Int 60: 1154–1163
5. Hotchkiss RS, Karl IE (2003) The pathophysiology and treatment of sepsis. N Engl J Med 348: 138–150
6. Ronco C, Bellomo R (2002) Acute renal failure and multiple organ dysfunction in the ICU: from renal replacement therapy (RRT) to multiple organ support therapy (MOST). Int J Artif Organs 25: 733–747
7. Ronco C, Tetta C, Mariano F, Wratten ML, Bonello M, Bellomo R (2003) Interpreting the mechanism of continuous renal replacement therapy in sepsis. The peak concentration hypothesis. Artif Organs 27: 792–801
8. Ronco C, Ricci Z, Bellomo R (2002) Importance of increased ultrafiltration volume and impact on mortality: sepsis and cytokine story and the role for CVVH. EDTRA ERCA J 2: 13–18
9. Honore PM, Joannes-Boyau O, Boer W, Gressens B (2007) High volume haemofiltration and hybrid techniques in sepsis: New insights into the rationale. Neth J Crit Care 11: 239–242
10. Honore PM, Joannes-Boyau O, Gressens B (2007) Blood and plasma treatments: the rationale of high-volume hemofiltration. Contrib Nephrol 156: 387–395
11. Di Carlo JV, Alexander SR (2005) Hemofiltration for cytokine-driven illness: the mediator delivery hypothesis. Int J Artif Organs 28: 777–786
12. Olszewski WL (2003) The lymphatic system in body homeostasis: physiological conditions. Lymphat Res Biol 1: 11–24
13. Klouche K, Cavadore P, Portales P, Clot J, Canaud B, Beraud JJ (2002) Continuous veno-venous hemofiltration improves hemodynamics in septic shock with acute renal failure without modifying TNF-α and IL-6 plasma concentrations. J Nephrol 15: 150–157
14. Seely AJ, Christou NV (2000) Multiple organ dysfunction syndrome: exploring the paradigm of complex nonlinear systems. Crit Care Med 28: 2193–2200
15. Mayer J, Rau B, Gansauge F, Beger HG (2000) Inflammatory mediators in human acute pancreatitis : clinical and pathopysiological implications. Gut 47: 542–552
16. Ertel W, Kremer JP, Kenney J, et al (1995) Down regulation of proinflammatory cytokine release in whole blood from septic patients. Blood 85: 1341–1347
17. Grootendorst AF, van Bommel EF, van der Hoeven B, van Leengoed LA, van Osta AL (1992)

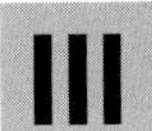

High volume hemofiltration improves right ventricular function in endotoxin-induced shock in the pig. Intensive Care Med 18: 235–240

18. Grootendorst AF, van Bommel EF, van Leengoed LA, Nabuurs M, Bouman CS, Groeneveld AB (1994) High volume hemofiltration improves hemodynamics and survival of pigs exposed to gut ischemia and reperfusion. Shock 2: 72–78
19. Rogiers P, Zhang H, Smail N, Pauwels D, Vincent JL (1999) Continuous venovenous hemofiltration improves cardiac performance by mechanisms other than tumor necrosis factor-alpha attenuation during endotoxic shock. Crit Care Med 27: 1848–1855
20. Honoré PM, Zydney AL, Matson JR (2003) High volume and high permeability haemofiltration in sepsis. The evidences and the key issues. Care Crit Ill 3: 69–76
21. Journois D, Israel-Biet D, Pouard P, et al (1996) High volume, zero-balanced hemofiltration to reduce delayed inflammatory response to cardiopulmonary bypass in children. Anesthesiology 85: 965–976
22. Honoré PM, Jamez J, Wauthier M, et al (2000) Prospective evaluation of short term high volume isovolemic haemofiltration on the haemodynamic course and outcome in patients with intractable circulatory failure resulting from septic shock. Crit Care Med 28: 3581–3587
23. Honoré PM, Joannes-Boyau O (2004) High volume hemofiltration (HVHF) in sepsis: a comprehensive review of rationale, clinical applicability, potential indications and recommendations for future research. Int J Artif Organs 27: 1077–1082
24. Matson JR, Zydney RL, Honoré PM (2004) Blood filtration : New opportunities and the implications on system biology. Crit Care Resusc;6: 209–218
25. Oudemans-van Straaten HM, Bosman RJ, van der Spoel JI, Zandstra DF (1999) Outcome of critically ill patients treated with intermittent high-volume haemofiltration: a prospective cohort analysis. Intensive Care Med 25: 814–821
26. Cole L, Bellomo R, Journois D, Davenport P, Baldwin I, Tipping P (2001) High-volume haemofiltration in human septic shock. Intensive Care Med 27: 978–986
27. Cornejo R, Downey P, Castro R, et al (2006) High-volume hemofiltration as salvage therapy in severe hyperdynamic septic shock. Intensive Care Med 32: 713–722
28. Joannes-Boyau O, Rapaport S, Bazin R, Fleureau C, Janvier G (2004) Impact of high volume hemofiltration on hemodynamic disturbance and outcome during septic shock. ASAIO J 50: 102–109
29. Piccinni P, Dan M, Barbacini S, et al (2006) Early isovolaemic haemofiltration in oliguric patients with septic shock. Intensive Care Med 32: 80–86
30. Ratanarat R, Brendolan A, Piccinni P, et al (2005) Pulse-high volume haemofiltration for treatment of severe sepsis: effects on hemodynamics and survival. Crit Care 9: 294–302
31. Bouman CS, Oudemans-Van-Straaten HM, Tijssen JG, Zandstra DF, Kosecioglu J (2002) Effects of early high-volume continuous venovenous hemofiltration on survival and recovery of renal function in intensive care patients with acute renal failure: a prospective, randomized trial. Crit Care Med 30: 2205–2211
32. Wang H, Zhang ZH, Yan XW, et al (2005)Amelioration of haemodynamics an oxygen metabolism by continuous veno venous hemofiltration in experimental pancreatitis. Word J Gastroenterol 11: 127–131
33. Wang H, Li WQ, Zhou W, Li N, Li JS (2003) Clinical effects of continuous high volume hemofiltration on severe acute pancreatitis complicated with multiple organ dysfunction syndrome. World J Gastroenterol 9: 2096–2099
34. Jiang HL, Xhue WJ,Li DK, et al (2005) Influence of continuous veno-venous hemofiltration on the course of acute pancreatitis. World J Gastroenterol 11: 4815–4821
35. Palevsky PM, Zhang JH, O'Connor TZ, et al (2008) Intensity of renal support in critically ill patients with acute kidney injury. N Engl J Med 359: 7–20
36. Ronco C, Honore PM (2008) Renal support in critically ill patients with acute kidney injury. N Engl J Med 359: 1959
37. Ronco C, Cruz D, Oudemans-van-Straaten HM, Honoré PM, House A, Bin D, Gibney N (2008) Dialysis dose in acute kidney injury: no time for therapeutic nihilism-a critical appraisal of the Acute Renal Failure Trial Network study. Crit Care 12: 308
38. Li CM, Chen JH, Zhang P, et al (2007) Continuous veno-venous haemofiltration attenuates myocardial mitochondrial respiratory chain complexes activity in porcine septic shock. Anaesth Intensive Care 35: 911–919

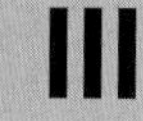

39. Mandolfo S, Galli F, Costa S, Ravani P, Gaggia P, Imbasciati E (2001) Factors influencing permanent catheter performance. J Vasc Access 2: 106–109
40. Ricci Z, Ronco C (2005) Pre- versus post-dilution CVVH. Blood Purif 23: 338–342
41. Nurmohamed SA, Vervloet MG, Girbes AR, Ter Wee PM, Groeneveld AB (2007) Continuous venovenous hemofiltration with or without predilution regional citrate anticoagulation: a prospective study. Blood Purif 25: 316–323
42. Ratanarat R, Cazzavillan S, Ricci Z, et al (2007) Usefulness of a molecular strategy for the detection of bacterial DNA in patients with severe sepsis undergoing continuous renal replacement therapy. Blood Purif 25: 106–111
43. Arzuaga A, Isla A, Gascon AR, Maynar J, Corral E, Pedraz JL (2006) Elimination of piperacillin and tazobactam by renal replacement therapies with AN69 and polysulfone hemofilters: evaluation of the sieving coefficient. Blood Purif 24: 347–354
44. Kooman JP, van der Sande FM, Beerenhout CM, Leunissen KM (2006) On-line filtration therapies: emerging horizons. Blood Purif 24: 159–162
45. Bellomo R, Honoré PM, Matson JR, Ronco C, Winchester J (2005) Extracorporeal blood treatment (EBT) methods in SIRS/Sepsis. Consensus statement. Position paper. ADQI III Conference. Int J Artif Organs 28: 450–458
46. Bellomo R, Kellum JA, Mehta R, Ronco C (2002) The Acute Dialysis Quality Initiative II: the Vicenza conference. Adv Ren Replace Ther 9 290–293
47. Tetta C, Bellomo R, Kellum J, et al (2004) High volume hemofiltration in critically ill patients: why, when and how? Contrib Nephrol 144: 362–375
48. Honore PM, Joannes-Boyau O, Gressens B (2007) Blood and plasma treatments: High-volume hemofiltration – A global view. Contrib Nephrol 156: 371–386
49. Honore PM, Joannes-Boyau O, Meurson L, et al (2006) The Big Bang of haemofiltration: the beginning of a new era in the third Millennium for extra-corporeal blood purification! Int J Artif Organs 2006 29: 649–659

Economic and Social Burden of Severe Sepsis

E. Silva and D.V. Araujo

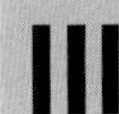

Introduction

Sepsis is highly prevalent within intensive care units (ICUs) and is associated with elevated rates of morbidity and mortality [1–3], and high costs [4–7]. For these reasons, healthcare providers, managers, government authorities, and insurance companies have focused their attention on strategies that could reduce the economic and social burden of sepsis. In the healthcare system, ICUs consume a considerable amount of resources and have frequently been considered the target for efforts to reduce escalating medical expenses.

The direct cost of caring for patients with sepsis has been shown to be 6-fold higher than caring for ICU patients without sepsis [8]. According to data from the US, each septic patient consumes, during hospitalization, about US$ 25,000, corresponding to approximately $ 17 billion annually [9]. These figures may increase when patients progress to septic shock and multiple organ dysfunction and require highly expensive therapeutic and diagnostic interventions, and a longer hospital stay [10].

In parallel, indirect costs have also been estimated as being excessively elevated. These costs, also called social costs, result from the productivity loss associated with absenteeism or early mortality. Indirect costs are those resulting from lack of productivity of an employee who is hospitalized or in ambulatory care or temporarily hindered from work. Indirect costs of sepsis have been estimated as 2–3 times the direct costs.

This chapter will describe the main studies addressing the direct and indirect costs of sepsis, as well as the cost and cost-effectiveness of sepsis treatment protocols.

Concepts

Before describing the main data regarding the cost of sepsis management, we will review some concepts related to health economic analyses which will be used in this chapter. The reason for this brief review is to standardize these concepts and to provide the reader with guidelines for reporting or interpreting economic analyses. This concern is not unfounded. Heyland and co-workers demonstrated that, from more than 1,000 studies that addressed intensive care costs, only three met minimal criteria for scientific rigor [11]. Many of the concepts and guidelines we will use were proposed in 1996 by the US Public Health Service Panel on Cost-effectiveness in Health and Medicine (PCEHM) for the conduct and reporting of economic analyses [12].

1) **Costs** – Usually expressed in monetary terms, costs are a measure of what we forfeit to achieve a utility or acquire an item.

2) **Direct costs** – Direct costs are those resulting directly from health interventions. They are divided into medical and non-medical costs. Direct medical costs stem from hospitalization, complementary exams, medications, prostheses and ortheses, among other products and services. Non-medical direct costs typically include the costs of transporting the patient to the hospital and fees for the temporary hiring of personnel to look after the patient during the recovery period

3) **Indirect costs** – As mentioned, indirect costs result from the productivity loss associated with absenteeism or early mortality. Indirect costs are those resulting from lack of productivity of an employee who is hospitalized or is in ambulatory care or temporarily hindered from work.

4) **Opportunity-cost** or economic opportunity loss – This represents the value of a product forgone to produce or obtain another product. Opportunity cost is a key concept in economics because it implies the choice between desirable, yet mutually exclusive results. The notion of opportunity cost plays a crucial part in ensuring that scarce resources are used efficiently.

5) **Top-down and bottom-up approaches** – There are two approaches to estimating unit costs: The top-down and the bottom-up approaches. The top-down approach divides the total expenditure on a service by units of activity. Units of activity are specific to the services for costing, for example, the cost per day of a hospital stay or the cost of a general practice consultation. The top-down approach also uses aggregated data along with a population-attributable fraction to calculate the attributable costs. The bottom-up approach is more comprehensive and involves more detailed costing of all the elements used to cost the service. The different resources used to deliver the service are identified and a value is assigned to each, these values are then summed and linked to an appropriate unit of activity to generate the unit cost. A number of reports and papers provide more details on how to measure and value costs [13–15].

6) **Developing the cost estimate (micro-costing)** – three basic steps are required to build a cost estimate (micro-costing) including identification, quantification, and valuation. The first step is building a resource use profile by determining which health care services are relevant for each therapy (identification). The next step is achieved by identifying the frequency of use and the proportion of users for each health care service in the profile (quantification). The last step is to apply a unit cost to each resource used (valuation).

7) **Quality-adjusted life-year (QALY)** - The QALY is a measure of health outcomes, known as a utility, which incorporates both the duration and quality of survival. Quality of life must be expressed as a numeric value ranging from 0 to 1, and the duration of time that a patient exists in that state is adjusted by the quality of life of being in that state.

8) **Efficacy versus effectiveness** – Efficacy describes the clinical effects under ideal circumstances (usually a controlled clinical trial). Effectiveness describes the clinical effects under typical 'real world' circumstances, where patients are not carefully selected and practice is not carefully monitored.

9) **Cost–effectiveness analysis** (CEA) – This produces a ratio, such as the cost per year of life gained, where the denominator reflects the gain in health from a specific intervention (e.g., life-years gained, number of additional survivors, or number of pneumonias averted) and the numerator reflects the cost in dollars of obtaining that gain [16].

10) **Cost utility** - This is a type of cost-effectiveness where effects are expressed as utilities, such as quality-adjusted survival, facilitating comparisons across different diseases and interventions (e.g., QALYs). From here forward, we use the standard terminology in which CEA refers to both cost-effectiveness and cost-utility analyses.

11) **Cost (burden) of illness** - Direct and indirect costs related to a specific disease.

12) **Budget impact analysis** - While economic evaluation of the efficient allocation of healthcare resources plays a useful role to healthcare purchasers, it is unable to address the issue of affordability. In addition to maximizing efficiency, healthcare purchasers must also strive to simply remain within their annual budgets.

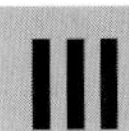

13) **Perspective** - It is important to know the perspective of an analysis in order to determine what the content of the cost profile will be. In many countries, the societal perspective is the one of choice for an economic analysis and indirect costs play a larger role in the decision-making process. In other countries the perspective of a third party payer responsible for the cost of comprehensive care is frequently the viewpoint of the analysis and direct medical costs are those that drive the decision process.

14) **Friction cost method** - This is a modification of the human capital method to calculate indirect costs. Whereas in the human capital method the economic costs (productivity losses) are calculated for the period from the beginning of the illness until the end of the age of gainful employment, this period is shortened in the friction cost method to the so called 'friction period', which corresponds to the length of time until the position in question is filled again.

Direct Costs of Sepsis Management

Direct medical costs associated with severe sepsis primarily consist of hospital costs. The main components of these costs can be divided into blocks according to the proposal by Edbrooke and co-workers [6]. These and other authors reported that personnel costs (for nurses, physicians, technicians, and assistants) consume from 45 to 60 % of the total ICU budget. Compared with the large proportion of personnel costs, other fixed costs (such as non-clinical support services, equipment, and rent and maintenance costs for building and properties) have a minor impact on the total costs of intensive care. Variable costs including drugs, other consumables, laboratory and diagnostic services, amounted to only 30 % of total costs [6].

Comparing this cost distribution per ICU patient-day with severe sepsis patient-day, personnel related costs are still extremely relevant. However, as demonstrated in **Figure 1**, drugs amount to 40 % of total costs [4]. Combining these data, we can easily conclude that an effective reduction in costs for a patient with severe sepsis in the ICU, could be achieved either by shortening length of stay, since a large proportion

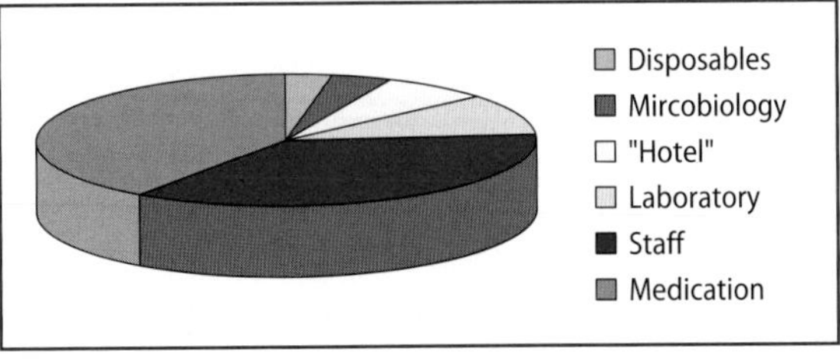

Fig. 1. Distribution of costs for intensive care unit (ICU) treatment of severe sepsis from three German university hospitals (1997–2000) [4].

of costs are fixed, or by reducing drug consumption. Later on, we will discuss how an integrated protocol of sepsis management could impact on those variables.

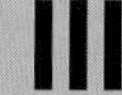

Some studies have reported the costs of sepsis management. For instance, Angus et al. [9] reported a total hospital cost of US$ 22,100 in a retrospective study in ICU and non-ICU septic patients in the United States. In this study, ICU septic patients were more severely ill, with longer lengths of stay (23.3 vs. 15.6 days, $p < 0.0001$) and cost more ($29,900 vs. $13,900, $p < 0.0001$) than non-ICU patients, In similar populations, Braun et al. [17] and Moerer et al. [4] reported even higher costs ranging from US$ 26,820 to €23,296 per patient. Costs have also varied depending on severity of the disease and outcome. Chalfin et al. [18] analyzed 1,405 patients and estimated mean total charges of $38,304 in survivors and $49,182 in non-survivors. Similarly, Brun-Buisson et al. [10], in an elegant study, reported costs from €26,256 to €35,185 depending on the severity of illness. However, a simple and direct comparison among all those studies is not feasible. Country-specific health care systems, reimbursement rates and regulations, as well as different cost and pricing factors prevent an easy comparison. Additionally, the case mix for sepsis should be taken into account. Therefore, in contrast to the findings of clinical studies, results of economic evaluations cannot be readily transferred from one country to another.

Direct Costs of Sepsis Management in Developing Countries: A Brazilian Experience

We performed a multicenter, prospective study to evaluate costs of septic patients in Brazilian ICUs [19]. Twenty-one ICUs and 524 septic patients were enrolled in this study. By using a bottom-up approach we collected every diagnostic and therapeutic intervention performed in these patients daily. Standard unit costs (year 2006 values) were based on the Brazilian Medical Association (AMB) price index for medical procedures and the BRASINDICE price index for medications, solutions and hospital consumables. Medical resource utilization was also assessed daily using the Therapeutic Intervention Scoring System (TISS)-28. Direct costs outside the ICU and indirect costs were not included.

The median total cost of sepsis was US$ 9632 (interquartile [IQ] range 4583–18387; 95 % CI 8657, 10672) per patient, while the median daily ICU cost per patient was $ 934 (IQ 735–1170; 95 % CI 897, 963). The median daily ICU cost per patient was significantly higher in non-survivors than in survivors ($ 1094 [IQ 888–1341; 95 % CI 1058, 1157] and $ 826 [IQ 668–982; 95 % CI 786, 854], $p < 0.001$). Interestingly in our study, the costs of non-survivors increased day-by-day while the costs of survivors decreased after the first few days (**Fig. 2**). In other words, we observed an increasing pattern in daily costs associated with death while survivors showed a decreasing pattern, indicating an increased use of resources in non-survivors. To our knowledge, this pattern of increasing daily costs has not previously been demonstrated. These data support that a surviving patient will use less sophisticated therapy upon his or her convalescence, as opposed to the non-survivors. This finding also suggests that those patients who receive effective treatment and respond to it will develop less organ dysfunction and consequently have reduced costs. In this context, an evidence-based approach can rationally provide the most effective management, increasing survival rates and, at the least, not increasing expenses.

For patients admitted to public and private hospitals, we found median sequential organ failure assessment (SOFA) scores at ICU admission of 7.5 and 7.1, respectively

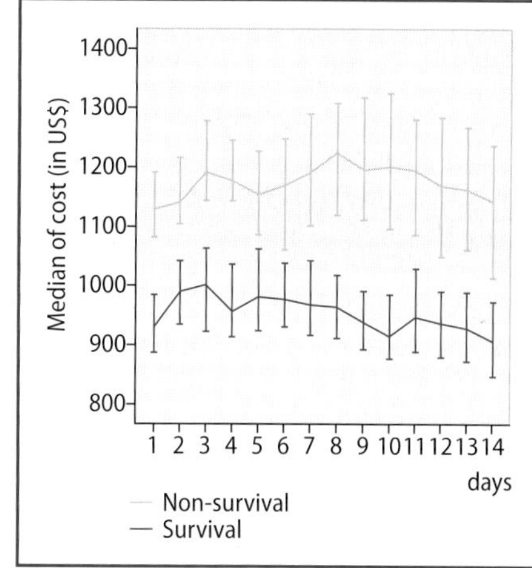

Fig. 2. Median daily ICU costs including error bars (95 % CI) for surviving and non-surviving septic patients. From [19] with permission

(p = 0.02), and the mortality rate was 49.1 % and 36.7 %, respectively (p = 0.006). Patients admitted to public and private hospitals had a similar length of stay of 10 (IQ 5–19) days versus 9 (IQ 4–16) days (p = 0.091), and the median total direct costs for public ($US 9773; IQR 4643–19 221; 95 % CI 8503, 10 818) versus private ($US 9490; IQR 4305–17 034; 95 % CI 7610, 11 292) hospitals did not differ significantly (p = 0.37).

This study provides the first economic analysis of the direct costs of sepsis in Brazilian ICUs and reveals that the cost of sepsis treatment is high and, despite similar ICU management and resource allocation, there was a significant difference regarding patient outcome between private and public hospitals [19]. These data reinforce the need for a national campaign in order to standardize management and decrease the heterogeneity with which these patients are treated in Brazilian institutions.

In another country, Cheng et al. [20] collected data from 10 Chinese ICUs and found a median length of stay of 7 days (3–14), with a mean hospital cost of US$ 11,390–11,455 per case of severe sepsis (mean cost per case per hospital day $ 502–401 USD).

Indirect Costs and Burden of Illness

Severe sepsis causes indirect costs as a consequence of productivity loss due to temporary unfitness for work, premature retirement, or premature death. All three kinds of work absenteeism are affected by severe sepsis [4]. Indirect costs of illness are calculated according to the human capital approach or friction cost approach (see these concepts above). Expected future productivity losses due to permanent morbidity or mortality could be discounted using a yearly discount rate of 5 %. Lower (0 %) and higher (10 %) discounting rates are tested in the scope of the sensitivity analysis [21].

In a retrospective study, using electronic charts from three German ICUs, Schmid and co-workers [21] reported the indirect costs associated with severe sepsis in that country. The annual prevalence of severe sepsis was considered to range from 44,000 to 95,000 cases. The productivity loss due to temporary morbidity ranged from 151 to 326 million Euros. Productivity loss due to permanent morbidity due to severe sepsis was 447–964 million Euros (upper and lower end of severe sepsis incidence).

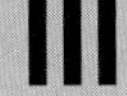

Premature death leads to a productivity loss between 2,024 and 4,370 million Euros, representing the largest proportion of the indirect costs. Assuming a reduced life expectancy for the surviving septic patient adds an additional 449–969 million Euros to these costs. The total indirect costs due to severe sepsis in Germany (without reduced life expectancy) ranged from 2,622 to 5,660 million Euros per year. In the same study, the authors calculated the burden of illness. The total costs of severe sepsis (burden of illness) in Germany were estimated to range from 3,647 to 7,874 million Euros per year. Productivity loss due to mortality represented the largest portion (56 %), followed by direct costs (28 %) and productivity loss due to permanent morbidity (12 %). Productivity loss due to temporary morbidity made up only 4 % of the total costs. To our knowledge this is the only study addressing cost-of-illness imposed by sepsis.

Impact of Therapeutic Strategies on Costs

As mentioned before, several factors can increase costs in the ICU, including length of stay (fixed costs mainly personnel), severity of disease, and drugs. Hence, interventions which could reduce length of stay and/or severity may attenuate costs. In general, cost-effective analyses are carried out to evaluate new interventions, such as drugs and devices. For example, there are several studies addressing the costs and cost-effectiveness of drotrecogin alfa (activated) [activated protein C] and evidence-based sepsis protocols, mainly based on the Surviving Sepsis Campaign guidelines [22].

Drotrecogin alfa (activated) has been indicated for patients with severe sepsis at high risk of death [22]. This recommendation is based on two randomized clinical trials (RCTs), PROWESS (Protein C Worldwide Evaluation in Severe Sepsis) [23] and ADDRESS (Administration of Drotrecogin Alfa [Activated] in Early Stage Severe Sepsis) [24]. There is an ongoing RCT evaluating the efficacy of this drug only in patients with septic shock (ClinicalTrials.gov Identifier: NCT00604214). The first economic evaluation of drotrecogin alfa (activated) treatment for severe sepsis was carried out by Manns et al. [25]. These authors collected clinical and cost information, including data from a three-year follow-up in a cohort of patients who had been admitted to an ICU with severe sepsis and had received conventional care. They estimated the cost-effectiveness of this drug for ICU patients with severe sepsis using a Markov analysis. For all patients, the cost per life-year gained by treating patients with drotrecogin alfa (activated) was $27,936; it was significantly more cost-effective to treat patients with an APACHE II score of 25 or more ($19,723 per life-year gained) than to treat those with an APACHE II score of 24 or less ($575,054 per life-year gained). However, the cost per quality-adjusted life-year gained was higher ($43,319 to $53,989) because of the reduction in ongoing health-related quality of life for survivors of sepsis. These authors concluded that the use of drotrecogin alfa (activated) in patients with severe sepsis, with greater severity of illness, and a reasonable life expectancy is cost effective (< 50 thousand dollars).

One year later, Angus et al. [26] also published a cost-effectiveness analysis based on data collected prospectively as part of a multicenter international trial. Analyses were conducted from the United States societal perspective, limited to healthcare costs, and using a 3 % annual discount rate. Over the first 28 days (short-term Base Case), drotrecogin alfa (activated) increased the costs of care by $9,800 and survival by 0.061 lives saved per treated patient. Projected to lifetime (lifetime Reference Case), drotrecogin alfa (activated) increased the costs of care by $16,000 and quality-adjusted survival by 0.33 quality-adjusted life-years per treated patient. Thus, drotrecogin alfa (activated) cost $48,800 per quality-adjusted life-year (with 82 % probability that the ratio is <$100,000 per quality-adjusted life-year). For more severely ill patients with APACHE II score higher 24, drotrecogin alfa (activated) cost $27,400 per quality-adjusted life-year. The authors concluded that this intervention had a cost-effectiveness profile similar to many well-accepted healthcare strategies.

More recently, Dhainaut et al. [27] reported another cost-effectiveness analysis in 'real life', by using an observational study design involving adult patients recruited before and after licensing of drotrecogin alfa (activated) in France. The incremental cost-effectiveness ratios gained were as follows: €20,278 per life-year gained and €33,797 per quality-adjusted life-year gained. There was a 74.5 % probability that this compound would be cost-effective if they were willing to pay €50,000 per life-year gained. An interesting commentary [28] accompanying this paper, highlighted some limitations of the study [27] that should be evaluated in every cost-effective analysis. First, the authors based their economic evaluation only on non-RCT data, even when RCT data [23] were available. Second, the study was only powered to find differences in costs, but not in effectiveness. Finally, they did not consider sensitivity analyses using the PROWESS data. Despite these limitations, the authors of the commentary concluded that the results appear to confirm that the use of drotrecogin alfa (activated) in the 'real world' is cost-effective [28].

Three other studies [29–31] have reported similar results regarding the cost-effectiveness ratio of drotrecogin alfa (activated). Importantly there is a consensus that this compound is only cost-effective in the more severely ill septic patients.

Taken together, these studies suggest that the use of drotrecogin alfa (activated) in severely ill septic patients is associated with a cost-effectiveness ratio in the range of other funded interventions. ICU managers and clinicians should decide if this intervention should or should not be incorporated in their units/institutions by considering the incremental costs and the opportunity cost of this intervention in relation to others not currently funded.

In contrast, there are some recent publications evaluating the costs and cost-effectiveness of integrated protocols using the Surviving Sepsis Campaign guidelines. Shorr et al. [32] evaluated the economic impact of an evidence-based sepsis protocol in their institutions. One hundred and twenty patients were assessed before (60) and after (60) the protocol implementation. In addition to increased survival rates, the median total hospital costs were significantly lower with use of the protocol ($16,103 vs. $21,985, $p = 0.008$), mainly because of shorter length of stay. They concluded that implementation of a sepsis management protocol was able both to improve mortality rate and to substantially save money.

Similarly, but using a cost-effectiveness analysis, Talmor et al. [33] carried out a cohort study evaluating the impact of the Multiple Urgent Sepsis Therapies (MUST) protocol (based on early goal-directed therapy [34]). These authors reported an association between adoption of this integrated sepsis protocol and increased in-patient survival at a moderate increase in treatment costs. The cost for treating a patient with an integrated sepsis protocol was approximately $8,800 greater than for treating patients before it. These increased costs in the study cohort were driven by higher ICU costs associated with increased ICU length of stay. The authors also plotted differences in costs versus differences in QALY (**Fig. 3**). They were able to demonstrate that the MUST protocol was largely localized in the upper-right quadrant, which means incremental increases in costs and in QALY, falling within acceptable standards for cost-effectiveness.

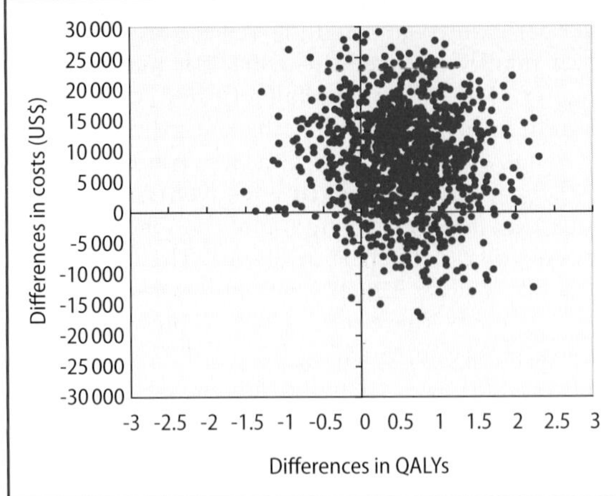

Fig. 3. Analysis of quality-adjusted life expectancy (QALY) versus cost. Base case cost-effectiveness distributions of the 1,000 simulations. Quadrants to the right of the y-axis represent regions where treating patients with the MUST protocol is associated with net QALYs gained. From [33] with permission

III

A recent systematic review was carried out to identify critical care interventions that are cost-effective [35]. The authors reviewed every cost-effectiveness analysis study related to this field. Methodological and analytical characteristics included the study perspective, discounting of future costs and life years, and performance of sensitivity analyses. They also converted all non-US currency ratios into US currency. Nineteen original cost-effectiveness studies (1993–2003) were included, which were directly related to the management of the critically ill patient in the ICU and presented cost per QALY or cost per life-year incremental cost-effectiveness ratios. Three interventions fell within accepted cost-effectiveness ratios including drotrecogin alfa (activated) for patients with sepsis, mechanical ventilation, and admission to the ICU itself. However, when selected populations were analyzed, such as drotrecogin alfa (activated) for septic patients and an APACHE score of < 25, mechanical ventilation in patients > 40 yrs old with stroke, and admission to the ICU for patients with hematologic malignancies, the cost-effectiveness ratio was unfavorable.

Conclusion

In summary, there is a relatively strong body of data demonstrating that the management of sepsis is costly. Cost-effectiveness analysis studies are crucial to evaluate the economic impact of critical care interventions. Although critical care support requires an expensive and complex structure, cost-effectiveness analyses are rare in the medical literature. This fact is largely because there is a scarcity of evidence of the effectiveness of critical care interventions and as a result of difficulty in measuring quality of life and utility, which are recommended for use in cost-effectiveness analyses. Additional well recognized obstacles include heterogeneic practice patterns, and the difficulty in measuring burden of critical illness. Despite these factors, managers and clinicians should be empowered by health economic studies before making decisions. Cost-effectiveness analyses are good examples of 'phase 4' studies which should be carried out in order to help us in the process of accepting different critical care interventions and/or incorporating a new drug or device into current practice.

References

1. Angus DC, Pereira CA, Silva E (2006) Epidemiology of severe sepsis around the world. Endocr Metab Immune Disord Drug Targets 6: 207–212
2. Silva E, Pedro MA (2004) Brazilian Sepsis Epidemiological Study (BASES study). Crit Care 8:R251–260
3. Martin G S, Mannino DM, Eaton S, Moss M (2003) The epidemiology of sepsis in the United States from 1979 through 2000. N Engl J Med 348: 1546–1554
4. Moerer O, Schmid A, Hofmann M, et al (2002) Direct costs of severe sepsis in three German intensive care units based on retrospective electronic patient record analysis of resource use. Intensive Care Med 28: 1440–1446
5. Burchardi H, Schneider H (2004) Economic aspects of severe sepsis. A review of intensive care unit costs, cost of illness and cost effectiveness of therapy. Pharmacoeconomics 22: 793–813
6. Edbrooke D, Hibbert C, Ridley S, Long T, Dickie H (1999) The development of a method for comparative costing of individual intensive care units. Anaesthesia 54: 110–120
7. Lee H, Doig CJ, Ghali WA, Donaldson C, Johnson D, Manns B (2004) Detailed cost analysis of care for survivors of severe sepsis. Crit Care Med 32: 981–985
8. Edbrooke DL, Hibbert CL, Kingsley JM, Smith S, Bright NM, Quinn JM (1999) The patient-related cost of care for sepsis patients in a United Kingdom adult general intensive care unit. Crit Care Med 27: 1760–1767
9. Angus DC, Linde-Zwirble WT, Lidicker J, et al (2001) Epidemiology of severe sepsis in the United States: Analysis of incidence, outcome, and associated costs of care. Crit Care Med 29: 1303–1310
10. Brun-Buisson C, Roudot-Thoraval F, Girou E, Grenier-Sennelier C, Durand-Zaleski I (2003) The costs of septic syndromes in the intensive care unit and influence of hospital-acquired sepsis. Intensive Care Med 29: 1464–1471
11. Heyland DK, Kernerman P, Gafni A, Cook DJ (1996) Economic evaluations in the critical care literature: do they help us improve the efficiency of our unit? Crit Care Med 24: 1591–1598
12. American Thoracic Society Workshop on Outcomes Research (2002) Understanding costs and cost-effectiveness in critical care. Am J Respir Crit Care Med 165: 540–550
13. Drummond MF, Sculpher MJ, Torrance GW, O'Brien BJ (2005) Methods for the Economic Evaluation of Health Care Programmes, 3rd ed. Oxford University Press, Oxford
14. Sefton T, Byford S, McDaid D, Hills J, Knapp M (2002) Making the Most of it: Economic Evaluation in the Social Welfare Field. Joseph Rowntree Foundation, York
15. References to obtain unit costs for pharmaceuticals and health care equipment Joint Formulary Committee. British National Formulary 52. British Medical Association and the Royal Pharmaceutical Society of Great Britain, London
16. Gold MR, Russell LB, Seigel JE, Weinstein MC (1996) Cost–effectiveness in Health and Medicine. Oxford University Press, New York
17. Braun L, Riedel AA, Cooper LM (2004) Severe sepsis in managed care: analysis of incidence, one-year mortality, and associated costs of care. J Manag Care Pharm 10: 521–530
18. Chalfin DB, Holbein ME, Fein AM, Carlon GC (1993) Cost-effectiveness of monoclonal antibodies to gram-negative endotoxin in the treatment of gram-negative sepsis in ICU patients. JAMA 269: 549–254
19. Sogayar AM, Machado FR, Rea-Neto A, et al (2008) A multicentre, prospective study to evaluate costs of septic patients in Brazilian intensive care units. Pharmacoeconomics 26: 425–434
20. Cheng B, Xie G, Yao S, et al (2007) Epidemiology of severe sepsis in critically ill surgical patients in ten university hospitals in China. Crit Care Med 35: 2538–2546
21. Schmid A, Burchardi H, Clouth J, Schneider H (2002) Burden of illness imposed by severe sepsis in Germany. Eur J Health Econ 3: 77–82
22. Dellinger, RP, Levy, MM, Carlet, JM, et al (2008) Surviving Sepsis Campaign: international guidelines for management of severe sepsis and septic shock: 2008. Intensive Care Med 34: 17–60
23. Bernard GR, Vincent JL, Laterre PF, et al (2001) Efficacy and safety of recombinant human activated protein C for severe sepsis. N Engl J Med 344: 699–709

III

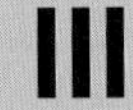

24. Abraham E, Laterre PF, Garg R, et al (2005) Drotrecogin alfa (activated) for adults with severe sepsis and a low risk of death. N Engl J Med 353: 1332–1341
25. Manns BJ, Lee H, Doig CJ, Johnson D, Donaldson C (2002) An economic evaluation of activated protein C treatment for severe sepsis. N Engl J Med 347: 993–1000
26. Angus DC, Linde-Zwirble WT, Clermont G, et al (2003) Cost-effectiveness of drotrecogin alfa (activated) in the treatment of severe sepsis. Crit Care Med 31: 1–11
27. Dhainaut JF, Payet S, Vallet B, et al (2007) Cost-effectiveness of activated protein C in real-life clinical practice. Crit Care 11:R99
28. Brar SS, Manns BJ (2007) Activated protein C: cost-effective or costly? Crit Care 11:164
29. Fowler RA, Hill-Popper M, Stasinos J, Petrou C, Sanders GD, Garber AM (2003) Cost-effectiveness of recombinant human activated protein C and the influence of severity of illness in the treatment of patients with severe sepsis. J Crit Care 18: 181–191
30. Neilson AR, Burchardi H, Chinn C, Clouth J, Schneider H, Angus D (2003) Cost-effectiveness of drotrecogin alfa (activated) for the treatment of severe sepsis in Germany. J Crit Care 18: 217–227
31. Betancourt M, McKinnon PS, Massanari RM, Kanji S, Bach D, Devlin JW (2003) An evaluation of the cost effectiveness of drotrecogin alfa (activated) relative to the number of organ system failures. Pharmacoeconomics 21: 1331–1340
32. Shorr AF, Micek ST, Jackson WL Jr, Kollef MH (2007) Economic implications of an evidence-based sepsis protocol: can we improve outcomes and lower costs? Crit Care Med 35: 1257–1262
33. Talmor D, Greenberg D, Howell MD, Lisbon A, Novack V, Shapiro N (2008) The costs and cost-effectiveness of an integrated sepsis treatment protocol. Crit Care Med 36: 1168–1174
34. Rivers E, Nguyen B, Havstad S, et al (2001) Early goal-directed therapy in the treatment of severe sepsis and septic shock. N Engl J Med 345: 1368–1377
35. Talmor D, Shapiro N, Greenberg D, Stone PW, Neumann PJ (2006) When is critical care medicine cost-effective? A systematic review of the cost-effectiveness literature. Crit Care Med 34: 2738–2747

IV Proposed Targets for New Therapies

Lymphocyte Apoptosis in Sepsis and Potential Anti-apoptotic Strategies

S. Weber, B. Baessler, and S. Schroeder

Introduction

Sepsis is a leading cause of death in many intensive care units [1]. The pathophysiology of sepsis is characterized by a dysregulation of the immune system in response to infection or secondary to trauma. Initial hyperinflammation often results in septic shock. Simultaneously, part of the immune system is deactivated leading to a temporary but often deadly immunosuppression. In attempting to arrive at a more detailed understanding of immunophysiological processes during sepsis over the last few years, apoptosis has been recognized as one of the key factors in the pathophysiology of sepsis [2]. As shown in several animal models, accelerated apoptosis seems to be induced in leukocytes and many immunocompetent cells during sepsis [3, 4]. Similar processes are involved in humans [5].

The mainstay of sepsis therapy remains symptomatic treatment with hemodynamic and organ support, as well as aggressive treatment of underlying infection with antibiotics or surgical intervention [6]. In addition, feasible therapeutic interventions that modulate the innate immune response may be beneficial [7]. Inhibition of apoptosis in a mouse model did dramatically improve survival [8], which demonstrates that the process of apoptosis is involved in the regulation of the immune response during sepsis. This might open up the way for new immunomodulating therapies. For many years, the predominant theory had been that sepsis represents an over-exuberant inflammatory response in which unbridled cytokine-mediated host defense mechanisms induce significant cell and organ injury [2]. However, in various clinical trials, cytokine or anti-inflammatory therapeutic agents either failed to improve survival in patients with sepsis or, in some cases, even exacerbated their condition [9]. These failures led to a reappraisal of the concept that death in sepsis is due to a hyperinflammatory response.

Many cell types are prone to apoptosis during sepsis with relevant consequences for organ function (reviewed in [10]). Many investigations over the last few years have demonstrated that apoptosis of lymphocytes is a major pathogenetic factor during sepsis [5]. Normally, apoptosis of immune cells is considered a vital process in counter-regulating an initial activation of the immune system. However, dysregulated apoptosis of immune cells results in secondary immunosuppression due to the transient loss of immune cells of the innate or adaptive immune system as well as to the immunosuppressive effect caused by apoptotic cells on surviving immune cells [2]. The severest form of this immunosuppression is termed 'immunoparalysis'. Most patients with sepsis will survive the initial few days of hyperinflammation and develop this protracted hypo-inflammatory, immunosuppressive state that is manifest by an inability to eradicate the primary infection, a predisposition to nosocomial infections, and a loss of delayed hypersensitivity. In this context, loss of immunocompetent cells due to apoptosis or reprogramming of cells by ingestion of apoptotic cells leading to an anti-inflammatory response may worsen the condition. In conclusion, the inhibition of accelerated apoptosis during sepsis is a promising target in the design of a novel and specific immunotherapy of sepsis.

Mechanisms of Apoptosis

Apoptosis, which is also referred to as programmed cell death, is an active, energy-dependent, well-defined process whereby cells carry out suicide. Apoptosis is crucial during embryonic and fetal tissue remodeling to maintain a balance between organized cell growth and death and it is responsible for the removal of interdigital webs, about 50 % of excess neurons, and interstitial lung fibroblasts after lung alveolarization. The lethal fate of most caspase-knockout mice demonstrates that controlled cell death is vital for life. The human body contains about 10^{14} cells, each of which is able to initiate apoptosis [2]. Every day, there are about 60×10^9 newly developing cells, whereas old ones are removed by programmed cell death and other processes. In the adult human organism, apoptosis plays an important role in the elimination of damaged, non-functional cells and is also a key factor during oncogenesis. Apoptosis should normally occur in mutated cells and eliminate potential tumor cells. Malignant cells, however, find many ways to circumvent those mechanisms and escape cell death [11]. Programmed cell death is characterized by sequential changes, including initial cell-volume reduction (whereas intracellular organelles as well as intracellular metabolism remain intact), shrinkage of the nucleus, chromatin condensation (pyknosis), DNA fragmentation, formation of nuclear fragments (apoptotic bodies), and zeiosis (dynamic plasma membrane blebbing). These morphological features represent a late/terminal stage of apoptosis. Another important biochemical change and an early event is the exposure of phosphatidylserine on the outside of the cell membrane, assigning the cell for phagocytosis by macrophages [12]. This mechanism forms the basis for selective organized elimination of cells, preventing a local inflammation of the surrounding tissue [11]. In apoptosis, potential pro-inflammatory molecules become compartmentalized so that there is no concurrent inflammatory response. There are many inducers of apoptosis, including steroids, cytokines such as tumor necrosis factor (TNF)-α, interleukin (IL)-1 and IL-6, FasL, heat shock proteins (HSPs), oxygen free radicals, nitric oxide (NO) and FasL-expressing cytotoxic T lymphocytes [11].

Pathways Involved in Apoptosis

There are two main pathways leading to apoptosis: A death-receptor-initiated caspase-8-mediated pathway (extrinsic pathway, **Fig. 1**) and a mitochondria-initiated caspase-9-mediated pathway (intrinsic pathway, **Fig. 1**) [13]. Some authors also describe a third pathway, the endoplasmatic reticulum or stress-induced pathway. This third pathway is the least understood of the apoptotic pathways and appears to involve activation of caspase 12 by Ca^{2+} and oxidant stress [14]. Caspases, a family of protein degrading enzymes, are the main effectors of apoptosis [11]. Fourteen human caspases have been described so far. They all have the amino acid cysteine in their active center and cleave off substrates after aspartate. The steric conformation in the active center determines their substrate specifity.

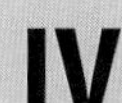

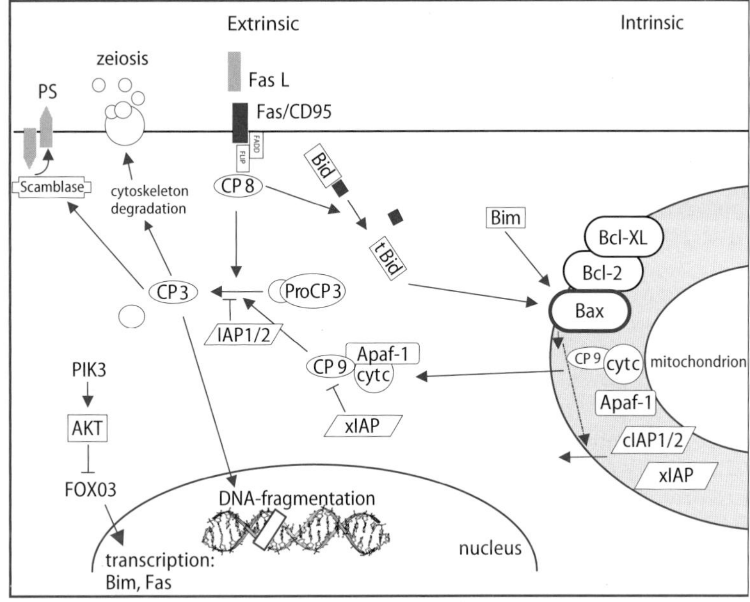

Fig. 1. Extrinsic and intrinsic pathways of apoptosis in sepsis. A simplified overview of apoptosis pathways during sepsis is displayed. Apoptosis is initiated via death receptors (e.g., Fas) or the mitochondrion. Both pathways converge on caspase-3 (CP 3) the main executioner of apoptosis. Caspase-3 leads to DNA-fragmentation, degradation of the cytoskeleton causing zeiosis, the blebbing of membranes, and to externalization of phosphatidyl serine (PS), which marks apoptotic cells for phagocytosis. Cyt c: cytochrome c; Apaf: apoptotic protease activating factor; FADD: Fas-associated death domain; FLIP: FADD-like IL-1β-converting enzyme inhibitory protein; PI3K: phosphoinositide 3-kinase

Extrinsic Pathway

CD95-initiated apoptosis is an illustrative example of the extrinsic pathway. Fas antigen (CD95), a major death receptor that belongs to the TNF superfamily of membrane receptors that is situated in the cell membrane, is the first component of this pathway to receive a death signal [11]. Fas is expressed on a variety of cell types, including thymocytes, activated B cells, T cells, monocytes, macrophages, and neutrophils, as well as on a variety of non-immune cells in the liver, lung, and heart [15]. When Fas binds to its ligand, FasL (which is located on the surface of lymphocyte subsets), it trimerises and creates a death-induced signaling complex (DISC) which recruits an adaptor molecule which also contains a death domain known as Fas-associated death domain (FADD) [12]. FADD binds to these activated death domains and to pro-caspase 8 through death effector domains (DEDs) to form the DISC. The death signal is then transduced from the DISC to a downstream caspase cascade when pro-caspase 8 is cleaved and becomes active caspase 8, which can, in turn, cleave and activate downstream effector caspases, such as caspase 3, 6, or 7 [2]. Caspase 3 cleaves inhibitors of caspase activated DNAse (ICAD) and cleaves DNA in the nucleus, which leads to apoptosis. Zeiosis is caused by digestion of the cytoskeleton through caspase-3. Caspases also activate an enzyme called scramblase, which externalizes phosphatidylserine onto the membrane surface and thus marks cells for phagocytosis [16]. Overall the Fas pathway is important in controlling apoptosis and the immune response, e.g., the activation-induced cell death of lymphocytes.

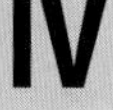

Intrinsic Pathway

In the intrinsic or mitochondrial pathway of apoptosis, almost no DISC is formed, but the mitochondrion contains multiple pro-apoptotic molecules that can amplify the incoming apoptotic signal [11]. The mitochondrion is essential for releasing cellular destruction molecules such as cytochrome c, which activates downstream caspases such as caspase 3 and caspase 9. The initiation of this pathway, however, is not well defined. The pathway can be activated by loss of growth factors, such as IL-2, IL-4 or granulocyte macrophage colony stimulating factor (GM-CSF), the addition of cytokines such as IL-1 and IL-6, or exogenous stressors such as steroids, reactive oxygen intermediates, peroxynitrite or NO, which in turn activate pro- or anti-apoptotic members of the Bcl-2 family. A caspase-8 mediated cleavage of the pro-apoptotic Bcl-2 family member, Bid (which normally exists in a quiescent state in the cytosol), to truncated protein Bid (tBid), transfers the signal to the mitochondrion where it acts to decrease mitochondrial membrane potential [12]. There are at least 25 members of the Bcl-2 family. Whereas group I molecules like Bcl-2 and Bcl-xL are anti-apoptotic, group II molecules like Bax and group III molecules like Bid are pro-apoptotic [13]. All proteins interact with each other and influence regulation and release of further signaling molecules. One possible mechanism for inducing apoptosis by the mitochondrial pathway is the opening and closure of the mitochondrial permeability transition pore complex [17]. This leads to the release of cytochrome c, second mitochondria-derived activator of caspase/direct inhibitor of apoptosis-binding protein with low pI (Smac/Diablo, also a mitochondrial protein) and the adaptor protein, apoptotic protease activating factor (Apaf)-1, into the cytosol. Together, they build a multienzyme complex, the so-called apoptosome [16]. This apoptosome interlinks with the caspase cascade by activating caspase-9, which can in turn activate downstream caspase-3. Studies indicate that both the death-receptor pathway and the mitochondrial pathway are likely to be involved in sepsis-induced lymphocyte apoptosis. Bcl-2 is an anti-apoptotic protein known to protect against apoptosis mediated through the mitochondrial pathway. However, it is important to note that in some cell types, Bcl-2 can also provide limited protection against apoptosis that is mediated by death receptors because of cross-talk between the two pathways.

Evidence in Animals

Apoptosis has been shown to be a major factor in several animal models of sepsis. To obtain an animal model of apoptosis, it is common practice to use ligation and perforation of the cecum to cause bacterial peritonitis (CLP model). Experimental studies looking at the septic animal suggest that loss of lymphocytes during sepsis may be due to dysregulated apoptosis and that this appears to be brought on by a variety of mediators effecting 'intrinsic' as well as 'extrinsic' cell death pathways. In addition, studies in recent years have suggested that the dysregulated apoptotic immune cell death may play a role in contributing to the immune dysfunction and multiple organ failure observed during sepsis, and blocking it can improve survival of animals in experimental sepsis. Immune cells most affected by this dysregulated apoptotic cell death appear to be lymphocytes [2].

Caspase-cascade

Several animal models have been used to examine the role of specific apoptotic signaling cascades. Inhibition of apoptosis confers a survival benefit in CLP-induced sepsis. Caspases are thought to be indispensable for apoptosis. Their overexpression seems to induce apoptosis, whereas certain caspase inhibitors are able to prevent apoptosis [2]. Therefore, one of the earliest anti-apoptotic approaches in sepsis research was the attempt to inhibit caspase activation using these caspase inhibitors. Braun and co-workers reported first that caspase inhibitors might be advantageous for the treatment of sepsis [18]. They showed that the broad spectrum caspase inhibitor, zVAD-fmk, provided significant neuroprotection by decreasing hippocampal neuronal death in a rabbit model of pneumococcal meningitis. Shortly after this report, Hotchkiss and colleagues demonstrated that survival was improved in the CLP model of sepsis using zVAD-fmk [19]. In a similar study, Neviere and colleagues observed that zVAD-fmk prevented cell apoptosis and improved myocardial contractility in a rat endotoxin model [20]. Subsequently, Hotchkiss and colleagues documented that the selective caspase-3 inhibitor, M-971, prevented lymphocyte apoptosis in sepsis, and in turn, improved survival by 40–45 % in septic animals [8, 21]. In addition, other caspase-specific inhibitors have been used including zDEVD-fmk (caspase 3 and 7) and AcYVAD-cmk (caspase 1) [22]. However, at high doses, caspase inhibitors can have non-specific effects and cause cytotoxicity. In this respect, a different kind of pan-caspase inhibitor called Q-VD.Oph has been studied, which potently inhibits apoptosis but is not toxic at high doses [23].

Preventing caspase-3 activation with genetic engineering shows similar effects as shown by using caspase inhibitors. Caspase-3-deficient mice have a significantly higher survival rate in CLP-induced sepsis [8]. The inhibition of caspase-11 by knock out improved survival from sepsis in a murine model [24]. Additional studies by Ayala and colleagues showed that small interfering RNA (siRNA) directed against the caspase-8 gene decreased apoptosis and improved survival in the CLP model of sepsis [25]. There is new evidence of a role for caspase-12 in opposing or counterbalancing the pro-inflammatory response [2]. Caspase-12 has an important role in regulating inflammation in humans [26]. The practical relevance of this finding is that patients of African descent who have the caspase-12L polymorphism might be more vulnerable to death during sepsis because they will mount a relatively poor pro-inflammatory response and rapidly progress to the immunosuppressive phase of sepsis [2]. Mice that are deficient in caspase-12 have marked differences in pro- versus anti-inflammatory cytokines and improved survival in sepsis [26].

Fas/CD95-induced apoptosis

There is evidence that the death receptor, Fas, plays an important role in accelerated leukocyte apoptosis during sepsis [25]. Increased inducible apoptosis in CD4+ T lymphocytes during polymicrobial sepsis is mediated by FasL [27] and FasL-deficient C3H/HeJ-FasL mice are more resistant to apoptosis after CLP. Blocking the Fas-FasL-system by application of Fas-receptor fusion protein prevented organ dysfunction and apoptosis in the liver and improved survival during polymicrobial sepsis [28]. More recently, interfering RNA technology has been utilized to target gene expression of members of the extrinsic death receptor/Fas pathway [23]. Double stranded siRNA against Fas and caspase 8 given 30 minutes after CLP improved survival by 50 %, while reducing indices of organ damage and apoptosis in both the liver and the spleen [23].

Mitochondrial Pathway

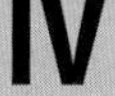

Several groups have shown that sepsis decreases the level of expression of Bcl-2 by lymphocytes [2]. Hotchkiss and colleagues demonstrated that lymphocytes from Bcl-2 transgenic mice were resistant to sepsis-induced apoptosis, and that these mice had a threefold improvement in survival compared with controls [29]. In addition, these authors showed that T-cells with overexpression of Bcl-2 were completely protected against sepsis-induced T-lymphocyte apoptosis in lymphatic tissue like thymus and spleen [29]. When a Bcl-XL fusion protein or a BH4-domain fusion protein was administered in the CLP-model, apoptosis was reduced and survival improved [30]. The survival kinase, Akt, can influence the transcription of proteins of the Bcl-2 family. Bommhardt and colleagues showed that overexpression of Akt decreased sepsis-induced lymphocyte apoptosis, improved survival [31] and boostered the T-helper (Th)-1 cytokine response [31].

Evidence in Humans

Elevated levels of nucleosomes, a sign of late apoptosis, were found in serum from patients with sepsis and systemic inflammatory response syndrome (SIRS) [32]. The mRNA-expression of the anti-apoptotic protein, bcl-2, was transiently downregulated in patients with severe sepsis [33]. These are strong arguments for the involvement of apoptosis in human sepsis.

A prospective study looking at 20 septic patients who died of multiple organ failure demonstrated ongoing apoptosis in all patients. Histopathophysiologically, apoptosis was predominantly found in the intestinal epithelium (colon, ileum) and spleen [5]. Almost all septic patients had significant peripheral lymphocytopenia and fewer lymphocytes in the spleen. The findings were interpreted as an indirect sign of lymphocytic apoptosis; as there was increased splenic caspase-3 activity, it was assumed to be caspase-3-mediated apoptosis. This leads to decreased immune defense in sepsis. Further investigations found focal apoptosis in gut tissue from ten trauma patients [34]. Apoptotic foci were seen shortly after the traumatic insult in intestinal lymphoid and epithelial tissue. A prospective study looking at 27 septic patients and 25 trauma patients demonstrated a caspase-9 mediated reduction of B-and CD4-Th cells. Interestingly there was no reduction in CD8-positive T-cells or natural killer cells [34]. In spleens of patients with sepsis and trauma, a profound loss of dendritic cells but not macrophages was observed [35]. Since dendritic cells constitute the main pool of antigen presenting cells, impaired activation of T- and B-cells may be expected.

Lymphocytes not only undergo accelerated apoptosis during sepsis. These cells are also more responsive to secondary induction of apoptosis. Lymphocytes are more sensitive to activation of induced cell death [36]. Increased apoptosis and subsequent loss of CD4-positive cells and B-cells seems paradoxical, as it occurs during a life threatening illness where an increase in all lymphocytes would rather be expected. Moreover, lymphocytes from septic patients proliferate less in response to lectins or CD3 [37].

Monocytes have been shown to respond with an increased expression of HSP70 in septic patients [38]. This study, looking at 18 septic patients and 17 healthy volunteers, also measured a reduced mitochondrial membrane potential which is an indicator of initiated irreversible monocyte apoptosis. Overall, no difference could be found with regards to Bcl-2 concentration in septic and healthy patients [38]. Sepsis survivors, however, had a significantly higher Bcl-2 concentration than non-survivors during the first 3 days.

Soluble modulators of apoptosis are markedly altered during sepsis. In pediatric sepsis, soluble Fas (sFas) was increased, whereas soluble FasL (sFasL) was not [39]. In adult patients with sepsis, sFas was elevated and was associated with poor survival [40]. In SIRS and sepsis, sFas was found to be elevated, but, in this study sFas did not correlate with outcome [41]. sFas is believed to act as a scavenger of sFasL or as a dummy receptor of FasL on apoptosis-inducing cells. In this regard, an increase in sFas during sepsis may be interpreted as a compensatory mechanism to limit increased apoptosis.

In a study by De Freitas and colleagues, serum levels of sFasL were elevated [42]. sFasL may act as an inducer of apoptosis in Fas bearing cells. This finding hints at the role of the Fas-FasL system in sepsis. The increase of soluble components may be due to endotoxemia, because an increase in sFAS as well as sFasL was detected after endotoxemia in healthy volunteers [43]. The expression of Fas on monocytes after endotoxemia was transiently downregulated but increased several fold within 24 hours. In sepsis, Fas and FasL were upregulated on lymphocytes in septic patients [44].

Therapeutic Molecular Targets

Despite the favorable results using caspase inhibitors in animal models of sepsis, a number of issues have arisen that have lead to caution in the development of caspase inhibitors as a potential therapy for treating human sepsis. It is necessary to have a high degree of inhibition of caspases to prevent cell death. This requirement presents great therapeutic challenges owing to the need for persistent and nearly complete caspase blockade. Third, there is increasing recognition that caspases have many functions in addition to their roles as cell-death proteases and regulators of inflammation, including being essential for lymphocyte activation, proliferation, and protective immunity [45]. Therefore, blocking caspases might have some beneficial effects in decreasing apoptosis in sepsis but these could be counterbalanced by their adverse effects on the ability of the patient to mount an effective immune response. Finally, there are recent reports indicating that inhibition of caspases might induce hyper-acute TNF-induced shock in certain situations [46]. In short, there are potential pitfalls of using caspase inhibitors to treat sepsis. The most effective therapeutic approach might be temporary inhibition of specific caspases, such as caspase-3 or caspase-12, timed to the appropriate phase of sepsis, i.e., the hyper-inflammatory phase or the hypo-inflammatory phase. Therefore, pharmacological manipulation of caspase-12 might represent a novel means of modulating the inflammatory response to sepsis or other inflammatory disorders. In addition to caspases, other proteases might also be involved in mediating apoptosis [47]. Treatment with protease inhibitors decreased lymphocyte apoptosis and improved survival in a mouse model [48]. It is unlikely that these drugs will exacerbate the immunosuppression that is a hallmark of patients with sepsis; they are thought to block apoptosis by preventing mitochondrial pore formation and subsequent loss of mitochondrial membrane potential.

Conclusion and Perspectives

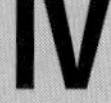

Although most studies have looked at small patient numbers, it can be argued that apoptosis plays an integral part in the pathophysiology of sepsis. A reduction in T-cell numbers caused by apoptosis may lead to immunosuppression, which is potentially fatal [1]. Furthermore, the presence of apoptotic cells in the circulation may elicit a Th2-response, which acts rather as an anti-inflammatory response. Specifically, apoptosis in immuncompetent cells opens capabilities for potential diagnostic and therapeutic interventions in the future [2]. Possible approaches include the use of caspase inhibitors, anti-apoptotic bcl-2 family fusion proteins [30], or an siRNA approach against caspases [25]. New concepts in the treatment of sepsis will only be successful if the exact time course of pro-and anti-inflammatory events is considered, as well as timely events during apoptosis and their pathophysiological relevance.

References

1. Hotchkiss RS, Karl IE (2003) The pathophysiology and treatment of sepsis. N Engl J Med 348: 138–150
2. Hotchkiss RS, Nicholson DW (2006) Apoptosis and caspases regulate death and inflammation in sepsis. Nat Rev Immunol 6: 813–822
3. Ayala A, Herdon CD, Lehman DL, Ayala CA, Chaudry IH (1996) Differential induction of apoptosis in lymphoid tissues during sepsis: variation in onset, frequency, and the nature of the mediators. Blood 87: 4261–4275
4. Wang SD, Huang KJ, Lin YS, Lei HY (1994) Sepsis-induced apoptosis of the thymocytes in mice. J Immunol 152: 5014–5021
5. Hotchkiss RS, Swanson PE, Freeman BD, et al (1999) Apoptotic cell death in patients with sepsis, shock, and multiple organ dysfunction. Crit Care Med 27: 1230–1251
6. Wheeler AP, Bernard GR (1999) Treating patients with severe sepsis. N Engl J Med 340: 207–214
7. Kox WJ, Volk T, Kox SN, Volk HD (2000) Immunomodulatory therapies in sepsis. Intensive Care Med 26 (Suppl 1):S124-S128
8. Hotchkiss RS, Chang KC, Swanson PE, et al (2000) Caspase inhibitors improve survival in sepsis: a critical role of the lymphocyte. Nat Immunol 1: 496–501
9. Fisher CJ, Jr., Agosti JM, Opal SM, et al (1996) Treatment of septic shock with the tumor necrosis factor receptor:Fc fusion protein. The Soluble TNF Receptor Sepsis Study Group. N Engl J Med 334: 1697–1702
10. Weber SU, Brummer-Smith S, Schroeder S (2008) Apoptosis in sepsis. In: Fenton RH, Burnside CB (eds) Cell Apoptosis Research Progress, 1st edn. Nova Science Publishers Inc, Hauppauge, pp 113–134
11. Hengartner MO (2000) The biochemistry of apoptosis. Nature 407: 770–776
12. Perl M, Chung CS, Ayala A (2005) Apoptosis. Crit Care Med 33: S526-S529
13. Green DR, Kroemer G (2004) The pathophysiology of mitochondrial cell death. Science 305: 626–629
14. Oyadomari S, Mori M (2004) Roles of CHOP/GADD153 in endoplasmic reticulum stress. Cell Death Differ 11: 381–389
15. Krammer PH (2000) CD95's deadly mission in the immune system. Nature 407: 789–795
16. Weber SU, Schewe JC, Putensen C, Stüber F, Schröder S (2004) [Apoptosis as a pathomechanism in sepsis]. Anaesthesist 53: 59–65
17. Zamzami N, Kroemer G (2001) The mitochondrion in apoptosis: how Pandora's box opens. Nat Rev Mol Cell Biol 2: 67–71
18. Braun JS, Novak R, Herzog KH, Bodner SM, Cleveland JL, Tuomanen EI (1999) Neuroprotection by a caspase inhibitor in acute bacterial meningitis. Nat Med 5: 298–302
19. Hotchkiss RS, Tinsley KW, Swanson PE, et al (1999) Prevention of lymphocyte cell death in sepsis improves survival in mice. Proc Natl Acad Sci USA 96: 14541–14546

20. Neviere R, Fauvel H, Chopin C, Formstecher P, Marchetti P (2001) Caspase inhibition prevents cardiac dysfunction and heart apoptosis in a rat model of sepsis. Am J Respir Crit Care Med 163: 218–225
21. Hotchkiss RS, Coopersmith CM, Karl IE (2005) Prevention of lymphocyte apoptosis-a potential treatment of sepsis? Clin Infect Dis 41 (Suppl 7):S465-S469
22. Rouquet N, Pages JC, Molina T, Briand P, Joulin V (1996) ICE inhibitor YVADcmk is a potent therapeutic agent against in vivo liver apoptosis. Curr Biol 6: 1192–1195
23. Wesche-Soldato DE, Swan RZ, Chung CS, Ayala A (2007) The apoptotic pathway as a therapeutic target in sepsis. Curr Drug Targets 8: 493–500
24. Kang SJ, Wang S, Kuida K, Yuan J (2002) Distinct downstream pathways of caspase-11 in regulating apoptosis and cytokine maturation during septic shock response. Cell Death Differ 9: 1115–1125
25. Wesche-Soldato DE, Chung CS, Lomas-Neira J, Doughty LA, Gregory SH, Ayala A (2005) In vivo delivery of caspase-8 or Fas siRNA improves the survival of septic mice. Blood 106: 2295–2301
26. Saleh M, Vaillancourt JP, Graham RK, et al (2004) Differential modulation of endotoxin responsiveness by human caspase-12 polymorphisms. Nature 429: 75–79
27. Ayala A, Chung CS, Xu YX, Evans TA, Redmond KM, Chaudry IH (1999) Increased inducible apoptosis in CD4+ T lymphocytes during polymicrobial sepsis is mediated by Fas ligand and not endotoxin. Immunology 97: 45–55
28. Chung CS, Yang S, Song GY, et al (2001) Inhibition of Fas signaling prevents hepatic injury and improves organ blood flow during sepsis. Surgery 130: 339–345
29. Hotchkiss RS, Swanson PE, Knudson CM, et al (1999) Overexpression of Bcl-2 in transgenic mice decreases apoptosis and improves survival in sepsis. J Immunol 162: 4148–4156
30. Hotchkiss RS, McConnell KW, Bullok K, et al (2006) TAT-BH4 and TAT-Bcl-xL peptides protect against sepsis-induced lymphocyte apoptosis in vivo. J Immunol 176: 5471–5477
31. Bommhardt U, Chang KC, Swanson PE, et al (2004) Akt decreases lymphocyte apoptosis and improves survival in sepsis. J Immunol 172: 7583–7591
32. Zeerleder S, Zwart B, Wuillemin WA, et al (2003) Elevated nucleosome levels in systemic inflammation and sepsis. Crit Care Med 31: 1947–1951
33. Bilbault P, Lavaux T, Lahlou A, et al (2004) Transient Bcl-2 gene down-expression in circulating mononuclear cells of severe sepsis patients who died despite appropriate intensive care. Intensive Care Med 30: 408–415
34. Hotchkiss RS, Tinsley KW, Swanson PE, et al (2001) Sepsis-induced apoptosis causes progressive profound depletion of B and CD4+ T lymphocytes in humans. J Immunol. 166: 6952–6963
35. Hotchkiss RS, Tinsley KW, Swanson PE, et al (2002) Depletion of dendritic cells, but not macrophages, in patients with sepsis. J Immunol. 168: 2493–2500
36. Schroeder S, Lindemann C, Decker D, et al (2001) Increased susceptibility to apoptosis in circulating lymphocytes of critically ill patients. Langenbecks Arch Surg. 386: 42–46
37. Roth G, Moser B, Krenn C, et al (2003) Susceptibility to programmed cell death in T-lymphocytes from septic patients: a mechanism for lymphopenia and Th2 predominance. Biochem Biophys Res Commun 308: 840–846
38. Adrie C, Bachelet M, Vayssier-Taussat M, et al (2001) Mitochondrial membrane potential and apoptosis peripheral blood monocytes in severe human sepsis. Am J Respir Crit Care Med 164: 389–395
39. Doughty L, Clark RS, Kaplan SS, Sasser H, Carcillo J (2002) sFas and sFas ligand and pediatric sepsis-induced multiple organ failure syndrome. Pediatr Res 52: 922–927
40. Papathanassoglou ED, Moynihan JA, Vermillion DL, McDermott MP, Ackerman MH (2000) Soluble fas levels correlate with multiple organ dysfunction severity, survival and nitrate levels, but not with cellular apoptotic markers in critically ill patients. Shock 14: 107–112
41. Torre D, Tambini R, Manfredi M, et al (2003) Circulating levels of FAS/APO-1 in patients with the systemic inflammatory response syndrome. Diagn Microbiol Infect Dis 45: 233–236
42. De Freitas I, Fernandez-Somoza M, Essenfeld-Sekler E, Cardier JE (2004) Serum levels of the apoptosis-associated molecules, tumor necrosis factor-alpha/tumor necrosis factor type-I receptor and Fas/FasL, in sepsis. Chest 125: 2238–2246
43. Marsik C, Halama T, Cardona F, et al (2003) Regulation of Fas (APO-1, CD95) and Fas ligand expression in leukocytes during systemic inflammation in humans. Shock 20: 493–496

44. Papathanassoglou ED, Moynihan JA, McDermott MP, Ackerman MH (2001) Expression of Fas (CD95) and Fas ligand on peripheral blood mononuclear cells in critical illness and association with multiorgan dysfunction severity and survival. Crit Care Med 29: 709–718
45. Perfettini JL, Kroemer G (2003) Caspase activation is not death. Nat Immunol 4: 308–310
46. Cauwels A, Janssen B, Waeytens A, Cuvelier C, Brouckaert P (2003) Caspase inhibition causes hyperacute tumor necrosis factor-induced shock via oxidative stress and phospholipase A2. Nat Immunol 4: 387–393
47. Kroemer G, Martin SJ (2005) Caspase-independent cell death. Nat Med 11: 725–730
48. Weaver JG, Rouse MS, Steckelberg JM, Badley AD (2004) Improved survival in experimental sepsis with an orally administered inhibitor of apoptosis. Faseb J 18: 1185–1191

The Pivotal Role of Beta-adrenoreceptors in Critical Illness Pathophysiology

G.L. Ackland and A.J. Patterson

Introduction

The coordinated, emergent regulation of nervous, endocrine, hemodynamic and metabolic processes in response to critical illness is characterized by marked release of catecholamines. Despite several-fold increases in circulating catecholamines, which correlate with clinical outcome, there is a limited understanding of the receptor and cellular consequences of this fundamental critical illness response. Beta-adrenoreceptors are pivotal in the response to this catecholamine surge, playing disparate roles in shaping physiological responses during different stages of critical illness. Here we review mechanisms and common disease processes through which acute and chronic alterations in β-adrenoreceptor physiology may affect important components of critical illness and discuss emerging therapeutic roles for beta-adrenoreceptor manipulation.

New Concepts in Adrenoreceptor Signaling Biology

The original concept for the consequences of activation of β_1- and β_2-adrenoreceptors by catecholamines involving a common linear signaling pathway has changed dramatically. The classic paradigm proposed that agonist binding induces conformational changes in both receptor subtypes. These conformational changes increase affinity for the stimulatory G protein (Gs, **Fig. 1**). Interaction with either the β_1 or β_2-adrenoreceptor causes Gs to disassemble into a $\beta\gamma$ subunit and an α subunit. The α subunit activates adenylate cyclase, that uses adenosine triphosphate (ATP) to generate cyclic adenosine monophosphate (cAMP). cAMP disinhibits protein kinase A (PKA), which in turn phosphorylates a variety of targets within the cytosol, including L-type calcium channels on the cell membrane and phospholamban and ryanodine receptors on the sarcoplasmic reticulum [1]. However, only β_2- and β_3-adrenoreceptors couple to inhibitory G protein (Gi). Selective stimulation of β_1- and β_2-adrenoreceptor subtypes elicits different physiological responses. β_1-adrenoreceptor stimulation, but not β_2-adrenoreceptor stimulation, induces cardiomyocyte hypertrophy [2, 3]. Transgenic mice with cardiomyocyte-specific over expression of the β_1-adrenoreceptor develop progressive cardiac hypertrophy and heart failure, whereas β_2-adrenoreceptor transgenic mice do not show such abnormalities [4, 5]. Isolated cardiomyocytes undergo apoptosis on β_1-selective stimulation, and β_2 stimulation may protect against this [6]. These β_1- and β_2-adrenoreceptor responses cannot be adequately explained by the classic concept of differential coupling of β_1- and β_2-adrenoreceptor to Gs and Gi proteins.

IV

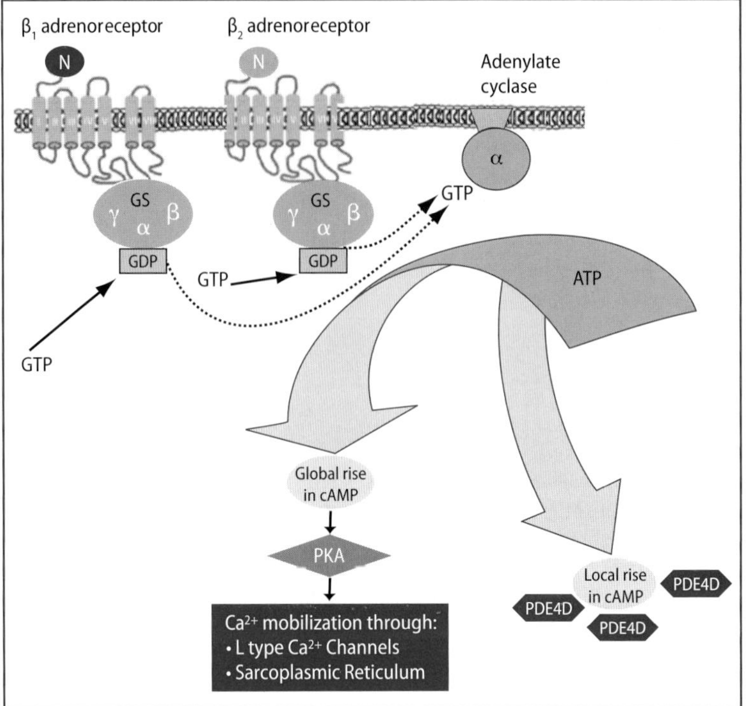

Fig. 1. During acute catecholaminergic stimulation, both beta-1 and beta-2 adrenoreceptor agonism results in the disassembly of stimulatory G-proteins (Gs) into $\beta\gamma$ and α subunits. Subsequently, the α subunit activates adenylate cyclase, generating cyclic adenosine monophosphate (cAMP)-mediated disinhibition of protein kinase A (PKA) and consequent calcium mobilization. PDE: phosphodiesterase

Hence, a new multidimensional signaling paradigm has emerged from recent data (simplified in **Fig. 2**) where β-adrenoreceptors dynamically couple to multiple G proteins, signaling and scaffold proteins in a temporally and spatially regulated manner. Differences between β_1- and β_2-adrenoreceptor signaling occur mainly through compartmentalization of signaling events, such as the formation of signalosomes [7] and the localized control of cAMP degradation through phosphodiesterases [8]. For example, local β_1-adrenoreceptor-mediated cAMP signals propagate over a distance involving multiple sarcomeres in adult cardiomyocytes through the activation of cyclic nucleotide-gated ion channels and the guanosine-5'-triphosphate exchange factor exchange protein activated cAMP. By contrast, the β_2-adrenoreceptor-evoked cAMP signal remains strictly confined by phosphodiesterase- and Gi-independent mechanisms within specific cellular sub domains [8]. It is now recognized that the switch in coupling from Gs to Gi that occurs with β_2-adrenoreceptors is a time-dependent process. Temporal regulation is also recognized as being important in the change of β_1-adrenoreceptor signaling from PKA activation to activation of calcium/calmodulin-dependent protein kinase II [7].

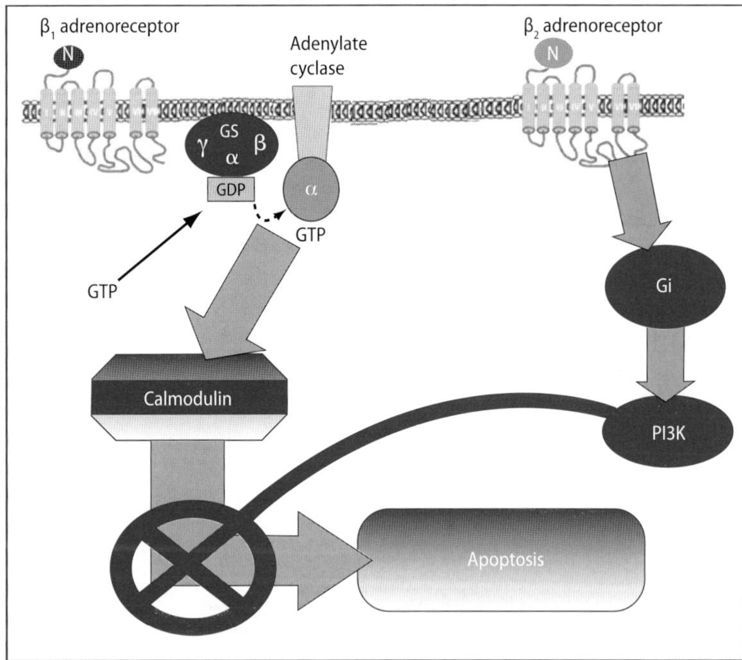

Fig. 2. Persistent activation of β-adrenoreceptors results in beta-subtype specific changes in cellular signaling. Continuous β_2 stimulation leads to inhibitory G protein (Gi) protective signaling pathways (e.g., phosphoinositide-3 kinase, PI3K) which reduces apoptosis. Temporal changes in β_1-adrenoreceptor stimulation lead to calmodulin mediated pathways associated with pro-apoptotic pathways.

Desensitization of Beta-adrenoreceptors

β_1- and β_2-adrenoreceptor subtypes also differ in terms of the processes by which they undergo desensitization during continuous and prolonged activation (**Fig. 3**). Two patterns of rapid desensitization have been characterized for G-protein-coupled receptors [9]. Homologous desensitization mainly involves G-protein-coupled receptor kinases and arrestins; heterologous desensitization is executed mainly through PKA and protein kinase C (PKC) [10]. Persistent agonist activation of β_1-adrenoreceptors results in desensitization by reducing the number of available receptors on the cell surface [10]. Degradation of receptors after internalization, together with a decrease in receptor mRNA provide the mechanisms whereby the reduction persists. β_1-adrenoreceptors are desensitized when agonist-occupied receptors are phosphorylated by PKA and by G protein-coupled receptor kinase 2 (GRK2), which is also called beta-adrenergic receptor kinase 1 (betaARK1) [10]. The cellular expression of GRK2 increases during continuous β_1-adrenoreceptor stimulation. Following receptor phosphorylation, binding of a small protein, known as β-arrestin, sterically blocks G protein activation; beta-arrestin binding also directs the internalization of desensitized receptors. Studies of mice over-expressing β_1-adrenoreceptors suggest that continuous β_1-adrenoreceptor stimulation leads to cardiomyocyte toxicity [4]. Studies in which the β_1/β_2 agonist, isoproterenol, was administered for prolonged periods of time to β_2-adrenoreceptor knockout mice also support this finding [11].

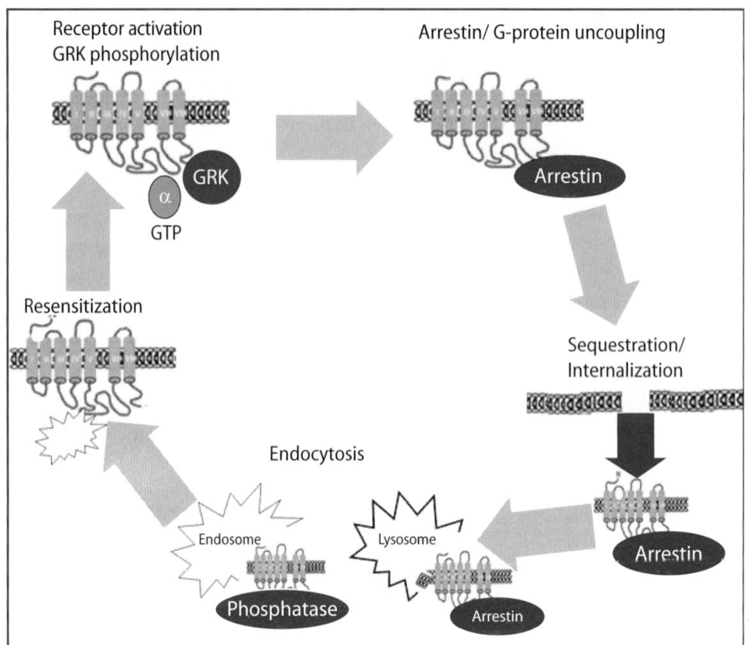

Fig. 3. The β_2-adrenoreceptor as a model for β-adrenoreceptor downregulation. Following binding of the β_2 agonist, G protein receptor kinases (GRKs) phosphorylate the receptor. Arrestin proteins bind to the phosphorylated β_2-adrenoreceptor, causing uncoupling from G proteins. Arrestins may also enable the delivery of the β_2-adrenoreceptor to clathrin-coated pits for endocytosis by endosomes or lysosomes. In endosomes, dissociation of arrestin and phosphatase mediated dephosphorylation resensitizes the β_2-adrenoreceptor, permitting it to recycle back to the plasma membrane. Alternatively, lysosomes degrade the β_2-adrenoreceptor arrestin complex.

The desensitization of β-adrenoreceptors during critical illness is associated with poorer clinical outcome. Preservation of cardiac and metabolic responses to exogenously administered dobutamine, dopamine, and epinephrine are associated with markedly better survival [12]. Experimental and clinical data have demonstrated that lactate production in the muscle is linked to epinephrine-β_2 receptor mediated stimulation of the Na^+, K^+-ATPase pump, independent of tissue hypoxia [13]. The ability to produce, and clear, more lactate following catecholamine administration in stable, non-lactatemic patients is associated with higher survival rates [14].

Catecholamine-induced Immune Dysregulation

Adrenoreceptor desensitization is a central mechanism involved in catecholamine-induced immune dysregulation. Sympathetic/adrenomedullary activity controls the expression of peripheral adrenoreceptors in target tissues, including immune cells [15]. Through direct communication via sympathetic nerve fibers that innervate lymphoid organs, catecholamines modulate mouse lymphocyte proliferation, differentiation, and cytokine production of rodent T cells and human peripheral blood mononuclear cells [15]. These interactions are facilitated by adrenergic receptors expressed on a range of immune cells, across species [15]. T cells, macrophages, and neutrophils, when stimulated, can synthesize and release catecholamines *de novo*. Catecholamines released from these immune cells act in a complex autocrine/paracrine manner to regulate cytokine mediator release differentially via the full complement of adrenergic receptors, including both β_1- and β_2-adrenoreceptor subtypes [16] .

At the onset of critical illness (sepsis, burns), pronounced increases in natural killer cells and CD8 lymphocytes occur, with moderate changes in B cells or CD4+lymphocytes [17]. An increasing body of evidence indicates that the prolonged neurohormonal response to critical illness contributes to the inhibition of pro-inflammatory/T-helper 1 (Th1) responses and up-regulation of anti-inflammatory/T-helper 2 (Th2) responses through complex effects on innate/adaptive immune cells [18]. Sustained catecholamine infusion in rats results in splenocyte apoptosis and decreases in natural killer cells, T and B lymphocytes. By contrast, acutely administered β-adrenoreceptor agonists, such as isoproterenol, suppress the expression of endotoxin-induced cytokines, experimental allergic encephalomyelitis and collagen/adjuvant-induced arthritis [18]. Although acutely administered non-specific β-blockers augment pro-inflammatory cytokine production in experimental studies, such responses are not seen in a variety of clinical, pro-inflammatory scenarios. Indeed, a direct, innate link between epinephrine and immune function has been demonstrated in both humans and rat strains with high and low endogenous basal levels of epinephrine. Lewis rats exhibit markedly lower baseline epinephrine levels and responsiveness to isoproterenol-induced cytokine inhibition compared to F344 rats [19]. Thus, low basal adrenomedullary activity confers enhanced immune responsiveness.

β-adrenoreceptor mediated immunosuppression by the sympathetic nervous system may also be dependent on the source of inflammation [20]. Under bacteria-free conditions, tumor necrosis factor (TNF)-α secretion is low, while interleukin (IL)-6 secretion is α_2-adrenoreceptor dependent. In the presence of *Pseudomonas* bacteria, TNF-α and IL-6 secretion increase, but IL-6 secretion is reduced by β-adrenoreceptor blockade with propranolol. This α- to β switch of IL-6 inhibition in the presence of bacteria adds a further layer of complexity to the immunomodulatory role of β-adrenoreceptors [20]. In addition to immunosuppression, catecholamine inotropes directly stimulate bacterial growth [21], mediated by removal of iron from lactoferrin and transferrin by the catechol moiety and its subsequent acquisition by bacteria.

Amelioration of lymphocyte apoptosis is a cardinal event in determining outcomes in experimental sepsis [22]. Catecholamines are likely to contribute to this during the systemic response to inflammation, since they directly increase apoptosis in various lymphoid populations [23], through both α- and β-adrenoreceptor subtypes. Treatment of splenic lymphocytes with a non-selective β-adrenoreceptor antagonist (propranolol) inhibited apoptosis as a consequence of hemorrhagic shock [24]. The precise contribution of each receptor subtype, and their roles in specific organs, is unclear with huge potential for intra- and inter-organ effects (**Fig. 4**).

IV

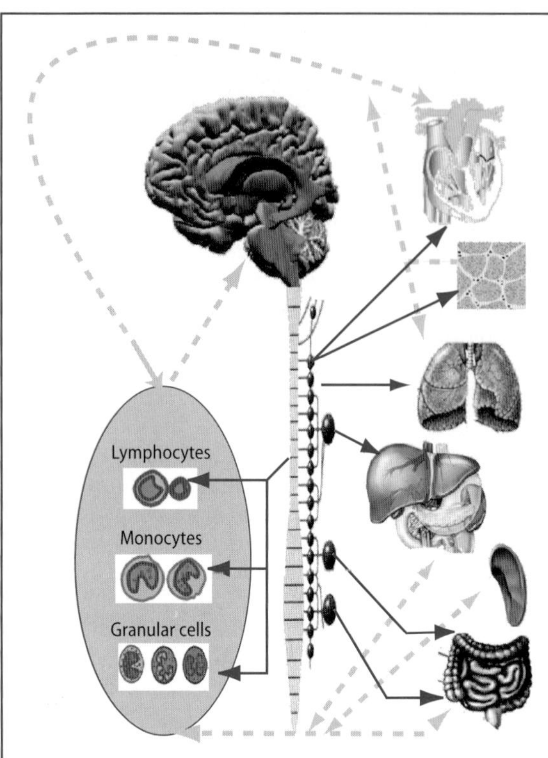

Fig. 4. Despite the intimate temporal, anatomical and physiological relationship between catecholamine release and key pathophysiological changes that occur during critical illness, the β-adrenoreceptor plays a largely ill-defined role in mediating the interaction between sympathetic nervous system outflow (solid blue lines), immune function (blue dotted lines), and organ dysfunction. Expression of β-adrenoreceptor on different lymphoid cells and their coupling to intracellular pathways is likely to differ according to their stage of maturation, differentiation, tissue localization and concurrent pathological changes. The bidirectional links (blue dotted lines/arrows) demonstrate potential links between β-adrenoreceptor-mediated catecholamine actions and inflammatory, neural, metabolic, and circulatory changes, which are likely to be compartmentalized between and perhaps within organs.

Beta-adrenoreceptor-mediated Metabolic Effects of Critical Illness

As well as impaired immune function, the metabolic hallmarks of critical illness physiology include hyperglycemia, marked net protein loss, insulin resistance, and peripheral lipolysis [25]. Excess catecholamines drive many of these processes directly through the stimulation of glycogenolysis in skeletal muscle and lipolysis in peripheral adipose tissue. The resultant increased production of lactate, alanine, glycerol, and free fatty acids, further fuels hepatic gluconeogenesis, augmenting glucose levels already driven higher through hepatic glycogenolysis triggered directly by higher circulating levels of norepinephrine and epinephrine. The seminal work of Herndon and colleagues has demonstrated in the pediatric burn population that administration of propranolol reduces energy expenditure, muscle protein catabolism, and peripheral lipolysis [26]. The reduction in peripheral lipolysis and free fatty acid oxidation shifts metabolism towards increased glucose oxidation. Human studies have revealed a net decrease in plasma glucose concentrations in patients receiving non-selective beta-blockade using propranolol during states of stress [27], due to a decrease in glucose production without any change in glucose clearance. Given the deleterious role of hyperglycemia in critically ill patients and the beneficial effects of glucose control [28], the targeting of β-adrenoreceptor mediated catecholamine-induced metabolic dysregulation is an attractive target to ameliorate the deleterious metabolic effects of critical illness.

Beta-adrenoreceptor-mediated Effects on Barrier Gut Function

There are compelling reasons to support the contention that the gut should be regarded as the motor of critical illness [29]. Loss of intestinal lymphocytes in the mucosal layer is likely to play a critical role in host defence [30] because these cells are exposed to a vast array of environmental antigens. Intestinal lymphocyte apoptosis triggered through the systemic release of catecholamines following sympathetic activation or tissue trauma may lead to the overgrowth of endogenous Gram-negative bacteria [31]. Catecholamines directly induce intestinal lymphocyte apoptosis [32], an effect that is ameliorated after exercise-induced lymphocytosis by nadolol, a non-specific β-adrenoreceptor antagonist [33].

Specific Beta-adrenoreceptor-mediated Roles in Common Critical Illness Pathophysiology

Traumatic Head Injury

Applied experimental critical illness models, such as head injury, where prolonged excessive catecholamine stimulation occurs, demonstrate the potential importance of β-adrenoreceptor biology in mediating clinical benefits. In a murine model of stroke, an immune deficient state characterized by the extensive apoptotic loss of lymphocytes and a shift from Th1 to Th2 cytokine production, rapidly leads to spontaneous systemic bacterial infection. Mortality and bacterial infections were prevented by propranolol-mediated inhibition of sympathetic nervous activity but not by steroid receptor blockade [34]. The positive effect of propranolol on immune profile and clinical outcome was identical to both the adoptive transfer of T and natural killer cells and administration of interferon (IFN)-γ, the archetypal Th1 cytokine. Recent clinical data support the idea that ß-blockade (albeit poorly defined) may be protective in isolated head trauma [35].

Cardiovascular Dysfunction during Critical Illness

The mammalian heart contains three β-adrenoreceptor subtypes: β_1-, β_2-, and β_3-adrenoreceptors. The β_1- and β_2-adrenoreceptor subtypes dominate the cardiac response to adrenergic stimulation. Differences in cell signaling between β_1- and β_2-adrenoreceptors with regard to activation of cytotoxic versus cytoprotective pathways (**Fig. 2.**) explain why continuous β_1-adrenoreceptor stimulation causes myocyte injury while continuous β_2-adrenoreceptor stimulation does not [36]. These differences may also help to explain why relatively β_1-adrenoreceptor selective antagonists produce favorable outcomes in ischemic heart disease and cardiac failure [37]. Both β_1- and β_2-adrenoreceptor polymorphisms are associated with an increased risk of adverse cardiovascular outcomes [38, 39].

Cardiac dysfunction during sepsis, though usually reversible, is associated with poorer clinical outcomes [40]. Sepsis induces a disruption at various levels of the β-adrenoreceptor signaling cascade. Since myocardial responses to increased extracellular calcium ion concentrations remain normal, disruption of G-protein signal transduction seems critical [41]. Gs proteins were decreased in endotoxemic rabbits [42], whereas Gi proteins were increased in non-survivors of septic shock [43]. These changes result in decreased activity of adenylyl cyclase and reduced levels of cAMP. β_3 receptors, linked to Gi proteins, are upregulated during human sepsis [44].

Clinically, a blunted contractile response to dobutamine during critical illness is associated with an increase in mortality (45).

Acute Lung injury

β_2-adrenoreceptors are expressed on different cell types in the lung, including respiratory epithelial cells, smooth muscle cells, and macrophages. Inhalation of propranolol enhances lipopolysaccharide (LPS)-induced lung inflammation and activation of coagulation pathways in mice, without altering neutrophil recruitment [46], suggesting a protective role for β-adrenoreceptors in lung injury. Experimental and preliminary clinical studies in acute lung injury (ALI) also support a therapeutic role for β_2 agonists [47], indicating multiple protective mechanisms, including an anti-inflammatory action [48].

Limitations of Current Experimental/clinical Data

Four important limitations preclude further interpretation of this literature with regard to the precise role of specific β-adrenoreceptor subtypes. First, most studies have employed non-specific β-blockers, thereby precluding specific insights into which subtype is important. Typically, propranolol has been used, which also possesses significant local anesthetic and serotonergic receptor actions that could contribute to immune regulation amongst other physiologic actions [49]. Second, both the timing and duration of administration, as well as agonist load, may influence the immune response through desensitization and switching of of subcellular mechanisms. Third, the uncontrolled systemic effects of β-adrenoreceptor agonism/antagonism on cardiac and peripheral vascular physiology may also introduce confounding factors that alter cytokine expression indirectly (e.g., hypotension). Lastly, tissue, pathogen and host (gender, age) specific differences in β-adrenoreceptor response in mediating inflammation may be important confounding factors. For example, experimental data suggest the route of administration of β-antagonists in ALI may be crucial in conferring protective β_2-mediated effects [46]. Furthermore, the recent Peri-Operative ISchemic Evaluation (POISE) trial, where perioperative cardiac injury was reduced yet overall mortality increased due to sepsis and stroke, provides a pivotal example as to how β-adrenoreceptor modulation may yield disparate clinical outcomes [50]. The apparently negative result of this landmark perioperative trial may be explained in part by the contention that the *acute* immuno-modulatory role of β_1-adrenoreceptor antagonism is detrimental, thereby influencing clinical outcome adversely independent of cardioprotective mechanisms.

Conclusion

β-adrenoreceptors play an important role in several pathophysiological processes familiar to critical care physicians. Nevertheless, the clinical utilization of β-adrenoreceptor agonists and antagonists is a mainstay of critical care, despite studies that highlight several potentially detrimental effects. The complex and apparently counteracting roles of catecholamines, either endogenous or exogenous, in different organs/systems demonstrates the further need to understand local and systemic consequences of critical illness on β-adrenoreceptor physiology. The roles of β-adrenoreceptor subtypes and β-adrenoreceptor downregulation/desensitization are central to an enhanced understanding of the complexity of the contribution of β-adrenoreceptors in critical illness.

References

1. Guimarães S, Moura D (2001) Vascular adrenoreceptors: an update. Pharmacol Rev. 53: 319–356
2. Xiao RP, Avdonin P, Zhou YY, et al (1999) Coupling of beta2-AR to Gi proteins and its physiological relevance in murine cardiac myocytes. Circ Res 84: 43–52
3. Xiao RP, Cheng H, Zhou YY, Kuschel M, Lakatta EG (1999) Recent advances in cardiac beta2-adrenergic signal transduction. Circ Res 85: 1092–1100
4. Engelhardt S, Hein L, Wiesmann F, Lohse MJ (1999) Progressive hypertrophy and heart failure in beta1-adrenergic receptor transgenic mice. Proc Natl Acad Sci USA 96: 7059 –7064
5. Milano CA, Allen LF, Rockman HA, et al (1994) Enhanced myocardial function in transgenic mice overexpressing the beta2-adrenergic receptor. Science 264: 582–586
6. Communal C, Singh K, Sawyer DB, Colucci WS (1999) Opposing effects of beta1-and beta2-adrenergic receptors on cardiac myocyte apoptosis: role of a pertussis toxin-sensitive G protein. Circulation 100: 2210 –2212
7. Xiao RP, Zhu W, Zheng M, et al (2006) Subtype-specific beta1 and beta2 adrenoreceptor Signaling in the Heart. Trends Pharmacol Sci 27: 330–337
8. Richter W, Day P, Agrawal R, et al (2008) Signaling from beta1 and beta2 adrenergic receptors is defined by differential interactions with PDE4. EMBO J 27: 384–393
9. Bünemann M, Lee KB, Pals-Rylaarsdam R, Roseberry AG, Hosey MM (1999) Desensitization of G-protein-coupled receptors in the cardiovascular system. Annu Rev Physiol 61: 169–192
10. Reiter E, Lefkowitz RJ (2006) GRKs and beta-arrestins: roles in receptor silencing, trafficking and signaling. Trends Endocrinol Metab 17: 159–165
11. Patterson AJ, Zhu W, Chow A, et al (2004) Protecting the myocardium: A role for the beta2 adrenergic receptor in the heart. Crit Care Med 32: 1041–1048
12. Collin S, Sennoun N, Levy B (2008) Cardiovascular and metabolic responses to catecholamine and sepsis prognosis: a ubiquitous phenomenon? Crit Care12: 118
13. Levy B, Gibot S, Franck P, Cravoisy A, Bollaert PE (2005) Relation between muscle Na+K+-ATPase activity and raised lactate concentrations in septic shock: a prospective study. Lancet 365: 871–875
14. Levraut J, Ichai C, Petit I, Ciebiera JP, Perus O, Grimaud D (2003) Low exogenous lactate clearance as an early predictor of mortality in normolactatemic critically ill septic patients. Crit Care Med 31: 705–710
15. Elenkov IJ, Wilder RL, Chrousos GP, Vizi ES (2000) The sympathetic nerve--an integrative interface between two supersystems: the brain and the immune system. Pharmacol Rev. 52: 595–638
16. Flierl MA, Rittirsch D, Huber-Lang M, Sarma JV, Ward PA (2008) Catecholamines-crafty weapons in the inflammatory arsenal of immune/inflammatory cells or opening pandora's box? Mol Med 14: 195–204
17. Sanders VM, Straub RH (2002) Norepinephrine, the beta-adrenergic receptor, and immunity. Brain Behav Immun 16: 290–332
18. Elenkov IJ, Chrousos GP (1999) Stress hormones, Th1/Th2 patterns, pro/anti-inflammatory cytokines and susceptibility to disease. Trends Endocrinol Metab 10: 359–368
19. Elenkov IJ, Kvetnansky R, Hashiramoto A, et al (2008) Low- versus high-baseline epinephrine output shapes opposite innate cytokine profiles: presence of Lewis- and Fischer-like neurohormonal immune phenotypes in humans? J Immunol 181: 1737–1745
20. Straub RH, Linde HJ, Männel DN, Schölmerich J, Falk W (2000) A bacteria induced switch of sympathetic effector mechanisms augments local inhibition of TNF-alpha and IL-6 secretion in the spleen. FASEB J 14: 1380–1388
21. Lyte M, Freestone PP, Neal CP, et al (2003) Stimulation of *Staph epidermidis* growth and biofi lm formation by catecholamine inotropes. Lancet 361: 130–135
22. Coopersmith CM, Stromberg PE, Dunne WM, et al (2002) Inhibition of intestinal epithelial

IV

apoptosis and survival in a murine model of pneumonia-induced sepsis. JAMA 287: 1716–1721
23. Stevenson JR, Westermann J, Liebmann PM, et al (2001) Prolonged alpha-adrenergic stimulation causes changes in leukocyte distribution and lymphocyte apoptosis in the rat. J Neuroimmunol 120: 50–57
24. Oberbeck R, van Griensven M, Nickel E, Tschernig T, Wittwer T, Pape HC (2002) Influence of beta-AR antagonists on hemorrhage-induced cellular immune suppression. Shock 18: 331–335
25. Norbury WB, Jeschke MG, Herndon DN (2007) Metabolism modulators in sepsis: propranolol. Crit Care Med 35: S616–620
26. Herndon DN, Hart DW, Wolf SE, Chinkes DL, Wolfe RR (2001) Reversal of catabolism by beta-blockade after severe burns. N Engl J Med 345: 1223–1229
27. Shaw JH, Holdaway CM, Humberstone DA (1988) Metabolic intervention in surgical patients: The effect of alpha- or beta-blockade on glucose and protein metabolism in surgical patients receiving total parenteral nutrition. Surgery 103: 520–525
28. Langouche L, Vanhorebeek I, Van den Berghe G (2007) Therapy insight: the effect of tight glycemic control in acute illness. Nat Clin Pract Endocrinol Metab 3: 270–278
29. Ackland G, Grocott MP, Mythen MG (2000) Understanding gastrointestinal perfusion in critical care: so near, and yet so far. Crit Care 4: 269–281
30. Husain KD, Coopersmith CM (2003) Role of intestinal epithelial apoptosis in survival. Curr Opin Crit Care 9: 159–163
31. Lyte M, Bailey MT (1997) Neuroendocrine-bacterial interactions in a neurotoxin-induced model of trauma. J Surg Res 70: 195–201
32. Marra S, Burnett M, Hoffman-Goetz L (2005) Intravenous catecholamine administration affects mouse intestinal lymphocyte number and apoptosis. J Neuroimmunol 158: 76–85
33. Marra S, Hoffman-Goetz L (2004) Beta-adrenergic receptor blockade during exercise decreases intestinal lymphocyte apoptosis but not cell loss in mice. Can J Physiol Pharmacol 82: 465–473
34. Prass K, Meisel C, Höflich C, et al (2003) Stroke-induced immunodeficiency promotes spontaneous bacterial infections and is mediated by sympathetic activation reversal by poststroke T helper cell type 1-like immunostimulation. J Exp Med 198: 725–736
35. Inaba K, Teixeira PG, David JS, et al (2008) Beta-blockers in isolated blunt head injury. J Am Coll Surg 206: 432–438
36. Patterson AJ, Zhu W, Chow A, et al (2004) Protecting the myocardium: a role for the beta2 adrenergic receptor in the heart. Crit Care Med 32: 1041–1048
37. Lohse MJ, Engelhardt S, Eschenhagen T (2003) What is the role of beta-adrenergic signaling in heart failure? Circ Res 93: 896–906
38. Small KM, Wagoner LE, Levin AM, Kardia SL, Liggett SB (2002) Synergistic polymorphisms of beta1- and alpha2C-adrenergic receptors and the risk of congestive heart failure. N Engl J Med 347: 1135–1142
39. Heckbert SR, Hindorff LA, Edwards KL, et al (2003) Beta2-adrenergic receptor polymorphisms and risk of incident cardiovascular events in the elderly. Circulation 107: 2021–2024
40. Rudiger A, Singer M (2007) Mechanisms of sepsis-induced cardiac dysfunction. Crit Care Med 35:1599–608
41. Matsuda N, Hattori Y, Akaishi Y, et al (2000) Impairment of cardiac [beta]-AR cellular signaling by decreased expression of Gs[alpha] in septic rabbits. Anesthesiology 93:1465–1473
42. Chung MK, Gulick TS, Rotondo RE, et al (1990) Mechanism of cytokine inhibition of beta-adrenergic agonist stimulation of cyclic AMP in rat cardiac myocytes. Impairment of signal transduction. Circ Res 67: 753–763
43. Böhm M, Kirchmayr R, Gierschik P, et al (1995) Increase of myocardial inhibitory G-proteins in catecholamine-refractory septic shock or in septic multiorgan failure. Am J Med 98: 183–186
44. Moniotte S, Belge C, Sekkali B, et al (2007) Sepsis is associated with an upregulation of functional beta3 ARs in the myocardium. Eur J Heart Fail 9: 1163–1171
45. Rhodes A, Lamb FJ, Malagon I, Newman PJ, Grounds RM, Bennett ED (1999) A prospective study of the use of a dobutamine stress test to identify outcome in patients with sepsis, severe sepsis, or septic shock. Crit Care Med 27: 2361–2366
46. Giebelen IA, Leendertse M, Dessing MC, et al (2008) Endogenous beta-adrenergic receptors

inhibit lipopolysaccharide-induced pulmonary cytokine release and coagulation. Am J Respir Cell Mol Biol 39: 373–379
47. Wiener-Kronish JP, Matthay MA (2006) Beta-2-agonist treatment as a potential therapy for acute inhalational lung injury. Crit Care Med 34: 1841–1842
48. Lovén J, Svitacheva N, Jerre A, Miller-Larsson A, Korn SH (2007) Anti-inflammatory activity of beta2-agonists in primary lung epithelial cells is independent of glucocorticoid receptor. Eur Respir J 30: 848–856
49. Green AR, Grahame-Smith DG (1976) (-)-Propranolol inhibits the behavioral responses of rats to increased 5-hydroxytryptamine in the central nervous system. Nature 262: 594–596
50. POISE Study Group (2008) Effects of extended-release metoprolol succinate in patients undergoing non-cardiac surgery (POISE trial): a randomized controlled trial. Lancet 371: 1839–1847

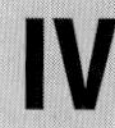

Non-septic Acute Lung Injury and Inflammation: Role of TLR4

E. Lorne, H. Dupont, and E. Abraham

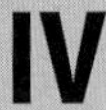

Introduction

Although the role of Toll-like receptor 4 (TLR4) in bacterial infection and sepsis is well characterized, recent studies have also shown that TLR4 can play an important role in contributing to acute inflammatory processes and organ dysfunction in settings in which lipopolysaccharide (LPS) or other bacterial products are not present. In particular, there is increasing evidence that TLR4 is not just a receptor for LPS, but can also transduce other pro-inflammatory signals and, thereby, contribute to cellular activation leading to acute lung injury (ALI) and other organ system dysfunction.

Participation of TLR4 in Ischemia-reperfusion Injury

Under physiological conditions, reactive oxygen species (ROS) participate in intracellular signaling pathways, transcriptional regulation, and other cellular events involved in maintaining homeostasis [1]. During pathophysiologic states associated with ischemia-reperfusion, there is increased production of ROS through the mitochondrial processes, the purine/xanthine oxidase system, and NADPH oxidase activation [2–4].

There is an increasing body of evidence showing that TLR4 can transduce proinflammatory signals produced by ROS. *In vivo* studies demonstrated that there is decreased organ dysfunction following hemorrhage, myocardial infarction, or kidney ischemia-reperfusion in transgenic mice lacking TLR4 or the TLR4-related scaffolding protein, MyD88 [5–7]. In these models of sterile inflammation, LPS is clearly not responsible for TLR4 activation. For example, TLR4 was shown to be a key receptor in neutrophil activation, increases in pulmonary concentrations of tumor necrosis factor (TNF)-α, and the development of ALI after hemorrhage, a situation in which circulating concentrations of xanthine oxidase and production of ROS are increased, even though there is no detectible LPS in plasma [5]. Similarly, infarction size after coronary ligation was decreased in C3H/HeJ mice that express non-functional TLR4, as compared to control C3H/HeN mice, showing that the entire TLR4 is required to transduce the cellular activation signal initiated by myocardial ischemia [6].

Extracellular superoxide appears to play a major role in TLR4 activation during ischemia-reperfusion injury. Unlike other ROS, which are able to rapidly diffuse across cell membranes, superoxide, as a charged species, is unable to transit from extracellular to intracellular sites. *In vivo* studies have demonstrated that superoxide generation in the extracellular milieu is pro-inflammatory. For example, excessive generation of extracellular superoxide through xanthine oxidase-dependent pathways or inhibition of dismutation of superoxide by the absence of extracellular superoxide dismutase (SOD) in extracellular-SOD knockout mice in the setting of severe hemorrhage leads to more severe organ dysfunction [8]. In contrast, enhanced removal of extracellular superoxide in mice overexpressing extracellular-SOD or through the administration of gene therapy resulting in increased expression of extracellular-SOD has beneficial effects on organ dysfunction induced by hemorrhage or other ischemic insults [9, 10].

During ischemia-reperfusion injury, xanthine oxidase and NADPH oxidase appear to be important sources of extracellular superoxide. We and others have demonstrated that inhibition of superoxide production either from xanthine oxidase using allopurinol or from NADPH oxidase by blocking translocation of NADPH phox 47 protected mice from organ injury, suggesting that superoxide rather than xanthine oxidase and NADPH oxidase *per se* is the major mediator of the pro-inflammatory processes initiated by hemorrhage or ischemia-reperfusion injury (**Fig. 1b**) [2–4, 11]. In addition, we have recently demonstrated that xanthine oxidase derived extracellular superoxide is able to activate TLR4 in neutrophils and that TLR4 is centrally involved in mediating the pro-inflammatory effects of extracellular superoxide [12]. Our studies show that xanthine oxidase can bind TLR4 [12], similarly to the NADPH subunit, NOX4 [13]. However, in order to activate TLR4, the catalytic ability of xanthine oxidase to produce superoxide is required [12]. In addition, we have shown that superoxide must be delivered by xanthine oxidase in close proximity to TLR4 in order to activate neutrophils. Heparin, which releases xanthine oxidase from association with the cell membrane, could be beneficial in disease states associated with increased circulating and cell-associated xanthine oxidase, such as hemorrhage or intestinal ischemia [12].

These recent findings suggest that interactions between TLR4 and extracellular superoxide generated during ischemia-reperfusion might contribute to the production of pro-inflammatory cytokines and tissue injury. It appears necessary that extracellular superoxide is delivered in close proximity to TLR4 in order to activate pro-inflammatory responses that occur through TLR4. The precise mechanism through which extracellular superoxide induces signaling through TLR4 is currently not well understood; because superoxide can react easily with nitric oxide (NO), forming peroxynitrite, future investigations to determine a potential contributory role for NO are necessary.

Hydrogen peroxide is produced by dismutation of superoxide, and has been shown to increase membrane lipid raft localization of TLR4 during hemorrhagic shock [14]. In contrast, carbon monoxide negatively affects the TLR4 signaling pathway by inhibiting translocation of TLR4 to lipid rafts through suppression of NADPH oxidase gp91phox subunit dependent ROS generation [15].

Heme Activates TLR4 by Different Mechanisms than does LPS

Heme is composed of an atom of iron linked to four ligand groups of porphyrin. Pathophysiologic conditions that induce hemolysis or extensive cell damage are associated with increased amounts of free heme. In particular, large amounts of free heme and heme proteins are found after hemolysis or rhabdomyolysis due to ischemia-reperfusion injury, hemoglobinopathies, resolution of hematomas, hemorrhage,

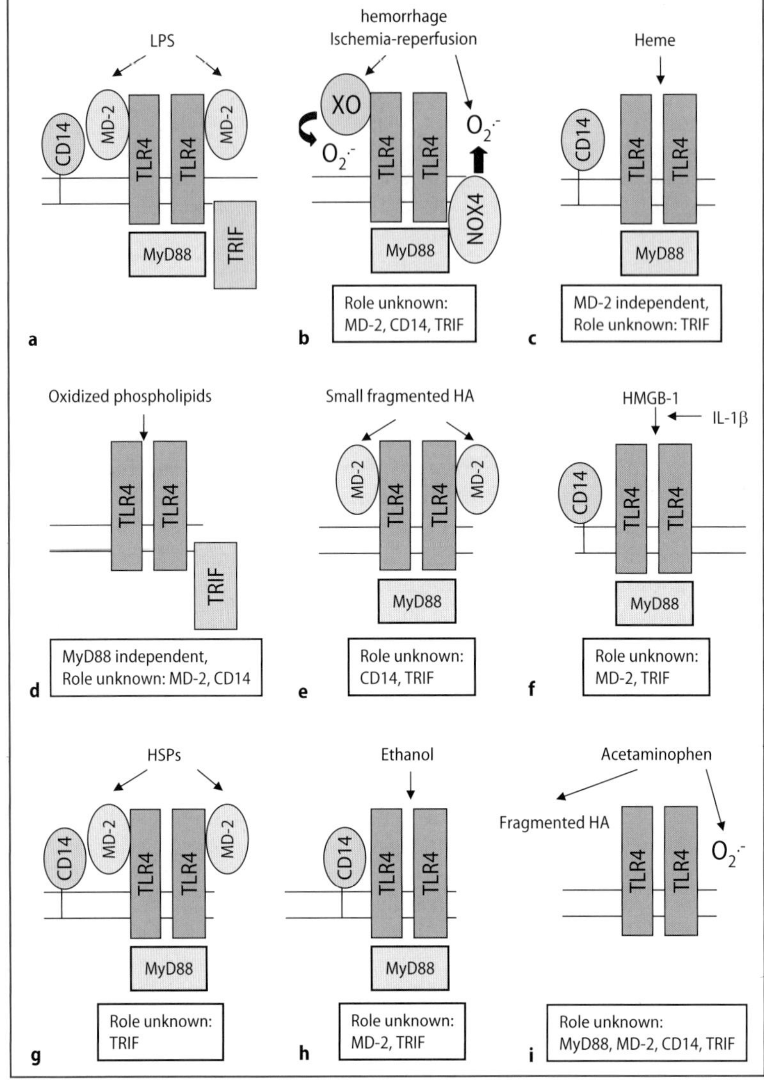

Fig. 1. Accessory proteins known to be necessary for the activation of TLR4 dependent inflammatory response. **a** Classical activation of TLR4 in Gram-negative bacterial infection or sepsis requires MD-2 and CD14, and activates two distinct pathways dependent on MyD88 or TRIF. **b** Hemorrhage and ischemia-reperfusion activate TLR4 by extracellular superoxide produced from xanthine oxidase (XO) or the NADPH NOX4 subunit. MyD88 is required to transduce such signaling. **c** Heme activation of TLR4 requires MyD88 and CD14, but not MD-2. **d** Oxidized phospholipids activate TLR4 through TRIF in a MyD88 independent manner. **e** TLR4 activation by small fragmented hyaluronic acid (HA) requires MD-2 and MyD88. **f** HMGB1 is able to activate TLR4 in a CD14 and MyD88 dependent manner. **g** TLR4 activation by heat shock proteins (HSPs) requires MD-2, CD14 and MyD88. Given the heterogeneous response of TLR4 activation by different HSPs, the accessory proteins are likely to be different between different HSPs. **h** Ethanol requires CD14 and MyD88 to activate TLR4. **i** Acetaminophen increases small fragmented hyaluronic acid (HA), and extracellular superoxide clearance by extracellular-SOD diminishes acetaminophen-induced pro-inflammatory responses.

or muscle injury [16, 17]. Free heme induces oxidative stress [18]. Exposure of macrophages to heme, but not its analogs/precursors, induced TNF-α secretion through a mechanism dependent on MyD88, TLR4, and CD14 (**Fig. 1c**) [19]. The activation of TLR4 by heme required the iron and the vinyl groups of the porphyrin ring [19]. Activation of TLR4-dependent signaling pathways by heme depended on an interaction distinct from the one between TLR4/MD2 and LPS (**Fig. 1a**) because anti-TLR4/MD2 antibodies or a lipid A antagonist inhibited LPS-induced TNF-α secretion but not TNF-α secretion induced by exposure of macropahges to heme. Conversely, protoporphyrin IX antagonized heme-induced activation of TLR4 without affecting that produced by LPS [19]. These results suggest that therapies targeted at TLR4 signaling during pathophysiologic processes associated with increased free heme may be beneficial in reducing organ injury.

Acute Lung Injury Produced by Avian Influenza Virus H5N1 or Acid Aspiration is Dependent on Activation of TLR4 By Oxidized Phospholipids

Oxidized phospholipids appear to play an important role in contributing to macrophage activation and ALI produced by acid aspiration or avian influenza virus H5N1 [20]. Oxidized phospholipids activate nuclear factor-kappa B (NF-κB) and lead to increased production of NF-κB dependent pro-inflammatory cytokines via the TLR4-Toll/interleukin-1 (IL-1) receptor-domain-containing adapter-inducing interferon-β (TRIF) pathway (**Fig. 1d**), instead of the classic cascade involving TLR4-MyD88 [20, 7].

Fragmented Hyaluronic Acid activates TLR4

Hyaluronic acid, a major extracellular matrix glycosaminoglycan, has been shown to be fragmented at sites of inflammation and during tissue damage [21, 22]. *In vivo*, high molecular weight hyaluronic acid ($2-6 \times 10^6$ Da) can be depolymerized to low molecular weight fragments (0.2×10^6 Da) via enzymatic degradation by hyaluronidase β-glucuronidase and hexosaminidase. The importance of hyaluronic acid fragments *in vivo* is highlighted by the fact that not only is lower molecular weight hyaluronic acid associated with active inflammation but also that decrease in CD44 dependent clearance of hyaluronic acid leads to enhanced inflammation-induced pathology [23–25]. Small molecular weight hyaluronic acid fragments were found to require TLR2 and TLR4 associated with MD-2, as well as MyD88 to stimulate mouse macrophages to produce inflammatory chemokines and cytokines (**Fig. 1e**) [26, 22].

TLR4 Participates in Inflammation Associated with Ventilator-induced Lung Injury or Cardiac Hypertrophy Produced by Aortic Stenosis

Mechanical ventilation can produce ventilator-induced lung injury (VILI). It has been suggested that pro-inflammatory pathways may contribute to VILI. A recent study found that TLR4 is involved in the primary inflammatory response induced in the lungs of mechanically ventilated mice, even at low tidal volumes. In contrast to wild type mice, the levels of TNF-α and IL-6 in the lung and the plasma were not increased after initiation of mechanical ventilation in TLR4 knockout mice [27].

Aortic stenosis results in increased pressure in the left ventricle and produces cardiac hypertrophy. TLR4 knockout mice subjected to aortic banding for 2 weeks have less cardiac hypertrophy than do wild type mice [28].

TLR4 Participates in Late Inflammatory Responses in which HMGB1 Plays a Contributory Role

High mobility group box-1 protein (HMGB1), originally described as a nuclear non-histone DNA-binding protein, has recently been shown to act as an extracellular participant in inflammation [29, 30]. Experiments in mice found that HMGB1 levels in serum are increased at late time points after endotoxin exposure [31, 30]. The pro-inflammatory effects of HMGB1 were demonstrated in mice by the ability of HMGB1 to produce ALI after direct intratracheal injection [32]. Administration of anti-HMGB1 antibodies protects mice from LPS-induced lethality even if the therapy is delayed several hours and is given after the appearance of the early pro-inflammatory cytokine response [30]. Administration of anti-HMGB1 antibodies also decreases the severity of LPS-induced ALI, even though pulmonary concentrations of pro-inflammatory cytokines, such as IL-1β or TNF-α remain elevated [32]. Similarly, in septic mice with peritonitis, mortality can be reduced if anti-HMGB1 antibodies are given as long as 24 hours after the initiation of infection with cecal ligation and perforation [33].

Transient transfection in immortalized human embryonic kidney-293 cells demonstrated that HMGB1 induced cellular activation and NF-κB-dependent transcription through TLR2 or TLR4. Co-immunoprecipitation studies showed interaction between HMGB1 and TLR2 as well as with TLR4. Such interactions between HMGB1 and TLR2 and TLR4 supply an explanation for the ability of HMGB1 to induce cellular activation and generate inflammatory responses that are similar to those initiated by LPS [34]. However, we and others have recently demonstrated that HMGB1 itself has weak pro-inflammatory activity, and only develops the ability to induce cytokine production from macrophages and other cell populations after binding to DNA or through binding to pro-inflammatory mediators, such as IL-1β (**Fig. 1f**) [35].

Heat Shock Proteins (HSP) Induce Pro-inflammatory Cytokine Release through TLR4

HSP60, HSP70, HSP90, and glycoprotein (Gp96) are capable of inducing the production of pro-inflammatory cytokines via CD14/TLR2 and CD14/TLR4 receptor complex-mediated signal transduction pathways (**Fig. 1g**) [36]. The primary function of the HSPs appears to be as molecular chaperones in which they recognize and bind to nascent polypeptide chains and partially folded protein intermediates, thereby preventing their aggregation and misfolding.

HSPs are expressed both constitutively and under stressful conditions. Upon necrotic cell death, HSPs are leaked into the extracellular compartment [37]. In addition, HSPs can be released extracellularly independent of necrotic cell death in response to a number of pathophysiologic conditions, including ischemia-reperfusion injury [38, 36]. However, the mechanism through which HSPs produce cellular activation through TLR4 dependent mechanisms is not well delineated and there is continuing controversy concerning the significance of interactions between HSPs and TLR4 [39, 40].

Recent studies have used recombinant HSP, which contains no LPS, to investigate the mechanism by which HSPs produce cellular activation. These studies demonstrate that exposure of cells to HSPs results in a specific pattern of pro-inflammatory cytokine expression, different from that induced by LPS, through a TLR4 dependent mechanism. For example, a recent study found that HSP72 is released by cells during hepatic ischemia-reperfusion injury [41], and stimulation of hepatocytes with purified human recombinant HSP72 did not induce production of TNF-α or IL-6, but did result in dose-dependent increases in macrophage inhibitory protein (MIP)-2 production. Hepatocyte production of MIP-2 was significantly decreased in hepatocytes obtained from TLR4 knockout mice [41]. A second study showed that HSP70 plays a role in ischemia-reperfusion injury by a TLR4 dependent mechanism and that recombinant HSP70 induced NF-κB activation as well as the expression of TNF-α, IL-1β, and IL-6, and depressed myocardial contractility in a TLR4-dependent manner [42].

IV

TLR4 Participates in Ethanol-induced Inflammation

TLR4 and MyD88 have been shown to have a central role in ethanol induced astrocyte activation and neuroinflammation (**Fig. 1h**). In macrophages and astrocytes, while high concentrations of ethanol (100 mM) inhibited TLR4 associated cellular activation, exposure of cells to lower concentrations (from 10 to 50 mM) resulted in TLR4 signaling, clustering of TLR4 in lipid rafts, NF-κB activation, and cytokine production [43]. Such ethanol associated cellular stimulation is dependent on the TLR4 extracellular domain as shown by inhibition when the cells are incubated with specific antibodies against the extracellular domain of TLR4 [43]. In addition, it has been demonstrated in astrocytes that ethanol is able to trigger endocytosis of TLR4 [44].

Acetaminophen-induced Liver Injury is TLR4-dependent

Acetaminophen-mediated liver damage was significantly greater in TLR4 +/+ wild type mice compared to C3H/HeJ mice with mutated TLR4 which is unable to transduce LPS signaling. Similarly, plasma alanine aminotrnsferase (ALT) levels were greater in wild type TLR4 +/+ mice compared to those found in transgenic mice with abnormal non-signaling TLR4 [45].

Serum hyaluronic acid is elevated in acetaminophen-mediated liver injury in humans and has been suggested as a prognostic indicator of survivability in acetaminophen overdose [46]. It is, therefore, possible that increased circulating levels of small molecular weight hyaluronic acid fragments could contribute to hepatic damage through a TLR4-dependent mechanism in the setting of acetaminophen overdose (**Fig. 1i**).

The role of ROS in acetaminophen-induced liver injury is well established. In acetaminophen hepatotoxicity, induction of inducible NO synthase (iNOS) is also thought to have a critical role in protecting hepatocytes [47]. NO delivery protected the liver against acetaminophen-associated toxicity, and treatment with inhibitors of iNOS enhanced acetaminophen hepatotoxicity, suggesting that the protective role of NO in this setting was by inactivating superoxide through formation of peroxynitrite [48, 49]. Supporting this hypothesis, removal of extracellular superoxide by extracellular-SOD gene therapy reduces acetaminophen-induced liver injury [50]. Such findings suggest that extracellular superoxide may participate in the genesis of acetaminophen-induced liver injury through interactions with TLR4 (**Fig. 1i**).

Conclusion

This chapter provides a review of the evidence that TLR4 is not only an 'LPS receptor', but also can be activated through other mechanisms relevant to the pathophysiology of critical illnesses. The consequences of TLR4 activation through ROS and other non-LPS dependent mechanisms may be different from those associated with binding of LPS to TLR4, and may produce different signatures of gene activation and release of pro-inflammatory mediators. Further investigation will be necessary to characterize more completely the nature of the interactions between TLR4 and non-LPS mediators of inflammation as well as their pathophysiologic significance in critical illness.

References

1. Droge W (2002) Free radicals in the physiological control of cell function. Physiol Rev 82: 47–95
2. Shenkar R, Abraham E (1999) Mechanisms of lung neutrophil activation after hemorrhage or endotoxemia: roles of reactive oxygen intermediates, NF-kappa B, and cyclic AMP response element binding protein. J Immunol 163: 954–962
3. Shiotani S, Shimada M, Taketomi A, et al (2007) Rho-kinase as a novel gene therapeutic target in treatment of cold ischemia/reperfusion-induced acute lethal liver injury: effect on hepatocellular NADPH oxidase system. Gene Ther 14: 1425–1433
4. Tan LR, Waxman K, Clark L, et al (1993) Superoxide dismutase and allopurinol improve survival in an animal model of hemorrhagic shock. Am Surg 59: 797–800
5. Barsness KA, Arcaroli J, Harken AH, et al (2004) Hemorrhage-induced acute lung injury is TLR-4 dependent. Am J Physiol Regul Integr Comp Physiol 287: R592–599
6. Oyama J, Blais C Jr, Liu X, et al (2004) Reduced myocardial ischemia-reperfusion injury in toll-like receptor 4-deficient mice. Circulation 109: 784–789
7. Wu H, Chen G, Wyburn KR, et al (2007) TLR4 activation mediates kidney ischemia/reperfusion injury. J Clin Invest 117: 2847–2859
8. Bowler RP, Arcaroli J, Abraham E, Patel M, Chang LY, Crapo JD (2003) Evidence for extracellular superoxide dismutase as a mediator of hemorrhage-induced lung injury. Am J Physiol Lung Cell Mol Physiol 284: L680–687
9. Bowler RP, Arcaroli J, Crapo JD, Ross A, Slot JW, Abraham E (2001) Extracellular superoxide dismutase attenuates lung injury after hemorrhage. Am J Respir Crit Care Med 164: 290–294
10. Li Q, Bolli R, Qiu Y, et al (2001) Gene therapy with extracellular superoxide dismutase protects conscious rabbits against myocardial infarction. Circulation 103: 1893–1898
11. Shenkar R, Abraham E (1997) Hemorrhage induces rapid in vivo activation of CREB and NF-kappaB in murine intraparenchymal lung mononuclear cells. Am J Respir Cell Mol Biol 16: 145–152
12. Lorne E, Zmijewski JW, Zhao X, et al (2008) Role of extracellular superoxide in neutrophil activation: interactions between xanthine oxidase and TLR4 induce proinflammatory cytokine production. Am J Physiol Cell Physiol 294: C985–993
13. Park HS, Jung HY, Park EY, Kim J, Lee WJ, Bae YS (2004) Cutting edge: direct interaction of TLR4 with NAD(P)H oxidase 4 isozyme is essential for lipopolysaccharide-induced production of reactive oxygen species and activation of NF-kappa B. J Immunol 173: 3589–3593

14. Powers KA, Szaszi K, Khadaroo RG, et al (2006) Oxidative stress generated by hemorrhagic shock recruits Toll-like receptor 4 to the plasma membrane in macrophages. J Exp Med 203: 1951–1961
15. Nakahira K, Kim HP, Geng XH, et al (2006) Carbon monoxide differentially inhibits TLR signaling pathways by regulating ROS-induced trafficking of TLRs to lipid rafts. J Exp Med 203: 2377–2389
16. Letarte PB, Lieberman K, Nagatani K, Haworth RA, Odell GB, Duff TA (1993) Hemin: levels in experimental subarachnoid hematoma and effects on dissociated vascular smooth-muscle cells. J Neurosurg 79: 252–255
17. Nath KA, Vercellotti GM, Grande JP, et al (2001) Heme protein-induced chronic renal inflammation: suppressive effect of induced heme oxygenase-1. Kidney Int 59: 106–117
18. Jeney V, Balla J, Yachie A, et al (2002) Pro-oxidant and cytotoxic effects of circulating heme. Blood 100: 879–887
19. Figueiredo RT, Fernandez PL, Mourao-Sa DS, et al (2007) Characterization of heme as activator of Toll-like receptor 4. J Biol Chem 282: 20221–20229
20. Imai Y, Kuba K, Neely GG, et al (2008) Identification of oxidative stress and Toll-like receptor 4 signaling as a key pathway of acute lung injury. Cell 133: 235–249
21. Agren UM, Tammi RH, Tammi MI (1997) Reactive oxygen species contribute to epidermal hyaluronan catabolism in human skin organ culture. Free Radic Biol Med 23: 996–1001
22. Termeer C, Benedix F, Sleeman J, et al (2002) Oligosaccharides of Hyaluronan activate dendritic cells via toll-like receptor 4. J Exp Med 195: 99–111
23. Teder P, Vandivier RW, Jiang D, et al (2002) Resolution of lung inflammation by CD44. Science 296: 155–158
24. Teriete P, Banerji S, Noble M, et al (2004) Structure of the regulatory hyaluronan binding domain in the inflammatory leukocyte homing receptor CD44. Mol Cell 13: 483–496
25. Wang Q, Teder P, Judd NP, Noble PW, Doerschuk CM (2002) CD44 deficiency leads to enhanced neutrophil migration and lung injury in Escherichia coli pneumonia in mice. Am J Pathol 161: 2219–2228
26. Jiang D, Liang J, Fan J, et al (2005) Regulation of lung injury and repair by Toll-like receptors and hyaluronan. Nat Med 11: 1173–1179
27. Vaneker M, Joosten LA, Heunks LM, et al (2008) Low-tidal-volume mechanical ventilation induces a toll-like receptor 4-dependent inflammatory response in healthy mice. Anesthesiology 109: 465–472
28. Ha T, Li Y, Hua F, et al (2005) Reduced cardiac hypertrophy in toll-like receptor 4-deficient mice following pressure overload. Cardiovasc Res 68: 224–234
29. Scaffidi P, Misteli T, Bianchi ME (2002) Release of chromatin protein HMGB1 by necrotic cells triggers inflammation. Nature 418: 191–195
30. Wang H, Bloom O, Zhang M, et al (1999) HMG-1 as a late mediator of endotoxin lethality in mice. Science 285: 248–251
31. Ulloa L, Batliwalla FM, Andersson U, Gregersen PK, Tracey KJ (2003) High mobility group box chromosomal protein 1 as a nuclear protein, cytokine, and potential therapeutic target in arthritis. Arthritis Rheum 48: 876–881
32. Abraham E, Arcaroli J, Carmody A, Wang H, Tracey KJ (2000) HMG-1 as a mediator of acute lung inflammation. J Immunol 165: 2950–2954
33. Yang H, Ochani M, Li J, et al (2004) Reversing established sepsis with antagonists of endogenous high-mobility group box 1. Proc Natl Acad Sci USA 101: 296–301
34. Park JS, Gamboni-Robertson F, He Q, et al (2006) High mobility group box 1 protein interacts with multiple Toll-like receptors. Am J Physiol Cell Physiol 290: C917–924
35. Sha Y, Zmijewski J, Xu Z, Abraham E (2008) HMGB1 develops enhanced proinflammatory activity by binding to cytokines. J Immunol 180: 2531–2537
36. Asea A, Rehli M, Kabingu E, et al (2002) Novel signal transduction pathway utilized by extracellular HSP70: role of toll-like receptor (TLR) 2 and TLR4. J Biol Chem 277: 15028–15034
37. Basu S, Binder RJ, Suto R, Anderson KM, Srivastava PK (2000) Necrotic but not apoptotic cell death releases heat shock proteins, which deliver a partial maturation signal to dendritic cells and activate the NF-kappa B pathway. Int Immunol 12: 1539–1546
38. Asea A (2007) Mechanisms of HSP72 release. J Biosci 32: 579–584

39. Osterloh A, Veit A, Gessner A, Fleischer B, Breloer M (2008) Hsp60-mediated T cell stimulation is independent of TLR4 and IL-12. Int Immunol 20: 433–443
40. Tsan MF, Gao B (2004) Cytokine function of heat shock proteins. Am J Physiol Cell Physiol 286: C739–744
41. Galloway E, Shin T, Huber N, et al (2008) Activation of hepatocytes by extracellular heat shock protein 72. Am J Physiol Cell Physiol 295: C514–520
42. Zou N, Ao L, Cleveland JC Jr, et al (2008) Critical role of extracellular heat shock cognate protein 70 in the myocardial inflammatory response and cardiac dysfunction after global ischemia-reperfusion. Am J Physiol Heart Circ Physiol 294: H2805–2813
43. Fernandez-Lizarbe S, Pascual M, Gascon MS, Blanco A, Guerri C (2008) Lipid rafts regulate ethanol-induced activation of TLR4 signaling in murine macrophages. Mol Immunol 45: 2007–2016
44. Blanco AM, Perez-Arago A, Fernandez-Lizarbe S, Guerri C (2008) Ethanol mimics ligand-mediated activation and endocytosis of IL-1RI/TLR4 receptors via lipid rafts caveolae in astroglial cells. J Neurochem 106: 625–639
45. Yohe HC, O'Hara KA, Hunt JA, et al (2006) Involvement of Toll-like receptor 4 in acetaminophen hepatotoxicity. Am J Physiol Gastrointest Liver Physiol 290: G1269–1279
46. Williams AM, Langley PG, Osei-Hwediah J, Wendon JA, Hughes RD (2003) Hyaluronic acid and endothelial damage due to paracetamol-induced hepatotoxicity. Liver Int 23: 110–115
47. Michael SL, Mayeux PR, Bucci TJ, et al (2001) Acetaminophen-induced hepatotoxicity in mice lacking inducible nitric oxide synthase activity. Nitric Oxide 5: 432–441
48. Hinson JA, Bucci TJ, Irwin LK, Michael SL, Mayeux PR (2002) Effect of inhibitors of nitric oxide synthase on acetaminophen-induced hepatotoxicity in mice. Nitric Oxide 6: 160–167
49. Knight TR, Ho YS, Farhood A, Jaeschke H (2002) Peroxynitrite is a critical mediator of acetaminophen hepatotoxicity in murine livers: protection by glutathione. J Pharmacol Exp Ther 303: 468–475
50. Laukkanen MO, Leppanen P, Turunen P, et al (2001) EC-SOD gene therapy reduces paracetamol-induced liver damage in mice. J Gene Med 3: 321–325

IV

Hydrogen Sulfide: A Metabolic Modulator and a Protective Agent in Animal Models of Reperfusion Injury

C. Szabó, P. Asfar, and P. Radermacher

Introduction

Hydrogen sulfide (H_2S), a gas with the characteristic odor of rotten eggs, is known for its toxicity and as an environmental hazard [1–5]. Recently H_2S has been recognized as a signaling molecule of the cardiovascular, inflammatory and nervous systems. Alongside with nitric oxide (NO) and carbon monoxide, it is now referred to as the "third endogenous gaseous transmitter" [6]. Inhalation of gaseous H_2S and administration of compounds that donate H_2S have been studied in various models of ischemia-reperfusion and circulatory shock [7–24].

The Biological Chemistry of Hydrogen Sulfide

In mammals, H_2S is synthesized from the sulfur containing amino acid, L-cysteine, by either cystathionine-β-synthase (CBS) or cystathionine-γ-lyase (CSE), both using pyridoxal 5'-phosphate (vitamin B_6) as a cofactor [1]. This results in low micromolar H_2S levels in the extracellular space, which can be rapidly consumed and degraded by various tissues. Similarly to NO and carbon monoxide, H_2S is a lipophilic compound, which easily permeates cell membranes without using specific transporters. H_2S undergoes rapid degradation via a variety of pathways, and the end products of this reaction are thiosulfate, sulfite and sulfate. Similar to NO and carbon monoxide, H_2S can also bind to hemoglobin, which is therefore now considered as a "common sink" for the three gaseous transmitters [6].

H_2S exerts its effects in biological systems through a variety of interrelated mechanisms (**Table 1**) [1]. Our knowledge of the biology of H_2S stems from *in vitro* studies in various cells and isolated organ systems, either using inhibitors of CSE and/or CBS such as DL-propargylglycine (PAG) and β-cyanoalanine (BCA), or administration of H_2S gas or H_2S donors such as sodium disulfide (Na_2S) and sodium hydrogen sulfide (NaHS). Lower (= physiologic, i.e., low micromolar) levels tend to exert cytoprotective (anti-necrotic or anti-apoptotic) effects in many studies, whereas higher (millimolar) levels are frequently accompanied with cytotoxic effects, which result from free radical generation, glutathione depletion, intracellular iron release and pro-apoptotic action through both the death receptor and mitochondrial pathways [1, 12–14, 25].

Cytochrome c oxidase, a component of the oxidative phosphorylation machinery within the mitochondrium, is one intracellular target of H_2S [4, 5]. Inhibition of cytochrome c oxidase has been implicated in the toxic effects of H_2S and in the induction of a so-called "suspended animation" [27, 28]. H_2S can, therefore, now be

Table 1. Selected biological effects of hydrogen sulfide (H_2S)

Environmental toxicology	Toxic gas originating from sewers, swamps, and putrefaction
Endogenous sources	Synthesized in various tissues from L-cysteine by cystathionine-β-synthase or cystathionine-γ-lyase
Pharmacological inhibitors	DL-propargylglycine and β-cyanoalanine (limited selectivity, non-specific side-effects)
Elimination kinetics	Half-life is less than 1 minute; main metabolites include thiosulfate, sulfite, and sulfate
Receptors and targets	K_{ATP} channels, cytochrome c oxidase
Vascular effects	Vasodilatation via multiple mechanisms (depending on local O_2 concentration)
Cellular effects	Antioxidant effects, free radical scavenging, upregulation of heme oxygenase-1, modulation of multiple signal transduction pathways

considered as an endogenous modulator of mitochondrial activity and cellular oxygen consumption [29, 30].

Potassium-dependent ATP (K_{ATP}) channels have also been implicated in the vasodilatory effects of H_2S [1, 7, 31, 32]. K_{ATP} channel blockers (sulfonylurea derivates), e.g., glibenclamide, attenuated H_2S-induced vasodilation both *in vivo* and *in vitro* [33, 34] and stimulation of K_{ATP} channels by H_2S was demonstrated in the myocardium, pancreatic β-cells, neurons, and the carotid sinus [7]. However, the role of these channels in vasodilatation may not be universal: In some experiments, inhibition of the channels did not attenuate the relaxation, and additional effects including an endothelium-dependent effect, inhibition of angiotensin-converting enzyme, enhancement of the vasorelaxation induced by NO, as well as direct metabolic effects within the vascular smooth muscle cell leading to vascular relaxation have been proposed [32–39]. Importantly, the local oxygen concentration modifies the vasomotor properties of H_2S [39, 40].

Due to its SH-group that allows reduction of disulfide bonds and radical scavenging, H_2S also exerts biological effects as an antioxidant [10], in particular as an endogenous peroxynitrite scavenger [41], which may account for some of its cytoprotective effects in various cell-based experiments [24, 42, 43]. There are also multiple effects of H_2S on multiple intracellular signaling pathways (including the mitogen-activated protein kinase [MAPK] and the phosphatidyinositol-3-kinase/Akt-pathway, the NF-kappa B [NF-κB] pathway, the stress-activated protein kinase c-Jun N-terminal kinase [JNK] pathway), which generally result in an anti-inflammatory cellular phenotype [1, 44, 45]. These effects may or may not be secondary to the effects of H_2S on intracellular redox processes.

H_2S as an Inducer of a State Resembling Suspended Animation

Suspended animation is a hibernation-like metabolic status characterized by a marked, yet reversible reduction of energy expenditure, which allows non-hibernating species to sustain environmental stress, such as extreme changes in temperature or oxygen deprivation [28]. In a landmark paper, Blackstone & Roth provided evidence that inhaled H_2S can induce such a suspended animation-like state [27, 28]: In awake mice breathing 80 ppm, H_2S caused a dose-dependent reduction in both respiratory and heart rate as well as oxygen uptake and carbon dioxide (CO_2) production, which was ultimately associated with a drop in body core temperature to levels ~ 2 °C above ambient temperature [27]. Follow-up studies have confirmed these observations and, using telemetry and echocardiography, it was shown that the bradycardia-related fall in cardiac output coincided with unchanged stroke volume and blood pressure. These physiologic effects of inhaled H_2S were present regardless of the body core temperature investigated (27 °C and 35 °C) [46]. In mechanically ventilated mice instrumented with left ventricular pressure volume conductance catheters and assigned to 100 ppm of inhaled H_2S, hypothermia alone (27 °C) but not normothermic H_2S inhalation (38 °C) decreased cardiac output due to fall in heart rate, whereas both stroke volume and parameters of systolic and diastolic function remained unaffected [47]. Inhaled H_2S in combination with hypothermia, however, was concomitant with the least stimulation of oxygen flux induced by addition of cytochrome-c during state 3 respiration with combined complex I and II substrates [48].

IV

In good agreement with the concept that a controlled reduction in cellular energetic expenditure would allow ATP homoeostasis to be maintained and thus outcome during shock states due to preserved mitochondrial function to be improved [28], the group of Roth subsequently demonstrated that pre-treatment with inhaled H_2S (150 ppm) for only 20 minutes markedly prolonged survival without any apparent detrimental effects in mice exposed to otherwise lethal hypoxia (5 % oxygen) [49]. Similarly, in a rat model of stroke, H_2S inhalation for 2 days after reperfusion resulted in a mild hypothermia and was protective in terms of infarct size and neurological outcome [50]. H_2S inhalation or parenteral administration was also protective in rats undergoing lethal hemorrhage (60 % of the calculated blood volume over 40 minutes) [9]. It is noteworthy that in the latter study the protective effect was comparable when using either inhaled H_2S or a single intravenous bolus of Na_2S: Parenteral sulfide administration has a number of practical advantages (ease of administration, no need for inhalation delivery systems, no risk of exposure to personnel, no issues related to the characteristic odor of H_2S gas) and, in particular, avoids the potential direct pulmonary irritant effects of inhaled H_2S. It is noteworthy that hypothermia is not an absolute pre-requisite of H_2S-related cytoprotection during hemorrhage: The H_2S donor, NaHS, improved hemodynamics, attenuated metabolic acidosis, and reduced oxidative and nitrosative stress in rats subjected to controlled hemorrhage at a mean blood pressure of 40 mmHg [10].

The clinical relevance of murine models may be questioned because, due to their large surface area/mass ratio, rodents can rapidly drop their core temperature. In fact, other authors failed to confirm the metabolic effect of inhaled H_2S in anesthetized and mechanically ventilated piglets (body weight ~ 6 kg) H_2S and sedated and spontaneously breathing sheep (body weight ~ 74 kg) exposed to up to 80 or 60 ppm of H_2S, respectively [51, 52]. This discrepancy most likely relates to a problem of dosing and/or timing of H_2S rather than to a lack of such an effect *per se*: In fact, we demonstrated in anesthetized and mechanically ventilated pigs (body weight ~ 45 kg), which underwent transient thoracic aortic balloon-occlusion, that infusing the intravenous H_2S donor, Na_2S, over 10 hours reduced heart rate and cardiac output without affecting stroke volume, and thereby allowed oxygen uptake and CO_2 production to be reduced and, ultimately core temperature [17]. The metabolic effect of H_2S coincided with an attenuation of the early reperfusion-related hyperlactatemia

– suggesting a reduced need for anaerobic ATP generation during the ischemia period – and improved norepinephrine responsiveness indicating both improved heart function and vasomotor response to catecholamine stimulation [17].

Protective Effects of H_2S in Local or Whole-body Ischemia or Ischemia-reperfusion

IV

Deliberate hypothermia is a cornerstone of the standard procedures to facilitate neurological recovery after cardiac arrest and improve post-operative organ function after cardiac and transplant surgery. Consequently, several authors have investigated the therapeutic potential of H_2S in treating ischemia-reperfusion injury. The results demonstrated that H_2S protected the lung [15], the liver [13], the kidney [18], and the heart [11, 12, 14, 16, 19, 26, 45]. Thus, H_2S administered prior to reperfusion limited infarct size and preserved left ventricular function in mice [11] and swine [12]. While these findings were obtained without induction of hypothermia, preserved mitochondrial function, documented by increased complex I and II efficiency, assumed major importance for the H_2S-induced cytoprotection [11]. The important role of preserved mitochondrial integrity was further underscored by the fact that 5-hydroxydeconoate, which is referred to as a mitochondrial K_{ATP}-channel blocker, abolished the anti-apoptotic effects of H_2S [19]. Clearly, anti-inflammatory and anti-apoptotic effects also contributed to the improved post-ischemic myocardial function: Treatment with H_2S was associated with reduced myocardial myeloperoxidase activity and absence of the increase in interleukin-1 beta (IL-1β) levels [11, 19], i.e., attenuated tissue inflammation, as well as complete inhibition of thrombin-induced leukocyte rolling, a parameter for leukocyte-endothelium interaction [11]. An improvement of myocardial contractile and vascular relaxant function by H_2S donor therapy was also noted in a model of cardiopulmonary bypass [26]. Moreover, the ischemia/reperfusion-induced activation of p38 MAPK, JNK and NF-κB was also attenuated by H_2S [19]. Finally, H_2S exerted anti-apoptotic effects as shown by reduced terminal deoxynucleotidyl transferase dUTP nick end labelling (TUNEL) staining [11, 12], expression of cleaved caspase-9 [19], caspase-3 [11, 12], activation of the nuclear enzyme poly-ADP-ribose-polymerase (PARP) [12], and activation of the cell death-inducing protooncogene, c-fos [14]. In various models of acute lung injury, parenteral H_2S donor therapy also improved oxygenation, reduced inflammatory mediator production and oxidative stress marker formation [22, 23]. We found, in anesthetized and mechanically ventilated mice undergoing sham-operation for surgical instrumentation, that normothermic H_2S (100 ppm) inhalation (38 °C) over five hours and hypothermia (27 °C) alone comparably attenuated inflammatory chemokine release (monocyte chemotactic protein-1, macrophage-inflammatory protein and growth related oncogen/keratinocyte-derived chemokine) in the lung tissue. While H_2S did not affect the tissue concentrations of tumor necrosis factor-alpha (TNF-α), combining hypothermia and inhaled H_2S significantly decreased tissue IL-6 expression [53].

Not only local ischemia-reperfusion responses, but also severe hemorrhage (or hemorrhagic shock – which has frequently been compared to as a 'whole-body' ischemia-reperfusion state) – has been shown to be beneficially affected by H_2S: In rats suffering from acute severe blood loss, treatment with H_2S or H_2S donors has been shown to provide a marked extension of survival [9]. **Table 2** and the references contained therein may be used to overview the various studies published so far with H_2S that demonstrate beneficial effects in various models of ischemia-reperfusion and shock.

Table 2. Beneficial effects of H_2S in animal models of critical illness

Experimental model	Effect of sulfide/sulfide donor	Reference
Myocardial ischemia/reperfusion models in the rat.	NaHS, given i.v. in various treatment paradigms (e.g., prior to the start of the coronary occlusion, or for 7 days prior to myocardial infarction, and continued for 2 days after infarction) reduced myocardial infarct size.	[14, 16, 19]
Myocardial ischemia/reperfusion in the mouse	IK-1001 (Na_2S) given as an i.v. bolus prior to the start of the reperfusion reduced myocardial infarct size.	[11]
Myocardial ischemia/reperfusion in the pig	IK-1001 (Na_2S) given as an i.v. infusion during reperfusion reduced myocardial infarct size, improved myocardial contractility and reduced neutrophil infiltration and myocardial cytokine expression.	[12]
A dog model of cardiopulmonary bypass	IK-1001 (Na_2S) given as an i.v. infusion during the procedure prevented the deterioration of cardiac function, improved hemodynamic parameters and coronary artery reactivity.	[26]
A pig model of thoracoabdominal aneurysm surgery	IK-1001 (Na_2S) given as an i.v. infusion improved hemodynamic parameters and reduced pressor agent requirement.	[17]
Hepatic ischemia/reperfusion injury in the mouse	IK-1001 (Na_2S) given as an i.v. bolus prior to the start of the reperfusion reduced hepatic enzyme release and improved histology.	[13]
Kidney ischemia/reperfusion injury in the rat	NaHS given i.v. during reperfusion reduced renal enzyme release and improved kidney histology.	[18]
Stroke in aged Sprague-Dawley rats	H_2S inhalation for 2 days, at a dose that induces mild hypothermia, reduced infarct size and improved neurological functions	[50]
Pulmonary ischemia/reperfusion injury in the rat	H_2S improved lung function and histology and attenuated pulmonary oxidative stress.	[15]
Smoke and burn injury-induced acute lung injury in the mouse	IK-1001 (Na_2S) improved survival and improved pulmonary markers of inflammation and oxidative stress.	[23]
Oleic acid-induced acute lung injury in the mouse	NaHS improved pulmonary gas exchange, reduced neutrophil infiltration, attenuated pro-inflammatory mediator production.	[24]
Lethal hypoxia (5 %) in mice	H_2S inhalation extended the survival of the mice subjected to lethal hypoxia.	[49]
Rapid lethal hemorrhage in the rat	H_2S inhalation or IK-1001 (Na_2S) extended survival during rapid severe blood loss.	[9]

i.v.: intravenous

IV

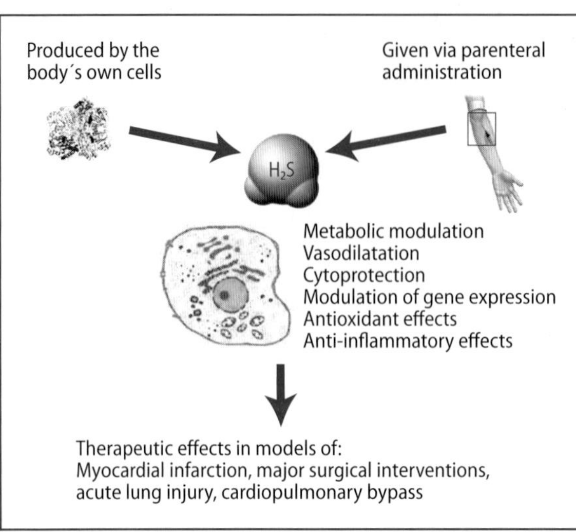

Fig. 1. The H_2S therapeutic concept. H_2S is produced by endogenous sources from L-cysteine via the enzymes, cystathionine-β-synthase or cystathionine-γ-lyase (top left). H_2S can also be administered via parenteral administration (top right) or via inhalation (not shown). By administering H_2S or its prodrugs, one can, in essence, 'substitute' an endogenous 'hormone', a mediator that the body is normally producing, in order to elicit pleiotropic biological effects (metabolic effects, effects on gene expression, effects on vascular tone, effects on oxidant and signal transduction pathways etc.) culminating in cytoprotection and improved outcome in various models of critical illness.

IV

Conclusion

Based on the concept that multiple organ failure secondary to shock, inflammation and sepsis may actually be an adaptive hypometabolic response to preserve ATP homoeostasis – such as was demonstrated for the septic heart – and, thus, represent one of the organism's strategies to survive under stress conditions, the interest of inducing a hibernation-like "suspended animation" with H_2S is obvious. By administering H_2S or its prodrugs, one can, in essence, 'substitute' an endogenous 'hormone', a mediator that the body is normally producing (**Fig. 1**), in order to elicit pleiotropic biological effects culminating in cytoprotection and improved outcome in various models of critical illness. It must be stressed, however, that only a relatively small proportion of the published studies was conducted in clinically relevant large animal models, and some of the findings reported are equivocal. In the rodent studies [11, 13, 19, 23], marked cytoprotective effects were apparent without a change in core body temperature, even though localized metabolic effects cannot be excluded [11]. There may be important issues to be considered in relation to the administration of H_2S: Inhalational route versus parenteral injection route, the question of dosing and timing, including bolus administration vs. continuous intravenous infusion, the establishment of target blood concentrations of reactive H_2S all need to be taken into account. There are, nevertheless, many lines of promising preclinical data to show that this approach merits further investigation as a potential future therapeutic agent for the management of critical illness.

References

1. Szabó C (2007) Hydrogen sulphide and its therapeutic potential. Nat Rev Drug Discov 6: 917–935
2. Beauchamp RO, Bus JS, Popp JA, Boreiko CJ, Andjelkovich DA (1984) A critical review of the literature on hydrogen sulfide toxicity. Crit Rev Toxicol 13: 25–97
3. Reiffenstein RJ, Hulbert WC, Roth SH (1992) Toxicology of hydrogen sulfide. Annu Rev Pharmacol Toxicol 32: 109–134

4. Khan AA, Schuler MM, Prior MG et al (1990) Effects of hydrogen sulfide exposure on lung mitochondrial respiratory chain enzymes in the rat. Toxicol Appl Pharmacol 103: 482–490
5. Dorman DC, Moulin FJM, McManus BE, Mahle KC, James RA, Struve MF (2002) Cytochrome oxidase inhibition induced by acute hydrogen sulfide inhalation: correlation with tissue sulfide concentrations in the rat brain, liver, lung, and nasal epithelium. Toxicol Sci 65: 18–25
6. Wang R (2002) Two's company, three's a crowd: Can H2S be the third endogenous gaseous transmitter? FASEB J 16: 1792–1798
7. Lowicka E, Beltowski J (2007) Hydrogen sulfide (H2S) – the third gas of interest for pharmacologists. Pharmacol Rep 59: 4–24
8. Mok YY, Atan MS, Yoke PC, et al (2004) Role of hydrogen sulphide in haemorrhagic shock in the rat: protective effect of inhibitors of hydrogen sulphide biosynthesis. Br J Pharmacol 143: 881–889
9. Morrison ML, Blackwood JE, Lockett SL, Iwata A, Winn RK, Roth MB (2008) Surviving blood loss using hydrogen sulfide. J Trauma 65: 183–188
10. Ganster F, Burban M, de la Bourdonnaye M, et al (2009) Intérêt d'un donneur de H2S (NaHS) dans le choc hémorragique chez le rat. Réanimation (in press)
11. Elrod JW, Calvert JW, Morrison J, et al (2007) Hydrogen sulfide attenuates myocardial ischemia-reperfusion injury by preservation of mitochondrial function. Proc Natl Acad Sci USA 104: 15560–15565
12. Sodha NR, Clements RT, Feng J, et al (2007) The effects of therapeutic sulfide on myocardial apoptosis in response to ischemia-reperfusion injury. Eur J Cardiothorac Surg 33: 906–913
13. Jha S, Calvert JW, Duranski MR, Ramachandran A, Lefer DJ (2008) Hydrogen sulfide attenuates hepatic ischemia-reperfusion injury: role of antioxidant and antiapoptotic signaling. Am J Physiol Heart Circ Physiol 295: H801-H806
14. Zhu XY, Yan XH, Chen SJ (2008) H2S protects myocardium against ischemia/reperfusion injury and its effect on c-Fos protein expression in rats. Sheng Li Xue Bao 60: 221–227
15. Fu Z, Liu X, Geng B, Fang L, Tang C (2008) Hydrogen sulfide protects rat lung from ischemia-reperfusion injury. Life Sci 82: 1196–1202
16. Ji Y, Pang QF, Xu G, Wang L, Wang JK, Zeng YM (2008) Exogenous hydrogen sulfide postconditioning protects isolated rat hearts against ischemia-reperfusion injury. Eur J Pharmacol 587: 1–7
17. Simon F, Giudici R, Duy CN, et al (2008) Hemodynamic and metabolic effects of hydrogen sulfide during porcine ischemia/reperfusion injury. Shock 30: 359–364
18. Tripatara P, Sa PN, Collino M, et al (2008) Generation of endogenous hydrogen sulfide by cystathionine lyase limits renal ischemia/reperfusion injury and dysfunction. Lab Invest 88: 1038–1048
19. Sivarajah A, Collino M, Yasin M, et al (2009) Antiapoptotic and anti-inflammatory effects of hydrogen sulfide in a rat model of regional myocardial I/R. Shock (in press)
20. Hu LF, Wong PT, Moore PK, Bian JS (2007) Hydrogen sulfide attenuates lipopolysaccharide-induced inflammation by inhibition of p38 mitogen-activated protein kinase in microglia. J Neurochem 100: 1121–1128
21. Zhang H, Moochhala SM, Bhatia M (2008) Endogenous hydrogen sulfide regulates inflammatory response by activating the ERK pathway in polymicrobial sepsis. J Immunol 181: 4320–4331
22. Tamizhselvi R, Moore PK, Bhatia M (2008) Inhibition of hydrogen sulfide synthesis attenuates chemokine production and protects mice against acute pancreatitis and associated lung injury. Pancreas 36: e24-e31
23. Esechie A, Kiss L, Olah G, et al (2008) Protective effect of hydrogen sulfide in a murine model of acute lung injury induced by combined burn and smoke inhalation. Clin Sci (Lond) 115: 91–97
24. Li T, Zhao B, Wang C, et al (2008): Regulatory effects of hydrogen sulfide on IL-6, IL-8 and IL-10 levels in the plasma and pulmonary tissue of rats with acute lung injury. Exp Biol Med (Maywood) 233: 1081–1087
25. Rose P, Moore PK, Ming SH, Nam OC, Armstrong JS, Whiteman M (2005) Hydrogen sulfide protects colon cancer cells from chemopreventative agent beta-phenylethyl isothiocyanate induced apoptosis. World J Gastroenterol 11: 3990–3997
26. Szabó C, Veres G, Radovits T, Karck M, Szabó G (2007) Infusion of sodium sulfide improves

myocardial and endothelial function in a canine model of cardiopulmonary bypass. Crit Care 11 (Suppl 2):S1 (abst)
27. Blackstone E, Morrison M, Roth MB (2005) H2S induces a suspended animation-like state in mice. Science 308: 518
28. Roth MB, Nystul T (2005) Buying time in suspended animation. Sci Am 292: 48–55
29. Hill BC, Woon TC, Nicholls P, Peterson J, Greenwood C, Thomson AJ (1984) Interactions of sulphide and other ligands with cytochrome c oxidase. An electron-paramagnetic-resonance study. Biochem J 224: 591–600
30. Leschelle X, Goubern M, Andriamihaja M, et al (2005) Adaptative metabolic response of human colonic epithelial cells to the adverse effects of the luminal compound sulfide. Biochim Biophys Acta 1725: 201–212
31. Zhang Z, Huang H, Liu P, Tang C, Wang J (2007) Hydrogen sulfide contributes to cardioprotection during ischemia-reperfusion injury by opening KATP channels. Can J Physiol Pharmacol 85: 1248–1253
32. Pryor WA, Houk KN, Foote CS (2006) Free radical biology and medicine: it's a gas, man! Am J Physiol Regul Integr Comp Physiol 291: R491-R511
33. Tang G, Wu L, Liang W, Wang R (2005) Direct stimulation of KATP channels by exogenous and endogenous hydrogen sulfide in vascular smooth muscle cells. Mol Pharmacol 68: 1757–1764
34. Zhao W, Zhang J, Lu Y, Wang R (2001) The vasorelaxant effect of H2S as a novel endogenous gaseous KATP channel opener. EMBO J 20: 6008–6016
35. Laggner H, Hermann M, Esterbauer H et al (2007) The novel gaseous vasorelaxant hydrogen sulfide inhibits angiotensin-converting enzyme activity of endothelial cells. J Hypertens 25: 2100–2104
36. Hosoki R, Matsuki N, Kimura H (1997) The possible role of hydrogen sulfide as an endogenous smooth muscle relaxant in synergy with nitric oxide. Biochem Biophys Res Commun 237: 527–531
37. Ali MY, Ping CY, Mok YY et al (2006) Regulation of vascular nitric oxide in vitro and in vivo; a new role for endogenous hydrogen sulphide? Br J Pharmacol 149: 625–634
38. Whiteman M, Li L, Kostetski I et al (2006) Evidence for the formation of a novel nitrosothiol from the gaseous mediators nitric oxide and hydrogen sulphide. Biochem Biophys Res Commun 343: 303–310
39. Kiss L, Deitch EA, Szabó C (2008) Hydrogen sulfide decreases adenosine triphosphate levels in aortic rings and leads to vasorelaxation via metabolic inhibition. Life Sci 83: 589–594
40. Koenitzer JR, Isbell TS, Patel HD, et al (2007) Hydrogen sulfide mediates vasoactivity in an O2-dependent manner. Am J Physiol Heart Circ Physiol 292: H1953-H1960
41. Whiteman M, Armstrong JS, Chu SH, et al (2004) The novel neuromodulator hydrogen sulfide: an endogenous peroxynitrite 'scavenger'? J Neurochem 90: 765–768
42. Kimura Y, Kimura H (2004) Hydrogen sulfide protects neurons from oxidative stress. FASEB J 18: 1165–1167
43. Wei HL, Zhang CY, Jin HF, Tang CS, Du JB (2008) Hydrogen sulfide regulates lung tissue-oxidized glutathione and total antioxidant capacity in hypoxic pulmonary hypertensive rats. Acta Pharmacol Sin 29: 670–679
44. Oh GS, Pae HO, Lee BS, et al (2006) Hydrogen sulfide inhibits nitric oxide production and nuclear factor-κB via heme oxygenase-1 expression in RAW264.7 macrophages stimulated with lipopolysaccharide. Free Radic Biol Med 41: 106–119
45. Hu Y, Chen X, Pan TT, et al (2008) Cardioprotection induced by hydrogen sulfide preconditioning involves activation of ERK and PI3K/Akt pathways. Pflugers Arch 455: 607–616
46. Volpato GP, Searles R, Yu B, et al (2008) Inhaled hydrogen sulfide: a rapidly reversible inhibitor of cardiac and metabolic function in the mouse. Anesthesiology 108: 659–668
47. Baumgart K, Simkova V, Weber S, et al (2008) Myocardial effects of hypothermia and inhaled H2S in ventilated mice. Shock 29 (Suppl 1):58 (abst)
48. Simkova V, Baumgart K, Barth E, et al (2008) Cytochrome c stimulated respiration in liver mitochondria of anesthetised mice: effects of body temperature and H2S. Shock 29 (Suppl 1):59 (abst)
49. Blackstone E, Roth MB (2007) Suspended animation-like state protects mice from lethal hypoxia. Shock 27: 370–372

50. Florian B, Vintilescu R, Balseanu AT, et al (2008) Long-term hypothermia reduces infarct volume in aged rats after focal ischemia. Neurosci Lett 438: 180–185
51. Li J, Zhang G, Cai S, Redington AN (2008) Effect of inhaled hydrogen sulfide on metabolic responses in anesthetized, paralyzed, and mechanically ventilated piglets. Pediatr Crit Care Med 9: 110–112
52. Haouzi P, Notet V, Chenuel B (2008) H2S induced hypometabolism in mice is missing in sedated sheep. Respir Physiol Neurobiol 160: 109–115
53. Gröger M, Simon F, Öter S, et al (2008) H2S attenuates oxidative DNA-damage during renal ischemia/reperfusion injury. Shock 29 (Suppl 1):57 (abst)

V Septic Shock

'Myocardial Depression' or 'Septic Cardiomyopathy'?

K. WERDAN, A. OELKE, and U. MÜLLER-WERDAN

Introduction

'Septic acute myocarditis' in the pre-antibiotic era was a purulent disease of the heart. Nowadays, non-specific pathomorphological and pathohistological alterations characterize the myocardium of patients whose hearts have failed in septic shock. For decades, septic myocardial depression in animal models was attributed to the release of cardiodepressant factors into the blood stream, while the existence of human septic myocardial depression was only unequivocally proven in the early 1980s by the group of Parrillo [1], who had examined patients in the ICU with nuclear imaging techniques. Since then, experimental and clinical evidence has accumulated arguing for a more complex alteration of the heart in sepsis than exclusive myocardial depression. The concept of a "septic cardiomyopathy" was proposed [2], which emphasizes alterations of cardiac cellular phenotype as a basis of organopathy in response to a variety of agents acting on heart cells, like bacterial toxins and endogenous cytokines, hormones, mediators, and cardiodepressant factors. Not only is impairment of complex intrinsic heart function a consequence, but regulation of cardiac function is also severely disturbed due to excessive autonomic dysfunction [3].

The intention of this chapter is to highlight newer aspects of cardiac involvement in severe sepsis and septic shock and its impaired regulation. Organ-related infectious heart diseases, like viral myocarditis or bacterial endocarditis, are not the focus of this article, rather the uniform reaction of the heart to the generalized inflammatory processes seen in sepsis.

Septic Cardiomyopathy: A Secondary Cardiomyopathy in the Scope of the Systemic Disease, 'Sepsis'

It had long been denied that cardiac involvement forms part of septic multiple organ dysfunction syndrome, as cardiac output values of septic patients are usually apparently normal or may even be enhanced in comparison to the physiological range (**Fig. 1**). However, heart failure becomes evident when cardiac output is considered in relation to the systemic vascular resistance (SVR), which is severely lowered due to sepsis-induced vasodilatation (**Fig. 2**). A healthy heart may compensate for the pathological decrease in afterload down to one-third or one-fourth of the normal value by an up to three- or fourfold increase in cardiac output (**Fig. 2**), while, very often, the observed values in our septic patients are considerably lower (**Fig. 2**); the compensatory increase in pump activity is not large enough to stabilize blood pres-

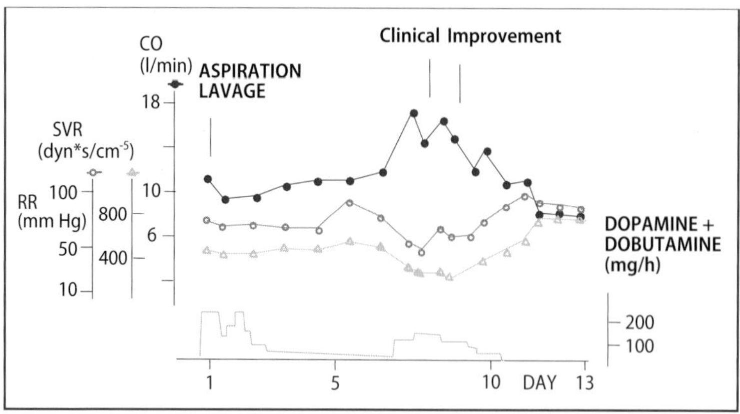

Fig. 1. Case report: Cardiovascular changes in *Pseudomonas* sepsis. This patient suffered from an aspiration pneumonia on day 1. After initial stabilization, cardiovascular deterioration occurred, resulting in septic shock around day 7. Thereafter, the patient had an uneventful recovery. CO: cardiac output.

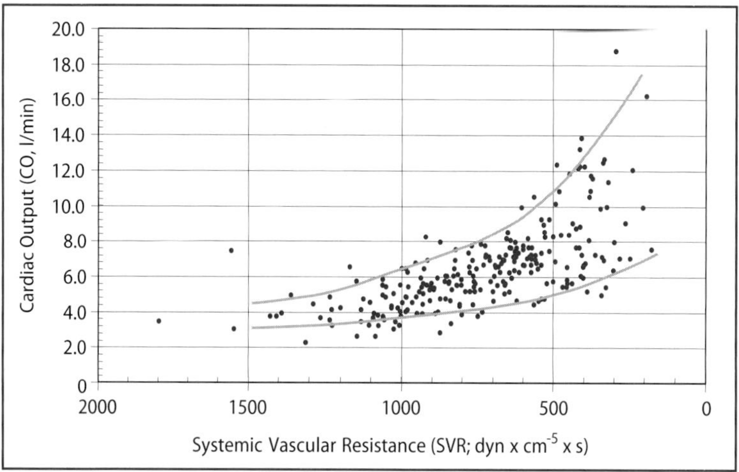

Fig. 2. Correlation of cardiac output and systemic vascular resistance (SVR) in patients with septic multiple organ dysfunction syndrome. In 31 patients with septic multiple organ dysfunction syndrome, cardiac output was measured repeatedly during the course of the disease and here is plotted against the respective SVR. With decreasing afterload (fall in SVR) cardiac output values increase, with considerable variation for any specific SVR value. The upper line represents the maximal cardiac output values achieved by hearts minimally or unimpaired related to the respective SVR, while the values below indicate reduced cardiac output values in the sense of more or less severe septic cardiomyopathy.

sure. This observation is the consequence of the complex pattern of septic cardiomyopathy and the impaired regulation of heart function (**Table 1**). Left ventricular stroke work indices were reported to be reduced to a similar degree in patients with various forms of Gram-negative, Gram-positive or fungal sepsis [2, 4], indicating that it is not so much bacterial virulence factors but rather the common mediator network that determines the occurrence and severity of the disease. Although septic cardiomyopathy is potentially completely reversible – described as myocardial hiber-

Table 1. Features of acute septic cardiomyopathy

Pump failure
- In relation to the lowered systemic vascular resistance
  - cardiac index not adequately increased
  - right and left ventricular ejection fractions and stroke work indices not enhanced or even decreased
  - pump volumes inadequately low
- Global and regional contractile disturbances
- Contraction and relaxation abnormalities
- Increase in ventricular compliance (shift of the pressure-volume-curves to the left)
- Considerable dilatation of the heart is possible
- Coronary arteries dilated, high coronary blood flow
- Impairment of coronary microcirculation?
- Myocardial hibernation: Reversible process

Right ventricular compromise and dilatation due to ARDS

Superimposed hypoxic heart damage
- Accentuated in preexisting coronary artery disease, particularly in shock: Steal syndrome

The heart as a 'cytokine producer'
- Pro-inflammatory cytokines not only depress myocardial depression, but also stimulate cytokine production in the heart
- (Excessive) stimulation of myocardial adrenoceptors induces the production of interleukin-6

Arrhythmias
- No specific 'sepsis arrhythmias' yet documented
- No higher rate of arrhythmias in septic multiple organ dysfunction syndrome compared to non-septic multiple organ dysfunction syndrome
- SIRS and sepsis are main triggers of postoperative tachyarrhythmias in surgical ICU patients

Impairment of cardiac regulation
- Endotoxin blocks pacemaker current I_f and sensitises I_f to sympathetic stimulation, thereby contributing to
  - inadequately high heart rate
  - strongly reduced heart rate variability related to severity of multiple organ dysfunction syndrome and to unfavorable prognosis
- Attenuation of the 'vagal anti-inflammatory reflex' means overshooting inflammation and further depression of cardiac function

nation [5] – it is still a condition of high prognostic importance and accounts for about 10 % of fatalities witnessed in sepsis and septic shock [1]. Moreover, it has only recently become evident that not only cardiac function, but also regulation of cardiac function is severely impaired in septic multiple organ dysfunction syndrome (see below).

In view of the complex pattern, cardiac impairment in severe sepsis and septic shock can be classified as 'septic cardiomyopathy'. This classification is well accepted by intensivists, less so by cardiologists: in the recent classification of cardiomyopathies [6], impairment of the heart in sepsis is neglected.

How to Quantify Septic Cardiomyopathy?

Septic cardiomyopathy occurs more often than presently diagnosed! In the strict sense, 30–80 % of patients with severe sepsis and septic shock formally suffer from a non-ST-elevation-myocardial infarction (NSTEMI), as serum troponin T/I values are above the normal range. Septic patients with elevated troponin levels need higher doses of norepinephrine and have an unfavorable prognosis [7, 8]. Elevated serum levels of natriuretic peptides also indicate cardiac impairment [7, 9–11]. Electrocardiographic (EKG) changes in septic patients can reveal signs of ischemia, but in most cases are non-specific.

Echocardiography [12], however, very often underestimates the severity of septic cardiomyopathy, due to the dramatic afterload reduction in sepsis. In clinical practice, the diagnosis of septic cardiomyopathy is frequently hampered by the fact that all reference values for cardiac function parameters are normalized to the normal afterload of about 1,000 dynes/s/cm^5, but that reference values, e.g., for echocardiography, for a SVR of 300 dynes/s/cm^5 have never been established. On the other hand, in at least about 50 % of all sepsis patients, systolic pump failure can be documented by echocardiography [10].

An interesting new approach to characterize myocardial depression is the calculation of the cardiac power output (Cpo)/cardiac power index (Cpi) as the product of mean arterial pressure (MAP) and cardiac flow as measured by cardiac output/cardiac index [Cpo/Cpi = MAP × CO/CI × 0,0022 (W × m^{-2})], in relation to the SVR [13]. Characteristic for septic shock are Cpi values of 0.5–1.0 W/m^2 and SVR index (SVRI) values of < 1,500 dyn/s/cm^5, while the normal range for Cpi is 0.5–0.7 W/m^2 and for SVRI 1,000–2,500 dyn/s/cm^5 [13].

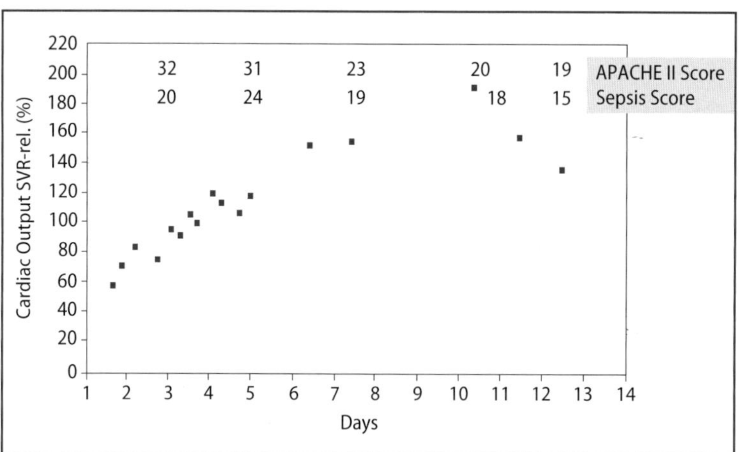

Fig. 3. Case report: Patient with pneumococcal-septic shock – Kinetics of recovery of impaired heart function. The patient was a survivor of pneumococcal septic shock. As a marker of the severity of sepsis, the sepsis score according to Elebute and Stoner [41] is given (sepsis: score ≥ 12), and as marker of the severity of disease, the APACHE II score is shown. As a marker of the severity of septic cardiomyopathy, systemic vascular resistance (SVR)-related cardiac output as a relative percentage of the normal value is given. As can be seen from the kinetics of SVR-related cardiac output, heart function is initially severely impaired (60 % of normal), but recovers early compared to the recovery from sepsis (sepsis score) and severity of disease (APACHE II score).

The method of choice for quantitating the severity of septic cardiomyopathy is measurement of cardiac output/cardiac index by a pulmonary artery catheter or PiCCO system and correlating these values to the SVR/SVRI data. According to **Figure 2**, an inverse correlation between afterload – represented best by the SVR – and cardiac performance could be demonstrated and quantitated. Quantitation assumes that the upper line in **Figure 2** resembles the cardiac output of those patients whose heart function is only minimally or even not impaired by the septic process (model calculation, Werdan et al, unpublished data). Taking these values as 100 %, the relative SVR-related cardiac output/cardiac index can be calculated from the value of cardiac output/cardiac index and the corresponding value of SVR. **Figure 3** shows the time course of recovery of septic cardiomyopathy in a patient with pneumococcal septic shock using the method of SVR-related cardiac output.

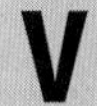

Septic Cardiomyopathy is of Prognostic Relevance

In our group of patients with septic multiple organ dysfunction syndrome (see legend to **Table 2**), only 42 % had normal or nearly normal SVR-related cardiac output values (**Table 2**), while in 38 %, cardiac function was moderately reduced, in 16 % severely reduced, and in 4 % very severely reduced (Werdan et al. unpublished data).

However, does quantification of septic cardiomyopathy really make sense? It would make sense, if the severity of septic cardiomyopathy correlated with an unfavorable prognosis of these septic patients; and this is indeed the case (**Table 2**). In our study group, 75 % of the surviving patients with septic multiple organ dysfunction syndrome had normal or nearly normal pump function (CO_{SVRrel} > 80 % of normal range), and only in 25 % could a moderate cardiac impairment (CO_{SVRrel} 60–80 % of expected value) be demonstrated. On the other hand, only 25 % of the non-surviving patients documented normal heart function (CO_{SVRrel} > 80 %), while 44 % had moderate (CO_{SVRrel} 60–80 % of expected value) and 31 % severe and very severe cardiac impairment (CO_{SVRrel} 60-< 40 % of normal value).

Raised serum levels of natriuretic peptides also document the cardiac impairment in sepsis: B-type natriuretic peptide (BNP) and N-terminal B-type natriuretic peptide (NT-proBNP) levels correlate inversely with left ventricular function [11] and discriminate very early between surviving and non-surviving patients [9,10]. Even in patients with normal echocardiographic findings, BNP levels can be astonishingly high [14].

Table 2. Incidence of septic cardiomyopathy in survivors and non-survivors of septic multiple organ dysfunction syndrome (Werdan et al. unpublished data)

$CO_{SVRrel.}$ % of normal	(Degree of failure)	Incidence (%) Total		Survivors		Non-Survivors	
> 80 %	(∅ or mild)	10/24	42 %	6/8	75 %	4/16	25 %
60 – 80 %	(moderate)	9/24	38 %	2/8	25 %	7/16	44 %
40 – 60 %	(severe)	4/24	16 %	0/8	0 %	4/16	25 %
< 40 %	(very severe)	1/24	4 %	0/8	0 %	1/16	6 %

Septic multiple organ dysfunction syndrome was defined by a pathologic sepsis score (≥ 12) according to Elebute and Stoner [41] and an APACHE II score ≥ 20.

Septic Cardiomyopathy: Triggers and Mechanisms

Many substances and mechanisms seem to be involved in myocardial depression in sepsis, with endotoxin, tumor necrosis factor (TNF)-α, interleukin (IL)-1, and nitric oxide (NO) being the most prominent players. These compounds interfere with the inotropic cascades of the cardiomyocyte (inhibiting the positive inotropic cyclic adenosine monophosphate [cAMP] system, stimulating the negative inotropic cyclic guanosine monophosphate [cGMP] system and disturbing the cellular Ca^{++} system), impair the mitochondrial function yielding to cytopathic hypoxia, activate the complement system, and trigger apoptosis [15–17]. Recently, our group demonstrated that endotoxin inhibits the pacemaker current, I_f, in atrial human cardiomyocytes and sensitizes I_f for sympathetic activation (**Fig. 4** [3,18]). Therefore, not only myocardial depressant factors but also substances impairing heart rhythm and autonomic cardiac regulation (see below) contribute to septic cardiomyopathy.

Pump Failure

Myocardial depression is the most prominent feature of septic cardiomyopathy, resulting in right and left ventricular pump failure (**Table 1**). In relation to the dramatic afterload reduction as seen by the lowered SVR, cardiac output/cardiac index, right and left ventricular ejection fractions as well as stroke volumes are not adequately increased or may even be depressed; global as well as regional contractile

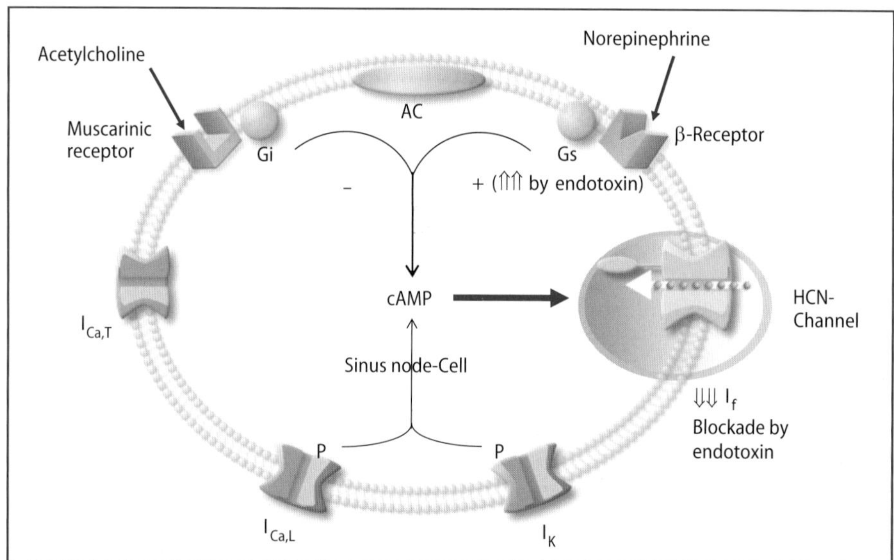

Fig. 4. Effects of endotoxin on pacemaker current I_f (HCN channels) and adrenergic I_f (HCN channel) stimulation in human atrial cardiomyocytes. Endotoxin inhibits I_f but also intensifies β-adrenoceptor-mediated stimulation of I_f [18]. I_f inhibition by endotoxin is not a non-specific effect, as the L-type calcium current ($I_{Ca,L}$) is not inhibited by endotoxin [18]. ⇑⇑ = stimulation; ⇓⇓ = inhibition; AC: adenylyl cyclase; cAMP: cyclic adenosine monophosphate; Gi: inhibitory G protein; Gs: stimulatory G protein; HCN channel: hyperpolarization-activated cyclic nucleotide-gated ion channel; I_f: 'funny' current (mediated by the HCN channels); $I_{Ca,T}$: T-type calcium channels; $I_{Ca,L}$: L-type calcium channels

disturbances can be found and not only systolic but also diastolic pump failure occurs [15–17]. Due to an increase in left ventricular compliance with a shift of the pressure-volume curve to the left, considerable dilatation of the left as well as the right heart can be seen, being a prognostically positive sign [1]. This pump failure is not primarily of hypoxic nature, because coronary arteries are vasoplegic and coronary blood flow in relation to MAP is higher than in non-septic patients [19]. However, one has to assume that at the coronary microcirculatory level similar disturbances may occur as generally seen in patients with sepsis. Fortunately, myocardial depression is potentially reversible, in agreement with a described myocardial hibernation in sepsis [5].

Additional right ventricular dysfunction essentially belongs to septic myocardial depression and can be accentuated in the presence of pulmonary hypertension due to acute respiratory distress syndrome (ARDS) [20]; right ventricular dilatation and a reduced right ventricular ejection fraction can further impair left ventricular performance by a decrease in left ventricular filling pressure and a mechanical compromise of the left ventricle by a septal shift.

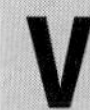

In patients with preexisting coronary artery disease, in particular, septic cardiomyopathy can be superimposed on further ischemic pump failure due to severe coronary artery stenoses, with the ischemic region getting even less blood flow due to steal phenomena because of the increased blood flow in the dilated non-stenosed coronary arteries, thus narrowing the coronary reserve. However, septic cardiomyopathy can be aggravated by myocardial ischemia, particularly in patients with preexisting coronary artery disease, as the increased coronary blood flow in sepsis narrows the coronary reserve.

The Role of Arrhythmias in Septic Cardiomyopathy

In contrast to the well-documented myocardial depression in sepsis, few experimental and clinical studies have described the occurrence of arrhythmias in sepsis. One case of the coincidence of long QT syndrome and torsade de pointes with septic cardiomyopathy was reported [21]. In a retrospective analysis of score evaluated patients, no increased incidence of ventricular and supraventricular arrhythmias was documented in 25 septic patients with multiple organ dysfunction syndrome compared to 15 non-septic multiple organ dysfunction syndrome patients [22]. There was no higher rate of arrhythmias in patients with septic multiple organ dysfunction syndrome compared to those with non-septic multiple organ dysfunction syndrome, while multiple organ dysfunction syndrome *per se* increased the risk of atrial fibrillation. At present, no specific arrhythmogenic sepsis profile has been identified. However, in postoperative intensive care unit (ICU) patients, sepsis and systemic inflammatory response syndrome (SIRS) have been identified as main triggers of tachyarrhythmias, with an adjusted odds ratio of 36 [23]!

The Heart as a 'Cytokine Producer'

Pro-inflammatory cytokines do not only depress contractility of the heart, they also get synthesized in the heart during the pro-inflammatory state and, thereby, intensify myocardial depression and cardiac impairment [24, 25]. In addition, stimulation of myocardial β-adrenoceptors and probably also of α-adrenoceptors by (excessive) catecholamines induces IL-6 production in the heart [25, 26]. Treatment with catecholamines can add to cytokine production in the heart, which can be blocked by the β/α-blocker, carvedilol [25, 26]. Consequently, all attempts to reduce catecholamine doses in sepsis treatment are welcome to reduce the pro-inflammatory burden on the heart.

Impaired Regulation of Cardiac Function in Septic Cardiomyopathy

At present, scientific research in the field of septic cardiomyopathy focuses on myocardial depression. However, it should not be forgotten that not only is myocardial depression a real problem in sepsis, but so too is the strongly impaired regulation of cardiac function, due to the extensive alterations of the cardiovascular autonomic nervous system [3, 27].

V

This cardiac autonomic dysfunction in sepsis and multiple organ dysfunction syndrome can be measured by parameters of 24-hour heart rate variability (HRV), which shows a very strong impairment in both the sympathetically and in the vagally mediated nervous signals (see Table 2 in [3]). While HRV measurement describes cerebral control of the heart, baroreflex sensitivity characterizes communication between the heart and the vascular system, whereas chemoreflex sensitivity represents the interaction between the respiratory system and the heart. All indicators of HRV, baroreflex sensitivity, and chemoreflex sensitivity are severely impaired in sepsis and multiple organ dysfunction syndrome (see Table 2 in [3], [28]).

The consequences of impaired regulation of cardiac function in sepsis and multiple organ dysfunction syndrome are manifold: In addition to impaired cardiac contractility (see above), the resultant chronotropic incompetence reduces HRV and increases heart rate, both of which are associated with an unfavorable prognosis [3, 28]. Finally, depression of the vagal cholinergic activity dampens the anti-inflammatory cholinergic reflex and consequently allows overshooting of inflammation, with all its detrimental consequences on prognosis [29].

Possible Mechanisms of Impaired Regulation of Cardiac Function in Sepsis: Pacemaker HCN Channels as Targets

Intravenously applied endotoxin induces reversible heart rate "stiffness" in healthy volunteers and thus causes myocardial autonomic dysfunction [30]. With this in mind, one can speculate that endotoxin contributes to the impaired cardiac autonomic function seen in patients with sepsis and multiple organ dysfunction syndrome. The decrease in HRV observed in these patients must be due to a mitigated heart rate regulation either by rate-increasing sympathetic activity, by rate-decreasing vagal activity, or both. The efferent sympathetic and vagal signals to the heart start in the brain, run through the sympathetic fibers and the vagus nerve, respectively, and finally use binding of the neurotransmitters norepinephrine to cardiac adrenoceptors and acetylcholine to muscarinic receptors (**Fig. 4**). Receptor binding triggers signal transduction pathways in the cardiac pacemaker cells which finally result in modulation of the pacemaker current. This pacemaker current is mainly carried by the I_f current ("funny" current) [31]. I_f is the result of ion flux through the hyperpolarization-activated cyclic nucleotide-gated (HCN) channel. The HCN channel is controlled by direct interaction with cAMP and, hence, contributes to sympathetic and parasympathetic regulation of heart rate [32]. Four HCN channels have been characterized so far (HCN 1–4) [32]. In the human sinus node, HCN 4 is the dominantly expressed HCN isoform.

In principle, cardiac autonomic impairment can occur at all levels: The brain, the autonomic nervous system, and the pacemaker cell. The endotoxin–heart rate stiffness experiments by Godin et al. [30] (see above), however, do not elucidate whether the heart rate "stiffness" observed is due to an endotoxin-induced alteration of the brain, the autonomic nervous system, or the pacemaker cell itself. As we were able to demonstrate that endotoxin also reduces beating rate variability in spontaneously beating cultured neonatal rat heart muscle cells [33], we hypothesized that endotoxin-induced heart rate "stiffness" is mediated, at least in part, by a direct impact of endotoxin on the cardiac pacemaker cells interfering with the signal transduction pathways and ion channels. A likely target for endotoxin is the pacemaker current I_f running through the HCN channels (see above), which is indicated by our study: In whole cell patch-clamp experiments by Zorn-Pauly et al. with isolated human myocytes from right atrial appendages, endotoxin (at concentrations of 1 and 10 μg/ml) significantly and specifically impaired I_f by suppressing the current at membrane potentials positive to -80 mV and slowing down current activation, but without affecting peak current [18, 33]. Furthermore, the response of I_f to β-adrenergic stimulation (1 μM isoproterenol) was significantly larger in endotoxin-incubated cells compared with control cells [18]. Using a spontaneously active sinoatrial cell model [34] we demonstrated that endotoxin-induced I_f impairment reduces the responsiveness of the model to fluctuations of autonomic input [18]. Therefore, our experiments demonstrate both a direct inhibitory effect of endotoxin on the cardiac pacemaker current I_f, and a sensitizing of I_f to β_1-adrenergic catecholamines (**Fig. 4**). These phenomena trigger a narrowing of HRV and, therefore, may contribute to the autonomic cardiac dysfunction (reduced HRV) seen in patients with severe sepsis and septic shock. Consequently, autonomic dysfunction is not only the result of an alteration of the autonomic nervous system reins, but also of an impairment in the signal transduction pathways/ion channels of the cardiac target cells mediating the autonomic nervous signals.

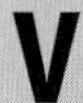

One point, however, needs clarification: Endotoxin-induced blockade of I_f lowers heart rate, while in patients with severe sepsis and septic shock, heart rate is usually inappropriately high. The combination of a markedly attenuated vagal tone, massive endogenous catecholamine release, exogenous catecholamine treatment, and the increased catecholamine sensitivity of HCN channels (**Fig. 4**) may override the bradycardic endotoxin blockade of I_f *in vivo* and thus account for this apparent discrepancy.

So, can we improve impaired cardiac regulation in septic cardiomyopathy? Today, we are still a long way from being able to answer this question in a positive manner. Experimental and clinical therapeutic approaches focus on improving the depressed vagal activity to strengthen the anti-inflammatory vagal reflex: Nicotine patches, acupuncture, and vagal stimulation devices have been suggested to stimulate the impaired anti-inflammatory vagal reflex [29], but have not been tested in clinical trials so far. It is interesting to note that drugs which show beneficial effects in septic and non-septic multiple organ dysfunction syndrome – statins, angiotensin converting enzyme (ACE) inhibitors and early treatment with β-blockers – also increase the reduced vagal activity [3].

Causal Approaches towards the Treatment of Acute Septic Cardiomyopathy

Current consensus guidelines to the therapy of sepsis give detailed recommendations for fluid resuscitation and vasopressor and inotropic therapy. If cardiovascular stabilization can be achieved within the first few hours, then the survival rate is relatively high. Dobutamine as inotrope and norepinephrine as vasopressor should be used if necessary, while dopamine use in patients with shock may be associated with an increased mortality [35]. Not (yet) part of the standard treatment of septic shock are phosphodiesterase inhibitors, vasopressin, and the calcium sensitizer, levosimendan [36]. NO inhalation therapy, sometimes used in the treatment of patients with ARDS, does not seem to have depressant effects on heart function.

Causal therapeutic strategies, aimed at interrupting mediator cascades, are being tested for use in septic cardiomyopathy and vasculopathy, but do not form part of the standard regimens. Modulation of cardiac inflammatory reactions by phosphodiesterase inhibitors [37] and adenosine [38] has also been reported. Present data [15] suggest that by antagonizing and eliminating pertinent pro-inflammatory mediators, septic vasculopathy is more approachable than septic cardiomyopathy.

The options for a causal therapy of septic cardiomyopathy are presently rather limited. In rats [39] the β_1-selective blocker, esmolol, improved septic myocardial dysfunction, with increased cardiac output and cardiac efficiency and improved myocardial oxygen utilization, parallel to a reduction in the systemic pro-inflammatory state as shown by a decrease in serum TNF-α levels.

Encouraging are findings in patients with severe sepsis and septic shock who are treated with activated protein C (drotrecogin alfa [activated]). Patients treated with activated protein C have lower troponin and NT-proBNP serum levels than those who are not treated [9]. This finding underscores the likely role of microcirculatory disturbances in sepsis [40] and especially in septic cardiomyopathy.

Conclusion

The original concept of septic myocardial depression proposing a negative inotropic blood factor has undergone an evolution in recent years. Heart failure in severe sepsis and septic shock is now regarded as a symptom of a – not yet classified – secondary cardiomyopathy, characterized by an altered cellular phenotype due to the impact of multiple mediators and toxins. Considerable progress has been made in characterizing the clinical spectrum of septic myocardial depression – including impaired regulation of heart function – and in elucidating the pathogenetic mechanisms underlying septic cardiomyopathy. However, trials to establish causal therapies have so far not yielded convincing results and continuing efforts are needed in both basic and clinical research. Better understanding and treatment of septic cardiomyopathy will be of benefit beyond the scope of sepsis, as pathogenetic mechanisms underlying septic heart failure may also be operative in non-septic heart failure, which is associated with a measurable systemic inflammatory response.

References

1. Parrillo JE (1989) The cardiovascular pathophysiology of sepsis. Ann Rev Med 40: 469–485
2. Müller-Werdan U, Reithmann C, Werdan K (1996) Cytokines and the Heart: Molecular Mechanisms of Septic Cardiomyopathy. Landes Bioscience, Austin
3. Schmidt H, Müller-Werdan U, Werdan K (2008) The consequences of cardiac autonomic dysfunction in multiple organ dysfunction syndrome. In: Vincent JL (ed) 2008 Yearbook of Intensive Care and Emergency Medicine. Springer, Heidelberg, pp 55–64
4. Pilz G, McGinn P, Boekstegers P, Kääb S, Weidenhöfer S, Werdan K (1994) Pseudomonas sepsis does not cause more severe cardiovascular dysfunction in patients than non-pseudomonas sepsis. Circ Shock 42: 174–182

5. Levy RJ, Piel DA, Acton PD, et al (2005) Evidence of myocardial hibernation in the septic heart. Crit Care Med 33: 2752–2756
6. Elliott P, Andersson B, Arbustini E, et al (2008) Classification of the cardiomyopathies: a position statement from the European Society Of Cardiology Working Group On Myocardial and Pericardial Diseases. Eur Heart J 29: 270–276
7. Spies C, Haude V, Fitzner R, et al (1998) Serum cardiac troponin T as a prognostic marker in early sepsis. Chest 113: 1055–1063
8. Wu AHB (2001) Increased troponin in patients with sepsis and septic shock: myocardial necrosis or reversible myocardial depression? Intensive Care Med 27: 959–961
9. Brueckmann M, Huhle G, Lang S, et al (2005) Prognostic value of plasma N-Terminal pro-brain natriuretic peptide in patients with severe sepsis. Circulation 112: 527–534
10. Charpentier J, Luyt C-E, Fulla Y, et al (2004) Brain natriuretic peptide: A marker of myocardial dysfunction and prognosis during severe sepsis. Crit Care Med 32: 660–665
11. Witthaut R, Busch C, Fraunberger P, et al K (2003) Plasma atrial natriuretic peptide and brain natriuretic peptide are increased in septic shock: impact of interleukin-6 and sepsis-associated left ventricular dysfunction. Intensive Care Med 29: 1696–1702
12. McLean AS, Huang SJ (2006) Intensive care echocardiography. In: Vincent JL (ed) 2006 Yearbook of Intensive Care and Emergency Medicine. Springer, Heidelberg, pp 131–141
13. Cotter G, Moshkovitz Y, Kaluski E, et al (2003) The role of cardiac power and systemic vascular resistance in the pathophysiology and diagnosis of patients with acute congestive heart failure. Eur J Heart Failure 5: 443–451
14. Maeder M, Ammann P, Kiowski W, Rickli H (2005) B-type natriuretic peptide in patients with sepsis and preserved left ventricular ejection fraction. Eur J Heart Fail 7: 1164–1167
15. Müller-Werdan U, Buerke M, Ebelt H (2006) Septic cardiomyopathy – A not yet discovered cardiomyopathy? Exp Clin Cardiol 11: 226–236
16. Levy RJ (2007) Mitochondrial dysfunction, bioenergetic impairment, and metabolic down-regulation in sepsis. Shock 28: 24–28
17. Cinel I, Nanda R, Dellinger RP (2008) Cardiac dysfunction in septic shock. In: Vincent JL (ed) Yearbook of Intensive Care and Emergency Medicine. Springer Heidelberg, pp 43–54
18. Zorn-Pauly K, Pelzmann B, Lang P, et al (2007) Endotoxin impairs the human pacemaker current I_f. Shock 28: 655–661
19. Dhainaut JF, Hughebaert M-F, Monsallier JF, et al (1987) Coronary hemodynamics and myocardial metabolism of lactate, free fatty acids, glucose, and ketones in patients with septic shock. Circulation 75: 533–541
20. Dhainaut J-F, Pinsky MR, Nouria S, Slomka F, Brunet F (1997) Right ventricular function in human sepsis – A thermodilution study. Chest 112: 1043–1049.
21. Varriale P, Ramaprasad S (1995) Septic cardiomyopathy as a cause of long QT syndrome. J Electrocardiology 28: 327–329
22. Prondzinsky R, Stache N, Witthaut R, et al (1997) Multiorgan-failure (MOF) with and without sepsis: differences in incidence and pattern of detected arrhythmias. Crit Care 1 (Suppl 1): P30
23. Knotzer H, Mayr A, Ulmer H, et al (2000) Tachyarrhythmias in a surgical intensive care unit: a case-controlled epidemiologic study. Intensive Care Med 26: 908–914
24. Müller-Werdan U, Engelmann H, Werdan K (1998) Cardiodepression by tumor necrosis factor α. Eur Cytokine Netw 9: 689–691
25. Müller-Werdan U, Werdan K (2000) Immune modulation by catecholamines – a potential mechanism of cytokine release in heart failure? Herz 25: 271–273
26. Müller-Werdan U, Jacoby J, Loppnow H, et al (1999) Noradrenaline stimulates cardiomyocytes to produce interleukin-6, indicative of a proinflammatory action, which is suppressed by carvedilol. Eur Heart J 20 (Suppl):P1721 (abst)
27. Godin P J, Buchman T G (1996) Uncoupling of biological oscillators: a complementary hypothesis concerning the pathogenesis of multiple organ dysfunction syndrome. Crit Care Med 24: 1107–1116
28. Schmidt H, Muller-Werdan U, Hoffmann T, et al (2005) Autonomic dysfunction predicts mortality in patients with multiple organ dysfunction syndrome of different age groups. Crit Care Med 33: 1994–2002
29. Tracey K J (2007). Physiology and immunology of the cholinergic antiinflammatory pathway. J Clin Invest 117: 289–296

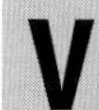

30. Godin P J, Fleisher L A, Eidsath A, et al (1996) Experimental human endotoxemia increases cardiac regularity: results from a prospective, randomized, crossover trial. Crit Care Med 24: 1117–1124.
31. Baruscotti M, Bucchi A, & Difrancesco D (2005) Physiology and pharmacology of the cardiac pacemaker ("funny") current. Pharmacol Ther 107: 59–79
32. Ludwig A, Zong X, Hofmann F, & Biel M (1999) Structure and function of cardiac pacemaker channels. Cell Physiol Biochem 9: 179–186
33. Schmidt H, Saworski J, Werdan K, Muller-Werdan U (2007) Decreased beating rate variability of spontaneously contracting cardiomyocytes after co-incubation with endotoxin. J Endotoxin Res 13: 339–342
34. Kurata Y, Hisatome I, Imanishi S, Shibamoto T (2002) Dynamical description of sinoatrial node pacemaking: improved mathematical model for primary pacemaker cell. Am J Physiol Heart Circ Physiol 283: H2074–2101
35. Sakr Y, Reinhart K, Vincent JL, et al (2006) Does dopamine administration in shock influence outcome? Results of the Sepsis Occurrence in Acutely Ill Patients (SOAP) Study. Crit Care Med 34: 589–597
36. Cunha-Goncalves D, Perez-de-Sa V, Dahm P, Grins E, Thörne J, Blomquist S (2007) Cardiovascular effects of levosimendan in the early stages of endotoxemia. Shock 28: 71–77
37. Takeuchi K, del Nido PJ, Ibrahim AE, et al (1999) Vesnarinone and amrinone reduce the systemic inflammatory response syndrome. J Thorac Cardiovasc Surg 117: 375–381
38. Wagner DR, McTiernan C, Sanders VJ, Feldman AM (1998) Adenosine inhibits lipopolysaccharide-induced secretion of tumor necrosis factor-α in the failing human heart. Circulation 97: 521–524
39. Suzuki T, Morisaki H, Serita R, et al (2005) Infusion of the beta-adrenergic blocker esmolol attenuates myocardial dysfunction in septic rats. Crit Care Med 33: 2294–2301
40. De Backer D, Creteur J, Preiser JC, Dubois MJ, Vincent JL (2002) Microvascular blood flow is altered in sepsis. Am J Respir Crit Care Med 166: 98–104
41. Elebute EA, Stoner HB (1983) The grading of sepsis. Br J Surg 70: 29–31

V

Determinants of Tissue PCO_2 in Shock and Sepsis: Relationship to the Microcirculation

A. Dubin, V.S.K. Edul, and C. Ince

V

Introduction

The development of gastrointestinal tonometry was an important step in the monitoring of tissue dysoxia. It rapidly became a useful tool in basic research. In addition, and for the first time, a regional parameter could be used to detect and to treat hypoperfusion. From an experimental point of view, tonometry adequately tracks intramucosal acidosis [1], i.e., the increase in intramucosal-arterial PCO_2 difference (ΔPCO_2). Likewise, the increase in ΔPCO_2 is better than other systemic and intestinal variables to show tissue hypoperfusion in normal volunteers [2] and in experimental models [3]. Intramucosal acidosis is a sensitive predictor of gastric [4] and colonic mucosal ischemia [5]. Furthermore, gastric tonometry is an insightful predictor of outcome. This usefulness has been shown in postoperative [6], critically ill [7], septic [8] and shock [9] patients. Gastric tonometry might also be used to assess the effect of vasoactive drugs [10, 11]. Finally, intramucosal pH (pHi) has been evaluated as a guide for resuscitation. Gutierrez et al. [12] demonstrated in a randomized controlled trial that pHi-guided therapy could decrease mortality in critically ill patients.

Despite having been the only clinically available approach to detect tissue hypoperfusion for many years and despite the scientific evidence supporting its usefulness, gastrointestinal tonometry is not commonly used. Various reasons may explain this issue, including that saline tonometry has poor reproducibility [13], although this was improved by the introduction of air tonometry [14]. Sublingual capnometry remains an attractive approach [15], but this technique has not yet been adequately validated.

Another source of uncertainty lies in the true significance of ΔPCO_2 elevation. In the last few years, new evidence has given a better understanding of the mechanisms underlying intramucosal acidosis. In this chapter, we will discuss the determinants of tissue and venous PCO_2 in shock and sepsis and their relationship to microcirculatory perfusion.

Mechanisms of Increase in Venous and Tissue PCO_2: The Basics

Increased mucosal intestinal PCO_2 has been mainly used to detect tissue dysoxia, the condition in which oxygen delivery (DO_2) can no longer sustain oxygen consumption (VO_2) [16]. Twenty years ago, Grum et al. [17] evaluated the adequacy of gut oxygenation by the tonometric measurement of pHi, during DO_2 reductions secondary to ischemia, hypoxemia, or a combination of both. pHi only decreased after crit-

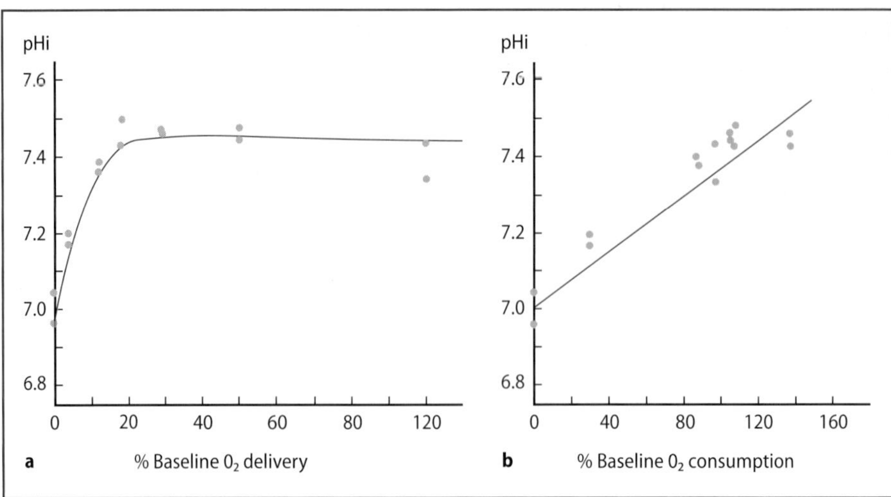

Fig. 1a. Intestinal intramucosal pH (pHi) as a function of oxygen (O_2) delivery. **b** Intestinal intramucosal pH as a function of intestinal O_2 consumption. Reductions of intramucosal pH are only present with critical reductions of O_2 delivery. From [17] with permission.

ical reductions of DO_2. Consequently, changes in VO_2 and pHi were closely correlated (**Fig. 1**). The authors concluded that pHi appears to be a sensitive indicator of tissue oxygenation, because it mirrors tissue VO_2. Nevertheless, critical DO_2 was only reached in ischemic experiments. In pure hypoxemic experiments, neither pHi nor VO_2 decreased.

Theoretically, PCO_2 can increase in the intestinal lumen by two mechanisms [18]: First, by bicarbonate buffering of the protons generated during the breakdown of high-energy phosphates and strong acids, in which case increased PCO_2 would represent tissue dysoxia; alternatively, PCO_2 can increase due to hypoperfusion and decreased washout of CO_2. The Fick Equation applied to CO_2, states that CO_2 production (VCO_2) is the product of cardiac output and venoarterial CO_2 content difference. Consequently, decreases in blood flow result in venous and tissue hypercarbia, regardless of the lack of change in VCO_2.

Trying to solve this controversy, Schlichtig and Bowles [18] presented evidence supporting intramucosal PCO_2 as a marker of dysoxia in extreme hypoperfusion when VO_2 decreases. In a dog model of cardiac tamponade, these authors demonstrated that below critical DO_2, mucosal PCO_2 increases because of anaerobic VCO_2. This conclusion was drawn using the Dill nomogram, which can, theoretically, detect anaerobic VCO_2 from the comparison of the measured ($\%HbO_{2v}$) vs. calculated ($\%HbO_{2v}{}^{DILL}$) venous oxyhemoglobin, within a given value of venous PCO_2. Since venous PCO_2 is considered representative of tissue PCO_2, the authors made the calculation with its intestinal equivalent, intramucosal PCO_2. Similar values of measured ($\%HbO_{2v}$) vs. calculated ($\%HbO_{2v}{}^{DILL}$) venous oxyhemoglobin would represent aerobic VCO_2. If $\%HbO_{2v}{}^{DILL}$ is lower than measured $\%HbO_{2v}$, anaerobic VCO_2 is then assumed. Using this approach, we identified an anaerobic source of gut intramucosal CO_2 during moderate hemorrhage [3]. Our $\%HbO_{2v}{}^{DILL}$ values obtained from gastric, jejunal, and ileal mucosal PCO_2 decreased markedly during ischemia, indicating the presence of anaerobia (**Fig. 2**). Notwithstanding the original contribu-

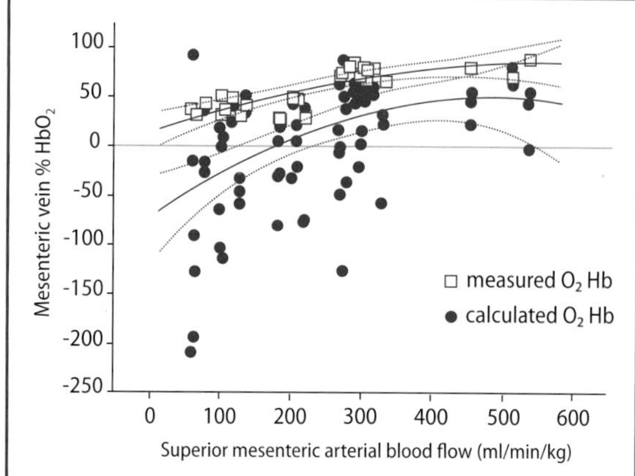

Fig. 2. Measured venous oxygen saturation ($\%HbO_{2v}$) (□) and venous oxygen saturation calculated from gut tissue PCO_2 ($\%HbO_{2v}^{DILL}$) (●) as a function of superior mesenteric artery blood flow. Since $\%HbO_{2v}^{DILL}$ is lower than measured $\%HbO_{2v}$, anaerobic production of CO_2 may be assumed. From [3] with permission.

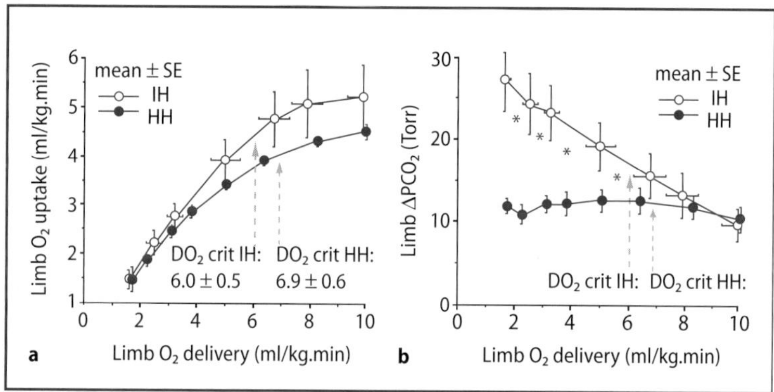

Fig. 3. a Hindlimb oxygen uptake as a function of limb oxygen delivery (DO_2) for ischemic hypoxia (IH) and hypoxic hypoxia (HH). There was no statistically significant difference at any DO_2. Critical DO_2 (DO_2crit) was not different in IH and HH. **b** Hindlimb venoarterial PCO_2 difference as a function of limb DO_2 for IH and HH. Despite similar degrees of tissue dysoxia, venoarterial PCO_2 difference remained constant in the HH group and increased more than twofold in the IH group. From [20] with permission.

tion of Schlichtig and Bowles [18] to the analysis of these topics, the use of low flow to produce critical DO_2 and decreased VO_2 may act as a potential confounder, given the impossibility of dissociating tissue dysoxia from hypoperfusion [19].

Vallet et al. [20] explored this issue by measuring venous PCO_2 in isolated dog hindlimb preparations subjected to comparable decreases in DO_2, produced by two mechanisms. In one group, blood flow was progressively decreased (ischemic hypoxia), whereas in the other, arterial PO_2 was lowered at constant perfusion flow (hypoxic hypoxia). Both groups experienced similar declines in DO_2 and VO_2, implying similar degrees of tissue dysoxia. The venoarterial PCO_2 difference, however, remained constant in the hypoxic hypoxia group, and increased more than twofold in the ischemic hypoxia group. The authors concluded that flow is the major determinant of venoarterial PCO_2 difference, not tissue dysoxia [20] (**Fig. 3**).

Nevière et al. assessed a similar hypothesis in pigs, comparing the effects of reduced inspired oxygen fraction (FiO_2) and decreased blood flow measured with

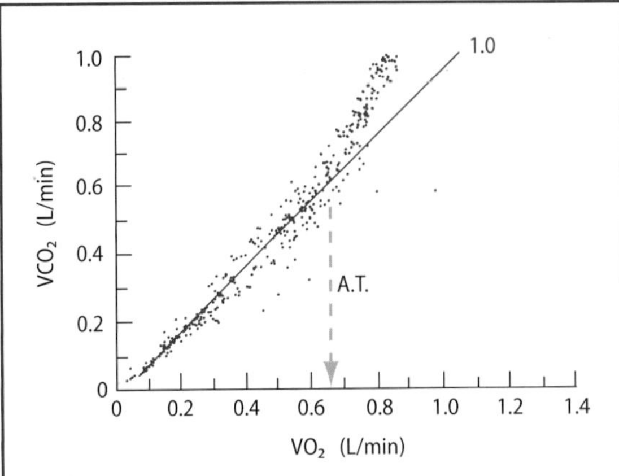

Fig. 4. Plot of carbon dioxide production (VCO_2) as a function of oxygen uptake (VO_2) in response to incremental work rate during a test of exercise. Line with slope 1.0 is the approximate mean of data points up to the point where VCO_2 breaks away and increases rapidly. When data points rise more steeply than a slope of 1.0 is theoretically the VCO_2 at which HCO_3^- starts buffering lactic acid (anaerobic threshold). From [22] with permission.

laser-Doppler [21]. In ischemic hypoxia, ΔPCO_2 rose to 60 mmHg. In hypoxic hypoxia, in which mucosal blood flow was maintained constant, ΔPCO_2 increase to 30 mmHg only with the lowest FiO_2 (0.06). The authors concluded that intramucosal PCO_2 elevation in hypoxic hypoxia denotes local CO_2 generation. Some flow heterogeneity could, however, have been present in their experiments that was not assessed by laser-Doppler, a method that only tracks global microvascular changes. In addition, in the two preceding steps of FiO_2 reduction, VO_2/DO_2 dependency had been reached, and ΔPCO_2 remained unchanged.

From a physiologic point of view, it is difficult to understand how VCO_2 might increase during oxygen supply dependency. During progressive exercise, there are corresponding increases in VO_2 and VCO_2 [22]. The slope of the VCO_2/VO_2 relationship is the respiratory quotient. When the exercise reaches the anaerobic threshold, there is an excess of VCO_2 to VO_2 due to the appearance of anaerobic VCO_2 from the bicarbonate buffering of lactic acid (**Fig. 4**). In this condition, both VCO_2 and respiratory quotient increase.

In the other extreme of physiology, during oxygen supply dependency, the respiratory quotient also increases [23]. This increase, however, occurs in the context of the reduction of total VCO_2 (**Fig. 5**). Anaerobic VCO_2 appears, but total VCO_2 decreases.

We further explored this issue in another model of hypoxic hypoxia [24]. In these experiments, venous and tissue PCO_2 increased during ischemic hypoxia, but not during hypoxic hypoxia. Therefore, ΔPCO_2 was unable to show the presence of tissue dysoxia during hypoxic hypoxia, in which blood flow is preserved (**Fig. 6a**). To confirm that blood flow is the main determinant of ΔPCO_2, we studied these relationships in another model of tissue dysoxia without hypoperfusion, anemic hypoxia [25] (**Fig. 6b**). We compared the effects of progressive bleeding to those of isovolemic exchange of blood with dextran. Our goal was to evaluate the behavior of CO_2 gradients as a function of systemic and intestinal blood flow, and also the other determinants, VCO_2 and the CO_2Hb dissociation curve. Tissue-arterial and venoarterial PCO_2 failed to reflect the dependence of VO_2 on DO_2. Nevertheless, these gradients increased by a few mmHg (**Figs. 6** and **7**). Conversely, however, venoarterial CO_2 content differences decreased. This apparent paradox might be explained by changes in the CO_2Hb dissociation curve induced by anemic hypoxia. The other determinant of PCO_2 differences, the VCO_2 remained unchanged, both at systemic and intestinal

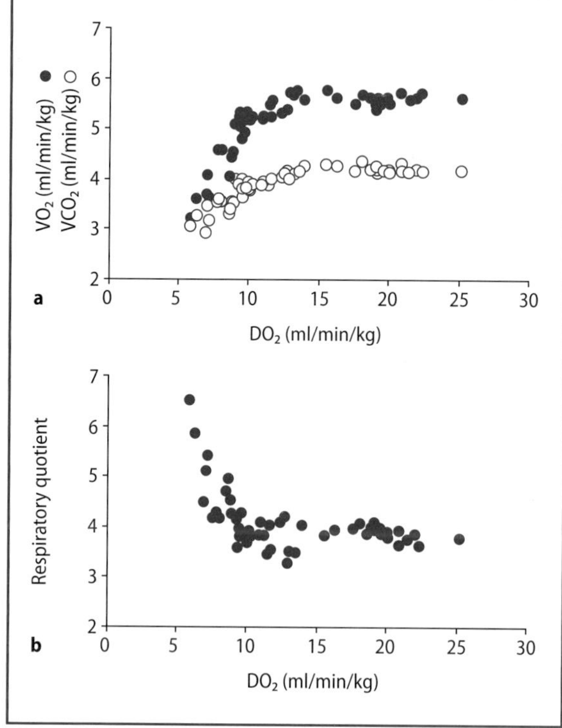

Fig. 5. Effects of progressive bleeding on oxygen consumption (VO_2), carbon dioxide production (VCO_2), and respiratory quotient. Panel **a**. After critical reductions in DO_2, VO_2 and VCO_2 decreased. Panel **b**. After critical reductions in DO_2, respiratory quotient increased [23].

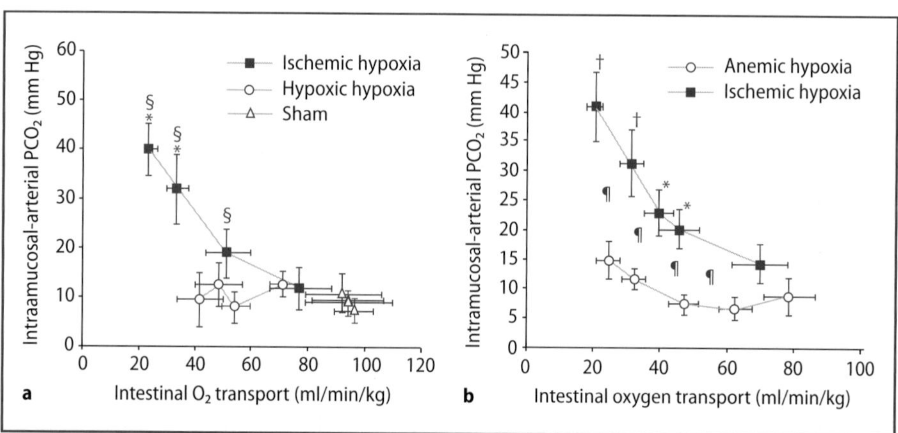

Fig. 6. a Ileal intramucosal-arterial PCO_2 difference (ΔPCO_2) as a function of intestinal oxygen transport in hypoxic and ischemic hypoxia. From [24] with permission. **b** ΔPCO_2 as a function of intestinal oxygen transport in anemic and ischemic hypoxia. From [25] with permission. In hypoxic and anemic hypoxia, ΔPCO_2 fails to reflect tissue dysoxia.

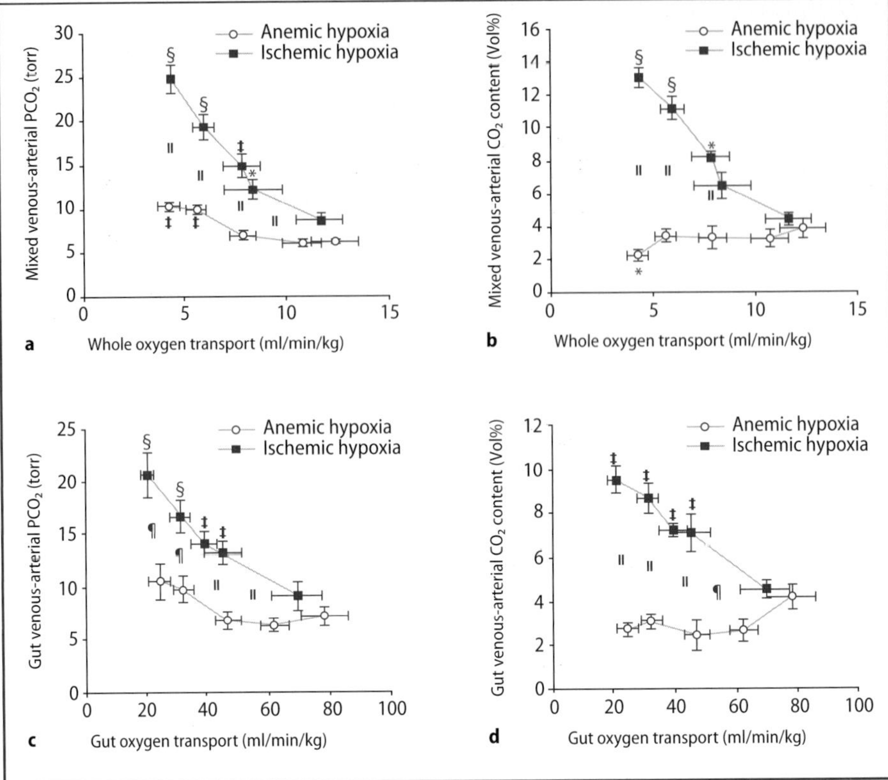

Fig. 7. a Mixed venous-arterial PCO_2 difference as a function of systemic oxygen transport (DO_2) in ischemic and anemic hypoxia. **b** Mixed venous-arterial CO_2 content difference as a function of systemic DO_2 in ischemic and anemic hypoxia. **c** Mesenteric venous-arterial PCO_2 difference as a function of intestinal DO_2 in ischemic and anemic hypoxia. **d** Mesenteric venous-arterial CO_2 content difference as a function of intestinal DO_2 in ischemic and anemic hypoxia. Differences were higher in ischemic than in anemic hypoxia. Venoarterial PCO_2 differences slightly increased while venoarterial CO_2 content differences decreased in anemic hypoxia, implying changes in the CO_2Hb dissociation curve. From [25] with permission.

levels. The systemic and intestinal respiratory quotient, however, increased because of VO_2 reductions.

In summary, our results [24, 25], together with those of Vallet et al. [20], support the concept that increases in tissue-arterial and venoarterial PCO_2 gradients reflect only microcirculatory stagnation, not tissue dysoxia. Tissue and venous PCO_2 are insensitive markers of dysoxia and merely indicate hypoperfusion. These experimental findings were confirmed by a mathematical model [26]. Gutierrez developed a two-compartment mass transport model of tissue CO_2 exchange for hypoxic hypoxia, to examine the relative contribution of blood flow and cellular dysoxia to the increases in tissue and venous PCO_2. The model assumed perfectly mixed homogeneous conditions, steady-state equilibrium, and VCO_2 occurring exclusively at the tissues. The results of the model supported the idea that changes in tissue and venous blood CO_2 concentrations during dysoxia reflect primarily alterations in vascular perfusion, and not shortage of energy supply.

Intramucosal Acidosis in Sepsis

Beyond the previous discussion, intramucosal acidosis is a common finding in clinical and experimental sepsis, conditions in which cardiac output is usually normal or increased. In resuscitated endotoxemic pigs, VanderMeer et al. found that intramucosal acidosis developed despite preserved mucosal oxygenation and blood flow measured only at the mucosa [27]. The underlying mechanism was attributed to metabolic disturbances, and led to the concept of "cytopathic hypoxia" [28]. Nevertheless, an important shortcoming of that study was the use of laser-Doppler flowmetry to measure tissue perfusion and the lack of measurement of tissue oxygenation at the serosal side of the intestines, an important source of gut CO_2 [31].

On the other hand, Vallet et al. studied dogs challenged with endotoxin, and then resuscitated them to normalize oxygen transport [29]. Intestinal VO_2 and mucosal PO_2 and pH, however, remained low. The authors ascribed these findings to blood flow redistribution from the mucosa toward the muscular layer. Nevertheless, Revelly et al. [30] described an inverse redistribution, with increased mucosal and decreased muscular blood flow, using dyed microspheres in endotoxemic pigs [30]. Paradoxically, pHi was inversely correlated with mucosal flow, though positively correlated with muscular perfusion. The authors concluded that intramucosal acidosis was not explained by mucosal hypoperfusion [30]. Siegemund et al. showed, in a similar model, reductions in mucosal and serosal microvascular PO_2, and an increase in ΔPCO_2 [31]. Fluid resuscitation normalized mucosal PO_2 but serosal PO_2 and ΔPCO_2 remained altered. Inhibition of inducible nitric oxide (NO) however restored serosal PO_2 and also ΔPCO_2 thereby identifying the source of intraluminal CO_2 measured in their model.

Conversely, Tugtekin et al. [32], in a porcine model of 24-hour endotoxin infusion, showed an association between intramucosal acidosis and severe hypoperfusion in ileal villi. In this study, about half of the evaluated villi were heterogeneously- or non-perfused, despite normal portal blood flow. Creteur et al. described, in septic patients, a correlation between sublingual ΔPCO_2 and microcirculatory blood flow [33]. In agreement with their results, results from our laboratory showed that endotoxic shock in sheep was associated with sublingual and intestinal microcirculatory alterations and intramucosal acidosis [34]. Fluid resuscitation normalized systemic and intestinal oxygen transport, as well as sublingual and intestinal serosal microcirculation. Nevertheless, a reduced number of perfused intestinal villi and increased ΔPCO_2 persisted. This led us to conclude that intramucosal acidosis was related to a persistent decrease in the mucosal microvascular flow index and a reduced number of perfused intestinal villi [34] (**Fig. 8**).

There are other studies further supporting the hypothesis that, in endotoxemia, changes in perfusion and not tissue dysoxia determine ΔPCO_2. We randomized endotoxemic sheep to saline solution resuscitation to maintain blood flow at baseline values or to increase it by 50 %. Increased perfusion prevented intramucosal acidosis, though metabolic acidosis continued due to increased anion gap [35]. Similarly, in endotoxemic sheep, the administration of levosimendan, an inotropic and vasodilator drug, precluded increases in ΔPCO_2 but hyperlactatemia was exacerbated [36] or unaffected [37]. The findings of these studies suggest that intramucosal acidosis is mainly related to local hypoperfusion and that metabolic disorders depend on a cellular mechanism which is unresponsive to changes in blood flow.

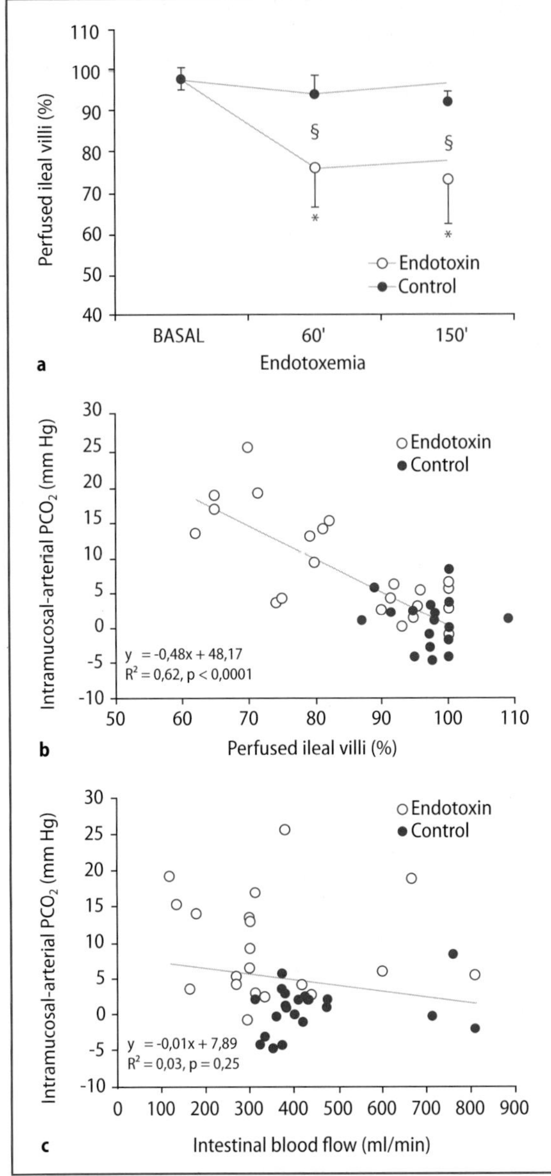

Fig. 8. Effects of endotoxic shock and resuscitation on the percentage of perfused ileal villi and intramucosal-arterial PCO_2 difference (ΔPCO_2). Endotoxic shock decreased the perfused intestinal villi and fluid resuscitation was unable to restore villus perfusion (**a**). ΔPCO_2 was correlated with perfused intestinal villi (**b**) but not with superior mesenteric artery blood flow (**c**). From [34] with permission.

Conclusion

Venoarterial and tissue-arterial PCO_2 gradients are the result of interactions in aerobic and anaerobic VCO_2, CO_2 dissociation curve, and blood flow to tissues. During VO_2/DO_2 dependency, opposite changes in aerobic and anaerobic VCO_2 occur. Aerobic VCO_2 decreases as a consequence of failing aerobic metabolism, but, at the same time, anaerobic VCO_2 starts due to bicarbonate buffering of protons derived from fixed acids. Total VCO_2 might not increase, as in our experiments. But as VO_2 falls, there is an increase in the respiratory quotient [27]. The relative increment of VCO_2 with respect to VO_2 can only cause venous and tissue hypercarbia during tissue hypoperfusion, in which CO_2 removal is reduced. These conditions can be present despite preserved systemic and regional blood flow.

Notwithstanding the fact that ΔPCO_2 is not a marker of dysoxia but of tissue perfusion, it remains a very useful clinical and experimental monitoring tool, particularly in clinical situations such as sepsis in which cardiac output is increased while microcirculatory flow can be impaired.

References

1. Antonsson JB, Boyle CC 3rd, Kruithoff KL, et al (1990) Validation of tonometric measurement of gut intramural pH during endotoxemia and mesenteric occlusion in pigs. Am J Physiol 259: G519-G523
2. Hamilton-Davies C, Mythen MG, Salmon JB, Jacobson D, Shukla A, Webb AR (1997) Comparison of commonly used clinical indicators of hypovolaemia with gastrointestinal tonometry. Intensive Care Med 23: 276-281
3. Dubin A, Estenssoro E, Murias G, et al (2001) Effects of hemorrhage on gastrointestinal oxygenation. Intensive Care Med 27: 1931-1936
4. Fiddian-Green R, McGough E, Pittenger G, Rothman E (1983) Predictive value of intramural pH and other risk factors for massive bleeding from stress ulceration. Gastroenterology 85: 613-620
5. Schiedler MG, Cutler BS, Fiddian-Green R (1987) Sigmoid intramural pH for prediction of ischemic colitis during aortic surgery. A comparison with risk factors and inferior mesenteric artery stump pressures. Arch Surg 122: 881-886
6. Mythen M, Webb A (1994) Intra-operative gut mucosal hypoperfusion is associated with increased post-operative complications and cost. Intensive Care Med 20: 99-104
7. Doglio G, Pusajo J, Egurrola M, et al (1991) Gastric mucosal pH as a prognostic index of mortality in critically ill patients. Crit Care Med 19: 1037-1040
8. Friedman G; Berlot G, Kahn R, Vincent JL (1995) Combined measurements of blood lactate concentrations and gastric intramucosal pH in patients with severe sepsis. Crit Care Med 23: 1184-1193
9. Maynard N, Bihari D, Beale R, et al (1993) Assessment of splanchnic oxygenation by gastric tonometry in patients with acute circulatory failure. JAMA 270: 1203-1210
10. Gutierrez G, Clark C, Brown SD, Price K, Ortiz L, Nelson C (1994) Effect of dobutamine on oxygen consumption and gastric mucosal pH in septic patients. Am J Respir Crit Care Med 150: 324-329
11. Nevière R, Mathieu D, Chagnon JL, Lebleu N, Wattel F (1996) The contrasting effects of dobutamine and dopamine on gastric mucosal perfusion in septic patients. Am J Respir Crit Care Med 154: 1684-1688
12. Gutierrez G, Palizas F, Doglio G, et al (1992) Gastric intramucosal pH as a therapeutic index of tissue oxygenation in critically ill patients. Lancet 339: 195-199
13. Oud L, Kruse J (1996) Poor in vivo reproducibility of gastric intramucosal pH determined by saline-filled balloon tonometry. J Crit Care 11: 144-150
14. Taylor D, Gutierrez G, Clark C, Hainley S (1997) Measurement of gastric mucosal carbon dioxide tension by saline and air tonometry. J Crit Care 12: 208-213
15. Toledo Maciel A, Creteur J, Vincent JL (2004) Tissue capnometry: does the answer lie under the tongue? Intensive Care Med 30, 2157-2165
16. Honig C, Connett R, Gayeski T, Brooks G (1990) Defining hypoxia: a systems view of VO_2, glycolysis, energetics, and intracellular PO_2. J Appl Physiol 68: 833-842
17. Grum C, Fiddian-Green R, Pittenger G, Grant B, Rothman E, Dantzker D (1984) Adequacy of tissue oxygenation in intact dog intestine. J Appl Physiol 56: 1065-1069
18. Schlichtig R, Bowles S (1994) Distinguishing between aerobic and anaerobic appearance of dissolved CO_2 in intestine during low flow. J Appl Physiol 76: 2443-2451

V

19. Vallet B, Tavernier B, Lund N (2000) Assessment of tissue oxygenation in the critically ill. In: Vincent JL (ed) Yearbook of Intensive Care and Emergency Medicine. Springer-Verlag, Heidelberg, pp 715–725
20. Vallet B, Teboul JL, Cain S, Curtis S (2000) Venoarterial CO_2 difference during regional ischemic or hypoxic hypoxia. J Appl Physiol 89: 1317–1321
21. Nevière R, Chagnon JL, Teboul JL, Vallet B, Wattel F (2002) Small intestine intramucosal PCO_2 and microvascular blood flow during hypoxic and ischemic hypoxia. Crit Care Med 30, 379–384
22. Wasserman K, Beaver WL, Whipp BJ (1990) Gas exchange theory and the lactic acidosis (anaerobic) threshold. Circulation 81 (1 Suppl):II14–30
23. Dubin A, Murias G, Estenssoro E, et al (2000) End-tidal CO_2 pressure determinants during hemorrhagic shock. Intensive Care Med 26: 1619–1623
24. Dubin A, Murias G, Estenssoro E, et al (2002) Intramucosal-arterial PCO_2 gap fails to reflect intestinal dysoxia in hypoxic hypoxia. Crit Care 6: 514–520
25. Dubin A, Estenssoro E, Murias G, et al (2004) Intramucosal-arterial PCO_2 gradient does not reflect intestinal dysoxia in anemic hypoxia. J Trauma 57: 1211–1217
26. Gutierrez G (2004) A mathematical model of tissue-blood carbon dioxide exchange during hypoxia. Am J Respir Crit Care Med 169: 525–533
27. VanderMeer T, Wang H, Fink M (1995) Endotoxemia causes ileal mucosal acidosis in the absence of mucosal hypoxia in a normodynamic porcine model of septic shock. Crit Care Med 23: 1217–1226
28. Fink M (2002) Bench-to-bedside review: Cytopathic hypoxia. Crit Care 6: 491–499
29. Vallet B, Lund N, Curtis S, Kelly D, Cain S (1994) Gut and muscle tissue PO_2 in endotoxemic dogs during shock and resuscitation. J Appl Physiol 76: 793–800
30. Revelly J-P, Ayuse T, Brienza N, Fessler H, Robotham J (1996) Endotoxic shock alters distribution of blood flow within the intestinal wall. Crit Care Med 24: 1345–1351
31. Siegemund M, van Bommel J, Schwarte L, et al (2005) Inducible nitric oxide synthase inhibition improves intestinal microcirculatory oxygenation and CO_2 balance during endotoxemia in pigs. Intensive Care Med 31: 985–992
32. Tugtekin IF, Radermacher P, Theisen M, et al (2001) Increased ileal-mucosal-arterial PCO2 gap is associated with impaired villus microcirculation in endotoxic pigs. Intensive Care Med 27: 757–766
33. Creteur J, De Backer D, Sakr Y, Koch M, Vincent JL (2006) Sublingual capnometry tracks microcirculatory changes in septic patients. Intensive Care Med 32: 516–523
34. Dubin A, Kanoore Edul V, Murias G, et al (2008) Persistent villi hypoperfusion explains intramucosal acidosis in sheep endotoxemia. Crit Care Med 36: 535–542
35. Dubin A, Murias G, Maskin B, et al (2005) Increased blood flow prevents intramucosal acidosis in sheep endotoxemia: a controlled study. Crit Care 9: R66–73
36. Dubin A, Maskin B, Murias G, et al (2006) Effects of levosimendan in normodynamic endotoxaemia: a controlled experimental study. Resuscitation 69: 277–286
37. Dubin A, Murias G, Sottile J; et al (2007) Effects of levosimendan and dobutamine in experimental acute endotoxemia: A preliminary controlled study. Intensive Care Med 33: 485–494

Refining the Tools for Early Goal-directed Therapy in Septic Shock

E. Kipnis, E. Robin, and B. Vallet

Introduction: Initial Management of Septic Shock

The cornerstone of septic shock treatment is initial therapy in the first hours to the extent that part of the therapy, response to fluid loading, is a diagnostic criterion for septic shock. Furthermore, owing to the lack of specificity of key clinical features in the classification of hypotension, diagnosis and treatment should be considered simultaneously since a good response to treatment confirms the working diagnosis. Immediate management includes ensuring oxygen supply, fluid therapy, assessment of the need for vasopressor or inotrope therapy, and specific treatments to control and treat the source of infection. In life-threatening situations, empirical treatment should not be delayed while monitoring devices are being inserted. Basic cardiorespiratory monitoring includes measurement of heart rate and blood pressure, and pulse oximetry. However, the new millenium has witnessed the emergence of a new paradigm in the resuscitation of septic shock: Early goal-directed therapy. Early goal-directed therapy is a therapeutic strategy integrating all the standard aspects of septic shock treatment such as fluid loading, vasopressor and inotrope use among others, into an algorithmic process in which each component has specific targets, and all are targeted to restored tissue perfusion. This strategy in itself has proved more successful in reducing mortality due to septic shock than any single pharmacologic treatment specifically targeting sepsis. However, there may be room for refining the steps, specific endpoints, and goals used in early goal-directed therapy in order to further reduce mortality in septic shock. This chapter will briefly overview early goal-directed therapy and its principles (**Fig. 1**) and, following the steps involved in early goal-directed therapy, will propose new tools or directions which could refine the strategy (**Fig. 2**).

Overview of Early Goal-directed Therapy

In a landmark study by Rivers et al [1], patients admitted to an emergency department with severe sepsis and septic shock were randomized to standard therapy (fluid loading targeted to central venous pressure [CVP] of 8–12 mmHg, mean arterial pressure [MAP] ≥ 65 mmHg, and urine output ≥ 0.5 ml/kg/h), or to early goal-directed therapy in which, in addition to the previous parameters, a central venous oxygen saturation ($ScvO_2$)2 ≥ 70 % was targeted through algorithmic management. Algorithm loops consisted of fluid loading titrated to CVP and MAP increase above thresholds, vasopressor initiation if fluid loading failed to increase MAP, transfusion-based maintenance of hematocrit ≥ 30 %, and/or incremental administration of

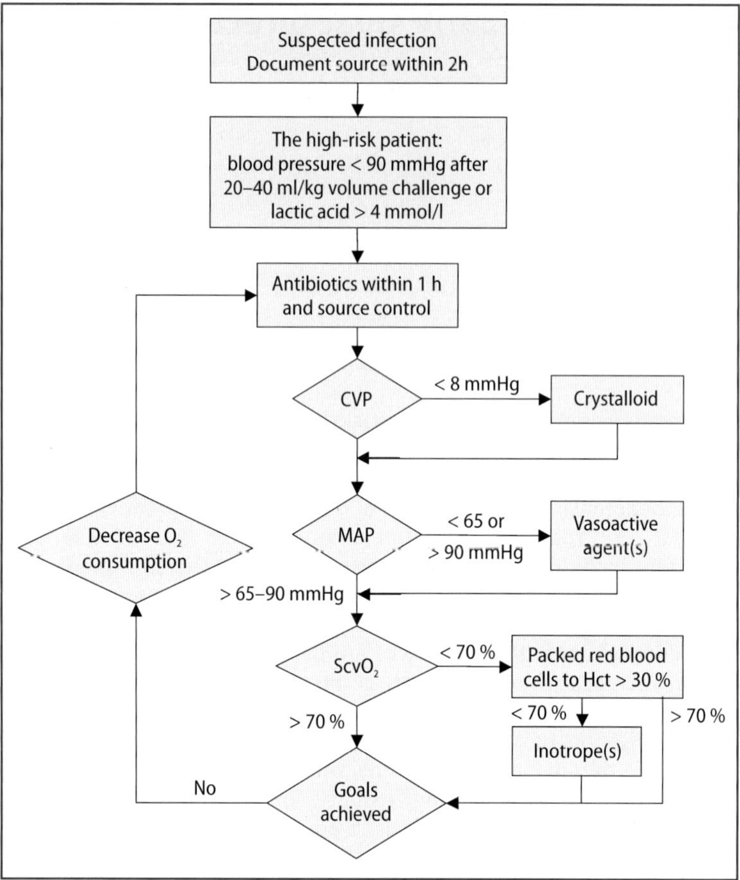

Fig. 1. Early goal-directed therapy (EGDT) in septic shock algorithm. Overview of the steps involved in the EGDT algorithm. Titration of fluids to central venous pressure (CVP) followed by mean arterial pressure (MAP). If MAP target is not met, use of vasopressors titrated to MAP. If perfusion goals assessed by central venous oxygen saturation ($ScvO_2$) are not met, maintenance of hematocrit (Hct) > 30 % with packed red blood cell transfusion. If target $ScvO_2$ is still not met, use of incremental doses of inotropes. Failure to meet perfusion goals should also lead to measures to decrease oxygen consumption. Going through any loop of the algorithm requires coming back to the initial starting point of CVP measurement.
Modified from Rivers et al. [32].

dobutamine to a maximum of 20 μg/kg/min and therapeutic measures to decrease oxygen consumption if perfusion goals were not met (**Fig. 1**). The initial $ScvO_2$ in both groups was low (49 ± 12 %), which serves as a reminder that severe sepsis is often a hypodynamic condition before fluid resuscitation is started, and that $ScvO_2$ indeed needed to be corrected. From the 1st to the 72nd hour, total fluid loading was not different between the two groups (≈13.4 l). However, in the earliest stage of management, from the 1st to the 7th hour, the amount of fluid received was significantly greater in the early goal-directed therapy patients (≈5000 ml vs. 3500 ml, p = 0.02). Conversely, from the 1st to the 72nd hour, the number of patients treated with vasopressors was significantly lower in the early goal-directed therapy group (36.8 %

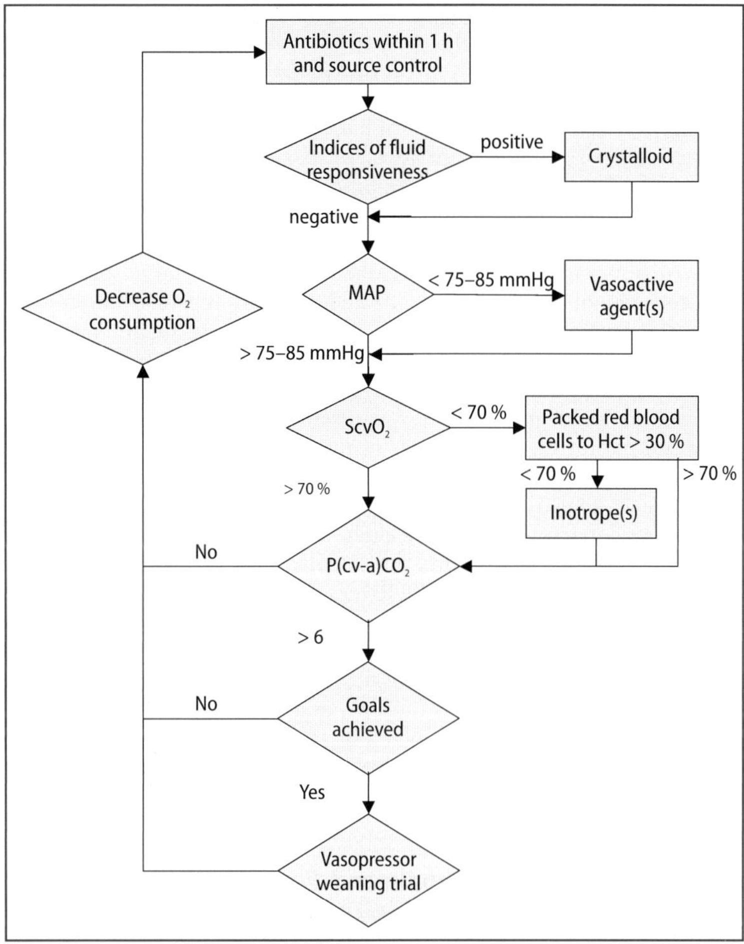

Fig. 2. Proposed tools for a refined early goal-directed therapy (EGDT) algorithm. Compared to the original algorithm (**Fig. 1**), new tools can replace or complement certain steps. Fluid responsiveness indices can replace central venous pressure (CVP) assessment as a first step. Mean arterial pressure (MAP) has the same importance albeit with different thresholds. Inotrope therapy should not be instituted without a full hemodynamic evaluation such as echocardiographic examination. If central venous oxygen saturation ($SvcO_2$) goals are achieved, tissue perfusion should be explored further through central venous-to-arterial carbon dioxide gap ($P(cv-a)CO_2$) as a last endpoint to be achieved. Modified From Rivers et al. [32].

vs. 51.3 %; $p = 0.02$). This was also the case from the 1st to the 7th hour although the difference was not significant (27.4 % vs. 30.3 %; $p = 0.62$). In the follow-up period between the 7th and the 72nd hour, in patients receiving early goal-directed therapy, mean $ScvO_2$ was higher (70.6 ± 10.7 % vs. 65.3 ± 11.4 %; $p = 0.02$), as was mean arterial pH (7.40 ± 0.12 vs. 7.36 ± 0.12; $p = 0.02$). Lactate plasma levels were lower in those receiving early goal-directed therapy (3.0 ± 4.4 mmol/l vs. 3.9 ± 4.4 mmol/l; $p = 0.02$), as was base excess (2.0 ± 6.6 mmol/l vs. 5.1 ± 6.7 mmol/l; $p = 0.02$). The organ failure score was also significantly altered in patients receiving standard therapy when compared with patients receiving early goal-directed therapy. Hospital mortality rates fell from 46.5 % (standard group) to 30.5 % in the early goal-directed therapy group (p = 0.009). Importantly, 99.2 % of patients receiving early goal-directed therapy achieved their hemodynamic goals within the first 6 hours compared with 86 % in the standard group. This was the first study demonstrating that early identification of patients with sepsis with early goal-directed therapy to achieve an adequate level of tissue oxygenation by oxygen delivery, as assessed by $ScvO_2$ monitoring, significantly improved mortality rates.

If the principles of early goal-directed therapy are to be summarized, they would first and foremost focus on the goal to be achieved, global tissue perfusion, and a stepwise approach to that means, each with its own target or threshold. First, rapid and consequent fluid loading titrated to fluid responsiveness and MAP; second, when the perfusion goal remains unattained, transfusion targeting a transfusion threshold; third, incremental inotrope therapy; and finally, a therapeutic decrease in oxygen consumption. These principles have been incorporated into recent national and international guidelines for the management of severe sepsis/septic shock [2] even though not under the form of the published early goal-directed therapy algorithm.

The early goal-directed therapy study by Rivers et al. [1] was conducted in the emergency department, appropriately when considering the emergency department is a point-of-entry of patients with septic shock thus allowing early therapy. Also appropriately for the setting, the Rivers study used targets and resuscitation parameters which could be easily obtained. However, an increasing number of hemodynamic monitoring techniques or bedside physiological explorations are available to intensivists which could allow physicians to delve deeper into the goals and stepwise targets of early goal-directed therapy, and hence refine the concept. We propose to review, following the steps involved in early goal-directed therapy, some monitoring techniques and applicable physiological explorations which might further advance early goal-directed therapy.

Therapeutic Steps and Goals and Proposed Refinements

Fluid Titration to Predictors of Fluid Responsiveness

In severe sepsis, and particularly in an early goal-directed therapy strategy, fluid loading is titrated to several targets. First, an indication of volume status, or more importantly of what effect fluid loading will have, or fluid responsiveness, is to be sought. Second, the macrocirculatory effect of the fluid loading has to be monitored and assessed.

To address volume status, the simplest but least reliable method is the CVP. Readily available as soon as a central venous line is in place, a prerequisite in any severely ill patient in whom venous access allowing vasopressor support must be secured, the measurement is simple. However, CVP values are 'static', and while very low values close to zero can be indicative of fluid responsiveness, and very high values over 20 indicate replete volume status, it is much harder to interpret other values even when considering 'dynamic' changes in CVP. Marik et al. recently conducted a systematic review of 24 studies of fluid responsiveness using CVP or dynamic variations in CVP and found a very poor correlation between either CVP or deltaCVP and fluid responsiveness [3]. Of course, the response to fluid loading, an increase in cardiac output, can be directly monitored through various techniques. A pulmonary artery catheter (PAC) equipped with continuous cardiac output and mixed venous oxygen saturation

(SvO_2) monitoring modalities and/or any less invasive flow assessment technique (e.g., transesophageal echocardiography [TEE], esophageal Doppler, LidCO or a peripheral transpulmonary dilution catheter) is recommended when hypotension persists or precise cardiac output optimization is required (e.g., for fluid loading). Fluid challenges should be repeated until the top of the Frank-Starling curve is reached – that is, when stroke volume does not increase > 10 % following a 250 ml colloid challenge. At this point, the ventricle becomes preload-independent [4]. In addition to providing the same information, echocardiography, transthoracic or transesophageal, may provide a rapid insight into differential diagnosis, particularly when the underlying problem is unclear [5]. For example, in the context of congestive heart failure, myocardial ischemia, or sudden collapse, echocardiography may diagnose any potentially reversible ventricular, valvular, or obstructive pathology. It provides information on both left and right ventricular function and can provide an initial assessment of preload and the presence of any regional wall-motion abnormalities. Echocardiography should not be considered simply within the context of cardiac output assessment, but within the context of global cardiac performance which can be altered in sepsis [6]. However, it is possible that bedside bidimensional echocardiography is still not available in all general intensive care units (ICUs).

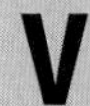

More interestingly than passively observing the cardiac output response to fluid loading, several monitoring techniques can provide indices which are predictive of the response to fluid loading [7]. Most are based upon the respiratory variations in preload in preload-dependent states and the measured translation on accessible parameters ranging from the complex, such as the variation in diameter of the superior vena cava in TEE [8], to the simple, such as the respiratory variance in pulse pressure (PPV) [9]. Some indices can even be automatically measured continuously, such as stroke volume variations through esophageal Doppler or similar indices from various hemodynamic monitoring devices [10].

However these measurements are only valid in certain conditions: Sedated, intubated, ventilated steady-state patients without severe valvular or rhythm problems. Unfortunately, arrhythmias or spontaneous breathing preclude this type of evaluation [11]. Other methods, such as observing the cardiac output response to passive leg raising have been proposed to determine fluid responsiveness in the spontaneously breathing patient [12, 13]. Assessing fluid responsiveness merely predicts the ability of a fluid challenge to induce an increase in cardiac output which cannot be a goal in itself as attested by the failure of many cardiac output-targeted studies in the past [14]. Indeed, the immediate target of fluid loading, even when guided by indices of fluid responsiveness, should be maintenance of a certain level of MAP.

Fluid Titration to Mean Arterial Pressure

With the possible exceptions of severe septic cardiac dysfunction or sepsis in a patient with pre-existing heart failure, the vast majority of hypotensive septic patients require fluid as first-line therapy because hypovolemia is nearly always present. Although experts argue over the advantages and disadvantages of particular colloid or crystalloid solutions, there is consensus on the need to administer enough fluid to restore an adequate circulation [2, 15]. Due to the underlying physiopathology of sepsis which leads to loss of vascular tone through vasodilatation (because of excessive activation of macrophages, neutrophils, or endothelium and over-production of pro-inflammatory mediators, such as prostanoids, nitric oxide [NO], kinins, and pyrogens) and loss of intravascular content (capillary leak, with additional fluid and electrolyte depletion from a variety of routes, e.g., sweat, vomit, diarrhea), fluid loading is a mainstay of management to the extent that it is a prerequisite to the diagnosis of septic shock. Indeed, in clinical practice, the terms 'hypotension' and 'shock' are often used interchangeably. Hypotension can be defined as a decrease in systolic blood pressure of > 40–50 mmHg from baseline, a systolic value of < 90 mmHg, or a MAP of < 65 mmHg. Most consensual definitions of septic shock incorporate the failure of an initial fluid loading to restore MAP > 65 mmHg as one of the diagnostic criteria [2, 15, 16]. Furthermore, it is important to stress that shock may be present despite a 'normal' blood pressure. Indeed, even though the definition of hypotension includes the decrease from baseline in order to include patients that are usually hypertensive, questions can be raised as to the significance of the definition itself. Indeed, a European study of severe sepsis progression to septic shock has shown that a systolic blood pressure (SBP) limit of 110 mmHg was predictive of progression towards septic shock [17]. Likewise, in a retrospective study of predictors of outcome in a database of 81,134 trauma patients, Eastridge et al. [18] found that at SBP < 110 mmHg there was an increase in mortality rate. Each further 10 mmHg decrement in SBP led to a 4.8 % increase in mortality, albeit all-cause and not limited to sepsis [18]. Therefore, close monitoring of MAP in patients with sepsis is highly valuable especially before the failure of fluid loading to restore MAP has established the diagnosis of septic shock. Arterial blood pressure should be recorded at a minimum of 5 min intervals but, ideally, it should be monitored continuously, and whenever possible invasively in the unstable patient [2]. Non-invasive measurements are often unreliable in shock states, and invasive arterial pressure monitoring should be instituted as soon as possible. Furthermore, invasive arterial pressure monitoring can assist in exploring fluid responsiveness. Once fluid loading has achieved a state in which there is no longer any potential fluid responsiveness, if target MAP is not restored, vasopressor therapy should be instituted.

Vasopressor Titration to MAP

After adequately restoring intravascular fluid volume, persistent hypotension requires the use of drugs that either improve myocardial contractility (to increase cardiac output) and/or increase vascular tone (to increase systemic vascular resistance [SVR]). Owing to their short half-life (minutes) and familiarity with their use, catecholamines are usually the preferred first-line agents. Taking into account their effects on cardiac contractility (inotropism) and vascular tone (constrictor or dilator effects), they can be separated into two major classes: Inodilators (inotrope plus vasodilator: Low-dose dopamine and any dose of dobutamine or dopexamine), or inoconstrictors (inotrope plus vasoconstrictor: High dose dopamine, any dose of norepinephrine, and moderate-to-high doses of epinephrine). Inodilators increase blood flow, but may actually have excessive vasodilating effects; inoconstrictors or vasopressors increase perfusion pressure and have variable effects on flow. Non-catecholamine vasopressor, such as vasopressin and its synthetic analogue, terlipressin, are now being evaluated in sepsis and other vasodilatory shock states.

The detection of a marked decrease in left ventricular ejection fraction using echocardiography can orient towards the use of dobutamine when signs of peripheral hypoperfusion persist despite volume resuscitation and restoration of perfusion pressure with vasopressors. However, given the predominance of relative and absolute hypovolemia and the extent of vascular tone loss during septic shock, it is recommended that vasopressor rather than inotropic therapy be initiated when MAP is not restored by fluid loading. Because of a highly variable individual sensitivity to these different catecholamine agents, dose titration is strongly recommended, ideally against measurement of cardiac output as well as MAP and other relevant variables, such as base deficit and urine output. The Surviving Sepsis Campaign recommends maintaining MAP at ≥ 65 mmHg in septic shock patients [2]. This titration of vasopressors to MAP is a Janus-like target. Indeed, the 65 mmHg threshold may be too low, just as higher thresholds may not be good surrogates of clinical benefit [19, 20]. Indeed, in a large, placebo-controlled, clinical trial, administration of the non-selective NO inhibitor, NG-methyl-l-arginine, in septic shock produced significant increases in both blood pressure and mortality rate [21]. This probably reflects the fact that MAP in itself cannot be a goal in early goal-directed therapy but rather a step in the strategy. Indeed, in the seminal early goal-directed therapy study of Rivers et al. [1], the group in which fluids and vasopressors were titrated to MAP had lower MAPs, closer to the 65 mmHg threshold than the group in which fluids and vasopressors were titrated to MAP and then to $ScvO_2$, which had MAPs approaching 85 to 95 mmHg [21]. Likewise, in a retrospective cohort study which found that predictors of survival in septic shock were the steps and goals of early goal-directed therapy (CVP, MAP and $ScvO_2$), the authors found that non-survivors had a MAP of 67 mmHg, again close to the 65 mmHg threshold, versus a significantly higher MAP of 76 mmHg for survivors [22]. Past studies of 'supranormal' or 'maximized' cardiac output in order to optimize oxygen delivery failed most probably because resulting tissue perfusion was not the targeted goal [14]. A recent study comparing different thresholds, 65 mmHg and 85 mmHg, as MAP targets for vasopressor titration found that $ScvO_2$ was higher in the high MAP group, although no other clinical benefit was apparent [20].

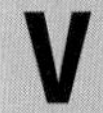

Apart from the controversy as to the optimal MAP threshold, the risk, when using vasopressors, is to vasoconstrict inadequately fluid-loaded patients and decrease tissue perfusion. This is the reason why fluid loading is the consensual first step in the management of septic shock and the first step in early goal-directed therapy. It is also the rationale for optimization of fluid loading through preload assessment as we have already discussed. However, vasopressor-increased vascular tone and vasopressor-induced reduced vascular compliance lead to 'masking' of fluid responsiveness. In a recent experimental study, Nouira et al. clearly demonstrated that preload independency could be artificially created, by infusing norepinephrine following hemorrhagic shock [23]. In hemorrhaged dogs (in which 35 ml/kg of blood was withdrawn), norepinephrine, in the absence of fluid or red blood cell infusion, resulted in a return of PPV from 28 % to a normal 12 %, while MAP and cardiac output were increased from 85 to 153 mmHg and from 1.98 to 3.08 l/min, respectively. Conversely, despite normalization of hemodynamics, pH fell from 7.29 to 7.24 and bicarbonate from 18.0 to 15.8 mmol/l. Given the variable intravascular half-life of various fluids, it is certain that the volume status of patients with septic shock changes dynamically over time even after vasopressor therapy has been initiated. Thus, it is probable that at an unpredicted time, a patient under vasopressor therapy with a no longer increasing MAP might benefit from fluid loading while fluid responsiveness, as assessed by dynamic indices such as PPV, will indicate a state of preload independence leading to an increase in vasopressor therapy and a vicious cycle possibly leading to deleterious effects on tissue perfusion. Therefore, it may be useful to 'test' this phenomenon in patients in whom vasopressors have been initiated for some hours by lowering their rate and reassessing fluid responsiveness through dynamic preload assessment.

V

The Goal: Tissue Perfusion

The originality of the study of Rivers et al. [1] is that both fluid loading titrated to CVP and vasopressors titrated to MAP are further titrated beyond CVP and MAP to tissue perfusion as assessed by a surrogate of the balance between oxygen delivery and oxygen consumption, $ScvO_2$.

SvO_2 explores the relationship between oxygen transport to tissues and oxygen use by tissues (VO_2) as attested by the relationship linking the two: $SvO_2 \approx SaO_2 - VO_2 / (Hb \times 1.34 \times \text{cardiac output})$ where SaO_2 represents arterial oxygen saturation, and Hb represents hemoglobin. Therefore, determinants of a decrease in SvO_2 (or $ScvO_2$) are, either alone or in combination, hypoxemia (decrease in SaO_2), an increase in VO_2 (sepsis, alert and awake distressed patient, work of breathing) without an increase in oxygen transport, a fall in cardiac output (decrease in MAP or myocardial depression), and a decrease in hemoglobin concentration. The normal range for SvO_2 is 68–77 % (+5 % for $ScvO_2$). An increase in VO_2 without an increase in cardiac output or oxygen transport, or a decrease in oxygen transport and no change in oxygen requirements, will result in an increase in oxygen extraction (O_2ER) and a fall in SvO_2. O_2ER2 and SvO_2 are linked by a simple equation: $O_2ER \approx 1 - SvO_2$, assuming $SaO_2 = 1$ [24]. Tissue dysoxia is usually present when SvO_2 falls below 40–50 %; however, this may also occur at higher levels of SvO_2, when O_2ER is impaired. Therefore, other markers of cellular oxygen inadequacy should be sought, such as hyperlactatemia. Usually, efforts to correct cardiac output (fluids or inotropes), hemoglobin level, SaO_2, VO_2, or a combination of the parameters, must target a return of SvO_2 ($ScvO_2$) from 50 to 65 % (70 % for $ScvO_2$).

However, it may be possible to further explore tissue perfusion in order to detect abnormalities undetected by $ScvO_2$. One approach is the bedside investigation of regional microcirculation, a field in itself [25]. Interference of sepsis-modified vasoactive drug properties by sepsis-induced microcirculatory disturbances has predominantly been investigated at the level of the splanchnic circulation, sublingual circulation, and skin using techniques such as regional capnometry, laser Doppler flowmetry, indocyanine green (ICG) dilution or orthogonal polarization spectroscopy (OPS) [25]. Besides the controversial measurement of lactate concentration in septic shock [26, 27], determination of gastric tonometer-to-arterial carbon dioxide pressure (PCO_2) remains the unique clinical monitoring tool that can aid in the assessment of the efficacy of fluid loading or catecholamine infusion on tissue perfusion [28].

The venous-to-arterial carbon dioxide difference [$P(v\text{-}a)CO_2$] can, to some extent, be proposed as a surrogate for tissue perfusion assessment, as suggested by Mekontso-Dessap et al. [29]. This approach does not depend on direct study of the microcirculation. We recently tested the hypothesis that, in resuscitated septic shock patients, central venous-to-arterial carbon dioxide difference [$P(cv\text{-}a)CO_2$] may serve as a global index of tissue perfusion when the $ScvO_2$ goal value has already been reached [30]. In a prospective observational study, 50 consecutive septic shock patients with $ScvO_2 > 70$ % were included immediately after their admission into the ICU (T0) following early resuscitation in the emergency unit. Patients were separated into Low $P(cv\text{-}a)CO_2$ (Low gap; n = 26) and High $P(cv\text{-}a)CO_2$ (High gap; n = 24) groups according to a threshold of 6 mmHg at T0. Measurements were performed every 6 hours for 12 hours (T0, T6, T12). At T0, there was a significant difference between the Low gap patients and the High gap patients for cardiac index (4.3 + 1.6 vs. 2.7 + 0.8 $l/min/m^2$, $p < 0.0001$) but not for $ScvO_2$ values (78 + 5 vs.

75 + 5 %, $p = 0.07$). From T0 to T12, the clearance of lactate was significantly larger for the Low gap group than for the High gap group ($p < 0.05$) as was the decrease in sequential organ failure assessment (SOFA) score after 24 hours ($p < 0.01$). At T0, T6 and T12, cardiac index and $P(cv\text{-}a)CO_2$ values were inversely correlated ($p < 0.0001$). Therefore, when the 70 % $ScvO_2$ goal is reached, the presence of a $P(cv\text{-}a)CO_2 > 6$ mmHg might be a useful tool to identify patients who remain inadequately resuscitated.

Red Blood Cell Transfusion

Hemoglobin is the oxygen transporter in blood. As such, it is the main determinant of oxygen content and the main determinant of oxygen transport aside from cardiac output. Therefore, for a constant cardiac output, such as that maintained by fluids and vasopressors in early goal-directed therapy, a decrease in hemoglobin will lead to a decrease in oxygen transport since oxygen transport = cardiac output × CaO_2, where CaO_2 is arterial oxygen content, with $CaO_2 \approx Hb \times SaO_2 \times 1.34$ (where SaO_2 is the arterial oxygen saturation; and 1.34 ml oxygen/g Hb is the oxygen-carrying capacity of Hb, and free soluble oxygen is discarded). Thus, in early goal-directed therapy, the decision to transfuse is based upon the hope of increasing oxygen transport to tissues and subsequently increasing cellular oxygen. However, transfusion thresholds, either hematocrit-based or hemoglobin-based, are arbitrary. In clinical practice, decisions to transfuse are usually based on consensual thresholds derived from epidemiologic studies showing benefit or lack of benefit of transfusion in certain populations at various thresholds. Even though these arbitrary levels take into account underlying diseases such as ischemic heart disease and acute coronary syndromes, it is hard to imagine that they are applicable in such a dynamically changing situation as sepsis. We, therefore, conducted a prospective study of recommendation-based transfusion in the post-operative setting compared to the resulting variation in $ScvO_2$ [31]. We found that 26 patients (49 %) were transfused in spite of recommendations, leading to an increase in $ScvO_2$ in 22.6 % of these patients with an initial $ScvO_2 < 70$ %. Conversely, 24.5 % of the patients fulfilled the recommendations and were transfused although $ScvO_2$ was ≥ 70 %.

Thus, $ScvO_2$, even outside of the situation of shock and very insufficient oxygen delivery, can probably be an interesting physiological trigger for transfusion. This may be even more valid in severe oxygen delivery dependent situations such as septic shock, as demonstrated by Rivers et al. [1] in which, in addition, volume loading leads to dilution and a relative decrease in hemoglobin.

Inotrope Therapy

In the early goal-directed therapy study of Rivers et al. [1], inotrope therapy using incremental doses of dobutamine involved few patients. It is also important to note that following each very progressive increment in dobutamine (2.5 mcg/kg/min), the whole algorithm of early goal-directed therapy was reassessed including fluid responsiveness due to the inodilator properties of dobutamine [32].

We shall not dwell on inotrope therapy since it is not the mainstay of early goal-directed therapy, rather a specific therapy addressing a specific subgroup of patients who do not restore tissue perfusion when volume status is corrected and minimal MAP attained, regardless of hemoglobin. In fact, rather than rely on the early goal-directed therapy algorithm to identify and treat this subgroup, it may be more relevant to include echocardiography to explore these fluid-loading, vasopressor and transfusion resistant situations which most probably have their origin in myocardial dysfunction.

Other Issues

Early Recognition of Severe Sepsis

There can be no conceivable early goal-directed therapy without efficient recognition of severe sepsis, as early as possible, even before septic shock or the accumulation of organ failures. In fact, the very implementation of guidelines for rapid recognition of severe sepsis might lead to increased survival by allowing patients to benefit from early goal-directed therapy early enough [33]. One such strategy, combining widespread institutional education geared towards early recognition of sepsis and septic shock combined with early goal-directed therapy protocols and a rapid response team led to a decrease in mortality from 40 % to 11 % over 5 years [33]. To this end, new tools such as scores predicting the evolutive risk of patients with systemic inflammatory response syndrome (SIRS) or sepsis have been proposed such as the Risk of Infection to Severe Sepsis and Shock Score [17]. Such concepts lead to a broader definition of severe sepsis which might also identify patients warranting close surveillance and monitoring allowing very early implementation of early goal-directed therapy [34].

Early Antimicrobials

Hemodynamic management and early goal-directed therapy are only one side of the battle against sepsis, the other being control of the source of infection and appropriate antimicrobial therapy. This is true to the extent that most studies of early goal-directed therapy have been conceived with concomittant institution of antimicrobial therapy as a prerequisite to enrollment. Studies have shown that there is a linear increase in mortality with each passing hour of delay in antimicrobial administration after the first episode of hypotension in severe sepsis [35]. This highlights the fact that the very technical and real-time aspects of hemodynamic management and early goal-directed therapy should in no case alter the focus on what is essentially an infection-related process and lead to delay in antimicrobial therapy.

Vasopressor Weaning

It must be remembered that in the Rivers early goal-directed therapy study [1], fluid loading titrated to CVP followed by vasopressor titration to MAP and both further titrated to $ScvO_2$ reduced vasopressor therapy and increased fluid loading when compared with a more conventional approach. This was followed by a net improvement in organ failure and survival rate. While not a vasopressor weaning protocol, these findings highlight that appropriate fluid management in septic shock can reduce possibly excessive and deleterious vasopressor use. Likewise, in two major randomized controlled trials in sepsis (using activated protein C or corticosteroids), successful therapeutic intervention led to a more rapid decrease in vasopressor therapy and an improvement in mortality rates [36, 37]. Taken together, this suggests that although vasopressors almost inevitably need to be rapidly introduced in the initial therapeutic strategy of septic shock, their benefit and especially the benefit/

current dose must be frequently questioned, and weaning must be rapidly considered or even tested as suggested above for vasopressor titration. Weaning from catecholamines is associated with the risk of inducing or 'unmasking' underlying preload dependency. Mallat et al. elegantly demonstrated that the decrease in catecholamine concentration during pheochromocytoma resection was associated with fluid responsiveness as assessed by increased systolic pressure variation, which was significantly reduced by fluid loading [38]. However, the authors also suggested that catecholamine reinstitution needed to be considered when the fluid loading that was titrated to reduce systolic pressure variation was not sufficient to correct MAP. Additionally to 'testing' an eventual benefit of further fluid loading by lowering vasopressor dose and measuring fluid responsiveness indices during early goal-directed therapy, as previously discussed in the section on vasopressor titration, it would be even more essential to 'test' vasopressor 'masking' of fluid responsiveness later on in the management of septic shock. Indeed, once early goal-directed therapy has run its course, no recommendations exist as to how fluid loading and vasopressors should be managed. When should fluids be administered again? Titrated to what goal? What to do with the vasopressors which have maintained the targeted MAP? When and how should they be weaned? We hypothesize that lowering the dose of a vasopressor such as norepinephrine could unmask preload dependency, and that a vasopressor weaning protocol based on MAP and systolic pressure variation, PPV, or stroke volume variation (SVV) should be considered (**Fig. 3**). This protocol could help in safely reducing norepinephrine dose. Moreover, it might be associated with improved organ perfusion and more rapid vasopressor withdrawal. As in early goal-directed therapy, biological parameters of organ perfusion should be assessed during the process (arterial and central venous blood gas analysis, with a special emphasis on SvO_2, pH and bicarbonate, and arterial lactate) in order to ascertain that the weaning process is not deleterious.

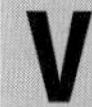

Conclusion

While tissue perfusion is clearly the goal in early goal-directed therapy, it may be possible to further detect abnormalities in either regional perfusion through bedside microcirculatory exploration or using the central venous-to-arterial carbon dioxide difference, $P(cv\text{-}a)CO_2$, in order to detect septic shock patients who currently may remain inadequately resuscitated. In order to achieve these perfusion goals, early goal-directed therapy remains the most attractive strategy in which each step may benefit from more complete approaches especially in the ICU. Fluid loading may be titrated to indices of fluid responsiveness rather than CVP. Testing the reappearance of fluid responsiveness by lowering vasopressor therapy and measuring the same indices may reveal further opportunities for fluid loading both in the initial phase of septic shock during early goal-directed therapy and particularly after early goal-directed therapy during the vasopressor weaning process which may be accelerated by such testing. Finally, early goal-directed therapy, whether, standard or refined using our proposed methods will only further reduce mortality if integrated into a broader strategy alongside early recognition of sepsis, early administration of antimicrobials, and control of infection source.

V

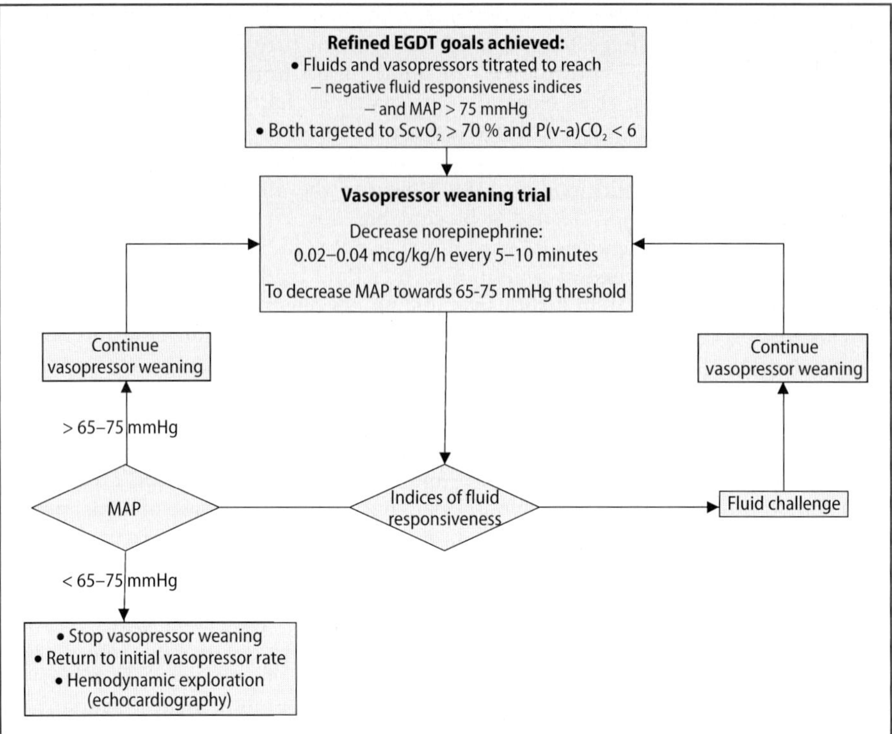

Fig. 3. Proposed protocol for vasopressor withdrawal or weaning trial. After reaching modified early goal-directed therapy (EGDT) goals, the reappearance of fluid responsiveness allowing vasopressor weaning should be tested. A prudent incremental decrease in vasopressors followed by assessment of fluid responsiveness will guide the process. A decrease in mean arterial pressure (MAP) towards 65–75 mmHg associated with positive fluid responsiveness indices allows the continuation of vasopressor weaning after fluid challenge. Maintained MAP above 65–75 mmHg after vasopressor decrease with negative fluid responsive indices allows continued weaning following regular reassessment of fluid responsiveness. Finally, a decrease in MAP upon a vasopressor weaning trial without reappearance of fluid responsiveness may indicate a status benefitting from the inotropic effects of vasopressors and justifies echocardiographic reassessment.

References

1. Rivers E, Nguyen B, Havstad S, et al (2001) Early goal-directed therapy in the treatment of severe sepsis and septic shock. N Engl J Med 345: 1368–1377
2. Dellinger RP, Levy MM, Carlet JM, et al (2008) Surviving Sepsis Campaign: international guidelines for management of severe sepsis and septic shock: 2008. Crit Care Med 36: 296–327
3. Marik PE, Baram M, Vahid B (2008) Does central venous pressure predict fluid responsiveness? A systematic review of the literature and the tale of seven mares. Chest 134: 172–178
4. Robin E, Costecalde M, Lebuffe G, Vallet B (2006) Clinical relevance of data from the pulmonary artery catheter. Crit Care 10 (Suppl 3): S3
5. Price S, Nicol E, Gibson DG, Evans TW (2006) Echocardiography in the critically ill: current and potential roles. Intensive Care Med 32: 48–59
6. Vieillard-Baron A, Prin S, Chergui K, Dubourg O, Jardin F (2003) Hemodynamic instability in sepsis: bedside assessment by Doppler echocardiography. Am J Respir Crit Care Med 168: 1270–1276

7. Pinsky MR, Teboul JL (2005) Assessment of indices of preload and volume responsiveness. Curr Opin Crit Care 11: 235–239
8. Vieillard-Baron A, Charron C, Chergui K, Peyrouset O, Jardin F (2006) Bedside echocardiographic evaluation of hemodynamics in sepsis: is a qualitative evaluation sufficient? Intensive Care Med 32: 1547–1552
9. Michard F, Teboul JL (2002) Predicting fluid responsiveness in ICU patients: a critical analysis of the evidence. Chest 121: 2000–2008
10. Pinsky MR, Brophy P, Padilla J, Paganini E, Pannu N (2008) Fluid and volume monitoring. Int J Artif Organs 31: 111–126
11. Michard F (2005) Changes in arterial pressure during mechanical ventilation. Anesthesiology 103: 419–428; quiz 449–415
12. Lamia B, Ochagavia A, Monnet X, Chemla D, Richard C, Teboul JL (2007) Echocardiographic prediction of volume responsiveness in critically ill patients with spontaneously breathing activity. Intensive Care Med 33: 1125–1132
13. Teboul JL, Monnet X (2008) Prediction of volume responsiveness in critically ill patients with spontaneous breathing activity. Curr Opin Crit Care 14: 334–339
14. Sharma VK, Dellinger RP (2003) The International Sepsis Forum's frontiers in sepsis: High cardiac output should not be maintained in severe sepsis. Crit Care 7: 272–275
15. Dellinger RP, Carlet JM, Masur H, et al (2004) Surviving Sepsis Campaign guidelines for management of severe sepsis and septic shock. Crit Care Med 32: 858–873
16. Abraham E, Matthay MA, Dinarello CA, et al (2000) Consensus conference definitions for sepsis, septic shock, acute lung injury, and acute respiratory distress syndrome: time for a reevaluation. Crit Care Med 28: 232–235
17. Alberti C, Brun-Buisson C, Chevret S, et al (2005) Systemic inflammatory response and progression to severe sepsis in critically ill infected patients. Am J Respir Crit Care Med 171: 461–468
18. Eastridge BJ, Salinas J, McManus JG, et al (2007) Hypotension begins at 110 mm Hg: redefining "hypotension" with data. J Trauma 63: 291–297
19. LeDoux D, Astiz ME, Carpati CM, Rackow EC (2000) Effects of perfusion pressure on tissue perfusion in septic shock. Crit Care Med 28: 2729–2732
20. Bourgoin A, Leone M, Delmas A, Garnier F, Albanese J, Martin C (2005) Increasing mean arterial pressure in patients with septic shock: effects on oxygen variables and renal function. Crit Care Med 33: 780–786
21. Lopez A, Lorente JA, Steingrub J, et al (2004) Multiple-center, randomized, placebo-controlled, double-blind study of the nitric oxide synthase inhibitor 546C88: effect on survival in patients with septic shock. Crit Care Med 32: 21–30
22. Varpula M, Tallgren M, Saukkonen K, Voipio-Pulkki LM, Pettila V (2005) Hemodynamic variables related to outcome in septic shock. Intensive Care Med 31: 1066–1071
23. Nouira S, Elatrous S, Dimassi S, et al (2005) Effects of norepinephrine on static and dynamic preload indicators in experimental hemorrhagic shock. Crit Care Med 33: 2339–2343
24. Rasanen J (1990) Mixed venous oximetry may detect critical oxygen delivery. Anesth Analg 71: 567–568
25. Trzeciak S, Cinel I, Phillip Dellinger R, et al (2008) Resuscitating the microcirculation in sepsis: the central role of nitric oxide, emerging concepts for novel therapies, and challenges for clinical trials. Acad Emerg Med 15: 399–413
26. Englehart MS, Schreiber MA (2006) Measurement of acid-base resuscitation endpoints: lactate, base deficit, bicarbonate or what? Curr Opin Crit Care 12: 569–574
27. Levy B (2006) Lactate and shock state: the metabolic view. Curr Opin Crit Care 12: 315–321
28. Levy B, Gawalkiewicz P, Vallet B, Briancon S, Nace L, Bollaert PE (2003) Gastric capnometry with air-automated tonometry predicts outcome in critically ill patients. Crit Care Med 31: 474–480
29. Mekontso-Dessap A, Castelain V, Anguel N, et al (2002) Combination of venoarterial PCO2 difference with arteriovenous O2 content difference to detect anaerobic metabolism in patients. Intensive Care Med 28: 272–277
30. Vallee F, Vallet B, Mathe O, et al (2008) Central venous-to-arterial carbon dioxide difference: an additional target for goal-directed therapy in septic shock? Intensive Care Med 34: 2218–2225

31. Vallet B, Adamczyk S, Barreau O, Lebuffe G (2007) Physiologic transfusion triggers. Best Pract Res Clin Anaesthesiol 21: 173–181
32. Rivers EP, McIntyre L, Morro DC, Rivers KK (2005) Early and innovative interventions for severe sepsis and septic shock: taking advantage of a window of opportunity. CMAJ 173: 1054–1065
33. Sebat F, Musthafa AA, Johnson D, et al (2007) Effect of a rapid response system for patients in shock on time to treatment and mortality during 5 years. Crit Care Med 35: 2568–2575
34. Groupe Transversal Sepsis (2007) Prise en charge initiale des états septiques graves de l'adulte et de l'enfant. Réanimation 16: S1-S21
35. Kumar A, Roberts D, Wood KE, et al (2006) Duration of hypotension before initiation of effective antimicrobial therapy is the critical determinant of survival in human septic shock. Crit Care Med 34: 1589–1596
36. Abraham E, Laterre PF, Garg R, et al (2005) Drotrecogin alfa (activated) for adults with severe sepsis and a low risk of death. N Engl J Med 353: 1332–1341
37. Annane D, Sebille V, Charpentier C, et al (2002) Effect of treatment with low doses of hydrocortisone and fludrocortisone on mortality in patients with septic shock. JAMA 288: 862–871
38. Mallat J, Pironkov A, Destandou MS, Tavernier B (2003) Systolic pressure variation (Delta-down) can guide fluid therapy during pheochromocytoma surgery. Can J Anaesth 50: 998–1003

VI Intravenous Fluids

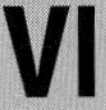

Hyperchloremic Metabolic Acidosis: More than Just a Simple Dilutional Effect

S.S. Abdel-Razeq and L.J. Kaplan

Introduction

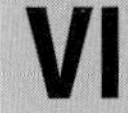

Fluid resuscitation lies at the heart of acute care medicine. Despite the central role occupied by plasma volume expansion therapeutics, there remains little consensus regarding the ideal fluid for plasma volume expansion. However, the unintended consequences of excessive plasma volume expansion as well as those untoward events directly ascribed to the prescribed fluids have come to the fore. Anasarca, pulmonary edema, myocardial stress, acute lung injury (ALI), acute kidney injury, as well as the secondary abdominal compartment syndrome have all been described as unintended consequences of plasma volume expansion following critical illness or injury [1–3]. It is important to note that these events occur with both crystalloid and colloid therapy, although at different rates.

Equally importantly, both crystalloids and colloid may create hyperchloremic metabolic acidosis. It is clear that colloids will do so at a slower rate than crystalloids principally related to their improved efficiency with regard to plasma volume expansion. Since colloid resuscitation generally requires less total volume, less total chloride is delivered and hyperchloremic metabolic acidosis occurs less rapidly. The genesis of hyperchloremic metabolic acidosis, as well as its significance, has been hotly debated over the last several decades [4–6]. Previously, the forces creating hyperchloremic metabolic acidosis were ascribed to simple dilution, and the significance of the acidosis minimized to a laboratory curiosity. Current investigations into hyperchloremic metabolic acidosis and its consequences embrace a diametrically opposed perspective. The focus of this chapter is to explore the mechanisms underpinning hyperchloremic metabolic acidosis as well as the impact of hyperchloremic metabolic acidosis on immunobiology, resuscitation, clotting, and oxygen delivery.

Mechanisms Underpinning pH Regulation: A Physico-chemical Approach

Plasma volume expansion impacts acid-base balance in predictable manners depending on the type and volume of infused fluid. The physical chemical approach articulated by Stewart provides a mechanistic means of understanding how plasma volume expansion alters pH by assessing changes in plasma charge [7–10]. The physico-chemical approach describes three independent variables that determine the pH in an aqueous milieu, such as human plasma: The strong ion difference (SID), the sum of associated and dissociated weak acid (A_{tot}), and CO_2.

Strong ions are cations and anions that are dissociated from their partner ions at physiologic pH. Examples of strong ions include Na^+, K^+, Ca^{2+}, Mg^{2+} and Cl^-. At physiologic pH, anions with pKa values < 4.0 including lactate, sulfate, and β-hydroxybutyrate also exist as strong ions. Strong cations predominate in the body leading to a net positive plasma charge that is described as the SID by the following formula:

$$SID\ (\sim^{+}40) = [Na^+ + K^+ + Ca^{2+} + Mg^{2+}] - [Cl^- + lactate^-]$$

This net positive charge must be counterbalanced with an equal negative charge to satisfy the Law of Electrical Neutrality.

The balancing negative charge derives from nonvolatile weak acids accounted for as A_{tot}. In plasma, these weak acids include albumin and inorganic phosphates. While the same is true of interstitial fluid, total concentrations in this compartment are very small. On the other hand, the predominant source of such acids in red cells is hemoglobin.

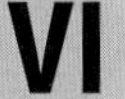

Non-volatile weak acids dissociate in body fluids as follows:

$$A_{tot} \leftrightarrow A^- + AH$$

A_{tot} reflects this dynamic equilibrium and provides the second independent control mechanism for pH as well, as approximately -40 mEq/l of anionic charge to maintain electrical neutrality. The vast majority of this charge stems from albumin and phosphate in patients without organ failure. Sulfates, β-hydroxybutyrate, and other anionic entities may contribute in those with organ failure.

Finally, the partial pressure of CO_2 (PCO_2) is a direct measure of blood-dissolved CO_2 versus pulmonary CO_2 clearance efficiency. The arterial PCO_2 ($PaCO_2$) is, therefore, an equilibrium value determined by the balance between CO_2 production (~15,000 mmol/day) and pulmonary CO_2 elimination (ventilation). In areas where PCO_2 is less directly controlled by alveolar ventilation (e.g., venous blood and interstitial fluid during low flow states), the total CO_2 concentration (TCO_2) becomes a significant independent variable [11]. The relative charge balance between SID and A_{tot} determines the direction of the following equation, which describes water dissociation in human plasma:

$$CO_2 + H_2O \leftrightarrow H_2CO_3 \leftrightarrow H^+ + HCO_3^-$$

Other nomenclatures that need to be recognized and understood are as follows:

- The *apparent* strong ion difference (SIDa) is the difference between the sums of *all* measured cations and strong anions.
- The *effective* strong ion difference (SIDe), on the other hand, represents the effect of the corrected PCO_2 and the non-volatile weak acids on the balance of electrical charges in plasma.
- The difference between the calculated SIDa and SIDe defines the strong ion gap (SIG). The calculated SIG is, therefore, an estimation of the *actual* SIG as only the most abundant ions are measured and used for its calculation.

In healthy humans, the SIG should equal zero, although ranges of ± 2 have been reported in healthy volunteers as well as hospitalized patients without critical illness [12, 13]. Increases or decreases in SIG occur with critical illness as well as with plasma volume expansion [12, 14]. For instance, an increased SIG, defined as > 2 mEq/l, indicates the accumulation of unmeasured anions in blood as a cause of acidosis [15]. A strong correlation between the SIG and the albumin- and lactate-corrected anion gap

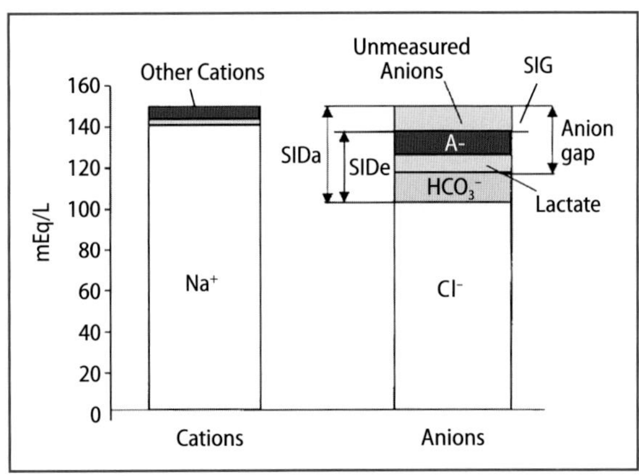

Fig. 1. Charge balance in blood plasma. "Other cations" include Ca^{++} and Mg^{++}. The strong ion difference (SID) is always positive (in plasma) and SID–SIDe (effective) should equal zero. Any difference between SIDe and apparent SID (SIDa) is the strong ion gap (SIG) and presents unmeasured anions. A- is the dissociated weak acids (mostly albumin and phosphates). From [55] with permission

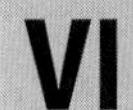

has been demonstrated [16]. It is unclear what species contribute to SIG elevation or depression and these species are therefore termed 'unmeasured ions' (**Fig. 1**).

Understanding the principles that govern the three independent pH control mechanisms allows one to explore how different fluids generate hyperchloremic metabolic acidosis.

Effects of Plasma Volume Expansion on pH

Commonly utilized fluids for plasma volume expansion are either absolutely or relatively hyperchloremic with regard to human plasma (**Table 1**). For instance, 0.9 % saline solution has 154 mEq/l of both sodium (Na^+) and chloride (Cl^-). This generates a SIDa of zero for saline. While the Na^+ is higher than plasma, the Cl^- is markedly higher, making saline absolutely hyperchloremic with regard to plasma. Lactated Ringer's solution has 130 mEq/l of Na^+ and 110 mEq/l of Cl^-. The Na^+ is below that of plasma while Cl^- is at the upper limit of many laboratory reference ranges. Thus, lactated Ringer's solution is relatively hyperchloremic since the Na^+ is much lower than normal. Delivering both of these fluids should predictably increase plasma Cl^- concentrations.

The net effect of hyperchloremia may be most easily understood by evaluating its impact on SIDa. As Cl^- concentration increases, the net positive charge of the SIDa diminishes. As a result, compensatory mechanisms designed to preserve plasma

Table 1. Composition of common crystalloids

	Na^+ (mEq/l)	K^+ (mEq/l)	HCO_3^- (mEq/l)	Cl^- (mEq/l)	Ca^{2+} (mEq/l)
0.9 % sodium chloride (normal saline)	154	–	–	154	–
0.45 % sodium chloride (half-strength normal saline)	77	–	–	77	–
Hartmann's solution	131	5	29	111	2
Lactated Ringer's solution	130	4	28	109	2.7

electrical neutrality act to increase the plasma positive charge. Humans are 55 molar with respect to water, providing a readily available and exchangeable pool of protons. By driving the following equation to the right, plasma positive charge increases as a result of increased proton concentration that one clinically detects as a diminished pH.

$$CO_2 + H_2O \leftrightarrow H_2CO_3 \leftrightarrow H^+ + HCO_3^-$$

Other compensation mechanisms similarly act to decrease the plasma negative charge, minimizing the absolute increase in proton concentration (and decreased pH) required to restore electrical neutrality. According to the Law of Conservation of Mass, the most readily available pool of negative charge that may be consumed to change the attributable charge is albumin; approximately 78 % of the negative charge stems from exposed histidine residues [17]. Thus, the decrease in albumin observed with plasma volume expansion, which is often attributed to simple dilution, truly reflects albumin consumption to decrease plasma negative charge. Moreover, since phosphate exists in small concentration in plasma, renal excretion as well as bone uptake will serve to decrease the negative charge of SIDe as well

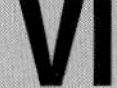

Thus, the genesis of hyperchloremic metabolic acidosis is readily understood based on changes in plasma charge as a result of electrolyte derangements, not just simple dilution. An in-depth analysis of the various permutations of pH derangements has been published previously [18]. The previously unanswered question is whether the decreased pH derived from hyperchloremia is clinically relevant or just an unimportant laboratory curiosity. Several lines of evidence highlight hyperchloremic metabolic acidosis as a clinically relevant entity that deserves therapeutic abrogation and, perhaps more importantly, conscious avoidance.

Clinical Consequences of Hyperchloremic Metabolic Acidosis

The clinical consequences of hyperchloremic metabolic acidosis may be conveniently grouped into several discrete domains, including fluid resuscitation and electrolyte manipulation, pulmonary compensation, ALI, coagulation cascade, microvascular flow, and immune activation or suppression. Exploring the data underpinning each of these areas will highlight the clinical relevance of hyperchloremic metabolic acidosis and the attendant therapeutic interventions available to the intensivist.

Fluid Resuscitation and Electrolyte Manipulation

It is clear that well-intentioned plasma volume expansion with sufficient volume of hyperchloremic solutions will lead to hyperchloremic metabolic acidosis. However, recognition of acidosis in the early phase of critical illness or injury often incorporates arterial blood gas analysis, or increasingly, venous blood gas analysis with some manipulation to correct for the expected increase in venous PCO_2 compared to the arterial side. These analyses are often accompanied by a lactate level, further enabling acid-base analysis. Later, especially for patients in the intensive care unit (ICU), arterial access is limited, and acid-base analysis hinges on the relationship between bicarbonate and standard base excess (SBE).

Metabolic acid-base disturbances arise from abnormalities in SID, A_{tot}, or both. Of note, neither SID nor A_{tot} need to be measured independently to quantify the metabolic acid-base status at the bedside: The SBE was developed to specifically address this situation [13, 14, 19, 20]. The SBE is calculated from buffer base offsets by assuming a mean extracellular hemoglobin concentration of 50 g/l and relies on the measured plasma bicarbonate level to arrive at its value according to the following formula:

$$SBE = 0.93 \times \{[HCO_3^-] + 14.84 \times (pH - 7.4) - 24.4\}$$

A standard reference range for SBE is ± 3.0 mEq/l. The range around zero reflects the change in extracellular SID needed to normalize metabolic acid-base status without changing A_{tot}. A negative deviation exceeding –3.0 mEq/l reflects the increase in extracellular SID needed to correct an existing metabolic acidosis. Likewise, if the SBE is greater than +3.0 mEq/l, a metabolic alkalosis exists and the positive deviation from zero represents the extracellular SID needed to correct this.

Given the reliance of the SBE on the measured plasma bicarbonate level, and understanding that bicarbonate is a dependent variable, hyperchloremic metabolic acidosis will necessarily decrease the plasma bicarbonate and, therefore, the SBE. If this relationship is not appreciated, a decreased bicarbonate and SBE may be misinterpreted for acidosis related to hypoperfusion [21]. Paradoxically, the prescription (plasma volume expansion) may worsen the underlying problem (acidosis) by further worsening hyperchloremia.

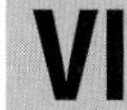

The clinician has several options open to correct a pre-existing hyperchloremic metabolic acidosis, usually related to plasma volume expansion. Since the underlying mechanism is providing a chloride excess (relative to sodium), providing fluids that are hypochloremic with regard to plasma creates a simply applied repair strategy. The authors employ the following fluids to achieve this goal:

- Maintenance*:* 5 % dextrose in water + 75 mEq/l $NaHCO_3$ at a body weight calculated rate
- Plasma volume expansion*:* half strength normal saline solution + 75 mEq/l $NaHCO_3$ provided at bolus fluid volumes.

Colloids are also used as another mechanism to decrease total chloride loading. Since the authors are constrained to use US Food and Drug Administration (FDA) approved plasma volume expanders, Hextend (6 % hydroxyethyl starch [HES] in a balanced salt solution; Hospira; Abbott Park, IL) is the fluid of choice as albumin is suspended in saline. Hextend is suspended in a less hyperchloremic solution (Cl^- = 120 mEq/l) than is 5 % albumin (Cl^- = 154 mEq/l).

Pulmonary Compensation/Acute Lung Injury

The most critically ill patients often require massive plasma volume expansion, especially in the current era heralded in by the sentinel early goal-directed therapy study in 2001 [22]. An emergency department study interrogating the interplay of plasma volume expansion and the onset of ALI for patients with non-pulmonary injury delineated a strong correlation between the post-resuscitation base deficit (more strongly than fluid volume or injury severity score [ISS]) and the likelihood of developing ALI [23]. Patients who developed ALI received approximately four additional liters of plasma volume expansion compared to those who did not. Those additional four liters of plasma volume expansion translated into a lower pH and a greater base deficit (SBE) that was judged to be due to hyperchloremic metabolic acidosis as lactate levels and organ failures were similar on arrival in the emergency room.

The juxtaposition of ALI and massive plasma volume expansion (with or without blood component transfusion) creates a vast potential for ventilator-induced lung injury (VILI). Since critical illness and injury commonly create a capillary leak syndrome, extravascular lung water accumulation is predictable, and contributes markedly to decreased compliance. As the pulmonary compensation for acute acidosis is an increased minute ventilation to deliberately decrease PCO_2 and increase pH, this strategy carries a significant risk of accelerated intra-tidal shear and biotrauma due to an increased frequency of gas exchange through swollen, narrowed airways and partly collapsed alveolar units [24, 25].

Furthermore, acidosis interacts with the inducible nitric oxide (NO) synthase (iNOS) enzyme pathway according to a rat model of pulmonary epithelium. Overactivity of iNOS can lead to peroxynitrite-induced protein destruction and provide an apototic trigger for endothelial cells. Rat lung function was assessed at two different pHs (7.36 and 7.14) [26]; acidotic rats demonstrated increased iNOS activity as well as lower PO_2 levels in the absence of another cause for ALI. Of note, interleukin (IL)-6 levels were also markedly increased in acidotic rats compared to their normal pH counterparts. Thus, acidosis of any cause impairs pulmonary function on multiple levels, providing a strong impetus for pH correction and avoidance of iatrogenically induced acidosis.

Coagulation Cascade

The 'lethal triad' of hypothermia, acidosis and coagulopathy is well described following injury [27]. The interplay of acidosis and coagulopathy is less well described, and often these entities are thought of as accompanying each other rather than having a causal relationship. Recall that the clotting cascade relies on both platelet conformational changes as well as the activity of serine proteases. As proteases, the clotting factors have pH optima and enzyme kinetics that are impaired by both acidosis and hypothermia [28, 29]. Since the dominant fluid utilized in conjunction with blood component therapy infusion is saline, careful attention should be paid to avoiding hyperchloremic metabolic acidosis in that setting. Clearly, relatively small volumes (< 2000 ml) will have little impact on pH. However, patients with exsanguinating hemorrhage often receive plasma volume expansion with large volumes of crystalloid fluids in addition to massive transfusion of blood component elements.

While enhanced survival is reported with massive transfusion protocol activation following near-exsanguination after injury, recent attention has focused on the ratio of packed red blood cells (RBCs) to units of fresh frozen plasma (FFP) citing improved survival with a 1:1 ratio [30]. While blood components generally have normal electrolytes, these components are transfused into patients who have already undergone plasma volume expansion with dilution of clotting cascade elements in the setting of lactic acidosis that is compounded by an iatrogenic hyperchloremic metabolic acidosis. Thus, avoiding hyperchloremic metabolic acidosis is an intelligent means of supporting the activity of the clotting cascade, which is already impaired from hypoperfusion-associated acidosis and further crippled by hypothermia [31].

A provocative operating room study assessed patients undergoing open abdominal aortic aneurysm repair as a model for large volume blood loss and resuscitation [32]. Patients were resuscitated intra-operatively with either saline or lactated Ringer's solution according to a pre-established protocol. The saline resuscitated patients demonstrated the predicted acidosis, received sodium bicarbonate infusion to correct the acidosis, and evidenced greater cell saver volumes of shed blood and required greater amounts of packed RBC, FFP, and platelet transfusion. The increased resource utilization and allogeneic exposure was linked to the induced acidosis in this study.

Microvascular Flow

While tremendous effort has been devoted to measuring and supporting cardiac performance as a means of providing oxygen delivery to support oxygen utilization, less effort is devoted to measuring microvascular flow at the organ level. Several studies have investigated microvascular flow in the buccal mucosa, and skeletal muscle domains [33–35].

Two important studies bear directly on this topic with regard to acidosis. The first study evaluated deltoid tissue oxygen by means of an implanted probe pre-, intra-, and post-operatively for the 1st 24 hours after elective major surgery [36]. Two groups were created based on the fluid choice for plasma volume expansion – one group received lactated Ringer's solution and one received a low molecular weight (130 kDa) and degree of molar substitution (0.4) HES. Resuscitation was performed according to a protocol including blood transfusion for hemoglobin concentration < 8 g/dl. While no demographic or care differences were noted between the groups, the deltoid tissue PO_2 was markedly decreased in the crystalloid group and enhanced in the colloid group by the end of surgery and was more pronounced by the following morning. The explanation for this observation stems from the second study.

Normal human RBC were assessed in media of different pH and queried for RBC volume and viscosity at low and high flow rates [37]. Importantly, acidosis predictably increased RBC volume by ~7 % (as assessed by hematocrit) – an effect that was reversed by acidosis abrogation with NaOH, akin to correction of pH with $NaHCO_3$ in the clinical circumstance. It is currently unclear whether the RBC volume increase is sufficient to impair spectrin function in supporting RBC rheology, but merits further investigation [38, 39]. Moreover, acidosis also resulted in an increase in viscosity at both low and high flow rates. These data support the need to correct hyperchloremic metabolic acidosis, and indeed any acidosis, as a means of supporting microvascular flow. Moreover, these data may provide an explanation for the 'no-reflow' phenomenon identified after tissue ischemia and oxygenated reperfusion.

The no-reflow phenomenon was comfortably attributed to lipid peroxidation and endothelial dysfunction as a result of toxic oxygen metabolites during oxygenated reperfusion of previously dysoxic tissue beds [40, 41]. However, it is important to recall that these beds are also vasodilated and acidic from anaerobic metabolism with high regional lactate concentrations [42]. Flow resumption directs RBCs into a zone of significant acidosis, which in turn leads to RBC swelling. If swollen RBCs are delivered to capillary beds that are in tissue beds swollen from edema accrued during plasma volume expansion, the capillary cross-sectional diameter may be narrowed leading to RBC sludging, capillary obstruction and rouleaux formation [43]. This hypothetical scheme is plausible based upon the above physiology, and would also help understand how restoration of systemic oxygen delivery may not meet oxygen utilization during the reperfusion phase after significant hypoperfusion [44, 45]. Hyperchloremic metabolic acidosis may also impair hemoglobin's ability to transport and unload oxygen at the tissue level as a result of the Haldane effect.

Initially articulated in 1914, the Haldane effect relates the interplay of hemoglobin with oxygen, chloride, and protons [46]. The Haldane effect hinges on the premise that the reduced (deoxygenated) form of hemoglobin is a better proton acceptor than the oxidized (oxygenated) form. Le Chatelier's principle is described by the following equation:

$$CO_2 + H_2O \rightarrow H_2CO_3 \rightarrow H^+ + HCO_3^-$$

Accordingly, it is apparent that deoxygenated hemoglobin will drive the reaction to the right as a result of the Law of Mass Action. Therefore, the enhanced affinity of deoxyhemoglobin for protons enhances the synthesis of bicarbonate, which is the major transport form that CO_2 assumes in blood. In essence, more HCO_3^- is carried in the RBC interior than would otherwise be possible, and consequently more H^+ binds to hemoglobin. Conversely, the Haldane effect promotes the dissociation of CO_2 from hemoglobin in the presence of oxygen. Thus, the summative equation for the Haldane effect may be best summarized as:

$$H^+ + HbO_2 \longleftrightarrow H^+ Hb + O_2$$

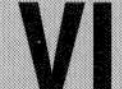

It has been demonstrated that the reversible binding of chloride to hemoglobin in deoxygenated blood occurs at those sites that have been newly protonated by the Haldane effect [47]. Accordingly, the converse may also be true: Cl^- binding enhances the Haldane effect, as Cl^- binding electrostatically stabilizes the deoxygenated state (with the effect that Cl^- decreases hemoglobin's oxygen affinity). Thus, hyperchloremic meta bolic acidosis may impair tissue level oxygen delivery by stabilizing hemoglobin in the deoxygenated state while enhancing hemoglobin's CO_2 transport ability [48].

Immune Activation or Suppression

Fluid resuscitation strategies have employed several different regimens spanning crystalloids and colloids including albumin, starches of different molecular weights and degrees of molar substitution as well as dextrans. When incubating human polymorphonuclear leukocytes (PMNs) with each of these different solutions, the most potent trigger of oxidative burst activity is crystalloids [49]. Thus, it would appear that standard US resuscitation strategies prime human neutrophils for immune activation and inflammation.

A rat cecal ligation and puncture model of intra-abdominal sepsis explored the immune activating effects of deliberate acidosis induction using a 0.1N HCl solution [50]. The more negative the SBE, the lower the achieved mean arterial pressure (MAP). Nitrite levels peaked in the group with SBE of -5 to -10 mEq/l and then decreased with progressive acid load. A separate study tied NO activity to lipopolysaccharide (LPS) stimulation as a necessary component to increase nitrite production in a RAW cell model [51]. In this model, NO production was maximal at a pH of 7.0 and then declined at a pH of 6.5, perhaps reflecting enzymatic derangements with progressive acidosis. Similar pH-linked effects were noted for IL-6 and IL-10 release in this model as well. However, when assessing the IL-6:IL-10 ratio as a measure of the intensity of inflammatory to anti-inflammatory influences, maximal pro-inflammatory activity was noted at the lowest pH range (6.5). These data support the notion that acidosis progressively and independently increases inflammation. The clinically relevant corollary is that acidosis merits correction as a means of potentially reducing inflammatory stimuli in an integrated approach to managing patients with severe sepsis and septic shock.

Nuclear factor-kappa B (NF-κB) activity has been hailed as a means of assessing subcellular triggering along inflammatory pathways. Similar to the IL-6:IL-10 ratio,

LPS-stimulated cells demonstrate enhanced NF-κB activity compared to unstimulated cells. Curiously, all acidoses do not appear similar with regard to immunomodulation (in this model). While a general pattern of decreased activity or production in a wide variety of inflammatory markers was demonstrated for decreased pH ranges from the addition of lactic acid to the media, a different pattern was observed when pH was decreased using HCl. In particular, increased NO activity and iNOS mRNA were noted with HCl (similar to hyperchloremic metabolic acidosis) while these were decreased at identically decreased pH ranges due to lactic acid.

Survival

Whether hyperchloremic metabolic acidosis impacts survival in an independent fashion has been assessed in a variety of pre-clinical and clinical studies. Using an *Escherichia coli* LPS (endotoxin) infusion sepsis model, rats were resuscitated with either saline, lactated Ringer's solution or Hextend to identical pre-determined goals. Predictable and anticipated changes in SID as a result of chloride loading were noted in the saline animals with concomitant decreased SBE and pH (i.e., hyperchloremic metabolic acidosis) [52]. Mean survival time inversely correlated with the absolute increase in Cl^- concentration and was, therefore, significantly reduced for the saline resuscitated animals compared to those resuscitated with Hextend (lowest total chloride delivery group).

VI

Lactic acid represents a readily measurable metabolic acid the absolute value of which as well as its trend over time has been utilized to predict outcome after injury [6, 53]. In a recent retrospective study of overall hospital mortality, lactic acidosis portended the worst prognosis (mortality rate = 56 %) compared to other forms of acidosis [54]. In this study, acidosis derived from unmeasured ions (i.e., SIG-associated) accrued a 39 % mortality rate, while that attributable to hyperchloremic metabolic acidosis was 29 % (**Fig. 2**). It is important to note that patients without acidosis who required critical care had a 26 % mortality rate.

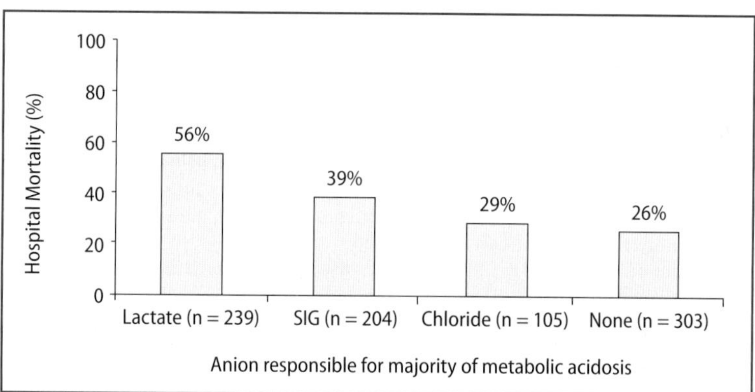

Fig. 2. Mortality associated with the major ion contributing to the metabolic acidosis [54]. Hospital mortality associated with the various etiologies of metabolic acidosis (standard base excess (SBE) < –2). Mortality percentage is mortality within each subgroup, not a percentage of overall mortality. 'Lactate' indicates that lactate contributes to at least 50 % of the SBE; 'SIG', SIG contributes to at least 50 % of SBE (and not lactate); 'hyperchloremic', absence of lactate or SIG acidosis and SBE < –2; 'none', no metabolic acidosis (SBE ≥ –2 mEq/l). SIG, strong ion gap. p < 0.001 for the four-group comparison.

Conclusion

It is increasingly clear that plasma volume expansion in sufficient quantity to alter plasma electrolyte concentrations may significantly impact plasma acid-base balance. As evidence mounts that iatrogenically driven electrolyte abnormalities create deleterious effects on diverse systems, it becomes increasingly incumbent upon the practitioner to regard plasma volume expanders as medications instead of as expected commensals of care. This chapter has explored how hyperchloremic metabolic acidosis influences the pulmonary system, coagulation, immune activation, and survival. Insufficiently explored aspects of electrolytically driven acidosis and immune activation includes how fluid selection drives unmeasured ion genesis and how those species influence survival [12, 14]. Early data suggest a negative impact upon survival, but longitudinal study is required. At present, the clinician can understand how hyperchloremic metabolic acidosis is generated, repair strategies once hyperchloremic metabolic acidosis is established, and the deleterious consequences of leaving hyperchloremic metabolic acidosis unrepaired.

References

1. Maerz L, Kaplan LJ (2008) Abdominal compartment syndrome. Crit Care Med 36 (Suppl 4): S212–215
2. Cope DK, Grimbert F, Downey JM, Taylor AE (1992) Pulmonary capillary pressure: a review. Crit Care Med 20: 1043–1056
3. Kalra PR, Anagnostopoulos C, Bolger AP, Coats AJ, Anker SD (2002)The regulation and measurement of plasma volume in heart failure. J Am Coll Cardiol 39: 1901–1908
4. Scheingraber S, Rehm M, Sehmisch C, Finsterer U (1999) Rapid saline infusion produces hyperchloremic acidosis in patients undergoing gynecologic surgery. Anesthesiology 90: 1265–1270
5. Healey MA, Davis RE, Liu FC, Loomis WH, Hoyt DB (1998) Lactated ringer's is superior to normal saline in a model of massive hemorrhage and resuscitation. J Trauma 45: 894–899
6. Kaplan LJ, Bailey H, Kellum JA (1999) The etiology and significance of metabolic acidosis in trauma patients. Curr Opin Crit Care 5: 458–463
7. Stewart PA (1981) How to Understand Acid-base. A Quantitative Acid-base Primer for Biology and Medicine. Elsevier, New York
8. Stewart PA (1983) Modern quantitative acid-base chemistry. Can J Physiol Pharmacol 61: 1444–1461
9. Kellum JA (2000) Determinants of blood pH in health and disease. Crit Care 4: 6–14
10. Wooten EW (2004) Science review: Quantitative acid-base physiology using the Stewart model. Crit Care 8: 448–452
11. Morgan TJ (2005) Clinical review: The meaning of acid-base abnormalities in the intensive care unit- effects of fluid administration. Crit Care 9: 204–211
12. Kaplan LJ, Kellum JA (2008) Comparison of acid-base models for prediction of hospital mortality after trauma. Shock 29: 662–666
13. Kellum JA, Pinsky MR (2002) Use of vasopressor agents in critically ill patients. Curr Opin Crit Care 8: 236–241
14. Kaplan LJ, Philbin N, Arnaud F, Rice J, Dong F, Freilich D (2006) Resuscitation from hemorrhagic shock: fluid selection and infusion strategy drives unmeasured ion genesis. J Trauma 61: 90–97
15. Kellum JA (2003) Closing the gap on unmeasured anions. Crit Care 7: 219–220
16. Moviat M, van Haren F, van der Hoeven H (2003) Conventional or pysiochemical approach in intensive care unit patients with meatabolic acidosis. Crit Care 7:R41-R45
17. Kellum JA, Kramer DJ, Pinsky MR (1995) Strong ion gap: a methodology for exploring unexplained anions. J Crit Care 10: 51–55
18. Kaplan LK, Kellum JA (2007) Acid-base disorders. In: Wilson W, Grande CM, Hoyt DB. Anesthesia, Trauma, and Intensive Care, 1st Edition. Informa Healthcare, New York, pp 793–810

19. Siggaard-Andersen O (1977) The Van Slyke equation. Scand J Clin Lab Invest Suppl 146: 15–20
20. Siggaard-Andersen O, Fogh-Andersen N (1995) Base excess or buffer base (strong ion difference) as measure of a non-respiratory acid-base disturbance. Acta Anesth Scand Suppl 107: 123–128
21. Brill SA, Stewart TR, Brundage SI, Schreiber MA (2002) Base deficit does not predict mortality when secondary to hyperchloremic acidosis. Shock 17: 459–462
22. Rivers E, Nguyen B, Havstad S, et al (2001) Early goal-directed therapy in the treatment of severe sepsis and septic shock. N Engl J Med 345: 1368–1377
23. Eberhard LW, Morabito DJ, Matthay MA, et al (2000) Initial severity of metabolic acidosis predicts the development of acute lung injury in severely traumatized patients. Crit Care Med 28: 125–131
24. dos Santos CC, Slutsky AS (2006) The contribution of biophysical lung injury to the development of biotrauma. Annu Rev Physiol 68: 585–618
25. Habashi NM (2005) Other approaches to open-lung ventilation: airway pressure release ventilation. Crit Care Med 33 (Suppl 3):S228–240
26. Haque IU, Huang CJ, Scumpia PO, Nasiroglu O, Skimming JW (2003) Intravascular infusion of acid promotes intrapulmonary inducible nitric oxide synthase activity and impairs blood oxygenation in rats. Crit Care Med 31: 1454–1460
27. Eddy VA, Morris JA Jr, Cullinane DC (2000) Hypothermia, coagulopathy, and acidosis. Surg Clin North Am 80: 845–854
28. Schreiber MA (2005) Coagulopathy in the trauma patient. Curr Opin Crit Care 11: 590–597
29. Martini WZ, Pusateri AE, Uscilowicz JM, Delgado AV, Holcomb JB (2005) Independent contributions of hypothermia and acidosis to coagulopathy in swine. J Trauma 58: 1002–1009
30. Holcomb JB, Jenkins D, Rhee P, et al (2007) Damage control resuscitation: directly addressing the early coagulopathy of trauma. J Trauma 62: 307–310
31. Johnston TD, Chen Y, Reed RL 2nd (1994) Functional equivalence of hypothermia to specific clotting factor deficiencies. J Trauma 37: 413–417
32. Waters JH, Gottlieb A, Schoenwald P, Popovich MJ, Sprung J, Nelson DR (2001) Normal saline versus lactated Ringer's solution for intraoperative fluid management in patients undergoing abdominal aortic aneurysm repair: an outcome study. Anesth Analg 93: 817–822
33. Cammarata GA, Weil MH, Castillo CJ, et al (2009) Buccal capnometry for quantitating the severity of hemorrhagic shock. Shock (in press)
34. Povoas HP, Weil MH, Tang W, Moran B, Kamohara T, Bisera J (2000) Comparisons between sublingual and gastric tonometry during hemorrhagic shock. Chest 118: 1127–1132
35. Weil MH, Nakagawa Y, Tang W, et al (1999) Sublingual capnometry: a new noninvasive measurement for diagnosis and quantitation of severity of circulatory shock. Crit Care Med 27: 1225–1229
36. Lang K, Boldt J, Suttner S, Haisch G (2001) Colloids versus crystalloids and tissue oxygen tension in patients undergoing major abdominal surgery. Anesth Analg 93: 405–409
37. Reinhart WH, Gaudenz R, Walter R (2002) Acidosis induced by lactate, pyruvate, or HCl increases blood viscosity. J Crit Care 17: 68–73
38. Hansen J, Skalak R, Chien S, Hoger A (1997) Spectrin properties and the elasticity of the red blood cell membrane skeleton. Biorheology 34: 327–348
39. Li J, Lykotrafitis G, Dao M, Suresh S (2007) Cytoskeletal dynamics of human erythrocyte. Proc Natl Acad Sci USA 104: 4937–4942
40. Kaplan LJ, Bellows CF, Blum H, Mitchell M, Whitman GJ (1994) Ischemic preconditioning preserves end-ischemic ATP, enhancing functional recovery and coronary flow during reperfusion. J Surg Res 57: 179–184
41. Kaplan LJ, Blum H, Bellows CF, Banerjee A, Whitman GJ (1996) Reversible injury: creatinine kinase recovery restores bioenergetics and function. J Surg Res 62: 103–108
42. Seal JB, Gewertz BL (2005) Vascular dysfunction in ischemia-reperfusion injury. Ann Vasc Surg 19: 572–584
43. Cicha I, Suzuki Y, Tateishi N, Maeda N (2003) Changes of RBC aggregation in oxygenation-deoxygenation: pH dependency and cell morphology. Am J Physiol Heart Circ Physiol 284: H2335–2342
44. Chiara O, Pelosi P, Segala M, et al (2001) Mesenteric and renal oxygen transport during hemorrhage and reperfusion: evaluation of optimal goals for resuscitation. J Trauma 51: 356–362

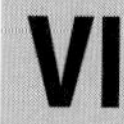

45. Kaplan LJ, Bellows CF, Carter S, Blum H, Whitman GJ (1995) The phosphocreatine overshoot occurs independent of myocardial work. Biochimie 77: 245–248
46. Benesch RE, Rubin H (1975) Interaction of hemoglobin with three ligans: organic phosphates and the Bohr effect. Proc Natl Acad Sci USA 72: 2465–2467
47. Giovannini I, Chiarla C, Boldrini G, Terzi R (1999) Quantitative assessment of changes in blood CO(2) tension mediated by the haldane effect. J Appl Physiol 87: 862–866
48. Prange HD, Schumaker Jr JL, Westen EA, Horstkotte DG, Pinshow B (2001) Physiological consequences of oxygen-dependent chloride binding to hemoglobin. J Appl Physiol 91: 33–38
49. Rhee P, Wang D, Ruff P, et al (2000) Human neutrophil activation and increased adhesion by various resuscitation fluids. Crit Care Med 28: 74–78
50. Kellum JA, Song M, Venkataraman R (2004) Effects of hyperchloremic acidosis on arterial pressure and circulating inflammatory molecules in experimental sepsis. Chest 125: 243–248
51. Kellum JA, Song M, Li J (2004) Lactic and hydrochloric acids induce different patterns of inflammatory response in LPS-stimulated RAW 264.7 cells. Am J Physiol Regul Integr Comp Physiol 286:R686–692
52. Kellum JA (2002) Fluid resuscitation and hyperchloremic acidosis in experimental sepsis: improved short-term survival and acid-base balance with Hextend compared with saline. Crit Care Med 30: 300–305
53. Abramson D, Scalea TM, Hitchcock R, Trooskin SZ, Henry SM, Greenspan J (1993) Lactate clearance and survival following injury. J Trauma 35: 584–589
54. Gunnerson KJ, Saul M, He S, Kellum JA (2006) Lactate versus non-lactate metabolic acidosis: a retrospective outcome evaluation of critically ill patients. Crit Care 10:R22
55. Gunnerson KJ, Kaplan JA (2003) Acid-base and electrolyte analysis in critically ill patients: are we ready for the new millennium? Curr Opin Crit Care 9: 468–473

Old versus New Starches: What do We Know about their Differences?

C. Hartog, F.M. Brunkhorst, and K. Reinhart

Introduction

Fluid therapy is the mainstay of critical care with the goal of restoring the circulating intravascular volume, maintaining organ perfusion, and reestablishing the balance between oxygen demand and delivery. Colloids are used as plasma expanders on the grounds that these macromolecules remain in the vasculature longer than crystalloids and, therefore, increase cardiac preload with less fluid needed than crystalloids. Hydroxyethyl starches (HES) are synthetic colloids which are popular plasma expanders in Europe [1–3]. However, evidence is accumulating that HES administration has adverse effects on kidney function, coagulation, and even may increase mortality in patients with severe sepsis [4–8]. Critics of these studies argue that outdated HES solutions were used and that 'new' HES solutions are safer and can be used without concern [9, 10]. HES 130/0.4 (tetrastarch) is the latest solution, available in Europe since 2000 and recently also in the US [11]. This chapter summarizes the evidence about the safety of 'old' and 'new' HES solutions.

Hydroxyethyl Starch Pharmacokinetics

HES solutions have been used in clinical practice since the 1970s. They are synthesized from plant starch and chemically modified by hydroxyethylation at the C2, C6, or C3 positions of the glucose molecules. The first number of the solution lists its molecular weight and the second the degree of substitution with hydroxyethyl moieties, e.g., 0.7 or 0.5. HES solutions can be classified according to high (450 kDA and above), medium (200–130 kDa), or low molecular weight (70 kDa or below) [12].

The pharmacokinetic properties of an HES solution are determined by its molecular weight, its molar substitution, and the substitution pattern or C2/C6 ratio (**Table 1**).

Table 1. Pharmacodynamics of different hydroxyethyl starch (HES) solutions

	Generation	Eponym	Molecular weight	Degree of substitution	Plasma clearance
HES 450/0.7 or 670/0.75[1]	'old'	Hetastarch	high	high	slow
HES 200/0.62	'old'	Hexastarch	medium	high	slow
HES 200/0.5	'old'	Pentastarch	medium	medium	medium
HES 70/0.5	'old'	Pentastarch	low	medium	medium
HES 130/0.4	'new'	Tetrastarch	medium	low	high

[1] HES 450/0.7 was relabeled 670/0.75 after revision of *in vivo* molecular weight

High molar substitution and high C2/C6 ratio decrease the intravascular hydrolysis of HES by α-amylase. HES molecules which pass the renal threshold (45 to 60 kDa) are mainly eliminated via glomerular filtration, but larger particles are phagocytosed and can be found in almost all organs of the body [13].

'New' HES 130/0.4 is of medium molecular weight with a low degree of substitution and high plasma clearance, which in volunteers was about 6-fold higher than that after HES 200/0.5 [11]. Hence, it is argued that HES 130/0.4 is associated with considerably fewer side effects than older HES. However, little is known about the metabolism of 'old' or 'new' HES solutions in critically ill patients with endothelial barrier dysfunction.

Volume Effects

Due to their intravascular persistence, HES solutions have a volume effect around 100 %. In a study of 10 patients undergoing acute normovolemic hemodilution before gynecological surgery, determination of plasma volume by the indocyanine green (ICG) dilution technique found that HES 130/0.4 had a volume effect of 102 ± 5 % [14]. Several clinical studies in the perioperative setting support the finding that the volume effects of HES 130/0.4 are comparable to HES 670/0.75 as well as HES 200/0.5 [15, 16].

Recent approval for HES 130/0.4 by the Food and Drug Administration (FDA), with publicly available documentation [11], was made on the basis of 21 clinical studies which were mostly non-inferiority studies with comparators HES 200 and HES 450 (hetastarch). The FDA concluded that "compared to hetastarch, 6 % HES 130/0.4 is just as effective in expanding plasma volume but is associated with fewer bleeding events and a lower incidence of (a) SAEs [serious adverse events] in the aggregate [i.e., the clinical trial roster provided by the manufacturer], (b) AEs of severe intensity (especially in the 65–75 and > 75 years old cohorts), and (c) AEs of the CNS, respiratory, and renal systems" [11].

However, it is disturbing that the issue of HES toxicity was not fully addressed. In the Pharmacology/Toxicology Review Memorandum included in the FDA approval material, the necessity for specific secondary safety pharmacology studies for HES 130/0.4 is waived on the grounds that both HES 200/0.5 and HES 450/0.7 have been used with relative safe clinical profiles. Surprisingly, the evidence for serious and long ranging adverse effects of 'older' HES products when used in higher cumulative doses over longer periods of time is not discussed [4–8, 17]. Although HES 130/0.4 is widely used in various clinical settings, there is unfortunately no clinical study in which HES 130/0.4 is used in higher cumulative doses and for longer periods of time.

The characteristics of the volume studies from which pooled analyses were derived are listed in Tables 2 a-c. They have several shortcomings: Short observation periods with a mean of 2 days, low cumulative doses less than the recommended daily dose limit, and mostly unsuitable comparators such as other HES solutions or the synthetic colloid gelatin, which have similar side effects (**Table 2a**). Mean duration of exposure was 9 hours [11]. In studies comparing HES 130/0.4 with other HES solutions, HES 130/0.4 was used in less amount in relation to the maximal daily dose limit (**Table 2b**). Furthermore, these trials included volunteers, low-risk non-surgical patients, and patients in whom HES was given for other indications such as hemodilution (**Table 2c**) but excluded patients with liver failure or dialysis-dependency.

Table 2 a–c. Methodological shortcomings of volume replacement studies submitted to the FDA for approval of hydroxyethyl starch (HES) 130/0.4 [11]

a Characteristics of volume studies

6 % HES 130/0.4	**N = 471**
Treatment days (mean ± SD)	2.0 (3.9 ± 3.3)
Cumulative dose (ml/kg body weight, mean ± SD)	41.9 (45.7 ± 47.8)
Percentage of recommended daily dose limit (50 ml/kg)	83.8 %
Comparators	**N = 547**
Other HES (6 % 200/0.5, 6 % 450/0.7)	328 (60.0 %)
Albumin	41 (7.5 %)
Crystalloids	56 (10.2 %)
Glucose	50 (9.1 %)

b Cumulative doses[1] in relation to daily dose limits

	6 % HES 130/0.4	6 % HES 200/0.5	6 % HES 450/0.7
Recommended daily dose limit	50 ml/kg	33 ml/kg	20 ml/kg
Cumulative dose in 2 studies (percentage of daily dose limit) N = 152	27 ml/kg (54 %)	27 ml/kg (81 %)	
Cumulative dose in 2 studies (percentage of daily dose limit) N = 159	12 ml/kg (24 %)		12 ml/kg (60 %)

[1] if not specified, cumulative dose was calculated by dividing the given mean total volume by 75 kg body weight

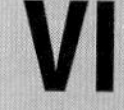

c Patient populations and indications

Population N (% of subjects)	HES 130/0.4 735 (100)	Comparator[1] 514 (100)
Volunteers, total	**67 (9)**	–
Non-surgical		
Stroke and brain injury	106 (14)	71 (14)
Sudden hearing loss	256 (34)	141 (28)
Total	362 (48)	212 (42)
Surgical		
Cardiac and major vascular surgery	87 (11)	86 (16)
Orthopedic surgery	127 (17)	125 (23)
Urologic surgery	20 (3)	20 (4)
Pediatric surgery	41 (5)	41 (8)
Cardiac and non-cardiac surgery	30 (4)	30 (5)
Total	306 (40)	302 (56)

[1] Including HES 200, 450, albumin, gelatin, normal saline

A diagnosis of renal and urinary disorders was uncommon. Exclusion criteria for many of these trials included a history of heart, liver, kidney, and severe infectious diseases, diabetes, and coagulation abnormalities [11].

It will be interesting to see the future results of post-marketing study commitments for HES 130/0.4 which are required by the FDA: "To perform a multiple-dose randomized controlled trial (RCT) to be conducted in subjects with severe sepsis including subjects with renal dysfunction and at risk for deterioration of renal dysfunction." [11].

Renal Effects

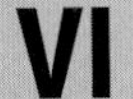

HES-induced effects on the kidney are deleterious and non-trivial and indicated by a growing body of evidence, initially in the form of observations and lately in randomized clinical trials. Following reports of renal failure in transplanted kidneys induced by HES administration to brain-dead donors [18], Schortgen et al. [4] conducted a prospective multicenter randomized study with 6 % HES 200/0.62 or 3 % modified gelatin in 129 patients with severe sepsis or septic shock. Acute renal failure, defined as a two-fold increase in serum creatinine from baseline or need for renal replacement therapy, occurred significantly more often in the HES group (27/65 [42 %] vs 15/64 [23 %], $p = 0.028$) and the use of HES constituted a risk factor for acute renal failure by multivariate analysis (odds ratio 2.57 [95 % CI 1.13–5.83], $p = 0.026$) [4]. Another multicenter study in 537 patients with severe sepsis (Efficacy of Volume Substitution and Insulin Therapy in Severe Sepsis, VISEP) by the German SepNet study group tested the hypothesis that resuscitation with 10 % HES 200/0.5 is superior to modified Ringer's lactate [7]. The investigators chose HES 200/0.5 which – at the time of study design – was considered to be a more modern solution with fewer nephrotoxic effects than HES 200/0.62 used by the French study group. However, the rate of acute renal failure was significantly higher after HES than after Ringer's lactate (34.9 % [95 % CI 29.1–40.7] vs 22.8 % [17.8–27.8]; $p < 0.002$). HES also increased the requirements for renal replacement therapy (31.0 % [25.4–36.7] vs 18.8 % [14.1–23.4]; $p < 0.001$). By post-hoc univariate analysis, the cumulative dose of HES (but not of Ringer's lactate) was directly associated with the need for renal-replacement therapy [7].

The VISEP study was criticized for using an 'old' HES solution. However, there is no evidence to support the claim that 'new' HES 130/0.4 is devoid of adverse renal effects in patients with sepsis. Plasma accumulation of HES 130/0.4 increases with severity of renal dysfunction in volunteers [19]. Most clinical studies on HES 130/0.4 that concluded a lack of negative renal effects were volume trials flawed by small sample size, too short observation periods, inadequate endpoints for renal dysfunction, and inadequate comparators [9, 11, 15, 20–23]. The adverse effects of HES are delayed and do not become apparent within a few hours or days. With observation periods of 5 days or less and creatinine serum levels as marker of renal dysfunction, neither the Schortgen [4] nor the VISEP [7] study would have revealed a higher incidence of renal failure after HES administration. Comparators such as other colloids or gelatins which themselves have adverse renal effects [24] should not be used.

Coagulation and Bleeding

The mechanisms by which HES impairs coagulation and increases bleeding are not fully understood. HES decreases factor VIII and von Willebrand factor, impairs platelet function, and leads to prolongation of partial prothrombin time and activated partial thromboplastin time (aPPT) [25]. The effects of HES on coagulation and fibrinolysis have also been studied using thromboelastography, suggesting prolonged clot formation time and increases in clot lysis after hemodilution with starch [26].

There is a large body of evidence that HES solutions are associated with severe bleeding events in susceptible patients. In patients with subarachnoid hemorrhage, HES 200/0.62 administration led to fatal cerebral hemorrhage and acquired von Willebrand's disease [6]. A recent prospective analysis of patients with subarachnoid hemorrhage showed that administration of the synthetic colloids, HES 200/0.5 (pentastarch) and 4 % gelatin, was associated with greater requirements for blood transfusion ($p = 0.003$) [27]. Patients with severe sepsis who were resuscitated with 10 % pentastarch had a significantly lower median platelet count and received more units of packed red cells than patients who had received Ringer's lactet (< 0.001) [7].

In the US, evidence for hetastarch-associated bleeding in comparison to albumin [5] led to withdrawal of approval for pump priming or volume expansion during cardiac surgery [28]. Of note, a meta-analysis of a total of 653 cardiac surgical patients showed that hetastarch (HES 450/0.7) and pentastarch (HES 200/0.5) had similar bleeding risks [5], suggesting that the impact of HES on coagulation in surgical patients may not only depend on different molecular weights or molar substitution.

VI

'New' HES 130/0.4 is suggested to have less negative effects on coagulation. Low cumulative doses of HES 130/0.4 as perioperative fluid therapy did not increase blood loss or transfusion of red blood cells (RBCs) compared to 5 % albumin in cardiac surgery [21] or compared to Ringer's or normal saline in abdominal surgery [29]. Higher cumulative doses (49 ml/kg) of HES 130/0.4 in cardiac surgery led to similar drainage losses, number of erythrocyte transfusions, and blood coagulation tests compared to HES 200/0.5. It is noteworthy that the HES 200/0.5 group had received three times as much additional gelatin as the HES 130/0.4 group [30]. Another perioperative study in cardiac surgery concluded that HES 130/0.4 was associated with less blood loss and less need for transfusion of RBCs than HES 200/0.5. However, administered total doses in relation to the upper daily dose limit were 62 % for HES 130/0.4 (31.0 ml/kg) but 93 % for HES 200/0.5 (30.6 ml/kg) and thus not comparable [15] (see **Table 2b** for recommended daily dose limits). In major orthopedic surgery, comparison of low cumulative doses of HES 130/0.4 with hetastarch did not result in significantly different estimated blood loss or need for allogeneic blood products, although there was a trend in favor of HES 130/0.4. Fewer patients given HES 130/0.4 than patients given hetastarch had factor VIII activity below the lower limit of normal at the end of surgery (5 vs. 13; $p < 0.031$) and 2 h after surgery (0 vs. 7; $p < 0.002$), but these analyses derived from post-hoc subgroups with a small sample size [16]. In a larger study with 100 patients undergoing orthopedic surgery and comparing low cumulative doses of HES 130/0.4 (22.2 ml/kg) to HES 200/0.5 (22 ml/kg), total blood loss at 5 hours after the end of surgery was similar, but factor VIII concentration was higher and partial thromboplastin time was lower ($p < 0.05$) in the HES 130/0.4 group [31]. HES 130/0.4 in a cumulative dose of 41 ml/kg compared to gelatin administration in cardiac surgery led to similar changes in thrombelastography data but patients with HES received more units of packed red cells [32]; in abdominal surgery, HES 130/0.4 in a cumulative dose of 32.4 ml/kg led to similar blood loss but platelet count was significantly lower than in the gelatin control group [33]. In comparison to crystalloids, HES 130/0.4 led to significantly greater *ex vivo* hemostatic changes [34] and to less stable *ex vivo* clot formation [35, 36].

A recent pooled analysis of data from selected studies in the surgical setting concluded that volume therapy with HES 130/0.4 in major surgery reduces blood loss

Table 3. Pooled analysis of coagulation effects of hydroxyethyl starch (HES) 130/0.4 versus HES 450/0.7 [11]

Estimated blood loss	**HES 130 total* (N = 768)**	**6 % HES 450/0.7 (N = 51)**
ml, mean ± SD	2115 ± 1888	1923 ± 2110
Transfusion of blood components	**6 % HES 130/.04 (N = 320)**	**6 % HES 450/0.7 (N = 51)**
RBC ml, mean ± SD	956 ± 954	1041 ± 759
N (% of subjects)	89 (28)	28 (55)
FFP ml, mean ± SD	1459 ± 1920	1830 ± 767
N (% of subjects)	59 (18)	4 (8)
RBC ml, mean ± SD	431 ± 348	452 ± 146
N (% of subjects)	14 (4)	4 (8)

* includes 2 %, 4 %, 6 %, and 10 % HES 130/0.4. RBC: red blood cell; FFP: fresh frozen plasma

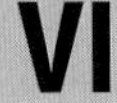

and transfusion requirements in comparison to 'older' HES 200/0.5 [37]. However, the derived differences were marginal and were not significant in the largest subgroup of cardiac surgical patients for estimated blood loss, calculated RBC loss, transfused RBC volumes, transfused platelets, and fresh frozen plasma. Another pooled analysis from the FDA website showed that estimated blood loss and transfusion of blood components was similar for HES 130/0.4 and HES 450/0.7 (**Table 3**) [11].

In summary, there is no conclusive evidence on the effects of HES 130/0.4 on coagulation from adequately performed studies with higher cumulative doses, large enough sample size, and suitable comparators, i.e., albumin or crystalloid solutions. Preliminary data suggest that 'new' HES 130/0.4 is not devoid of adverse effects on coagulation although there may be some gradual differences.

Tissue Storage

It has long been known that HES is taken up and stored in the body for considerable periods of time [38]. In patients who were re-admitted after previous HES administration and underwent operations for reasons such as malignancy or orthopedic disorders, biopsies revealed that HES was present in all organs investigated including liver, spleen, intestine, muscle, and skin up to 54 months after HES administration [13]. HES has been found in endothelial cells of blood and lymphatic vessels, basal keratinocytes, epithelia of sweat glands and in small peripheral nerves, the latter being responsible for HES-associated pruritus [39]. Uptake of HES into renal tubules leads to osmotic nephrosis-like lesions [40] which can persist for as long as 10 years after initial use [8].

In a model of acute hemodilution in pigs, different HES solutions (HES 200/0.62, 200/0.5, and 100/0.5) were stored rapidly and independently of molecular weights in liver, kidney, lung, spleen, and lymph nodes already after 6 hours [41]. When storage of radioactively labeled HES 130/0.4 and 200/0.5 in rat tissue was compared, storage of HES 130/0.4 at 52 days was several-fold lower in most organs but, interestingly, the amounts stored in the kidney were equal to HES 200/0.5 [42].

Pruritus

Protracted pruritus after chronic HES administration is related to storage of the starch in skin [39]. It is increasingly being recognized as a common major adverse effect of HES administration which is generally refractory to available therapies and can persist for up to 12–24 months [43]. Again, HES 130/0.4 is not completely devoid of this side effect. Three out of 12 healthy volunteers reported itching which lasted up to 16 days after administration of 10 consecutive daily units of 10 % HES 130/0.4 [44]. 10 % HES 130/0.4 led to increased incidence of itching compared to HES 200/0.5 [11].

Long-term Survival

In critically ill patients, HES administration may be associated with increased mortality, possibly through tissue storage in the immune system and other organs. Chronic HES administration in critically ill patients can result in massive HES storage in macrophages, bone marrow, and liver cells with the aspect of a storage disease, manifesting as foamy macrophage syndrome, acquired lysosomal storage disease, hydrops lysosomalis generalisatus, liver failure, or worsening of liver disease with ascites [17, 45–47]. Autopsy of a patient who succumbed to sepsis after receiving large doses of HES and dextran revealed widespread colloid uptake in reticuloendothelial cells of liver, lung, kidney, and spleen with massive vacuolization and change of organ morphology [46]. In patients with acute ischemic stroke, hemodilution therapy with pentastarch (HES 200/0.5) significantly increased mortality related to cerebral edema [48]. A post-hoc analysis of data from the VISEP study showed that patients with severe sepsis receiving high cumulative doses of 10 % pentastarch (median 136.0 ml/kg vs. 48.3 ml/kg) had a considerably increased mortality rate compared to patients receiving Ringer's lactate (57.6 % vs. 30.9 %, $p < 0.001$) [7]. The cumulative dose of HES (not of Ringer's lactate) was directly associated with the rate of death at 90 days by logistic regression analysis. In an earlier retrospective analysis of discharge data of approximately 20,000 patients after coronary artery bypass surgery, HES administration was associated with a significantly higher mortality rate than albumin (2.47 vs 3.03 %, $p = 0.02$) [49]. In a recent prospective analysis of patients receiving fluid therapy after subarachnoid hemorrhage, patients receiving the synthetic colloids, HES 200/0.5 and 4 % gelatin, had an increased and dose-related risk of unfavorable neurological outcome at 6 months (OR 2.53 [95 % CI 1.13–5.68]; $p = 0.025$), while crystalloids decreased the risk [27].

How HES impairs survival remains speculative. There are no studies with high cumulative doses of HES in critically ill patients to judge its impact on outcome. It could be that uptake of HES results in impairment of immune function. For example, bled mice resuscitated with HES were more susceptible to an intraperitoneal LPS challenge [50].

Conclusion

HES solutions are popular colloids in some parts of the world. 'Old' HES solutions, including pentastarch HES 200/0.5, hexastarch HES 200/0.62, and hetastarch HES 450/0.7 or 670/0.75 have adverse and potentially detrimental effects on renal function, coagulation, and mortality when given in higher cumulative doses. A 'new' HES 130/0.4 (tetrastarch) has been available for several years in Europe and has recently been introduced in the US. It has been suggested that this latest HES solution has a more favorable risk profile; however, this has only been shown in low risk patients and with low cumulative doses. No studies exist to show that HES 130/0.4 is safe in critically ill patients and nothing is known about its safety in higher cumulative doses and over longer periods of time. There are indications that HES 130/0.4 may have comparable adverse effects to 'older' starches, including impairment of renal function and coagulation, tissue uptake, and pruritus although there may be gradual differences. Unless adequately designed clinical studies with non-colloid comparators, large enough sample size, higher cumulative doses, and longer observation periods in patients with vascular leakage and systemic inflammation show that HES 130/0.4 is safe, the 'new' HES should be treated with as much caution as the 'old'.

References

1. Schortgen F, Deye N, Brochard L (2004) Preferred plasma volume expanders for critically ill patients: results of an international survey. Intensive Care Med 30: 2222–2229
2. FLUIDS study investigators for the Scandinavian Critical Care Trials Group (2008) Preferences for colloid use in Scandinavian intensive care units. Acta Anaesthesiol Scand 52: 750–758
3. Basora M, Moral V, Llau JV, Silva S (2007) [Perioperative colloid administration: a survey of Spanish anesthesiologists' attitudes]. Rev Esp Anestesiol Reanim 54: 162–168
4. Schortgen F, Lacherade JC, Bruneel F, et al (2001) Effects of hydroxyethylstarch and gelatin on renal function in severe sepsis: a multicentre randomised study. Lancet 357: 911–916
5. Wilkes MM, Navickis RJ, Sibbald WJ (2001) Albumin versus hydroxyethyl starch in cardiopulmonary bypass surgery: a meta-analysis of postoperative bleeding. Ann Thorac Surg 72: 527–533
6. Jonville-Bera AP, Autret-Leca E, Gruel Y (2001) Acquired type I von Willebrand's disease associated with highly substituted hydroxyethyl starch. N Engl J Med 345: 622–623
7. Brunkhorst FM, Engel C, Bloos F, et al (2008) Intensive insulin therapy and pentastarch resuscitation in severe sepsis. N Engl J Med 358: 125–139
8. Pillebout E, Nochy D, Hill G, et al (2005) Renal histopathological lesions after orthotopic liver transplantation (OLT). Am J Transplant 5: 1120–1129
9. Godet G, Lehot JJ, Janvier G, Steib A, De Castro V, Coriat P (2008) Safety of HES 130/0.4 (Voluven(R)) in patients with preoperative renal dysfunction undergoing abdominal aortic surgery: a prospective, randomized, controlled, parallel-group multicentre trial. Eur J Anaesthesiol 25: 986–994
10. Jungheinrich C, Sauermann W, Bepperling F, Vogt NH (2004) Volume efficacy and reduced influence on measures of coagulation using hydroxyethyl starch 130/0.4 (6 %) with an optimised in vivo molecular weight in orthopaedic surgery : a randomised, double-blind study. Drugs R D 5: 1–9
11. Department of Health and Human Services, FDA NDA review memo (mid-cycle). 6-Mar-2007. Available at: http://www.fda.gov/CbER/nda/voluven/voluvenmidmem.pdf. Accessed on 9 November, 2008
12. Treib J, Baron JF, Grauer MT, Strauss RG (1999) An international view of hydroxyethyl starches. Intensive Care Med 25: 258–268
13. Sirtl C, Laubenthal H, Zumtobel V, Kraft D, Jurecka W (1999) Tissue deposits of hydroxyethyl starch (HES): dose-dependent and time-related. Br J Anaesth 82: 510–515
14. Jacob M, Rehm M, Orth V, et al (2003) [Exact measurement of the volume effect of 6 % hydoxyethyl starch 130/0.4 (Voluven) during acute preoperative normovolemic hemodilution]. Anaesthesist 52: 896–904
15. Gallandat Huet RC, Siemons AW, Baus D, et al (2000) A novel hydroxyethyl starch (Voluven) for effective perioperative plasma volume substitution in cardiac surgery. Can J Anaesth 47: 1207–1215
16. Gandhi SD, Weiskopf RB, Jungheinrich C, et al (2007) Volume replacement therapy during major orthopedic surgery using Voluven (hydroxyethyl starch 130/0.4) or hetastarch. Anesthesiology 106: 1120–1127

17. Auwerda JJ, Leebeek FW, Wilson JH, van Diggelen OP, Lam KH, Sonneveld P (2006) Acquired lysosomal storage caused by frequent plasmapheresis procedures with hydroxyethyl starch. Transfusion 46: 1705–1711
18. Cittanova ML, Leblanc I, Legendre C, Mouquet C, Riou B, Coriat P (1996) Effect of hydroxyethylstarch in brain-dead kidney donors on renal function in kidney-transplant recipients. Lancet 348: 1620–1622
19. Jungheinrich C, Scharpf R, Wargenau M, Bepperling F, Baron JF (2002) The pharmacokinetics and tolerability of an intravenous infusion of the new hydroxyethyl starch 130/0.4 (6 %, 500 mL) in mild-to-severe renal impairment. Anesth Analg 95: 544–551
20. Boldt J, Brenner T, Lehmann A, Lang J, Kumle B, Werling C (2003) Influence of two different volume replacement regimens on renal function in elderly patients undergoing cardiac surgery: comparison of a new starch preparation with gelatin. Intensive Care Med 29: 763–769
21. Boldt J, Scholhorn T, Mayer J, Piper S, Suttner S (2006) The value of an albumin-based intravascular volume replacement strategy in elderly patients undergoing major abdominal surgery. Anesth Analg 103: 191–199
22. Boldt J, Brosch C, Ducke M, Papsdorf M, Lehmann A (2007) Influence of volume therapy with a modern hydroxyethylstarch preparation on kidney function in cardiac surgery patients with compromised renal function: a comparison with human albumin. Crit Care Med 35: 2740–2746
23. Blasco V, Leone M, Antonini F, Geissler A, Albanese J, Martin C (2008) Comparison of the novel hydroxyethylstarch 130/0.4 and hydroxyethylstarch 200/0.6 in brain-dead donor resuscitation on renal function after transplantation. Br J Anaesth 100: 504–508
24. Hussain SF, Drew PJ (1989) Acute renal failure after infusion of gelatins. BMJ 299: 1137–1138
25. Levi M, Jonge E (2007) Clinical relevance of the effects of plasma expanders on coagulation. Semin Thromb Hemost 33: 810–815
26. Egli GA, Zollinger A, Seifert B, Popovic D, Pasch T, Spahn DR (1997) Effect of progressive haemodilution with hydroxyethyl starch, gelatin and albumin on blood coagulation. Br J Anaesth 78: 684–689
27. Tseng MY, Hutchinson PJ, Kirkpatrick PJ (2008) Effects of fluid therapy following aneurysmal subarachnoid haemorrhage: a prospective clinical study. Br J Neurosurg 22: 257–268
28. Haynes GR, Havidich JE, Payne KJ (2004) Why the Food and Drug Administration changed the warning label for hetastarch. Anesthesiology 101: 560–561
29. Boldt J, Ducke M, Kumle B, Papsdorf M, Zurmeyer EL (2004) Influence of different volume replacement strategies on inflammation and endothelial activation in the elderly undergoing major abdominal surgery. Intensive Care Med 30: 416–422
30. Kasper SM, Meinert P, Kampe S, et al (2003) Large-dose hydroxyethyl starch 130/0.4 does not increase blood loss and transfusion requirements in coronary artery bypass surgery compared with hydroxyethyl starch 200/0.5 at recommended doses. Anesthesiology 99: 42–47
31. Langeron O, Doelberg M, Ang ET, Bonnet F, Capdevila X, Coriat P (2001) Voluven, a lower substituted novel hydroxyethyl starch (HES 130/0.4), causes fewer effects on coagulation in major orthopedic surgery than HES 200/0.5. Anesth Analg 92: 855–862
32. Haisch G, Boldt J, Krebs C, Suttner S, Lehmann A, Isgro F (2001) Influence of a new hydroxyethylstarch preparation (HES 130/0.4) on coagulation in cardiac surgical patients. J Cardiothorac Vasc Anesth 15: 316–321
33. Haisch G, Boldt J, Krebs C, Kumle B, Suttner S, Schulz A (2001) The influence of intravascular volume therapy with a new hydroxyethyl starch preparation (6 % HES 130/0.4) on coagulation in patients undergoing major abdominal surgery. Anesth Analg 92: 565–571
34. Mittermayr M, Streif W, Haas T, et al (2007) Hemostatic changes after crystalloid or colloid fluid administration during major orthopedic surgery: the role of fibrinogen administration. Anesth Analg 105: 905–917
35. Mittermayr M, Streif W, Haas T, et al (2008) Effects of colloid and crystalloid solutions on endogenous activation of fibrinolysis and resistance of polymerized fibrin to recombinant tissue plasminogen activator added ex vivo. Br J Anaesth 100: 307–314
36. Nielsen VG (2006) Hemodilution modulates the time of onset and rate of fibrinolysis in human and rabbit plasma. J Heart Lung Transplant 25: 1344–1352
37. Kozek-Langenecker SA, Jungheinrich C, Sauermann W, Van der Linden P (2008) The effects

of hydroxyethyl starch 130/0.4 (6 %) on blood loss and use of blood products in major surgery: a pooled analysis of randomized clinical trials. Anesth Analg 107: 382–390
38. Thompson WL, Fukushima T, Rutherford RB, Walton RP (1970) Intravascular persistence, tissue storage, and excretion of hydroxyethyl starch. Surg Gynecol Obstet 131: 965–972
39. Stander S, Szepfalusi Z, Bohle B, et al (2001) Differential storage of hydroxyethyl starch (HES) in the skin: an immunoelectron-microscopical long-term study. Cell Tissue Res 304: 261–269
40. Legendre C, Thervet E, Page B, Percheron A, Noel LH, Kreis H (1993) Hydroxyethylstarch and osmotic-nephrosis-like lesions in kidney transplantation. Lancet 342: 248–249
41. Eisenbach C, Schonfeld AH, Vogt N, et al (2007) Pharmacodynamics and organ storage of hydroxyethyl starch in acute hemodilution in pigs: influence of molecular weight and degree of substitution. Intensive Care Med 33: 1637–1644
42. Leuschner J, Opitz J, Winkler A, Scharpf R, Bepperling F (2003) Tissue storage of 14C-labelled hydroxyethyl starch (HES) 130/0.4 and HES 200/0.5 after repeated intravenous administration to rats. Drugs R D 4: 331–338
43. Bork K (2005) Pruritus precipitated by hydroxyethyl starch: a review. Br J Dermatol 152: 3–12
44. Waitzinger J, Bepperling F, Pabst G, Opitz J (2003) Hydroxyethyl starch (HES) [130/0.4], a new HES specification: pharmacokinetics and safety after multiple infusions of 10 % solution in healthy volunteers. Drugs R D 4: 149–157
45. Schmidt-Hieber M, Loddenkemper C, Schwartz S, Arntz G, Thiel E, Notter M (2006) Hydrops lysosomalis generalisatus – an underestimated side effect of hydroxyethyl starch therapy? Eur J Haematol 77: 83–85
46. Ginz HF, Gottschall V, Schwarzkopf G, Walter K (1998) [Excessive tissue storage of colloids in the reticuloendothelial system]. Anaesthesist 47: 330–334
47. Christidis C, Mal F, Ramos J, et al (2001) Worsening of hepatic dysfunction as a consequence of repeated hydroxyethylstarch infusions. J Hepatol 35: 726–732
48. The Hemodilution in Stroke Study Group (1989) Hypervolemic hemodilution treatment of acute stroke. Results of a randomized multicenter trial using pentastarch. Stroke 20: 317–323
49. Sedrakyan A, Gondek K, Paltiel D, Elefteriades JA (2003) Volume expansion with albumin decreases mortality after coronary artery bypass graft surgery. Chest 123: 1853–1857
50. van Rijen EA, Ward JJ, Little RA (1998) Effects of colloidal resuscitation fluids on reticuloendothelial function and resistance to infection after hemorrhage. Clin Diagn Lab Immunol 5: 543–549

VI

Impact of Hydroxyethyl Starch on Renal Function

G. Marx, L. Hüter, and T. Schuerholz

Introduction

Adequate volume replacement to restore and maintain circulating plasma volume appears to be fundamental to improve organ perfusion and nutritive microcirculatory flow in critically ill patients [1]. A variety of pharmaceutical preparations are available that can be used to replace or compensate for lost extracellular fluids in different clinical settings, including colloid and crystalloid solutions. Circulatory stability following fluid resuscitation is usually achieved at the expense of tissue edema formation, which may significantly influence vital organ function. The question of which type of solution should be used as volume replacement remains controversial [2]. Clinically, colloids are frequently used for volume replacement when attempting to maintain or improve tissue perfusion in patients experiencing infection, sepsis, trauma, shock, or surgical stress [3]. Compared to crystalloids, colloids have the advantage of maintenance of an increased colloid osmotic pressure (COP). Thus, fluid is retained in the intravascular space, even in the presence of increased permeability, thereby minimizing edema formation and improving oxygen delivery and organ function [4, 5].

Hydroxyethyl starch (HES) solutions are one group of volume replacement solutions with which one can approach the hemodynamically unstable patient. HES soultions are among the most widely used compounds because their volume-expanding effect is both large and long-lasting. Furthermore, there are recent developments including the introduction of new formulations and newly available HES products. On the other hand, the adverse effects discussed in association with HES administration include anaphylactic reactions, storage, pruritus, and interference with hemostasis and renal dysfunction.

The problem of HES-induced adverse effects on renal function [6] has stimulated ongoing extensive research into the pathological mechanisms. This chapter will consider critically the clinical and experimental available data assessing the current status of the impact of HES on renal dysfunction based on important information on the pharmacokinetic profile of different HES solutions.

Pharmacokinetic Profile of HES Solutions

HES is a branched polymer of amylopectin with hydroxyethyl groups substituted for hydrogen atoms on the glucose ring. Pharmaceutical-grade HES is manufactured by subjecting starch, typically from a potato or maize source, to hydrolysis followed by reaction with ethylene oxide under alkaline conditions at 25–50 °C. Three aspects of the chemical composition of HES are important to the physicochemical properties and clinical effects of the agent when used as a volume expander: Molecular weight, the level of molar substitution, and the C2/C6 substitution ratio. Chemical modifications to both HES molecules and to carrier solutions have continued to improve efficacy and safety.

The molecular weight of currently available products ranges from 450–670 kDa (high molecular weight) to 70–130 kDa (low molecular weight); HES with a molecular weight of approximately 200 kDa is classified as a medium molecular weight product. Pre-clinical studies have examined the effects of high molecular weight HES preparations in the range of 650–900 kDa [7–9]. The level of molar substitution is defined by the average number of hydroxyethyl groups per glucose unit and ranges from 0.75 (high molar substitution) to approximately 0.4 (low molar substitution), in currently available products. The pattern of hydroxyethyl group substitution is described using the ratio of substitution within the glucose unit at carbon position C2 and C6. The majority of commercially available products include C2/C6 ratios in the range of 5:1–9:1. Pre-clinical studies have explored the effect of C2/C6 ratios in the range of 2.7:1–14:1 [8]. The molecular weight and molar substitution of HES solutions are generally shown as suffixes, e.g., HES 200/0.5; the C2/C6 ratio is added less frequently as a third suffix.

After being infused into the blood, HES is metabolized to smaller molecular weight molecules. This *in vivo* molecular weight is a key determinant of the subsequent therapeutic (and other) effects of the HES solution. The rate of metabolism is dependent on both the level of hydroxyethyl substitution and the C2/C6 ratio; HES molecules with a high substitution level and a high C2/C6 ratio are degraded slowly [10], have prolonged intravascular persistence and a sustained volume replacement effect. As with other colloids, HES is stored in the body. Approximately one-third to two-thirds of administered HES is excreted in the urine over the first 24 hours after infusion [11]. Administering 1000 ml of high molecular and highly substituted HES 450/0.7 in 10 patients, intracellular vacuoles of HES were demonstrated by histopathology 6 to 28 days after infusion in parenchymal liver cells, Kupffer's cells, interstitial histiocytes, and, to a lesser degree, in the cells of the small bile ducts [12]. Multiple doses of 10 % HES 130/0.4 and 10 % HES 200/0.5 were investigated in rats [13]. After 52 days, HES 130/0.4 compared to HES 200/0.5 total body ^{14}C-activity was decreased by 75 % with no difference in the kidney storage (HES 130/0.4: 0.019 ± 0.006 % of the dose versus HES 200/0.5: 0.019 ± 0.005 % of the dose) [13]. In patients discharged from the ICU, HES was shown to be deposited and stored in many tissues in a dose-dependent manner, although the amounts accumulated were depleted over time [14, 15]. The issue of HES storage seems to be most likely dose dependent [16].

Low molecular weight HES solutions were developed aimed at optimizing pharmacokinetics and retaining volume replacement effect, but avoiding the adverse effects of accumulation. In healthy volunteers, HES 130/0.42/6:1 was investigated using a crossover design with HES 200/0.5/5:1 serving as control [17]. Fifty grams of either HES solution was administered in 4 hour per day for a period of five consecutive days. Although the circulation was freed of the load with HES 130/0.42/6:1 within 20 hours after the end of the previous infusion, the amount of HES 200/0.5/5:1 increased continuously from one administration to the other indicating accumulation. The area under the curve (AUC) and elimination half-life were significantly lower with HES 130/0.42. The AUC and elimination half-life of HES 200/0.5 showed an increase between the first and the fifth administration whereas only a minimal shift was present with HES 130/0.42. Thus, repeated administration of HES 130/0.42/6:1 showed no accumulation and fewer tendencies to time-dependent changes in pharmacokinetic parameters than HES 200/0.5/5:1. The improved reproducibility suggests improved drug safety, particularly as the accumulation of residual starch with HES 200/0.5/5:1 did not contribute to the colloid's volume effect, but may rather increase the risk of undesired reactions. The authors compared further the bioequivalence of HES 130/0.42/6:1 to HES 130/0.4/9:1 in healthy volunteers using a randomized, crossover design [18]. Using non-compartmental analysis, significant differences were found for AUC24 (45.97 ± 8.97 mg h/ml vs 58.32 ± 9.23 mg h/ml; HES 130/0.42/6:1 vs HES 130/0.4/9:1) and total apparent clearance (1.14 ± 0.4 l/h vs 0.81 ± 0.34 l/h). Maximum serum concentration and elimination half-life were similar. These data suggest that the pharmacokinetic coefficients of HES respond very sensitively to differences in the pharmaceutical specifications of the colloid. Even minute differences between the pharmaceutical specifications of HES 130/0.42/6:1 and HES 130/0.4/9:1 (as compared to the much larger deviation from HES 200/0.5) still result in significantly different pharmacokinetic properties. Being equivalent with HES 200/0.5/5:1 and HES 130/0.4/9:1 in terms of colloid osmotic and hemodilution effect, HES 130/0.42/6:1 showed the fastest clearance from the circulation. Compared with middle molecular and middle substituted HES solutions, such as HES 200/0.5/5:1, the low substituted HES preparations with their lower molecular weight and molar substitution show approximately 50–60 % of the former solution's AUC, i.e., 50–60 % of its presence over time in the circulation. The elimination half-lives of the low substituted HES solutions are likewise diminished by similar degrees, whereas their hemodilution effect is equal to that of HES 200 in terms of degree and duration.

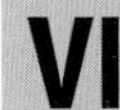

Pathomechanisms of HES-induced Renal Dysfunction

The effects of HES administration on renal function are under continuous discussion. HES is partly eliminated by the reticuloendothelial system, and a dose dependent uptake in macrophages, endothelial and epithelial cells has been detected [19]. Various investigations reported vacuoles in different human tissue specimens [14, 20]. Tissue deposition of HES seems to be transitory and dose-dependent [15, 19]. These HES containing vacuoles in the kidneys are called osmotic-like lesions. It was suggested that these osmotic-like lesions explained the adverse renal effects of HES, although nobody has demonstrated a pathophysiologic relationship between the vacuoles and renal dysfunction. In kidney transplantation, osmotic-like histological lesions of the tubules were noticed retrospectively in kidney transplant recipients when HES was used for fluid resuscitation of brainstem-dead donors [21]. However, these lesions had no significant effect on the occurrence of delayed graft function and serum creatinine at 3 and 6 months post-transplantation. A prospective trial using HES 200/0.62 demonstrated a detrimental effect on initial graft function [22]. In two other studies, HES 200/0.5 did not impair early graft function after kidney transplantation [23, 24]. Recently, Blasco et al. compared the effects of 6 % HES 130/0.4 or 6 % HES 200/0.6 used for the resuscitation of brain-dead donors [25]. They demonstrated a non-significant difference in the rate of delayed graft function when using 6 % HES 130/0.4 versus 6 % HES 200/0.6 (22 % versus 33 %), but significantly lower serum creatinine levels up to 1 year post-transplantation in the 6 % HES 130/0.4 group. Serum creatinine levels were 128 ± 36 mmol/l when the donors had been treated with 6 % HES 130/0.4, and 147 ± 43 mmol/l when they had been treated with 6 % HES 200/0.6 ($p < 0.005$) suggesting that HES preparations with a low degree of substitution seem to be associated with a better effect on the renal function of recipients.

On the other hand, an *in vitro* sepsis model using proximal tubular epithelial cells following inflammatory stimulation showed that the presence of HES 130/0.42 and HES 200/0.5 attenuated cell injury [26] suggesting that HES solutions provide immune modulatory potential. Interestingly, HES 200/0.5 was found to be more protective than HES 130/0.42 in this *in vitro* sepsis model.

Hauet et al. compared a non-specified HES solution to sodium chloride, gelatin, and albumin in an isolated, renal whole blood model over two hours [27]. The authors concluded from their results that HES induces osmotic nephrosis. Injury mechanisms remain unclear but the oncotic force of the volume replacement solution seems to be important, because when the oncotic pressure is so high that it offsets the hydraulic pressure of glomerular filtration it may suppress urine output [28]. Furthermore, glomerular filtration of hyperoncotic molecules from colloids causes hyperviscous urine and a stasis of tubular flow, resulting in obstruction of tubular lumen [29].

In order to evaluate possible pathomechanisms of HES-induced adverse effects on renal function, we also compared 6 % HES 130/0.42, 10 % HES 200/0.5, and Ringer's lactate in an isolated porcine kidney perfusion model [30]. Interestingly, we identified vacuolization of tubular epithelial cells in all groups; they were significantly more present after the application of 10 % HES 200/0.5 or 6 % HES 130/0.42 compared to Ringer's lactate but were also present after Ringer's lactate infusion (**Fig. 1**). The question remains whether these tubular epithelial vacuoles represent renal injury or may be an epiphenomenon without clinical importance. There was an increase in N-acetyl-ß-D-glucosaminidase (NAG) levels in all groups indicating that tubular injury had occurred. Using Ringer's lactate, diuresis and creatinine clearance were significantly higher and ß-NAG levels significantly lower compared to both 10 % HES 200/0.5 and 6 % HES 130/0.42 indicating HES-induced adverse renal effects. On histological investigation, we identified renal interstitial proliferation, macrophage infiltration, and tubular damage as structural alterations of the kidney associated with HES-induced adverse renal effects [31]. Interstitial cell proliferation was higher with the 10 % HES 200/0.5 than the 6 % HES 130/0.42 indicating more pronounced cell activation by 10 % HES 200/0.5. In addition, significant differences between the two HES solutions with respect to macrophage infiltration could be

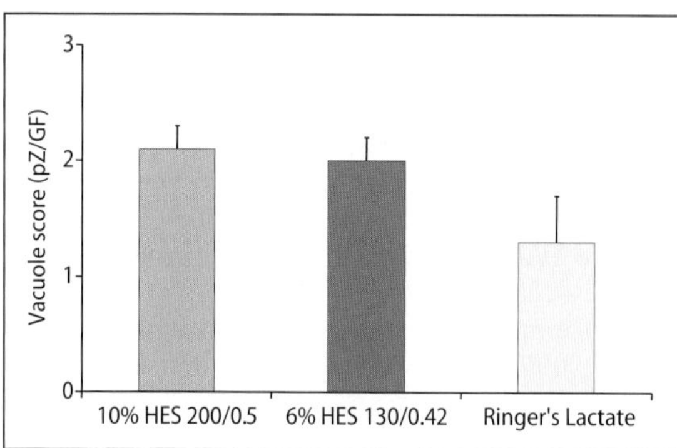

Fig. 1. Osmotic-like lesions due to infusion of 10 %HES 200/0.5 compared to 6 %HES 130/0.42 and Ringer's lactate in an *ex vivo* renal perfusion model. There were statistically more osmotic nephrosis-like lesions in the HES 200/0.5 and 130/0.42 groups compared to the Ringer's lactate group. Original magnification: × 200 [30].

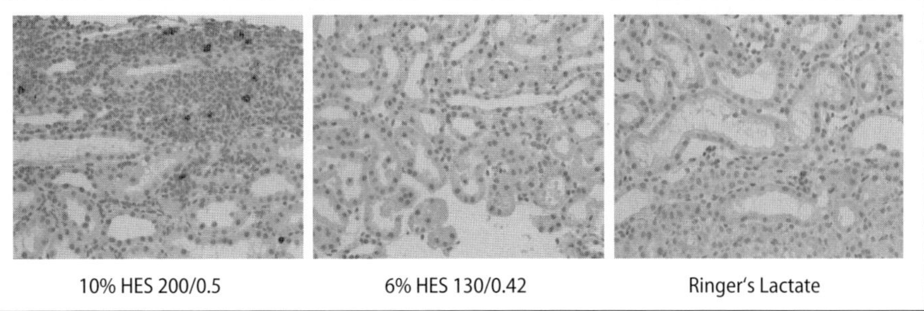

Fig. 2. Macrophage infiltration as a potential pathomechanism of HES-induced renal injury in an *ex vivo* renal perfusion model. Immunohistological staining of ED-1 positive interstitial macrophages. There was a significantly higher number of infiltrating macrophages and also of other inflammatory cells with 10 % HES 200/0.5 compared to 6 % HES 130/0.42 and Ringer's lactate using an *ex vivo* renal perfusion model. Original magnification: × 200 [31].

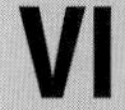

identified (**Fig. 2**), indicating that interstitial inflammation was more pronounced with 10 % HES 200/0.5 than with 6 % HES 130/0.42. Of note, macrophage infiltration also tended to be higher in the Ringer's lactate group compared to the 6 % HES 130/0.42 suggesting that infusion of a crystalloid solution may not be without associated inflammation in this model either. In this context, it is interesting to notice that large amounts of HES 200/0.5 aggravated macrophage enzyme release in patients with impaired renal function possibly resulting in an acquired lysosomal storage disease [14]. As an isooncotic solution, 6 % HES 130/0.42, was compared with a hyperoncotic solution, 10 % HES 200/0.5, it cannot be differentiated whether the oncotic force, the molecular weight, the degree of molar substitution, molecular size, or all these factors together were determining factors of the HES-induced adverse effects on renal function and structure. The underlying link between macrophages and HES-induced renal failure needs to be elucidated further.

Clinical Evidence of HES-induced Renal Dysfunction

There have been numerous studies published on the effects of HES administration on renal function [6]. In the perioperative situation, studies investigate renal effects of HES traditionally over a short period of time only, i.e., 2–5 days. Boldt et al. compared 6 %HES 130/0.4 with gelatin for pump priming and volume expansion in a randomized trial of 40 patients over 70 years of age undergoing first time cardiopulmonary bypass (CPB) surgery [32]. Four sensitive markers of renal impairment, NAG, α1-microglobulin, glutathione transferase-π, and glutathione transferase-α, indicated perioperative renal dysfunction for both solutions. On the 2nd postoperative day, kidney-specific proteins had returned almost to normal values and none of the patients developed acute renal failure. Thus, 6 % HES 130/0.4 and gelatin did not differ with regard to kidney integrity in elderly patients undergoing cardiac surgery. In patients undergoing major abdominal surgery, patients > 65 years were compared to patients < 65 years without previous renal dysfunction using 6 % HES 70/0.5, 6 % HES 200/0.5, and until the 3rd postoperative day [33]. Using similar, sensitive markers of renal function, no negative influence on renal function was detected and there was no difference between the colloid solutions. Of note, patients in this study received approximately 3 l of crystalloids in addition to colloid volume replacement until the first postoperative day. None of the patients developed acute renal failure requiring hemodialysis or hemofiltration during the investigation period. Wiesen et al. collected data retrospectively in 3,124 patients who underwent coronary artery bypass and/or valvular surgery [34]. Three fluid regimens were used for priming the bypass circuit and for postoperative fluid resuscitation, including HES 200/0.5, gelatin, and a combination of the two fluids. From this analysis, no significant differences in postoperative serum creatinine concentrations or adverse renal function among the three groups were observed.

Recent studies have taken into account the potential long-term renal effects of colloids [35, 36]. Boldt et al. compared 6 % HES 130/0.4 and 5 % albumin in 50 patients with comprised renal function undergoing cardiac surgery [37]. A follow-up after discharge from the hospital was performed showing that none of the patients developed acute renal failure requiring renal replacement therapy during the hospital stay and up to 60 days thereafter. The methodology of this postal survey has been questioned, because no response was received for approximately one third of the patients [38]. Over the 48-hour study period patients received 2500 ± 500 ml 6 % HES 130/0.4 and 2350 ± 430 ml 5 % human albumin, respectively. Glutathione transferase-α and NAG increased significantly in both groups without a difference between the two colloids. Neutrophil gelatinase-associated lipocalin (NGAL) increased significantly more in the albumin group compared to the 6 % HES 130/0.4 group. In a multicenter randomized controlled trial in 65 patients with preoperative renal dysfunction undergoing abdominal aortic surgery, 6 % HES 130/0.4 and 3 % gelatin were compared [39]. Oliguria was encountered in three patients in the HES and four in the gelatin treatment group. One patient receiving gelatin required dialysis secondary to surgical complications. Two patients in each treatment group died. Patients received a cumulative dose of 32.3 ± 17.3 ml/kg body weight 6 % HES 130/0.4 and 29.4 ± 15.6 ml/kg body weight 3 % gelatin over 6 days. Serum creatinine increased by 26.3 ± 55.3 μmol/l (median 4.5; range –47 to 222) in the HES treatment group and by 36.5 ± 103.3 μmol/l (median 4.0; range –22 to 561) in the gelatin treatment group. Non-inferiority of 6 % HES 130/0.4 could be statistically shown after exclusion of outliers (one patient per treatment group). Comparing 4 % gelatin and 6 % HES 130/0.4 in cardiac surgical patients older than 80 years, volume therapy with 6 % HES 130/0.4 was associated with less marked changes in kidney function and a less marked endothelial inflammatory response than 4 % gelatin [36]. Serum creatinine was higher and creatinine clearance was lower in the gelatin group compared to the HES group during the initial 48 hour postoperative period. Kidney function did not differ between the groups up to 60 days. Hence, in the perioperative situation, no HES-specific renal dysfunction has so far been evidenced following HES administration with a low molecular weight (130 kDa) and molar substation of 0.4/0.42. Interestingly, in this clinical area an adequately powered prospective clinical study comparing crystalloids and HES and including long-term (90 days) observations is still lacking.

In severe sepsis and septic shock, Schortgen and colleagues showed that 6 % HES200/0.62 compared to 3 % gelatin was an independent risk factor for acute kidney injury (AKI) [40]. The methodology of this study, however, has been questioned although it was randomized and controlled [41–43]. Despite randomization, the baseline creatinine was higher in the HES group compared to the gelatin group. Furthermore, a valid criticism made at the time underlined the inadequate provision of crystalloids in the HES group, possibly resulting in dehydration, a hyperoncotic state and subsequent compromise of renal function.

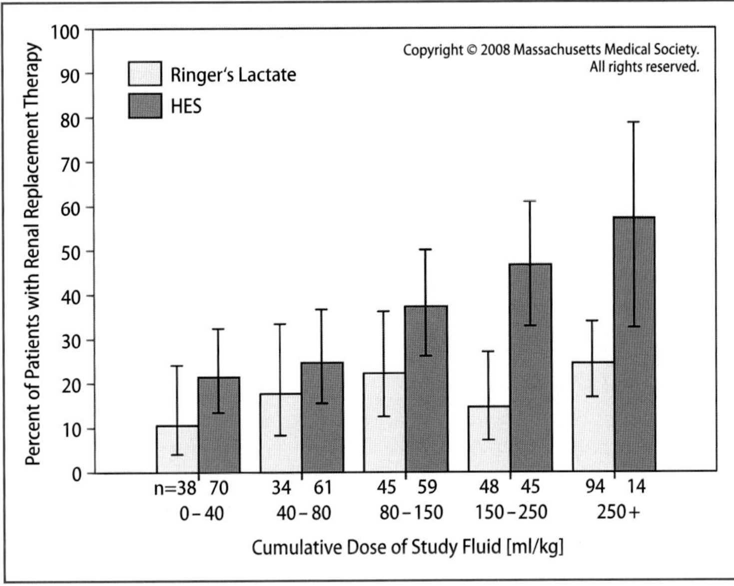

Fig. 3. VISEP-study: Cumulative effect of volume resuscitation with 10 % HES 200/0.5 or Ringer's lactate on the need for renal-replacement therapy at 90 days. The need for renal-replacement therapy was significantly correlated with the cumulative dose of HES ($p < 0.001$) but not with the dose of Ringer's lactate. From [35] with permission.

In the recent German multicenter controlled efficacy of volume substitution and insulin therapy in severe sepsis (VISEP) trial it was shown that the use of 10 % HES 200/0.5 compared to Ringer's lactate in patients with severe sepsis or septic shock was associated with an increased need for renal replacement therapy [35], although mortality rates at 28 and 90 days were not significantly different in the two groups. In this study, the cumulative dosage of 10 % HES200/0.5 was significantly correlated with the need for renal replacement therapy (**Fig. 3**). The VISEP study has been criticized for the use of a hyperoncotic HES with a COP of 68 mmHg rather than a 6 % HES (COP: 36 mmHg); a much more hyperoncotic colloid was, therefore, used in comparison to the high molecular weight 6 % HES (200/0.62) used in the first Schortgen study [44]. On the other hand, a recent large prospective observational study (sepsis occurrence in acutely ill patients, SOAP) in 3147 critically ill patients of whom 1075 received HES treatment showed that in those with ICU stays of > 24 hours, sepsis, heart failure and hematological cancer were all significantly associated with the need for dialysis or hemofiltration therapy, but volume replacement with HES was not [45]. Even in the subgroup of patients with severe sepsis and septic shock (n = 822), HES was not associated with an increased risk for renal replacement therapy. Unfortunately, this study did not distinguish between different HES solutions. Comparing the result from this study [45] with the data from the VISEP study [35], one important difference is the total amount of HES administered. In the VISEP study, patients received HES for up to 21 days with a median cumulative dose of 70.4 ml/kg body weight (interquartile range: 33.4–144.2 ml/kg), whereas in the observational SOAP study the median total amount of HES per patient was lower: 1000 ml or approximately 13 ml/kg body weight (interquartile range: 500–2250 ml). In the VISEP trial, 160 out of the 275 patients in the Ringer's lactate group received a median amount of 725 ml colloids (interquartile range: 500–1000 ml) as volume resuscitation in the 12 hour period prior to inclusion and randomization in the study. These data support the importance of time and dose of fluid resuscitation.

Recently, the occurrence of renal adverse events after resuscitation of shock in 822 ICU patients using crystalloids, hypooncotic (gelatin and 4 % albumin) and hyperoncotic (HES and dextran) colloids, and hyperoncotic 20 % albumin has been investigated in an observational multicenter cohort study [46]. The occurrence of renal adverse events was more frequent in both hyperoncotic groups compared to crystalloids and normo-oncotic colloids, suggesting that the hyperoncocity was more relevant than the nature of the product itself. When the volume of artificial hyperoncotic colloids was over 2 l within 36 hours it was significantly associated with a higher incidence of renal adverse events. The type of HES used was 6 % 130/0.4 as well as older starches. Surprisingly, the modern 6 % 130 HES used, though expected to be less hyperoncotic, did not reduce the risk of adverse renal adverse events [44]. Still, there are some criticisms: The patients receiving hyperoncotic fluid had a significantly higher number of organ dysfunctions. One cannot rule out inadequate rehydration and volume loading since hemodynamics were monitored using a central venous pressure (CVP) in only 64 % of the patients. Furthermore, plasma was administered to 169 patients in addition to other fluids and these patients were still included in the groups of patients receiving hyperoncotic colloids; 113 of 401 in the artificial hyperoncotic colloids group and 56 of 105 in the hyperoncotic albumin group. The authors pooled all artificial colloids and did not provide sufficient information to distinguish between different HES solutions. However, this study reemphasizes the need to be cautious using hyperoncotic fluid in critically ill patients in order to avoid damage to the kidney.

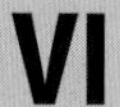

Conclusion

There remains little doubt that guaranteed rehydration and adequate volume loading are more important than the type of fluid used. Whether different HES products affect kidney function in patients with pre-existing kidney failure or at risk of developing renal failure remains unclear. Based on the experimental and clinical evidence available regarding the impact of HES on renal function it seems important to differentiate and be precise:

- The use of any hyperoncotic solutions should be avoided because this may produce hyperoncotic kidney failure.
- Recent data suggest the cumulative dose of HES is an important factor in association with the induction of renal injury.
- HES does not equal HES: It is necessary to distinguish between different HES products and specifications, and between different clinical scenarios.
- In the perioperative situation, no HES-specific renal dysfunction has so far been evidenced following 6 % HES administration with a low molecular weight (130 kDa) and molar substation of 0.4/0.42.
- 10 % HES 200/0.5 and 6 % HES 200/0.6–0.66 are associated with an increased incidence of acute renal failure and renal replacement therapy in patients with severe septic patients and should not be used in this group of patients.

- Whether 6 % HES 130/0.4 or 0.42 can be used safely in septic patients or patients with pre-existing kidney failure or at risk of developing renal failure remains to be elucidated in adequately powered, long-term (90 days) clinical studies.
- Mechanisms of HES-induced renal injury remain unclear, although recent experimental data using an *ex vivo* renal perfusion model suggest renal interstitial proliferation, macrophage infiltration, and tubular damage as potential pathological mechanisms of HES-induced adverse effects on renal function. In this experimental setting, 10 % HES 200/0.5 had more pro-inflammatory effects compared to 6 % HES 130/0.42 and caused more pronounced tubular damage than 6 % HES 130/0.42.

As so often, further research is needed to elucidate the potential impact of HES in the development of renal injury.

References

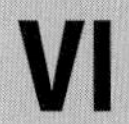

1. Boldt J (2000) Volume therapy in the intensive care patient--we are still confused, but. Intensive Care Med 26: 1181–1192
2. Marx G (2003) Fluid therapy in sepsis with capillary leakage. Eur J Anaesthesiol 20: 429–442
3. Groeneveld AB (2000) Albumin and artificial colloids in fluid management: where does the clinical evidence of their utility stand? Crit Care 4:S16–20
4. Carlson RW, Rattan S, Haupt M (1990) Fluid resuscitation in conditions of increased permeability. Anesth Rev 17 (Suppl 3):14
5. Rackow EC, Falk JL, Fein IA, et al (1983) Fluid resuscitation in circulatory shock: a comparison of the cardiorespiratory effects of albumin, hetastarch, and saline solutions in patients with hypovolemic and septic shock. Crit Care Med 11: 839–850
6. Davidson IJ (2006) Renal impact of fluid management with colloids: a comparative review. Eur J Anaesthesiol 23: 721–738
7. Madjdpour C, Thyes C, Buclin T, et al (2007) Novel starches: single-dose pharmacokinetics and effects on blood coagulation. Anesthesiology 106: 132–143
8. von Roten I, Madjdpour C, Frascarolo P, et al (2006) Molar substitution and C2/C6 ratio of hydroxyethyl starch: influence on blood coagulation. Br J Anaesth 96: 455–463
9. Madjdpour C, Dettori N, Frascarolo P, et al (2005) Molecular weight of hydroxyethyl starch: is there an effect on blood coagulation and pharmacokinetics? Br J Anaesth 94: 569–576
10. Treib J, Haass A, Pindur G, Grauer MT, Wenzel E, Schimrigk K (1996) All medium starches are not the same: influence of the degree of hydroxyethyl substitution of hydroxyethyl starch on plasma volume, hemorrheologic conditions, and coagulation. Transfusion 36: 450–455
11. Waitzinger J, Bepperling F, Pabst G, Opitz J (2003) Hydroxyethyl starch (HES) [130/0.4], a new HES specification: pharmacokinetics and safety after multiple infusions of 10 % solution in healthy volunteers. Drugs R D 4: 149–157
12. Jesch F, Hubner G, Zumtobel V, Zimmermann M, Messmer K (1979) Hydroxyethyl starch (HAS 450/0.7) in human plasma and liver. Course of concentration and histological changes. Infusionsther Klin Ernahr 6: 112–117
13. Leuschner J, Opitz J, Winkler A, Scharpf R, Bepperling F (2003) Tissue storage of 14C-labelled hydroxyethyl starch (HES) 130/0.4 and HES 200/0.5 after repeated intravenous administration to rats. Drugs R D 4: 331–338
14. Auwerda JJ, Leebeek FW, Wilson JH, van Diggelen OP, Lam KH, Sonneveld P (2006) Acquired lysosomal storage caused by frequent plasmapheresis procedures with hydroxyethyl starch. Transfusion 46: 1705–1711
15. Sirtl C, Laubenthal H, Zumtobel V, Kraft D, Jurecka W (1999) Tissue deposits of hydroxyethyl starch (HES): dose-dependent and time-related. Br J Anaesth 82: 510–515
16. Kimme P, Jannsen B, Ledin T, Gupta A, Vegfors M (2001) High incidence of pruritus after large doses of hydroxyethyl starch (HES) infusions. Acta Anaesthesiol Scand 45: 686–689
17. Lehmann GB, Asskali F, Boll M, et al (2007) HES 130/0.42 shows less alteration of pharmacokinetics than HES 200/0.5 when dosed repeatedly. Br J Anaesth 98: 635–644

18. Lehmann G, Marx G, Forster H (2007) Bioequivalence comparison between hydroxyethyl starch 130/0.42/6:1 and hydroxyethyl starch 130/0.4/9:1. Drugs R D 8: 229–240
19. Stander S, Szepfalusi Z, Bohle B, et al (2001) Differential storage of hydroxyethyl starch (HES) in the skin: an immunoelectron-microscopical long-term study. Cell Tissue Res 304: 261–269
20. Jamal R, Ghannoum M, Naud J-F, Turgeon P-P, Leblanc M (2008) Permanent renal failure induced by pentastarch. Nephrol Dial Transplant Plus 5: 322–325
21. Legendre C, Thervet E, Page B, Percheron A, Noel LH, Kreis H (1993) Hydroxyethylstarch and osmotic-nephrosis-like lesions in kidney transplantation. Lancet 342: 248–249
22. Cittanova ML, Leblanc I, Legendre C, Mouquet C, Riou B, Coriat P (1996) Effect of hydroxyethylstarch in brain-dead kidney donors on renal function in kidney-transplant recipients. Lancet 348: 1620–1622
23. Coronel B, Mercatello A, Colon S, Martin X, Moskovtschenko J (1996) Hydroxyethylstarch and osmotic nephrosis-like lesions in kidney transplants. Lancet 348:1595
24. Deman A, Peeters P, Sennesael J (1999) Hydroxyethyl starch does not impair immediate renal function in kidney transplant recipients: a retrospective, multicentre analysis. Nephrol Dial Transplant 14: 1517–1520
25. Blasco V, Leone M, Antonini F, Geissler A, Albanese J, Martin C (2008) Comparison of the novel hydroxyethylstarch 130/0.4 and hydroxyethylstarch 200/0.6 in brain-dead donor resuscitation on renal function after transplantation. Br J Anaesth 100: 504–508

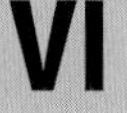

26. Wittlinger M, De Conno E, Schläpfer M, Spahn DR, Beck-Schimmer B (2008) Effect of different HES preparations (HES 130/0.42; HES 200/0.5) on activated proximal tubular epithelial cells in vitro. Eur J Anaesthesiol 25 (Suppl 44):173 (abst)
27. Hauet T, Faure JP, Baumert H, et al (1998) Influence of different colloids on hemodynamic and renal functions: comparative study in an isolated perfused pig kidney model. Transplant Proc 30: 2796–2797
28. Barron J (2000) Pharmacology of crystalloids and colloids. In: Transfusion Medicine and Alternative to Blood Transfusion. R&J-Editions Medicales, Paris, pp 123–137
29. Chinitz JL, Kim KE, Onesti G, Swartz C (1971) Pathophysiology and prevention of dextran-40-induced anuria. J Lab Clin Med 77: 76–87
30. Hueter L, Simon T, Weinmann L, Marx G (2008) Osmotic nephrosis is not the exclusive HES associated phenomenon but occurs also after Ringers lactate infusion in an isolated renal perfusion model. Eur J Anaesthesiol 25 (Suppl 44):165–166 (abst)
31. Hueter L, Simon T, Weinmann L, Marx G (2008) HES200/0.5 induces more renal macrophage infiltration than HES 130/0.42 in an isolated renal perfusion model. Crit Care 12 (Suppl 2):S90 (abst)
32. Boldt J, Brenner T, Lehmann A, Lang J, Kumle B, Werling C (2003) Influence of two different volume replacement regimens on renal function in elderly patients undergoing cardiac surgery: comparison of a new starch preparation with gelatin. Intensive Care Med 29: 763–769
33. Kumle B, Boldt J, Piper S, Schmidt C, Suttner S, Salopek S (1999) The influence of different intravascular volume replacement regimens on renal function in the elderly. Anesth Analg 89: 1124–1130
34. Wiesen P, Canivet JL, Ledoux D, Roediger L, Damas P (2005) Effect of hydroxyethylstarch on renal function in cardiac surgery: a large scale retrospective study. Acta Anaesthesiol Belg 56: 257–263
35. Brunkhorst FM, Engel C, Bloos F, et al (2008) Intensive insulin therapy and pentastarch resuscitation in severe sepsis. N Engl J Med 358: 125–139
36. Boldt J, Brosch C, Rohm K, Papsdorf M, Mengistu A (2008) Comparison of the effects of gelatin and a modern hydroxyethyl starch solution on renal function and inflammatory response in elderly cardiac surgery patients. Br J Anaesth 100: 457–464
37. Boldt J, Brosch C, Ducke M, Papsdorf M, Lehmann A (2007) Influence of volume therapy with a modern hydroxyethylstarch preparation on kidney function in cardiac surgery patients with compromised renal function: a comparison with human albumin. Crit Care Med 35: 2740–2746
38. Davidson IJ (2008) Hydroxyethyl starch 130/0.4: safe in cardiac surgery? Crit Care Med 36: 1695–1696
39. Godet G, Lehot JJ, Janvier G, Steib A, De Castro V, Coriat P (2008) Safety of HES 130/0.4 (Voluven(R)) in patients with preoperative renal dysfunction undergoing abdominal aortic

surgery: a prospective, randomized, controlled, parallel-group multicentre trial. Eur J Anaesthesiol 25: 986–994
40. Schortgen F, Lacherade JC, Bruneel F, et al (2001) Effects of hydroxyethylstarch and gelatin on renal function in severe sepsis: a multicentre randomised study. Lancet 357: 911–916
41. Gosling P, Rittoo D, Manji M, Mahmood A, Vohra R (2001) Hydroxyethylstarch as a risk factor for acute renal failure in severe sepsis. Lancet 358:582
42. Godet G (2001) Hydroxyethylstarch as a risk factor for acute renal failure in severe sepsis. Lancet 358: 582–583
43. Boldt J (2001) Hydroxyethylstarch as a risk factor for acute renal failure in severe sepsis. Lancet 358: 581–583
44. Honore PM, Joannes-Boyau O, Boer W (2008) Hyperoncotic colloids in shock and risk of renal injury: enough evidence for a banning order? Intensive Care Med 34: 2127–2129
45. Sakr Y, Payen D, Reinhart K, et al (2007) Effects of hydroxyethyl starch administration on renal function in critically ill patients. Br J Anaesth 98: 216–224
46. Schortgen F, Girou E, Deye N, Brochard L (2008) The risk associated with hyperoncotic colloids in patients with shock. Intensive Care Med 34: 2157–2168

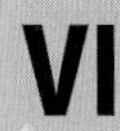

Rational Approach to Fluid Therapy in Acute Diabetic Ketoacidosis

J. Ochola and B. Venkatesh

Introduction

Diabetic ketoacidosis remains one of the most serious acute complications of diabetes mellitus. The mortality rate is < 5 % with modern management strategies. The mainstay of treatment for this condition includes the following: Hydration, insulin therapy, correction of electrolyte abnormalities, and treatment of the underlying precipitating factors. While several advances have been made with the type and delivery of insulins, controversy and confusion surround the prescription of optimal fluid therapy in diabetic emergencies. The focus of this commentary is to examine the evidence base for the choice of resuscitation and maintenance fluid in diabetic ketoacidosis.

Historical Perspective

The classic study by Atchley et al. in two diabetic volunteers formed one of the original reports on metabolic derangement in diabetic ketoacidosis [1]. In these subjects, a comprehensive study of electrolyte and water balance was undertaken following withdrawal and reestablishment of insulin therapy. The reported fluid deficit was of the order of 5–10 liters and appeared to approximate half from the extracellular compartment and the remainder from the intracellular space. Nabarro et al. extended the observations of Atchley; in adults with diabetic ketoacidosis, they showed fluid deficits of approximately 5 liters with an associated 20 % total body sodium and potassium loss [2]. Hartmann independently verified these findings in children [3]. It is generally agreed that the average water loss is about 5–10 liters, and sodium and potassium losses range between 250–500 mmol/l. A knowledge of the pathophysiology of diabetic ketoacidosis formed the basis for the development of a variety of fluid regimes.

As early as the 1930s, several fluid regimes were trialled in the management of diabetic ketoacidosis. Hartmann performed one of the early trials comparing three different crystalloids [3]. Eighty-six patients were divided into three groups: Group 1 received dextrose and Ringer's solution, Group 2 received dextrose, Ringer's solution, and sodium bicarbonate and Group 3 received dextrose, Ringer's solution and sodium lactate. Hartmann concluded that the use of alkali either as sodium bicarbonate or sodium lactate resulted in a more rapid and better resolution of acidosis (**Fig. 1**) and that the use of sodium lactate obviated the need for using supplemental dextrose.

The findings of this study [3] were also in accord with the prevailing view that in cases of acidosis due to diarrhea, where there was bicarbonate loss, "salt administra-

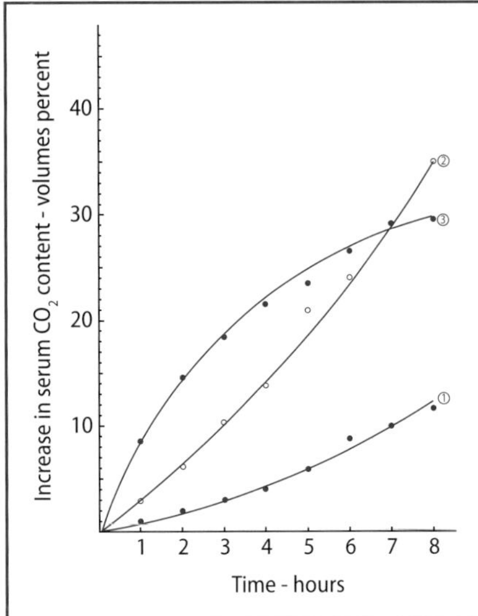

Fig. 1. Changes in serum CO_2 during resuscitation of patients with diabetic acidosis. A comparison of three different fluid regimes. This figure shows the mean increases in total serum CO_2 content over time in the three groups: Group 1 – Dextrose and Ringer's solution; Group 2 – Dextrose, Ringer's solution, and sodium bicarbonate; and Group 3 – dextrose, Ringer's solution and sodium lactate. From [3] with permission.

tion was considered contraindicated in the presence of high plasma chloride and low bicarbonate [4]." However, Joslin's group advocated caution in the use of alkali. In a series of 70 cases of diabetic ketoacidosis treated without alkali, only one death was reported. In view of such a low mortality in the absence of alkali, there was no compelling need to change protocol. The case for non-alkali management was further reinforced when the same group reported adverse outcomes in two other patients who received bicarbonate [3].

In the 1950s, the practice of combining sodium lactate with sodium chloride in various formulations for the treatment of diabetic ketoacidosis was popularized with the use of Butler's solution [5]. However, concerns regarding glucose regeneration, excessive alkalinization and hypokalemia from the lactate resulted in a resurgence in the use of 0.9 % saline for the management of diabetic ketoacidosis. Diabetic ketoacidosis trials in the 1970s were performed largely with the use of saline. Current American and British guidelines also recommend 0.9 % saline as the initial resuscitation fluid of choice [6, 7]. Of note, however, there are no randomized controlled trials supporting the use of one fluid over another in diabetic ketoacidosis. The varied recommendations over the last 50 years (**Table 1**) for fluid therapy in diabetic ketoacidosis stand as a testament to the uncertainty in this area.

Pathophysiology

The underlying pathogenesis of this condition is a relative or absolute deficiency of circulating insulin coupled with a concomitant elevation of counterregulatory hormones, catecholamines, glucagon, growth hormone, and cortisol. The hallmark of diabetic ketoacidosis is its hyperglycemic, hyperketotic, hyperosmolar state which is predominantly responsible for fluid and electrolyte losses. The increased filtered load of glucose overwhelms the renal tubular reabsorptive capacity resulting in marked glycosuria and osmotic diuresis. This urinary water loss is accompanied by

Table 1. Fluid therapy used in the treatment of diabetic ketoacidosis over the last 50 years.

Author	Fluid composition
Butler (1950) [5]	Butler solution: 100 mEq/l Na, 60 mEq/l Cl, 45 mEq/l lactate or bicarbonate
Williams (1968) [37]	After initial bicarb., 100 mEq Na, 60 mEq C1, 40 mEq HCO_3 or lactate/l, for 1–3 h. Then 0.42 % or 0.85 % saline.
London (1970) [38]	1 l 0.85 % saline in 1st h, with added alkali 4 l in 1st 12 h.
Hardwick (1970) [39]	1 /h 0.85 % saline
Steinke and Thorn (1970) [40]	0.85 % saline, 4–8 l fluid in 24 h.
Bondy (1971) [41]	0.42 % saline with 2.5 % fructose. Rate not specified.
Kolb (1971) [42]	0.45 % saline
Petrides (1971) [43]	1 l in 1 h of 33 % 'N' saline, 33 % 'N' bicarb., 33 % water. 4–6 l per 24 h by age and severity.
Duncan (1971) [44]	1–1.5 l 0.85 % saline in 30 min. 0.5 l. alternating 1:2 with 5 % dextrose, 1–2 l per h for 2–3 h, then less.
American Diabetes Association (2006) [6]	0.9 % saline

This table was partially adapted from [36]

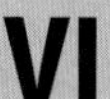

a disproportionately lower amount of electrolyte losses further contributing to the rising serum osmolality. In addition, hyperketonemia causes osmotic diuresis and obligatory losses of cations that accompany the ketoanions, further aggravating the electrolyte deficit.

One third of total body water content is normally distributed in the extracellular space and the remaining two thirds in the intracellular space. In diabetic ketoacidosis, the osmotic diuresis coupled with hyperosmolality-induced intracellular dehydration leads to water losses from both the intravascular and the intracellular compartment. The water loss, therefore, is more hypotonic, equivalent in osmolality to that of 0.45 % saline. Other factors contributing to fluid and electrolyte losses include vomiting and acute gastric dilatation. In diabetic ketoacidosis, water losses have been estimated to range between 30 to 100 ml/kg with an associated elevated serum osmolality of 320 to 340 msom/l [8].

There are wide variations in the severity of fluid and electrolyte deficits. At presentation, the magnitude of these deficits depends on the severity and duration of illness and the extent to which the patient was able to maintain oral intake of fluids and electrolytes.

Aims of Fluid Therapy

The therapeutic goals of fluid management are directed at:

- expanding both intracellular and extracellular fluid compartments to restore circulating volume and tissue perfusion over the first 24–48 hours [9]
- reducing serum osmolality and plasma glucose concentrations towards normal levels
- improving glomerular filtration rate to enhance the clearance of ketones and glucose from the blood
- correcting electrolyte imbalances
- limiting the risk of complications such as cerebral edema

Volume replacement is an independent factor in determining survival. Adequate hydration with subsequent correction of the hyperosmolar state augments the response to insulin therapy. One study of patients with diabetic ketoacidosis demonstrated the critical importance of adequate hydration by documenting that hydration alone (without insulin administration) reduced hyperglycemia, acidosis, hyperosmolality, and insulin counterregulatory hormone levels [10].

Optimal Management

How best to achieve the fluid treatment aims remains contentious with particular controversy revolving around the optimal initial fluid. Both crystalloids and colloids have been considered as potential agents in the management of diabetic ketoacidosis.

Evidence Base for 0.9 % Saline

0.9 % saline is commonly used as the initial fluid of choice for resuscitation [11, 12]. As noted, the use of saline is largely historically based (**Table 1**). Of interest, despite absence of sound evidence, it is also the recommended fluid of choice in the American Diabetes Association Guidelines [6]. The arguments for the use of isotonic saline as the initial fluid include: a) It achieves the desired restoration and maintenance of the intravascular space while counteracting the contraction of the extracellular compartment when the serum glucose falls rapidly during treatment; b) it is still hypotonic to the extracellular and intracellular fluid of the severely dehydrated patient with diabetic ketoacidosis.

Problems with 0.9 % Saline

The rationale for using 0.9 % saline as the initial fluid for resuscitation is based on its more efficacious ability to restore the circulating volume and improve tissue perfusion, as compared to hypotonic solutions. However, only a quarter of this crystalloid remains in the intravascular compartment or even less if hypovolemia is present [13]. The remainder is distributed in the interstitial space. Therefore, administering large volumes of 0.9 % saline and titrating its effect to surrogates of intravascular volume may result in fluid overload in the form of interstitial edema. This may present as cerebral or pulmonary edema in the absence of cardiac dysfunction.

Non-cardiogenic pulmonary edema is a potential complication of overzealous rehydration with crystalloids. Special care must be taken in those with renal failure or congestive cardiac failure. Colloid oncotic pressure (COP) initially increases in diabetic ketoacidosis following marked diuresis and electrolyte losses. During rehydration, there is a gradual decline in COP to levels that have been associated with a progressive decrease in arterial PO_2 and a concomitant increase in the alveolar-arterial gradient [14]. Patients with an increased alveolar-arterial gradient and those with crepitations on initial auscultation may be at increased risk of acute respiratory distress syndrome (ARDS) [15].

Resuscitation with 0.9 % saline can also cause sodium overload secondary to an increase in serum sodium and osmolality in the absence of free water required to replace intracellular losses. Hypovolemia-induced sodium retention and the anti-natriuretic effects of insulin therapy are also contributory.

Finally, the use of 0.9 % saline is associated with the development of a hyperchloremic acidosis. Oh et al. were one of the first groups of investigators to describe the development of hyperchloremic acidosis during the recovery phase of diabetic ketoacidosis in patients treated with 0.9 % saline [16]. Adrogue et al. [17] extended this concept by dichotomizing diabetic ketoacidosis patients into those with pure raised anion gap acidosis and those with coexisting normal anion gap acidosis. When patients were treated with 0.9 % saline, the recovery of total CO_2 was much slower in those with concomitant normal anion gap acidosis [17]. In another study, the incidence of hyperchloremic acidosis was shown to progressively increase from 6 % at the start of treatment to 94 % after 20 hours of treatment [18]. In diabetic ketoacidosis, there is an increase in chloride reabsorption in the proximal renal tubule in response to decreased bicarbonate generation secondary to the loss of ketone substrates in urine. 0.9 % saline has a strong ion difference (SID) of zero, which on administration in large quantities will tend to produce a dilutional acidosis [19]. Although the normal anion gap acidosis is attributed to excretion of ketoanions in the urine and, therefore, unavailability of substrate for regeneration of bicarbonate, Stewart's physico-chemical approach also provides a framework for understanding the mechanism of development of hyperchloremic acidosis during saline therapy (see below).

VI

Hyperchloremic acidosis may not be as innocuous as one is led to believe [20]. Hyperchloremia *per se* may be associated with increased morbidity. One obvious concern is the misinterpretation of the cause of acidosis. For example, the persistent base deficit during fluid resuscitation in diabetic ketoacidosis may be interpreted as an indication of ongoing ketosis. Such a presumption may result in inappropriate increments or prolongation of insulin administration. It is also known be related to renal dysfunction and in association with acidosis, may increase the risk of hemorrhage and acute lung injury (ALI) [21, 22]. Human volunteers experienced mental changes, abdominal discomfort, and relative oliguria after receiving 50 ml/kg of 0.9 % saline over 1 hour but not following the same volume of Hartmann's solution [23].

Evidence Base for 0.45 % Saline

Studies have shown that hyperglycemic-induced osmotic diuresis produces urine that contains about 70 millimoles of sodium per liter [24]. Therefore, from a physiological perspective, the ideal fluid for accurate replacement of losses from all compartments would be 0.45 % saline (half-normal saline). However, because of its large volume of distribution, the rate of restoration of the circulating volume may be protracted.

If the corrected serum sodium is normal or exceeds 155 mmol/l, the American Diabetes Association recommends that 0.45 % saline is commenced at a rate of 4 to 14 ml/kg/h [6]. Potential advantages include the correction of dehydration with the avoidance of sodium overload and hyperchloremia. However, the evidence for this recommendation is limited.

It has been suggested that very hypotonic solutions (< 75 mmol/l of sodium) may result in a decline in plasma osmolality and hyponatremia predisposing to cerebral edema [25]. The etiology of cerebral edema remains poorly understood. A number of mechanisms have been postulated and primarily suggest that the treatment of diabetic ketoacidosis is causally related to its development. Bello and Sotos [26] retrospectively analyzed 11 patients with diabetic ketoacidosis associated with cerebral edema and noted that a declining serum sodium concentration was ominous. In addition, a decrease in serum osmolality was identified as a risk factor for development of cerebral edema. In a review by Duck and Wyatt involving diabetic ketoacidosis patients with associated cerebral edema, rapid fluid administration was associated with an increased risk of developing cerebral edema and a shortening of time to herniation. These authors, therefore, recommended limiting the rate of rehydration therapy [27]. On the other hand, Azzopardi et al. [28] demonstrated that there was no clinical or subclinical occurrence of cerebral edema in adult patients with diabetic ketoacidosis who received isotonic (150 mmol/l of sodium) or hypotonic (120 mmol/l of sodium) solutions as part of their fluid regimen.

There are significant limitations in the methodology of these studies. In particular, the majority are retrospective and lack a control group. Furthermore, the small sample size of patients with cerebral edema means that these studies are significantly underpowered.

Evidence Base for Hartmann's Solution

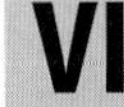

The use of Hartmann's solution in diabetic ketoacidosis dates back to the 1950s. Nabarro et al. [29] noted that the retention of extracellular electrolytes during the recovery phase of diabetic ketoacidosis was in a sodium to chloride ratio of 1.3:1.0 mEq. These authors, therefore, suggested that this represented the optimal composition of the fluid most appropriate for initial resuscitation and restoration of the extracellular compartment [29]. A retrospective-prospective study comparing Ringer's lactate, 0.9 % saline or 0.45 % saline for initial therapy in diabetic ketoacidosis reported no differences in mortality between the three groups [30].

More recently, Stewart's physical chemical analysis of biological acid-base [31] has been used to provide a framework to explaining how Hartmann's is the best known balanced physiological solution commercially available and results in minimal disturbance of the acid-base status.

In the Stewart analysis, there are three independent variables determining acid-base balance: PCO_2, the total weak acid concentration $[A_{tot}]$ and the SID. A_{tot} in plasma is largely albumin and inorganic phosphate, whereas erythrocytic A_{tot} is comprised primarily of hemoglobin. Raising and lowering $[A_{tot}]$ while holding the SID constant causes a metabolic acidosis and alkalosis respectively. Strong ions are chemical entities that remain fully dissociated at physiological concentration under all acid-base conditions compatible with life. Examples include Na^+, K^+, Cl^- and lactate. Quantitatively, their unionized concentrations are so minute they can be disregarded. In biological fluids, total strong cation concentrations exceed strong anion concentrations. The surfeit is quantified by the SID concentration ([SID]), for which, because this is a charge difference, the units are mEq/l. In normal plasma the [SID] is approximately 42 mEq/l. Lowering and raising plasma [SID] in isolation causes metabolic acidosis and alkalosis respectively.

In the Stewart paradigm, crystalloids administered in large volumes bring about acid-base changes in two ways. By simply causing hemodilution, $[A_{tot}]$ is lowered, causing a metabolic acidosis. Simultaneously, plasma [SID] is altered towards that of the infused fluid. Depending on the composition of the crystalloid, plasma [SID] can thus be raised, lowered, or left unaltered. The final outcome represents a combination of balance between reduced $[A_{tot}]$ metabolic alkalosis and [SID] effects. It follows that the metabolic acidosis associated with the use of saline preparations (in which [SID] = 0) occurs because the resultant [SID] reduction overwhelms the metabolic alkalosis of $[A_{tot}]$ dilution.

To prevent acid-base disturbances during crystalloid fluid loading, Morgan et al. demonstrated from their *in vitro* and hemodilution data that the balanced crystalloid should have a SID of 24 mEq/l to prevent a rapid fall in extracellular SID at a rate sufficient to counteract the progressive A_{tot} dilutional alkalosis [32]. In other words, 0.9 % saline can be 'balanced' by replacing 24 mEq/l of chloride with bicarbonate, or alternatively with anions which are metabolized to bicarbonate on infusion, such as lactate, citrate or acetate.

On the other hand, because Hartmann's solution contains 29 millimoles of racemic lactate per liter of solution, concerns have been raised as to whether this may result in hyperlactatemia. However, this concern is more theoretical than real in diabetic ketoacidosis, as hepatic dysfunction, a prerequisite for the development of hyperlactemia, is not usually present. There is also the potential for this lactate to be metabolized to glucose and potentially exacerbate the hyperglycemic state. Thomas and Alberti found that the use of 1 to 1.5 liters of Hartmann's solution post-operatively was associated with a 7.5 mmol/l increase in plasma glucose concentration compared to an increase of 2.1 mmol/l in diabetic patients who received no intravenous fluids. They therefore concluded that Hartmann's solution may have an adverse metabolic effect in diabetic patients [33].

Because Hartmann's solution is more hypotonic compared to extracellular fluid, it has been postulated that this may increase the risk of cerebral edema in patients with diabetic ketoacidosis. Finally, concerns have been raised about the possibility of hyperkalemia due to the presence of 5 millimoles of potassium in every liter of Hartmann's solution. Frequently however, potassium supplementation is the norm in diabetic ketoacidosis and, therefore, the small concentration of potassium is unlikely to pose a serious risk during its administration to patients with diabetic ketoacidosis. There are no randomized controlled studies to resolve any of these issues and inferences can only be drawn from historical data.

Evidence Base for Colloids

Traditionally, colloids have been advocated as the most effective fluids at restoring hemodynamic stability in the context of shock [34]. The oversimplistic view that they are mainly confined to the intravascular space provides a theoretical advantage during the resuscitation of patients presenting with acute diabetic ketoacidosis. Titrating their rate of infusion to hemodynamic endpoints, can lead to rapid restoration of the circulatory volume. At least three times the volume of crystalloid has historically been quoted as achieving the same effect as colloids although this ratio was recently refuted in the Saline versus Albumin Fluid Evaluation (SAFE) study where the ratio of crystalloid to colloid required to achieve treatment goals was only 1:1.4 over the first 4 days of the trial [35]. Fein et al. [14] postulated that large volumes of crystalloid were responsible for a rapid decline in plasma oncotic pressure which in turn contributed to the development of cerebral and pulmonary edema [14]. They performed serial measurements of arterial blood gases, cerebral ventricular width and COP and showed a direct correlation between declining COP and respiratory function and ventricular width.

However, no data in the form of a clinical trial exist to support the use of colloids in preference to crystalloids in the treatment of diabetic ketoacidosis.

Conclusion

In view of the inconclusive nature of current literature, there can be no definitive recommendations on fluid therapy in the management of acute diabetic ketoacidosis. There is level I evidence that fluid replacement is mandatory. However, the type and the volume of fluid therapy required remains an unanswered question. The American Diabetes Association recommends 0.9 % saline at an initial rate of 15 to 20 ml/kg body weight per hour in the absence of cardiac dysfunction (level III evidence). Subsequent fluid therapy to replace deficits is determined by the corrected serum sodium. 0.45 % saline is recommended if the corrected serum sodium is normal or greater than 155 mmol/l (level III evidence). Fluid therapy should correct estimated deficits within the first 24 hours. It has, however, been highlighted that the average rate of change in serum osmolality ideally should not exceed 3 mosm/kg of water per hour (level III evidence) [5]. As noted above, low levels of evidence exist for many of these recommendations. These questions can be answered reliably only in multicenter trials.

References

1. Atchley D, Loeb R, Richards D, et al (1933) On diabetes acidosis. A detailed study of electrolyte balances following the withdrawal and re-establishment of insulin therapy. J Clin Invest 12: 297–326
2. Nabarro J, Spencer A, Stowers J (1952) Metabolic studies in severe diabetic ketosis. Quart. J Med 21: 225–248
3. Hartmann A (1935) Treatment of severe diabetic ketoacidosis. A comparison of methods with particular preference to the use of racemic sodium lactate. Arch Intern Med 56: 413–434
4. Hartmann A, Darrow D, Morton M (1928) Chemical changes in the body as the result of certain diseases. III The composition of the plasma in severe diabetic acidosis and the changes taking place during recovery. J Clin Invest 6: 257–276
5. Butler A (1950) Diabetic coma. N Engl J Med 243 17: 648–659
6. Kitabchi A, Umpierrez G, Murphy M et al (2006) Hyperglycemic crises in adult patients with diabetes. A consensus statement from the American Diabetes Association. Diabetes Care 29:2739 -2749
7. Wolfsdorf J, Craig M, Daneman D, et al (2007) ISPAD Clinical Practice Consensus Guidelines. Diabetic Ketoacidosis. Paediatr Diabetes 8: 28–43
8. Trachtenbarg D (2005) Diabetic ketoacidosis. Am Fam Physician 71: 1705–1714
9. Kitabchi A, Umpierrez G, Murphy M, et al (2001) Management of hyperglycaemic crisis in patients with diabetes. Diabetes Care 24: 131–153
10. Waldhausl W, Kleinberger D, Korn A, et al (1979) Severe hyperglycemia: effects of rehydration on endocrine derangements and blood glucose concentration. Diabetes 28: 577–584
11. Henriksen O, Prahl J, Roder M, Svendsen O (2007) Treatment of diabetic ketoacidosis in adults in Denmark: A national survey. Diabetes Res Clin Pract 77: 113–119
12. Savage M, Mah P, Weetman A, Newell-Price J (2004) Endocrine emergencies. Postgrad Med J 80: 506–515
13. Pain R (1977) Body fluid compartments. Anaesth Intensive Care 5:284
14. Fein I, Rachow E, Sprung C, Grodman R (1982) Relation of colloid osmotic pressure to arterial hypoxemia and cerebral edema during crystalloid volume of patients with diabetic ketoacidosis. Ann Intern Med 96: 570–575
15. Carroll P, Matz R (1982) Adult respiratory distress syndrome complicating severely uncontrolled diabetes mellitus: report of nine cases and a review of the literature. Diabetes Care 5: 574–580
16. Oh MS, Banerji MA, Carroll H (1981) The mechanism of hyperchloremic acidosis during the recovery phase of diabetic ketoacidoais. Diabetes 30: 310–313

17. Adrogue H, Wilson H, Boyd A, et al (1982) Plasma acid-base patterns in diabetic ketoacidosis. N Engl J Med 307: 1603–1610
18. Taylor D, Durward A, Tibby S, et al (2006) The influence of hyperchloraemia on acid base interpretation in diabetic ketoacidosis. Intensive Care Med 36: 295–301
19. Morgan T, Venkatesh B (2003) Designing 'balanced' crystalloids. Crit Care Resusc 5: 284–91
20. Dhatariya K (2007) Diabetic ketoacidosis. BMJ 334:1284
21. Kaplan L, Frangos S (2005) Clinical review: Acid-base abnormalities in the intensive care unit. Crit Care 9: 198–203
22. Wilcox C (1983) Regulation of renal blood flow by plasma chloride. J Clin Invest 71: 726–735
23. Williams EL, Hildebrand KL, McCormick SA, Bedel MJ (1999) The effect of intravenous lactated Ringer's solution versus 0.9 % sodium chloride solution on serum osmolality in human volunteers. Anesth Analg 88: 999–1003
24. Arieff A, Carroll H (1972) Nonketotic hyperosmolar coma with hyperglycaemia: clinical features, pathophysiology, renal function and acid-base balance, plasma cerebrospinal fluid equilibria and the effects of therapy in 37 cases. Medicine (Baltimore) 51: 73–94
25. Winegrad A, Kern E, Simmons D (1985) Cerebral edema in diabetic ketoacidosis. N Engl J Med 312: 1184–1185
26. Bello F, Sotos J (1990) Cerebral oedema in diabetic ketoacidosis in children. Lancet 336:64
27. Duck S, Wyatt D (1988) Factors associated with brain herniation in the treatment of diabetic ketoacidosis. J Pediatr 113: 10–14
28. Azzopardi J, Gatt A, Zammit A, Alberti G (2002) Lack of evidence of cerebral oedema in adults treated for diabetic ketoacidosis with fluids of different tonicity. Diabetes Res Clin Pract 57: 87–92
29. Nabarro J, Spencer A, Stowers J (1952) Treatment of diabetic ketoacidosis. Lancet 1: 983–989
30. Wagner A, Risse A, Brill H, et al (1999) Therapy of severe diabetic ketoacidosis. Zero-mortality under very low dose insulin application. Diabetes Care 22: 674–677
31. Stewart PA (1981) How to Understand Acid-base. A Quantitative Acid-base Primer for Biology and Medicine. Elsevier, New York
32. Morgan TJ, Venkatesh B, Beindorf A, Andrew I, Hall J (2007) Acid-base and bio-energetics during balanced versus unbalanced normovolaemic haemodilution. Anaesth Intensive Care 35: 173–179
33. Thomas D, Alberti G (1978) Hyperglycaemic effects of Hartmann's solution during surgery in patients with maturity onset diabetes. Br J Anaesth 50: 185–187
34. Shoemaker W (1976) Comparison of the relative effectiveness of whole blood transfusions and various types of fluid therapy in resuscitation. Crit Care Med 4:71
35. Finfer S, Bellomo R, Boyce N, French J, Myburgh J, Norton R (2004) A comparison of albumin and saline for fluid resuscitation in the intensive care unit. N Engl J Med 350: 2247–2256
36. Hockaday T, Alberti K (1972) Diabetic coma. Clin Endocrinol Metab 1: 751–788
37. Williams R (1968) Textbook of Endocrinology. WB Saunders, Philadelphia
38. London D (1970) Therapy of common diseases. In: Cranston W, Gunn A (eds) The International Handbook of Medical Science. Medical and Technical Publishing Company, Aylesbury pp 488–498
39. Hardwick C (1970) Diabetes mellitus. In: Havard CWH (ed) Current Medical Treatment, 3rd Edition, Staples Press, London, pp 430–434
40. Steinke J, Thorn GW (1970) Diabetes mellitus. In: Wintrobe M (ed) Harrison's Principles of Internal Medicine. Mcgraw-Hill, New York, pp 523–539
41. Bondy P (1971) Disorders of carbohydrate metabolism. In: Beeson P, McDermott W (eds) Textbook of Medicine. Saunders, Philadelphia, pp 1639–1664
42. Kolb F (1971) In: Krupp M, Chatton M, Margen S (eds) Current Diagnosis and Treatment. Blackwell, Oxford, pp 637–639
43. Petrides P (1971) Diabetes Mellitus. Urban & Schwazenberg, Munich
44. Duncan L (1971) In: Macgregor A, Girdwood R (eds) Textbook of Medical Treatment, 12th Edition. Churchill Livingstone, Edinburgh, pp 332–335

VI

VII Hemodynamic Support

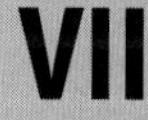

Cardiac Filling Volumes and Pressures in Assessing Preload Responsiveness during Fluid Challenges

R.-M.B.G.E. Breukers, R.J. Trof, and A.B.J. Groeneveld

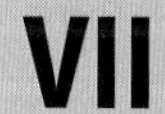

Introduction

Heart-lung interactions, loss of circulating blood volume and fluid loading are accompanied by changes in cardiac output, mainly as a consequence of changes in cardiac preload. However, hypotension and oliguria do not necessarily indicate hypovolemia, for instance during cardiogenic shock. During increased airway pressures, i.e., positive end-expiratory pressure (PEEP), thereby decreasing venous return, cardiac preload may fall, at an unchanged blood volume. Nevertheless, fluid loading for treatment of circulatory insufficiency, irrespective of its cause, is probably the earliest and most common step in the treatment of critically ill patients, and perhaps also the most controversial one. Controversies include the reasons, types, and amounts of fluid to be given and the end-points of resuscitation during shock, hypotension, oliguria, or combinations. The importance of prediction and careful monitoring of fluid therapy is the prevention of under- and overfilling [1]. Tailored therapy is more likely to be adequate in individual patients than the use of fixed volumes, for instance given peri-operatively, in clinical trials of 'liberal' versus 'restrictive' fluid regimens in surgical patients.

In the last few decades, another controversy has evolved concerning the value of indicators for preload responsiveness of stroke volume and cardiac output, such as static filling pressures and volumes of the heart, to predict effect and monitor fluid therapy [2–4]. This narrative chapter summarizes the physiology of static indicators used to predict and monitor preload responsiveness in critically ill patients on mechanical ventilation. We will not address pressure and stroke volume variations and other dynamic indicators of preload responsiveness, since these measures, influenced by tidal volume and transmitted airway pressure, are only meaningful in patients on controlled mechanical ventilation and in sinus rhythm [3, 5–11]. We first summarize the goals and effects of fluid loading.

Goals and Effects of Fluid Loading: Defining Preload and Fluid Responsiveness

The goals of fluid therapy in the critically ill patient with circulatory insufficiency and impaired tissue oxygenation, regardless of (plasma) volemic status, is to optimize cardiac output and, thereby, tissue oxygen delivery to the point that tissue oxygen requirements are met. Withholding fluid challenges in patients with a predicted low increase in stroke volume or cardiac output may carry the risk of undertreatment. On the other hand, continued fluid loading beyond optimal stroke volume or cardiac output may only increase filling pressures and deleterious overfilling and pulmonary edema may ensue, thereby threatening arterial oxygenation and thus tissue oxygen delivery [1, 12, 13]. Of note, a positive fluid response can be encountered in normal healthy volunteers [14], and is, therefore, not necessarily a sign of hypovolemia. Conversely, the mere presence of predictors of a positive fluid response should not automatically prompt for fluid administration, unless there is a clinical problem associated with impaired tissue oxygenation and likely ameliorated by an increase in cardiac output and thereby oxygen delivery following fluid infusion. Preload responsiveness of cardiac output does not necessarily imply a positive fluid response, i.e., fluid responsiveness, when infused fluids do not reach the heart to increase preload. For instance, saline loading may be less effective than colloid loading in boosting cardiac output and, also, cardiac output may increase during fluid loading through other mechanisms than a rise in blood volume and cardiac preload [12–16]. Indeed, a fall in afterload resulting from decreased viscosity or increased contractility upon fluid loading may contribute to a rise in cardiac output that may surpass the expected effect for a given volume infused [14, 15]. Finally, a rise in plasma volume and subsequent hemodilution may prevent a rise in tissue oxygen delivery during fluid loading, even when cardiac output increases. Nevertheless, arterial blood pressure may increase and, thereby, improve regional, perfusion pressure-dependent blood flow, as in the kidneys.

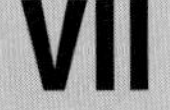

Fluid challenges consisting of rapid infusions of small volumes of (colloid) solutions can be regarded as physiological experiments, and the response can help to decide whether patients may benefit from further fluid loading or not [17]. Standard boluses of 100–500 ml or 7–10 ml/kg of non-crystalloid solutions infused over 10–30 min are commonly used, and stroke volume or cardiac output increases of 5–20 % measured some time after the challenge are taken as clinically relevant, positive responses, i.e. fluid responsiveness [2–4, 6, 7, 9–11, 15–26].

The question is whether absolute increases are clinically less important than relative increases and how defining fluid responsiveness relates to the measurement error inherent to the cardiac output measurement technique to assess it. Moreover, the fractional increase in cardiac output may depend on the volume of fluid administered. The use of stroke volume, although more appropriate to assess cardiac function, may differ somewhat from that of cardiac output when heart rate changes, while, on the other hand, cardiac output is a major determinant of tissue oxygenation. Effect of fluid loading can be transient, so that the time interval between loading and measurements influences the observed effect.

Filling Pressures and Volumes of the Heart

Classically, filling pressures have been recommended to guide fluid challenges of the heart and to avoid harmful (pulmonary) fluid overloading when rapid increases in pressures may augment fluid filtration into the lungs. The central venous pressure (CVP) and the pulmonary artery occlusion pressure (PAOP) are taken as indicators of right and left ventricular end-diastolic, i.e., filling, pressure, respectively, in the absence of valvular abnormalities. Interruption of the fluid column by high airway pressures or venous obstruction may confound PAOP. Filling pressures are measured with help of a properly positioned fluid-filled central venous or pulmonary artery catheter, at the end of expiration and referenced to atmospheric pressure and the mid-chest level (in supine position). When PEEP is transmitted during mechanical ventilation, atmospheric pressure-referenced filling pressures do not reflect cardiac transmural pressures, while ventricular preload may depend on transmural pressure [7]. Absolute filling pressures as indicators of cardiac preload and preload responsiveness have been discredited by the increasingly accepted notion that their value, particularly in mechanically ventilated patients, in predicting and monitoring fluid responses is low, as compared to cardiac volumes/dimensions, for instance [26, 27]. This may only partly relate to the propensity for measurement errors and the low range of observed pressures.

A guideline published more than 30 years ago and recently validated [13, 17, 18] recommends that fluid loading should be tapered or discontinued when filling pressures rise abruptly and greatly, indicating that the limits of cardiac dilatation have been reached. Of note, changes in filling pressures employed in this guideline are independent of PEEP. Delta filling pressure-guided fluid loading may increase end-diastolic volume in parallel with increased filling pressures, during clinical hypovolemia after cardiovascular surgery, for instance [13, 17]. By prompting to stop fluid therapy upon severe increases in filling pressures, a delta filling pressure-guided fluid challenge may thus help to increase cardiac output, when clinically needed, and at the same time prevent overfilling and development of pulmonary edema, irrespective of ventilator settings [13, 17]. Nevertheless, filling pressures may increase, depending on baseline values, during both preload responsiveness (small increases of pressures) as well as unresponsiveness (large and rapid increases) and, as such, may thus have little predictive value for the change in cardiac output.

VII

In contrast to pressure measurements, volume measurements are not confounded by transmitted airway pressure during mechanical ventilation. (Transesophageal) echocardiography allows assessment of venous, atrial, and ventricular dimensions, regional systolic and diastolic function, ventricular interaction, valvular blood flow (velocities) and preload responsiveness [5, 8, 9, 12, 14, 19, 23, 24, 28–32]. Changes in ejection fraction and regional wall motion may indeed not be easily detected by pulmonary artery catheter-derived parameters [31]. The technique carries the disadvantage of need for extensive experience thereby hampering, together with patient intolerance, the potential for continuous monitoring.

The bolus thermodilution technique in combination with a rapid response thermistor, allows evaluation of right ventricular volumes and ejection fraction [16, 20, 33–38]. These measures appear relatively accurate, as compared to echocardiographic and nuclear angiographic techniques, even though the evaluation of right ventricular volume is hampered by its conformation and some doubts remain about the confounding effects of tricuspid regurgitation and the respiratory cycle [39]. The latter problem is probably circumvented by the continuous right ventricular end-diastolic volume measurement technique, which evolved from semicontinuous cardiac output monitoring with the help of a pulmonary artery catheter [23, 24, 39].

The (double and single) transpulmonary thermodilution techniques involve right atrial injection of cold saline solution and thermal detection at the level of the femoral arteries. This allows reproducible determinations of intrathoracic blood volume (ITBV) and global (i.e., right and left heart chambers together) end-diastolic volume (GEDV). Volumes derived from single transpulmonary thermal dilution are similar to those obtained by double thermal-dye dilution and reproducibility may be around 10 % [2, 4, 6, 8, 10, 21–23, 29, 40–42]. Of note, right and left heart dilatation cannot be separated by these measurements and pulmonary emboli or other causes of right ventricular dilatation may surpass detection when left ventricular volume decreases by ventricular interaction. Thoracic aortic aneurysms and shunts may also confound measurements. The virtual volumes showed good relations with left ventricular dimensions and function on echocardiography, thus likely in the absence of right ventricular overload [5, 8, 9, 19, 22, 23, 43]. In some studies, however, the correlation between transpulmonary or right-sided volumes and left or right ventricular echocardiographic dimensions was less obvious [10, 22, 24, 38].

An alternative method applicable at the bedside is biventricular nuclear angiography but this method necessitates additional expertise and equipment and is therefore rarely used nowadays at the bedside in the intensive care unit (ICU) [14, 15, 44–46]. Volumes may hardly relate, particularly in mechanically ventilated patients [15, 16, 44, 45], to filling pressures, even when changes in individual patients are considered, and this may reflect measurement errors or widely varying ventricular compliances. The observation does not necessarily favor pressures or volumes as true indicators of ventricular preload (responsiveness).

Physiological Considerations and Clinical Implications

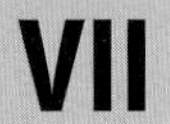

In muscle physiology, preload is the resting muscle length and this can be approximated by end-diastolic wall tension or stress for intact cardiac ventricles [48]. According to La Place's law for a sphere, end-diastolic wall stress (s) is determined by PR/2w, where P is pressure, R is radius and w is wall thickness [47, 48]. Consequently, both pressures and volumes contribute (but do not equate) to ventricular preload. For instance, right ventricular output after cardiovascular surgery is better predicted by elastic energy incorporating right ventricular end-diastolic pressure and volume, rather than by either factor alone [36]. Right ventricular preload can also vary independently of volume, when shape changes, for instance during fluid loading, while the left ventricle is more spherical or ellipsoid, therefore, perhaps, better obeying La Place's law.

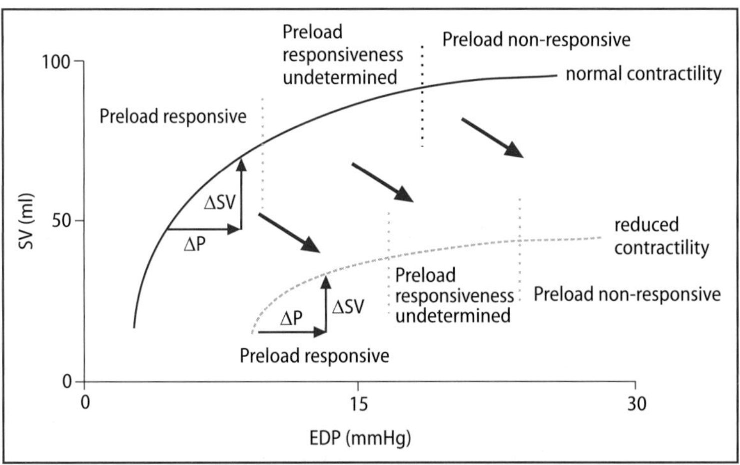

Fig. 1. Schematic representation of the classical cardiac function curve: Stroke volume (SV) versus end-diastolic filling pressure (EDP). The dashed line denotes reduced cardiac contractility (or increased afterload). The domains of preload responsiveness and non-responsiveness are indicated. For the undetermined domain, the increase in SV for a given preload is determined by cardiac function (or afterload).

Figure 1 depicts the classical cardiac function curve relating cardiac output (stroke volume/work) to end-diastolic filling pressure (of either ventricle). This relation depends on contractility and afterload. In hearts with impaired (ventricular) contractility and systolic dysfunction, the function curve is displaced downward and to the right. The plateau of the curve is thus displaced also. Indeed, the idea that hearts with systolic dysfunction need relatively high filling pressures to optimize their output is widely accepted. **Figure 2** schematically depicts the relationship between end-diastolic filling pressure and volume, i.e., compliance, according to two states of diastolic function. As indicated, the volume domain (A) is associated with a low but increasing preload of the heart, while in the pressure domain (B), pressures will rise more than volumes when overfilling the heart at high and further increasing preload. The range of volumes versus those of pressures and their relative predictive values for changes in cardiac output depends on the position on the compliance curve (i.e., cardiac size) and the position and shape of the curve (i.e., diastolic function). In other words, low volumes and changes thereof may better predict and monitor preload responsiveness and operation in the steep part of the cardiac function curve than (changes in) pressures, particularly in (near-) normal hearts. The curvilinearity of the cardiac function curve relating cardiac output (stroke volume) to filling pressure and of the diastolic pressure-volume curve contribute to the linearity of the relationship between cardiac output (stroke volume) on the one hand and filling volume on the other in the steep part of the function curve (**Fig. 3**). Indeed, the relation between ventricular stroke work or power, i.e., stroke volume or cardiac output multiplied by mean arterial pressure, respectively, to ventricular end-diastolic volumes is linear and reflects one contractile status, independently of afterload (and heart rate) [13, 36, 45]. This is termed preload-recruitable stroke work or preload-adjusted maximal power, respectively. The relation between end-diastolic volume and stroke volume or cardiac output alone is also linear in most circumstances, as demonstrated in healthy volunteers or critically ill patients [16, 28] and can be denoted as preload-recruitable stroke volume or cardiac output. This has not been widely appreciated, however, when stroke volume/cardiac output to end-diastolic volume relations have been depicted as curvilinear relationships. Nevertheless, the indices can be modified by changes in arterial pressure and thus afterload. The linear relation implies that at low volumes, in the steep part of the cardiac function curve, fractional increases in volumes and blood flow are greater than at higher fill-

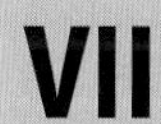

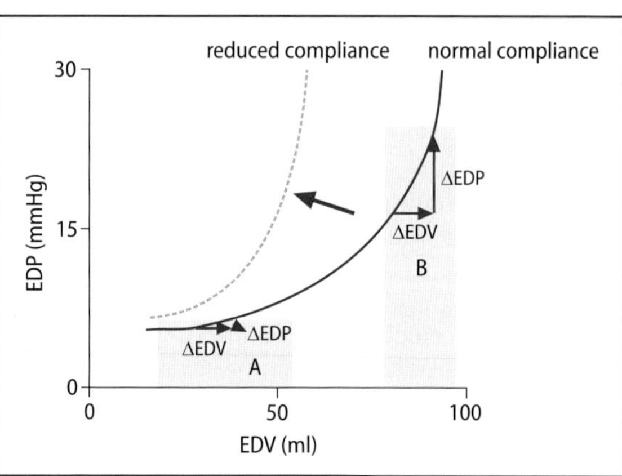

Fig. 2. Schematic representation of cardiac compliance: Diastolic pressure-volume curve. A denotes the volume domain (see text) and B the pressure domain in a normally compliant heart. For a given rise in end-diastolic volume (EDV), the end-diastolic pressure (EDP) will increase to a lesser degree in the volume domain compared to the pressure domain. Dashed line denotes a heart with diastolic dysfunction and reduced compliance.

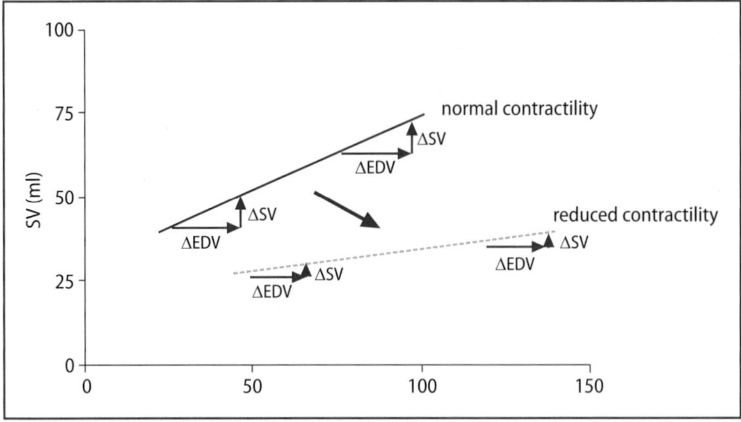

Fig. 3. Schematic representation of ventricular recruitable stroke volume (SV): A linear relation with end-diastolic volume (EDV). The dashed line denotes a state of impaired contractility or increased afterload. With increasing volume, the fractional rise in stroke volume decreases.

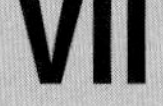

ing volumes, in the plateau of the classical cardiac function curve, until the heart cannot further dilate (and filling pressures rapidly rise). Following systolic dysfunction, the curve is displaced downward and to the right, suggesting that dilated hearts need more volume to attain the plateau cardiac output.

The relations between volumes and pressures may have consequences for the predictive and monitoring value of either type of variable for preload responsiveness in normal and abnormal hearts with systolic or diastolic dysfunction. The graphs may help to understand these relative merits (and detriments). Indeed, despite numerous clinical studies over the last few decades, the controversy between pressures and volumes has not been solved yet. In (near) normally functioning hearts of healthy volunteers, septic patients, or patients after uncomplicated coronary artery surgery, for example, filling volumes proved better predictors and monitors of preload responsiveness than filling pressures [2, 4, 6, 14, 15, 19, 21, 22, 24, 25, 29, 46]. This may have contributed to the lack of demonstrable effect of pulmonary artery catheterization on morbidity and outcome of (groups of) critically ill patients. In dilated hearts following systolic dysfunction, however, pressure (changes) may better predict preload responsiveness than volume (changes), when rightward displacement of the function curve has shifted preload into the pressure domain of the pressure-volume curve. Thus, cardiac dilation increases the value of pressures over volumes in predicting operation in the (less than normal) steep part of the cardiac function curve [48]. Wagner and Leatherman [20] found that the PAOP was a better predictor of preload responsiveness in critically ill (septic) patients than the right ventricular end-diastolic volume, suggesting predominant left ventricular dysfunction in their study population rendering the PAOP of greater value than end-diastolic volume [20]. Mundigler et al. [49] found, in non-surgical cardiac patients, that pressures better predicted preload responsiveness upon fluid loading than volumes, when the left ventricular ejection fraction was $< 35\,\%$. We found that after valvular surgery compared to coronary surgery, pressures were of greater value than volumes in predicting and monitoring preload responsiveness to fluid loading, whereas after coronary surgery volumes were of greater value than pressures [50]. The predictive value for fluid responsiveness of the PAOP, in particular associated with a low ejection fraction, suggested that left ventricular dysfunction and dilatation had rendered preload responsiveness more dependent on left ventricular end-diastolic pressure than volume. This could imply greater (monitoring) benefit of pulmonary artery catheters after valvular than coronary artery surgery [50]. The relevance for other types of systolic (left ventricular) dysfunction, in the course of cardiogenic or septic shock, for instance remains to be studied. In subnormally compliant hearts, in the course of ventricular hypertrophy for instance, pressures may also better predict preload responsiveness in the steep portion of the cardiac function curve, than volumes. Swenson et al. [30] observed that hypertrophied left ventricles indeed need higher than normal PAOP to optimize output.

A final factor that may determine the relative value of pressures and volumes in assessing preload responsiveness is ventricular interaction, when loading of right and left ventricles is dissimilar and dysfunction of the right ventricle becomes the limiting factor in the response to fluid loading [21, 24, 25, 34, 36, 45]. This may also explain in part the varying predictive values of left and right-sided measurements, including volumes, among studies and populations [5, 10, 20, 22–24, 33–35, 37, 38, 46]. Indeed, mild pulmonary hypertension is a frequent complication of sepsis, trauma, burns, cardiac valvular disease and surgery, thereby placing a load on the right ventricle [15, 16, 34, 37, 46]. The right ventricle dilates and is less capable of accommodating fluid and responding by an increase in cardiac output, even in view of normal left ventricular function. The series effect can be supplemented by a leftward shift of the septum that may decrease left ventricular compliance [16, 35, 46]. Particularly during hypotension and resultant right coronary hypoperfusion, the right ventricle may further fail, dilate upon fluid loading, and preclude a rise in cardiac output, as demonstrated in patients with septic shock [46].

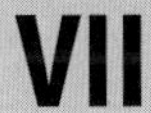

A large PEEP-induced increase in expiratory lung volume may increase right ventricular afterload to the extent that a fall in venous return, by an increase in transmitted airway pressure, is overwhelmed and the right ventricle enlarges, while left ventricular dimensions and cardiac output fall. This type of ventricular interaction may respond less well to fluid loading to restore cardiac output than when biventricular dimensions fall following a predominant decrease in venous return with increasing transmitted PEEP. Biventricular filling volumes may then better help to explain hemodynamic changes than pressures, since atmospheric pressure-referenced filling pressures increase with PEEP [37].

The consequences of pressure- versus volume-guidance of fluid therapy for patient-centered outcomes are unclear. Paradoxically, volume-guided treatment may result in more positive fluid balances than pressure-guided treatment, even though the former is supposedly more accurate and thus better capable of limiting overhydration than the latter, after cardiac surgery or burn injury [1, 42].

Conclusion

The relative predictive value of static filling pressures and volumes for the cardiac output response to preload changes depends on biventricular systolic and diastolic function. This implies that both pressures and volumes may be needed to predict and monitor fluid responses, but pressure monitoring (by pulmonary artery catheter) could suffice in some and volume monitoring (for instance by transpulmonary thermodilution) in other patients. In the absence of volume measurements, a delta filling pressure protocol may be both effective and safe, irrespective of ventilator settings in mechanically ventilated patients. The ultimate guide to fluid therapy, when clinically needed may, however, be frequently intermittent or, preferably, continuous and reliable cardiac output monitoring to prevent fluid overloading by discontinuing fluid infusions when cardiac output does not further increase.

References

1. Goepfert MS, Reuter DA, Akyol D, Lamm P, Kilger E, Goetz AE (2007) Goal-directed fluid management reduces vasopressor and catecholamine use in cardiac surgery patients. Intensive Care Med 33: 96–103
2. Brock H, Gabriel C, Bibi D, Necek S (2002) Monitoring intravascular volumes for postoperative volume therapy. Eur J Anaesthesiol 19: 288–294
3. Bendjelid K, Romand JA (2003) Fluid responsiveness in mechanically ventilated patients: a review of indices used in intensive care. Intensive Care Med 29: 352–360
4. Michard F, Alaya S, Zarka V, Bahloul M, Richard C, Teboul JL (2003) Global end-diastolic volume as an indicator of cardiac preload in patients with septic shock. Chest 124: 1900–1908
5. Reuter DA, Felbinger TW, Schmidt C, et al (2002) Stroke volume variations for assessment of cardiac responsiveness to volume loading in mechanically ventilated patients after cardiac surgery. Intensive Care Med 28: 392–398
6. Marx G, Cope T, McCrossan L, et al (2004) Assessing fluid responsiveness by stroke volume variation in mechanically ventilated patients with severe sepsis. Eur J Anaesthesiol 21: 132–138
7. De Backer D, Heenen S, Piagnerelli M, Koch M, Vincent JL (2005) Pulse pressure variations to predict fluid responsiveness: influence of tidal volume. Intensive Care Med 31: 517–523
8. Hofer CK, Müller SM, Furrer L, Klaghofer R, Genoni M, Zollinger A (2005) Stroke volume and pulse pressure variation for prediction of fluid responsiveness in patients undergoing off-pump coronary artery bypass grafting. Chest 128: 848–854
9. Preisman S, Kogan S, Berkenstadt H, Perel A (2005) Predicting fluid responsiveness in patients undergoing cardiac surgery: functional haemodynamic parameters including the respiratory systolic variation test and static preload indicators. Br J Anaesth 95: 746–755
10. Reuter DA, Goepfert MS, Goresch T, Schmoeckel M, Kilger E, Goetz AE (2005) Assessing fluid responsiveness during open chest conditions. Br J Anaesth 94: 318–323
11. Wiesenack C, Fiegl C, Keyser A, Prasser C, Keyl C (2005) Assessment of fluid responsiveness in mechanically ventilated cardiac surgical patients. Eur J Anaesthesiol 22: 658–665
12. Axler O, Tousignant C, Thompson CR, et al (1997) Small hemodynamic effect of typical rapid volume infusion in critically ill patients. Crit Care Med 25: 965–970
13. Verheij J, van Lingen A, Beishuizen A, et al (2006) Cardiac response is greater for colloid than saline fluid loading after cardiac or vascular surgery. Intensive Care Med 32: 1030–1038
14. Kumar A, Anel R, Bunnell E, et al (2004) Pulmonary artery occlusion pressure and central venous pressure fail to predict ventricular filling volume, cardiac performance, or the response to volume infusion in normal subjects. Crit Care Med 32: 691–699
15. Calvin JE, Driedger AA, Sibbald WJ (1981) The hemodynamic effect of rapid fluid infusion in critically ill patients. Surgery 90: 61–76
16. Reuse C, Vincent JL, Pinsky MR (1990) Measurements of right ventricular volumes during fluid challenges. Chest 98: 1450–1454
17. Vincent JL, Weil MH (2006) Fluid challenge revisited. Crit Care Med 34: 1333–1337
18. Weil MH, Henning RJ (1979) New concepts in the diagnosis and fluid treatment of circulatory shock. Thirteenth annual Becton, Dickinson and Company Oscar Schwidetsky memorial lecture. Anesth Analg 58: 124–132
19. Hinder F, Poelaert JL, Schmidt C, et al (1998) Assessment of cardiovascular volume status by transoesophageal echocardiography and dye dilution during cardiac surgery. Eur J Anaesthesiol 15: 633–640
20. Wagner JG, Leatherman JW (1998) Right ventricular end-diastolic volume as a predictor of the hemodynamic response to a fluid challenge. Chest 113: 1048–1054
21. Wiesenack C, Prasser C, Keyl C, Rödig G (2001) Assessment of intrathoracic blood volume as an indicator of cardiac preload: single transpulmonary thermodilution technique versus

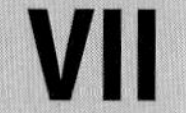

assessment of pressure preload parameters derived from a pulmonary artery catheter. J Cardiothorac Vasc Anesth 15: 584–588
22. Reuter DA, Felbinger TW, Moerstedt K, et al (2002) Intrathoracic blood volume index measured by thermodilution for preload monitoring after cardiac surgery. J Cardiothorac Vasc Anesth 16: 191–195
23. Hofer CK, Furrer L, Matter-Ensner S, et al (2005) Volumetric preload measurement by thermodilution: a comparison with transoesophageal echocardiography. Br J Anaesth 94: 748–755
24. Wiesenack C, Fiegl C, Keyser A, Laule S, Prasser C, Keyl C (2005) Continuously assessed right ventricular end-diastolic volume as a marker of cardiac preload and fluid responsiveness in mechanically ventilated cardiac surgical patients. Crit Care 9:R226-R233
25. Osman D, Ridel C, Ray P, et al (2007) Cardiac filling pressures are not appropriate to predict hemodynamic response to volume challenge. Crit Care Med 35: 64–68
26. Marik PE, Baram M, Vahid B (2008) Does central venous pressure predict fluid responsiveness? A systematic review of the literature and the tale of seven mares. Chest 134: 172–178
27. Magder S, Bafaqeeh F (2007) The clinical role of central venous pressure measurements. J Intensive Care Med 22: 44–51
28. Nixon JV, Murray RG, Leonard PD, Mitchell JH, Blomqvist CG (1982) Effect of large variations in preload on left ventricular performance characteristics in normal subjects. Circulation 65: 698–703
29. Lichtwarck-Aschoff M, Zeravik J, Pfeiffer UJ (1992) Intrathoracic blood volume accurately reflects circulatory volume status in critically ill patients with mechanical ventilation. Intensive Care Med 18: 142–147
30. Swenson JD, Bull D, Stringham J (2001) Subjective assessment of left ventricular preload using transesophageal echocardiography: corresponding pulmonary artery occlusion pressures. J Cardiothorac Vasc Anesth 15: 580–583
31. Bouchard MJ, Denault A, Couture P, et al (2004) Poor correlation between hemodynamic and echocardiographic indexes of left ventricular performance in the operating room and intensive care unit. Crit Care Med 32: 644–648
32. Veillard-Baron A, Charron C, Chergui K, Peyrouset O, Jardin F (2006) Bedside echocardiographic evalation of hemodynamics in sepsis: is a qualitative evaluation sufficient ? Intensive Care Med 32: 1547–1552
33. Yu M, Takiguchi S, Takanishi D, Myers S, McNamara JJ (1995) Evaluation of the clinical usefulness of thermodilution volumetric catheters. Crit Care Med 23: 681–686
34. Chang MC, Blinman TA, Rutherford EJ, Nelson LD, Morris JA Jr (1996) Preload assessment in trauma patients during large-volume shock resuscitation. Arch Surg 131: 728–731
35. Kraut EJ, Owings JT, Anderson JT, Hanowell L, Moore P (1997) Right ventricular volumes overestimate left ventricular preload in critically ill patients. J Trauma 42: 839–846
36. Squara P, Journois D, Estagnasié P, et al (1997) Elastic energy as an index of right ventricular filling. Chest 111: 351–358
37. Cheatham ML, Nelson LD, Chang MC, Safcsak K (1998) Right ventricular end-diastolic volume index as a predictor of preload status in patients on positive end-expiratory pressure. Crit Care Med 26: 1801–1806
38. Spöhr F, Hettrich E, Bauer H, Haas U, Martin E, Böttiger BW (2007) Comparison of two methods for enhanced continuous circulatory monitoring in patients with septic shock. Intensive Care Med 33: 1805–1810
39. De Simone R, Wolf I, Mottl-Link S, et al (2005) Intraoperative assessment of right ventricular volume and function. Eur J Cardiothorac Surg 27: 988–993
40. Gödje O, Peyerl M, Seebauer T, Lamm P, Mair H, Reichart B (1998) Central venous pressure, pulmonary capillary wedge pressure and intrathoracic blood volumes as preload indicators in cardiac surgery patients. Eur J Cardiothorac Surg 13: 533–540
41. Gödje O, Peyerl M, Seebauer T, Dewald O, Reichart B (1998) Reproducibility of double indicator dilution measurements of intrathoracic blood volume compartments, extravascular lung water and liver function. Chest 113: 1070–1077
42. Holm C, Melcer B, Hörbrand F, Wörl HH, Henckel von Donnersmarck G, Mühlbauer W (2000) Intrathoracic blood volume as an end point in resuscitation of the severely burned: an observational study of 24 patients. J Trauma 48: 728–734

43. Combes A, Berneau JB, Luyt CE, Trouillet JL (2004) Estimation of left ventricular systolic function by single transpulmonary thermodilution. Intensive Care Med 30: 1377–1383
44. Calvin JE, Driedger AA, Sibbald WJ (1981) Does the pulmonary capillary wedge pressure predict left ventricular preload in critically ill patients? Crit Care Med 9: 437–443
45. Hansen RM, Viquerat CE, Matthay MA, et al (1986) Poor correlation between pulmonary arterial wedge pressure and left ventricular end-diastolic volume after coronary artery bypass graft surgery. Anesthesiology 64: 764–770
46. Schneider AJ, Teule GJ, Groeneveld AB, Nauta J, Heidendal GA, Thijs LG (1988) Biventricular performance during volume loading in patients with early septic shock, with emphasis on the right ventricle: a combined hemodynamic and radionuclide study. Am Heart J 116: 103–112
47. Norton JM (2001) Toward consistent definitions for preload and afterload. Adv Physiol Educ 25: 53–61
48. Cheung AT, Savino JS, Weiss SJ, Aukburg SJ, Berlin JA (1994) Echocardiographic and hemodynamic indexes of left ventricular preload in patients with normal and abnormal ventricular function. Anesthesiology 81: 376–387
49. Mundigler G, Heinze G, Zehetgruber M, Gabriel H, Siostrzonek P (2000) Limitations of the transpulmonary indicator dilution method for assessment of preload changes in critically ill patients with reduced left ventriuclar function. Crit Care Med 28: 2231–2237
50. Breukers RMBGE, Trof RJ, de Wilde RBP, et al (2009) Relative value of pressures and volumes in assessing fluid responsiveness after valvular and coronary artery surgery. Eur J Cardiothorac Surg 35: 62–68

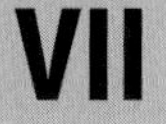

Update on Preload Indexes: More Volume than Pressure

G. Della Rocca, M.G. Costa, and L. Spagnesi

Introduction

Hemodynamic assessment is of primary importance in guiding volume therapy and vasoactive drug administration to optimize organ perfusion and to avoid fluid overload with lung edema in critically ill patients [1, 2]. Clinical examination has been shown to be of minimal value in detecting inadequate cardiac preload [3]. Several methods for preload determination, such as central venous pressure (CVP) and pulmonary artery occlusion pressure (PAOP), have been widely used [4]. Cardiac filling pressures are not always accurate indicators of ventricular preload because of erroneous readings of pressure tracings, discrepancy between measured and transmural pressures, and changes in ventricular compliance [5]. In recent years, right ventricular end-diastolic volume (RVEDV) evaluated by fast response pulmonary artery catheters (PACs), left ventricular end-diastolic area (LVEDA) measured by echocardiography, and the intrathoracic blood volume (ITBV) evaluated by the transpulmonary indicator dilution technique, have been proposed to assess cardiac preload at the bedside [6–8].

Filling Pressures (CVP and PAOP)

It is reasoned that cardiac output ultimately depends on stroke volume from the left heart and, based on the Frank-Starling relationship, the better the filling of the left heart, the better the forward output. Since left heart dysfunction can occur without major right heart dysfunction, it is argued that it is important to evaluate left-sided rather than right-sided pressures when determining optimal cardiac filling. This reasoning, however, ignores some important physiological considerations and can potentially lead to errors in clinical management. First, in the steady state, cardiac output must equal venous return. Second, it needs to be appreciated that the heart does not control cardiac output by creating an arterial pressure which pushes the blood around the body, but rather maintains cardiac output by lowering right atrial pressure and allowing blood to drain back to the heart so it can be pumped out again [9–11].

CVP is the pressure recorded from the right atrium or superior vena cava. It is measured in almost all patients in intensive care units (ICU) throughout the world. CVP is frequently used to make decisions regarding the administration of fluids and international clinical guidelines recommended the use of CVP as an endpoint for fluid resuscitation [12]. The basis for using CVP to guide fluid management comes from the dogma that it reflects intravascular volume; it is widely believed that patients with a low CVP are volume depleted while patients with a high CVP level are volume overloaded. Since CVP plays such a central role in the fluid management strategy of critically ill patients, Marik and colleagues recently systematically reviewed the evidence that supports this practice [5]. The results of this systematic review are first, that there is no association between CVP and circulating blood volume, and second that CVP does not predict fluid responsiveness across a wide spectrum of clinical conditions. In none of the studies included in the systematic review, was CVP able to predict these variables. It is important to note that none of the studies included in the analysis took the positive end-expiratory pressure (PEEP) levels or changes in intrathoracic pressure into account when recording CVP. This is important because right ventricular filling is dependent on the transmural right atrial pressure gradient rather than on the CVP alone [13]. However, in clinical daily practice, transmural filling pressures are rarely if ever calculated. Based on their findings, the authors affirmed that if fluid resuscitation is guided by CVP, it is likely that patients will have volume overload and pulmonary edema [5]. It is possible, however, that resuscitation guided by CVP will result in inadequate volume replacement. The Surviving Sepsis Campaign guidelines for management of severe sepsis and septic shock recommend a CVP of 8 to 12 mmHg as the "goal of the initial resuscitation of sepsis induced hypoperfusion" and "a higher targeted CVP of 12–15 mmHg" in patients receiving mechanical ventilation [14]. Based on results from their systematic review, Marik and co-workers suggest that these recommendations should be revisited [5].

The PAOP is obtained following inflation of the balloon at the tip of the PAC. In theory, after inflation of the balloon there is a continuous column of blood from the pulmonary artery to the left ventricle during diastole. The end of diastole can be identified by the 'a' wave of the PAOP curve which coincides with the 'p' wave on the electrocardiogram (EKG). Consequently, PAOP is considered an approximation of the left ventricular end-diastolic pressure (LVEDP). For a given left ventricular compliance, LVEDP is proportional to the left ventricular end-diastolic volume (LVEDV). As described by the Frank-Starling relationship, the force of ventricular contraction is proportional to the length of the myocardial fibers, as determined by LVEDV. Therefore, PAOP can be considered an indicator of preload. However, the assumption that PAOP always induces a continuous blood column may not be valid in some cases. First, when the catheter tip is in West zone 1 or 2, the increase in alveolar pressure interrupts the blood column. Consequently, PAOP is higher than end-diastolic pulmonary pressure and pulmonary venous pressure. To address this problem, the catheter tip must be in West zone 3. If this is the case, then the following relationship will be present during the respiratory cycle in mechanically ventilated patients: End-diastolic pulmonary pressure > PAOP, and ΔPAOP/ΔPAP> 1.5 (where PAP is the pulmonary artery pressure). Second, in mitral valve disease, PAOP reflects the increase in left atrial pressure and not the LVEDP. Finally, all changes in ventricular compliance (the LVEDP/LVEDV relationship) induce overestimation of preload by PAOP. Modification of left ventricular compliance may result from numerous pathologies, including myocardial ischemia and failure, myocardial hypertrophy or dilatation, septic shock, aortic disease, and pericardial disease [15].

It is well known that an increased gradient between PAOP and diastolic PAP indicates increased pulmonary resistance or increased pulmonary blood flow, or both. In these settings, pulmonary capillary pressure (Pcp) may exceed PAOP [16]. Therefore, an increased gradient between diastolic PAP and PAOP is considered a valuable indicator of increased Pcp. The resistance between pulmonary artery and left atrium can be simply modelled as one artery resistance and one venous resistance in series, with a capacitance located in the capillary bed. Because of this series resistance with a capillary capacitance, the Pcp can be measured from the pressure decay profile after occlusion of the balloon. After occlusion of the pulmonary artery, the downstream blood is discharged into the capillary across venous resistance [16]. The initial rapid drop in pressure reflects the Pcp as the downstream blood is trapped in the capillary bed and equilibrates with the Pcp. The following slower drop in pressure is determined by the discharge of blood across the pulmonary venous resistance and tends toward the PAOP. Using a graphical method, the Pcp is estimated at the bedside as the point at which the pressure curve deviates from the slope of the first decay.

Because Pcp is the main determinant of efflux between capillary lumen and alveolar space, whether the integrity of alveolar-capillary barrier is impaired or not, its measurement may be of interest in pathologies such as acute respiratory distress syndrome (ARDS) to guide fluid loading [17]. A Pcp threshold value must be determined above which pulmonary edema develops, and pulmonary compliance and gas exchange are impaired. Fluid loading should then be limited to this threshold value as much as possible, taking into consideration the perfusion of other organs. Further studies are necessary to explore the utility of such a strategy and to develop new tools for automatic measurement of Pcp.

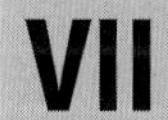

Kumar et al. [18] tried to assess the relationship between pressure estimates of ventricular preload (PAOP and CVP), end-diastolic ventricular volumes, and cardiac performance in healthy volunteers. These investigators collected data before and after the infusion of a large volume (3 l) of saline solution over 3 hours. They used radionuclide cineangiography and volumetric echocardiography to determine cardiac output and stroke volume. They concluded that cardiac compliance was highly variable and as a consequence, neither CVP nor PAOP appeared to be a useful predictor of ventricular preload with respect to optimizing cardiac performance.

The main reason for the lack of correlation between values of CVP and blood volume is that the body does everything possible to maintain homeostasis; an adequate transmural CVP is a must for cardiovascular function. The most accurate measurement of 'volume status' would be the mean cardiac filling pressure, which cannot be measured in a clinical setting [9].

Continuous Right Ventricular End-diastolic Volume (cRVEDV)

According to the Frank-Starling principle, the vigor of cardiac contraction relates directly to muscle fiber length at end-diastole. While monitoring of muscle fiber length would be ideal, it has been shown that end-diastolic volume of the left ventricle is a better indicator of muscle fiber length than PAOP [19, 20]. These relationships are also valid for the right ventricle. Current technology, based on echocardiography or thermodilution, allows us to estimate ventricular end-diastolic volume [7, 21–22]. There is indeed a renewed interest in PAC-related bedside devices that allow calculation of right ventricular volumes based on the thermodilution technique. The first generation of such catheters was introduced in the 1980s, and the current generation, introduced in the late 1990s, allows continuous monitoring of cardiac output or index, right ventricular ejection fraction (cRVEF), and right ventricular end-diastolic volume index (cRVEDVI).

The new cRVEF algorithm generates a relaxation waveform resembling the bolus thermodilution washout decay curve. The waveform is based on the repeating On-

Off input signal and is generated by accumulating the temperature change for each Of and Off segment of the input signal. cRVEF is calculated based on the estimation of the exponential decay time constant (τ) of this curve and heart rate (HR):

$$cRVEF = 1 - \exp[-60 / (\tau \times HR)].$$

cRVEDV is calculated as (cardiac output/HR) / cRVEF.

Several studies have confirmed that RVEDVI shows higher correlation with cardiac output than CVP and PAOP [22–24]. De Simone and colleagues demonstrated that intraoperative assessment of right ventricular volumes by means of thermodilution and transesophageal three-dimensional echocardiography (TEE) is feasible [23]; they reported that RVEDVI by thermodilution was larger than that determined by echocardiography, mainly due to the geometry of the right ventricle and the differences in technique. Despite these different results, the presence of significant agreement in measuring RVEF confirmed that these two methods can be reliably used for serially measuring RVEDVI and right ventricular function during surgery [23]. Recently Wiesenack and co-workers showed that cardiac preload is more reliably reflected by cRVEDVI than by CVP, PAOP or LVEDA index (LVEDAI), but that cRVEDVI could not predict the response to a fluid challenge in patients undergoing elective coronary surgery [24].

VII

Hofer and colleagues compared volume preload monitoring using two different thermodilution techniques with left ventricular preload assessment by TEE [22]. They studied 20 patients undergoing elective cardiac surgery with preserved left-right ventricular function after induction of anesthesia. Global end diastolic volume index (GEDVI), cRVEDVI, LVEDAI, and stroke volume index (SVI) increased significantly after fluid loading. The correlation coefficient for ΔGEDVI and ΔSVI was stronger ($r^2 = 0.576$) than for ΔcRVEDVI and ΔSVI ($r^2 = 0.267$). The authors concluded that GEDVI assessed by the PiCCO system gives a better reflection of echocardiographic changes in left ventricular preload in response to fluid replacement therapy, than cRVEDVI measured by a modified PAC.

More recently, in a multicenter study performed during liver transplantation, we found that cRVEDVI was a better reflection of preload than CVP and PAOP, based on the strong correlation between SVI and cRVEDVI [25]. We observed that an increase in cRVEDVI of 1 ml/m^2 led to an increase in SVI of 0.25 ml/m^2 while the correlations between SVI and CVP and PAOP were less strong. The correlations between SVI and cRVEDVI, PAOP, CVP, and cRVEF were similar at different stages of the procedure, and the correlations between SVI and cRVEDVI, PAOP, and CVP were not influenced by cRVEF [25].

Some limitations have to be considered for cRVEDVI monitoring: cRVEDVI shows a delayed reactivity to rapid changes in intravascular volume; also, inaccuracies in measurement of cRVEDVI can result from poor positioning of the injectate port in relation to the tricuspid valve and of the thermistor in relation to the pulmonary valve. Additionally, sinus tachycardia and cardiac arrhythmias can also affect the accuracy of measurements. Finally, mathematical coupling (due to the fact that cRVEDVI is calculated by using the SVI that, in turn, is derived from cardiac index [CI] measurements) is a potential problem, although Chang et al. and Nelson et al. concluded that this was not a real concern [26, 27].

Global-end Diastolic Volume and Intrathoracic Blood Volume

A transpulmonary indicator dilution technique obtained with the injection done through a central venous line and the change in temperature detected in a thermistor embedded in an arterial catheter is now available (PiCCO System, Pulsion Medical System, Munich, Germany). Cardiac output can be measured by the transpulmonary indicator dilution technique and, after calibration, the system also provides a continuous pulse contour derived cardiac output, a method which was first described by Wesseling et al. [28]. The transpulmonary indicator dilution technique allows estimations of intrathoracic volumes (GEDV, ITBV) and extravascular lung water (EVLW). Experimental and clinical data have demonstrated that single arterial thermodilution-derived ITBV correlates well with the respective values measured by the double indicator technique [29, 30]. The commercially available device currently using this technology uses a linear equation with a coefficient of 1.25 and an intercept of 0 to estimate ITBV from measured GEDV values: ITBVI= 1.25 x GEDV (ml).

ITBV has been suggested as a sensitive indicator of cardiac preload as volume changes preferentially alter the volume in the intrathoracic compartment which serves as the primary reservoir for the left ventricle. In the last few years many papers have confirmed the ability of the ITBVI to predict preload in various clinical settings [31–34] (**Table 1**).

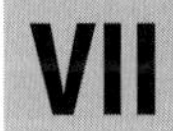

Table 1. Relationships between intravascular volume and filling pressures and stroke volume index (SVI)/ cardiac index (CI).

Authors	Year	Clinical Setting	Patients	Data analyzed	r
Gödje [35]	1998	CABG	30	GEDVI vs SVI	0.82
Sakka [31]	1999	ICU (septic shock)	57	ΔITBVI vs ΔSVI	0.67
Gödje [36]	2000	Cardiac surgery	40	GEDVI vs SVI	0.73
Buhre [39]	2000	Neurosurgery	10	ΔITBVI vs ΔSVI	0.78
Bindels [41]	2000	Critically ill patients	45	ΔITBVI vs ΔSVI	0.81
Holm [45]	2000	Burn patients	24	ITBVI vs CI	0.45*
Della Rocca [33]	2002	Orthotopic liver transplantation	60	ITBVI vs SVI	0.55*
Della Rocca [34]	2002	Lung transplantation	50	ITBVI vs SVI	0.41*
Hofer [40]	2002	Pneumoperitoneum	30	ITBVI vs SVI	0.79
Schiffman [43]	2002	Pediatric ICU	10	GEDVI vs SVI	0.76
Reuter [37]	2002	ICU cardiac surgery	19	ΔITBVI vs ΔSVI	0.85
Michard [21]	2003	Septic shock	36	ΔGEDVI vs ΔSVI	0.72
Kuntscher [43]	2003	Burn patients	18	ITBVI vs CI	0.74
Neumann [48]	2005	Spontaneous breathing	15	ΔGEDVI vs ΔSVI	0.34*
Hofer [22]	2005	CABG	20	ΔGEDVI vs ΔSVI ΔcRVEDVI vs ΔSVI	0.576* 0.267
Huber [32]	2008	Pancreatitis	24	ITBVI vs CI CVP vs CI	0.566 0.089

* = r^2; CABG: coronary artery bypass graft; cRVEDVI: continuous right ventricular end-diastolic volume index; CVP: central venous pressure; GEDVI: global end-diastolic volume index; ICU: intensive care unit; ITBVI: intrathoracic blood volume index; LVEDAI: left ventricular end-diastolic area index

The accuracy of ITBV as a measure of preload was prospectively assessed by Lichtwarck-Aschoff et al. in 1992 [8] in a group of ventilated patients with acute respiratory failure. This study demonstrated a much tighter correlation between changes in ITBVI and CI than between changes in either CVP or PAOP and cardiac index.

In the last ten years, many authors have described their experience with the transpulmonary indicator dilution technique in cardiac surgical patients, both intra- and post-operatively [35–38]. Gödje and colleagues compared filling pressures with ITBV and GEDV in 30 patients after coronary artery by-pass grafting (CABG) [35]. The linear regression analysis was computed between changes in preload-dependent left ventricular SVI and cardiac index and the corresponding, presumably preload-indicating, parameters, CVP, PAOP, ITBV, and GEDV. No correlation was found between ΔCVP compared with ΔSVI or ΔCI, and ΔPAOP compared with ΔSVI or ΔCI. ΔITBVI correlated well with ΔSVI and ΔCI: coefficients were 0.76 and 0.83, respectively. Correlation coefficients of ΔGEDVI compared with ΔSVI/ΔCI were 0.82 and 0.87, respectively. Gödje and co-workers also performed a study focused on preload in heart-transplanted patients in whom ITBVI and GEDVI were significantly correlated with changes in SVI ($r = 0.65$ and $r = 0.73$, respectively), while CVP and PAOP failed ($r = 0.23$ and $r = 0.06$, respectively) [36].

VII

In cardiac surgery patients, Goepfert and colleagues applied a goal-directed therapy based on volumetric data (GEDVI) [38]. These authors observed that catecholamine and vasopressor dependence was shorter than in the control group managed according to CVP, mean arterial pressure (MAP), and clinical evaluation (187 ± 70 vs 1458 ± 197 min). The goal-directed therapy group received more colloids (6918 ± 242 vs 5514 ± 171 ml) and less vasopressor (0.73 ± 0.32 vs 6.67 ± 1.21 mg) and catecholamine (0.01 ± 0.01 vs 0.83 ± 0.27 mg) than the control group. The duration of mechanical ventilation (12.6 ± 3.6 vs 15.4 ± 4.3 h) and time to achieve a fit for ICU discharge status was also shorter in the goal-directed therapy group (25 ± 13 vs 33 ± 17 h). The authors concluded that perioperative hemodynamic management based on early optimization of preload and cardiac output using the transpulmonary indicator dilution technique led to improved treatment of patients undergoing cardiac surgery [38].

Other studies on the PiCCO system have been performed during neurosurgery, laparoscopic procedures, major abdominal surgery in the Trendelenburg position, and in critically ill patients [39–42]. A significant increase in ITBV was observed after induction of pneumoperitoneum, persisting in the supine, head-up and head-down positions [40]. The authors concluded that the onset of pneumoperitoneum, even with moderate intra-abdominal pressures, is associated with an increased ITBV in American Society of Anesthesiologists (ASA) I-II patients.

We investigated pressure and volume preload indexes during anesthesia in patients undergoing double lung transplantation. The main finding of this study was a fairly good correlation between ITBVI and SVI ($r^2 = 0.41$, $p < 0.0001$), while PAOP correlated poorly with SVI ($r^2 = 0.01$, not significant) [33]. We also found that ITBV better reflected preload in hyperdynamic patients receiving liver transplantation (ITBVI vs SVI, $r^2 = 0.55$) [34].

Sakka and colleagues, comparing each preload variable (CVP, PAOP, and ITBVI) under clinical routine conditions, in the early phase of hemodynamic stabilization of 57 critically ill patients with sepsis or septic shock, found a significant correlation between ITBVI and SVI, while CVP and PAOP did not correlate [31]. The authors, confirming results obtained by Lichtwarck-Aschoff and co-workers under controlled conditions [8], concluded that ITBVI is also a more reliable preload indicator than cardiac filling pressures in critically ill patients with sepsis or septic shock.

Michard and co-workers studied 36 patients with septic shock and evaluated GEDV and CVP after fluid challenge and dobutamine tests [21]. GEDV, CVP, SVI, and CI significantly increased after volume loading and changes in GEDVI were correlated with changes in SVI ($r = 0.72$, $p < 0.001$), while changes in CVP were not. Dobutamine infusion induced an increase in SVI and CI but no significant changes in CVP and GEDVI. The authors concluded that in patients with septic shock, in contrast to CVP, the transpulmonary thermodilution GEDVI behaves as an indicator of cardiac preload.

The transpulmonary indicator dilution technique was also applied by Huber and colleagues in critically ill patients with necrotizing pancreatitis [32]. They evaluated the predictive value of CVP and hematocrit with regard to ITBVI, and correlated these parameters to CI. They reported that absolute values and changes in ITBVI correlated with CI (ITBVI vs CI $r = 0.566$, $p < 0.001$, ΔITBVI vs ΔCI $r = 0.603$, $p < 0.001$) while absolute values as changes in CVP failed to correlate. In this clinical condition, the volumetric preload indicator was also confirmed to be more appropriate for volume management than CVP or hematocrit.

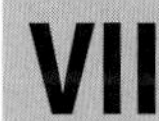

Schiffmann and co-workers demonstrated that the transpulmonary indicator dilution technique enabled the measurement of cardiac output and intravascular volume status in critically ill neonates and infants at the bedside, whereas CVP was not indicative of changes in intravascular volume status [43]. Cecchetti and colleagues investigated the possible correlations between GEDVI and CI and SVI in critically ill pediatric patients to assess whether GEDVI may help in the decision-making process concerning volume loading [44]. They divided the patients into six groups, according to the kind of illness. They reported that GEDVI correlated with CI and SVI in the hemorrhagic shock group ($r^2 = 0.647$ and $r^2 = 0.738$, respectively), and in the cardiogenic shock group ($r^2 = 0.645$ and $r^2 = 0.841$, respectively), and concluded that GEDV may potentially be a useful guide for treating pediatric patients in preload-dependent conditions, such as hemorrhagic and cardiogenic shock.

Further investigation is needed in the burn population as different results have been reported with the transpulmonary indicator dilution technique [45, 46]. Holm et al. introduced ITBVI as a possible endpoint to guide major burn fluid resuscitation [45] while Kuntscher and co-workers found that the transpulmonary indicator dilution technique performed with a single indicator was not suitable to assess ITBV and EVLW in burn shock, although the method was suitable for assessing cardiac output and its derived parameters in this population [46].

Hofer and colleagues studied the new volumetric ejection fraction monitoring system (VoLEF) combined with the PiCCO system for measurements of left and right heart end-diastolic volume by thermodilution in 20 cardiac surgical patients [47]. In this study, both LVEDAI and GEDVI increased significantly after fluid administration, while left heart end-diastolic volume index failed to correlate. The authors concluded that only GEDVI can be recommended as an estimate of left ventricular preload.

Neumann and colleagues demonstrated that changes in GEDV were also linearly correlated with changes in cardiac index in spontaneously breathing patients as 34 % of the changes in cardiac index were explained by changes in the GEDV [48].

Uchino and colleagues conducted a prospective multicenter, multinational study in a cohort of 331 critically ill patients who received hemodynamic monitoring by PAC or PiCCO, according to physician preference, in ICUs from eight hospitals in four countries [49]. Direct comparison showed that the use of PiCCO was associated with a greater positive fluid balance and fewer ventilator-free days. After correcting for confounding factors, the choice of monitoring did not influence major outcomes, while a positive fluid balance was a significant independent predictor of outcome. Future studies may best be targeted at understanding the effect of pursuing different fluid balance regimens rather than different monitoring techniques.

The transpulmonary indicator dilution technique method has some limitations as it is not suitable for patients with severe peripheral vascular disease, those undergoing vascular surgery, or those with other contraindications for femoral artery cannulation.

Conclusion

GEDV, ITBV, and cRVEDV seem to reflect preload in different clinical settings better than filling pressures. CVP and PAOP are not able to identify volume status as the first depends on the relationship between cardiac pump function and venous return and the second is an indicator of pulmonary back pressure rather than of volume status. GEDV and ITBV associated with EVLW give a 'picture' of the critically ill patient, identifying intravascular volume status and lung edema. The last generation of PACs, equipped with cRVEDV and cRVEF monitoring, still remains the only bedside device to evaluate right ventricular function.

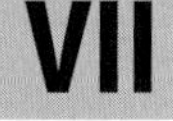

References

1. Slinger PD (1995) Perioperative fluid management for thoracic surgery: the puzzle of postpneumonectomy pulmonary edema. J Cardiothorac Vasc Anesth 9: 442–451
2. Connors AF, Mc Caffee DR, Gray RA (1983) Evaluation of right heart catheterization in the critically ill patient without myocardial infarction. N Engl J Med 308: 263–267
3. Shippy CR, Appel PL, Shoemaker WC (1984) Reliability of clinical monitoring to assess blood volume in critically ill patients. Crit Care Med 12: 107–112
4. Teboul JL, Pinsky MR, Mercat A, et al (2000) Estimating cardiac filling pressure in mechanically ventilated patients with hyperinflation. Crit Care Med 28: 3631–3636
5. Marik PE, Baram M, Vahid B (2008) Does central venous pressure predict fluid responsiveness? A systematic review of the literature and the tale of seven mares. Chest 134: 172–178
6. Reuse C, Vincent JL, Pinsky MR (1990) Measurements of right ventricular volumes during fluid challenge. Chest 98: 1450–1454
7. Tousignant CP, Walsh F, Mazer CD (2000) The use of transesophageal echocardiography for preload assessment in critically ill patients. Anesth Analg 90: 351–355
8. Lichtwarck-Aschoff M, Zeravik J, Pfeiffer UJ (1992) Intrathoracic blood volume accurately reflects circulatory volume status in critically ill patients with mechanical ventilation. Intensive Care Med 18: 142–147
9. Gelman S (2008) Venous function and central venous pressure. A physiologic story. Anesthesiology 108: 735–748
10. Urbanowicz JH, Shaaban MJ, Cohen NH, et al (1990) Comparison of transesophageal echocardiographic and scintigraphic estimates of left ventricular end-diastolic volume index and ejection fraction in patients following coronary artery bypass grafting. Anesthesiology 72: 607–612
11. Magder S, De Varennes B (1998) Clinical death and the measurement of stressed vascular volume. Crit Care Med 26: 1061–1064
12. Boldt J, Lenz M, Kumle B, et al (1998) Volume replacement strategies on intensive care units: results from a postal survey. Intensive Care Med 24: 147–151
13. Magder S (2006) Central venous pressure monitoring. Curr Opin Crit Care 12: 219–227
14. Dellinger RP, Carlet JM, Masur H, et al (2004) Surviving Sepsis Campaign guidelines for management of severe sepsis and septic shock. Crit Care Med 32: 858–873

15. Robin E, Costecalde M, Lebuffe G, Vallet B (2006) Clinical relevance of data from the pulmonary artery catherer. Crit Care 10 (suppl 3):S3
16. Takala J (2003) Pulmonary capillary pressure. Intensive Carte Med 29: 890–893
17. Pinsky MR (2003) Clinical significance of pulmonary artery occlusion pressure. Intensive Care Med 29: 175–178
18. Kumar A, Anel R, Bunnell E et al (2004) Pulmonary artery occlusion pressure and central venous pressure fail to predict ventricular filling volume, cardiac performance, or the response to volume infusion in normal subjects. Crit Care Med 32: 691–699
19. Diebel LN, Wilson RF, Tagett MG, Kline RA (1992) End-diastolic volume: a better indicator of preload in the critically ill. Arch Surg 127: 817–822
20. Diebel L, Wilson RF, Heins J, Larky H, Warsow K, Wilson S (1994) End-diastolic volume versus pulmonary artery wedge pressure in evaluating cardiac preload in trauma patients. J Trauma 37: 950–955
21. Michard F, Alaya S, Zarka V, Bahoul M, Richard C, Teboul JL (2005) Global end-diastolic volume as an indicator of cardiac preload in patients with septic shock. Chest 124: 1900–1908
22. Hofer CK, Furrer L, Matter-Ensner S, et al (2005) Volumetric preload measurement by thermodilution: a comparison with transoesophageal echocardiography. Br J Anaesthesia 94: 748–755
23. De Simone R, Wolf I, Mottl-Link S et al (2005) Intraoperative assessment of right ventricular volume and function. Eur J Cardiothorac Surg 27: 988–933
24. Wiesenack C, Fiegl C, Keyser A, Laule S, Prasse C, Keyl C (2005) Continuously assessed right ventricular end-diastolic volume as a marker of cardiac preload and fluid responsiveness in mechanically ventilated cardiac surgical patients. Crit Care 9:R226-R233
25. Della Rocca G, Costa MG, Feltracco P, et al (2008) Continuous right ventricular end diastolic volume and right ventricular ejection fraction during liver transplantation: A multicentre study. Liver Transplantation 14: 327–332
26. Chang MC, Black CS, Meredith JW (1996) Volumetric assessment of preload in trauma patients: addressing the problem of the mathematical coupling. Shock 6: 326–329
27. Nelson LD, Safcsak K, Cheatham ML, Block EF (2001) Mathematical coupling does not explain the relationship between right ventricular end-diastolic volume and cardiac output. Crit Care Med 29: 940–943
28. Wesseling KH, de Wit B, Weber JAP, et al (1983) A simple device for the continuous measurement of cardiac output. Adv Cardiovasc Physiol 5: 16–52
29. Sakka SG, Rühl CC, Pfeiffer UJ, et al (2000) Assessment of cardiac preload and extravascular lung water by single transpulmonary thermodilution. Intensive Care Med 26: 180–187
30. Neumann P (1999) Extravascular lung water and intrathoracic blood volume: double versus single indicator dilution technique. Intensive Care Med 25: 216–219
31. Sakka SG, Bredle DL, Reinhart K, Meier-Hellmann A (1999) Comparison between intrathoracic blood volume and cardiac filling pressures in the early phase of hemodynamic instability of patients with sepsis and septic shock. J Crit Care 14: 78–83
32. Huber W, Umgelter A, Reindl W, et al (2008) Volume assessment in patients with necrotizing pancreatitis: A comparison of intrathoracic blood volume index, central venous pressure, and hematocrit, and their correlation to cardiac index and extravascular lung eater index. Crit Care Med 36: 2348–2354
33. Della Rocca G, Costa MG, Coccia C, Pompei L, Di Marco P, Pietropaoli P (2002) Preload index: pulmonary artery occlusion pressare versus intrathoracic blood volume monitoring during lung transplantation. Anesth Analg 95: 835–43
34. Della Rocca G, Costa MG, Coccia C, Pompei L, Pietropaoli P (2002) Preload and haemodynamic assessment during liver transplantation. A comparison between pulmonary artery catheter and transpulmonary indicator dilution technique. Eur J Anaesthesiol 19: 868–875
35. Gödje O, Peyerl M, Seebauer T, Lamm P, Mair H, Reichart B (1998) Central venous pressure, pulmonary capillary wedge pressure and intrathoracic blood volumes as preload indicators in cardiac surgery patients. Eur J Cardiothoracic Surg 13: 533–539
36. Gödje O, Peyerl M, Seebauer T, Dewald O, Reichart B (2000) Hemodynamic monitoring by double-indicator dilution technique in patients after orthotopic heart transplantation. Chest 118: 775–781
37. Reuter DA, Felbinger TW, Moerstedt K, et al (2002) Intrathoracic blood volume index mea-

sured by thermodilution for preload monitoring after cardiac surgery. J Cardiothorac Vasc Anesth 16: 191–195

38. Goepfert MSG, Reuter DA, Akyol D, Lamm P, Kilger E, Goetz AE (2007) Goal directed fluid management reduces vasopressor and catecholamine use in surgery patients. Intensive Care Med 33: 96–103
39. Buhre W, Weyland A, Bhure K, et al (2000) Effects of the sitting position on the distribution of the blood volume in patients undergoing neurosurgical procedures. Br J Anaesth 84: 354–357
40. Hofer CK, Zalunardo MP, Klaghofer R, Spahr T, Pasch T, Zollinger A (2002) Changes in intrathoracic blood volume associated with pneumoperitoneum and positioning. Acta Anaesthesiol Scand 46: 303–308
41. Bindels AJGH, van der Hoeven JG, Graafland AD, de Konig J, Meinders AE (2000) Relationships between volume and pressure measurements and stroke volume in critically ill patients. Crit Care 4: 193–199
42. Reuter DA, Felbinger TW, Schmidt C, et al (2003) Trendelenburg positioning after cardiac surgery: effects on intrathoracic blood volume index and cardiac performance. Eur J Anaesthesiol 2003 20: 17–20
43. Schiffmann H, Erdlenbruch B, Singer D, et al (2002) Assessment of cardiac output, intravascular volume status, and extravascular lung water by transpulmonary indicator dilution in critically ill neonates and infants. J Cardiothorac Vasc Anesth 16: 592–559
44. Cecchetti C, Lubrano R, Cristaldi S, et al (2008) Relationship between global end diastolic volume and cardiac output in critically ill infants and children. Crit Care Med 36: 928–932
45. Holm C, Melcer B, Horbrand F, et al (2000) Intrathoracic blood volume as an end point in resuscitation of the severely burned: an observational study of 24 patients. J Trauma 48: 728–734
46. Kuntscher MV, Czermak C, Blome-Eberwein S, Dacho A, Germann G (2003) Transcardiopulmonary thermal dye versus single thermodilution methods for assessment of intrathoracic blood volume and extravascular lung water in major burn resuscitation. J Burn Care Rehabil 24: 142–147
47. Hofer CK, Ganter MT, Matter-Enser S, et al (2006) Volumetric assessment of left heart preload by thermodilution: comparing the PiCCO–VoLEF system with transoesophageal echocardiography. Anaesthesia 61: 316–321
48. Neumann P, Schubert A, Heuer J, Hinz J, Quintel M, Klockgether-Radke A (2005) Hemodynamic effects of spontaneous breathing in the postoperative period. Acta Anaesthesiol Scand 49: 1443–1448
49. Uchino S, Bellomo R, Morimatsu H, et al (2006) Pulmonary artery catheter versus pulse contour analysis: a prospective epidemiological study. Crit Care 10:R174

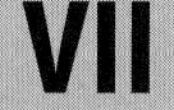

Monitoring Arterial Blood Pressure and Cardiac Output using Central or Peripheral Arterial Pressure Waveforms

J. Smith, L. Camporota, and R. Beale

Introduction

Arterial blood pressure and cardiac output are the two most important and frequently measured hemodynamic parameters in critically ill patients as they provide indirect information on global tissue perfusion and oxygen delivery, and can guide fluid management and vasoactive drug use [1, 2]. Inaccurate measurement of these parameters, both in the intensive care unit (ICU) and the operating room (OR), can lead to misdiagnosis and inappropriate treatment, potentially impacting on patient morbidity and mortality. In the ICU, arterial blood pressure is commonly measured invasively via a peripheral artery (e.g., radial) or less frequently via a central artery (e.g., femoral). However, because the arterial blood pressure is not constant throughout the arterial tree – as a consequence of changes in hydrostatic pressure, arterial stiffness, and pressure wave reflection that are dependent on individual characteristics (e.g., age, height, gender), disease state (e.g., sepsis), and the administration of vasoactive drugs – the site of arterial blood pressure measurement may not faithfully reflect organ perfusion pressure.

Cardiac output is routinely measured using a variety of methods [3–5], but increasingly popular are those that use an indicator dilution technique to calibrate a continuous cardiac output measurement which is based on the analysis of the arterial pressure waveform obtained through a radial or a femoral arterial catheter [6–11]. Several different commercially available systems give a continuous cardiac output value based on an arterial waveform, but these differ considerably from one another in the way they relate changes in arterial blood pressure to changes in stroke volume [1, 2]. One approach is to calculate continuous cardiac output from the analysis of the area under the systolic portion of the arterial waveform, which is therefore pressure waveform morphology dependent (pulse-contour method) (i.e., PiCCO, PiCCO*plus* [Pulsion, Munich, Germany]) [12]; another approach is to calculate stroke volume from the entire arterial waveform (not just the systolic area), which is therefore not pressure morphology based (i.e., not a pulse contour method, PulseCO; LiDCO, Cambridge, UK) [13–15]. This latter system uses autocorrelation (a time-based system), rather than Fourier transform (frequency based system) to calculate the net power of the nominal stroke volume (to be converted in actual stroke volume after multiplying by a calibration factor), with the theoretical advantage of being less influenced by the timing of the reflected wave and the degree of damping of the arterial waveform. Other commercially available systems require no initial calibration with bolus indicator dilution technique ('uncalibrated systems') and give information on the changes in continuous cardiac output over time (FloTrac™, Vigileo™; Edwards Lifesciences, Irvine, CA, USA, Pressure Recording Analytical Method – PRAM, Vytech Health, Padova, Italy and LiDCO*rapid*, LiDCO, Cambridge, UK). Since all the methods that calculate continuous cardiac output rely on the analysis of the arterial waveform, it seems clear that obtaining an accurate arterial blood pressure waveform is crucial not only for the appropriate titration of vasopressors, but also for an accurate estimation and correct interpretation of continuous cardiac output measurement.

The translation of arterial pressure into stroke volume and then into cardiac output is mainly influenced by the following factors: 1) damping and resonance of the system; 2) the non-linearity of the relationship between the change in arterial pressure and the change in stroke volume in the arterial system (i.e., compliance of the system), which mandates a compliance correction to linearize a pressure signal into a arterial volume change; 3) the presence, size and timing of the reflected waves with effects that vary depending on the distance of the measurement site from the heart and on the vascular compliance. Therefore, the site where an arterial waveform is recorded (central versus peripheral) will determine the absolute value of blood pressure and the shape of the arterial pulse, and ultimately the dose of vasopressors and the estimation of cardiac output. In this chapter, we discuss the effects of the site of measurement of arterial blood pressure on continuous cardiac output values and arterial pressure which, if not considered in clinical practice, may lead to important misuse of fluids and vasoactive drugs.

Wave Contour in the Central and Peripheral Arteries

At each systole, the heart ejects a volume of blood into the aorta (stroke volume) and generates a forward pressure wave which then travels along the arterial tree. During this transit, the mean arterial pressure (MAP) progressively falls by 1–3 mmHg between the ascending aorta and brachial or radial artery, but the systolic and pulse pressure progressively increase and at the extremities the systolic blood pressure (SBP) can be twice the SBP in the ascending aorta [16], with absolute differences (radial-aortic) of up to 40 mmHg [17]. The contour of the pressure wave is modified as it travels from the central arteries to the peripheral vessels. This is accepted as being a consequence of the duration of systole, MAP, vasomotor tone, pulse wave velocity and 'pressure augmentation' by wave reflection and resonance arising from reflection and re-reflection of the pulse between the upper and lower part of the body. In the proximal aorta, the arrival of the reflected wave is in early diastole and if the velocity of the waveform increases, the reflected wave will arrive earlier in systole with the effect of increasing the systolic pressure. The major sites of wave reflection in the circulatory system are the points of impedance discontinuity, such as arterial branching and arterial-arteriolar junctions and particularly high-resistance arterioles where a pulse waveform entering the aorta is exposed to a sudden impedance change, resulting in a large increment in resistance and producing reflected pulse waveforms [18]. Morphologically, the amplified peripheral pressure wave has a shorter interval between the initial systolic peak and diastolic wave suggesting 'resonance' in a shorter system [19] and is displayed as a sharp narrow arterial wave, which usually contains the summation of two systolic peaks: One represents the 'forward pressure' wave generated by the heart, and the second, a superimposed wave, is the 'backward pressure' wave reflected from the peripheries [18]. The contribution of the reflected wave to the measured SBP occurs earlier in the periphery, where the SBP may be up to 35 mmHg higher than the central aortic pressure [17]. This distal pulse amplification by wave reflection is always present when peripheral vascular resistance is high [20] and is most marked in young adults, in whom the amplitude of the radial pulse pressure may be 50 % greater than that in the ascending aorta, but is reduced during a Valsalva maneuver, hypotension, hypovolemia, and in the presence of vasodilatation. The latter is particularly well documented after administration of nitrates, when a significant reduction in aortic systolic pressure may not be appreciated by recording brachial or radial artery pressure (reviewed in [16]). In the contrary situation, during intense vasoconstriction, an increased wave reflection in the peripheries can lead to an underestimation of central aortic pressure if the SBP is measured in the radial artery [19]. Drug-induced alteration in central blood pressure and wave contours may be explained on the basis of change in arterial caliber, arterial stiffness and wave reflection.

A similar mechanism can occur also in the absence of drugs, in any clinical condition that leads to vasodilatation, such as in septic shock where radial systolic pressure may grossly overestimate by up to 20 mmHg the pressure in the central arteries as a result of a decreased wave reflection from the lower body which contributes to the reduced SBP in the central arteries but does not influence SBP in distal peripheral arteries to the same degree [19, 21]. The appreciation of this phenomenon is important because clinicians target a blood pressure value as though this was constantly the same, under all conditions and in all arteries. Even more therapeutically important is the situation that occurs during intense vasoconstriction (i.e., high doses of vasopressors or after cardiac surgery). While the arterial pressure is normally amplified in the radial artery and, therefore, is higher than the central arterial pressure, under conditions of excess vasoconstriction (typically high dose vasopressor use and relative hypovolemia) the radial pressure may underestimate central systolic and organ perfusion pressure, to the extent that it can grossly misguide the requirement of fluid and vasoactive agents (reviewed in [19]). The effect of vasoconstriction (e.g., during norepinephrine use) on the pressure waveform or flow wave contours is much less the more centrally the measurements are made (even if this can reduce mean flow), and this is explained by the fact that in the femoral artery the arteriolar tone is already high, and so the reflection coefficient (the ratio between the reflected wave and the incident wave in the frequency domain) already generated from this point in the circulation can be increased only marginally by intense vasoconstriction [19].

Being aware of these potential differences between central and peripheral arterial waveforms is important clinically for two main reasons: First, it is the central pressure and not the radial pressure that more directly determines organ perfusion; second, the degree to which radial pressure is variably affected by the pressure amplification that occurs in the peripheries means that it does not always accurately reflect the central pressure, which is usually the intended target of any therapeutic interventions aimed at achieving a particular blood pressure target. These principles emphasize the importance of monitoring central arterial pressure when perfusion pressure and cardiac afterload have to be determined precisely, as in shock states, during high doses of vasoactive drugs, or in the presence of an intra-aortic balloon pump (IABP) [19].

Agreement between Central and Peripheral Blood Pressure in Specific Clinical Situations

Invasive blood pressure measurement is performed through a catheter placed most commonly in the radial artery as it is easy to cannulate and has a low risk of complications. The femoral artery is one of several alternatives [22, 23]. Although the agreement between pressure obtained from a peripheral and central artery has been evaluated by many authors, the degree to which these two measures are interchangeable clinically is still a matter of debate. Some studies have shown a good correlation between the site measurements. Mignini et al. [24], in a recent trial in 55 medical and surgical patients requiring high dose of vasopressors (dopamine = 10 μg/kg/min or epinephrine or norepinephrine = 0.1 μg /kg/min) or low dose of vasopressor, compared simultaneous measurements of arterial pressure in peripheral and central arteries. The study showed no significant difference between the femoral and the radial artery in SBP (135 ± 31 vs 126 ± 30 mmHg), diastolic blood pressure (DBP, 63 ± 14 vs 62 ± 13 mmHg) or MAP (85 ± 17 vs 82 ± 17 mmHg). No difference was found either between the group on high doses of vasoactive drugs versus the group on low doses with a bias ± precision in the blood pressure of 3 ± 4 mmHg and 3 ± 4 mmHg, respectively, showing that the radial and femoral measurement of the blood pressure agreed well regardless of the dose of vasoactive drug used, and the authors suggested that these two measurements are interchangeable. Similarly, Yazigi et al. [25] found that the radial arterial pressure seemed an accurate measure of the central arterial pressure as there was no statistically significant difference between peripheral and central arterial pressures either before, during or after controlled hypotension by vasodilatation in 10 healthy patients undergoing surgery. However, discrepancies between central to peripheral blood pressures have been reported to occur in a number of clinical circumstances such as after cardiopulmonary bypass (CPB) [26–28], during deep hypothermic circulatory arrest [29], cardiopulmonary resuscitation (CPR) [30], isofluorane anesthesia [31], in patients with sepsis treated with high dose vasoconstrictors [32], and in patients during reperfusion post-liver transplant [33].

Kanazawa et al. [26], in patients after CPB, showed the presence of a pressure gradient between central and peripheral sites and changes in the pulse wave velocity (PWV). Of the 12 patients, seven had a pressure gradient and a difference of 27 ± 11 mmHg in the SBP between the aorta and the radial artery and the PWV gradually decreased from the central to peripheral artery. The occurrence of a pressure gradient after CPB was due to a decrease in arterial elasticity from the aorta to the radial artery. Similar blood pressure differences have been described by Baba et al. who reported that 38/75 patients undergoing CPB displayed a gradient (femoral-radial) in MAP > 5 mmHg and radial artery constriction could be responsible for the pressure gradient [27] and Chauhan et al. who showed that femoral artery perfusion pressures were higher and more reliable during the initial part of CPB [28]. Similarly, Gravlee et al. [34] showed that a clinically important (> 10 mmHg) underestimation of systolic aortic pressures occurred in 52 % of radial artery catheters and radial artery MAP underestimated aortic MAP by > 5 mmHg in 61 % of the patients two minutes after CPB. In a different setting, Manecke et al. [29] showed that 76 % of the patients receiving CPB with profound hypothermia and circulatory arrest exhibited a mean arterial gradient of at least 10 mmHg either during or after CPB, with femoral readings being higher. Clinically significant gradients were noted throughout the CPB period and the post-CPB period in these patients. In the 54 patients studied, the SBP gradient was 32 ± 19 mmHg after CPB and the MAP gradient was 6.3 ± 4.9 mmHg. The duration of clinically significant SBP (> 10 mmHg) and MAP (> 5 mmHg) gradients in the postoperative period were 5.2 ± 5.7 hours and 5.8 ± 7.2 hours, respectively, making the recommendation for the use of central arterial pressure monitoring for intraoperative and postoperative care [29]. Similarly, Arnal et al. [33] in 72 patients undergoing liver transplantation found that femoral SBP was significantly higher than radial SBP only during liver reperfusion (92 ± 22 vs 76 ± 22 mmHg, $p < 0.01$); the DBP and MAP did not differ in two sites. In 27 of 72 patients who required vasopressors for hemodynamic instability, there was a statistically significant difference between femoral and radial systolic arterial pressure during the reperfusion period. Taken together, these findings suggest that this is a real and important phenomenon, but only occurs in some patients in some circumstances, and so may be underestimated if evaluated solely by the use of statistics applied to a whole study population.

A systematic discrepancy between radial and central blood pressure measurement has also been demonstrated in an important paper by Dorman et al. [32] on 14 post-operative patients with septic shock requiring high doses of norepinephrine – a situation highly relevant to current critical care practice. In these patients, a consistent underestimation of peripheral blood pressure was observed in the radial measurement. Femoral artery systolic pressures were significantly higher than radial artery systolic pressures (143 ± 8.9 vs 86 ± 4.5 mmHg), but, what is more pertinent is that the MAPs were also higher in the femoral artery than in the radial artery (81 ± 2.5 vs 66 ± 2.2 mmHg). The difference between the two sites was large enough to allow a reduction in vasopressor support in 11 (79 %) of 14 patients (85.6 ± 25.3 to 57.2 ± 16.4 μg /min, $p < 0.05$), even discontinuing it in two patients. These data strongly suggest that in hemodynamically unstable patients requiring large amounts of vasoactive drugs, monitoring arterial pressure from the femoral site seems preferable, as the radial site may significantly underestimate not only SBP but also MAP, with important repercussions on fluid and vasoactive drug use.

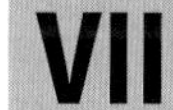

Influence of the Site of Blood Pressure Measurement on Continuous Cardiac Output Estimation

The increasingly routine use of continuous cardiac output monitoring derived from the arterial pressure wave (pulse contour analysis), in place of the more invasive pulmonary artery catheter (PAC) [35, 36], makes obtaining an accurate arterial waveform and the understanding of the factors influencing the shape of the waveform essential for the correct clinical interpretation of the cardiac output [37]. Studies comparing continuous cardiac output measurements derived from the peripheral and central artery have shown that the quality of the pressure waveform obtained from the radial artery is accurate also for pulse contour analysis. de Wilde et al. [38] compared femoral and radial artery pressure measurement signals as inputs for the PiCCO system in 14 patients following cardiac surgery. The study showed a high level of agreement between cardiac output in the femoral artery and cardiac output in the radial artery (bias -0.01, SD [0.31] l/min), which suggests the interchangeability of radial and femoral arterial pressure signals for continuous cardiac output monitoring. Similarly, Orme et al. [39] and Wouters et al. [40] studied the accuracy of using the brachial artery to measure cardiac output. The values obtained from the brachial artery agreed with the values obtained from the PAC (bias 0.38, SD 0.77 l/min and bias

0.91, SD 0.41 l/min for the two studies, respectively). Moreover, the pulse contour analysis using a brachial artery catheter was in agreement with pulmonary artery thermodilution, concluding that thc brachial artery is a valid alternative to the femoral artery when the femoral approach is not desirable. However, in spite of the reassuring tenor of these studies, since arterial blood pressure and arterial waveform measured at the radial artery can differ significantly from those measured simultaneously in the central arteries particularly during the administration of vasoactive drugs, continuous cardiac output measured at the two sites can vary in a proportion of critically ill patients. In our experience, in patients requiring high doses of vasopressors, femoral arterial pressure is generally higher than radial arterial pressure (**Figs. 1–3**), and

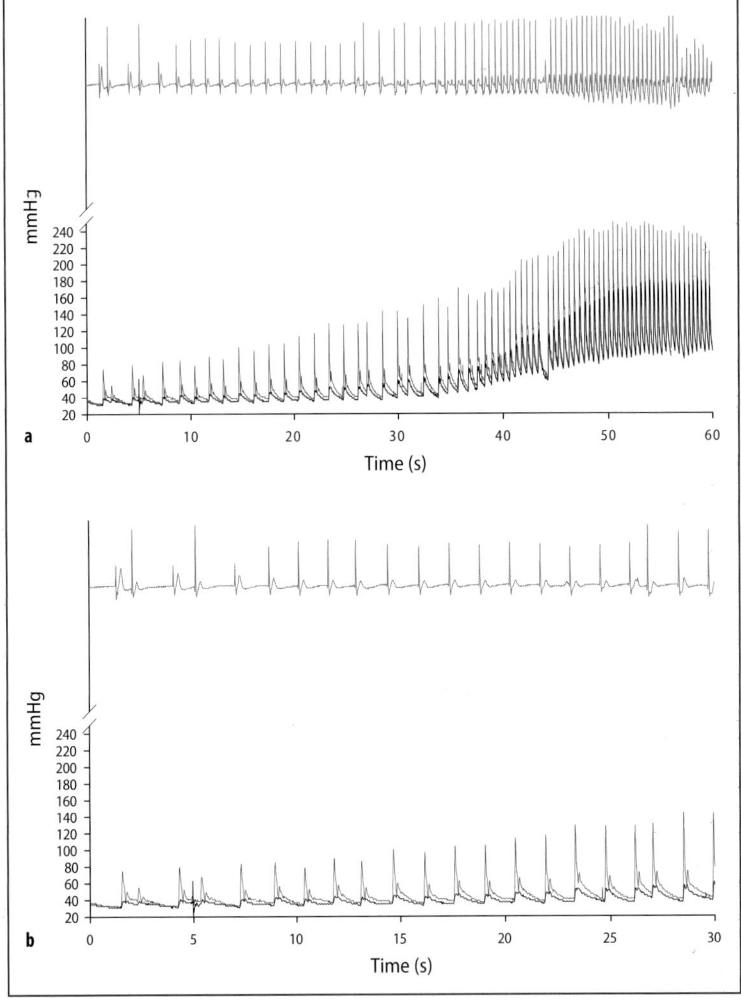

Fig. 1. During extreme hemodynamic conditions, a bolus of epinephrine was administered and the radial (black line) and femoral (blue line) arterial pressures were evaluated. The femoral arterial blood pressure was higher than the radial arterial blood pressure. Panel **a** shows the first 30 seconds of the recording in **b**.

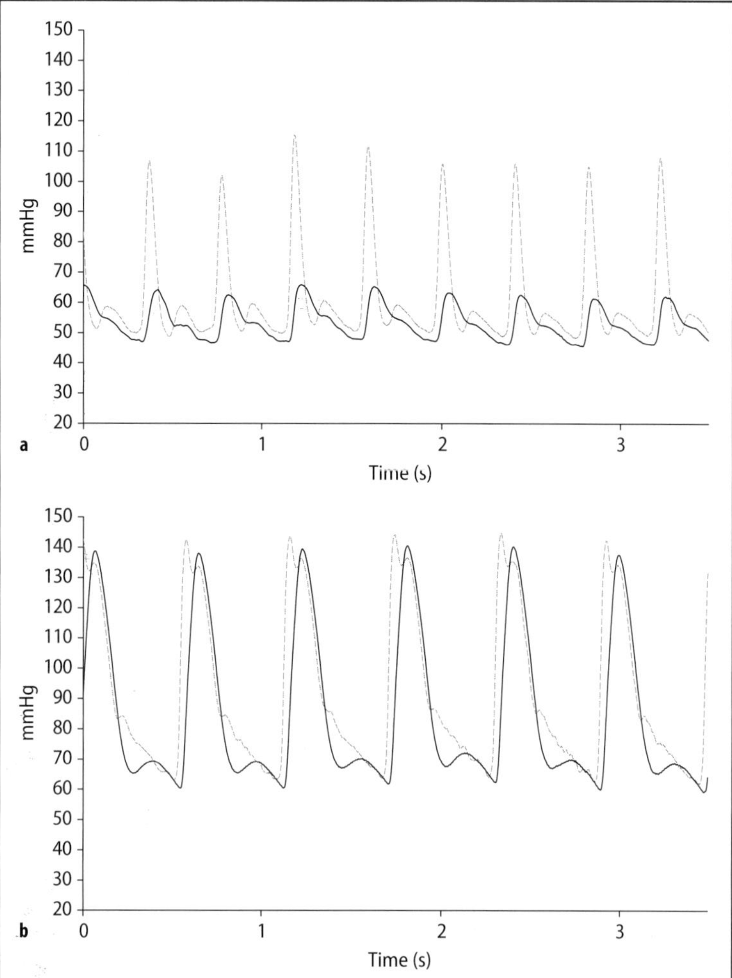

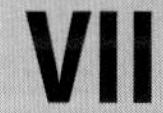

Fig. 2a. A patient with septic shock post bowel resection for fecal peritonitis in hypovolemic state requiring vasopressors (norepinephrine 0.7 μg/kg/min). The discrepancy between radial (solid line) and femoral (dashed line) arterial blood pressure measurement is evident. **b** agreement between the two arterial blood pressure measurements is seen after vasopressor reduction and fluid resuscitation.

this discrepancy can be even more dramatic under extreme hemodynamic conditions (**Fig. 1**). The difference in arterial blood pressure is then reflected in a large difference in the continuous cardiac output value at the two arterial sites (**Fig. 4**) leading to a difference in cardiac output between the two sites of up to 3 l/min [41]. This suggests that radial and femoral artery are not automatically interchangeable sites for cardiac output monitoring anymore than they are for blood pressure monitoring, and there may be important differences in various physiological conditions (e.g., age, aortic compliance) or in association with low flow/cardiac output states, particularly during rapid changes in hemodynamics as a consequence of the use of fluids and high doses of vasoactive agents in shock.

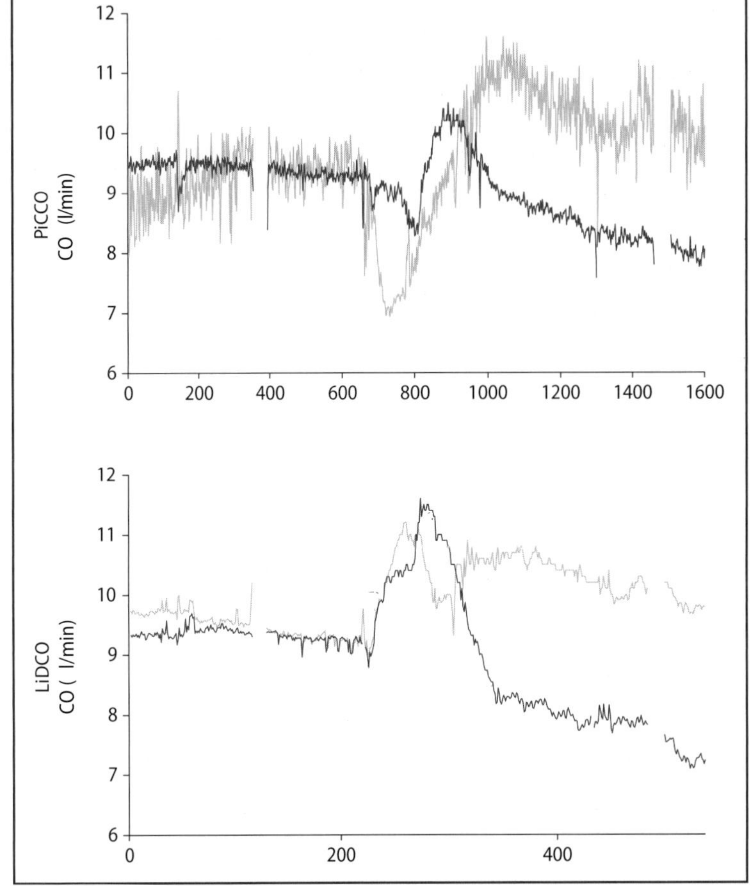

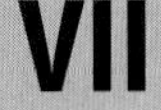

Fig. 3. Continuous cardiac output recording with the PiCCO system and the LiDCO system in radial (pale blue line) and femoral (dark blue line) arteries. The discrepancy between the two sites is evident.

The question therefore arises as to when it is reasonable to assume that the peripheral (radial) pressure measurement is a faithful reflection of the central pressure, either for blood pressure targeting *per se*, or for cardiac output derivation. In our view, the safest option is to use radial pressure if the radial pressure is in the "normal" range, if the pulse wave morphology is well defined, and if peripheral perfusion is clinically good or if a vasopressor is being used at a moderate and/or decreasing dose.

▷

Fig. 4. Top: Cardiac output (CO) ratio between radial and femoral site in 17 ICU patients [40]. The median value of the cardiac output ratio was 0.95 (IQR 0.88 to 1.02), with a high variability among the patients, ranging from 0.3 to 1.41, whereas intra-patient variability was low, with a median CV of 3.26 % (IQR 1.1 to 5.3 %). Bottom: Cardiac output measurement derived from simultaneous radial (pale blue line) and femoral (dark blue line) blood pressures in a single patient. When evaluating the data by individual time point pairs,

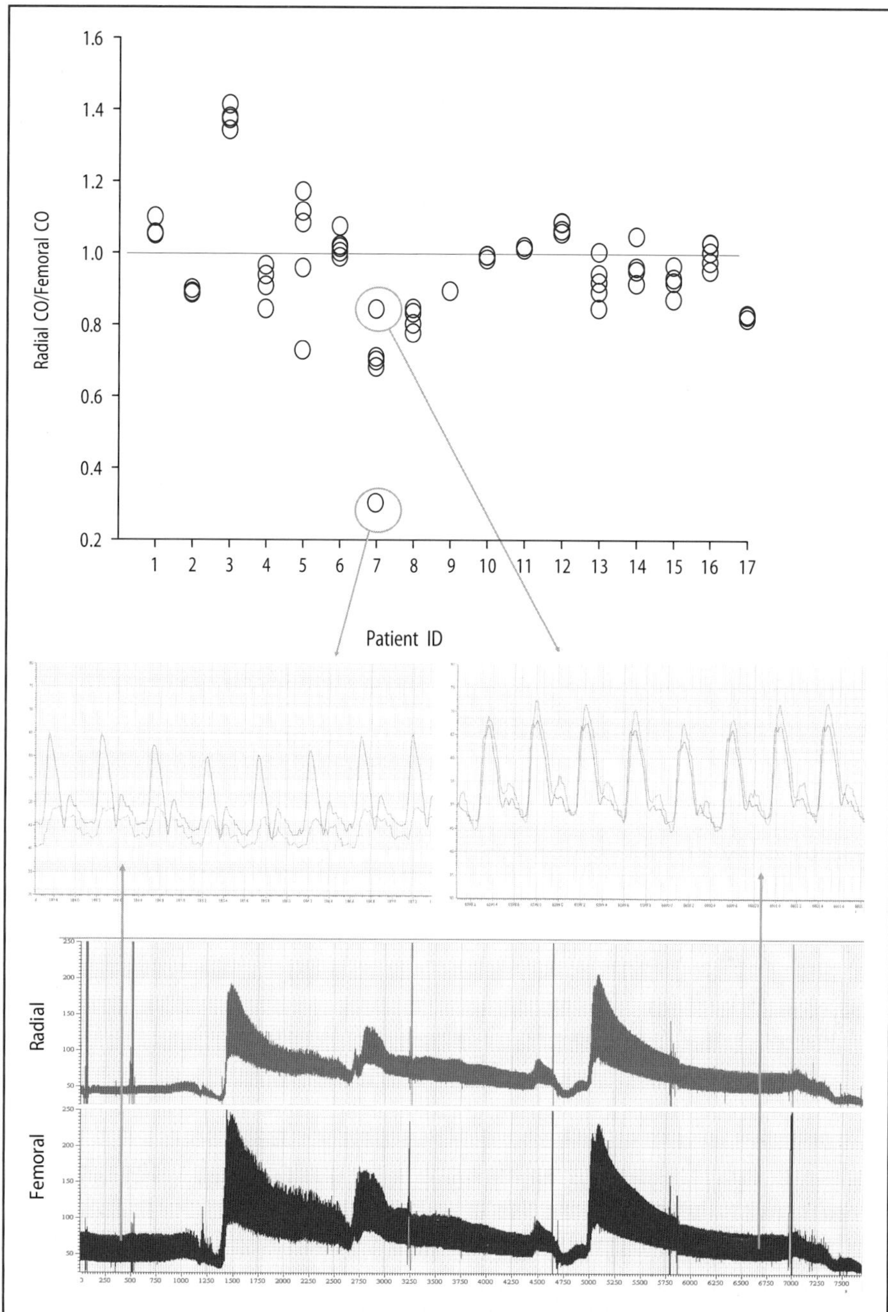

the ratio of cardiac outputs between the two sites varied greatly. The difference between the median (range) arterial pressures was 2 mmHg (–3 to 8 mmHg), however, the pulse pressure difference was generally large with a median (range) of 2 mmHg (–26 to 44 mmHg). The difference between the two sites is large enough to be clinically unacceptable without a site-specific recalibration.

In these situations the peripheral blood pressure is assumed to be equivalent to the central pressure. In situations where the radial pressure is low, the pulse wave morphology is 'damped' but technical problems with the arterial catheter or the tubing system cannot be identified (i.e., normal damping and resonance of the system after a 'flush test'), peripheral perfusion is clinically poor and the vasopressor dose is high and increasing, central pressure measurement is preferable and more likely to accurately reflect the 'true' organ perfusion pressure.

Conclusion

There may be a dramatic pressure gradient between femoral and radial arterial pressure in several conditions which are either physiological (e.g., age, aortic compliance) or in association with low flow/cardiac output state, particularly during rapid changes in hemodynamics as a consequence of vasoactive agents in shock. This is especially the case with high doses of vasopressors and hypovolemia. Peripheral pressure waveform may underestimate or overestimate central blood pressure depending on the type of vasoactive drugs (vasoconstrictors or vasodilators) used and the degree of blood flow limitation (cardiac output). It follows that using the peripheral arterial pressure may occasionally lead to false assumptions about the correct therapeutic intervention under these circumstances.

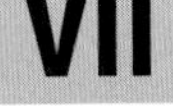

Acknowledgement: The authors would like to thank Drs Eleonora Corno and Eleonora Menaldo for their contributions to the preparation of this manuscript.

References

1. Pinsky MR (2002) Functional hemodynamic monitoring. Intensive Care Med 28: 386–388
2. Hofer CK, Ganter MT, Zollinger A (2007) What technique should I use to measure cardiac output? Curr Opin Crit Care 13: 308–317
3. Cholley BP, Payen D (2005) Noninvasive techniques for measurements of cardiac output. Curr Opin Crit Care 11: 424–429
4. Berton C, Cholley B (2002) Equipment review: new techniques for cardiac output measurement – oesophageal Doppler, Fick principle using carbon dioxide, and pulse contour analysis. Crit Care 6: 216–221
5. Della Rocca G, Costa MG (2005) Volumetric monitoring: principles of application. Minerva Anestesiol 71: 303–306
6. Rodig G, Prasser C, Keyl C, Liebold A, Hobbhahn J (1999) Continuous cardiac output measurement: pulse contour analysis vs thermodilution technique in cardiac surgical patients. Br J Anaesth 82: 525–530
7. Tannenbaum GA, Mathews D, Weissman C (1993) Pulse contour cardiac output in surgical intensive care unit patients. J Clin Anesth 5: 471–478
8. Weissman C, Ornstein EJ, Young WL (1993) Arterial pulse contour analysis trending of cardiac output: hemodynamic manipulations during cerebral arteriovenous malformation resection. J Clin Monit 9: 347–353
9. Gratz I, Kraidin J, Jacobi AG, deCastro NG, Spagna P, Larijani GE (1992) Continuous noninvasive cardiac output as estimated from the pulse contour curve. J Clin Monit 8: 20–27
10. Linton NW, Linton RA (2001) Estimation of changes in cardiac output from the arterial blood pressure waveform in the upper limb. Br J Anaesth 86: 486–496
11. Jansen JR, Wesseling KH, Settels JJ, Schreuder JJ (1990) Continuous cardiac output monitoring by pulse contour during cardiac surgery. Eur Heart J 11 (Suppl I):26–32
12. Godje O, Hoke K, Goetz AE, et al (2002) Reliability of a new algorithm for continuous cardiac output determination by pulse-contour analysis during hemodynamic instability. Crit Care Med 30: 52–58

13. Band DM, Linton RA, O'Brien TK, Jonas MM, Linton NW (1997) The shape of indicator dilution curves used for cardiac output measurement in man. J Physiol 498 (Pt 1):225–229
14. Linton RA, Band DM, Haire KM (1993) A new method of measuring cardiac output in man using lithium dilution. Br J Anaesth 71: 262–266
15. Linton R, Band D, O'Brien T, Jonas M, Leach R (1997) Lithium dilution cardiac output measurement: a comparison with thermodilution. Crit Care Med 25: 1796–1800
16. O'Rourke MF, Seward JB (2006) Central arterial pressure and arterial pressure pulse: new views entering the second century after Korotkov. Mayo Clin Proc 81: 1057–1068
17. Pauca AL, Wallenhaupt SL, Kon ND, Tucker WY (1992) Does radial artery pressure accurately reflect aortic pressure? Chest 102: 1193–1198
18. Hirata K, Kawakami M, O'Rourke MF (2006) Pulse wave analysis and pulse wave velocity: a review of blood pressure interpretation 100 years after Korotkov. Circ J 70: 1231–1239
19. Nichols WW, O'Rourke MF (2005) McDonald's Blood Flow in Arteries, Fifth edn. Hodder Arnold, London
20. O'Rourke MF, Blazek JV, Morreels CL Jr, Krovetz LJ (1968) Pressure wave transmission along the human aorta. Changes with age and in arterial degenerative disease. Circ Res 23: 567–579
21. Kelly RP, Gibbs HH, O'Rourke MF, et al (1990) Nitroglycerin has more favourable effects on left ventricular afterload than apparent from measurement of pressure in a peripheral artery. Eur Heart J 11: 138–144
22. Slogoff S, Keats AS, Arlund C (1983) On the safety of radial artery cannulation. Anesthesiology 59: 42–47
23. Soderstrom CA, Wasserman DH, Dunham CM, Caplan ES, Cowley RA (1982) Superiority of the femoral artery of monitoring. A prospective study. Am J Surg 144: 309–312
24. Mignini MA, Piacentini E, Dubin A (2006) Peripheral arterial blood pressure monitoring adequately tracks central arterial blood pressure in critically ill patients: an observational study. Crit Care 10:R43
25. Yazigi A, Madi-Jebara S, Haddad F, Hayek G, Jawish D (2002) Accuracy of radial arterial pressure measurement during surgery under controlled hypotension. Acta Anaesthesiol Scand 46: 173–175
26. Kanazawa M, Fukuyama H, Kinefuchi Y, Takiguchi M, Suzuki T (2003) Relationship between aortic-to-radial arterial pressure gradient after cardiopulmonary bypass and changes in arterial elasticity. Anesthesiology 99: 48–53
27. Baba T, Goto T, Yoshitake A, Shibata Y (1997) Radial artery diameter decreases with increased femoral to radial arterial pressure gradient during cardiopulmonary bypass. Anesth Analg 85: 252–258
28. Chauhan S, Saxena N, Mehrotra S, Rao BH, Sahu M (2000) Femoral artery pressures are more reliable than radial artery pressures on initiation of cardiopulmonary bypass. J Cardiothorac Vasc Anesth 14: 274–276
29. Manecke GR, Jr., Parimucha M, Stratmann G, et al (2004) Deep hypothermic circulatory arrest and the femoral-to-radial arterial pressure gradient. J Cardiothorac Vasc Anesth 18: 175–179
30. Rivers EP, Lozon J, Enriquez E, et al (1993) Simultaneous radial, femoral, and aortic arterial pressures during human cardiopulmonary resuscitation. Crit Care Med 21: 878–883
31. Pauca AL, Wallenhaupt SL, Kon ND (1994) Reliability of the radial arterial pressure during anesthesia. Is wrist compression a possible diagnostic test? Chest 105: 69–75
32. Dorman T, Breslow MJ, Lipsett PA, et al (1998) Radial artery pressure monitoring underestimates central arterial pressure during vasopressor therapy in critically ill surgical patients. Crit Care Med 26: 1646–1649
33. Arnal D, Garutti I, Perez-Pena J, Olmedilla L, Tzenkov IG (2005) Radial to femoral arterial blood pressure differences during liver transplantation. Anaesthesia 60: 766–771
34. Gravlee GP, Wong AB, Adkins TG, Case LD, Pauca AL (1989) A comparison of radial, brachial, and aortic pressures after cardiopulmonary bypass. J Cardiothorac Anesth 3: 20–26
35. Wheeler AP, Bernard GR, Thompson BT, et al (2006) Pulmonary-artery versus central venous catheter to guide treatment of acute lung injury. N Engl J Med 354:2213–2224
36. Shah MR, Hasselblad V, Stevenson LW, et al (2005) Impact of the pulmonary artery catheter in critically ill patients: meta-analysis of randomized clinical trials. JAMA 294: 1664–1670

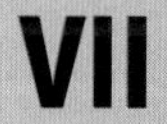

37. Hirschl MM, Binder M, Gwechenberger M, et al (1997) Noninvasive assessment of cardiac output in critically ill patients by analysis of the finger blood pressure waveform. Crit Care Med 25: 1909–1914
38. de Wilde RB, Breukers RB, van den Berg PC, Jansen JR (2006) Monitoring cardiac output using the femoral and radial arterial pressure waveform. Anaesthesia 61: 743–746
39. Orme RM, Pigott DW, Mihm FG (2004) Measurement of cardiac output by transpulmonary arterial thermodilution using a long radial artery catheter. A comparison with intermittent pulmonary artery thermodilution. Anaesthesia 59: 590–594
40. Wouters PF, Quaghebeur B, Sergeant P, Van Hemelrijck J, Vandermeersch E (2005) Cardiac output monitoring using a brachial arterial catheter during off-pump coronary artery bypass grafting. J Cardiothorac Vasc Anesth 19: 160–164
41. Smith J, Wolff C, Mills E, et al (2007) Comparison between uncalibrated cardiac output using the femoral and radial arterial pressure waveform in critically ill patients. Crit Care 11 (Suppl 2): P296 (abst)

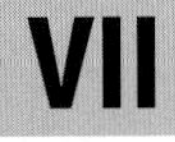

Intrathoracic Pressure Regulation for the Treatment of Hypotension

I. Cinel, A. Metzger, and R.P. Dellinger

VII

Introduction

Intrathoracic pressure regulation therapy is based upon the physiological principles of the inspiratory impedance threshold device which was developed to increase the return of venous blood back to the heart for treatment of a number of different clinical conditions associated with clinically significant hypotension, including cardiac arrest [1–9]. Intrathoracic pressure regulation therapy works by modulating pressures inside the thorax to augment circulation in states of low blood pressure. This technology was first used in the setting of cardiopulmonary resuscitation (CPR). In the non-spontaneously breathing patient, by harnessing the chest wall recoil with a device that prevents air from entering the lungs each time the chest re-expands after a chest compression, an impedance threshold device (ResQPOD®, Advanced Circulatory Systems, Minneapolis, MN) lowers intrathoracic pressures, enhancing blood return to the heart while lowering intracranial pressures (drop in internal jugular vein pressure). In spontaneously breathing patients, inspiration through a differently configured impedance threshold device (ResQGard®) lowers intrathoracic pressures and similarly enhances cardiac preload and lowers intracranial pressures. Both mechanisms contribute to increases in cerebral perfusion during CPR and in spontaneously breathing patients. Based upon collaborative research with the National Aeronautics and Space Administration (NASA) and the United States Army Institute for Surgical Research, the impedance threshold device has recently been recommended in spontaneously breathing patients for treatment of hypotension due to multiple potential causes, including blood loss, intradialytic hypotension, perioperative hypotension, orthostatic hypotension, and hypotension associated with labor and delivery [10–16]. The technology was evaluated by NASA, as some astronauts develop severe orthostatic hypotension after space flight. It is now used as part of the care for astronauts after prolonged space flights. In this chapter, the potential use of intrathoracic pressure regulation for the treatment of hypotension will be discussed, including preliminary preclinical data on use of this approach to treat hypotension in pigs secondary to *Escherichia coli* peritonitis.

Active Intrathoracic Pressure Regulation Therapy for Apneic Hypotension Patients

The active intrathoracic pressure regulation device for non-breathing patients is called the CirQlator®. Whereas the ResQPOD requires complete chest wall recoil during CPR in order to generate negative intrathoracic pressures, the CirQlator

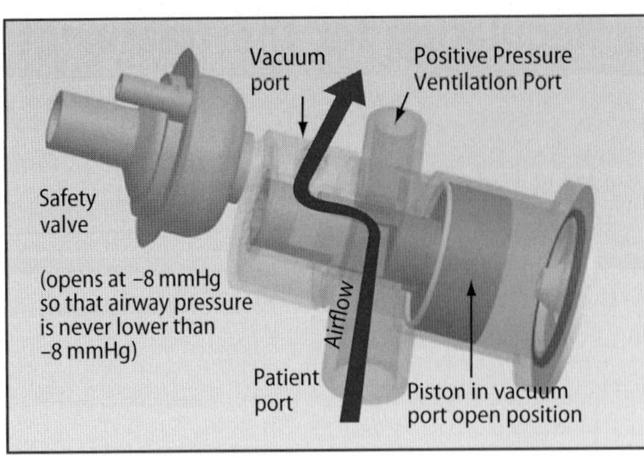

Fig. 1. Function of intrathoracic pressure regulation device (when airway pressure is negative).

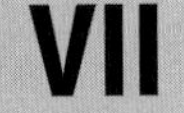

requires an external regulated vacuum source to actively increase negative intrathoracic pressure in apneic patients. The CirQlator is used to treat hypotensive patients requiring positive pressure ventilation to maintain adequate respiration and generates an intrathoracic vacuum during the expiratory phase of ventilation to enhance venous blood flow back to the heart and to simultaneously lower intracranial pressures. The CirQlator was approved by the United States Food and Drug Administration (FDA) in 2007 and is illustrated in **Figure 1**. The device works in a biphasic manner: First, a positive pressure ventilation breath from a manual resuscitator or ventilator is delivered and then the device rapidly draws respiratory gases out of the thorax until a predetermined vacuum develops inside the thorax. The currently available device generates a vacuum of –12 cmH_2O in between positive pressure breaths. The positive and negative intrathoracic pressures are instantaneously transmitted throughout the intrathoracic cavity and the physiological effects of the resultant pressure changes impact cardiovascular hemodynamics.

While this novel approach has recently been applied to patients in cardiac arrest and to those with hypotension secondary to low intravascular volume who are able to breathe spontaneously, the sickest patients in shock are usually not able to breathe independently. This is particularly true for patients who have suffered significant traumatic injury, and those with septic shock. The CirQlator was developed specifically to improve blood pressure for any non-breathing patient with significant hypotension secondary to a decrease in cardiac preload or central blood volume. In cardiac arrest, it provides a more continuous and controlled negative intrathoracic vacuum between positive pressure ventilations, potentially improving circulation to the heart and brain. In non-cardiac arrest applications, it actively lowers intrathoracic pressure continuously when a positive pressure ventilation is not being delivered, thereby enhancing the gradient for venous blood flow back to the heart while lowering intracranial pressure. Combined, these mechanisms offer potential to exploit normal physiological processes to enhance circulation in hypotensive non-breathing patients.

Intrathoracic Pressure Regulation Therapy in Cardiac Arrest with CPR

Since its discovery, there have been more than fifteen published studies using the impedance threshold device in animal models of cardiac arrest from multiple animal laboratories and seven published clinical randomized prospective studies with the impedance threshold device in patients in cardiac arrest [1–7, 17–25]. These studies have demonstrated that use of the impedance threshold device with either conventional manual CPR alone or active compression-decompression (ACD) CPR resulted in increased blood pressure, increased circulation of drug therapies, and increased survival rates. With conventional manual CPR, double blinded randomized clinical trials with the impedance threshold device showed that systolic blood pressures were twice as high when the active impedance threshold device was used (85 mmHg compared to 44 mmHg in sham-treated controls, $p < 0.001$) and short-term survival rates were also doubled in patients who presented with an initial rhythm of either ventricular fibrillation (VF) or pulseless electrical activity [17, 19]. As a result of the multiple, published, clinical outcomes-based trials involving nearly 1000 patients, the impedance threshold device was given a level 2a recommendation in the 2005 American Heart Association Guidelines for CPR [26]. Aufderheide et al. showed that treatment using the combination of the impedance threshold device and application of the new CPR Guidelines, compared to historical controls, doubled survival to hospital discharge rates for patients with an out-of-hospital cardiac arrest, regardless of the initial presenting rhythm [27].

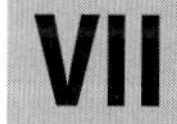

Intrathoracic Pressure Regulation Therapy and CPR

The effects of intrathoracic pressure regulation therapy using the CirQlator have been studied in pigs in VF during CPR. In this setting, an early prototype of the CirQLator was used to lower intrathoracic pressures. This change in intrathoracic pressure resulted in: 1) Enhancement of venous return to the heart to refill the heart with blood after each compression; 2) an increase in cardiac output with each compression; and 3) lowering of intracranial pressure linked directly to the lowering of intrathoracic pressure, which reduces the resistance for blood flow from the brain. The newly discovered benefit of lowering intracranial pressures by lowering intrathoracic pressures during CPR and other states of low blood pressure is one of the more unique aspects of this new technology as it provides potential to enhance cerebral circulation and increase CPR efficacy [28].

In a porcine model of cardiac arrest, after 8 minutes of untreated cardiac arrest, CPR was performed on 20 pigs for 6 minutes at 100 compressions/min with positive pressure ventilation (100 % O_2) and a compression:ventilation ratio of 15:2 [28]. In a second protocol, 6 animals were bled 50 % of their blood volume. After 4 minutes of untreated VF, interventions were performed for 2 minutes with standard-CPR (Std-CPR) and 2 minutes with intrathoracic pressure regulator-CPR (ITPR-CPR). Vital organ perfusion pressures and end tidal carbon dioxide ($ETCO_2$) were significantly improved with ITPR-CPR in both protocols. Survival rates were 100 % (10/10) with ITPR-CPR versus 10 % (1/10) with Std-CPR. Oxygen saturation was 100 % throughout the study in both protocols. Compared to Std-CPR, use of ITPR-CPR improved hemodynamics, vital organ perfusion pressures, and carotid blood flow in both VF and hypovolemic cardiac arrest. **Figure 2** demonstrates the significant hemodynamic differences seen when using the intrathoracic pressure regulation device during standard CPR in the animal model of cardiac arrest.

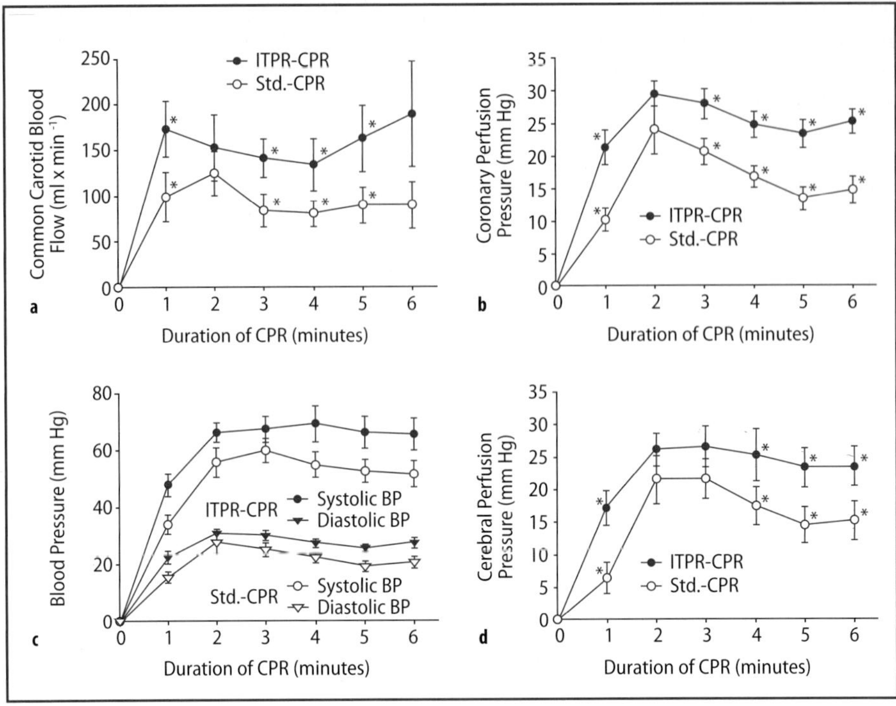

Fig. 2. Effect of intrathoracic pressure regulation-cardiopulmonary resuscitation (ITPR-CPR) on carotid blood flow, coronary perfusion pressure, blood pressure, and cerebral perfusion pressure compared to standard CPR (Std-CPR) [28]. *$p < 0.05$

Intrathoracic Pressure Regulation Therapy and Survival Outcomes in Hemorrhagic Shock

To test the hypothesis that intrathoracic pressure regulation therapy using the CirQLator would demonstrate significantly increased mean arterial pressures and 24-hour survival rates when compared with no intervention in a fixed bleed model of controlled and severe hemorrhagic shock, a prospective trial randomizing two groups of pigs after a fixed bleed to receive: 1) no resuscitation, or 2) resuscitation with the intrathoracic pressure regulation device was conducted [29].

After an acute 55 % blood loss and 5 minutes of stabilization, 18 pigs with an average weight of 28 ± 1.2 kg were prospectively randomized to either a CirQLator intervention group, with the device set to maintain intrathoracic pressures of -8 mmHg in between positive pressure ventilations, or a control group treated only with positive pressure ventilation (plus 3 cmH_2O positive end-expiratory pressure [PEEP]). After 90 minutes, surviving animals received intravenous fluid resuscitation and were followed for 24-hours to evaluate survival and neurological outcomes. There were no differences in the average blood loss in each group. After 55 % blood loss, the application of a negative airway pressure of –8 mmHg resulted in a significant increase in mean arterial pressure for the entire 90 minutes of treatment as compared with the control group (**Fig. 3**). Mean arterial blood pressure returned to normal after blood re-infusion at 90 minutes. Arterial blood gases showed progres-

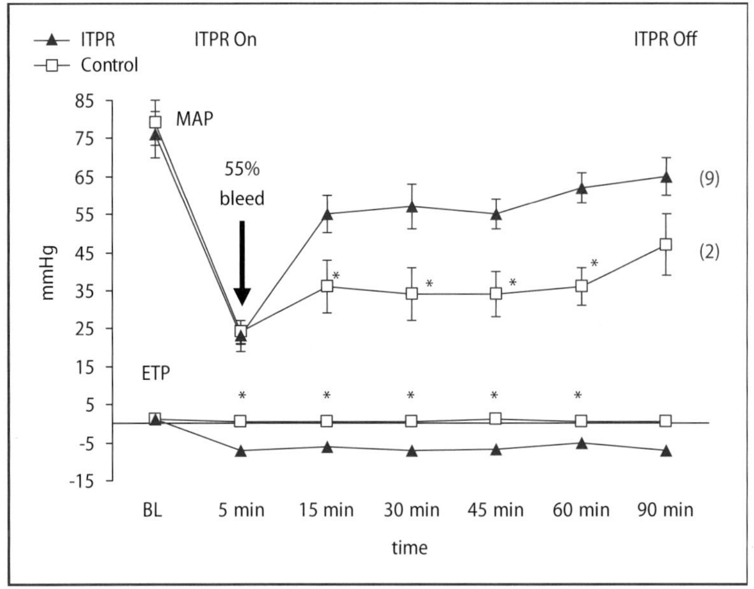

Fig. 3. Following controlled blood loss (55 %), the intrathoracic pressure regulator (ITPR), set at -8 mmHg, resulted in a significant decrease in endotracheal pressure (ETP) and a significant increase in mean arterial blood pressure (MAP), compared to controls [29]. BL: pre-bleed baseline; $*p < 0.05$ between groups. The numbers in parentheses are the animals alive at the end of 90 minutes.

sive metabolic acidosis with increasing base deficit in the control group whereas in the intrathoracic pressure regulation device group metabolic acidosis was maintained to a level compatible with life. The only two animals that survived the 90 minute period of time in the control group had a less severe metabolic acidosis compared to the rest of the control group animals. There was a significant increase in $ETCO_2$ throughout the 90 minutes of CirQLator application compared to the control group. The difference between $PaCO_2$ and $ETCO_2$ was consistently lower in the intrathoracic pressure regulation device group as well. Oxygenation was adequate in both groups without significant differences. Nine animals survived to blood re-infusion at 90 minutes in the intrathoracic pressure regulation device treatment group and only two animals survived in the control group. After 24 hours, all animals were alive in the intrathoracic pressure regulation device group but only 1/9 (11 %) was alive in the control group ($p < 0.01$). Eight of 9 animals in the intrathoracic pressure regulation device group had normal neurological function after 24 hours, 1/9 had a Cerebral Performance Score of 4 using a well established porcine neurological scoring system [30]. The sole survivor in the control group had normal neurological function after 24 hours.

These results supported prolonged application of the intrathoracic pressure regulation device with intermittent positive pressure ventilation during hypovolemic hypotension as a route to increased blood pressure and improved survival rates compared with untreated controls. The data support the use of the intrathoracic pressure regulation-CirQLator to increase survival rates by enhancing perfusion pressures and preventing the development of severe metabolic acidosis in the setting of severe hypotension [29].

Intrathoracic Pressure Regulation Therapy and Sepsis

Treatment of sepsis is a critically time-sensitive emergency; patients stand the best chance for survival when effective therapeutic interventions are delivered as early as possible [31, 32]. Cellular injury and organ injury have been shown to occur rapidly, as a direct consequence of both the inflammatory response and hypoperfusion in sepsis [33, 34]. Rapid stabilization of the patient's hemodynamic status, including volume expansion and administration of combined vasopressors/inotropes titrated to selected physiological endpoints of resuscitation, is critically important to limit further cell death and to optimize the chances for organ function restoration [35, 36]. To further improve survival, there is a need for novel therapeutic interventions which target the critical initial resuscitation phase in sepsis.

A series of pilot studies were performed in order to examine the effects of the CirQlator on cardiac output and stroke volume in porcine peritonitis and septic shock. The goal of these pilot studies was to determine whether pulsed intrathoracic pressure regulation device therapy could alter progressive hypotension in a well accepted, well characterized, reproducible animal model. Seven pigs were subjected to the previously published peritonitis protocol [37, 38] and treated with the CirQlator starting 30 minutes after *E. coli* clot implantation (5–7 x 10^{-9} cfu/kg *E. coli O111.B4*). In untreated animals, this produces cardiovascular collapse within 6 hours in > 60 % of all animals [37, 38]. Each animal was then followed for six hours and the intrathoracic pressure regulation device therapy was cycled 30 min on and then 30 min off [39]. Two control animals were not treated with the intrathoracic pressure regulation device to confirm the basic time course of the hemodynamic changes of this model. These control pigs responded in a similar fashion to the numerous other control pigs that have been previously recorded using the same pig model.

Application of the intrathoracic pressure regulation device (28 times in 7 animals) in the absence of fluid resuscitation consistently caused a marked increase in cardiac index, stroke volume and mean arterial pressure, consistent with the mechanism of action of the intrathoracic pressure regulation device to increase venous return and cardiac preload (Cinel et al., unpublished data). These changes occurred in the absence of fluid resuscitation, within 2–5 minutes. Importantly, in these pigs, normal saline infusion was restricted to 1 ml/kg/hour to replace insensible losses. There was no statistical change in heart rate and oxygen saturation stayed above 90 % during the entire treatment course. Pulmonary artery pressures decreased. The data from this preclinical study are supportive that intrathoracic pressure regulation device therapy will provide a significant hemodynamic benefit in the early treatment phase of sepsis.

Some might argue that current fluid resuscitation measures are acceptable during the early resuscitative phase of septic shock and that an alternate therapy is not needed. However, we hypothesize that intrathoracic pressure regulation therapy provides a number of advantages, especially when considered as a complementary therapy to the current standards of care. These include: 1) the intrathoracic pressure regulation device can be used when fluids are not available or in complement with a reduced amount of fluids and the device can be simply added in line to an endotracheal tube as long as the patient is intubated; 2) the current pig data suggest that the circulation can be increased faster with intrathoracic pressure regulation therapy then with traditional fluid therapy alone and certainly when central venous access is not available; 3) the intrathoracic pressure regulation device may also buy time to insert a central line in a more controlled and less hurried manner; 4) in contrast to fluids, intrathoracic pressure regulation therapy appears to reduce pulmonary artery capillary pressures, at least when administered in pulse doses of 30 minutes each; 5) intrathoracic pressure regulation therapy may reduce or avoid the need for vasopressor therapy which might have detrimental effects on renal function and cardiac function (ischemia) and rhythms (atrial and ventricular dysrhythmias); 6) finally, even if the intrathoracic pressure regulation device is used in conjunction with fluids or vasopressors, we speculate that less fluid resuscitation therapy would be required for the same hemodynamic benefit and less vasopressor therapy may be required. In many ways, intrathoracic pressure regulation therapy functions like a mechanical drug, except that it provides its therapeutic benefit non-invasively.

Potential Adverse Consequences and Limitations of Intrathoracic Pressure Regulation Therapy

While studies to date have shown that application of intrathoracic pressure regulation in cardiac arrest and hypovolemic shock results in a marked improvement in hemodynamics and survival rates, the longer-term potential consequences of intrathoracic pressure regulation therapy remain unknown. One can speculate that with more negative intrathoracic pressures there may be greater flow/perfusion mismatch within the lungs, the potential for shunting, and the potential for pulmonary atelectasis. Another potential limitation is that in order for this technology to be of clinical benefit, the thorax must be intact and the patient needs to be intubated. Otherwise it is not possible to consistently generate expiratory phase negative intrathoracic pressures. While this limitation can be overcome by paralyzing and intubating a patient, some patients may at present not warrant endotracheal intubation but develop significant hypotension. As such, a minor paradigm shift may be necessary once the diagnosis of sepsis has been confirmed by currently recommended clinical criteria.

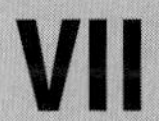

Another potential limitation is that it is not possible to lower the expiratory phase intrathoracic pressures and concurrently use PEEP, unless the intrathoracic pressure regulation device is used as a pulsed therapy, which is under evaluation. Thus, the benefit of circulatory enhancement with the intrathoracic pressure regulation therapy must be balanced clinically with the need to provide PEEP. Animal studies to date suggest that intrathoracic pressure regulation therapy can provide both circulatory and ventilatory support for up to 6 hours.

Conclusion

The significance of this innovative approach rests in its simplicity, the anticipated significant enhancement in blood pressure and circulation, and the ability to harness the body's natural response mechanism to hypotensive stress to improve circulation and blood pressure. Analogous to optimizing the heart rate on an implantable pacemaker based upon the patient's underlying medical condition, different patients will respond differently to different levels of negative intrathoracic pressure based upon their overall condition, the amount of central volume, their starting venous pressure, and other co-existing medical conditions. To date, preclinical and clinical data using intrathoracic pressure regulation therapy to treat cardiac arrest and hypotension in spontaneously-breathing patients confirm that this innovative approach provides an important new therapeutic option for the hypotensive patient population where increased cardiac preload would be beneficial.

References

1. Lurie K, Voelckel W, Plaisance P, et al (2000) Use of an inspiratory impedance threshold valve during cardiopulmonary resuscitation: a progress report. Resuscitation 44: 219–230
2. Lurie KG, Coffeen P, Shultz J, McKnite S, Detloff B, Mulligan KA (1995) Improving active compression-decompression cardiopulmonary resuscitation with an inspiratory impedance valve. Circulation 91: 1629–1632
3. Lurie KG, Mulligan KA, McKnite S, Detloff B, Lindstrom P, Lindner KH (1998) Optimizing standard cardiopulmonary resuscitation with an inspiratory impedance threshold valve. Chest 113: 1084–1090
4. Lurie KG, Voelckel WG, Zielinski T, et al (2001) Improving standard cardiopulmonary resuscitation with an inspiratory impedance threshold valve in a porcine model of cardiac arrest. Anesth Analg 93: 649–655
5. Lurie KG, Zielinski T, McKnite S, Aufderheide T, Voelckel W (2002) Use of an inspiratory impedance valve improves neurologically intact survival in a porcine model of ventricular fibrillation. Circulation 105: 124–129
6. Lurie KG, Zielinski TM, McKnite SH, et al (2004) Treatment of hypotension in pigs with an inspiratory impedance threshold device: a feasibility study. Crit Care Med 32: 1555–1562

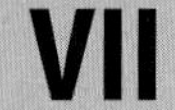

7. Plaisance P, Lurie KG, Payen D (2000) Inspiratory impedance during active compression-decompression cardiopulmonary resuscitation: a randomized evaluation in patients in cardiac arrest. Circulation 101: 989–994
8. Samniah N, Voelckel WG, Zielinski TM, et al (2003) Feasibility and effects of transcutaneous phrenic nerve stimulation combined with an inspiratory impedance threshold in a pig model of hemorrhagic shock. Crit Care Med 31: 1197–1202
9. Sigurdsson G, Yannopoulos D, McKnite SH, et al (2006) Effects of an inspiratory impedance threshold device on blood pressure and short term survival in spontaneously breathing hypovolemic pigs. Resuscitation 68: 399–404
10. Convertino VA, Cooke WH, Lurie KG (2005) Inspiratory resistance as a potential treatment for orthostatic intolerance and hemorrhagic shock. Aviat Space Environ Med 76: 319–325
11. Convertino VA, Ratliff DA, Crissey J, Doerr DF, Idris AH, Lurie KG (2005) Effects of inspiratory impedance on hemodynamic responses to a squat-stand test in human volunteers: implications for treatment of orthostatic hypotension. Eur J Appl Physiol 94: 392–399
12. Convertino VA, Ratliff DA, Ryan KL, et al (2004) Effects of inspiratory impedance on the carotid-cardiac baroreflex response in humans. Clin Auton Res 14: 240–248
13. Convertino VA, Ratliff DA, Ryan KL, et al (2004) Hemodynamics associated with breathing through an inspiratory impedance threshold device in human volunteers. Crit Care Med 32 (Suppl 9): S381–386
14. Marino BS, Yannopoulos D, Sigurdsson G, et al (2004) Spontaneous breathing through an inspiratory impedance threshold device augments cardiac index and stroke volume index in a pediatric porcine model of hemorrhagic hypovolemia. Crit Care Med 32 (Suppl 9): S398–405
15. Melby DP, Lu F, Sakaguchi S, et al (2007) Increased impedance to inspiration ameliorates hemodynamic changes associated with movement to upright posture in orthostatic hypotension: a randomized blinded pilot study. Heart Rhythm 4: 128–135
16. Walcott GP, Killingsworth CR, Smith WM, Ideker RE (2002) Biphasic waveform external defibrillation thresholds for spontaneous ventricular fibrillation secondary to acute ischemia. J Am Coll Cardiol 39: 359–365
17. Aufderheide TP, Pirrallo RG, Provo TA, et al (2005) Clinical evaluation of an inspiratory impedance threshold device during standard cardiopulmonary resuscitation in patients with out-of-hospital cardiac arrest. Crit Care Med 33: 734–740
18. Lurie KG, Barnes TA, Zielinski TM, McKnite SH (2003) Evaluation of a prototypic inspiratory impedance threshold valve designed to enhance the efficiency of cardiopulmonary resuscitation. Respir Care 48: 52–57

19. Pirrallo RG, Aufderheide TP, Provo TA, et al (2005) Effect of an inspiratory impedance threshold device on hemodynamics during conventional manual cardiopulmonary resuscitation. Resuscitation 66: 13–20
20. Plaisance P, Lurie KG, Vicaut E, et al (2004) Evaluation of an impedance threshold device in patients receiving active compression-decompression cardiopulmonary resuscitation for out of hospital cardiac arrest. Resuscitation 61: 265–271
21. Plaisance P, Soleil C, Lurie KG, et al (2005) Use of an inspiratory impedance threshold device on a facemask and endotracheal tube to reduce intrathoracic pressures during the decompression phase of active compression-decompression cardiopulmonary resuscitation. Crit Care Med 33: 990–994
22. Raedler C, Voelckel WG, Wenzel V, et al (2002) Vasopressor response in a porcine model of hypothermic cardiac arrest is improved with active compression-decompression cardiopulmonary resuscitation using the inspiratory impedance threshold valve. Anesth Analg 95: 1496–1502
23. Wolcke BB, Mauer DK, Schoefmann MF, et al (2003) Comparison of standard cardiopulmonary resuscitation versus the combination of active compression-decompression cardiopulmonary resuscitation and an inspiratory impedance threshold device for out-of-hospital cardiac arrest. Circulation 108: 2201–2205
24. Yannopoulos D, Sigurdsson G, McKnite S, et al (2004) Reducing ventilation frequency combined with an inspiratory impedance device improves CPR efficiency in swine model of cardiac arrest. Resuscitation 61: 75–82
25. Yannopoulos D, Tang W, Roussos C, et al (2005) Reducing ventilation frequency during cardiopulmonary resuscitation in a porcine model of cardiac arrest. Respir Care 50: 628–635
26. American Heart Association (2005) Guidelines for Cardiopulmonary Resuscitation and Emergency Cardiovascular Care. Circulation 112 (Suppl 24): IV1–203
27. Aufderheide T, Birnbaum M, Lick C, et al (2007) A tale of seven EMS systems: an impedance threshold device and improved CPR techniques double survival rates after out-of-hospital cardiac arrest. Circulation 116: II-936
28. Yannopoulos D, Nadkarni VM, McKnite SH, et al (2005) Intrathoracic pressure regulator during continuous chest-compression advanced cardiac resuscitation improves vital organ perfusion pressures in a porcine model of cardiac arrest. Circulation 112: 803–811
29. Yannopoulos D, McKnite S, Metzger A, Lurie KG (2007) Intrathoracic pressure regulation improves 24-hour survival in a porcine model of hypovolemic shock. Anesth Analg 104: 157–162
30. Bircher N, Safar P (1985) Cerebral preservation during cardiopulmonary resuscitation. Crit Care Med 13: 185–190
31. Cinel I, Dellinger RP (2006) Current treatment of severe sepsis. Curr Infect Dis Rep 8: 358–365
32. Cinel I, Dellinger RP (2007) Advances in pathogenesis and management of sepsis. Curr Opin Infect Dis 20: 345–352
33. Cinel I, Opal S (2009) Molecular biology of inflammation and sepsis: A primer. Crit Care Med 37: 291–304
34. Treziack S, Cinel I, Dellinger RP, et al (2008) Resuscitating the microcirculation in severe sepsis and septic shock: Emerging concepts, challenges, and future directions. Acad Emerg Med 15: 1–15
35. Dellinger RP, Levy MM, Carlet JM, et al (2008) Surviving Sepsis Campaign: international guidelines for management of severe sepsis and septic shock: 2008. Crit Care Med 36: 296–327
36. Dellinger RP, Levy MM, Carlet JM, et al (2008) Surviving Sepsis Campaign: international guidelines for management of severe sepsis and septic shock: 2008. Intensive Care Med 34: 17–60
37. Goldfarb RD, Glock D, Johnson K, et al (1998) Randomized, blinded, placebo-controlled trial of tissue factor pathway inhibitor in porcine septic shock. Shock 10: 258–264
38. Goldfarb RD, Dellinger RP, Parrillo JE (2005) Porcine models of severe sepsis: emphasis on porcine peritonitis. Shock 24 (Suppl 1): 75–81
39. Cinel I, Goldfarb R, Metzger A, et al (2009) Intrathoracic pressure regulation stimulates cardiac index in porcine peritonitis. Crit Care Med (abst, in press)

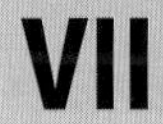

Functional Hemodynamic Monitoring: A Personal Perspective

M.R. Pinsky

Introduction

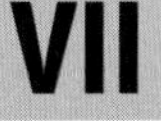

Hemodynamic monitoring is a central component of the overall management approach to the critically ill patient. Hemodynamic monitoring of critically ill patients has a dual function. First, it can be used to document hemodynamic stability and the lack of need for acute therapeutic interventions. Second, through monitoring we can measure variables and define the degree to which they vary from their baseline values. Thus, hemodynamic monitoring must be able to define both stability and change.

The utilization of different monitoring techniques, procedures and devices is essential for the effective assessment and management of the critical care patient. The utilization of hemodynamic monitoring is not only vital in assessing the patient's condition but also for close titration of therapies whose treatment is guided by these data. Implicit in this approach are the assumptions that physiological assessment of the subject's cardiopulmonary status can be made, and that its trends over time reflect known pathophysiological processes and the impact of treatment on these processes. Regrettably, this is the step upon which most treatments fail to make the correct linkage of monitoring to implication.

As a generic and pragmatic statement, hemodynamic monitoring is used to assess cardiovascular insufficiency and sufficiency and to direct therapies to maintain adequate tissue perfusion and organ system function. A fundamental means to attain tissue wellness is to sustain adequate amounts of oxygen delivery (DO_2) to the tissues. Since there is no clear evidence that maintaining target levels of DO_2 will insure adequate delivery of oxygen to all tissues in critically ill patients, the justification for the use of specific types of monitoring has been grouped into three levels of defense based on their level of validation, as described by Bellomo and Pinsky [1]. The basic level of defense argues from the basis of historical controls where prior experience using similar monitoring was traditionally used and presumed to be beneficial. The mechanism by which the benefit is achieved need not be understood or even postulated. The second level of defense uses arguments based on an understanding of the pathophysiology of the process being treated. This physiological argument is stated as: "Knowledge of how a disease process creates its effect and thus preventing the process from altering measured bodily functions should prevent the disease process from progressing or injuring remote physiological functions." Most of the rationale for hemodynamic monitoring resides at this level. The third level of defense is based on documentation that the monitoring device, by altering therapy in otherwise unexpected ways, improves outcome in terms of survival and quality of life. In reality, few therapies used in medicine can claim benefit at this level. Thus, we are left with the physiological rationale as the primary defense of monitoring of critically ill patients.

Regrettably, the physiological interpretation of traditional monitoring is often inaccurate, not supported by clinical data or simply incorrect. I previously examined in depth the limitations of present hemodynamic monitoring [2], and the reader is referred to that paper for further discussion. Suffice it to say that the present use of static hemodynamic variables, no matter what their nature – pressures, flow, O_2 or CO_2 levels, etc. – will greatly improve diagnosis, treatment, or outcome from critical illness beyond where we are today without a completely different perspective as to their application.

Use of Dynamic Responses to Identify Nascent Cardiovascular States

Few static hemodynamic variables describe well the response of the subject to stress. However, by using dynamic variables, one can understand much more about the responsiveness and reserve of the subject than can ever be defined by static variables. Although recent interest in the stroke volume variation (SVV) and pulse pressure variation (PPV) as markers of volume responsiveness has emerged [3], they are only examples of functional hemodynamic monitoring, not the initial ones nor probably the best examples.

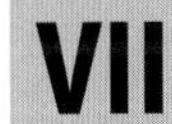

Two classic examples of functional markers follow that serve to illustrate this point. Subjects presenting with hypovolemic shock often have normotension owing to intact baroreceptor activity increasing vasomotor tone to sustain cardiac output despite a decreasing blood volume. One may elicit occult hypovolemia by performing a hydrostatic test. If one measures blood pressure and heart rate in the supine and then sitting position, hypovolemia will often manifest itself as increasing heart rate and hypotension. These 'postural' signs of functional hypovolemia also may occur in subjects with dysautonomia, dehydration, and excessive sympathetic blockade. Still, there is nothing special about the measures of blood pressure or pulse that are made, just their dynamic change induced by the maneuver of sitting up. Similarly, the electrocardiogram (EKG) is useful in identifying arrhythmias and the existence of ventricular hypertrophy, ischemia, and prior myocardial infarctions, but it predicts poorly the existence of asymptomatic coronary artery disease, even if high grade coronary stenosis is present. However, by examining the effect of graded exercise on the EKG, emergent parameters develop, such as ST segment depression, T wave inversion, and arrhythmias that are highly sensitive and specific for clinically relevant coronary artery disease. Again, as in the above example of the postural challenge, there is nothing new or special about the EKG, it is the way in which the data from the EKG changes in response to the test that allows its sensitivity and specificity to be increased. Accordingly, using dynamic stressors, one creates emergent novel parameters that can greatly improve the sensitivity and specificity of existing and new monitoring techniques.

Preload Responsiveness

Since one of the primary therapeutic questions in hemodynamically unstable patients is their ability to increase cardiac output and DO_2 in response to volume loading, it is reasonable to start our analysis of the studies by assessing the measures of preload responsiveness. Positive pressure ventilation alters venous return and induces several predictable changes in vena caval diameters, pulmonary blood flow and left ventricular output. In the volume responsive subject, increasing intrathoracic pressure during positive-pressure inspiration will decrease venous return by decreasing the pressure gradient for venous return. One will see narrowing of the superior and inferior vena cava, inspiration-associated decreases in pulmonary blood flow and a three to four beat phase lag decrease in left ventricular stroke volume and arterial pulse pressure. These studies have been recently reviewed [4, 5]. In fact, one can fluid resuscitate high risk surgery patients until PPV decreases $< 10\,\%$ and demonstrate improved outcomes [6]. These techniques are limited however, because of the need to have the patient fully in synchrony with the positive pressure breaths and without vigorous spontaneous breathing [7]. Still, as a means to assess volume responsiveness in the sedated and ventilated patient, for whom most of anesthesiology is its field, this is a major advance in monitoring potential.

To address assessment of volume responsiveness in spontaneously breathing subjects and those with arrhythmias, clinicians have returned to the classic hydrostatic challenges of sitting up and passive leg raising. Postural changes such as passive leg raising have been used for many years as a means to transiently increase venous return. Not surprisingly numerous studies have demonstrated that the dynamic changes in cardiac output induced by passive leg raising are as sensitive and specific to predicting volume responsiveness as are PPV and SVV during positive pressure breathing [8] (reviewed in [5]).

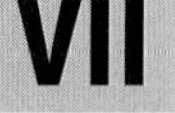

Thus, the bedside clinician now has several means to assess preload responsiveness in all patients if he or she only tries and also uses functional hemodynamic monitoring.

Cardiovascular Sufficiency

Although assessing preload responsiveness is a useful and important tool, critically ill patients in circulatory shock can also be non-responsive to fluid administration and still need to be resuscitated. Similarly, knowing when increasing DO_2 has restored tissue perfusion and no further increase is necessary is an important question to ascertain because over resuscitation also carries risks. Unfortunately, indirect measures of flow are not readily available at the bedside and those that have been developed have not yet been used in clinical trials. Perhaps the most commonly used methods to assess circulatory sufficiency are mixed venous oxygen saturation (SvO_2) and its surrogate, central venous oxygen saturation ($ScvO_2$). We previously suggested using SvO_2 to drive resuscitation and determine physiologic end-points [9], and $ScvO_2$ may also be useful, though in a diminished capacity owing to the streaming of venous blood and the problems with venous blood sampling.

One new technology that has recently become available is the measurement of tissue oxygen saturation (StO_2) using near infrared spectroscopy. Again, static measures of StO_2 are not very useful in defining resuscitation outcomes [10] but the dynamic StO_2 response to a defined vascular occlusion test allows the measure of reoxygenation rates upon vascular occlusion release [11] (**Fig. 1**). Again, the StO_2 value by itself is not sensitive or specific to identify occult tissue hypoperfusion, but its reoxygenation slope is. Although more new clinical data need to be acquired on this vascular occlusion technique, it is emblematic of the approaches which need to be considered in going forward.

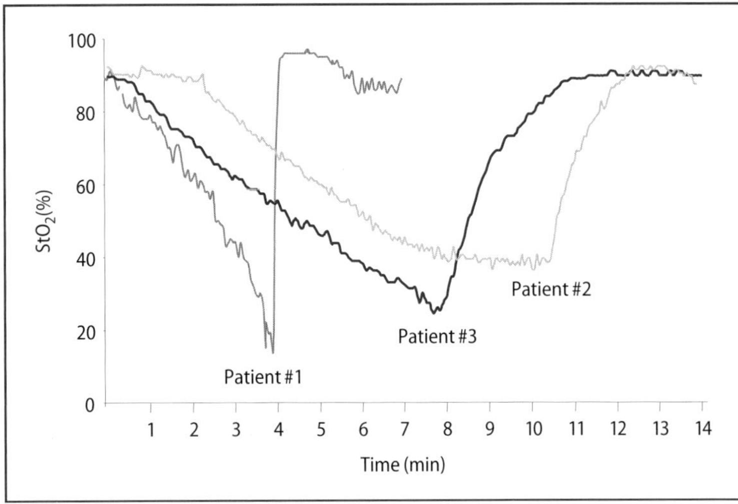

Fig. 1. Representative values of tissue O_2 saturation (StO_2) during a vascular occlusion test wherein release was started after StO_2 decreased to < 20 %. Note that patient #1 has a more rapid oxygen consumption and reoxygenation rate than the other two with patient #3 having the slowest rates and patient #2 having only a selective decrease in oxygen consumption with an intermediate reoxygenation rate compared to the other two patients.

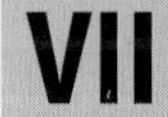

Future Trends

The academic community is encouraged to take a leadership role in this evolving field of functional monitoring. Clinicians have always used such approaches in their bedside titration of care, including assessing the impact of a volume challenge or other specific controlled clinical trials [12]. In all cases, the bedside clinician makes a specific hypothesis, then performs a maneuver, and then assesses the dynamic response, whether it be a spontaneous breathing trial, fluid challenge, or drug infusion. However, where these trials become functional is when the subject's response is determined by their underlying physiological state and reserve. For example, one can examine the pulse oximetry oxygen saturation (SpO_2) response to sitting up and taking deep breaths in a chronic obstructive pulmonary disease (COPD) patient on low flow oxygen and with existing hypoxemia (SpO_2 < 90 %). If the cause of the hypoxemia is a poor ventilation/perfusion match, then the effect of increasing blood flow associated with sitting up and minor alveolar recruitment will improve SpO_2. If, however, the cause of the hypoxemia is pneumonia or complete lung collapse then the associated fall in SvO_2 induced by the exercise of sitting up will cause SpO_2 to fall. Thus, by simply examining the dynamic response to SpO_2 one may identify the causes of hypoxemia at the bedside in COPD patients. In fact, there are probably no monitoring devices present today that cannot be used in a dynamic way to assess physiological status and reserve. We need only see them within this framework and start to collectively move forward toward a more interactive and specific assessment of our patient's health status and response to therapy. The advantages of these approaches are that they require no new technologies, are essentially free, and will have immediate and direct patient benefit.

Acknowledgement: This work was supported in part by NIH grants HL007820 and HL067181

References

1. Bellomo R, Pinsky MR (1996) Invasive monitoring. In: Tinker J, Browne D, Sibbald W (eds) Critical Care – Standards, Audit and Ethics. Arnold Publishing Company, London, pp 82–104
2. Pinsky MR (2007) Hemodynamic evaluation and monitoring in the ICU. Chest 123: 2020–2029
3. Michard F, Boussat S, Chemla D, et al (2000) Relation between respiratory changes in arterial pulse pressure and fluid responsiveness in septic patients with acute circulatory failure. Am J Respir Crit Care Med 162: 134–138
4. Pinsky MR, Payen D (2005) Functional hemodynamic monitoring. Crit Care 9: 566–572
5. Hadian M, Pinsky MR (2007) Functional hemodynamic monitoring. Curr Opin Crit Care 13: 318–323
6. Lopes MR, Oliveira MA, Pereira VO, Lemos IPB, Auler JO Jr, Michard F (2007) Goal-directed fluid management based on pulse pressure variation monitoring during high-risk surgery: a pilot randomized controlled trial. Crit Care 11:R100–107
7. Pinsky MR (2002) Functional hemodynamic monitoring. Intensive Care Med 28: 386–388
8. Monnet X, Rienzo M, Osman D, et al (2006) Response to leg raising predicts fluid responsiveness in critically ill. Crit Care Med 34: 1402–1407
9. Pinsky MR, Vincent J-L (2005) Let us use the pulmonary artery catheter correctly and only when we need it. Crit Care Med 33: 1119–1122
10. Skarda DE, Mulier KE, Myers DE, Taylor JH, Beilman GJ (2007) Dynamic near-infrared spectroscopy measurements in patients with severe sepsis. Shock 27: 348–353
11. Gómez H, Torres A, Zenker S, et al (2008) Use of non-invasive NIRS during a vascular occlusion test to assess dynamic tissue O(2) saturation response. Intensive Care Med 34: 1600–1607
12. Pinsky MR (1998) Controlled observations in critical care medicine: The therapeutic trial. Ann Acad Med Singapore 27: 387–396

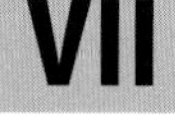

VIII Airway Management

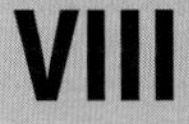

Endotracheal Intubation in the ICU

S. Jaber, B. Jung, and G. Chanques

Introduction

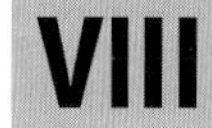

Patients admitted to the intensive care unit (ICU) often have acute respiratory failure and/or cardiovascular collapse. In addition, reserves of oxygenation and organ perfusion are limited in ICU patients in contrast to non-critically ill patients. Endotracheal intubation, which is one of the most commonly performed procedures in the ICU, is associated with a high incidence of complications because of the precarious hemodynamic and respiratory status of critically ill patients [1–3]. The incidence of life-threatening complications associated with endotracheal intubation (severe hypoxemia, cardiovascular collapse, cardiac arrest, death) in ICU patients ranges from 25 to 39 % [1, 3, 4]. Severe but non life-threatening complications, including cardiac arrhythmia, difficult endotracheal intubation, esophageal and/or traumatic endotracheal intubation, aspiration, and patient agitation [1] generally occur in 10 to 30 % of endotracheal intubations [1, 3, 4].

Contrary to airway management performed in the operating room and pre-hospital conditions, few studies designed to improve endotracheal intubation safety in the ICU have been published [5]. The objectives of this chapter are to describe the complications associated with the endotracheal intubation procedure performed in the ICU and to propose a 10-point care management bundle for endotracheal intubation in the ICU to reduce the incidence of severe and life-threatening complications occurring immediately after the procedure. We have divided the care bundle into three phases: pre-, per-, and post-intubation (**Table 1**). We do not include airway management in the pediatric ICU, impending cardiac arrest, or emergency surgical procedures performed in the operating room.

Care Management Bundle to Increase the Safety of Endotracheal Intubation in the ICU

Pre-intubation Period

Endotracheal intubation in the ICU is rarely a real emergency. In the majority of cases, the ICU team therefore has a few minutes to prepare the procedure in order to improve safety. Each time they are confronted with a patient needing endotracheal intubation, clinicians must assess for signs predictive of difficult intubation. Several predictive scores have been reported and are of great value for clinicians (**Table 2**). Indeed, mouth opening to accommodate less than two fingers, invisible uvula, thyromental distance less than 65 mm, short thick neck, interincisor gap < 5 cm with mandibular luxation < 0, head and neck movement < 90° and Mallampati

Table 1. Proposed care bundle for intubation management

Pre-Intubation
1. Presence of two operators
2. Fluid loading (isotonic saline 500 ml or starch 250 ml) in absence of cardiogenic edema
3. Preparation of long-term sedation
4. Pre-oxygenate for 3 min with non-invasive positive pressure ventilation in case of acute respiratory failure (FiO_2 100 %, pressure support ventilation level between 5 and 15 cmH_2O to obtain an expiratory tidal volume between 6 and 8 ml/kg and PEEP of 5 cmH_2O)

Per-Intubation

5. Rapid sequence induction: etomidate 0.2–0.3 mg/kg or ketamine 1.5–3 mg/kg associated with succinylcholine 1–1.5 mg/kg in absence of allergy, hyperkalemia, severe acidosis, acute or chronic neuromuscular disease, burns patient for more than 48 h and medullar trauma
6. Sellick maneuver

Post-Intubation

7. Immediate confirmation of tube placement by capnography
8. Norepinephrine if diastolic blood pressure remains < 35 mmHg
9. Initiate long-term sedation
10. Initial 'protective ventilation': tidal volume 6–8 ml/kg, PEEP < 5 cmH_2O and respiratory rate between 10 and 20 cycles/min, FiO_2 100 % with a plateau pressure < 30 cmH_2O

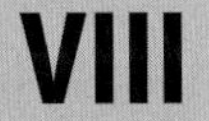

Table 2. Components of the pre-operative physical airway examination, adapted from [6] and [10]

Airway Examination Component	Non-reassuring Findings
Length of upper incisors	Relatively long
Relation of maxillary and mandibular incisors during normal jaw closure	Prominent 'overbite' (i.e., maxillary incisors anterior to mandibular incisors)
Relation of maxillary and mandibular incisors during voluntary protrusion	Patient cannot bring mandibular incisors anterior to (in front of) maxillary incisors
Interincisor distance	< 3 cm
Visibility of uvula	Not visible when tongue is protruded with patient in sitting position (e.g., Mallampati class ≥ II)
Shape of palate	Highly arched or very narrow
Compliance of mandibular space	Stiff, indurated, occupied by mass, or nonresilient
Thyromental distance	Less than three ordinary finger breadths
Length of neck	Short
Thickness of neck	Thick
Range of motion of head and neck	Patient cannot touch tip of chin to chest or cannot extend neck

score > 2 (**Fig. 1**) are all signs that must alert the clinician in charge of the endotracheal intubation [6]. Other clinical situations, such as facial trauma or burns, X-ray therapy of the upper body must also alert the clinician. Furthermore, the presence of at least two of the following signs – age above 55 years, body mass index > 26 kg/m^2, beard, lack of teeth, history of snoring – is associated with manual ventilation difficulties [7]. When a clinician suspects difficulties with manual ventilation and/

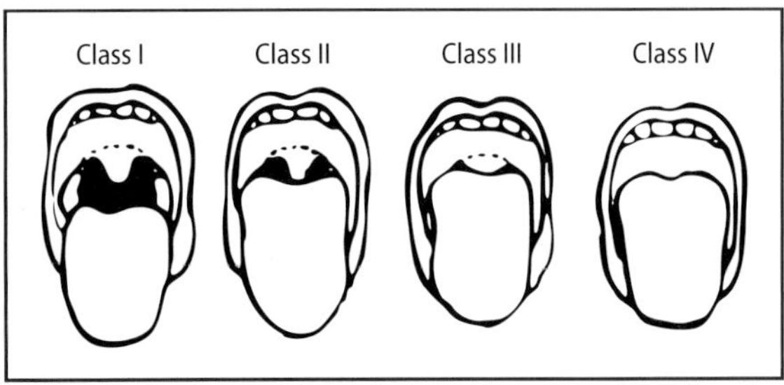

Fig. 1. Mallampati classification for grading airways from the least difficult airway (I) to the most difficult airway (IV). Class I = visualization of the soft palate, fauces, uvula, and anterior and posterior pillars; class II = visualization of the soft palate, fauces, and uvula; class III = visualization of the soft palate and the base of the uvula; and class IV = soft palate is not visible at all.

or endotracheal intubation, he/she should call for assistance in order to manage the airway of the patient using alternative techniques (**Fig. 2**). The main difference between airway management in the ICU and in the operating room is that intensivists cannot wake the critically ill patient to propose an alternative awake intubation, such as fibroscopic intubation; the patient must be oxygenated and ventilated quickly. Hence, in this situation, difficult airway management is much more restricted than in anesthesia care. Furthermore, it is important to remember that the ultimate objective of airway management is to ventilate and oxygenate the patient, not to intubate them.

Optimization of pre-oxygenation can lead to improved procedure safety. In a hypoxic patient, pre-oxygenation is mandatory so as to limit the risk of severe desaturation during the laryngoscopy. Our group reported that non invasive ventilation (NIV) is more effective in reducing arterial oxyhemoglobin desaturations than other methods [8]. We also reported similar results for the pre-oxygenation of very obese patients in the operating room [9]. We then proposed that all hypoxemic ICU patients should be systematically pre-oxygenated with NIV using a face mask present at the head of each ICU bed, with an FiO_2 equal to 1, low to moderate pressure support levels (PSV 5 to 15 cmH_2O) and 5 cmH_2O of positive end-expiratory pressure (PEEP) to obtain an expiratory tidal volume (V_T) between 6 to 10 ml/kg of ideal body weight. Pre-oxygenation NIV is administered during the time required to prepare induction drugs and the intubation device (**Table 1**). A multiple center study is ongoing to evaluate the impact of pre-oxygenation NIV on the outcome of ICU patients intubated for acute respiratory distress (clinicaltrials.gov identifier NCT00472160).

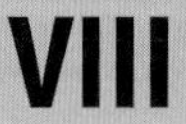

Cardiovascular collapse frequently occurs within a few minutes following intubation [1, 4]. The additive effects of hypovolemia, the suppression of the endogenous activation of sympathetic response by the anesthetic drugs [10, 11], and the intrathoracic positive pressure due to mechanical ventilation are implicated in cardiovascular collapse after endotracheal intubation in critically ill patients. The impact of fluid loading to prevent cardiovascular collapse after endotracheal intubation in the ICU has never been specifically studied, but we speculate that it could limit its occurrence, except in the case of cardiogenic edema.

Per-intubation Period

Choice of drugs should take into account the hemodynamic and neurologic status of patients and should have specific pharmacokinetic properties for induction of anesthesia and long-term sedation [11]. To limit the effects of drugs on cardiovascular status, we believe that clinicians should avoid agents such as propofol or thiopental,

Airway management necessary
Call senior physician für assistance
Invasive airway management
Non-invasive airway management
Fails
NIPPV
Potential for DMV and/or DI
Yes, adequate physiologic reserve
Primary awake technique (FOI, nasotracheal)
No
Yes, pt in respiratory arrest
Supralaryngeal ventilation as conduit for intubation
Direct Laryngoscopy Ablation vs preservation of SB. With or without NMBA
No
Yes
Fails, mask ventilation inadequate
Fails, mask ventilation inadequate
Intubating-, video-assisted-, or classic LMA as bridge for definitive airway mgt
ASA DAA emergency pathway

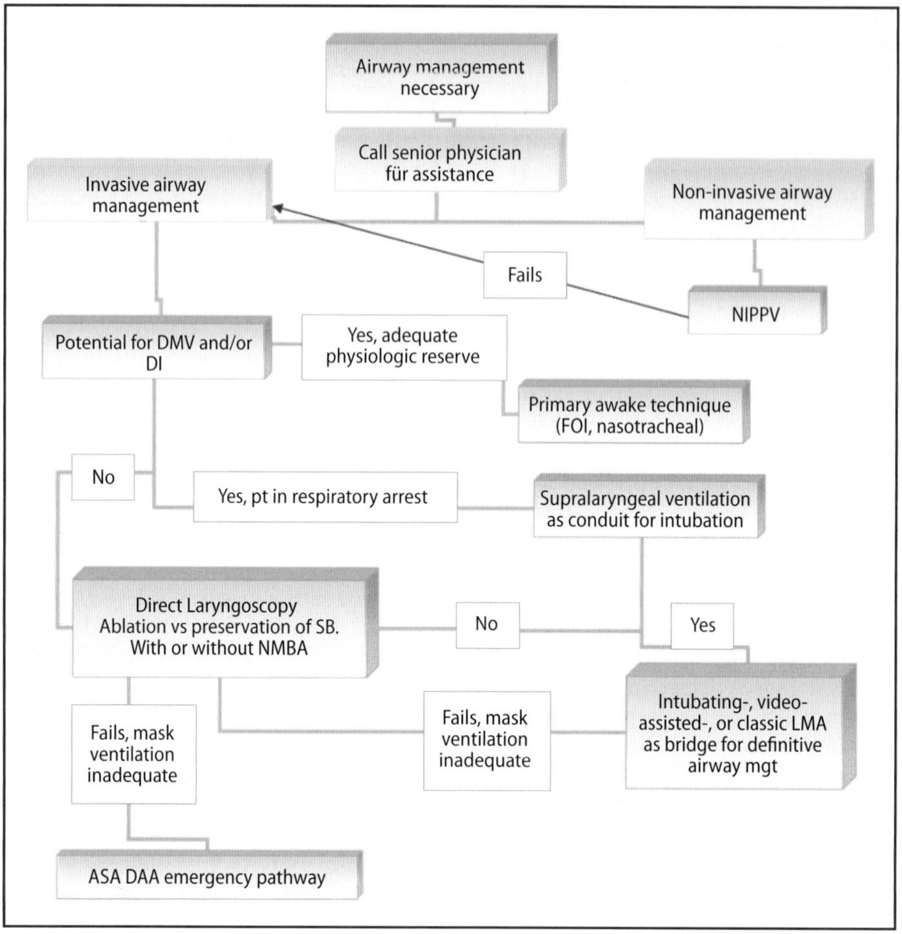

Fig. 2. Algorithm for airway management in the ICU, adapted from [10]. SB: spontaneous breathing; NMBA: neuromuscular blocking agent; DMV: difficult mask ventilation; pt: patient; NIPPV: non-invasive positive pressure ventilation; DI: difficult intubation

VIII

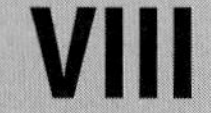

and propose a rapid sequence induction with ketamine or etomidate and succinylcholine, unless contraindicated [11] (**Table 1**). Ketamine (1–2 mg/kg), and etomidate (0.3–0.5 mg/kg) are anesthetic agents widely used in pre-hospital or emergency room conditions because they have a rapid onset, short half-life, are well tolerated hemodynamically, and improve intubation conditions [10–12].

Several studies have recently shown that even a single administration of etomidate could have a negative effect on adrenal function, especially in septic shock patients [13–15]. However, other recently published studies could not confirm this adverse effect of etomidate [16, 17] and/or showed that this impairment was reversible 12 h after administration [18]. Furthermore, the international consensus conference on adrenal function in intensive care reported controversial definitions of adrenal insufficiency [19]: Should an ACTH test use 1 or 250 μg of synacthen? Should albumin-bound cortisol or the free blood portion be measured? What is the definition of adrenal insufficiency in septic patients? To our knowledge, there is no published study comparing the potentially deleterious effect of etomidate on adrenal function versus its hemodynamic tolerability in critically ill patients. Therefore, we believe that etomidate or ketamine are elective hypnotic agents for endotracheal intubation in the ICU. A French multicenter study evaluating the use of ketamine and etomidate as hypnotic drugs in the pre-hospital setting has recently been completed (clinicaltrials.gov identifier NCT00440102).

Succinylcholine is a rapid onset, short-term myorelaxant agent recommended for rapid sequence induction [11]. Succinylcholine does improve intubation conditions but its use should be avoided in certain cases (**Table 1**) [11]. Indeed, pre-existing hyperkalemia, severe acidosis or previous myogenic disease are well known contraindications to succinylcholine [20]. Other conditions also increase the risks of life-threatening complications with succinylcholine in ICU patients, including burns, rhabdomyolysis or chronic (spine trauma, myopathy, Charcot's disease) and acute (long-term immobilization, denervation of muscles or ICU-acquired paresis) neuromuscular disease. Rocuronium may be an alternative to succinylcholine when faced with these contraindications. Rocuronium is a non-depolarizing myorelaxant with rapid onset of action, but a long plasma half-life (45 minutes) that may be dangerous in the case of non-anticipated airway management difficulties. Sugammadex is a chelating agent which reduces the rocuronium half-life from 45 to 1 min. Following its introduction in the USA, it will soon be available on the European market and may allow rocuronium to become a real alternative to succinylcholine in ICU patients.

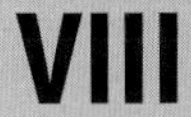

The Sellick maneuver is a part of rapid sequence induction which should be systematically performed to prevent gastric contents from leaking into the pharynx and the associated inhalation of substances into the lungs, as well as vomiting into an unprotected airway. This maneuver is contraindicated in unstable cervical spine trauma [21].

Although, no randomized controlled study has been performed to evaluate intubation performed systematically with or without rapid sequence induction with a myorelaxant, pooling results from ICU studies suggests that the proportion of difficult intubations is inversely correlated to the proportion of intubations performed with rapid sequence induction in critically ill patients (**Fig. 3**).

Being prepared for unforeseen complications during endotracheal intubation is of prime importance when instrumenting the airways of a critically ill patient. Furthermore, conditions for intubation should be as close to ideal as possible in a hectic ICU environment and should include adequate personnel, optimal patient positioning and lighting, and the necessary equipment for endotracheal intubation. For the management of difficult intubations, a supply of devices and an algorithm must be available in every ICU (**Fig. 2**).

Post-intubation Period

Capnography allows confirmation of the endotracheal position of the tube and can verify the absence of esophageal placement [22]. Although capnography is widely used and strictly recommended in the operating room, no studies have evaluated its impact in the ICU [22–25]. We proposed a care management bundle (with capnography) of endotracheal intubation in the ICU which improved the safety of the procedure [26]. Although we could not demonstrate an independent positive action of capnography, we believe that its systematic use could improve the safety of endotracheal intubation because of the rapid recognition of esophageal intubation [27].

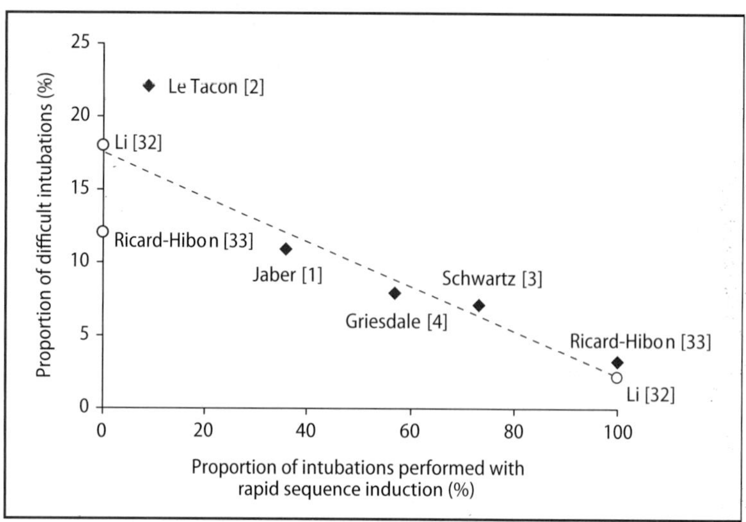

Fig. 3. Proportion of difficult intubations according to the proportion of intubations performed with rapid sequence induction in studies in critically ill patients

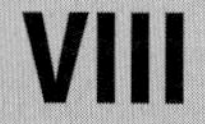

After intubation, it is recommended that the cuff pressure be verified so as to avoid excessive pressure on the trachea and associated risk of tracheal ischemia [28].

The rapid introduction of sedation could also improve the safety of endotracheal intubation by decreasing the agitation rate in an unstable intubated patient [26, 29]. Although no study has evaluated the impact of protective ventilatory settings, we propose ventilating critically ill patients with 'protective parameters', such as a V_T of 6–8 ml/kg, a PEEP less than 5 cmH_2O, a respiratory rate between 10 and 20 cycles/min, an FiO_2 initially at 100 %, and a plateau pressure less than 30 cmH_2O (**Table 1**), because high V_T (> 12 ml/kg) may worsen re-ventilation collapse in unstable ICU patients, may promote inflammatory cytokines even in healthy lungs [30], and is known to be deleterious for patients with acute respiratory distress syndrome (ARDS) [31].

We reported in a multiple center study that the implementation of an endotracheal intubation management protocol can reduce immediate severe life-threatening complications subsequent to intubation of ICU patients [26] **Figs. 4** and **5**). All endotracheal intubations performed during two consecutive 6-month phases, before (control phase) and after (intervention phase) the implementation of an endotracheal intubation management protocol were evaluated. Six of the ten recommendations (non-invasive positive pressure ventilation for pre-oxygenation, presence of two operators, rapid sequence induction with Sellick maneuver, capnography, and protective ventilation) have been shown to be individually efficacious in critical and/or anesthesia care. Four recommendations were developed on the basis of the clinical experience (fluid loading, preparation and early administration of sedation, and vasopressor use if needed). The primary end-points were the incidence of life-threatening complications occurring within 60-mins after endotracheal intubation (cardiac arrest or death, severe cardiovascular collapse, and hypoxemia). Other complications (moderate) were also evaluated. The endotracheal intubation procedure in the intervention phase (n = 121) was associated with significant decreases in life-threatening complications (21 vs 34 %, p = 0.04) and in moderate complications (9 vs 21 %, p = 0.02) compared to the control phase (n = 123) (**Figs. 4** and **5**).

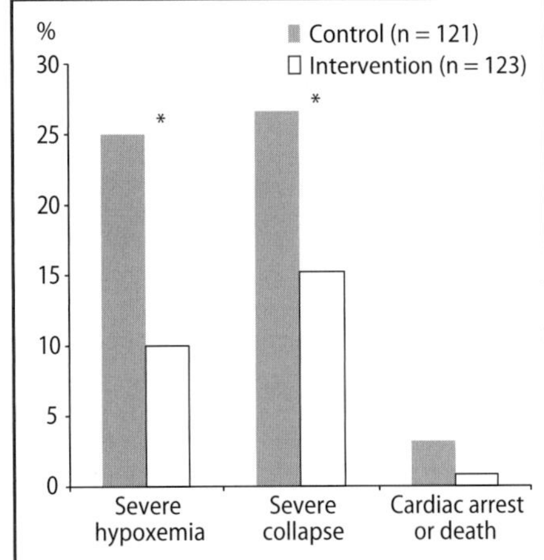

Fig. 4. Life-threatening complications occurring after all intubations performed during the control (n = 121) and the intervention (n = 123) phases [26]. Severe hypoxemia and hemodynamic collapses were significantly lower in the interventional phase than in the control phase. *p < 0.05

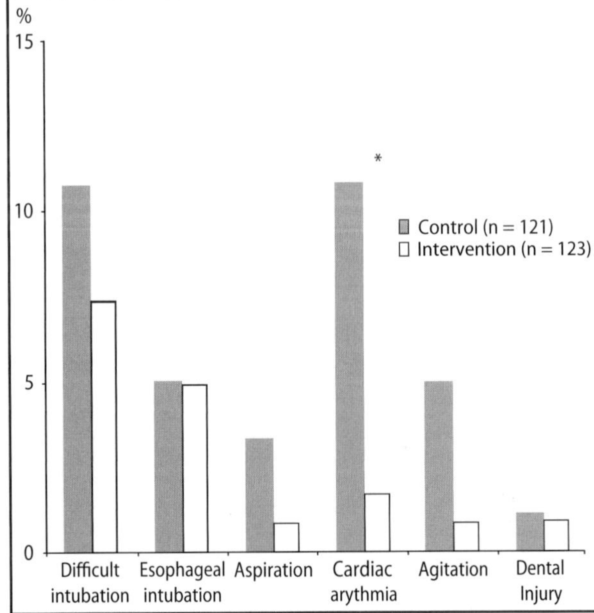

Fig. 5. Mild to moderate complications occurring after all intubations performed during the control (n = 121) and the intervention (n = 123) phases [26]. No significant difference was observed between the two phases for the overall mild to moderate complications except for cardiac arrhythmias which occurred less frequently after the implementation of the protocol. *p < 0.05

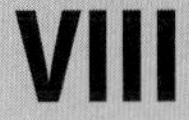

Conclusion

Managing the airway of a critically ill patient poses some unique challenges for the intensivist. The combination of a limited physiologic reserve in the patient and the potential for difficult mask ventilation and intubation mandates careful planning with a good working knowledge of alternative tools and strategies, should conventional attempts at securing the airway fail. To limit the incidence of severe complications associated with this hazardous procedure, we believe that endotracheal intubation should be directed by developing protocols with safety procedures for pre-, per- and post-intubation management.

References

1. Jaber S, Amraoui J, Lefrant JY, et al (2006) Clinical practice and risk factors for immediate complications of endotracheal intubation in the intensive care unit: a prospective, multiple-center study. Crit Care Med 34: 2355–2361
2. Le Tacon S, Wolter P, Rusterholtz T, et al (2000) [Complications of difficult tracheal intubations in a critical care unit]. Ann Fr Anesth Reanim 19: 719–724
3. Schwartz DE, Matthay MA, Cohen NH (1995) Death and other complications of emergency airway management in critically ill adults. A prospective investigation of 297 tracheal intubations. Anesthesiology 82: 367–376
4. Griesdale DE, Bosma TL, Kurth T, Isac G, Chittock DR (2008) Complications of endotracheal intubation in the critically ill. Intensive Care Med 34: 1835–1842
5. Leibowitz AB (2006) Tracheal intubation in the intensive care unit: extremely hazardous even in the best of hands. Crit Care Med 34: 2497–2498
6. Arne J, Descoins P, Fusciardi J, et al (1998) Preoperative assessment for difficult intubation in general and ENT surgery: predictive value of a clinical multivariate risk index. Br J Anaesth 80: 140–146
7. Langeron O, Masso E, Huraux C, et al (2000) Prediction of difficult mask ventilation. Anesthesiology 92: 1229–1236
8. Baillard C, Fosse JP, Sebbane M, et al (2006) Noninvasive ventilation improves preoxygenation before intubation of hypoxic patients. Am J Respir Crit Care Med 174: 171–177
9. Delay J, Sebbane M, Jung B, et al (2008) The effectiveness of non invasive positive pressure ventilation to enhance preoxygenation in morbidly obese patients: a randomized controlled study. Anesth Analg 107: 1707–1713

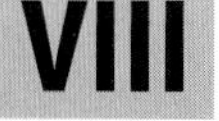

10. Walz JM, Heard SO (2005) Making tracheal intubation safer in the critically ill patient. Crit Care Med 33: 2716–2717
11. Walz JM, Zayaruzny M, Heard SO (2007) Airway management in critical illness. Chest 131: 608–620
12. Smith DC, Bergen JM, Smithline H, Kirschner R (2000) A trial of etomidate for rapid sequence intubation in the emergency department. J Emerg Med 18: 13–16
13. den Brinker M, Hokken-Koelega AC, Hazelzet JA, de Jong FH, Hop WC, Joosten KF (2008) One single dose of etomidate negatively influences adrenocortical performance for at least 24h in children with meningococcal sepsis. Intensive Care Med 34: 163–168
14. Lipiner-Friedman D, Sprung CL, Laterre PF, et al (2007) Adrenal function in sepsis: the retrospective Corticus cohort study. Crit Care Med 35: 1012–1018
15. Mohammad Z, Afessa B, Finkielman JD (2006) The incidence of relative adrenal insufficiency in patients with septic shock after the administration of etomidate. Crit Care 10:R105
16. Ray DC, McKeown DW (2007) Effect of induction agent on vasopressor and steroid use, and outcome in patients with septic shock. Crit Care 11:R56
17. Riche FC, Boutron CM, Valleur P, et al (2007) Adrenal response in patients with septic shock of abdominal origin: relationship to survival. Intensive Care Med 33: 1761–1766
18. Schenarts CL, Burton JH, Riker RR (2001) Adrenocortical dysfunction following etomidate induction in emergency department patients. Acad Emerg Med 8: 1–7
19. Marik PE, Pastores SM, Annane D, et al (2008) Recommendations for the diagnosis and management of corticosteroid insufficiency in critically ill adult patients: consensus statements from an international task force by the American College of Critical Care Medicine. Crit Care Med 36: 1937–1949
20. Martyn JA, Richtsfeld M (2006) Succinylcholine-induced hyperkalemia in acquired pathologic states: etiologic factors and molecular mechanisms. Anesthesiology 104: 158–169
21. Kabrhel C, Thomsen TW, Setnik GS, Walls RM (2007) Videos in clinical medicine. Orotracheal intubation. N Engl J Med 356:e15
22. O'Connor M (1998) Airway management. In: Hall JB, Schmidt GA, Wood LDH (eds) Principles of Critical Care, 2nd ed. McGraw Hill, New York, pp 111–119
23. American Society of Anesthesiologists Task Force on Management of the Difficult Airway (2003) Practice guidelines for management of the difficult airway. Anesthesiology 98: 1269–1277
24. Langeron O, Amour J, Vivien B, Aubrun F (2006) Clinical review: management of difficult airways. Crit Care 10:243

25. Donald MJ, Paterson B (2006) End tidal carbon dioxide monitoring in prehospital and retrieval medicine: a review. Emerg Med J 23: 728–730
26. Jaber S, Jung B, Corne P, et al (2007) Intubation protocol in ICU decrease the incidence of life-threatening complications. Intensive Case Med 33 (Suppl 2):S140 (abst)
27. Grmec S (2002) Comparison of three different methods to confirm tracheal tube placement in emergency intubation. Intensive Care Med 28: 701–704
28. Jaber S, Chanques G, Matecki S, et al (2003) Post-extubation stridor in intensive care unit patients. Risk factors evaluation and importance of the cuff-leak test. Intensive Care Med 29: 69–74
29. Chanques G, Jaber S, Barbotte E, et al (2006) Impact of systematic evaluation of pain and agitation in an intensive care unit. Crit Care Med 34: 1691–1699
30. Schultz MJ, Haitsma JJ, Slutsky AS, Gajic O (2007) What tidal volumes should be used in patients without acute lung injury? Anesthesiology 106: 1226–1231
31. The Acute Respiratory Distress Syndrome Network (2000) Ventilation with lower tidal volumes as compared with traditional tidal volumes for acute lung injury and the acute respiratory distress syndrome. N Engl J Med 342: 1301–1308
32. Li J, Murphy-Lavoie, H, Bugas C, Martinez J, Preston C (1999) Complications of emergency intubation with and without paralysis. Am J Emerg Med 17: 141–143
33. Ricard-Hibon A, Chollet C, Leroy C, Marty J (2002) Succinylcholine improves the time of performance of a tracheal intubation in prehospital critical care medicine. Eur J Anaesthesiol 19: 361–367

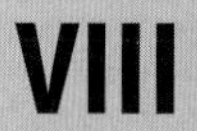

Pediatric Advanced Airway Management Training for Non-anesthesia Residents

A. Nishisaki, V.M. Nadkarni, and R.A. Berg

Introduction

Tracheal intubation procedures are common, high risk events for critically ill children. Although tracheal intubation is infrequently performed by resident trainees, the Accreditation Committee for Graduate Medical Education (ACGME) in the United States mandates that pediatric residents gain tracheal intubation procedural competency during clinical rotations in the delivery room, neonatal ICU (NICU), and pediatric ICU (PICU) [1]. We will review current issues regarding tracheal intubation training and skill acquisition, as well as the effects of this training on patient outcomes.

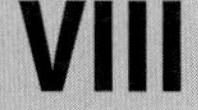

Risks associated with Tracheal Intubation and Provider Competence

Non-neonatal Intubation

The hazards and performance measures of pediatric advanced airway management have been characterized in several out-of-hospital, emergency department, or in-patient settings. Gausche et al. reported that out-of-hospital pediatric intubation by emergency medical personnel may worsen patient outcomes [2]. After providing two rigorous 3-hour pediatric airway management educational sessions for more than 3000 paramedics, they randomized 830 pediatric patients to either bag-valve-mask ventilation or to orotracheal intubation by even or odd days. The overall likelihood of survival and neurological outcome were not statistically different between these two groups. Survival to discharge was attained in 123/404 (30 %) of children randomized to bag-mask ventilation compared with 110/416 (23 %) of children randomized to tracheal intubation (OR 0.82; 95 %CI, 0.61 – 1.11). Unexpectedly, respiratory arrest patients were less likely to survive to hospital discharge in the tracheal intubation than the bag-valve-mask ventilation group (33/54 [61 %] versus 46/54 [85 %], OR 0.27; 95 % CI, 0.11 – 0.69). When endotracheal intubation was attempted, it was successful in only 174/305 (57 %) of the patients. Not surprisingly, emergency medical personnel spent more time in the field with children randomized to tracheal intubation compared to those randomized to bag-valve-mask ventilation (median 11 min vs. 9 min, $p < 0.001$). In addition, the endotracheal intubation group suffered from frequent intubation complications. For example, 33 (18 %) had mainstem intubations and 44 (24 %) were intubated with an incorrect size endotracheal tube. Most importantly, some of the endotracheal intubation group had life-threatening complications: Three (2 %) had esophageal intubations, 12 (6 %) had unrecognized dislodgement of endotracheal tubes, 15 (8 %) had recognized dislodgement of endotracheal tubes. Among these 30 patients with esophageal intubation or with unrecognized tube dislodgement, 29/30 died. This study established that pediatric advanced airway management in the out-of-hospital setting can be dangerous.

Sagarin et al. evaluated the safety and effectiveness of pediatric intubation attempts by physicians in the Emergency Department [3]. Of 1288 intubations at 11 Emergency Departments from June 1996 to September 1997, 156 (17 %) were pediatric intubations (0 – 18 years old). Emergency medicine residents and pediatric emergency medicine fellows each had overall success rates for pediatric tracheal intubations of 89 %, whereas pediatric residents were only successful in 69 % of cases ($p < 0.05$). Both emergency medicine residents and pediatric emergency medicine fellows successfully intubated 77 % of the children on their first attempt, whereas pediatric residents were only successful on 50 % of their first attempts ($p < 0.05$). In addition, 27/156 (17 %) of these children experienced adverse events in association with their advanced airway management. Of these adverse events, 19/27 (70 %) were technical problems, such as esophageal intubation, mainstem intubation, wrong drug dose, or air leak due to uncuffed tube or inappropriate tube size.

Easley and colleagues also evaluated pediatric advanced airway management by physicians in the Emergency Department [4]. These authors studied 250 consecutive patients who were admitted to the PICU after tracheal intubation was performed in an Emergency Department (60 % at an outside facility, 40 % at the Emergency Department in their own hospital). They defined major practice variances as technical problems resulting in a significant risk for airway trauma and increased morbidity, such as mainstem intubation or multiple attempts (> 2 attempts). Minor variances were defined as problems of airway management that should be avoided but do not significantly increase the immediate risk to the patient, such as inappropriate sizing of endotracheal tube or excessive cuff volume. Major or minor variances were documented in 136/250 (54 %) of these children. Major variances were observed in 93/250 (37 %) of the children, and minor variances in 43/250 (17 %) (**Table 1**). The

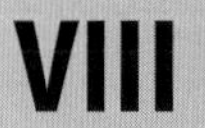

Table 1. Major and minor practice variances in tracheal intubation before PICU admission. From [4] with permission

Overall results (n = 250)		
No. of patients with variances (%)	136	54
Major	93	37
Minor	43	17
Total no. of variances	244	(average of 1.79 variances per patient)
Major Variances	138	(60 % of variances) (%)
Mainstem intubations	70	51
Multiple attempts	51	37
Airway trauma	11	8
Dental damage	2	1
Barotrauma	3	2
Minor Variances	106	(40 % of variances) (%)
Incorrect sized ET tube	41	39
No NG/OG placed	29	27
Improperly secured ET tube	17	16
Cuffed tube (< 6 yrs old)	4	4
Gastric distention	15	14

ET: endotracheal, NG/OG: nasogastric/orogastric tube

most common major variance was mainstem bronchus intubation, documented in 70/250 (28 %) patients. Major and minor variances occurred much more commonly among children who had advanced airway management at an outside institution compared with their own children's hospital Emergency Department ($p < 0.00097$). Their study did not address the training status or discipline (e.g., emergency medicine versus pediatrics) of the intubators.

There is no multicenter study demonstrating the success rate and the incidence of complications of pediatric advanced airway management in PICUs. A few investigators have described the success rate and incidence of complications in pediatric advanced airway management from single institutions. Nishisaki et al. reported on 254 orotracheal intubations from a single PICU in a tertiary care children's hospital in the USA [5]. The participation rate of residents for tracheal intubation was only 22 %, and the participation rate for pediatric critical care fellows was 81 %. The residents were able to successfully intubate 53 % of these children compared with the fellows' success rate of 93 % ($p < 0.001$). The residents' first attempt success rate was only 40 % compared with the fellows' first success rate of 77 % ($p < 0.001$). The pre-defined unwanted tracheal intubation-associated event (major and minor potential complications) rate was 26 % with the first attempt by a resident versus 16 % with the first attempt by a fellow ($p = 0.11$).

Orlowski et al. reported that 12/100 (12 %) of children had major complications associated with tracheal intubation in a single center PICU (10 % infection or tracheitis, 6 % post-extubation stridor, 5 % pneumothorax) [6]. Rivera and Tibballs also reported that 110/500 (24 %) children had complications associated with tracheal intubations in a single center PICU [7]. Most of these complications were associated with prolonged intubation and mechanical ventilation, and were not linked with advanced airway management itself.

VIII

Neonatal Intubation

Recently several groups of investigators have reported the incidence rates of complications associated with neonatal intubations. O'Donnell et al. reported the success rate and time to neonatal intubation in the labor and delivery room of a single institution [8]. Residents successfully intubated 24 % of the babies with a mean time to intubation of 49 ± 13 seconds. In contrast, fellows successfully intubated 78 % of the babies with a mean time to intubation of 32 ± 13 seconds, and consultants (attending physicians) successfully intubated 86 % of the babies with a mean time to intubation of 25 ± 17 seconds (**Table 2**) [8]. In their study, no infants deteriorated (saturation or heart rate decrease more than 10 %) when intubation attempts were < 20 seconds. However, 33 % (4/12) of infants deteriorated when intubation attempts were 20–29 seconds, and 20/27 (74 %) deteriorated when intubation attempts were ≥ 30 seconds.

Table 2. Success rate and duration of attempts according to the grade of doctor attempting intubation. From [8] with permission

	Total	Residents	Fellows	Consultants
No. of attempts	60	21	18	21
No. (%) of successful attempts	37 (62)	5 (24)	14 (78)	18 (86)
Duration of attempts, mean (SD), s	33 (19)	38 (20)	36 (16)	28 (19)
Duration of successful attempts, mean (SD), s	31 (17)	51 (13)	32 (13)	25 (17)

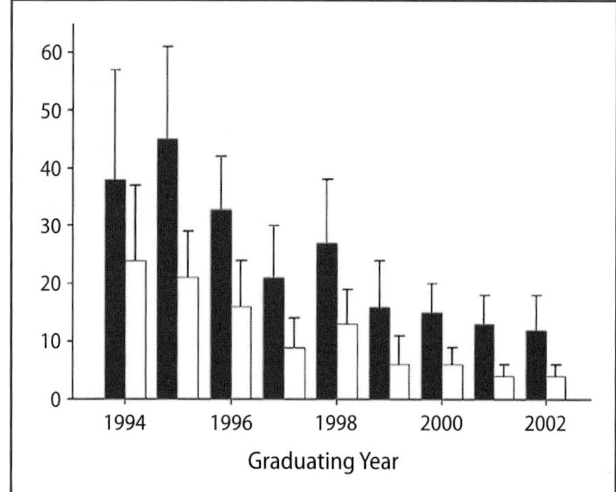

Fig. 1. Mean number of intubation attempts (blue bars) and mean number of successful intubations (white bars) by pediatric trainees during their residency program plotted against the year of training completion (with standard deviations). From [10] with permission

Falck et al. evaluated the success rate of neonatal intubations by pediatric residents at various training levels [9]. Post-graduate year 1 (PGY-1) residents successfully intubated 49.7 % of the neonates, compared with 54.8 % by PGY-2 residents ($p = 0.41$), and 62.3 % by PGY-3 residents ($p = 0.006$). The proportion of successful intubations with the first attempt was 35.1 % for the PGY-1 group, 33.4 % for the PGY-2 group, and 45.4 % for the PGY-3 group (PGY-1 vs. PGY-2, $p = 0.81$; PGY-1 vs. PGY-3, $p = 0.06$). It is striking that despite more than two years of pediatric residency training, PGY-3 pediatric residents were unable to intubate > 1/3 of these neonates within 2 attempts, and they were never able to successfully intubate > 1/4 of the neonates.

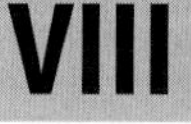

Leone et al. noted that over the last 10 years, pediatric residents are having fewer neonatal tracheal intubation experiences in the Delivery Room during their training [10]. These authors examined trends in pediatric resident experience in tracheal intubation from 1992–2002. **Figure 1** demonstrates the decrease in both the number of tracheal intubation attempts and the success rate per attempt over time (**Fig. 1**). Their overall success rates (intubation success within 2 attempts) were 49.6 % for PGY-1 and 67.4 % for PGY-2 and PGY-3, similar to the observations by Falck [9]. Leone and colleagues [10] attributed the decline in the number of intubation attempts to changes in the approach to newborns with meconium-staining in the revised Neonatal Resuscitation Program Guidelines [11].

All three of these studies [8–10] raise important concerns about the tracheal intubation skills of pediatric residents. Clearly, these observations establish that third year residents often have inadequate performance, challenging the ACGME expectation that pediatric residents should be competent in tracheal intubation by the end of their pediatric residency program (see below).

Demand for Pediatric Airway Management Competence in Pediatric Resident Trainees

The ACGME mandates that pediatric residents should gain procedural competency during their residency training [1]. Moreover, pediatric program directors believe that tracheal intubation is an important procedural skill that pediatric residents should attain during their training. In a survey of the Association of Pediatric Program Directors (including 112/139 program directors), > 80 % considered neonatal intubations to be an important procedure for their residents to learn and 65 % considered non-neonatal intubations an important procedure for their residents to learn [12]. Interestingly, 60 % of program directors believed that almost all of their residents were competent in neonatal intubations, whereas only 30 % believed that almost all of their residents were competent in non-neonatal intubations.

Process of Acquisition and Retention of Pediatric Tracheal Intubation Competence

Acquisition of Intubation Skill Competence

The acquisition of this complex psychomotor skill requires substantial training. Furthermore, continued excellence requires frequent performance. In fact, the most competent providers (e.g., anesthesiologists) perform these procedures on a nearly daily basis.

Plummer and Owen evaluated medical students' manikin-based learning of tracheal intubation [13, 14]. They concluded that 15 trials of intubation are necessary for an 80 % success rate, a 'cut-off' often used in other tracheal intubation studies [9] (**Fig. 2**). These authors also reported that the rate of successful intubation decreased substantially when students switched to different intubation manikins compared with re-intubating the same mankin (adjusted odds ratio 0.5; 95 % CI, 0.4–0.7). They emphasized the importance of students' exposure to different manikins in order to broaden the training experience. This varied experience slowed the time to achieve competence, but seemed to enhance both skill retention and transfer of the skills to new settings. These investigations re-enforced two important additional general observations about educational processes: 1) Students learn best from successful experiences, and 2) students learn little from performing these skills incorrectly (i.e., they do not learn much from their psychomotor skill 'mistakes').

Konrad et al. studied the acquisition of technical skills among 11 first year anesthesiology residents at a single institution (**Fig. 3**) [15]. The 80 % success rate goal was achieved after 30–40 attempts, and their more ambitious goal of 90 % was attained after 57 attempts. Other skills assessed were arterial line placement, epidural anesthesia, brachial plexus anesthesia, and spinal anesthesia. The general learn-

VIII

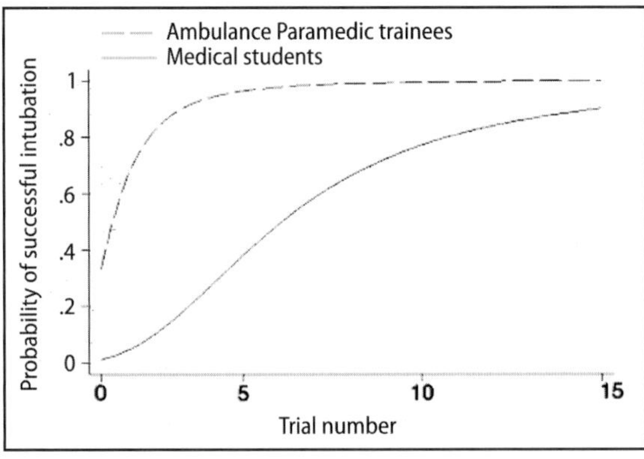

Fig. 2. Estimated learning curves for two groups of trainees: Ambulance paramedic trainees and medical students. Ambulance paramedic trainees, who generally had considerable prior experience in clinical procedures, were successful in approximately 30 % of initial endotracheal intubation attempts and improved rapidly approaching 100 % success rates after around 6 attempts. Medical students, who had more limited prior experience, began with a lower success rate and learned more slowly. From [14] with permission

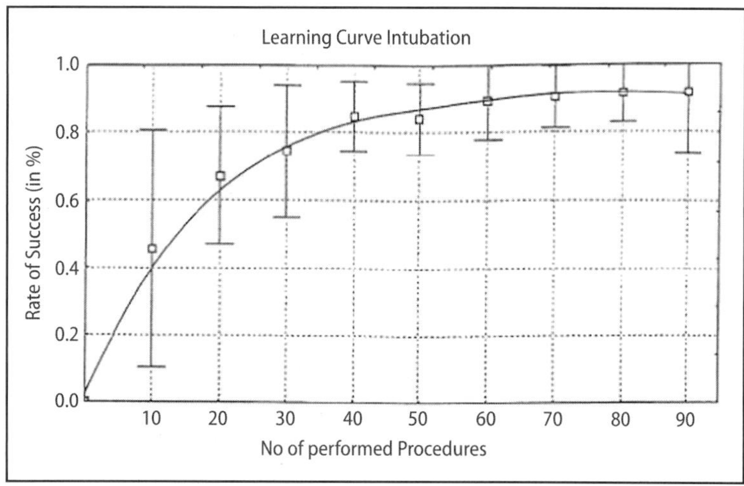

Fig. 3. Intubation learning curve for anesthesiology residents in the operating room. From [15] with permission

ing curve was different for each technical skill, and the specific learning curve for individual residents varied greatly.

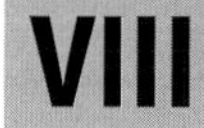

Retention of Intubation Skill Competence

Retaining competence in complex technical skills that are infrequently performed typically requires rigorous refresher training. This is particularly true for tracheal intubation in pediatric trainees, because each trainee practices this psychomotor skill infrequently in actual clinical settings. However, the optimal schedule for refresher training is not known. Issues that would impact on the optimal schedule include: 1) How rapidly pediatric tracheal intubation psychomotor skills decline, 2) how often the refresher training needs to be conducted to maintain a high level competence, and 3) what factors are associated with refresher training effectiveness.

Kovacs et al. studied various aspects of airway management skill retention among emergency medicine residents [16]. They provided an initial 2-day intensive airway training course, followed by subsequent weekly practice session for 3 weeks. Then they randomized participants to one of three groups: 1) one group without feedback at the time of testing or further practice sessions, 2) the second group with feedback at follow-up testing without further practice sessions, and 3) the third group with feedback at follow-up testing and eight practice sessions over a 10-month period. The first two groups exhibited rapid decay in airway management skills 16 weeks after initial training. In contrast, the group with feedback and subsequent practice sessions maintained the airway skills without decay over the 10-month study period. Frequent refresher training was remarkably effective.

We studied the effect of previous pediatric tracheal intubation training on effectiveness during refresher manikin-based tracheal intubation training [17]. We evaluated the time to successful intubation of an infant manikin among 26 non-anesthesiology providers (pediatric critical care fellows, pediatric emergency medicine fellows, and transport team nurses who are trained and credentialed to perform intubation) using three different simulation conditions with an infant simulator (tracheal intubation with no cervical restrictions, tracheal intubation with a rigid cervical collar, tracheal intubation with manual in-line stabilization). Time to successful intubation was 33.8 ± 9.4 seconds(s) for the first manikin intubation (T1), and decreased to 29 ± 6.4 seconds at the second intubation (T2). The times for the next four intubations were: 27.4 ± 5.6 seconds, 29.8 ± 9.2 seconds, 28 ± 5.4 seconds, and 25.6±5.1 seconds. Clearly, repeated training resulted in shorter time to intubation, and the largest improvement occurred between the first and second training sessions.

Immediate refresher training effectiveness was calculated as the proportion of time taken for intubation at the second session to the time for intubation at the first session (T2/T1). This was significantly associated with recent intubation training ≤ 3 months (74 ± 17 % when recent training occurred ≤ 3 months versus 98 ± 26 % without recent training, p = 0.025 [the smaller number is 'better']). However, training effectiveness was not associated with the intubator trainee's discipline (80 ± 29 % among pediatric critical care fellows, 81 ± 18 % among pediatric emergency medicine fellows, and 94 ± 24 % among transport team nurses, p = 0.40). Interestingly, training effectiveness was not associated with years of clinical intubation experience. For example, training effectiveness was 89 ± 26 % among providers with ≤ 3 years of previous intubation experience versus 88 ± 23 % among providers with > 3 years of previous intubation experience, p = 0.93). After controlling for these potential confounding factors, recent training (within 3 months) remained significant (p = 0.017). Surprisingly, the number of intubation attempts and the number of tracheal intubation associated events did not differ among trainee groups with or without recent training, trainees from the different disciplines, or trainees with varied years of clinical experience.

VIII

These two studies [16, 17] suggest that intubation refresher training may be necessary at least every 3–4 months to maintain competence. Because the boost effect of refresher training is large with recent previous training, refresher training may not have to be as intense as the initial training. Interestingly, studies of cardiopulmonary resuscitation (CPR) training have reported similar findings [18]. We clearly need more studies to evaluate the timing and intensity of refresher tracheal intubation training on maintenance of competence in order to develop optimal training schedules.

Validation of and Evidence for Simulation in Tracheal Intubation Training

Medical simulation is an exciting new educational modality for individual skill training and for team training (e.g., crisis resource management) [19]. Simulation-based training can effectively improve clinical performance and decrease the incidence of adverse events [20, 21]. The US Food and Drug Administration (FDA) now requires simulation-based training for certain intravascular surgery devices [22].

Medical simulation has long been utilized to evaluate competence and training for emergencies [23, 24]. Objective competence measurement through simulation is more reliable compared to self-efficacy (confidence level of trainees). Trainees' self-assessments typically over-estimate their skill performance [25, 26]. Importantly, competence measurement through simulation translates into operational performance in clinical settings [25–27].

Medical simulation is particularly well suited to test or train a high risk, low incidence situation repeatedly [21, 22]. Highly sophisticated simulator function with realistic anatomy and simulated physiology has been utilized to enhance clinical education and training effectiveness. Moreover, the clinical relevance of airway management simulation has been validated through several studies. Overly et al. showed that the success rate for pediatric resident intubation attempts on manikins was 56 %, and the success rate for these residents on children in the Emergency Department was 50 % [28].

The fidelity of manikin-based simulation is validated by other similar clinical results such as the rate of intubation associated events (mainstem bronchial intubation, esophageal intubation). The incidence of mainstem bronchus intubation with delayed recognition in one manikin study (2 %) [15] was comparable to Sagarin's report from the clinical National Emergency Airway Registry (7 %) [3]. The incidence of esophageal intubation was also similar: 1.3 % versus 3.2 %, respectively [15]. In addition, the overall rate of tracheal intubation-associated adverse events in our manikin study was 33 % [17], similar to the overall adverse event rate of 16–25 % in one clinical study [3] and 54 % in another [4].

Hall et al. demonstrated that intense manikin intubation training was as effective as training on actual patients [29]. Thirty-six paramedic students without previous experience were randomized to either: 1) Simulation group with a didactic session and 10 hours of manikin-based skill training plus 10 hours of simulation training, or 2) operating room (OR) group with a didactic session and 10 hours manikin-based skill training plus 15 actual tracheal intubations in the OR. They then evaluated each trainee during 15 post-training actual OR intubations. Despite the apparent advantage for the OR group because the environment of training was similar to the evaluation setting, the overall intubation success rates were 87.8 % after manikin training and 84.8 % after OR training ($p = 0.42$). Furthermore the first attempt success was 84.4 % in the simulation group versus 80.0 % first attempt success in the OR group ($p = 0.27$). This study provides further validation of the effectiveness of simulation-based training.

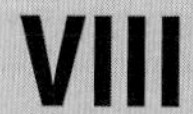

Future Directions

Recently, more emphasis has been placed on outcome-based education [30]. Technical skills training for tracheal intubation needs to be based on sound science. We need to learn more about the optimal timing and intensity of initial technical skill training to achieve clearly defined competence. In addition, we also need to learn more about the optimal timing and intensity of refresher training to achieve and maintain pre-defined competence [17]. Little is known about the non-technical aspects (behavioral skills) of tracheal intubation. We developed an evaluation tool for team performance of basic and advanced airway management in an infant with impending respiratory failure through healthcare failure mode and effect analysis [31]. Based on our preliminary results, non-technical skills are at least as important as technical skills for safe and competent tracheal intubation practice in PICUs.

Conclusion

Pediatric tracheal intubation is considered an important skill for pediatric resident trainees. Unfortunately, many pediatric residents are unable to perform this skill. Academic pediatric critical care physicians have a dilemma: How can we provide safe, high-quality care for sick children and yet provide ample learning opportunities for resident trainees to achieve and maintain competence in high risk skills, such as tracheal intubation. Simulation-based tracheal intubation skill training is a promising approach to teach this important skill without harming patients. More research is necessary to evaluate initial and refresher training effectiveness in complex psychomotor skills such as tracheal intubation.

References

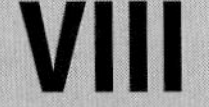

1. ACGME Program Requirements for Graduate Medical Education in Pediatrics. Available at: http://www.acgme.org/acWebsite/downloads/RRC_progReq/320pediatrics07012007.pdf. Accessed October 2008.
2. Gausche M, Lewis RJ, Stratton SJ, et al (2000) Effect of out-of-hospital pediatric endotracheal intubation on survival and neurological outcome: A controlled clinical trial. JAMA; 283: 783–790
3. Sagarin MJ, Chiang V, Sakles JC, et al (2002) Rapid sequence intubation for pediatric emergency airway management. Pediatr Emerg Care 18: 417–423
4. Easley RB, Segeleon JE, Haun SE, et al (2000) Prospective study of airway management of children requiring endotracheal intubation before admission to a pediatric intensive care unit. Crit Care Med 28: 2058–2063
5. Nishisaki A, Ferry S, Kalsi M, et al (2007) Who actually performs tracheal intubation in an academic Pediatric Intensive Care Unit? Crit Care Med 35 (Suppl):A128 (abst)
6. Orlowski JP, Ellis NG, Amin NP, Crumrine RS (1980) Complications of airway intrusion in 100 consecutive cases in a pediatric ICU. Crit Care Med 8: 324–331
7. Rivera R, Tibballs J (1992) Complications of endotracheal intubation and mechanical ventilation in infants and children. Crit Care Med 20: 193–199
8. O'Donnell CP, Kamlin CO, Davis PG, et al (2006) Endotracheal intubation attempts during neonatal resuscitation: Success rates, duration and adverse effects. Pediatrics 117: e16-e21
9. Falck AJ, Escobedo MB, Baillargeon JG, Villard LG, Gunkel JH (2003) Proficiency of pediatric residents in performing neonatal endotracheal intubation. Pediatrics 112: 1242–1247
10. Leone TA, Rich W, Finer NN (2005) Neonatal intubation: Success of pediatric trainees. J Pediatr 146: 638–641
11. Kattwinkel J (2000) The Textbook of Neonatal Resuscitation. 4th edition. American Academy of Pediatrics and American Heart Association, Elk Glove Village
12. Gaies MG, Landrigan CP, Hafler JP, et al (2007) Assessing procedural skills training in pediatric residency programs. Pediatrics 120: 715–722
13. Plummer JL, Owen H (2001) Learning endotracheal intubation in a clinical skills learning center: A quantitative study. Anesth Analg 93: 656–662
14. Owen H, Plummer JL (2002) Improving learning of a clinical skill: the first year's experience of teaching endotracheal intubation in a clinical simulation facility. Med Educ 36: 635–642
15. Konrad C, Schüpfer G, Wietlisbach M, Gerber H (1998) Learning manual skills in anesthesiology: Is there a recommended number of cases for anesthetic procedures? Anesth Analg 86: 635–639
16. Kovacs G, Ackroyd-Stolarz S, Cain E, et al (2000) A randomized controlled trial on the effect of educational interventions in promoting airway management skill maintenance. Ann Emerg Med 36: 301–309
17. Nishisaki A, Scrattish L, Boulet J, et al (2008) Effect of recent refresher training on in situ simulated pediatric tracheal intubation psychomotor skill performance. In Henriksen K, Battles JB, Keyes MA, Grady ML (eds) Advances in Patient Safety: New Directions and Alternative Approaches, Vol. 3. Performance and Tools. Agency for Healthcare Research and Quality, Rockville
18. Niles D, Sutton R, Donoghue A, et al (2007) "Rolling Refreshers": A novel approach to maintain CPR psychomotor skill competence. Pediatr Crit Care Med 8 (Suppl): A243 (abst)
19. Hunt EA, Shilkofski NA, Stavroudis TA, Nelson KL (2007) Simulation: translation to improved team performance. Anesthesiol Clin 25: 301–319
20. Seymour NE, Gallagher AG, Roman SA, et al (2002) Virtual reality training improves operating room performance. Ann Surg 236: 458–464

21. Grantcharov TP, Kristiansen VB, Bendix J, et al (2004) Randomized clinical trial of virtual reality simulation for laparoscopic skills training. Br J Surg 91: 146–150
22. Dawson DL (2006) Training in carotid artery stenting: do carotid simulation systems really help? Vascular 14: 256–263
23. DeVita MA, Schaeffer J, Lutz J, Dongilli T, Wang H (2004) Improving medical crisis team performance. Crit Care Med 32 (Suppl 2):S61–65
24. Zirkle M, Blum R, Raemer DB, Healy G, Roberson DW (2005) Teaching emergency airway management using medical simulation: a pilot program. Laryngoscope 115: 495–500
25. Nishisaki A, Keren R, Nadkarni V (2007) Does simulation improve patient safety? Self-efficacy, competence, operational performance, and patient safety. Anesthesiol Clin 25: 225–236
26. Moorthy K, Munz Y, Adams S, et al (2006) Self-assessment of performance among surgical trainees during simulated procedures in a simulated operating theater. Am J Surg 192: 114–118
27. Mayo PH, Hackney JE, Mueck T, et al (2004) Achieving house staff competence in emergency airway management: results of a teaching program using a computerized patient simulator. Crit Care Med 32: 2422–2427
28. Overly FL, Sudikoff SN, Shapiro MJ (2007) High-fidelity medical simulation as an assessment tool for pediatric residents' airway management skills. Pediatr Emerg Care 23: 11–15
29. Hall RE, Plant JR, Bands CJ, et al (2005) Human patient simulation is effective for teaching paramedic students endotracheal intubation. Acad Emerg Med 12: 850–855
30. Harden RM (2007) Learning outcomes as a tool to assess progression. Med Teach 29: 678–682
31. Nishisaki A, Donoghue A, Bishnoi R, et al (2007) Validation of an in situ ICU technical and behavioral simulation scoring tool: Just in Time Pediatric Airway Provider performance Scale. Crit Care Med 35 (Suppl):A122 (abst)

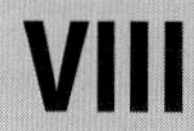

Automatic Tube Compensation in the Weaning Process

J. Cohen, M. Shapiro, and P. Singer

Introduction

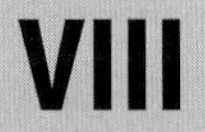

Unnecessarily prolonging or prematurely discontinuing mechanical ventilation may result in significant morbidity and even mortality. In order to optimize the timing of ventilation discontinuation, evidence-based guidelines suggest that patients undergo a daily screen (for measures of oxygenation, cough and secretions, adequate mental status, and hemodynamic stability) to assess weaning readiness [1]. For patients meeting the criteria, a spontaneous breathing trial is then performed in order to assess their ability to breathe unaided. The way the trial is tolerated, determined by both objective (respiratory and hemodynamic parameters) and subjective (evidence of increased work of breathing and distress) criteria, determines whether extubation is performed.

Spontaneous breathing trials have traditionally been performed while the patient receives varying levels of ventilatory support, including continuous positive airway pressure (CPAP) [2], a T-tube circuit [3], or low-level pressure support ventilation (PSV) [4]. The level of support may be relevant to whether the breathing trial is tolerated, since it has been argued that for some patients, weaning failure may be attributable to the respiratory load imposed by the endotracheal tube [5], what might be termed 'iatrogenic' weaning failure. In support of this, Koksal et al. demonstrated a significant increase in the endocrine stress response, as assessed by plasma levels of cortisol, insulin, and glucose, and by urinary levels of vanilmandelic acid (VMA) during a spontaneous breathing trial [6]. The magnitude of the response was influenced by the mode used, being significantly greater at the end of a breathing trial with a T-tube than with either CPAP or PSV. A particularly interesting finding was the fact that 48 hours after extubation, the levels of VMA had returned to normal in the PSV group but remained elevated in the CPAP and T-tube group (being highest in the latter group). Significantly, all patients requiring reintubation were in the T-tube group. In addition, in a randomized trial comparing trials of spontaneous breathing performed with either a T-tube or PSV, Esteban et al. showed that significantly more patients failed the breathing trial in the T-tube compared with the PSV group ($p = 0.03$) [7]. While the difference in the percentage of patients who remained extubated after 48 hours was not statistically significant between the two groups (T-tube, 63 % vs. PSV, 70 %; $p = 0.14$), this represented an absolute benefit increase of 7 % and a relative benefit increase of 11 % when the breathing trial was performed with PSV. Taken together, these studies suggest that minimizing work of breathing during a spontaneous breathing trial may positively influence extubation outcome, at least in some patients.

For these reasons, PSV or CPAP are often used during a breathing trial. CPAP may improve lung mechanics and reduce the effort required by mechanically ventilated patients with airflow obstruction and enhance breath triggering in patients with significant auto-PEEP [8]. PSV, by supporting the patient's inspiration, has been shown to compensate for the additional work of breathing imposed by the endotracheal tube [9]. However, PSV provides constant inspiratory support and so is unable to compensate for the non-linear, flow dependent, resistive workload imposed by the endotracheal tube [10]. The result may be either inadequate support (under-compensation) when inspiratory flow is high, or over assistance (over-compensation) when inspiratory flow is low.

Automatic Tube Compensation

Automatic tube compensation (ATC) has been designed to overcome the imposed work of breathing due to artificial airways [11]. The resistance of the endotracheal tube is flow dependent. Therefore, as inspiratory gas flow changes constantly throughout each breath during spontaneous breathing, the tube resistance also varies considerably [11]. With ATC, the ventilator regulates to the tracheal pressure (at the distal tracheal end of the tube) rather than to airway pressure (at the proximal end of the tube). Compensation for endotracheal tube resistance is achieved via closed loop control of calculated tracheal pressure. By using the known resistive coefficients of the tracheal tube and measurement of instantaneous flow, pressure is applied proportionally to resistance throughout the total respiratory cycle. The amount of ventilatory support is, therefore, continuously and automatically adapted to match the changing flow rate and the related pressure drop across the endotracheal tube, without affecting the patient's breathing pattern [12]. ATC thus provides dynamic ventilatory support for each spontaneous breath, so-called variable pressure support.

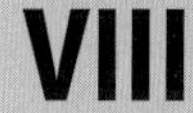

Numerous studies have shown that ATC is able to decrease the work of breathing necessary to overcome endotracheal tube resistance more effectively than either PSV or CPAP [10]. Normal volunteers perceived ATC as more comfortable than PSV; the discomfort of PSV being associated with a substantial increase in tidal volume, minute ventilation, gas flow, and pressure [13]. In addition, the natural breathing pattern may be better preserved and synchronization between the patient and ventilator improved with ATC [14]. Finally, ineffective ventilator-triggering as a result of auto-PEEP appears to be less common with ATC than with PSV [15]. For these reasons, ATC has been designated as 'electronic extubation' and seems ideally suited for use in the weaning process.

Commercially available Automatic Tube Compensation Systems

All the initial studies of ATC in the clinical setting [10, 13–15] were performed with prototype ATC software. This allows for continuous adjustment of the pressure assist during the ventilatory cycle, being increased during inspiration and lowered during expiration [16]. Commercially available ATC systems are present in the Evita XL and Evita-4 ventilators (Drager Medical AG, Lubeck, Germany) and Puritan-Bennett 840 ventilator (Puritan-Bennett Corporation, Pleasanton, CA, USA). The difference between the commercial and original ATC systems is related to the negative pressure source incorporated only in the original ATC system. Under these circumstances, the pressure available for expiratory tube compensation is not limited to a preset PEEP level. The performance of the commercially available ventilators has recently been formally assessed [16]. It was found that, compared with the original system, the simplified commercially available ATC systems may be adequate for inspiratory but probably not for expiratory tube compensation. It should be stated, however, that the lack of expiratory assist may, in fact, be advantageous for certain groups of patients, such as those with chronic obstructive pulmonary disease (COPD), as expiratory ATC may result in an increased tendency for airway closure of the small airways.

Potential Clinical Uses of Automatic Tube Compensation

Increasing the Predictive Potential of a Spontaneous Breathing Trial

Studies using prototype ATC software

The first systematic, randomized study of ATC in the weaning period was conducted by Haberthur et al. [17]. Patients receiving mechanical ventilation for acute respiratory failure for > 24 hours were randomized to undergo a 2-hour spontaneous breathing trial with a T-tube, PSV of 5 cmH_2O, or ATC (30 patients in each group). While more patients in the ATC group tolerated the breathing trial (ATC, 97 %; PSV, 83 %; T-tube 80 %), this difference did not reach statistical significance. Patients failing the breathing trial were then ventilated with the two remaining modes of ventilation in random order. The authors found that 50 % of the patients who had failed the breathing trial with either T-tube or PSV were subsequently successfully extubated after a trial with ATC. However, there was no advantage shown for patients failing a trial with ATC who were subsequently ventilated with either a T-tube or PSV. No significant differences in extubation outcome were observed among the three groups. The fact that extubation was inappropriately withheld in a number of patients undergoing the trial with a T-tube or PSV, but not with ATC, suggests that tube resistance may well be a significant factor in some patients who do not tolerate a breathing trial and that ATC may be particularly useful in these difficult to wean patients.

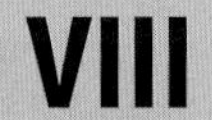

Studies using commercially available ATC systems

In a recent study published in abstract form, the authors assessed the accuracy of the compensation provided by PSV and ATC relative to endotracheal tube-related pressure dissipation [18]. They showed that the difference between the theoretical pressure required to overcome the endotracheal tube resistive properties and the actual pressure delivered by the ventilator was lower, always positive and negligible when ATC was applied during a spontaneous breathing trial when compared to PSV (higher difference, and frequently negative). The authors suggested that the use of ATC more closely simulates the state after extubation, and might improve the specificity and sensitivity of the breathing trial in predicting successful extubation.

We have recently conducted two prospective, randomized, controlled trials comparing ATC to other modes of ventilation, namely CPAP and PSV, during a spontaneous breathing trial. In both studies, the primary outcome was the ability to maintain spontaneous breathing for > 48 hours after removal of the endotracheal tube.

a) ATC versus CPAP: In the first study, 99 consecutive patients requiring mechanical ventilation in our adult, general ICU for > 24 hours were entered into the study [19]. After passing a daily screen, patients were randomly assigned to undergo a

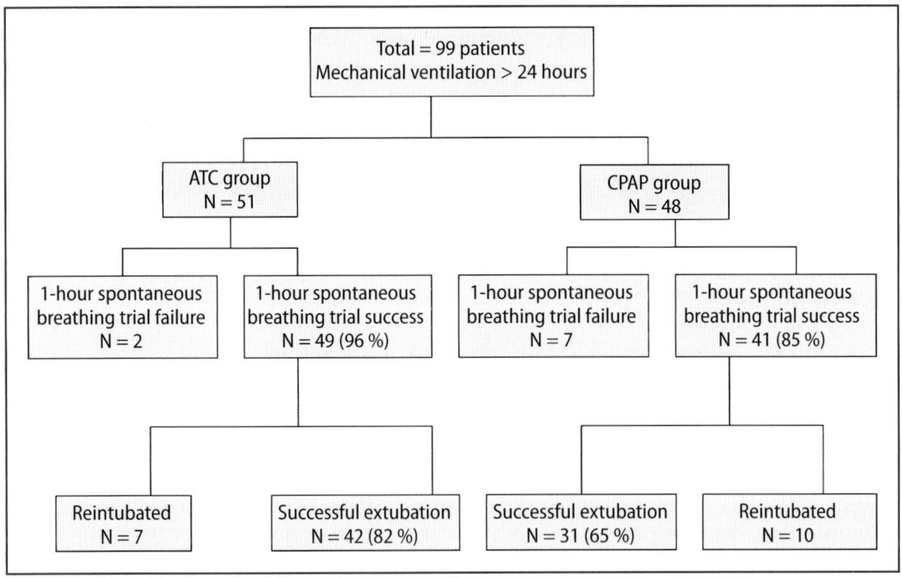

Fig. 1. Course and outcome for patients in the automatic tube compensation (ATC) group vs. the continuous positive airway pressure (CPAP) group. From [19] with permission.

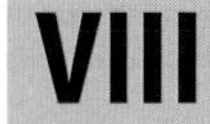

1-hour spontaneous breathing trial using CPAP alone (CPAP of 5 cmH_2O, n = 48) or CPAP with ATC (CPAP of 5 cmH_2O, with inspiratory ATC set at 100 %, n = 51). Extubation was performed immediately for those tolerating the trial. There were no significant differences between the treatment groups regarding baseline demographics or respiratory or hemodynamic parameters. The results of the trial are shown in **Figure 1**. There was a trend for more patients in the ATC group to tolerate the breathing trial (49/51 vs. 41/48, p = 0.08). A total of 17 patients (17 %) required reintubation, 7 (14 %) in the ATC group and 10 (24 %) in the CPAP group; this difference was not statistically significant (p = 0.28). Overall, significantly more patients in the ATC group met the primary outcome measure (p = 0.04). This represented an absolute risk reduction in favor of ATC of 17.7 % (95 % confidence interval, 0.67–35 %) and a number needed to treat of 6.

b) ATC versus PSV: In the second study (Cohen et al, unpublished data), using the same methodology, we compared extubation outcome following a spontaneous breathing trial with either ATC (n = 87) or low-level PSV (n = 93). In the ATC group, 81/87 (94 %) of patients tolerated the breathing trial and underwent extubation, compared to 80/93 (86 %) in the PSV group; this observed 10 % difference was not, however, statistically significant (p = 0.12). A total of 28 patients (17.3 %) required reintubation: 16 (18.4 %) in the ATC group and 12 (12.9 %) in the PSV group (p = 0.43). Reasons for reintubation were similar in both groups. There was no significant difference between the two groups in the number of patients who remained extubated after 48 hours (ATC, 65/87 [74.7 %] vs. PSV, 68/93 [73.1 %]; p = 0.81).

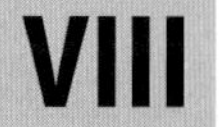

Potential Disadvantage of Reducing Imposed Workload

A concern has been expressed that decreasing the work of breathing during a spontaneous breathing trial by providing respiratory support would allow more marginal patients to tolerate the breathing trial who would then develop ventilatory failure after extubation [20]. However, this concern has not been realized in clinical practice. In both our studies, the reintubation rates did not differ significantly between the ATC and PSV or CPAP groups (see above), and the rates were comparable to those in the literature. This has also been the case in other studies comparing varying levels of respiratory support during a breathing trial, including that of Haberthur et al. [17] comparing ATC, PSV and T-tube, and that of Esteban et al. comparing PSV with a T-tube [7].

Use of Automatic Tube Compensation as a Weaning Predictor

As about 15–20 % of patients who tolerate a breathing trial subsequently undergo reintubation, which is associated with significant morbidity and mortality, the search for additional parameters which may improve extubation outcome continues. While no index has proven to be highly predictive of weaning, the frequency to tidal volume ratio (f/V_T), expressed as breaths per minute per liter, is a simple bedside test, not dependent on patient cooperation and effort, and which has been shown to be most consistently and powerfully predictive of extubation outcomes [21]. Indeed, recent reviews continue to include the f/V_T as an integral part of weaning protocols [20]. In addition, a recent study showed that the best predictors of extubation failure included the f/V_T, a positive fluid balance 24 hours prior to extubation, and pneumonia as the cause for initiating mechanical ventilation [22]. However, although the test is sensitive, the reported specificities are much lower (11 to 64 %) [23, 24]. The f/V_T is typically measured 1 min after the patient is allowed to breathe spontaneously prior to the start of a spontaneous breathing trial. However, Chatila et al. [25] suggested that this may not be enough time for the respiratory drive to fully develop or to reflect respiratory muscle endurance, and this factor may account for the lack of specificity. They showed, in a prospective study of 100 patients undergoing weaning trials, that the f/V_T measured after 30 to 60 min of a breathing trial was a better predictor than that measured after 1 min. Since ATC has been designated as 'electronic extubation', we hypothesized that measuring the f/V_T with ATC (ATC-assisted f/V_T) would provide a 'resistance-free' value more closely approximating the state after extubation. In a prospective study [26], we found that the ATC-assisted f/V_T measured at 60 minutes was in fact a better predictor of successful extubation (area under the curve [AUC], 0.81 ± 0.03) compared to the unassisted-f/V_T (AUC, 0.69 ± 0.05).

In our more recent study comparing ATC to PSV during a breathing trial (Cohen et al, unpublished data), we included the assessment of the ATC-assisted f/V_T, measured at the start of a breathing trial, as an additional predictor of extubation outcome. Our results showed this parameter to have a significant contribution in predicting successful extubation at 48 hours beyond the non-significant contribution of the unassisted f/V_T (unassisted f/V_T: $p = 0.19$; vs. ATC-assisted f/V_T: $p = 0.006$, odds ratio = 0.94).

The ATC-assisted f/V_T ratio thus appears to be a better pretrial predictor of successful extubation, whether assessed before or after a spontaneous breathing trial.

Practical Aspects of using Automatic Tube Compensation

In order to achieve the required effect, it is important to enter appropriate data into the ventilator when ATC is being used [27]. These include whether the patient is ventilated via an endotracheal tube or tracheostomy, the internal diameter of the endotracheal tube or tracheostomy, and the percentage of support required (recommended support is 100 %). It is also important to be aware that secretions and kinks in the endotracheal tube or tracheostomy may result in narrowing of the internal tube diameter to a value that is less than that originally entered. This may result in inaccuracies in the calculation of the variable pressure required to overcome tube resistance and may affect the magnitude of the tube compensation. As no effective method for detecting such tube narrowing presently exists, the tube should be periodically assessed for any airway obstructions which should be appropriately removed.

Conclusion

ATC is a relatively new mode of ventilation designed to overcome the imposed work of breathing due to artificial airways. The mode appears to increase the comfort of ventilated patients while preserving the natural breathing pattern and synchronization between the patient and ventilator. Clinical studies using ATC suggest that providing adequate ventilatory support during a spontaneous breathing trial in order to overcome the resistance of the endotracheal tube, allows more patients to tolerate a spontaneous breathing trial and thus undergo extubation. This does not appear to be associated with an increased rate of re-intubation. In addition this mode may more accurately predict successful extubation outcome following a spontaneous breathing trial and improve the predictive value of the f/V_T. ATC thus appears to be a valuable additional ventilatory mode ideally suited for use during the weaning process.

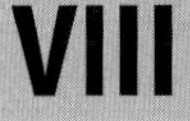

References

1. MacIntyre NR, Cook DJ, Ely EW Jr, et al (2001) Evidence-based guidelines for weaning and discontinuing ventilatory support: a collective task force facilitated by the American College of Chest Physicians; the American Association for Respiratory Care; and the American College of Crit Care Med. Chest 120 (Suppl 6):375S-395S
2. Seymour CW, Halpern S, Christie JD, Gallop R, Fuchs BD (2008) Minute ventilation recovery time measured using a new simplified methodology predicts extubation outcome. J Intensive Care 23: 52–60
3. Chien J, Lin M, Huang YT, Chien Y, Yu C, Yang P (2008) Changes in B-type natriuretic peptide improve weaning outcome predicted by spontaneous breathing trial. Crit Care Med 36: 1421–26
4. Robertson E, Sona C, Schallom L, et al (2008) Improved extubation rates and earlier liberation from mechanical ventilation with implementation of a daily spontaneous-breathing trial protocol. J Am Coll Surg 206: 489–95
5. Frutos-Vivar F, Esteban A (2003) When to wean from a ventilator: an evidence-based strategy. Clev Clin J Med 70: 389–400
6. Koksal GM, Sayilgan C, Sen O, Oz H (2004) The effects of different weaning modes on the endocrine stress response. Crit Care 8: R31–34
7. Esteban A, Alia I, Gordo F, et al (1997) Extubation outcome after spontaneous breathing trials with T-tube or pressure support ventilation. Am J Respir Crit Care Med 156: 459–465

8. Petrof BJ, Legare M, Goldberg P, Milic-Emili J, Gottfried SB (1990) Continuous positive airway pressure reduces the work of breathing and dyspnea during weaning from mechanical ventilation in severe chronic obstructive pulmonary disease. Am Rev Respir Dis 141: 281–289
9. Brochard L, Rua F, Lorino H, Lemaire F, Harf A (1991) Inspiratory pressure support compensates for the additional work of breathing caused by the endotracheal tube. Anaesthesiology 75: 739–745
10. Fabry B, Guttman J, Eberhard L, Wolff G (1994) Automatic tube compensation of endotracheal tube resistance in spontaneously breathing patients. Tech Health Care 1: 281–291
10. Haberthur C, Elsasser S, Eberhard L, Stocker R, Guttmann J (2000) Total versus tube-related additional work of breathing in ventilator-dependent patients. Acta Anaesthesiol Scand 44: 749–757
11. Guttmann, J, Eberhard, L, Fabry, B, et al (1993) Continuous calculation of intratracheal pressure in tracheally intubated patients. Anaesthesiology 79: 503–513
12. Fabry, B, Haberthur, C, Zappe, D, et al (1997) Breathing pattern and additional work of breathing in spontaneously breathing patients with different ventilatory demands during inspiratory pressure support and automatic tube compensation. Intensive Care Med 23: 545–552
13. Guttmann J, Bernhard H, Mols G, et al (1997) Respiratory comfort of automatic tube compensation and inspiratory pressure support in conscious humans. Intensive Care Med 23: 1119–1124
14. Haberthur C, Fabry, Zappe D, et al (1998) Effects of mechanical unloading and mechanical loading on respiratory loop gain and periodic breathing in man. Respir Physiol 112: 23–36
15. Stocker R, Fabry B, Haberthur C (1997) New modes of ventilatory support in spontaneously breathing intubated patients. In: Vincent JL (ed) Yearbook of Intensive Care and Emergency Medicine. Springer, Heidelberg, pp 514–533

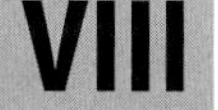

16. Elsasser S, Guttmann J, Stocker R, Mois G, Priebe HJ, Haberthur C (2003) Accuracy of automatic tube compensation in new-generation mechanical ventilators. Crit Care Med 31: 2619–2626
17. Haberthur C, Mols G, Elsasser S, Bingisser R, Stocker R, Guttmann J (2002) Extubation after breathing trials with automatic tube compensation, T-tube or pressure support ventilation. Acta Anaesthesiol Scand 46: 973–979
18. Ferreyra G, Weber-Cartens S, Aquadrone V, et al (2007) Comparison of automatic tube compensation (ATC) with pressure support ventilation (PSV) during spontaneous breathing trials. Intensive Care Med 33: s57 (abst)
19. Cohen J, Shapiro M, Grozovski E, Lev S, Fisher H, Singer P (2006) Extubation outcome following a spontaneous breathing trial with automatic tube compensation versus continuous positive airway pressure. Crit Care Med 34: 682–686
20. Eskandar N, Apostolakos MJ (2007) Weaning from mechanical ventilation. Crit Care Clin 23: 263–274
21. Siner JM, Manthous CA (2007) Liberation from mechanical ventilation: what monitoring matters? Crit Care Clin 23: 613–638
22. Frutos-Vivar F, Ferguson ND, Esteban A, et al (2006) Risk factors for extubation failure in patients following a successful spontaneous breathing trial. Chest 130: 1664–1671
23. Ely W, Baker AM, Dunagan DP, et al (1996) Effect on the duration of mechanical ventilation of identifying patients capable of spontaneous ventilation. N Eng J Med 335: 1864–1869
24. Lee KH, Hui KP, Chan TB, et al (1994) Rapid shallow breathing (frequency to tidal volume ratio) did not predict extubation outcome. Chest 105: 540–543
25. Chatila, W, Jacob, B, Guanglione, D, et al (1996) The unassisted respiratory rate: tidal volume ratio accurately predicts weaning outcome. Am J Med 101: 61–67
26. Cohen JD, Shapiro M, Grozovski E, Singer P (2002) Automatic tube compensation-assisted respiratory rate to tidal volume ratio improves the prediction of weaning outcome. Chest 122: 980–984
27. Unoki T, Serita A, Grap MJ (2008) Automatic tube compensation during weaning from mechanical ventilation. Evidence and clinical implications. Crit Care Nurse 28: 34–42

IX Mechanical Ventilation

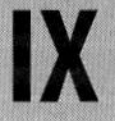

Extracorporeal Membrane Oxygenation for Cardiac and Pulmonary Indications: Improving Patient Safety

R. Kopp, S. Leonhardt, and S. Kowalewski

Introduction

Extracorporeal membrane oxygenation (ECMO) is used for patients with the most severe acute respiratory distress syndrome (ARDS) or for cardiopulmonary assist due to cardiogenic shock, cardiac arrest, or low cardiac output after cardiac surgery. Most centers use modified cardiopulmonary bypass (CPB) devices without automated control or safety concepts (**Fig. 1**), although there is no continuous observation by a perfusionist on the intensive care unit (ICU).

In this chapter, control and safety concepts are discussed for veno-venous or veno-arterial ECMO in case of severe ARDS or cardiac failure.

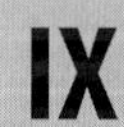

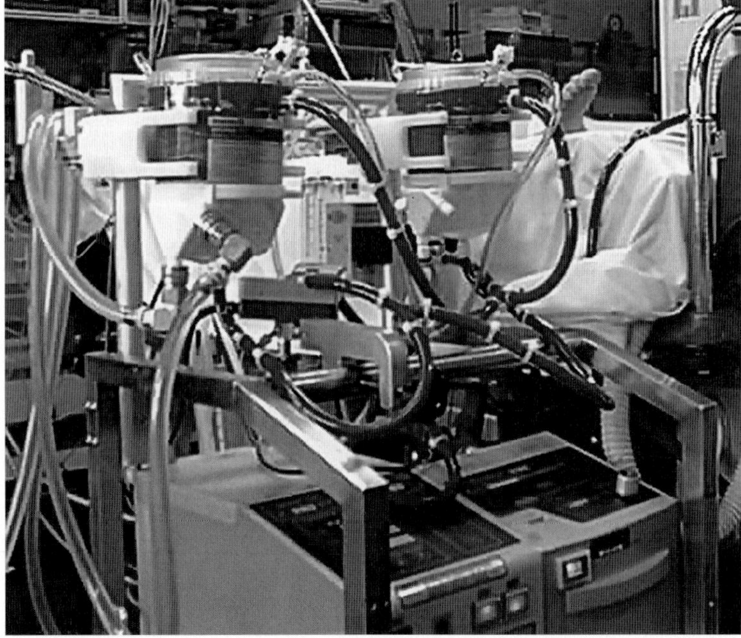

Fig. 1. Example of an ECMO system.

Application of ECMO Today

Indications for ECMO

ECMO is used to manage severe cardiac, pulmonary, or combined cardiopulmonary failure due to different diseases (**Table 1**). In the most severe cases of ARDS, patients frequently die because conservative strategies, e. g., prone position, inhaled vasodilators, or lung protective ventilation with permissive hypercapnia, are not sufficient to prevent life threatening hypoxemia. However, the survival rate of patients with severe hypoxemic ARDS is similar to overall survival rates in ARDS when extracorporeal gas exchange is used to facilitate oxygenation and decarboxylation in these patients [1].

In cases of severe refractory low cardiac output after cardiac surgery, veno-arterial ECMO is used to achieve sufficient organ perfusion and oxygenation with unloading of the heart. When recovery of cardiac function occurs after up to 5 days, the patient is weaned from ECMO or ECMO has to be changed to a long-term cardiac assist. About 60 % of patients can be weaned from ECMO, but hospital mortality rate is 76 % [2]. For refractory cardiogenic shock with or without in-hospital cardiac arrest, ECMO with femoral cannulation can also be used to preserve blood perfusion and gas exchange. In an observational study of 81 patients, change to long-term assist (left or biventricular assist) was necessary in 17 cases, 31 % received heart transplantation, and 42 % survived to hospital discharge [3].

Components of ECMO Devices

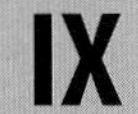

Today a typical ECMO circuit consists of a blood pump (centrifugal or roller pump), an oxygenator, and cannulas as well as connecting tubes. Cannulas are usually placed percutaneously, but sometimes the atrial and aortic cannulas of CPB are used for post-cardiotomy ECMO. Monitoring is limited to blood flow, gas flow, oxygen fraction, and blood pressure before and after the blood pump and oxygenator. Typical technical and device related complications are cannula problems, oxygenator failure, clotting, pump failure, air in circuit, tubing/circuit disruption, bleeding, hemolysis, disseminated intravascular coagulation (DIC), or hemorrhage with an incidence of 3–30 % for each complication [4].

Table 1. Indications for extracorporeal membrane oxygenation

Acute respiratory distress syndrome	**Cardiac failure**
Pneumonia	Dilated cardiomyopathy
Aspiration	Pulmonary embolism
Sepsis	Acute myocardial infarction
Trauma	Myocarditis
	Post-cardiotomy
Lung transplantation	Post-heart-transplantation
Bridge to transplant	
Post-lung-transplantation	**Miscellaneous**

Further Development of ECMO

Oxygenator

In the past, silicone and microporous membranes were used for oxygenators. Most European centers preferred microporous oxygenators because of the higher gas transfer rate leading to a smaller surface area and less heparin coating of the blood-contacting ECMO surfaces to increase hemocompatibility. Veno-venous ECMO with heparin coating requires less heparinization thus decreasing the risk of bleeding complications [5].

A severe complication of microporous membranes is 'plasma leakage', when large amounts of blood plasma pass through the pores of the membranes. Because of the dramatically reduced gas transfer, the affected oxygenators have to be immediately changed [6]. Risk factors for 'plasma leakage' are increased blood concentrations of lipids or phospholipids, liver failure, younger patient age, and the number of oxygenators already replaced. Newly developed fibers combine a microporous texture with a thin closed layer on the surface to prevent plasma leakage and to extend the running-time of the oxygenators (**Fig. 2**) [7]. Oxygenators with a plasma resistant polymethylpentene fiber have been successfully used for long term ECMO [8].

Blood Pump

Roller pumps have been standard for ECMO, but continuous mechanical stress can result in rupture and embolism of tube particles. This requires that the tubes in roller pumps are changed regularly. Although centrifugal pumps avoid these complications, blood depositions on centrifugal pumps may increase damage to blood cells and hemolysis requiring regular exchange of the pump head. Contactless magnetic bearing of the rotor seems to reduce platelet deposition and increase run-time. Additionally a considerable length of tubing is needed to connect the patient to the ECMO device, when the roller pump and centrifugal console with pump head are placed beside the bed of the patient [9].

IX

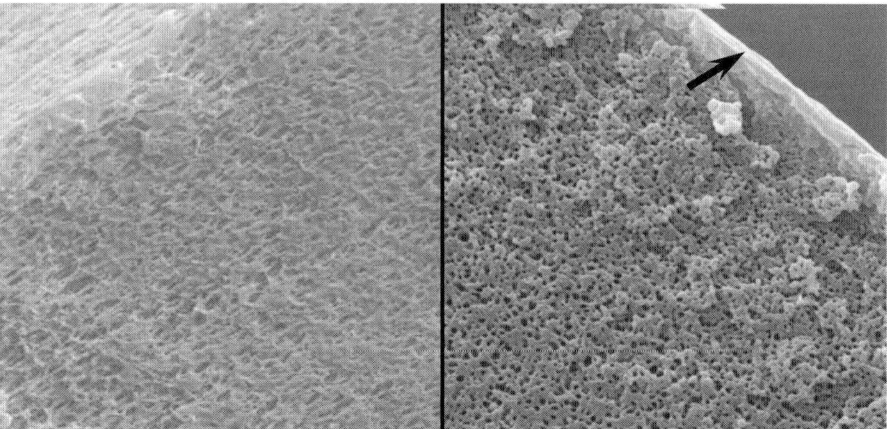

Fig. 2. Characteristics of microporous polypropylene membrane (left) and polymethylpentene composite membranes (right) with a closed layer on the outside (arrow).

Modifications of ECMO Console and Circuit

Uncoupling of console and pump head allows the ECMO circuit to be placed beside the patient with reduced filling volume due to the shorter tubing. In particular during intra- or interhospital transfer of the patient, risk of disconnection and dislocation is reduced [10]. New concepts for highly integrated venovenous ECMO during ARDS include coupling of the oxygenator and blood pump to reduce foreign surface area and priming volume even more and to use the waste heat of the pump motor housing instead of a heat exchanger to keep blood temperature constant (**Fig. 3**). This compact design should further simplify clinical management [11].

Pumpless Extracorporeal Lung Assist

In the past, a blood pump was necessary to overcome flow resistance of cannulas and oxygenators and to achieve sufficient blood flow for extracorporeal lung support. Using newly designed oxygenators and cannulas with reduced pressure drop, mean arterial blood pressure becomes sufficient to achieve adequate extracorporeal blood flow. Mathematical analysis demonstrated for the pumpless arterio-venous extracorporeal lung assist (ECLA) device, that total extracorporeal CO_2-removal is possible with a blood flow of 10–15 % cardiac output, a gas flow ≥ 5 l/min and a sufficient diffusing capacity of the oxygenator [12]. The oxygen transfer is limited due to the oxygenated blood coming into the membrane lung. ECLA can be placed between the legs of the patients. Proof of concept was demonstrated in a case series with 90 patients [13]. Reduced priming volume and lack of a blood pump simplified control and monitoring of the device for blood flow, mean arterial pressure, and perfusion of the leg after cannulation of the femoral artery. Low oxygen transfer and arterio-venous shunt limit the clinical application of this technique to patients with decompensated hypercapnia and without severe cardiac failure and hypoxia.

IX

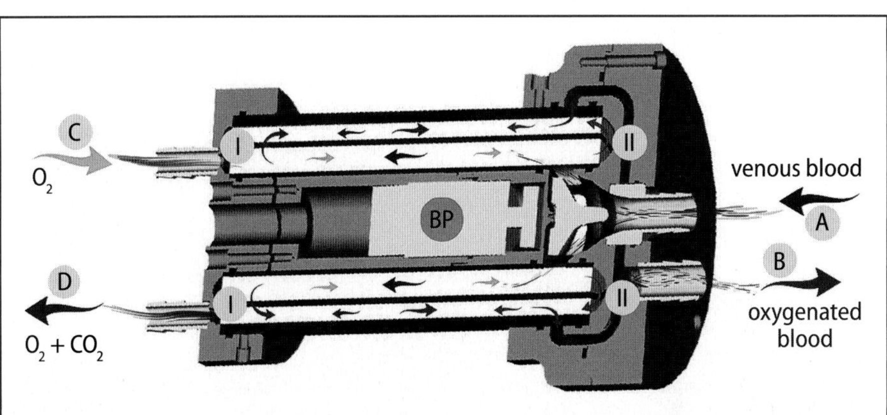

Fig. 3. Scheme of highly integrated extracorporeal membrane oxygenator (HEXMO) with rotary blood pump. Blood in (A); change in direction of blood stream (I); blood out (B), integrated blood pump (BP); gas in (C); change in direction of gas stream (II); gas out (D)

Control and Safety

Automation for Related Applications

Initial efforts were made to integrate basic automated pump control in CPB. For example, the Deltastream pump (Medos, Stolberg, Germany) offers the possibility to limit extracorporeal blood flow depending on the preload, for example when suctioning the venous cannula, and to stop the pump automatically in case of bubble detection after the oxygenator or low level in the venous reservoir (**Fig. 4**) [14]. Additionally temperature and humidity in the pump housing are continuously measured to detect failure of motor and seal status. With new models, automated control of gas transfer for CPB [15] as well as control of pulsatile and continuous extracorporeal blood flow [16] seems possible. These systems have been tested in different *in vitro* models and demonstrated robustly stable performances.

For patients with left or biventricular cardiac assist devices, automated control could optimize safety and performance. Adaptation of blood flow is mostly controlled by the operator or by venous filling of devices performing in asynchronous mode: For example, with increased venous return and faster filling of the assist, pump rate increases resulting in higher cardiac output [17]. Another approach is control of left cardiac assist with rotary blood pumps to changing physiological demands by measuring the pressure differences between the left ventricle and the aorta [18]. Since implantation of two pressure sensors limits the application of these systems, a model was developed to calculate blood flow from the pump parameters: voltage, current, and speed. Pressure differences can then be estimated from calcu-

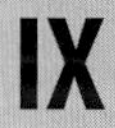
IX

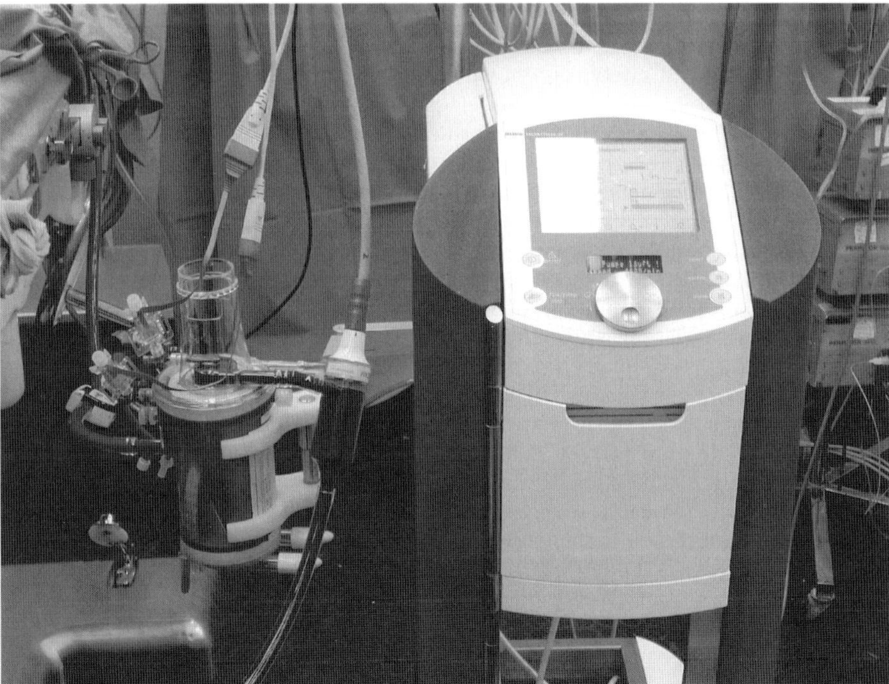

Fig. 4. Miniaturized ECMO with deltastream console and pump.

lated blood flow and speed [19]. Experience with this system is still limited to simulation.

Available Control and Safety Concepts for ECMO

For ECMO, the implementation of control and safety concepts is limited to commercially available blood pumps with basic control mechanisms, such as the Deltastream console (see above).

For short-term CPB support, the Lifebridge system has been developed with automated priming and air elimination (Lifebridge Medizintechnik AG, Ampfing, Germany). Additionally, venous drainage is controlled by a venous reservoir with a low-level detector and an automated pump stop [20]. Indications for this system are cardiopulmonary support during high-risk percutaneous cardiac intervention as well as intra- and interhospital transfer of patients with low cardiac output for further therapy, such as cardiac surgery or implantation of long-term cardiac assist.

However, control and safety concepts for ECMO require additional efforts to increase patient safety. For patients with veno-venous lung support or partial veno-arterial assist, in particular, measuring outflow oxygen and carbon dioxide content is not sufficient to control gas exchange as described for full CPB during cardiac surgery [15]. It seems necessary to integrate patient blood gas status into the control of ECMO.

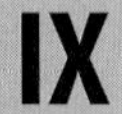

New Control and Safety Concepts

More sophisticated automation solutions for control of medical devices must always address two equally important issues: Appropriate control of internal and physiological values as well as a safety concept which prevents patient injury from device malfunction and operator error. Both targets need specific device properties and dedicated software and algorithms. **Figure 5** shows a possible setup for such an advanced ECMO system. Basic therapy is performed by the standard equipment (blood pump, gas dosage, and oxygenator) which is in use today. This standard setup is extended by introducing additional sensors (e.g., continuous blood gas, hemodynamic monitoring) and actuators (electronic gas mixer, externally adjustable pump) as well as a network infrastructure with local security nodes, serial bus system (CAN), and a central automation platform (dSPACE). The main therapy goal is sufficient oxygenation and decarboxylation with minimal blood cell damage. In order to achieve this goal, a cascading control structure is chosen (**Fig. 6**). The inner loop controls parameters locally at the oxygenator. The outer control loop controls the physiological target values. By choosing such control structures, side conditions and physiological constraints can be implemented easily at the interface between inner and outer control loop by design. The global control is implemented at a central level processing unit. In contrast, the safety concept is distributed in decentralized local security nodes. Apart from providing measurement data in the local network, the translation units contain security nodes which ensure functionality and data integrity of the connected devices locally. Additional redundant and secondary information, which is available in the network, is used to create extra safety information, e.g., data integrity and validity can be improved by model based virtual sensors. A superior hierarchy integrates the fault decision knowledge which can be implemented in a rule based system. This security layer collects occurring faults, rates their severity and

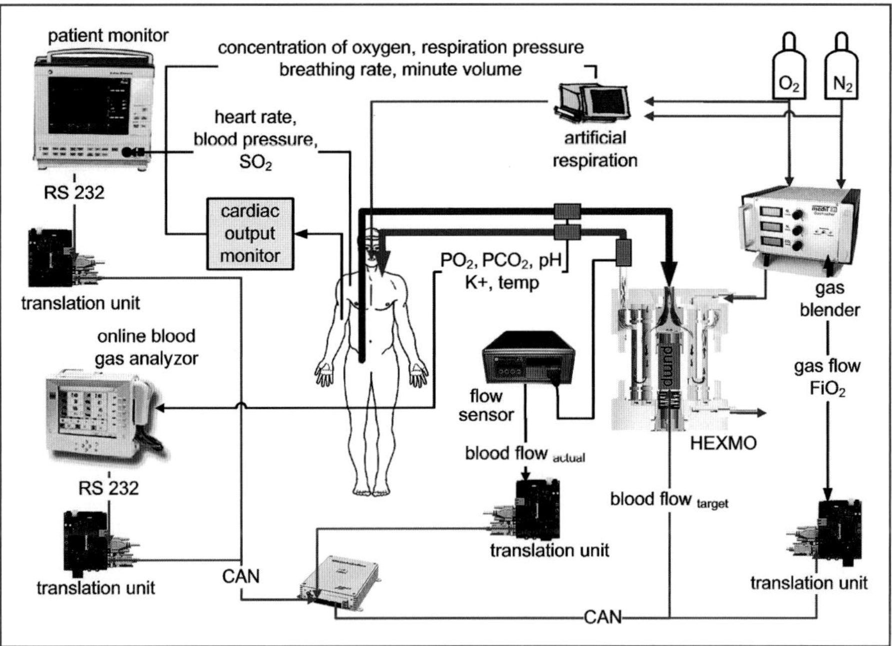

Fig. 5. Possible setup for an advanced ECMO system integrating appropriate control of internal and physiological values as well as a safety concept to prevent patient injury from device malfunctions and operator errors.

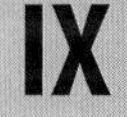

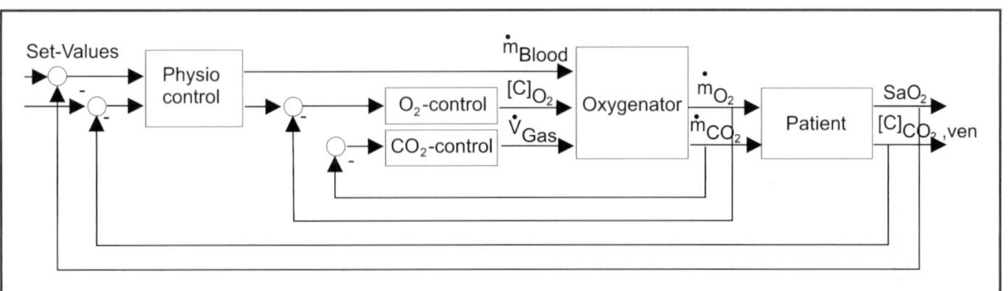

Fig. 6. Scheme of a cascading control structure with an inner loop to control parameters locally at the oxygenator and an outer control loop for the physiological target values. $\dot{m}$: mass flow; $\dot{V}$: volume flow; [C]: concentration

initiates appropriate reactions like alarms, security function, machine reconfiguration, etc.

Conclusion

ECMO is used for pulmonary, cardiac, and cardiopulmonary support in cases of severe ARDS, cardiogenic shock, or low cardiac output after cardiac surgery. To increase the safety and reliability of devices, oxygenator design has been optimized by integrating new plasma-resistant composite membranes. Additionally, new blood pumps are used with longer durability and reduced blood cell damage. Another approach is the use of an arterio-venous pumpless perfusion without a blood pump (pumpless ECLA) to simplify management and to avoid pump related complications.

Initial attempts were made to integrate basic control and safety concepts into ECMO circuits, but these seemed not to be sufficient to overcome the specific problems of ECMO (long term use and limited supervision on the ICU). The integration of sophisticated automated control and safety concepts in combination with revised ECMO circuits could allow the more reliable application of ECMO on the ICU without continuous observation by a perfusionist. Easier intra- and interhospital transfer of patients receiving ECMO would be another advantage.

References

1. Kopp R, Dembinski R, Kuhlen R (2006) Role of extracorporeal lung assist in the treatment of acute respiratory failure. Minerva Anestesiol 72: 587–595
2. Doll N, Kiaii B, Borger M, et al (2004) Five-year results of 219 consecutive patients treated with extracorporeal membrane oxygenation for refractory postoperative cardiogenic shock. Ann Thorac Surg 77: 151–157
3. Combes A, Leprince P, Luyt CE, et al (2008) Outcomes and long-term quality-of-life of patients supported by extracorporeal membrane oxygenation for refractory cardiogenic shock. Crit Care Med 36: 1404–1411
4. Hemmila MR, Rowe SA, Boules TN, et al (2004) Extracorporeal life support for severe acute respiratory distress syndrome in adults. Ann Surg 240: 595–605
5. Murphy JA, Savage CM, Alpard SK, Deyo DJ, Jayroe JB, Zwischenberger JB (2001) Low-dose versus high-dose heparinization during arteriovenous carbon dioxide removal. Perfusion 16: 460–468

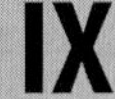

6. Meyns B, Vercaemst L, Vandezande E, Bollen H, Vlasselaers D (2005) Plasma leakage of oxygenators in ECMO depends on the type of oxygenator and on patient variables. Int J Artif Organs 28: 30–34
7. Eash HJ, Jones HM, Hattler BG, Federspiel WJ (2004) Evaluation of plasma resistant hollow fiber membranes for artificial lungs. ASAIO J 50: 491–497
8. Khoshbin E, Roberts N, Harvey C, et al (2005) Poly-methyl pentene oxygenators have improved gas exchange capability and reduced transfusion requirements in adult extracorporeal membrane oxygenation. ASAIO J 51: 281–287
9. Lewandowski K (2000) Extracorporeal membrane oxygenation for severe acute respiratory failure. Crit Care 4: 156–168
10. Arlt M, Philipp A, Zimmermann M, et al (2008) First experiences with a new miniaturised life support system for mobile percutaneous cardiopulmonary bypass. Resuscitation 77: 345–350
11. Cattaneo G, Strauss A, Reul H (2004) Compact intra- and extracorporeal oxygenator developments. Perfusion 19: 251–255
12. Conrad SA, Brown EG, Grier LR, et al (1998) Arteriovenous extracorporeal carbon dioxide removal: a mathematical model and experimental evaluation. ASAIO J 44: 267–277
13. Bein T, Weber F, Philipp A, et al (2006) A new pumpless extracorporeal interventional lung assist in critical hypoxemia/hypercapnia. Crit Care Med 34: 1372–1377
14. Gobel C, Arvand A, Rau G, et al (2002) A new rotary blood pump for versatile extracorporeal circulation: the DeltaStream. Perfusion 17: 373–382
15. Hexamer M, Misgeld B, Prenger-Berninghoff A, et al (2004) Automatic control of the extracorporal bypass: system analysis, modelling and evaluation of different control modes. Biomed Tech (Berl) 49: 316–321
16. Misgeld BJ, Werner J, Hexamer M (2005) Robust and self-tuning blood flow control during extracorporeal circulation in the presence of system parameter uncertainties. Med Biol Eng Comput 43: 589–598
17. Samuels LE, Holmes EC, Garwood P, Ferdinand F (2005) Initial experience with the Abiomed AB5000 ventricular assist device system. Ann Thorac Surg 80: 309–312

18. Giridharan GA, Pantalos GM, Gillars KJ, Koenig SC, Skliar M (2004) Physiologic control of rotary blood pumps: an in vitro study. ASAIO J 50: 403 – 409
19. Giridharan GA, Skliar M (2006) Physiological control of blood pumps using intrinsic pump parameters: a computer simulation study. Artif Organs 30: 301 – 307
20. Mehlhorn U, Brieske M, Fischer UM, et al (2005) LIFEBRIDGE: a portable, modular, rapidly available "plug-and-play" mechanical circulatory support system. Ann Thorac Surg 80: 1887 – 1892

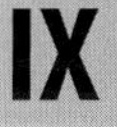

Patient-ventilator Interaction during Non-invasive Ventilation

P. Jolliet, D. Tassaux, and L. Vignaux

Introduction

Over the years, non-invasive ventilation (NIV) has evolved into becoming a standard of care in both hypercapnic and non-hypercapnic acute respiratory failure [1–3]. However, its success in avoiding intubation is largely determined by patient tolerance to the technique [4]. The optimal combination of the patient's spontaneous breathing activity and the ventilator's set parameters, known as 'patient-ventilator interaction', depends on numerous factors, and can prove very difficult to achieve [5, 6]. If patient ventilator asynchrony is present, the work of breathing can increase [5, 6]. Further complicating the matter, leaks at the patient-mask interface during NIV can interfere with various aspects of ventilator function, thereby increasing the risk of patient-ventilator asynchrony [7–10]. As an illustration, a recent study documented that severe asynchrony was present in 43 % of patients undergoing NIV for acute respiratory failure [11]. Consequently, when applying NIV the clinician must pay close attention to both the proper setting of ventilator parameters and the avoidance of excessive leaks at the patient-mask interface.

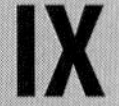

The purpose of this chapter is to review the basic mechanisms involved in patient-ventilator interaction, and their possible solutions, focusing on the specific modes and aspects used during NIV.

NIV in Acute Respiratory Failure

Several recent publications have outlined the key role played by NIV as a first-line technique to avoid endotracheal intubation in patients with acute respiratory failure [1–3]. Initially considered as more helpful in patients with chronic obstructive pulmonary disease (COPD) presenting with hypercapnic acute respiratory failure [1], NIV has also proved its value in various groups of patients with non-hypercapnic acute respiratory failure [3, 12, 13]. One important aspect in NIV is the choice of ventilator mode, the two most common options being pressure support and assist-control [14, 15]. Very few studies have compared these modes in patients with acute respiratory failure. Overall, however, there is evidence that although assist-control can prove more effective in terms of reducing respiratory muscle workload, this advantage comes at the price of lesser patient tolerance [16–18]. The lack of hard evidence favoring one mode over another probably accounts for the fact that most published recommendations suggest that the choice of NIV mode be guided mainly by local expertise [19, 20]. Nonetheless, improved patient tolerance has probably been a key element behind the more widespread use of pressure support, which has become the mode of choice in most patients with acute respiratory failure [2]. Therefore, the focus of the next paragraphs will be placed on pressure support ventilation.

Pressure support is a spontaneous-assisted mode in which every breath is triggered by the patient, each breath being assisted by a set amount of inspiratory pressure provided by the ventilator [21]. Once the pressure level has been reached, the ventilator cycles into expiration, letting the patient exhale passively. Thus, four key phases of pressure support can be identified: Triggering, slope of pressurization, level of pressure support, and cycling. Each phase can be a source of patient-ventilator asynchrony, due to patient characteristics (e.g., insufficient inspiratory effort, tachypnea, agitation), improper ventilator settings, and leaks around the mask. Indeed, while studies have reported the use of bilevel-type home ventilation devices and intensive care unit (ICU) ventilators, the latter are often used most often when NIV is applied in the ICU setting. The problem is that these machines are designed for the mostly leak-free ventilation of intubated patients, and often have difficulties adjusting to usually leak-rich NIV conditions [22].

We will now briefly review the main issues associated with each pressure support phase during NIV and discuss the implications of leaks in these conditions on ICU ventilator function.

Triggering of the Ventilator

When the patient performs an inspiratory effort, the ventilator detects either a decrease in circuit pressure (pressure trigger) or an inspiratory flow (flow trigger). Considerable progress has been made in the overall sensitivity of ventilators' triggering mechanisms, in terms of both the inspiratory effort required and initial delay; triggering thereby adding little to the overall work of breathing [23]. In a study comparing flow- and pressure triggering on a bench lung model and in intubated patients, Aslanian et al. showed that flow triggering was associated with a lower work of breathing [24]. Similar results were reported by Nava et al. in COPD patients undergoing NIV [25]. These results suggest that flow-triggering should be preferred. However, during NIV, leaks can be erroneously detected by the ventilator as an inspiratory effort, thereby triggering the ventilator in the absence of patient inspiratory effort. This problem is known as auto-triggering (**Fig. 1a**), and the frequency of its occurrence has been shown to correlate with the magnitude of the leak [7]. Therefore, the sensitivity of the flow trigger should be set high enough to avoid increasing the respiratory muscle workload, but low enough to avoid auto-triggering [26]. Alternatively, pressure triggering can be used, but at the cost of a slight increase in inspiratory effort [24, 25]. Leak control is in any case important, a significant correlation having been found between leak volume and the number of ineffective breaths [11]. The use of the NIV mode on ICU ventilators can partly alleviate the triggering issue caused by leaks, the efficacy of this mode varying between machines [22].

One problem often facing clinicians is that of trigger asynchrony [27], i.e., the presence of inspiratory efforts that do not succeed in triggering the ventilator (**Fig. 1b**). The most common cause of these ineffective inspiratory attempts is the presence of intrinsic positive end-expiratory pressure (PEEPi) in patients with obstructive airways disease [27, 28]. PEEPi acts as an inspiratory threshold load which the patient often cannot offset with each breath. This situation can markedly increase

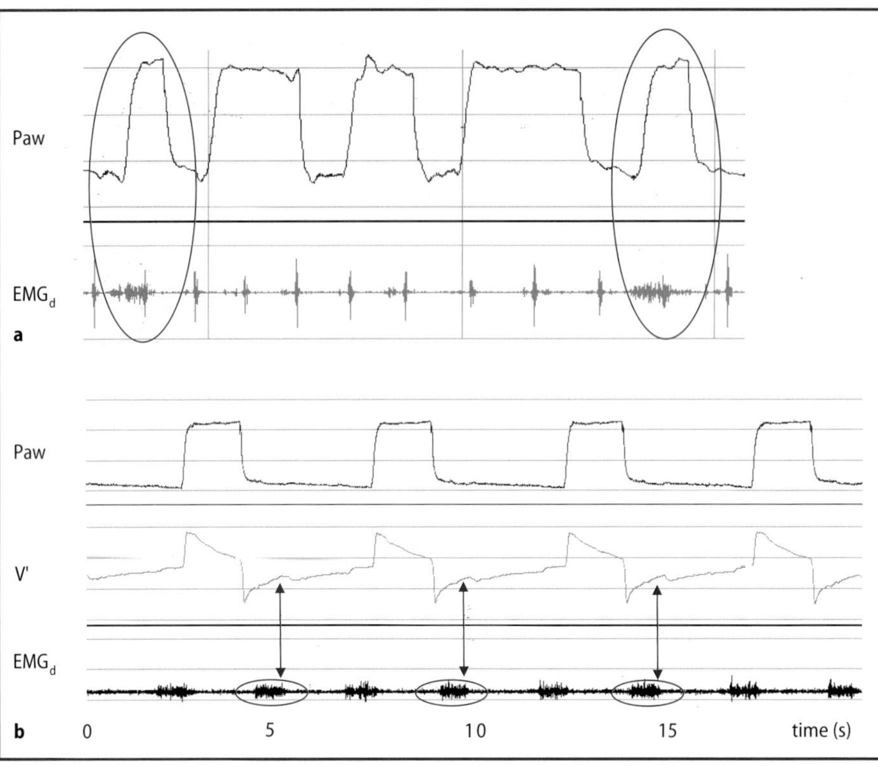

Fig. 1. Representative tracings of triggering asynchrony during NIV. **a** Auto-triggering: Only the first and last cycles (circled) are triggered by the patient, as shown by the concomitant diaphragmatic electromyogram (EMG$_d$) activity. The other cycles show no such activity (the visible spikes are due to the cardiac electrical activity). **b** Ineffective inspiratory efforts: The three circled inspiratory efforts are not followed by a pressurization response from the ventilator. A detectable deflection of the expiratory portion of the instantaneous flow curve is observed (arrow), which is a consequence of the inspiratory effort. Paw: airway pressure; V': instantaneous flow.

the work of breathing [28], even if maximum trigger sensitivity is set, since the offsetting of PEEPi is still necessary for the trigger to react [27]. Adding external PEEP (PEEPe) has been shown to decrease both the number of ineffective breaths and the associated work of breathing [28]. No validated approach to determine the optimal level of PEEPe has been described yet. Our pragmatic approach is to start at zero end-expiratory pressure (ZEEP), and to titrate PEEPe upwards by 1–2 cmH_2O increments, until ineffective inspiratory attempts markedly decrease or disappear. During NIV, one must, however, remember that increasing PEEPe is likely to increase leaks around the mask, which in turn can lead to auto-triggering and other problems which will be described in the following sections.

Another option is to reduce the level of pressure support, given that insufflation of a high tidal volume can increase dynamic hyperinflation and PEEPi, thereby worsening trigger asynchrony [29].

Pressurization Slope

The slope of pressurization, i.e., the incremental increase in airway pressure per time unit, can be adjusted on most ventilators [23]. In intubated patients with both restrictive and obstructive respiratory system mechanics, a steep slope is associated with a lower work of breathing – the steeper the slope the lower the work of breathing [30, 31]. A study performed in COPD patients undergoing NIV has yielded similar results, the diaphragmatic pressure-time product being significantly lower at the fastest pressurization rate [9]. However, the same study also showed the limits of how fast the pressurization ramp can be set. Indeed, the fastest rate was associated with a significant increase in air leaks and proved to be the most uncomfortable for the patients [9]. This issue is certainly of importance, given that in at least one large multicenter study, patients who failed NIV and required intubation had larger air leaks than those not requiring intubation [4]. Therefore, it is probably wise not to decrease the pressure support rise time to < 100 ms, and, if a patient exhibits discomfort, to increase the time up to 200 ms.

Level of Pressure Support

Pressure support can decrease the load imposed on respiratory muscle in a titrable manner, i.e., the higher the level of applied pressure support, the more unloading is provided to these muscles [32]. Respiratory muscle unloading is one of the key mechanisms by which NIV helps to avoid intubation [14, 33, 34], and, therefore, one might be tempted to reason that the higher the level of pressure support, the higher the efficacy of NIV to attain that goal. However, several limitations should be kept in mind. First, excessive levels of pressure support can result in the insufflation of a large tidal volume, which in turn can worsen dynamic hyperinflation and PEEPi in obstructive patients, resulting in an increase in the number of ineffective inspiratory attempts [29]. Second, a high inspiratory pressure is expected to increase the risk of gastric air intake, thereby increasing discomfort and the risk of vomiting and aspiration. Third, a high level of pressure support coupled with leaks can worsen the delayed cycling phenomenon which will be described in the next section. Finally, leaks increase in proportion to the pressure generated inside the mask. In a bench model study, Schettino et al. showed that leaks around the mask were minor up to a pressure support of 16 cmH_2O and could be compensated for by the ventilator, whereas above that level most of the flow delivered by the ventilator was lost in leaks [10]. This last mechanism probably provides some safeguard against excessive tidal volume insufflation and gastric intake of air, but can lead to delayed cycling, as will be discussed below. Furthermore, given that ventilators differ markedly in their capacity to compensate for leaks [35], any increase in pressure support might paradoxically lead to a decrease in delivered tidal volume due to the increase in leaks. As an illustration of the consequences of excessive levels of pressure support, it has been recently shown that the higher the pressure support, the more likely it was that severe asynchrony was present [11]. There are no published practice guidelines on the titration of the optimal level of pressure support during NIV. However, a reasonable approach is to start with a pressure support of 8–10 cmH_2O, titrated upwards to maintain an expired tidal volume of around 6–8 ml/kg, while minimizing leaks as much as possible. Automated modes designed to pursue the optimal titration of pressure support [36] could also prove useful during NIV, and preliminary results

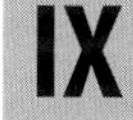

suggest the feasibility of this approach [37]; however, this path has yet to be explored more fully.

Cycling

In pressure support mode, the transition from inspiration to expiration, known as cycling, occurs when instantaneous inspiratory flow (V'_{insp}) decreases to a predetermined fraction of peak inspiratory flow (V'_{insp}/V'_{peak}) [21]. This threshold value of V'_{insp} is often referred to as the 'expiratory trigger'. In an ideal situation, cycling coincides with the end of the patient's inspiratory effort. Prolonged pressurization by the machine into the patient's expiratory phase is known as delayed cycling (**Fig. 2a**), whereas premature cycling describes the cessation of pressurization before the end of the patients inspiratory effort (**Fig. 2b**). Delayed cycling can lead to

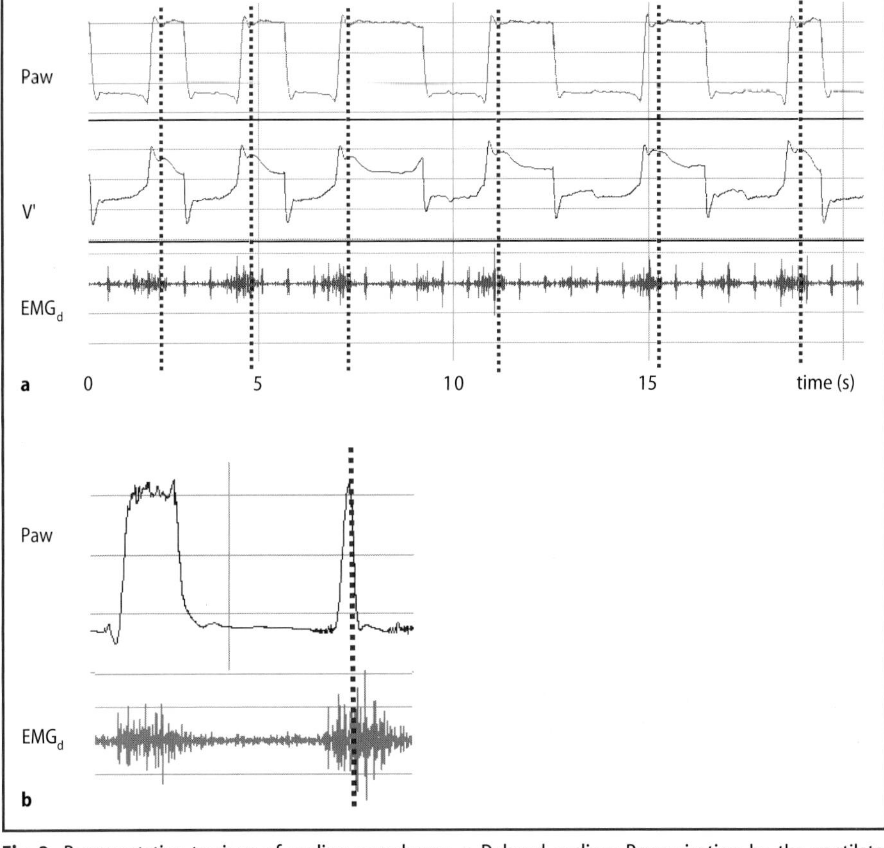

Fig. 2. Representative tracings of cycling asynchrony. **a** Delayed cycling: Pressurization by the ventilator extends well beyond the end of the patient's inspiratory time (dotted vertical line), determined from the surface diaphragmatic electromyographic recording (EMG_d). **b** Premature cycling: Pressurization by the ventilator stops well before the end of the patient's inspiratory time (dotted vertical line), determined from the surface EMG_d. Paw: airway pressure; V': instantaneous flow.

expiratory asynchrony and increased work of breathing [38, 39]. Delayed cycling has been shown to occur mostly in patients with obstructive airways disease [40–42], mainly because as obstruction becomes more severe the V'_{insp} profile changes, the instantaneous V' curve plotted against time becoming more spread-out, resulting in the 25 % cut-off value being reached later [41]. However, in a recent study, delayed cycling was the most prevalent type of asynchrony during NIV [11]. Indeed, additional factors can contribute to delayed cycling during NIV. Calderini et al. showed that leaks around the mask led to a prolonged pressurization by the ventilator, in turn leading to an insufficient decrease in V'_{insp} to the cycling threshold [8]. Consequently, cycling was considerably delayed, the patients were attempting to cycle the ventilator by active expiration [39], and work of breathing was increased [8]. Relying on time rather than on flow cycling, i.e., by limiting the maximum inspiratory time, can reduce delayed cycling, the magnitude of inspiratory efforts and the work of breathing [8].

Another possible solution comes from the NIV modes of ICU ventilators, which can to a variable extent correct for the presence of leaks and reduce the duration of delayed cycling [22]. Naturally, reducing leaks can also contribute to alleviating this problem, but tight-fitting masks are a source of discomfort for patients, which can lead to overall intolerance to NIV and reduce its chances of success. Finally, delayed cycling can also occur as a result of increased leaks caused not by an insufficient mask seal but by a high pressurization rate [9].

In addition to ensuring minimal leaks through the proper choice of mask, reducing excessive pressurization rates, and resorting to time-cycled ventilation, it is also possible to reduce the magnitude of delayed cycling by increasing the level of expiratory triggering. Indeed, increasing expiratory triggering from its default 25 % value to 50 % has been shown to reduce the magnitude of delayed cycling and inspiratory muscle workload in intubated COPD patients ventilated with pressure support [43]. Whether the same result could be obtained during NIV remains to be determined.

Masks

An in-depth discussion of masks is beyond the scope of the present chapter. Suffice it to say that, given the issues outlined above, two aspects of this subject are important regarding patient-ventilator interaction. The first is minimizing leaks to avoid loss of pressure support [10] and delayed cycling [8]. The second goal should be to avoid patient discomfort as much as possible, given the impact of patient tolerance on the success rate of NIV [4]. Few studies have compared nasal and full face masks in patients with acute respiratory failure. Kwok et al. reported comparable efficacy in improving clinical signs of respiratory distress and gas exchange in a group of 70 patients in whom the predominant causes of acute respiratory failure were acute cardiogenic pulmonary edema and decompensated COPD, but mask intolerance was significantly higher with the nasal mask [44]. On the other hand, Navalesi et al. studied 26 stable hypercapnic patients and found that the nasal mask was better tolerated, while the full face mask led to a greater improvement in hypercapnia [45]. Differences between these two studies probably stem from the difference in studied populations and acute versus chronic respiratory failure. From a practical point of view, and given the large number of masks on the market, each presenting distinct features, any center using NIV on a regular basis should have several types of mask readily available, the goal being to generate minimal leaks while avoiding excessive discomfort [15]. Finally, recent studies on the use of the helmet device for NIV have shown encouraging results, both in improving gas exchange and in reducing the rate of complications such as pressure sores, eye irritation, and gastric distension associated with conventional mask NIV [46, 47]. Further evaluations of this technique should determine its impact on other aspects of patient-ventilator interaction, especially given the differences in characteristics between the various types of helmets available [48].

Conclusion

Increase in our knowledge of patient-ventilator interactions over the years has highlighted the complexity of an apparently simple mode such as pressure support [49, 50]. It is clear that the various key phases and pitfalls of this mode should be understood by ICU physicians and caregivers, to reduce unnecessary respiratory muscle workload and improve patients comfort. While this assertion holds true for both invasive and non-invasive ventilation, leaks and patient intolerance in acutely decompensated patient present an added challenge to the clinician during NIV. Meeting this challenge requires further knowledge of those aspects of patient-ventilator interactions specific to the setting of NIV, the goal being to administer the technique safely and possibly to reduce the intubation rate further. To help in this task, ventilator manufacturers have developed specific NIV modes and automated ventilator setting algorithms. However, these new technologies now need thorough testing in patients to determine their precise role in performing NIV in acutely decompensated patients.

References

1. Peter J, Moran J, Hughes J (2002) Noninvasive mechanical ventilation in acute respiratory failure – a meta-analysis update. Crit Care Med 30: 555–562
2. Liesching T, Kwok H, Hill N (2003) Acute applications of noninvasive positive pressure ventilation. Chest 124: 699–713
3. Ferrer M, Esquinas A, Leon M, Gonzalez G, Alarcon A, Torres A (2003) Noninvasive ventilation in severe hypoxemic respiratory failure. Am J Respir Crit Car Med 168: 1438–1444
4. Carlucci A, Richard J, Wysocki M, Lepage E, Brochard L (2001) Noninvasive versus conventional mechanical ventilation. An epidemiologic survey. Am J Respir Crit Care Med 163: 874–880
5. Tobin M, Jubran A, Laghi F (2001) Patient-ventilator interaction. Am J Respir Crit Care Med 163: 1059–1063
6. Kondili E, Prinianakis G, Georgopoulos D (2003) Patient-ventilator interaction. Br J Anaesth 91: 106–119
7. Bernstein G, Knodel E, Heldt GP (1995) Airway leak size in neonates and autocycling of three flow-triggered ventilators. Crit Care Med 23: 1739–1744
8. Calderini E, Confalonieri M, Puccio P, Francavilla N, Stella L, Gregoretti C (1999) Patient-ventilator asynchrony during noninvasive ventilation: the role of expiratory trigger. Intensive Care Med 25: 662–7
9. Prinianakis G, Delmastro M, Carlucci A, Ceriana P, Nava S (2004) Effect of varying the pressurisation rate during noninvasive pressure support ventilation. Eur Respir J 23: 314–320
10. Schettino G, Tucci M, Sousa R, Valente Barbas C, Passos Amato M, Carvalho C (2001) Mask mechanics and leak dynamics during noninvasive pressure support ventilation: a bench study. Intensive Care Med 27: 1887–1891
11. Vignaux L, Vargas F, Roeseler J, et al (2009) Patient-ventilator interaction during non-invasive ventilation for acute respiratory failure: a multicenter study. Intensive Care Med (in press)

12. Martin T, Hovis JD, Costantino J, et al (2000) A randomized, prospective evaluation of noninvasive ventilation for acute respiratory failure. Am J Respir Crit Care Med 161: 807–813
13. Nava S, Gregoretti C, Fanfulla F, et al. (2005) Noninvasive ventilation to prevent respiratory failure after extubation in high-risk patients. Crit Care Med 33: 2465–2470
14. Mehta S, Hill N (2001) Noninvasive ventilation. Am J Respir Crit Care Med 163: 540–577
15. Schönhofer B, Sortor-Leger S (2002) Equipment needs for noninvasive mechanical ventilation. Eur Respir J 20: 1029–1036
16. Cinnella G, Conti G, Lofaso F, et al (1996) Effects of assisted ventilation on the work of breathing: volume-controlled versus pressure-controlled ventilation. Am J Respir Crit Care Med 153: 1025–1033
17. Girault C, Richard J, Chevron V, et al (1997) Comparative physiologic effects of noninvasive assist-control and pressure support ventilation in acute hypercapnic respiratory failure. Chest 111: 1639–1648
18. Vitacca M, Rubini F, Foglio K, Scalvini S, Nava S, Ambrosino N (1993) Non-invasive modalities of positive pressure ventilation improve the outcome of acute exacerbations in COLD patients. Intensive Care Med 19: 450–455
19. British Thoracic Society Standards of Care Committee (2002) Non-invasive ventilation in acute respiratory failure. Thorax 57: 192–211
20. Evans T (2001) International Consensus Conference in Intensive Care Medicine: Noninvasive positive pressure ventilation in acute respiratory failure. Intensive Care Med 27: 166–178
21. Brochard L (1994) Inspiratory pressure support. Eur J Anesthesiol 11: 29–36
22. Vignaux L, Tassaux D, Jolliet P (2007) Performance of noninvasive ventilation modes on ICU ventilators during pressure support: a bench model study. Intensive Care Med 33: 1444–1451
23. Richard JC, Carlucci A, Breton L, et al (2002) Bench testing of pressure support ventilation with three different generations of ventilators. Intensive Care Med 28: 1049–1057
24. Aslanian P, El Atrous S, Isabey D, et al (1998) Effects of flow triggering on breathing effort during partial ventilatory support. Am J Respir Crit Care Med 157: 135–143
25. Nava S, Ambrosino N, Bruschi C, Confalonieri M, Rampulla C (1997) Physiological effects of flow and pressure triggering during non-invasive mechanical ventilation in patients with chronic obstructive pulmonary disease. Thorax 52: 249–254
26. Hill LL, Pearl R (2000) Flow triggering, pressure triggering, and autotriggering during mechanical ventilation. Crit Care Med 28: 579–581
27. Chao D, Scheinhorn D, Stearn-Hassenpflug M (1997) Patient-ventilator trigger asynchrony in prolonged mechanical ventilation. Chest 112: 1592–1599
28. Nava S, Bruschi C, Rubini F, Palo A, Iotti G, Braschi A (1995) Respiratory response and inspiratory effort during pressure support ventilation in COPD patients. Intensive Care Med 21: 871–879
29. Leung P, Jubran A, Tobin M (1997) Comparison of assisted ventilator modes on triggering, patient effort, and dyspnea. Am J Respir Crit Care Med 155: 1940–1948
30. Bonmarchand G, Chevron V, Chopin C, et al (1996) Increased initial flow rate reduces inspiratory work of breathing during pressure support ventilation in patients with exacerbation of chronic obstructive pulmonary disease. Intensive Care Med 22: 1147–1154
31. Bonmarchand G, Chevron V, Ménard J, et al (1999) Effects of pressure ramp slope values on the work of breathing during pressure support ventilation in restrictive patients. Crit Care Med 27: 715–722
32. Brochard L, Harf A, Lorino H, Lemaire F (1989) Inspiratory pressure support prevents diaphragmatic fatigue during weaning from mechanical ventilation. Am Rev Respir Dis 139: 513–521
33. Brochard L, Isabey D, Piquet J, et al (1990) Reversal of acute exacerbations of chronic obstructive lung disease by inspiratory assistance with a face mask. N Engl J Med 323: 1523–1530
34. L'Her E, Deye N, Lellouche F, et al (2005) Physiologic effects of noninvasive ventilation during acute lung injury. Am J Respir Crit Care Med 172: 1112–1118
35. Mehta S, McCool F, Hill NS (2001) Leak compensation in positive pressure ventilators: a lung model study. Eur Respir J 17: 259–267
36. Dojat M, Harf A, Touchard D, Lemaire F, Brochard L (2000) Clinical evaluation of a computer-controlled pressure support mode. Am J Respir Crit Care Med 161: 1161–6
37. Battisti A, Roeseler J, Tassaux D, Jolliet P (2006) Automatic adjustment of pressure support by

a computer-driven knowledge based system during noninvasive ventilation: a feasibility study. Intensive Care Med 33: 632–638
38. Jubran A, Van de Graaf W, Tobin M (1995) Variability of patient-ventilator interactions with pressure support ventilation in patients with chronic obstructive pulmonary disease. Am J Respir Crit Care Med 152: 129–136
39. Parthasarathy S, Jubran A, Tobin M (1998) Cycling of inspiratory and expiratory muscle groups with the ventilator in airflow limitation. Am J Respir Crit Care Med 158: 1471–1478
40. Nava S, Bruschi C, Fracchia C, Braschi A, Rubini F (1997) Patient-ventilator interaction and inspiratory effort during pressure support ventilation in patients with different pathologies. Eur Respir J 10: 177–183
41. Tassaux D, Michotte J, Gainnier M, Gratadour P, Fonseca S, Jolliet P (2004) Expiratory trigger setting in Pressure Support Ventilation: from mathematical model to bedside. Crit Care Med 32: 1844–1850
42. Tokioka H, Tanaka T, Ishizu T, et al (2001) The effect of breath termination criterion on breathing patterns and the work of breathing during pressure support ventilation. Anesth Analg 92(1):161–5
43. Tassaux D, Gainnier M, Battisti A, Jolliet P (2005) Impact of expiratory trigger setting on delayed cycling and inspiratory muscle workload. Am J Respir Crit Care Med 172: 1283–1289
44. Kwok H, McCormack J, Cece R, Houtchens J, Hill NS (2003) Controlled trial of oronasal versus nasal mask ventilation in the treatment of acute respiratory failure. Crit Care Med 31: 468–473
45. Navalesi P, Fanfulla F, Frigerio P, Gregoretti C, Nava S (2000) Physiologic evaluation of noninvasive mechanical ventilation delivered with three types of masks in patients with chronic hypercapnic respiratory failure. Crit Care Med 28: 1785–1790
46. Antonelli M, Conti G, Pelosi P, et al (2002) New treatment of acute hypoxemic respiratory failure: noninvasive pressure support ventilation delivered by helmet – a pilot controlled trial. Crit Care Med 30: 602–608
47. Antonelli M, Pennisi MA, Pelosi P, et al (2004) Noninvasive positive pressure ventilation using a helmet in patients with acute exacerbation of chronic obstructive pulmonary disease: a feasibility study. Anesthesiology 100: 16–24
48. Costa R, Navalesi P, Spinazzola G, et al (2008) Comparative evaluation of different helmets on patient-ventilator interaction during noninvasive ventilation. Intensive Care Med 34: 1102–1108
49. Brochard L (1996) Inspiratory pressure support: still a simple mode? Intensive Care Med 22: 1137–1138
50. Mancebo J (2003) Triggering and cycling off during pressure support ventilation: simplicity or sophistication? Intensive Care Med 29: 1871–1872

Variable Mechanical Ventilation: Breaking the Monotony

M. Gama de Abreu, P.M. Spieth, and P. Pelosi

Introduction

Healthy biological systems are characterized by intrinsic variability of their function even during conditions of apparent steady state, i.e., conditions that do not require major adaptation to the external environment. The most impressive example is the heart, exhibiting large variability of cardiac rhythm over short and long time scales at rest [1]. The respiratory system behaves similarly, with fluctuations of respiratory rate and/or tidal volumes observed in resting subjects [2, 3]. Such intrinsic variability, however, can be diminished or even abolished in diseased biological systems. For instance, heart rate variability may be impaired in patients with coronary heart disease even before symptoms appear [4]. A decrease of variability in respiratory rate and/or tidal volumes has been also reported in patients with chronic obstructive pulmonary disease (COPD) [5] and in those who failed to wean from mechanical ventilation [6]. In addition, the use of sedative drugs, which is commonly required during mechanical ventilation, may impair the natural variation of the respiratory pattern [7].

Differently from other organs, the variability of respiratory parameters can be easily modulated. The respiratory pattern during controlled or assisted mechanical ventilation can be fully or partially determined by the ventilator which in turn can be programmed to enhance the fluctuations of respiratory rate and/or tidal volume, mimicking spontaneous breathing variability.

In this chapter, we will give an overview of the state of the art of variable controlled and assisted mechanical ventilation, focusing on: 1) Current terms and definitions; 2) physiological rationale; 3) mechanisms of action; and 4) clinical and experimental evidence.

Patterns of Variability and their Characterization

A system is said to have variability when its output changes over time. Variability can be regular or deterministic, irregular, or a combination of the two. Deterministic variability occurs when the output changes in a predictable way, while irregular variability is when the variability follows an unpredictable pattern. Regular variability is usually seen when the pattern of output changes is not complex, as for instance in a sinus wave. Conversely, in irregular variability the pattern of change among levels is complex. For example, tidal breathing has a regular component and an irregular component that changes from cycle to cycle.

The variability is commonly expressed by the coefficient of variation, which represents the ratio of the standard deviation and the mean. However, this parameter

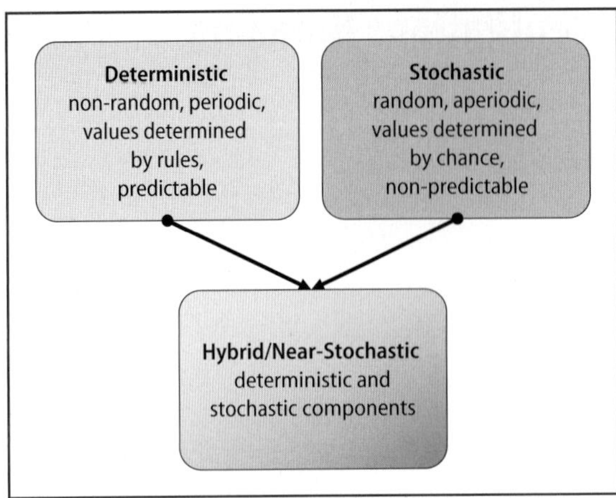

Fig. 1. Types of variable systems according to the variability of their outputs.

has some important limitations. For example, heart rate time series of healthy individuals and patients with obstructive sleep apnea can have nearly identical means and standard deviations [8]. However, the analysis of raw time series of the heart rate in both groups reveals important differences in their temporal structure. Differently from healthy subjects, diseased individuals show regular oscillations, with minor irregularities superimposed [9]. Therefore, when analyzing the patterns of variability in the output of biological systems, the use of conventional statistical measures or simple frequency domain Fourier analysis may be insufficient for classification and comparison purposes.

A system can be deterministic (i.e., non random) when it works according to predefined rules without random components and the output of the system can be predicted by these rules. Furthermore, systems can show a hybrid or near-deterministic behavior, when both deterministic and stochastic components are present (**Fig. 1**). Healthy biological systems usually underlie such simple rules. In the case of the respiratory system, this becomes evident when the variability of the time series of tidal volumes and/or respiratory frequency are carefully analyzed at different time scales. By so-doing, similar patterns can be recognized at different time scales. This phenomenon is called self-similarity or scale-invariance and is typically seen in geometric structures where small parts resemble larger parts. Such structures are called fractals. Time series can also display fractal properties: Fractal dynamics in tidal volume and/or respiratory frequency means an irregular and non-stationary behavior, where the values of the time series at a given scale correlate with the values at different scales. From a practical perspective for the respiratory system, fractal dynamics permits adaptation of the lungs to sudden and unexpected changes, making them physiologically more efficient. Complex mathematical approaches known as scale invariant analysis have been developed for the characterization of the time correlations of complex systems. For instance, the 'detrended fluctuation analysis' has been developed for quantifying the long-range correlations within a times series coming from a biological system. Also, approximate entropy analysis can measure the degree of randomness. Such tools may be useful to identify loss of complexity or irregularity in the dynamics of biological systems.

Different terms have been used to classify variable mechanical ventilation in the current literature: Biological, fractal, chaotic, naturally noisy, and noisy. While noisy ventilation is related to patterns that have been randomly generated by computers, the other terms are related to recordings of tidal volume and/or respiratory rate measured mainly in healthy animals. Thus, biological, fractal, chaotic, and naturally noisy ventilation refer to non-random, periodic patterns, whereas noisy ventilation refers to random ones.

Besides the fact that patterns from biological systems can have deterministic components, i.e., non random, the frequency distribution of many physiological variables often follows a power-law, which has a long tail compared to a Gaussian distribution. In other words, lower and higher tidal volumes are observed more frequently than would be expected in a normal distribution. In contrast, random ventilation patterns commonly, but not necessarily, follow a normal Gaussian distribution.

Irrespective of the nature of variability used in the different works, we will use the more general term 'variable mechanical ventilation' throughout this text. Also, we will differentiate between variable controlled and variable assisted mechanical ventilation, as appropriate.

Rationale for the Use of Variable Patterns in Mechanical Ventilation

There is a considerable body of evidence showing that healthy subjects have irregular respiratory patterns and that loss of irregularity accompanies lung disease and impairment of organ function [10]. However, the main question is whether external modulation of tidal volume and/or respiratory frequency during mechanical ventilation may improve respiratory function and/or contribute to the healing process. The appropriate degree of variability of respiratory pattern may improve: 1) Gas-exchange mixing; 2) recruitment and maintenance of airways patency.

The airways and the pulmonary circulation represent branching trees with typical fractal structures, where lower airway generations closely resemble higher generations and small branches of the pulmonary circulation are similar to larger ones [11, 12]. This fractal structure maximizes the area for gas exchange and supports irregular gas-mixing at lower branches [13].

One of the most common problems observed in mechanically ventilated lungs is the closure of peripheral airways during expiration [14]. Failure of reopening of those airways during inspiration may lead to atelectasis with consequent deterioration of gas exchange and respiratory mechanics. On the other hand, cyclic closing/reopening can increase the shear-stress and trigger the inflammatory response, worsening or leading to lung injury [15]. Suki et al. [16] showed that once the critical opening pressure ($P_{critical}$) of collapsed airways/alveoli has been exceeded, all subtended or daughter airways/alveoli with lower $P_{critical}$ will be opened in an 'avalanche'. Since the $P_{critical}$ values of closed airways as well as the time to achieve these values may differ across the lungs, mechanical ventilation patterns that produce different airway pressures and inspiratory times may be advantageous to maximize lung recruitment and stabilization, as compared to regular patterns.

History of Variable Mechanical Ventilation

The concept of variable mechanical ventilation was first proposed by Wolff et al. [17] in 1992. They suggested that breath-by-breath variation of inspiratory to expiratory ratios and positive end-expiratory pressure (PEEP) levels could be more effective than conventional mechanical ventilation for emptying lung regions with different expiratory time constants, and speculated that gas exchange and lung mechanics would improve. In 1996, Mutch's group introduced the first mode of controlled mechanical ventilation based on variation of respiratory rate and tidal volume that mimicked the variability of spontaneous breathing. Since the respiratory pattern was derived from healthy animals, this mode was named biological variable ventilation [18]. In an oleic acid-induced acute lung injury (ALI) model, the authors found that biological variable ventilation was superior to conventional controlled mechanical ventilation for improving arterial oxygenation and respiratory system compliance. In 1998, Suki et al. [19] offered a theoretical basis to explain why variability may be beneficial during controlled mechanical ventilation. Using a computer model of collapsed lungs with an S-shaped volume-pressure curve, they suggested that mechanical ventilation is usually performed in a range where recruitment of lung volume following a small increase in peak airway pressure is significantly higher than the loss of lung volume resulting from a comparable decrease in airway pressure. Accordingly, these authors showed that random variability, or noise, around a given mean peak airway pressure is able to recruit lungs and improve gas exchange. On the other hand, excessive variability deteriorated oxygenation in their model.

The increasing interest in permitting spontaneous breathing activity even in the early phase of ALI, added to the observation that the breathing patterns of patients under assisted mechanical ventilation has less variability than spontaneous breathing, led our group to introduce noisy pressure support ventilation (noisy PSV) in 2008 [20]. Noisy PSV represents the random variation of PSV, which provides higher variability of the respiratory pattern independently from the inspiratory effort.

Variable Controlled Mechanical Ventilation

Most experience with variable ventilation has been obtained from studies on controlled mechanical ventilation in ALI models, mainly with volume control. In **Figure 2**, we show a pattern of tidal volume variability randomly generated for variable controlled mechanical ventilation (values between 16 ml/kg and 1.6 ml/kg; mean 6 ml/kg and coefficient of variation 40 %). When the sequence is completed, it loops itself.

Since the first description of biological variable ventilation by Lefevre et al. [18], different authors have confirmed that variable controlled mechanical ventilation can improve lung mechanics and arterial oxygenation compared to monotonic, regular controlled ventilation in experimental ALI [21–29], although this claim has been challenged [30]. However, apart from the improvement in lung function, the most striking and common finding during variable controlled mechanical ventilation across different studies was the reduction of mean peak airway and mean airway pressures. Also of note is the fact that variable controlled mechanical ventilation improves lung function not only when compared to the lung protective strategies of the acute respiratory distress syndrome (ARDS) Network [23, 26], but also with the open lung approach [26, 27].

Variable controlled mechanical ventilation has also been reported to improve lung function in experimental models of asthma [31] and atelectasis [32], as well as during one-lung ventilation [33]. Unfortunately, however, to date there are only two reports on the use of variable controlled mechanical ventilation in humans. Boker et al. [34] reported improved arterial oxygenation and compliance of the respiratory system in patients ventilated with biological variable ventilation compared to con-

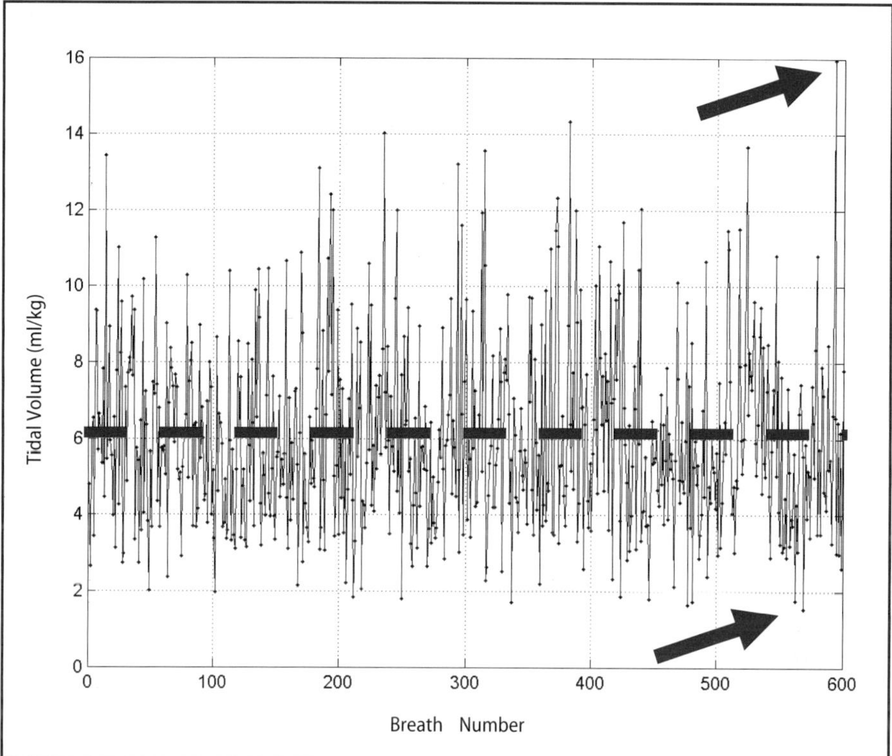

Fig. 2. Set of tidal volumes (n = 600) used by the authors in different studies with variable controlled mechanical ventilation. The dashed line represents the mean value (6 ml/kg). Arrows indicate the maximum and minimum values of the series (16 and 1.6 ml/kg, respectively). After completion of one cycle of 600 values, the system loops itself.

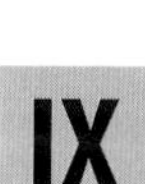

ventional mechanical ventilation during surgery for repair of abdominal aorta aneurysms. Currently, Taccone et al. [35] are conducting a prospective randomized trial of variable versus controlled mechanical ventilation in patients with ARDS. Preliminary results seem to indicate beneficial effects of variable controlled mechanical ventilation on arterial oxygenation, but it is still uncertain whether the compliance of the respiratory system also improves.

Variable Assisted Mechanical Ventilation

Due to the activity of the respiratory center, breathing patterns during assisted ventilation are considerably more irregular than during controlled mechanical ventilation. Nowadays, different modes of assisted mechanical ventilation are able to support such variability. Although during PSV each breath is supported by the same level of pressure at the airway (Paw), independently from the patient's drive, breath-by-breath differences in the inspiratory effort and inspiratory time may generate oscillations in tidal volume and/or respiratory rate. As compared to PSV, the variability of the breathing pattern may be reduced during assist pressure control ventilation, due to the fixed inspiratory time. In contrast, proportional assist ventilation (PAV) generates positive pressure throughout inspiration in proportion to the patient's generated flow and volume. In other words, PAV adapts to changes in a patient's demand of ventilation, and may result in higher variability of the respiratory pattern [36].

Recently, an innovative approach to assisted mechanical ventilation was proposed that can also increase the variability of the respiratory pattern. Neurally adjusted ventilatory assist (NAVA) uses the electrical activity of the diaphragm as indicator of the respiratory drive to guide ventilatory support. This method seems to be advantageous to improve patient-ventilator synchrony, since neural drive permits differences in the magnitude of the inspiratory effort and the beginning of relaxation of the diaphragm to be detected more rapidly than other methods. Similar to the other modes, however, the variability of the respiratory pattern during NAVA depends on the intrinsic variability of the respiratory center.

In contrast with previously described forms of assisted mechanical ventilation where every triggered breath is supported by positive pressure, biphasic intermittent positive airway pressure (BiPAP) and airway pressure release ventilation (APRV) allow non-supported spontaneous breathing at two continuous positive airway pressure (CPAP) levels, and higher variability in the respiratory pattern may result.

Clearly, in all these forms of assisted mechanical ventilation, the variability of the respiratory pattern corresponds to the intrinsic variability from the patient. Thus, lower intrinsic variability of respiratory drive, for instance due to sedation or disease [5, 7], results in a less complex respiratory pattern independent of the type of assisted mechanical ventilation. Noisy PSV is able to overcome such limitation. Following the patient's triggering, pressure support varies breath-by-breath, leading to variation in tidal volume and respiratory rate, even if the respiratory center and muscles are not able to generate enough variability. Since noisy PSV is delivered in pressure limited mode, the variability of tidal volume may depend on different factors: 1) The pattern of variability of pressure support; 2) the mechanical properties of the respiratory system, i.e., elastance, resistance and volume-pressure curve; and 3) the breath-by-breath inspiratory effort.

Preliminary results, in surfactant depleted pigs, suggest that noisy PSV is superior to conventional PSV and BIPAP/APRV combined with spontaneous breathing to improve arterial oxygenation and reduce the work of breathing [37, 38]. The pressure support was randomly varied following a normal distribution, with a coefficient of variation 30 %, which we found gave the best compromise between arterial oxygenation and elastance of the respiratory system [39]. Curiously, this is approximately the coefficient of variation reported for tidal volume in healthy, spontaneously breathing young subjects [2], and is much higher than the coefficients of variation during PSV or PAV with automatic tube compensation in patients with ALI/ARDS (7.6 % and 12.0 % mean values, respectively) [36].

Why does Respiratory Function Improve during Variable Mechanical Ventilation?

Five different mechanisms have been suggested to explain the beneficial effects of variable ventilation on respiratory function (**Table 1**).

Since higher tidal volumes are generated intermittently during variable ventilation, the $P_{critical}$ of different closed airways and alveoli is reached and deep regions of

Table 1. Putative mechanisms for improvement in lung function with variable mechanical ventilation

Putative Mechanism	Evidence/Theoretical basis
1. Lung recruitment: Airway pressure exceeds opening critical pressures across different lung regions.	Suki et al. [19], Mutch et al. [21, 32]; Bellardine et al. [28], Gama de Abreu et al. [26]
2. Jensen's inequality: The convex lower part of the pressure-volume curve favors lower mean airway pressures in the presence of variation of tidal volume.	Suki et al. [19], Brewster et al. [40]
3. Surfactant release: Alveolar type II cells are stimulated by stretching and variable stretching seems to be advantageous.	Arold et al. [42]
4. Improved ventilation-perfusion matching through:	
a) enhanced respiratory sinus arrhythmia: Possible increase in heart rate during inspiration.	a) Mutch et al. [43]
b) redistribution of pulmonary blood flow: Lower airway pressures in better ventilated zones may favor improved redistribution of blood flow.	b) Gama de Abreu et al. [37]
5. Stochastic resonance: The level of variability of the input of a system (e.g., tidal volume) can be tuned to achieve maximal amplitude of the output (e.g., oxygenation). Too low and too high variability may be deleterious.	Suki et al. [19]

the lung pop open in avalanches [16]. Thus, lung recruitment can play an important role in improving gas-exchange during variable ventilation. This hypothesis is supported not only by theoretical models [19], but also by experimental studies. Bellardine et al. [28] showed that recruitment following high tidal volumes lasts longer with variable than monotonic ventilation in excised calf lungs. In addition, Thammanomai et al. [29] showed that variable ventilation improves recruitment in both normal and injured lungs in mice. Indirect evidence for lung recruitment as a mechanism to improve respiratory function can be inferred from studies that compared variable mechanical ventilation with strategies based on lung recruitment and stabilization of the lungs. The beneficial effects of variable mechanical ventilation when used in combination with the open lung approach are less pronounced than during permissive atelectasis strategies [26].

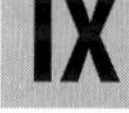

Due to the S-shaped relationship of the volume-pressure curve of the respiratory system, variable pressures applied at the convex, lower portion of the curve, result in variable tidal volumes with a different distribution. It is important to note that, for the same mean airway pressure, the mean tidal volume with variation is higher than it would be observed if less or no variation in pressure is used (Jensen's inequality) [19, 40]. In turn, variable tidal volumes applied at lower portion of the volume-pressure curve will reduce mean peak and mean airway pressures.

Variable mechanical ventilation may also enhance the release of lung surfactant. Stretch is an important trigger for release of surfactant from alveolar type II cells [41]. However, variable stretching of the alveolar epithelium has been shown to improve surfactant release and composition in rodents compared to stretching resulting from conventional mechanical ventilation [42].

Improved ventilation-perfusion matching has been also proposed to explain better respiratory function with variable mechanical ventilation by two different mechanisms: Respiratory sinus arrhythmia and redistribution of regional perfusion. In spontaneously breathing subjects, the heart frequency during inspiration is higher than during expiration, a phenomenon known as respiratory sinus arrhythmia. However, during mechanical ventilation, respiratory sinus arrhythmia may be abolished or even inverted. Assuming that heart frequency can be used as a surrogate for perfusion, in conventionally mechanically ventilated lungs blood flow is higher when the ventilation is lower and vice-versa, leading to deterioration of gas exchange. Mutch et al. [43] observed that during variable mechanical ventilation, respiratory sinus arrhythmia was enhanced compared to regular ventilation.

We demonstrated that during assisted mechanical ventilation with PSV, blood flow redistributed from dorsal to ventral lung zones in pigs with ALI lying in the supine position, compared to controlled mechanical ventilation [37]. The redistribution of pulmonary blood flow tended to be more pronounced during noisy PSV than with PSV. In ALI, the shift of pulmonary blood flow from dependent to non-dependent lung zones is mediated by the hypoxic pulmonary vasoconstriction effect [44]. Therefore, variable mechanical ventilation, by reducing the mean airway pressures in ventilated areas, may reduce the vascular impedance and, consequently, contribute to improved ventilation-perfusion matching.

Finally, the phenomenon of stochastic resonance could also explain the effects of variable mechanical ventilation. In non-linear systems, like the respiratory system, the amplitude of the output can be modulated by the noise in the input. Typical inputs are respiratory rate and tidal volumes, while outputs are mechanical properties and gas exchange. Thus, by choosing appropriate level variability (noise) in tidal volumes and/or respiratory frequency, the output can be maximized. Accordingly, too less or too much variability in the input reduces the amplitude of the output (e.g., oxygenation) [19]. Indeed, this is exactly what has been reported for both controlled and assisted noisy ventilation [24, 39]. Conceptually, the stochastic resonance behavior of the lungs does not correspond to one specific mechanism of action, but rather to a possible complex interaction among the different physiological phenomena discussed above.

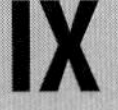

Is Variable Mechanical Ventilation Equivalent to Regular Ventilation with Intermittent Sighs?

Sigh is defined as an increase in total lung volume above average values for only a few seconds and can be observed in healthy spontaneously breathing subjects. Sighs have been used to counteract progressive lung de-recruitment during both controlled and assisted mechanical ventilation, showing moderate success for improving lung mechanics and gas exchange in ALI/ARDS [45, 46]. During variable mechanical ventilation, sigh-like tidal volumes occur at intervals. Using a porcine model of lung atelectasis, Mutch et al. [32] showed that variable controlled mechanical ventilation was superior to conventional ventilation combined with intermittent sighs to improve gas exchange and respiratory system compliance. In experimental ALI, we found that the variability of tidal volumes was higher with noisy PSV than with PSV and sighs (19.1 % vs. 7.8 %, median values). Accordingly, noisy PSV resulted in better oxygenation and reduced venous admixture than PSV and sighs [37]. Recently, Thammanomai et al. [29] showed that variable mechanical ventilation improved the inflammatory lung response of mice with ALI, as compared to regular ventilation with periodic sighs.

These data, therefore, suggest that the complex pattern of breathing during noisy ventilation cannot be considered equivalent to the use of periodic intermittent sighs.

Can Variable Mechanical Ventilation be Injurious?

Patients with ALI/ARDS who had been mechanically ventilated with tidal volumes of 12 ml/kg exhibited higher levels of inflammatory cytokines in plasma and had a higher mortality rate than those ventilated with 6 ml/kg [47]. There is also considerable experimental and clinical evidence that proportionally higher tidal volumes and inspiratory pressures may worsen lung injury [48], a phenomenon that is usually known as ventilator-associated lung injury (VALI). Some authors have even claimed that mechanical ventilation with higher tidal volumes may initiate lung injury in previously healthy lungs [49]. Thus, variable mechanical ventilation with tidal volumes exceeding 12 ml/kg could, at least theoretically, trigger or aggravate the inflammatory lung response. Nonetheless, this is not what has been observed in experimental studies on variable mechanical ventilation.

Boker et al. [23] have claimed that variable ventilation may be more protective than the ARDS Network mechanical ventilation protocol. In an oleic acid model of ALI, they found that the concentration of interleukin (IL)-8 in tracheal aspirates was lower with variable ventilation than during conventional protective mechanical ventilation, at comparable degrees of lung edema. Funk et al. [25], showed that respiratory function was better with variable ventilation compared to a lower tidal volume strategy combined to recruitment maneuvers and moderate levels of PEEP. In addition, lung histology, counts of inflammatory cells, and cytokine levels in the bronchoalveolar lavage (BAL) fluid, did not differ significantly between modes. Arold et al. [42] found that variable mechanical ventilation in normal guinea pigs, reduced IL-6 and tumor necrosis factor (TNF)-α in the BAL fluid, as compared to conventional controlled mechanical ventilation. These authors also observed that variable mechanical ventilation led to a lipid composition index similar to unventilated lungs, while conventional ventilation increased that index significantly, suggesting a potential role for variable mechanical ventilation to protect against VALI.

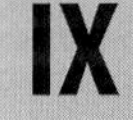

In a surfactant depletion pig model of ALI, we showed for the first time that variable mechanical ventilation combined with either the ARDS Network mechanical ventilation protocol or the open lung approach improved not only functional lung parameters, but also reduced histological damage [26]. When variable ventilation was used in combination with the ARDS Network protocol, we found a reduction in interstitial edema, hemorrhage, and epithelial destruction, mainly in dependent zones. In contrast, when variable ventilation was used in combination with the open lung approach, it resulted in reduced overdistension, mainly in non-dependent regions [26]. This finding is particularly interesting, since the potential for overdistension during the open lung approach precludes its widespread use in some centers. Therefore, variable controlled mechanical ventilation with maximum tidal volumes as high as 16 ml/kg once every 20–30 min and with a mean of 6 ml/kg seems not to trigger more inflammatory lung response than conventional protective mechanical ventilation.

Taken together, these data suggest that variable mechanical ventilation is not injurious and may even be more protective and beneficial than conventional strategies. But how can we explain this finding in light of the current evidence on mechanical stress-induced lung injury? There are different possible explanations. First, variable mechanical ventilation may lead to proportionally higher lung stretching, but as many as 50 % of tidal volumes are less than the mean target of 6 ml/kg when power-law or Gaussian distributions of the tidal volume time series are used. Further reduction of the mechanical stress caused by tidal excursions can be achieved when other distributions are used, for instance high order polynomial transformations of normal distributed values [19], based on Jensen's inequality. Second, alveolar recruitment results in more homogenous distribution of ventilation and improved mechanical properties during variable mechanical ventilation. Third, during variable ventilation mean and peak airway pressures may be decreased as a result of lower elastance of the respiratory system and peak airway pressures at comparable mean tidal volume. Fourth, it is possible that monotonic and variable lung stress and straining have different impacts on plasma membrane failure, but this issue is highly speculative.

Limitations of Variable Mechanical Ventilation

Although variable mechanical ventilation seems to be a promising ventilator strategy, several limitations must be addressed. First, most of the data come from animal studies conducted over short periods of time. Second, the different ALI models used, namely surfactant depletion and oleic acid, do not reproduce the much more complex clinical ALI/ARDS. Third, the optimal setting of variability, i.e., the distribution pattern, for large animals and humans has not been determined yet. Fourth, the mechanisms leading to the improvement in respiratory function and reduced lung damage have not been fully elucidated. Fifth, previous studies were performed with subjects in a supine position and the interactions of variable mechanical ventilation with body position are unknown. Caution must, therefore, be taken when directly extrapolating these findings to the clinical scenario.

Conclusion

Variable mechanical ventilation is technically easy to implement in most mechanical ventilators and has an attractive physiological rationale. It can be used in combination with both controlled and assisted mechanical ventilation to increase the variability of the respiratory pattern to levels comparable with those observed during spontaneous breathing in normal subjects. In ALI/ARDS, variable mechanical ventilation seems to lead to improved respiratory function, without further damaging the lungs. The reduction in airway pressures achieved during variable mechanical ventilation may even reduce VALI. Thus, variable mechanical ventilation has the potential to improve outcome, shorten the duration of mechanical ventilation, and reduce the costs involved with intensive care therapy. Further studies are warranted to define the role and potentials of variable mechanical ventilation in critically ill patients.

Acknowledgements: We are indebted to Dr. B. Suki, from the Department of Biomedical Engineering, Boston University, Boston, MA, USA, for his suggestions on the manuscript. We are also grateful to Mr. T. Handzsuj, from Dräger medical (Lübeck, Germany) for technical support with the controller for variable mechanical ventilation. We acknowledge invaluable financial support from the European Society of Anaesthesiology (ESA), Brussels, Belgium, and the German Research Council (DFG), Bonn, Germany, for some of the studies addressed herein.

References

1. Ivanov PC, Amaral LAN, Goldberger AL, et al (1999) Multifractality in human heartbeat dynamics. Nature 399: 461–465
2. Tobin MJ, Mador MJ, Guenther SM, Lodato RF, Sackner MA (1988) Variability of resting respiratory drive and timing in healthy subjects. J Appl Physiol 65: 309–317
3. Frey U, Silverman M, Barbási AL, Suki B (1998) Irregularities and power law distributions in the breathing pattern in preterm and term infants. J Appl Physiol 85: 789–797
4. Huikuri HV, Mäkikallio TH (2001) Heart rate variability in ischemic heart disease. Auton Neurosci 90: 95–101
5. Brack T, Jubran A, Tobin MJ (2002) Dyspnea and decreased variability of breathing in patients with restrictive lung disease. Am J Respir Crit Care Med 165: 1260–1264
6. Wysocki M, Diehl JL, Lefort Y, Derenne JP, Similowski T (2006) Reduced breathing variability as a predictor of unsuccessful patient separation from mechanical ventilation. Crit Care Med 34: 2078–2083
7. Galletly D, Larsen P (1999) Ventilatory frequency variability in spontaneously breathing anaesthetized subjects. Br J Anaesth 83: 552–563
8. Goldberger AL (2006) Complex systems. Proc Am Thorac Soc 3: 467–472
9. Goldberger AL, Amaral LAN, Hausdorff JM, Ivanov PC, Peng CK, Stanley HE (2002) Fractal dynamics in physiology: Alterations with disease and aging. Proc Natl Acad Sci USA 99 (Suppl 1):2466–2472
10. Goldberger AL (1996) Non-linear dynamics for clinicians: chaos theory, fractals, and complexity at the bedside. Lancet 347: 1312–1314
11. Nelson TR, West BJ, Goldberger AL (1990) The fractal lung: universal and species-related scaling patterns. Experientia 46: 251–254
12. Boxt LM, Katz J, Liebovitch LS, Jones R, Esser PD, Reid L (1994) Fractal analysis of pulmonary arteries: the fractal dimension is lower in pulmonary hypertension. J Thorac Imaging 9: 8–13
13. Tsuda A, Rogers RA, Hydon PE, Butler JP (2008) Chaotic mixing deep in the lung. Proc Natl Acad Sci USA 99: 10173–10178
14. Hughes JM, Rosenzweig DY, Kivitz PB (1970) Site of airway closure in excised dog lungs: histologic demonstration. J Appl Physiol 29: 340–344
15. dos Santos CC, Slutsky AS (2000) Invited review: mechanisms of ventilator-induced lung injury: a perspective. J Appl Physiol 89: 1645–1655
16. Suki B, Barabási AL, Hantos Z, Peták F, Stanley HE (1994) Avalanches and power-law behavior in lung inflation. Nature 368: 615–618
17. Wolff G, Eberhard L, Guttmann J, Bertschmann W, Zeravik J, Adolph M (1992) Polymorphous ventilation: A new ventilation concept for distributed time constants. In: Rügheimer E, Mang H, Tchaikowsky K (eds) New aspects on respiratory failure, Springer-Verlag, Berlin, pp 235–252
18. Lefevre GR, Kowalski SE, Girling LG, Thiessen DB, Mutch WA (1996) Improved arterial oxygenation after oleic acid lung injury in the pig using a computer-controlled mechanical ventilator. Am J Respir Crit Care Med 154: 1567–1572
19. Suki B, Alencar AM, Sujeer MK, et al (1998) Life-support system benefits from noise. Nature 393: 127–128
20. Gama de Abreu M, Spieth P, Pelosi P, et al (2008) Noisy pressure support ventilation: a pilot study on a new assisted ventilation mode in experimental lung injury. Crit Care Med 36: 818–827
21. Mutch WAC, Harms S, Lefevre GR, Graham MR, Girling LG, Kowalski SE (2000) Biologically variable ventilation increases arterial oxygenation over that seen with positive end-expiratory pressure alone in a porcine model of acute respiratory distress syndrome. Crit Care Med 28: 2457–2464
22. Mutch WAC, Lefevre GR, Cheang MS (2001) Biologic variability in mechanical ventilation in a canine oleic acid lung injury model. Am J Respir Crit Care Med 163: 1756–1757
23. Boker A, Graham MR, Walley KR, et al (2002) Improved arterial oxygenation with biologically variable or fractal ventilation using low tidal volumes in a porcine model of acute respiratory distress syndrome. Am J Respir Crit Care Med 165: 456–462

24. Arold SP, Mora R, Lutchen KR, Ingenito EP, Suki B (2002) Variable tidal volume ventilation improves lung mechanics and gas exchange in a rodent model of acute lung injury. Am J Respir Crit Care Med 165: 366–371
25. Funk DJ, Graham MR, Girling LG, et al (2004) A comparison of biologically variable ventilation to recruitment manoeuvres in a porcine model of acute lung injury. Respir Res 5: 22
26. Gama de Abreu M, Spieth P, Hoehn C, et al (2007) Chaotic variation of tidal volume improves different protective mechanical ventilation strategies. Am J Respir Crit Care Med 175: A788 (abst)
27. Spieth P, Meissner C, Kasper M, Koch T, Gama de Abreu M (2007) Chaotic variation of tidal volumes adds further benefit to the open lung approach in experimental lung injury. Eur J Anaesthesiol 24 (Suppl):146 (abst)
28. Bellardine CL, Hoffman AM, Tsai L, et al (2006) Comparison of variable and conventional ventilation in a sheep saline lavage lung injury model. Crit Care Med 34: 439–445
29. Thammanomai A, Hueser E, Majumdar A, Bartolák-Suki E, Suki, B (2008) Design of a new variable-ventilation method optimized for lung recruitment in mice. J Appl Physiol 104: 1329–1340
30. Nam AJ, Brower RG, Fessler HE, Simon BA (2000) Biologic variability in mechanical ventilation rate and tidal volume does not improve oxygenation or lung mechanics in canine oleic acid lung injury. Am J Respir Crit Care Med 161: 1797–1804
31. Mutch WAC, Buchman TG, Girling L, Walker E, McManus BM, Graham MR (2007) Biologically variable ventilation improves gas exchange and respiratory mechanics in a model of severe bronchospasm. Crit Care Med 35: 1749–1755
32. Mutch WAC, Harms S, Graham MR, Kowalski SE, Girling LG, Lefevre GR (2000) Biologically variable or naturally noisy mechanical ventilation recruits atelectatic lung. Am J Respir Crit Care Med 162: 319–323
33. McMullen MC, Girling LG, Graham MR, Mutch WAC (2006) Biologically variable ventilation improves oxygenation and respiratory mechanics during one-lung ventilation. Anesthesiology 105: 91–97
34. Boker A, Haberman CJ, Girling L, et al (2004) Variable ventilation improves perioperative lung function in patients undergoing abdominal aortic aneurysmectomy. Anesthesiology 100: 608–616
35. Taccone P, Polli F, Chiumello D, Vespro V, Gattinoni L (2008) Effects of variable ventilation during lung protective mechanical ventilation strategy in ALI/ARDS patients. Am J Respir Crit Care Med 177: A765 (abst)
36. Varelmann D, Wrigge H, Zinserling J, Muders T, Hering R, Putensen C (2005) Proportional assist versus pressure support ventilation in patients with acute respiratory failure: cardiorespiratory responses to artificially increased ventilatory demand. Crit Care Med 33: 1968–1975
37. Gama de Abreu M, Spieth P, Pelosi P, et al (2008) Noisy pressure support ventilation: A pilot study on a new assisted ventilation mode in experimental lung injury. Crit Care Med 36: 818–827
38. Gama de Abreu M, Spieth PM, Carvalho AR, Pelosi P, Koch T (2008) Pressure support ventilation is superior to pressure controlled ventilation in experimental lung injury and can be further improved by noise. Am J Respir Crit Care Med 177: A385 (abst)
39. Spieth PM, Carvalho AR, Güldner A, et al (2009) Effects of different levels of pressure support variability in experimental lung injury. Anesthesiology (in press)
40. Brewster JF, Graham MR, Mutch WAC (2005) Convexity, Jensen's inequality and benefits of noisy mechanical ventilation. J R Soc Interface 2: 393–396
41. Wirtz HR, Dobbs LG (1990) Calcium mobilization and exocytosis after one mechanical stretch of lung epithelial cells. Science 30: 1266–1269
42. Arold SP, Suki B, Alencar AM, Lutchen KR, Ingenito EP (2003) Variable ventilation induces endogenous surfactant release in normal guinea pigs. Am J Physiol – Lung Cell Mol Physiol 285: L370-L375
43. Mutch WAC, Graham MR, Girling LG, Brewster JF (2005) Fractal ventilation enhances respiratory sinus arrhythmia. Respir Res 6: 41
44. Brimioulle S, Julien V, Gust R, Kozlowski JK, Naeije R, Schuster DP (2002) Importance of hypoxic vasoconstriction in maintaining oxygenation during acute lung injury. Crit Care Med 30: 874–880

45. Pelosi P, Bottino N, Chiumello D, et al (2003) Sigh in supine and prone position during acute respiratory distress syndrome. Am J Respir Crit Care Med 167: 521–527
46. Patroniti N, Foti G, Cortinovis B, et al (2002) Sigh improves gas exchange and lung volume in patients with acute respiratory distress syndrome undergoing pressure support ventilation. Anesthesiology 96: 788–794
47. The Acute Respiratory Distress Syndrome Network (2000) Ventilation with lower tidal volumes as compared with traditional tidal volumes for acute lung injury and the acute respiratory distress syndrome. N Engl J Med 342: 1301–1308
48. Oeckler RA, Hubmayr RD (2007) Ventilator-associated lung injury: a search for better therapeutic targets. Eur Respir J 30: 1216–1226
49. Dreyfuss D, Saumon G (1998) Ventilator-induced lung injury. Am J Respir Crit Care Med 157: 294–323

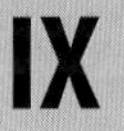

Life-threatening Asthma: Focus on Lung Protection

H. Quiroz Martínez and N.D. Ferguson

Introduction

Acute asthma exacerbation is a common medical emergency; approximately 10 % of asthma related hospital admissions will require intensive care and, despite aggressive medical therapy, 4 % will develop life-threatening asthma requiring endotracheal intubation and mechanical ventilation for persistent respiratory failure. Not surprisingly, patients with life-threatening asthma have high morbidity and mortality. In this chapter, we will review the pathophysiology of dynamic hyperinflation and respiratory failure in asthma, and armed with this knowledge we describe how to provide lung protective mechanical ventilation while delivering adequate oxygenation and maximizing medical therapy. We will also comment on the different rescue therapies available for patients with refractory respiratory failure who fail mechanical ventilation.

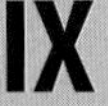

Epidemiology

Asthma is the most common chronic lung disease worldwide, and its prevalence has been increasing over the past decades. Four to five percent of patients with asthma are considered to have severe asthma. An acute exacerbation of asthma is a common medical emergency, and about 20–30 % of asthmatics presenting to the emergency department (ED) will require hospitalization. Of these, approximately 10 % of asthmatics admitted to the hospital will require intensive care and 4 % will warrant endotracheal intubation and mechanical ventilation [1]. These interventions can be life saving but they are associated with significant morbidity and mortality [2, 3]. The complications found in the group of patients who require intensive care unit (ICU) admission include: Hypotension, pneumothorax, pneumomediastinum, atelectasis, nosocomial infections, arrhythmias, sepsis, gastrointestinal bleeding, and anoxic brain injury.

Worldwide, the reported mortality rate from an exacerbation of asthma that requires intubation varies widely, from 1.50 to 86.92 deaths per million population, with a weighted average of 22.0 deaths per million population. Krishnan et al. reported an overall in-hospital mortality rate for all asthmatics admitted of 0.5 % in the United States [1]. Historical cohorts and case series published since 1990 have reported mortality rates of 2.7 % of all asthmatics admitted to ICU and 6.9–26.7 % for patients requiring intubation and mechanical ventilation [1, 4, 5]. The mortality rates in children and adults have remained fairly constant since 1996, after several decades of steady rise. The economic impact of asthma is difficult to measure, nevertheless the hospital costs for a patient admitted to the ICU range from 34 to 55 thousand US dollars [1].

Definitions

An acute asthma exacerbation is defined by the presence of one or more of the following features: Accessory muscle activity, paradoxical pulse exceeding 25 mmHg, heart rate > 100 beats/min, respiratory rate > than 25–30 beats/min, limited ability to speak, peak expiratory flow rate (PEF) or forced expiratory volume in 1 second (FEV_1) < 50 % of predicted, and an arterial oxygen saturation 90–92 % [6]. Most patients will improve with intensive inhaled bronchodilators and systemic corticosteroids. Life-threatening asthma is defined as an acute asthma exacerbation that progresses to respiratory failure despite aggressive medical therapy and requires life-sustaining therapies to get through the acute attack. Mechanical ventilation is reserved for this group of patients. The decision to intubate is often delayed and is used mostly as a last resort when all conventional medical treatments have failed. Although life saving, mechanical ventilation and its associated interventions can also cause significant morbidity and increase the risk of death.

Risk Factors

The identified risk factors associated with life-threatening asthma and death from asthma can be divided into major and minor risk factors. The major risk factors include:

1. Recent history of poorly controlled asthma manifested by the need of more than two beta-agonist metered does inhaler (MDI) canisters per month, systemic corticosteroid dependency, non-compliance with therapy, inconsistent medical follow-up, delayed medical care, denial of or failure to perceive the severity of illness [7, 8].
2. Prior history of near fatal asthma exacerbation characterized by previous ICU admissions with or without endotracheal intubation and mechanical ventilation, previous episodes of rapidly progressing respiratory distress or sudden respiratory deterioration, decreased level of consciousness or seizures during the exacerbation [9–11].

The minor risk factors include:

3. Food-induced asthma exacerbations, exercise, respiratory viruses, aspirin sensitivity, aeroallergens, cigarette smoking, inhaled or smoked drug abuse, long duration of asthma, older age, depression (or other psychiatric disorder) and poor socioeconomic conditions [11–14].

Pathophysiology of the Acute Asthma Attack

Two subtypes of life-threatening asthma have been described in the literature, according to onset, progression, pathophysiology, and response to therapy (**Table 1**) [15, 16]. However, while the presenting history and time to resolution may be different, once in the throes of an exacerbation the signs and symptoms are indistinguishable and the therapeutic approach is similar for both subtypes.

Table 1. Life-threatening asthma subtypes

	Slow Onset	Rapid Onset
Frequency	80–85 %	< 20 %
Triggers	Respiratory tract infection	Allergen exposure Fume or irritant inhalation Exercise or emotional stress Aspirin and NSAIDs
Symptoms	Symptoms for more than 12 hours and sometimes for one to three weeks	2–6 hour of onset of symptoms
Pathology	Eosinophilic inflammation Airway obstruction due to edema and impacted secretions (mucus and desquamated epithelial cells)	No eosinophils or mucus plugs Neutrophil-predominant Airway obstruction is due to smooth muscle spasm
Recovery	Slow	Rapid

NSAID: non-steroidal anti-inflammatory drugs

Airflow limitation due to airway narrowing is the key abnormality behind an acute asthma exacerbation. The reduction in airway caliber is due in part to bronchial hyper-responsiveness, but the most important reasons are airway edema and increased mucus production related to airway inflammation. The inflammation results from an immune reaction triggered by respiratory viruses, allergens, or inhaled irritants. Recent studies have shown that this phenomenon is not homogeneous throughout the lungs, so there are some lung areas with patent airways and near normal ventilation, while others are underventilated with severe obstruction.

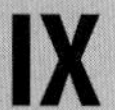

During an acute asthma exacerbation, inspiration is not initially affected but lung emptying is impaired; expiration becomes an active process, thus increasing the work of breathing. If the airflow obstruction is severe enough, the expiration is interrupted by the next inspiratory effort before the end-expiratory lung volume has reached a static equilibrium or functional residual capacity (FRC). There are three factors involved in the development of air trapping or hyperinflation: Tidal volume, expiratory flow limitation, and expiratory resistance [17, 18]. In asthma, expiratory resistance results from airway narrowing due to dynamic collapse secondary to increased intrathoracic pressure during expiration, bronchospasm, inflammation, or remodeling and expiratory glottic constriction [19]. The expiratory flow limitation becomes critical due to low pulmonary elastic recoil and high outward recoil of the chest wall generated by the persistent activation of the inspiratory muscles [20]. In addition, the mechanical load to the inspiratory respiratory muscles progressively increases as the end–expiratory volume increases because of shift along the volume-pressure relationship and a subsequent decrease in compliance. As the resistive and elastic work of breathing rises, the inspiratory muscles must generate more force to offset the rise in the end-expiratory pressure.

When the next inspiration begins before a return to FRC and inspired gas volume (and therefore pressure) remains in the chest, this phenomenon is known as auto-positive end-expiratory pressure (PEEP) (**Fig. 1**) [21]. As previously mentioned, this process may be extremely heterogeneous. The asthmatic lung behaves as a small functional lung overdistended by large tidal volume with contiguous hypoventilated areas due to significant hyperinflation and alveolar collapse (**Fig. 2**) [22]. The cyclic

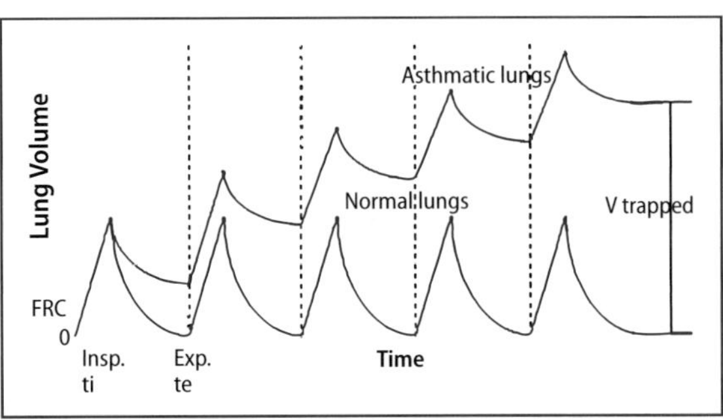

Fig. 1. In patients with severe airway obstruction during an acute asthma attack there is a dynamic hyperinflation of the lungs characterized by an increase in the end-expiratory lung volume due to severe expiratory flow limitation. FRC: Functional residual capacity; Vtrapped: volume trapped above FRC. From [36] with permission

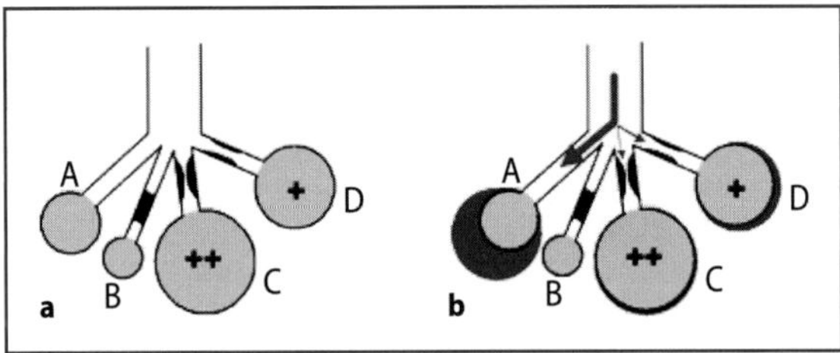

Fig. 2. a Effect of varying amounts of airway obstruction on end-expiratory alveolar volumes and pressures; **b** Expected distribution of the tidal volume during positive-pressure mechanical ventilation in the context of inhomogeneous obstruction.

overdistention of 'normally ventilated areas' will cause further increase in dead space due to compression of alveolar capillaries and increase the risk of barotrauma in those areas. As the lung volume increases, the intrathoracic pressure rises, increasing pulmonary vascular resistance and decreasing venous return, which in turn results in a lower cardiac output and hypotension [23].

Therapeutic Approach

Patients with severe asthma exacerbation (peak expiratory flow rate [PEFR] < 50 % predicted or personal best) who show a poor response to initial therapy (e.g., less than 10 % increase in PEFR) or whose condition deteriorates during therapy should be admitted to an ICU. Admission is also warranted for respiratory arrest, altered mental status, myocardial injury, and when there is need for frequent nebulizer treatments.

Pharmacological Therapy

Pharmacological therapy in the patient with life-threatening asthma is a continuation of the emergency department regimen which includes inhaled bronchodilators, systemic corticosteroids, and magnesium sulfate. The use of high dose albuterol (salbutamol) and ipratropium bromide in extremely ill patients on first presentation or not responding to albuterol alone within 30 minutes is recommended. During mechanical ventilation, bronchodilators should be delivered preferentially with a pressurized MDI (pMDI) and a spacer. High dose corticosteroids should be administered intravenously early in the course of the attack because there is a significant delay in the onset of action (> 6 hours). The routine use of magnesium sulfate is not justified but it appears safe, is inexpensive, and may be beneficial in severe exacerbations. Indepth discussion about the pharmacological approach to acute severe asthma is out of the scope of this chapter. Please refer to the following comprehensive reviews [24, 25] for further reading.

Non-Invasive Ventilation

Martin et al. in 1982 showed that continuous positive airway pressure (CPAP) decreased the work of breathing without causing further hyperinflation in 8 patients with induced bronchospasm [26]. In 1993, Shivaram and colleagues published the cardiopulmonary responses to CPAP in 21 patients with acute asthma. These authors showed that CPAP reduced respiratory rate and dyspnea with no untoward effects on gas exchange, expiratory airflow, or hemodynamics [27].

Evidence from one retrospective study and two small randomized controlled trials supports the use of non-invasive ventilation (NIV) in patients with acute severe asthma. Face-mask NIV improves alveolar ventilation and gas exchange, alleviates respiratory distress, prevents exhaustion, and can reduce the need for intubation. Concurrently it improves hemodynamics without increasing the risk of barotrauma or complications associated with delayed intubation [28, 29]. Finally, in selected patients, NIV can shorten the attack, improve lung function, and prevent hospitalization [30]. A systematic review concluded that current evidence supports the use of NIV in acute asthma exacerbation but it is not strong enough to recommend its use and further studies are required to determine the role of NIV in these patients [31].

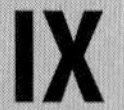

We suggest that in centers with good NIV experience, patients with acute severe asthma with mild to moderate respiratory distress who have an increased work of breathing despite the initial medical therapy, and are not in imminent cardiorespiratory collapse could be managed in a closely monitored setting with NIV. The ventilator of choice should be able to provide leak compensation and some degree of respiratory monitoring (e.g., NIV mode on a critical care ventilator or a portable non-invasive ventilator, such as the bi-level positive airway pressure [BiPAP] Vision ventilatory support system). The inspiratory pressure should be limited to 20 cmH_2O and titrated to patient comfort. PEEP should be adjusted to facilitate triggering and the inspired fraction of oxygen (FiO_2) titrated to achieve an oxygen saturation (SO_2) $\geq$ 90 %. A respiratory therapist, nurse or physician (familiar with NIV) should be at the bedside to reassure and monitor the patient and adjust the ventilator (**Table 2**).

Table 2. Benefits and limitations of non-invasive ventilation in asthma

Benefits	Limitations
Decreases airflow obstruction	Requires patient cooperation
Reduces trans-diaphragmatic pressure	May impair ability to clear secretions and deliver medications
Re-expands atelectasis	Does not provide definitive control of the airway
Improves comfort and provides assistance with work of breathing	May cause gastric distention and increase the risk of aspiration
	May increase the sense of air hunger
	Patients may feel claustrophobic

Intubation

The absolute indications for intubation are coma and respiratory arrest. Relative indications for intubating the trachea of the acute asthmatic include worsening pulmonary function and increased work of breathing leading to exhaustion and ventilatory failure despite aggressive treatment, and altered mental status. Rapid sequence intubation is usually the method of choice, although some advocate for an awake intubation. Manipulation of the airway can increase airway responsiveness and, thus, aggravate the airflow obstruction. Because intubation of a patient with status asthmaticus has several serious potential consequences, it should be performed by the most experienced intubator available. The crucial objective is to prevent any further increase in lung hyperinflation during and just after the intubation. Approximately 25 to 35 % of patients develop postintubation hypotension, which is due to loss of vascular tone related to the induction drugs, relative hypovolemia, dynamic hyperinflation, or tension pneumothorax. Pulseless electrical activity associated with intermittent positive pressure ventilation in patients with asthma has been described. Hypovolemia and sedatives can potentiate the effects of dynamic hyperventilation [32, 33]. The patient should be adequately fluid resuscitated prior to the intubation to minimize the risk of postintubation hypotension.

Mechanical Ventilation

Fortunately, less than 1 % of asthmatics require intubation and mechanical ventilation. These interventions are associated with hypotension, barotrauma, infection, and myopathy, especially when prolonged administration of both muscle relaxants and systemic corticosteroids is required. Evidence from cohort studies and case series support the use of invasive ventilation, despite a high level of morbidity related to the intervention, based on the assumption that without this intervention further fatalities would ensue. Adverse effects reported in one retrospective study of 88 episodes of mechanical ventilation were hypotension (20 %), barotrauma (14–27 %), and arrhythmias (10 %). Animal studies suggest that controlled hypercapnia is safe. Cohort studies and one case series found fewer deaths and complications with controlled hypoventilation using smaller tidal volumes with lower airway pressures compared with ventilation in which carbon dioxide levels were normalized [34, 35].

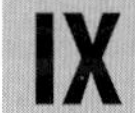

The initial goals of mechanical ventilation in life-threatening asthma are to correct the hypoxia with higher FiO_2 without attempting to restore normal alveolar ventilation (**Table 3**). It is also crucial to maximize secretion clearance and bronchodilator administration during mechanical ventilation. Correction of hypercapnia is obtained later when bronchial obstruction is relieved, a better ventilation-perfusion distribution is re-established and the risks of barotrauma and cardiocirculatory failure appear to be significantly decreased [34]. These are the basic concepts of a lung protective ventilation strategy in an asthmatic. The goals of such a strategy are to reduce the work of breathing, provide adequate oxygenation and sufficient ventilation, minimize the lung damage induced by hyperinflation and positive pressure ventilation, and avoid complications associated with intubation and mechanical ventilation. Tolerating high levels of PCO_2 (or low blood pH) from deliberate hypoventilation to mitigate the damage induced by high positive pressure mechanical ventilation is known as permissive hypercapnia or controlled hypoventilation [34, 36]. The most important objectives are to prevent further hyperinflation, allow lung defla-

Table 3. Initial ventilator settings

Low respiratory rate (8–16 breaths/min)
Small tidal volume 6–8 ml/kg of predicted body weight
Plateau pressure < 30 cmH_2O
High peak inspiratory flow (70–100 l/min)
Prolonged expiratory time (inspiratory:expiratory ratio 1:3–1:4)
Positive-end expiratory pressure (PEEP) to compensate for intrinsic PEEP (PEEPi) if patient is breathing spontaneously (80 % of auto-PEEP) Zero end-expiratory pressure (ZEEP) if patient is sedated, paralyzed and on controlled mechanical ventilation to maximize exhalation
FiO_2 to achieve $SO_2 \geq 88$ %

tion, and limit alveolar pressures to prevent barotrauma and circulatory collapse from decreased venous return [37]. Severe acute hypercapnia can lead to severe acidemia with neurologic dysfunction and death so it should be avoided if possible in patients with intracranial disease, particularly recent anoxic brain injury following cardiorespiratory arrest. It has been shown that $PaCO_2$ up to 90 mmHg and/or a pH ≥ 7.2 are generally well tolerated and without any long term sequelae, when adequate oxygenation is achieved, and indeed more extreme values than these are frequently experienced. Frequently, patients with acute respiratory failure due to severe airway obstruction refractory to medical management may need deep sedation with or without neuromuscular paralysis in order to achieve the goals of a lung protective ventilation strategy.

There is no particular benefit related to the mode of mechanical ventilation used in life-threatening asthma as long as a lung protective ventilation strategy is used. After intubation the FiO_2 should be titrated to achieve at least 88 % blood SO_2 and the respiratory rate on the ventilator should be set to 8–16 breaths per minute with a tidal volume 6–8 ml/kg of predicted body weight, avoiding plateau pressures (Pplat) higher than 35 cmH_2O. High peak inspiratory flow (and a short inspiratory time) should be used to maximize the expiratory time. It has been shown that there is no additional benefit in reducing hyperinflation by prolonging the expiratory time beyond 4 seconds [37]. The use of PEEP in patients with asthma is controversial and setting it can be challenging. In patients sedated and paralyzed on a controlled mode of ventilation, zero end-expiratory pressure (ZEEP) should be used to maximize exhalation and minimize regional overdistention. If the patient is breathing spontaneously, PEEP should be set to compensate for intrinsic PEEP (PEEPi) and allow adequate triggering of the ventilator (~80 % of auto-PEEP) [38, 39]. A recent study has shown three different responses to the application of external-PEEP in patients with acute airway obstruction during controlled mechanical ventilation. The application of external PEEP was shown to relieve hyperinflation in some patients, but these patients were only recognizable in retrospect – baseline information was not useful to distinguish them from the rest of the patients. The authors suggest that an empirical PEEP trial investigating Pplat response to identify who would benefit from external-PEEP may a reasonable strategy with minimal side effects [40].

Assessing Lung Inflation

Hyperinflation can be assessed in the paralyzed patient by measuring the volume at end-inspiration (V_{EI}), which is determined by collecting expired gas from total lung capacity to FRC during 40 to 60 seconds of apnea. A V_{EI} greater than 20 ml/kg has been correlated with barotrauma [41]. Similarly, Pplat and auto-PEEP can only be reliably measured when the patient is not breathing spontaneously (**Fig. 3**). Pplat is a surrogate of the end-inspiratory lung volume, which correlates with the risk of barotrauma. Auto-PEEP is a surrogate of the end-expiratory lung volume (hyperinflation) that correlates with the degree of airway obstruction and hemodynamic effects. Ideally, we would like to see Pplat kept below 30 cmH_2O and auto-PEEP below 5 cmH_2O; however, this is frequently not possible. In addition, in patients with high Pplat and low measured auto-PEEP, the presence of occult auto-PEEP should be suspected because measured auto-PEEP may not reflect the alveolar pressure behind areas of completely obstructed airway [42].

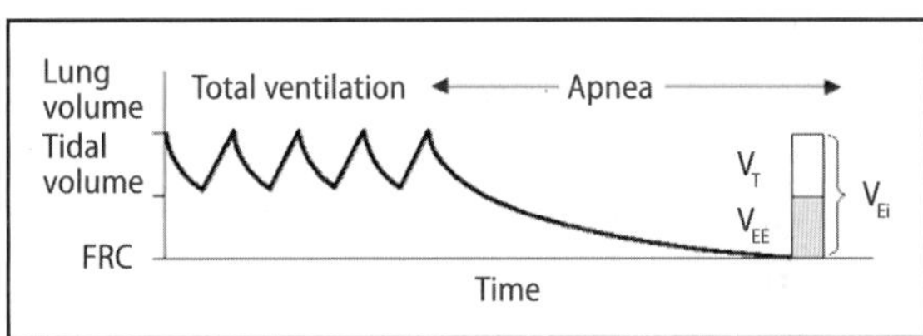

Fig. 3. Hyperinflation can be assessed in the paralyzed patient by measuring the volume at end-inspiration (V_{EI}). V_{EI} is determined by collecting expired gas from total lung capacity to functional residual capacity (FRC) during 40 to 60 seconds of apnea. V_{EI} = end-expiratory lung volume (V_{EE}) + tidal volume (V_T)

IX

Analgesia, Sedation, Paralysis, and Inhaled Anesthetics

Opiates, and particularly fentanyl, are the drugs of choice to suppress the respiratory drive. Morphine can cause hypotension and may worsen bronchoconstriction due to histamine release. Propofol is a potent hypnotic with rapid onset of action and short half-life, that suppresses the respiratory drive and has potent bronchodilator properties; however, it has the inconvenient side-effect of causing hypotension, which may at times be profound. Its use is recommended for short-term intubations. Benzodiazepines (i.e., midazolam and lorazepam) are widely used for sedation during mechanical ventilation in the ICU with minimal adverse effects but are usually not enough to suppress the respiratory drive and they have no identified bronchodilator effect. Ketamine is an intravenous anesthetic with sedative, analgesic, and bronchodilating properties. It indirectly stimulates catecholamine release and, in a dose of up to 2 mg/kg, will produce bronchodilation in the critically ill asthmatic [43]. It is suitable as an induction agent and for intubated patients with severe bronchospasm refractory to aggressive conventional therapies. It is contraindicated in ischemic heart disease, severe hypertension, pre-eclampsia, and increased intracranial pressure. Side effects include hallucinations, increased secretions, and, on rare occasions, laryngospasm. Short-term neuromuscular paralysis after intubation is warranted when safe and effective mechanical ventilation cannot be achieved with sedation alone.

The use of inhalational anesthetics (halothane, isoflurane and enflurane) in patients with status asthmaticus requiring mechanical ventilation refractory to intensive conventional bronchodilator therapy has been repeatedly reported in the literature. These agents produce a dramatic reduction in bronchospasm, dynamic hyperinflation, and the associated the risk of barotrauma. There is a concurrent improvement in arterial blood gases with minimal hemodynamic adverse effects. The bronchodilator effect of inhalational anesthetics is short lived and interruption is associated with rebound bronchospasm. Medical therapy should be maximized before discontinuing the administration of the gas. Inhalation anesthesia may be useful in the treatment of refractory cases of asthma but should be used carefully because it may be hazardous owing to poor flow capabilities of most anesthesia ventilators [44–46].

Heliox

Helium is a low-density inert gas that lowers airway resistance and decreases respiratory work. Heliox, an 80:20 mixture of helium and oxygen, can be considered in patients with respiratory acidosis who fail conventional therapy. A systematic review of the pediatric and adult literature showed that heliox is safe and well tolerated but no significant differences were demonstrated between heliox or oxygen/air group. The authors concluded that there are not enough data to make a strong recommendation but the existing evidence does not provide support for the administration of helium-oxygen mixtures to patients with moderate-to-severe acute asthma [47].

Rescue Therapies

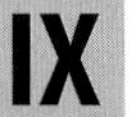

There are a few case reports where extracorporeal life support has been used successfully in patients with persistent respiratory failure due to refractory life threatening asthma. Perfusionist-driven veno-venous and veno-arterial extracorporeal membrane oxygenation (ECMO) and pumpless Novalung have been reported [48–50]. Novalung is an extra-corporeal lung assist device with a low resistance and high efficiency gas exchange membrane that can be used pumpless reliant on arteriovenous shunt and a sweep flow of oxygen to ensure diffusion of oxygen and carbon dioxide. Patients with acute severe asthma often will have sufficient cardiac output and blood pressure to maintain an arteriovenous shunt across the membrane. Extracorporeal life support should be considered as a rescue therapy for patients with intractable respiratory failure secondary to refractory bronchospasm, who have failed all usual interventions, or patients who develop cardiorespiratory arrest and controlled hypoventilation is not recommended due to anoxic brain injury. Large bore arterial and venous cannulation is required and systemic anticoagulation is warranted during the use of extracorporeal life support.

Conclusion

Life-threatening asthma is the most severe presentation of an acute asthma exacerbation. Early identification and a full understanding of the mechanisms of airway obstruction and the resultant hyperinflation are crucial to provide a comprehensive therapeutic approach. A lung protective mechanical ventilation strategy will not relieve the underlying airway obstruction but it will provide adequate oxygenation and prevent further complications and perhaps death. A few rescue therapies can be considered in patients who have failed to respond to aggressive medical therapy and have persistent respiratory failure despite mechanical ventilation.

References

1. Krishnan V, Diette GB, Rand CS, et al (2006) Mortality in patients hospitalized for asthma exacerbations in the United States. Am J Respir Crit Care Med 174: 633–638
2. Anzueto A, Frutos-Vivar F, Esteban A, et al (2004) Incidence, risk factors and outcome of barotrauma in mechanically ventilated patients. Intensive Care Med 30: 612–619
3. Mansel JK, Stogner SW, Petrini MF, Norman JR (1990) Mechanical ventilation in patients with acute severe asthma. Am J Med 89: 42–48
4. Gupta D, Keogh B, Chung KF, et al (2004) Characteristics and outcome for admissions to adult, general critical care units with acute severe asthma: a secondary analysis of the ICNARC Case Mix Programme Database. Crit Care 8: R112–121
5. McFadden ER Jr (2003) Acute severe asthma. Am J Respir Crit Care Med 168: 740–759
6. National Asthma Education and Prevention Program (2007) Expert Panel Report 3 (EPR-3): Guidelines for the Diagnosis and Management of Asthma-Summary Report 2007. J Allergy Clin Immunol 120: S94–138
7. McFadden ER Jr, Warren EL (1997) Observations on asthma mortality. Ann Intern Med 127: 142–147
8. Eisner MD, Lieu TA, Chi F, et al (2001) Beta agonists, inhaled steroids, and the risk of intensive care unit admission for asthma. Eur Respir J 17: 233–240
9. Turner MO, Noertjojo K, Vedal S, Bai T, Crump S, Fitzgerald JM (1998) Risk factors for near-fatal asthma. A case-control study in hospitalized patients with asthma. Am J Respir Crit Care Med 157: 1804–1809
10. Dhuper S, Maggiore D, Chung V, Shim C (2003) Profile of near-fatal asthma in an inner-city hospital. Chest 124: 1880–1884
11. Marquette CH, Saulnier F, Leroy O, et al (1992) Long-term prognosis of near-fatal asthma. A 6-year follow-up study of 145 asthmatic patients who underwent mechanical ventilation for a near-fatal attack of asthma. Am Rev Respir Dis 146: 76–81
12. Becker JM, Rogers J, Rossini G, Mirchandani H, D'Alonzo GE Jr (2004) Asthma deaths during sports: report of a 7-year experience. J Allergy Clin Immunol 113: 264–267
13. Levine M, Iliescu ME, Margellos-Anast H, Estarziau M, Ansell DA (2005) The effects of cocaine and heroin use on intubation rates and hospital utilization in patients with acute asthma exacerbations. Chest 128: 1951–1957
14. Tan WC, Xiang X, Qiu D, Ng TP, Lam SF, Hegele RG (2003) Epidemiology of respiratory viruses in patients hospitalized with near-fatal asthma, acute exacerbations of asthma, or chronic obstructive pulmonary disease. Am J Med 115: 272–277
15. de Magalhaes Simoes S, dos Santos MA, da Silva Oliveira M, et al (2005) Inflammatory cell mapping of the respiratory tract in fatal asthma. Clin Exp Allergy 35: 602–611
16. James AL, Elliot JG, Abramson MJ, Walters EH (2005) Time to death, airway wall inflammation and remodelling in fatal asthma. Eur Respir J 26: 429–434
17. McCarthy DS, Sigurdson M (1980) Lung elastic recoil and reduced airflow in clinically stable asthma. Thorax 35: 298–302
18. Cormier Y, Lecours R, Legris C (1990) Mechanisms of hyperinflation in asthma. Eur Respir J 3: 619–624
19. Collett PW, Brancatisano T, Engel LA (1983) Changes in the glottic aperture during bronchial asthma. Am Rev Respir Dis 128: 719–723
20. Peress L, Sybrecht G, Macklem PT (1976) The mechanism of increase in total lung capacity during acute asthma. Am J Med 61: 165–169
21. Pepe PE, Marini JJ (1982) Occult positive end-expiratory pressure in mechanically ventilated patients with airflow obstruction: the auto-PEEP effect. Am Rev Respir Dis 126: 166–170
22. Harris RS, Winkler T, Tgavalekos N, et al (2006) Regional pulmonary perfusion, inflation, and ventilation defects in bronchoconstricted patients with asthma. Am J Respir Crit Care Med 174: 245–253
23. Tuxen DV, Lane S (1987) The effects of ventilatory pattern on hyperinflation, airway pressures, and circulation in mechanical ventilation of patients with severe air-flow obstruction. Am Rev Respir Dis 136: 872–879
24. Rodrigo GJ, Rodrigo C, Hall JB (2004) Acute asthma in adults: a review. Chest 125: 1081–1102
25. Shapiro JM (2002) Management of respiratory failure in status asthmaticus. Am J Respir Med 1: 409–416

26. Martin JG, Shore S, Engel LA (1982) Effect of continuous positive airway pressure on respiratory mechanics and pattern of breathing in induced asthma. Am Rev Respir Dis 126: 812–817
27. Shivaram U, Miro AM, Cash ME, Finch PJ, Heurich AE, Kamholz SL (1993) Cardiopulmonary responses to continuous positive airway pressure in acute asthma. J Crit Care 8: 87–92
28. Fernandez MM, Villagra A, Blanch L, Fernandez R (2001) Non-invasive mechanical ventilation in status asthmaticus. Intensive Care Med 27: 486–492
29. Meduri GU, Cook TR, Turner RE, Cohen M, Leeper KV (1996) Noninvasive positive pressure ventilation in status asthmaticus. Chest 110: 767–774
30. Soroksky A, Stav D, Shpirer I (2003) A pilot prospective, randomized, placebo-controlled trial of bilevel positive airway pressure in acute asthmatic attack. Chest 123: 1018–1025
31. Ram FS, Wellington S, Rowe B, Wedzicha JA (2005) Non-invasive positive pressure ventilation for treatment of respiratory failure due to severe acute exacerbations of asthma. Cochrane Database Syst Rev CD004360
32. Rosengarten PL, Tuxen DV, Dziukas L, Scheinkestel C, Merrett K, Bowes G (1991) Circulatory arrest induced by intermittent positive pressure ventilation in a patient with severe asthma. Anaesth Intensive Care 19: 118–121
33. Kollef MH (1992) Lung hyperinflation caused by inappropriate ventilation resulting in electromechanical dissociation: a case report. Heart Lung 21: 74–77
34. Darioli R, Perret C (1984) Mechanical controlled hypoventilation in status asthmaticus. Am Rev Respir Dis 129: 385–387
35. Bidani A, Tzouanakis AE, Cardenas VJ Jr, Zwischenberger JB (1994) Permissive hypercapnia in acute respiratory failure. JAMA 272: 957–962
36. Tuxen DV (1994) Permissive hypercapnic ventilation. Am J Respir Crit Care Med 150: 870–874
37. Leatherman JW, McArthur C, Shapiro RS (2004) Effect of prolongation of expiratory time on dynamic hyperinflation in mechanically ventilated patients with severe asthma. Crit Care Med 32: 1542–1545

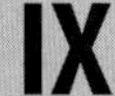

38. Smith TC, Marini JJ (1988) Impact of PEEP on lung mechanics and work of breathing in severe airflow obstruction. J Appl Physiol 65: 1488–1499
39. Tan IK, Bhatt SB, Tam YH, Oh TE (1993) Effects of PEEP on dynamic hyperinflation in patients with airflow limitation. Br J Anaesth 70: 267–272
40. Caramez MP, Borges JB, Tucci MR, et al (2005) Paradoxical responses to positive end-expiratory pressure in patients with airway obstruction during controlled ventilation. Crit Care Med 33: 1519–1528
41. Williams TJ, Tuxen DV, Scheinkestel CD, Czarny D, Bowes G (1992) Risk factors for morbidity in mechanically ventilated patients with acute severe asthma. Am Rev Respir Dis 146: 607–615
42. Leatherman JW, Ravenscraft SA (1996) Low measured auto-positive end-expiratory pressure during mechanical ventilation of patients with severe asthma: hidden auto-positive end-expiratory pressure. Crit Care Med 24: 541–546
43. Hemming A, MacKenzie I, Finfer S (1994) Response to ketamine in status asthmaticus resistant to maximal medical treatment. Thorax 49: 90–91
44. Maltais F, Sovilj M, Goldberg P, Gottfried SB (1994) Respiratory mechanics in status asthmaticus. Effects of inhalational anesthesia. Chest 106: 1401–1406
45. Mutlu GM, Factor P, Schwartz DE, Sznajder JI (2002) Severe status asthmaticus: management with permissive hypercapnia and inhalation anesthesia. Crit Care Med 30: 477–480
46. Saulnier FF, Durocher AV, Deturck RA, Lefebvre MC, Wattel FE (1990) Respiratory and hemodynamic effects of halothane in status asthmaticus. Intensive Care Med 16: 104–107
47. Rodrigo GJ, Rodrigo C, Pollack CV, Rowe B (2003) Use of helium-oxygen mixtures in the treatment of acute asthma: a systematic review. Chest 123: 891–896
48. Elliot SC, Paramasivam K, Oram J, Bodenham AR, Howell SJ, Mallick A (2007) Pumpless extracorporeal carbon dioxide removal for life-threatening asthma. Crit Care Med 35: 945–948
49. Kukita I, Okamoto K, Sato T, et al (1997) Emergency extracorporeal life support for patients with near-fatal status asthmaticus. Am J Emerg Med 15: 566–569
50. Shapiro MB, Kleaveland AC, Bartlett RH (1993) Extracorporeal life support for status asthmaticus. Chest 103: 1651–1654

X Respiratory Monitoring

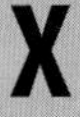

Bedside Monitoring of Diaphragm Electrical Activity during Mechanical Ventilation

C. Sinderby, L. Brander, and J. Beck

Introduction and Background

Mechanical ventilation is a life saving treatment applied in about one third of all critically ill patients [1, 2]. Although a large proportion of patients receive mechanical ventilation, it is still poorly understood how the ventilator settings should be adjusted to meet the demands of each individual patient. Consequently, many patients suffer from patient-ventilator asynchrony [3], because of a mismatch between the timing of inspiration and expiration, or the delivery of too much or too little assist in relation to the patient's inspiratory efforts and respiratory load.

The term poor patient-ventilator interaction can be defined as poor synchronization between: i) the onset of patient inspiratory effort and the start of assist delivery; ii) the adjustment of assist delivery in relation to patient inspiratory effort; and iii) the end of inspiratory effort and termination of inspiratory assist. How to determine, at the bedside, that the ventilator delivers assist in synchrony to the patient's breathing efforts has been troublesome in the past when it was limited to waveform analysis using airway flow, volume and pressure [4]. As illustrated in **Figure 1**, for a patient in pressure control mode, monitoring of only airway pressure, flow and volume makes it difficult to determine whether or not each inspiratory effort is assisted by the ventilator. Recently, the clinical introduction of neurally-adjusted ventilatory assist (NAVA) has allowed quantitative determination of neural respiratory drive to the diaphragm by measuring the electrical activity of the diaphragm (EAdi), and presenting it as a waveform. Thus, what previously was considered a research tool can now be used for bedside monitoring of patient-ventilator asynchrony in mechanically ventilated patients.

There is growing evidence that poor patient-ventilator interaction may have adverse consequences for mechanically ventilated patients. Poor patient-ventilator interaction is associated with increased duration of mechanical ventilation [3, 5]. Prolonged exposure to mechanical ventilation increases the probability of complications, for example, acquiring ventilator-associated pneumonia (VAP) [6]. In addition, the probability of survival has been shown to be related to the number of days on ventilation [2]. Since patients who 'fight' the ventilator require increased levels of sedation, they are more prone to respiratory muscle inactivity, which likely plays a role in prolongation of weaning from mechanical ventilation. Extensive research in animals and more recently in humans has conclusively demonstrated that inactivation of the diaphragm is associated with severe atrophy of the muscular fibers within just a few days [7]. Further evidence for diaphragm 'degeneration' during mechanical ventilation was shown in a study by Laghi et al. [8] who demonstrated pronounced reduction in diaphragm contractility.

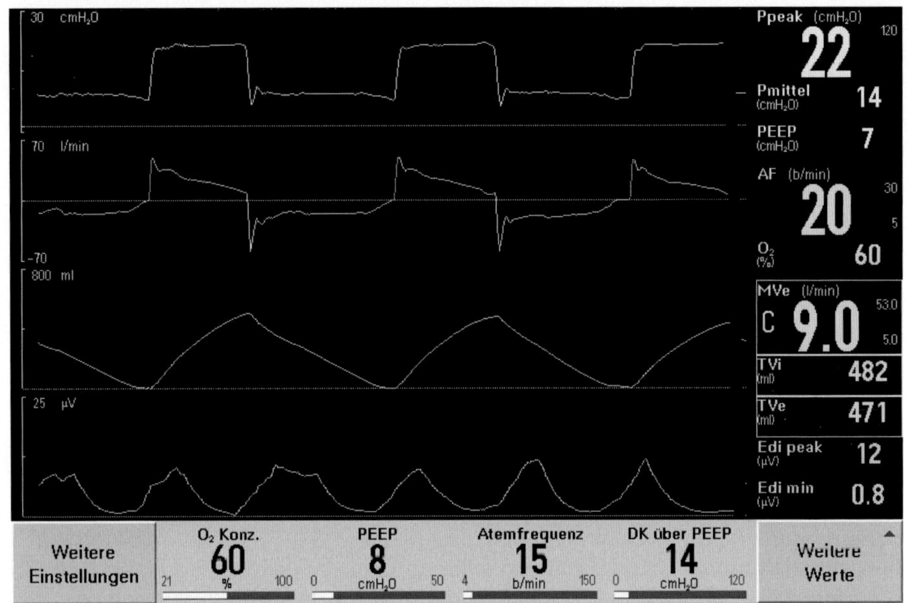

Fig. 1. Example of tracings (from top to bottom) of airway pressure, flow, volume, and diaphragm electrical activity in one patient ventilated in pressure control mode. The trigger indicator of the ventilator, and waveform analysis of the top three pneumatic tracings, reveal that the patient is triggering the ventilator assist in every breath. However, except for very slight upward deflection of the flow curve immediately after the assist cycles-off, there are no pneumatic indications of patient-ventilator asynchrony. Analysis of the bottom tracing (EAdi) shows that: a) the ventilator assist is triggered when neural inspiratory effort and EAdi have reached 50 % of its peak; b) the duration of inspiratory assist extends well beyond the duration of neural inspiration; and c) the neural respiratory rate is twice the ventilator rate.

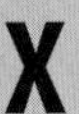

Numerous studies have shown that daily interruption of sedation and/or reduced levels of sedation can decrease the duration of mechanical ventilation [9, 10]. When paired with daily spontaneous breathing trials, the time on mechanical ventilation can be further reduced, as well as reducing 6-month mortality [11]. It should be noted that patient-ventilator interaction was not monitored in the studies of sedation interruption or daily spontaneous breathing trials, nor was there any emphasis on how or whether patients were kept spontaneously breathing (e.g., in pressure support ventilation mode). Impaired patient-ventilator synchrony also affects the quality of sleep, a factor that is also associated with a poorer outcome in critically ill patients [12].

Intuitively, the above discussion suggests that in order to achieve a reduced time on mechanical ventilation and possibly improve outcome, it is important to maintain intrinsic breathing function, i.e., patients need to engage their respiratory muscles while being mechanically ventilated. This however, requires that the applied assist does not exceed the patient's respiratory demand and hence suppress his/her own respiratory activity and that the application of mechanical ventilation does not disturb or agitate the patient, such that increased sedation is necessary.

With few exceptions, the literature on patient-ventilator-interaction only addresses issues related to the timing of assist delivery, i.e., the study of delays between onset and end of patient inspiratory effort and the ventilator's start and termination of the assist, of inspiratory efforts that the ventilator does not respond to (so called wasted inspiratory efforts), and of assist delivered even if there is no patient effort (so called auto triggering).

It has been demonstrated that increasing levels of pressure delivered with pneumatically controlled modes of assist worsen patient-ventilator synchrony [13, 14]. Since excessive levels of pressure support are quite common and cause patient-ventilator asynchrony, it was recently suggested and demonstrated that targeting lower tidal volumes (~6 ml/kg of predicted body weight) significantly reduces the number of wasted inspiratory efforts [15]. Although, such an approach may mend some problems related to timing asynchrony, it will, similar to modes automatically regulating pressure to maintain a target tidal volume, not facilitate the patient's ability to vary volumes in response to respiratory demand as with neurally controlled mechanical ventilation [16].

However, poor patient-ventilator interaction is not only about poor timing, and this suggests a need for ventilator modes that adequately adjust assist in tandem with changes in patient demand. Currently there are two modes of mechanical ventilation that adapt the assist level in relation to patient respiratory demand on a breath-by-breath basis. Proportional assist ventilation (PAV) uses the flow and volume measured by the ventilator and repeated measurements of the elastic and resistive properties of the respiratory system to determine the amount of assist to be delivered [17]. NAVA measures the EAdi and regulates assist in response to this signal [18]. Other modes, such as Smartcare [19] and adaptive support ventilation [20], adjust pressure support level from time-to-time based on assumptions of breathing comfort and optimal breathing patterns, i.e., they are not able to adapt support during, for example, a sigh. Other modes regulate pressure to ensure a target volume, which may result in a reduced assist in response to increasing patient efforts, which is paradoxical if the increased effort represents progressive respiratory failure. Apart from NAVA, there are no means of monitoring the patient's neural respiratory drive or patient-ventilator asynchrony during ventilation with these modes.

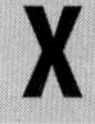

Bedside Monitoring of EAdi

Neural respiratory drive to the diaphragm can be quantified by means of EAdi [21]. Clinically, the EAdi signal can be measured via electrodes mounted on a nasogastric tube if the electrode array is located at the level where the esophagus passes through the diaphragm [22, 23]. Since nasogastric tubes are frequently used to feed or evacuate the stomach in critically ill patients, the measurement of EAdi, although invasive, does not necessarily add complexity to the patient's treatment. In fact, information from electro-cardiac waveforms, an actual disturbance to the EAdi signal, can help to ensure that the electrode array is correctly positioned and that the tip of the nasogastric catheter is located in the stomach. Moreover, the retrocardially measured electro-cardiac signal may, for example, reveal rhythm disturbances (e.g., differentiate atrial fibrillation from atrial flutter), which may be more difficult to diagnose when examining the standard 3 or 5 lead surface electrocardiogram (EKG) typically obtained in critical care patients.

Given that the EAdi comprises the temporal and spatial summation of neural impulses that are translated into diaphragm fiber action potentials, its amplitude relates to changes in motor unit firing rate and recruitment [24]. Thus, a low respiratory drive during resting breathing will produce a small amplitude of the EAdi waveform, whereas, increased respiratory drive will increase the amplitude of the EAdi waveform [25]. Due to anatomical differences, the peak EAdi, if measured in absolute terms, is not reliable for comparison between individuals, however if normalized to, e.g., maximal efforts, EAdi can be used to compare subjects [26]. The EAdi expressed in absolute values, e.g., μV, can however be used to perform repeated measurements in the same individual such that it is possible to monitor changes in neural drive to the diaphragm over time or with a specific intervention [26].

Although it may sound redundant, monitoring the EAdi in order to ensure that patients on partial ventilatory assist are actually breathing can be of great value. Often, patients in pneumatic modes receive too much assist [3], which may be due to any of the following, alone or in combination: Auto-triggering caused by leaks [27], cardiac oscillations [28], excessive and fixed levels of assist, and poorly adjusted flow off-cycling criteria. In the worst case scenario, poor combinations of ventilator settings and sedation level may cause complete inactivation of the diaphragm [29], which, as mentioned above, may lead to inactivation atrophy [7]. Newer modes of mechanical ventilation that deliver assist in proportion to patient effort, such as PAV and NAVA, minimize or eliminate the risk of diaphragm inactivity due to poor setting of the assist. However, neither NAVA nor PAV are immune to the impact of excessive sedation on respiratory drive. A simple illustration of this is presented in **Figure 2**,

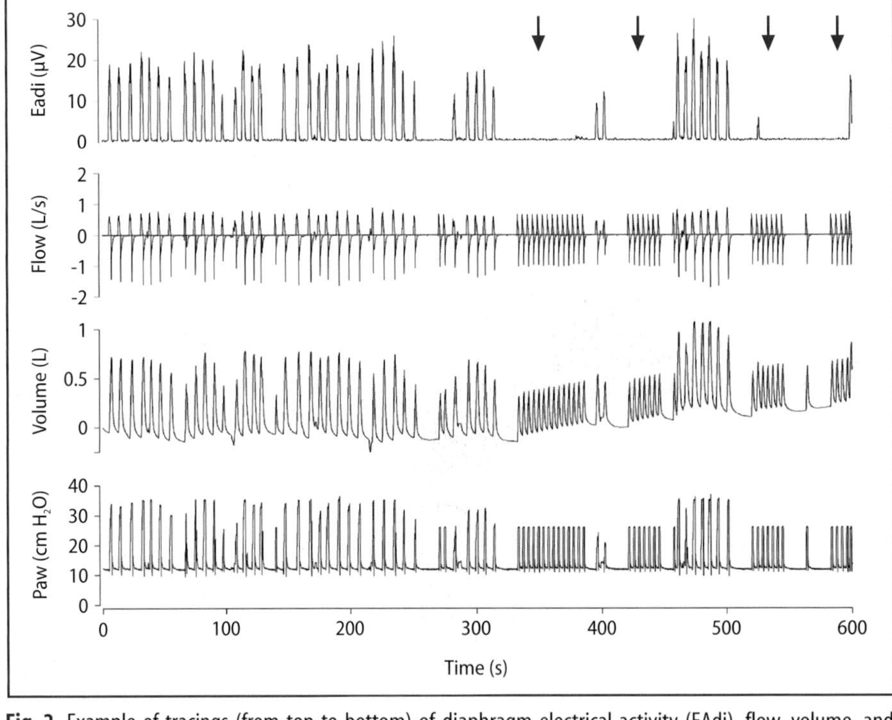

Fig. 2. Example of tracings (from top to bottom) of diaphragm electrical activity (EAdi), flow, volume, and airway pressure (Paw) in one patient ventilated in NAVA. The tracings illustrate the patient's response to bolus administration of sedatives, which initially results in short intermittent interruptions of the neural respiratory drive, followed by more prolonged apneic periods, causing the ventilator to go into backup mode, as indicated by the arrows.

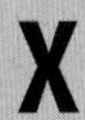

where a patient received sedatives during NAVA, abolishing the EAdi, such that the ventilator switched to the backup pressure control mode. Absence of EAdi can also be due to impaired central respiratory drive, nerve transmission, and neuromuscular junction due to, e.g., trauma, intoxication or neuromuscular disorders. In addition, the actual EAdi waveform by itself (i.e., the shape of the waveform) will describe whether or not the patient has a chaotic/agitated breathing pattern or a stable, regular pattern. Thus, bedside monitoring of EAdi is not only helpful to ensure that the patient is spontaneously breathing, but may also be of diagnostic value.

EAdi has been shown to be the most reliable variable to determine patient inspiratory effort and patient-ventilator interaction [14, 30], in modes designed and assumed to be synchronous with patient inspiratory effort. **Figure 3** illustrates severe patient-ventilator asynchrony due to poor trigger and off-cycling functions, and too high assist delivery in a patient ventilated in pressure support mode, a well described phenomena [14, 31]. Similar to **Figure 1**, the pneumatic waveforms by themselves do not reveal the severity of the asynchrony, whereas implementation of the EAdi (lowest waveform) clearly facilitates bedside detection of the impaired patient-ventilator interaction, and thus could aid in adjusting the ventilator settings. Hence, unwanted negative consequences of poor timing between assist and the patient's inspiratory effort, e.g., impaired sleep quality, prolonged time on mechanical ventilation, can hence be minimized by monitoring EAdi.

In terms of setting the level of assist, EAdi makes it possible to quantify the reduction of neural inspiratory effort with increasing assist [14, 16, 32–34]. If a

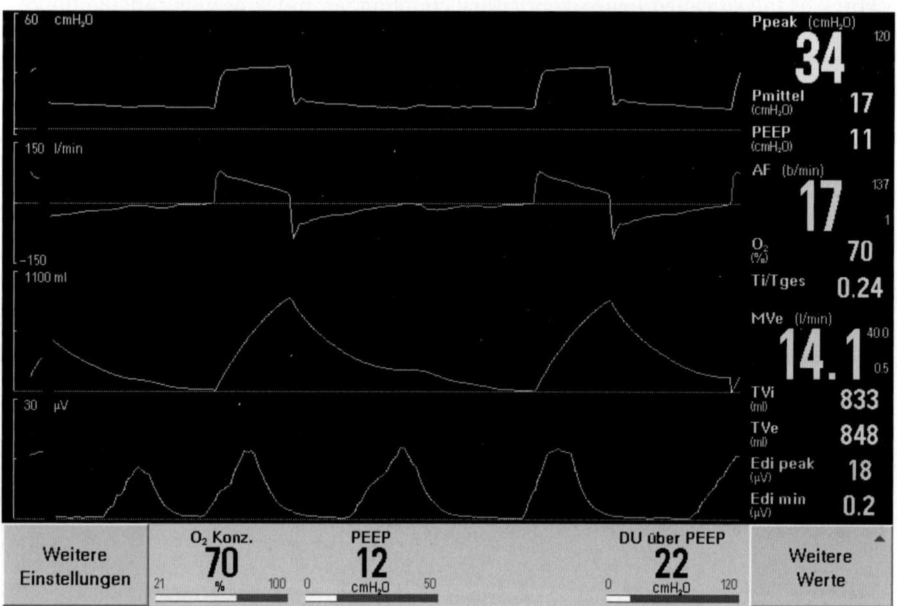

Fig. 3. Example of tracings (from top to bottom) of airway pressure, flow, volume, and diaphragm electrical activity in one patient ventilated in pressure support mode. This example demonstrates a ventilator respiratory rate of 17, where it is clear from the EAdi waveform that the patient's true respiratory rate is about two times higher. Moreover, for the triggered breaths, it is easy to see at the bedside that the patient effort ceases long before the end of the ventilator's assist, revealing that the patient has too much assist with inappropriate off-cycling.

patient with acute respiratory failure that is primarily caused by increased inspiratory load and/or inspiratory muscle weakness receives increased levels of assist, this should at some point result in a decrease in respiratory drive (and therefore EAdi amplitude) due to the unloading of inspiratory muscles [14, 16, 35]. If a reduction in EAdi is not observed one has to also consider underlying causes other than inspiratory muscle weakness and loading. Conversely, a decrease of the ventilatory support from a comfortable level of assist should result in an increased respiratory drive and EAdi.

Obtaining EAdi values with and without assist and calculating the ratio between EAdi during assist and without assist will provide an index for the relative reduction in respiratory drive at a given level of assist. If the measurements of the EAdi are repeated at the same level of assist or during spontaneous breathing trials (i.e. without assist) this will provide information about the patient's progress. For example a progressive decrease of EAdi over time would suggest that the patient either needs less neural drive to breathe or is becoming more unresponsive, e.g., due to sedation or hyperventilation. In fact, monitoring of EAdi in association with delivery of sedatives and analgesics could prove useful in terms of individual bedside monitoring to ensure comfort while ensuring adequate neural respiratory drive.

Another method to monitor whether a patient's ability to generate a breath actually changes over time, while avoiding confounding interference of sedation and assist levels, is by studying the tidal volume (V_T) in relation to the EAdi. The easiest approach is by simply dividing V_T by EAdi, whereas a more accurate approach would be to compare the inspiratory volume at a given EAdi. The V_T to EAdi ratio expresses the so called neuro-ventilatory coupling, an index of how capable the diaphragm is to generate inspiratory volume [26]. An increased V_T to EAdi ratio suggests that the patient is improving the ability to generate a volume due to improved inspiratory muscle function and/or reduced inspiratory load, whereas a decreasing V_T to EAdi ratio suggests the opposite.

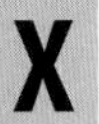

If there is an interest in evaluating whether muscle function in itself is a factor contributing to altered neuro-ventilatory coupling (V_T to EAdi ratio), it is possible to monitor so called neuro-mechanical coupling, which is an index of the patient's ability to generate inspiratory pressure for a given neural drive [24]. The pressure measured at the airways during an occlusion is associated with the pressure in the lower third of the esophagus, which in turn is a representation of the pleural pressure acting to expand the lungs [36]. The neuro-mechanical coupling can thus be obtained by measuring the peak deflection in the airway pressure and the corresponding EAdi during an end-expiratory occlusion. It is also possible, and likely more reliable, to measure the inspiratory airway pressure deflection for a given EAdi. The steps of transformation from neural input to pressure generation (neuro-mechanical coupling) to ventilation (neuro-ventilatory coupling) are illustrated in **Figure 4**. For more extensive review on the topic of neuro-ventilatory and neuro-mechanical coupling, please see references [32, 37].

Conclusion

Recent studies have clearly shown the importance of maintaining spontaneous breathing and patient-ventilator synchrony in mechanically ventilated patients. Until recently, it was not possible to monitor the presence of spontaneous diaphragm activity, nor its response to the assist delivered by mechanical ventilators. The avail-

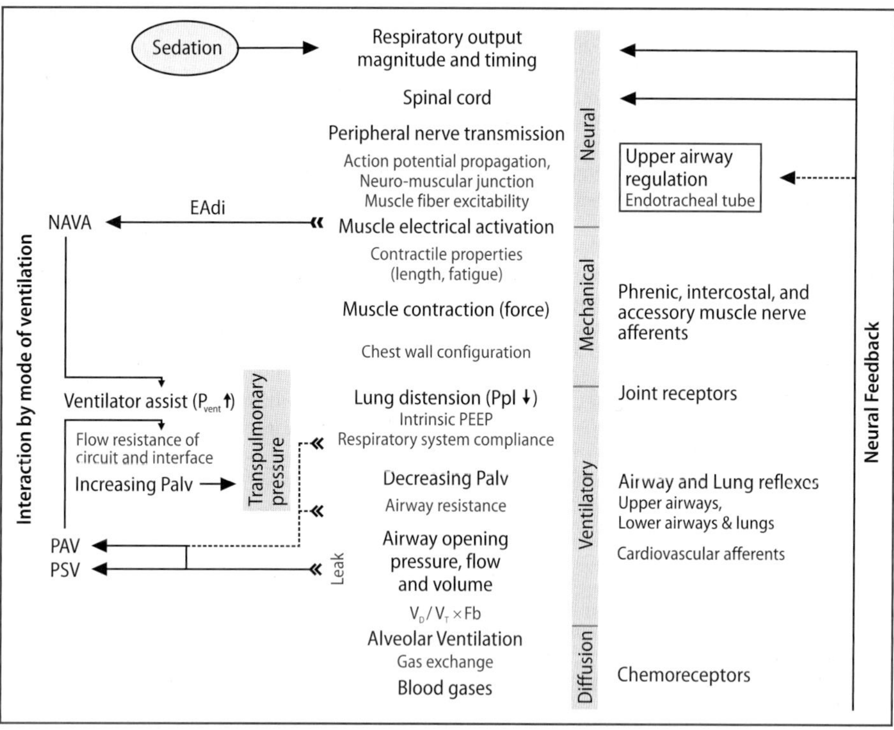

Fig. 4. Schematic description of the chain of events during spontaneous breathing and interaction to mechanical ventilation. The center panel describes the transformation steps from central initiation of a breath to the generation of airway pressure, flow, and volume. The blue vertical bar indicates the steps related to neural, mechanical, and ventilatory energy transformation taking place during a breath. The right panel indicates the neural feedback systems involved in the control of breathing. The left panel shows at which level and how different modes of mechanical ventilation interact during spontaneous breathing. EAdi: electrical activity of the diaphragm; Fb: breathing frequency; Palv: alveolar pressure; Ppl: pleural pressure; NAVA: neurally-adjusted ventilatory assist; PAV: proportional assist ventilation; PSV: pressure support ventilation; Pvent: ventilator pressure; V_D: dead space; V_T: tidal volume.

ability of EAdi at the bedside now provides us with the tools necessary to monitor neural respiratory drive and its response to changes in clinical interventions and/or the patient's status. In fact, monitoring the EAdi not only helps to better understand patient-ventilator interactions on a breath-by-breath basis but may also provide useful information when monitored on an hour-to-hour or day-to-day basis.

References

1. Esteban A, Anzueto A, Alía I, et al (2000) How is mechanical ventilation employed in the intensive care unit? An international utilization review. Am J Respir Crit Care Med 161: 1450–1458
2. Esteban A, Anzueto A, Frutos F, et al (2002) Characteristics and outcomes in adult patients receiving mechanical ventilation: a 28-day international study. JAMA 287: 345–355
3. Thille AW, Rodriguez P, Cabello B, Lellouche F, Brochard L (2006) Patient-ventilator asynchrony during assisted mechanical ventilation. Intensive Care Med 32: 1515–1522

X

4. Nilsestuen JO, Hargett KD (2005) Using ventilator graphics to identify patient-ventilator asynchrony. Respir Care 50: 202–234
5. Chao DC, Scheinhorn DJ, Stearn-Hassenpflug M (1997) Patient-ventilator trigger asynchrony in prolonged mechanical ventilation. Chest 112: 1592–1599
6. Tejerina E, Frutos-Vivar F, Restrepo MI, et al (2006) Incidence, risk factors, and outcome of ventilator-associated pneumonia. J Crit Care 21: 56–65
7. Levine S, Nguyen T, Taylor N, et al (2008) Rapid disuse atrophy of diaphragm fibers in mechanically ventilated humans. N Engl J Med 358: 1327–1335
8. Laghi F, Cattapan SE, Jubran A, et al (2003) Is weaning failure caused by low-frequency fatigue of the diaphragm? Am J Respir Crit Care Med 167: 120–127
9. Kress, JP, Pohlman, AS, O'Connor, MF, Hall JB (2000) Daily interruption of sedative infusions in critically ill patients undergoing mechanical ventilation. N Engl J Med 342: 1471–1414
10. de Wit M, Gennings C, Jenvey WI, Epstein SK (2008) Randomized trial comparing daily interruption of sedation and nursing-implemented sedation algorithm in medical intensive care unit patients. Crit Care 12: R70
11. Girard TD, Kress JP, Fuchs BD, et al (2008) Efficacy and safety of a paired sedation and ventilator weaning protocol for mechanically ventilated patients in intensive care (Awakening and Breathing Controlled trial): a randomised controlled trial. Lancet 371: 126–134
12. Bosma K, Ferreyra G, Ambrogio C, et al (2007) Patient-ventilator interaction and sleep in mechanically ventilated patients: pressure support versus proportional assist ventilation. Crit Care Med 35: 1048–1054
13. Leung P, Jubran A, Tobin MJ (1997) Comparison of assisted ventilator modes on triggering, patient effort, and dyspnea. Am J Respir Crit Care Med 155: 1940–1948
14. Beck J, Gottfried SB, Navalesi P, et al (2001) Electrical activity of the diaphragm during pressure support ventilation in acute respiratory failure. Am J Respir Crit Care Med 164: 419–424
15. Thille AW, Cabello B, Galia F, Lyazidi A, Brochard L (2008) Reduction of patient-ventilator asynchrony by reducing tidal volume during pressure-support ventilation. Intensive Care Med 34: 1477–1486
16. Colombo D, Cammarota G, Bergamaschi V, De Lucia M, Corte FD, Navalesi P (2008) Physiologic response to varying levels of pressure support and neurally adjusted ventilatory assist in patients with acute respiratory failure. Intensive Care Med 34: 2010–2018
17. Younes M (1992) Proportional assist ventilation, a new approach to ventilatory support. Theory. Am Rev Respir Dis 145: 114–120
18. Sinderby C, Navalesi P, Beck J, et al (1999) Neural control of mechanical ventilation in respiratory failure. Nat Med 5: 1433–1436
19. Dojat M, Harf A, Touchard D, Lemaire F, Brochard L (2000) Clinical evaluation of a computer-controlled pressure support mode. Am J Respir Crit Care Med 161: 1161–1166
20. Brunner JX, Iotti GA (2002) Adaptive Support Ventilation (ASV). Minerva Anestesiol 68: 365–368
21. Lourenço RV, Cherniack NS, Malm JR, Fishman AP (1966) Nervous output from the respiratory center during obstructed breathing. J Appl Physiol 21: 527–533.
22. Sinderby CA, Beck JC, Lindström LH, Grassino AE (1997) Enhancement of signal quality in esophageal recordings of diaphragm EMG. J Appl Physiol 82: 1370–1377
23. Aldrich T, Sinderby C, McKenzie D, Estenne M, Gandevia S (2002) Electrophysiologic techniques for the assessment of respiratory muscle function. Am J Respir Crit Care Med 166: 518–624
24. Beck J, Sinderby C, Lindström L, Grassino A (1998) Effects of lung volume on diaphragm EMG signal strength during voluntary contractions. J Appl Physiol 85: 1123–1134
25. Sinderby C, Spahija J, Beck J, et al (2001) Diaphragm activation during exercise in chronic obstructive pulmonary disease. Am J Respir Crit Care Med 163: 1637–1641
26. Sinderby C, Beck J, Spahija J, Weinberg J, Grassino A (1998) Voluntary activation of the human diaphragm in health and disease. J Appl Physiol 85: 2146–2158.
27. Nava S, Ceriana P (2005) Patient-ventilator interaction during noninvasive positive pressure ventilation. Respir Care Clin N Am 11: 281–293
28. Imanaka H, Nishimura M, Takeuchi M, Kimball WR, Yahagi N, Kumon K (2000) Autotriggering caused by cardiogenic oscillation during flow-triggered mechanical ventilation. Crit Care Med 28: 402–407

29. Sinderby C, Brander L, Beck J (2007) Is one fixed level of assist sufficient to mechanically ventilate spontaneously breathing patients? In: Vincent JL (ed) Yearbook of Intensive Care and Emergency Medicine. Springer, Heidelberg, pp 348–357
30. Parthasarathy S, Jubran A, Tobin MJ (1998) Cycling of inspiratory and expiratory muscle groups with the ventilator in airflow limitation. Am J Respir Crit Care Med. 158: 1471–1478
31. Tassaux D, Gainnier M, Battisti A, Jolliet P (2005) Impact of expiratory trigger setting on delayed cycling and inspiratory muscle workload. Am J Respir Crit Care Med 172: 1283–1289.
32. Beck J, Spahija J, Sinderby C (2003) Respiratory muscle unloading during mechanical ventilation. In: Vincent JL (ed) Yearbook of Intensive Care and Emergency Medicine. Springer, Heidelberg, pp 280–287
33. Allo JC, Beck JC, Brander L, Brunet F, Slutsky AS, Sinderby CA (2006) Influence of neurally adjusted ventilatory assist and positive end-expiratory pressure on breathing pattern in rabbits with acute lung injury. Crit Care Med 34: 2997–3004
34. Beck J, Brander L, Slutsky AS, Reilly MC, Dunn MS, Sinderby C (2008) Non-invasive neurally adjusted ventilatory assist in rabbits with acute lung injury. Intensive Care Med 34: 316–323
35. Sinderby C, Beck J, Spahija J, et al (2007) Inspiratory muscle unloading by neurally adjusted ventilatory assist during maximal inspiratory efforts in healthy subjects. Chest 131: 711–717
36. Baydur A, Behrakis PK, Zin WA, Jaeger M, Milic-Emili J (1982) A simple method for assessing the validity of the esophageal balloon technique. Am Rev Respir Dis 126: 788–791
37. Sinderby C, Beck J (2008) Proportional assist ventilation and neurally adjusted ventilatory assist – better approaches to patient ventilator synchrony? Clin Chest Med 29: 329–342

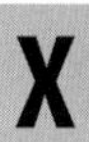

Electrical Impedance Tomography

E.L.V. Costa, R. Gonzalez Lima, and M.B.P. Amato

Introduction

Electrical impedance tomography (EIT) is a non-invasive, radiation-free monitoring tool that allows real-time imaging of ventilation [1–3]. EIT was first used to monitor respiratory function in 1983 and remains the only bedside method that allows repeated, non-invasive measurements of regional changes in lung volumes [4, 5]. For this reason, EIT has been used as a monitoring tool in a variety of applications in critical care medicine, including monitoring of ventilation distribution [3, 6], assessment of lung overdistension [7] and collapse [8, 9], and detection of pneumothorax [10, 11], among others. In this chapter, we will provide a brief overview of the fundamentals of the EIT technique and review the use of EIT in critical care patients in the light of recent literature.

How Electrical Impedance Tomography Works

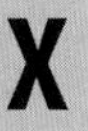

EIT uses injection of electricity in the thorax to obtain images of a cross section of the lungs. Typically, the EIT device uses 16 or 32 electrodes distributed circumferentially around the thorax to inject high-frequency and low-amplitude alternating electrical currents (**Fig. 1**) [2, 10]. These currents travel through the thorax following pathways that vary according to chest wall shape and distribution of impeditivities inside the thorax. The resulting intrathoracic current densities determine electrical potentials on the surface of the chest wall. The electrical potentials are measured and used to obtain the electrical impedance distribution within the thorax using an estimation algorithm that solves an ill-posed non-linear problem. Ill-posedness means that, given a set of measured voltages on the chest-wall surface, the solution for intrathoracic impedances may not be unique or may be extremely unstable: Small errors in voltage measurements may lead to drastically different solutions. This problem is aggravated by the relatively small number of measurements made at the body surface (because of limitations in the current technology, there is a minimum requirement for electrode size and it is only possible to fit a relatively small number of electrodes along the thoracic perimeter). In order to overcome the ill-posed nature of impedance estimation, most EIT imaging algorithms make use of additional assumptions, known as regularizations, such as smoothness of the intrathoracic impedance distribution [12, 13]. These regularizations help the estimation algorithm to decide between competing solutions, producing an image that is a reasonable estimation of the true impedance distribution within the thorax, but at the expense of some degraded spatial resolution or some attenuation of the maximum perturbation.

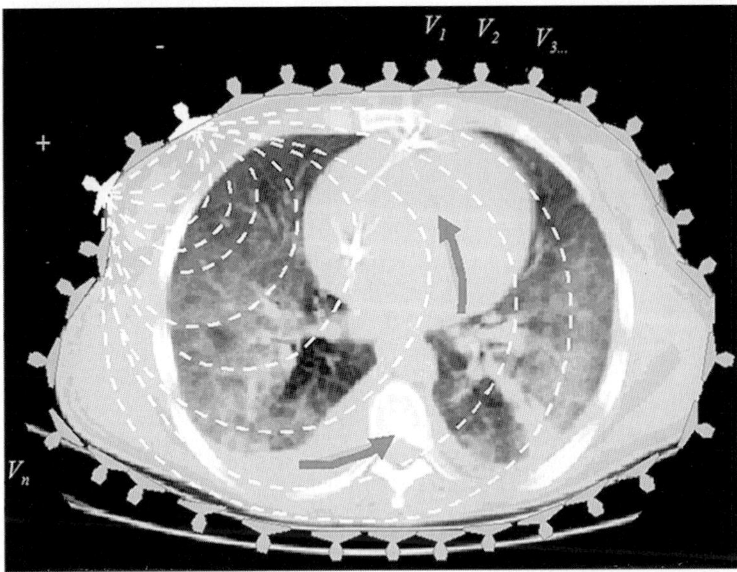

Fig. 1. Computed tomographic axial slice of the thorax of a patient with schematically drawn electrodes and electrical current pathways through the thorax. One pair of electrodes injects electrical current at a time while the remaining electrodes read the voltages produced as a result of electrical current passing through the thorax. The injecting pair is alternated sequentially so that after a full cycle, all possible adjacent electrodes serve as injectors. Each full cycle results in an image and 50 images are produced each second.

Reconstruction Algorithms

Reconstruction or estimation algorithms refer to the computations that transform the acquired voltages at the surface of the thorax into a cross-sectional image of impedances (**Fig. 2**). To get a grasp of the complexity of EIT reconstruction algorithms, it helps to compare EIT with X-ray computed tomography (CT). The reconstruction of a CT image is relatively simple because X-rays pass through the thorax as a straight beam, with negligible scattering of the energy. Thus, a localized change in tissue density affects a few measurements (only the measures taken from the detectors at the projection of the line connecting the X-ray beamer and the tissue perturbation). In contrast, when an electrical current passes through the thorax, the current spreads out in three dimensions, following a complex path that is determined by the place of current injection and also by the three-dimensional distribution of tissue impedances. Any local change in tissue impedance will affect all voltage measurements at the surface of the thorax in a non-linear fashion, producing a voltage gradient that will depend on the complex distribution of current densities across the thorax. Thus, the relationship between tissue impedance and voltages is extremely complex, essentially non-linear, and depends on non-local phenomena.

The first algorithm used to generate images of ventilation using EIT was called filtered backprojection [2], and used a linear approximation to solve the EIT problem. This approximation imposes some constraints in terms of the maximum impedance variation that can be reliably measured. Many other linearized algorithms have been developed since then in pursuit of an algorithm that is at the same time fast and capable of providing images with good spatial resolution [14–16]. No

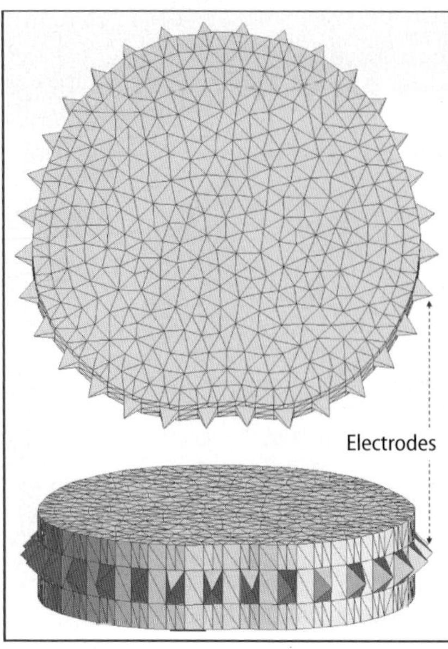

Fig. 2. Finite element mesh used for image reconstruction. From [10] with permission

single algorithm, however, stood out in terms of spatial resolution or speed, and different linearized algorithms are used in different EIT devices. For imaging the functional changes in organs like the heart and lung, speed is important because the ability of EIT to collect repeated data in time is one of the advantages of EIT over other available imaging modalities with higher spatial resolution, such as CT. Therefore, iterative algorithms, although yielding more precise results because they take into account the non-linearity of the EIT problem, have too high computational costs and, at the moment, are not suitable for fast online imaging [13]. The two types of algorithm are not mutually exclusive, though, and the output of iterative algorithms could be used to improve the accuracy of linearized algorithms.

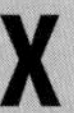

Patterns of Applying the Electrical Current

There are two general approaches for applying the electrical current. According to the first approach, electrical current is injected simultaneously by all electrodes, and the electrodes read the voltages produced at the same time electrical current is being injected [13]. While this method tends to produce higher current densities inside the thorax and thus higher signal-to-noise ratio, it has the drawback of introducing the necessity to deal with skin-electrode contact impedances. In the ideal scenario, contact impedance can be easily modeled [17], but when electrodes are not in perfect contact with the skin, or when they partly come off during deep breaths, contact impedance might become an important part of the impedance being measured.

The second approach consists of applying electrical current at one electrode pair at a time, while the remaining electrodes function as voltage readers. The most common design injects electrical current at adjacent electrodes, but many other designs are possible, including injection in every other electrode (**Fig. 1**) or in diametrically opposite electrodes. The pair of active electrodes is alternated sequentially until all possible pairs are used (according to the application pattern used). At the end of one full cycle, there are N × (N-3) voltage measurements (N being the number of electrodes) and these are used to feed the estimation algorithm and produce one image. This approach has the advantage of not having to take into account skin-electrode contact impedances because all voltage readings occur at near-zero current. Most systems used for the study of lung function have used this second approach.

Absolute versus Difference Images

Thoracic shape can contribute as much as internal thoracic impedances to the measured voltages at the chest wall surface [13]. Consequently, reconstruction of the absolute impedance distribution, albeit feasible, requires knowledge of the shape of the thorax. To avoid taking thoracic geometry into account, Barber and Brown suggested an approach based on the dynamic changes in impedance, i.e., relative changes in impedance from time to time or during respiration [2], assuming that the shape of the thorax did not change between measurements. This relative or differential approach cancels out most errors related to wrong assumptions about true thoracic shape (the same error is equally present in both images) and has proven its validity in recent years. The use of normalized voltage measurements further improves the robustness of such solution, which completely ignores the absolute values of impedance at the beginning of measurements. Typically, at a frequency of 10 KHz, the electrical impedance of the chest tissues is in the order of 2 – 4 Ωm, and the average impedance of the lung is around 10 Ωm [18]. During respiration, while lung impedance changes up to 300 % (from 7.2 to 23.6 Ωm in one report) [18], chest wall impedance remains relatively constant.

Most currently available EIT devices and most publications in the field use the relative approach and thus calculate difference impedance images in relation to a reference. The output image of such algorithms is a 32 × 32 array from which each element corresponds to a pixel on the image and contains the change in impedance in relation to a reference frame, expressed as a percentage. The baseline impedance cannot be recovered. Thus, breaths producing a change in lung impedance from 5 to 10 Ωm, or from 10 to 20 Ωm will produce exactly the same relative image. As we will see below, this limitation is not worrisome as far as clinical applications are concerned, because there is a well described and linear relationship between the amount of air entering the voxel and the percent change in lung impedance [19].

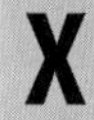

One drawback of the use of difference images is that only regions of the thorax that change their impedance over time are represented in EIT images. Consequently, pre-existing consolidated areas of the lung (e.g., pneumonia or atelectasis), pleural effusions or large bullae are not represented in difference EIT images. For this reason, absolute images have the potential to bring additional and important information and there is continuing research using iterative algorithms to improve the quality of absolute images. Although some progress has been made, with promising results having been presented by Hahn et al. [11], the quality of the images is still not good enough for meaningful clinical use. Further development in this area, using estimations of electrode position and taking thoracic shape into account will enable precise absolute image reconstruction.

Spatial and Temporal Resolution

Spatial resolution of EIT depends on the accuracy and noise of the measurements, the number of electrodes, and the regularization used. For this reason, spatial resolution varies from one EIT device to another, and varies even within a single device depending on the settings employed. In bench tests using tanks or phantoms, the resolution is usually optimized because less regularization is required. At the bedside, however, noise and wrong assumptions about thoracic shape require stronger regularizations and resolution is compromised. On average, for a 16-electrode system, resolution is about 12 % of the thoracic diameter for regions in the periphery of the lung and 20 % for central regions. By using a 32-electrode system, this resolution could be improved to 6 – 10 % of the thoracic diameter (Turri F, personal communication). In a typical adult patient, this resolution corresponds to approximately 1.5 – 3 cm in the cross-sectional plane. The spatial resolution in the craniocaudal direction is even lower, the slice thickness amounting to approximately 7 – 10 cm. In fact, this characteristic is not necessarily a limitation; such thick slices are potentially useful for representing lung behavior during mechanical ventilation, when the detection of heterogeneities along the gravitational axis is the main target [20, 21].

Although it is possible to improve resolution, for example by increasing the number of electrodes or by improving hardware performance, it is unlikely that EIT will ever reach the resolution of CT or magnetic resonance imaging (MRI) [22]. On the other hand, modern EIT devices are characterized by high temporal resolution, with some generating up to 50 images/s. It is thus possible to follow closely and on a regional basis the time pattern of inflation and deflation of the lung. For example, it is possible to show that some areas start to inflate after the others, reflecting either tidal recruitment [23] or local auto-positive end-expiratory pressure (PEEP). Additionally, by use of brief periods of apnea or by filtering out ventilation [24], it is now possible to monitor changes in intrathoracic impedance caused by perfusion. This opens new horizons for the use of EIT with the perspective of studying at the bedside the intricate relationships between ventilation and perfusion in real-time.

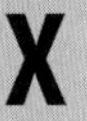

Clinical Applications

The body of literature on EIT has increased steadily over the last years. In the last 5 years, more than 200 papers have been published, representing an increase of almost 100 % in relation to the previous 5-year period. Initial EIT applications in critical care medicine focused mainly on ventilation and its distribution; now other applications are being explored such as detection of pneumothorax, assessment of lung recruitment and collapse, and lung perfusion. In this section, we will review the literature pertaining to respiratory and critical care medicine.

Assessment of Lung Recruitment and Lung Collapse

Careful titration of PEEP is of utmost importance for the success of ventilatory strategies based on the open lung approach. Traditionally, global lung parameters, such as pressure-volume curves [25, 26] or respiratory system compliance [27], have been used, but they fail to represent what is happening to the lung on a regional basis [28]. Collapsed and overdistended lung compartments commonly coexist, and a method capable of assessing both, simultaneously, would be invaluable as a tool to titrate PEEP. Our group described an EIT-based method for estimating alveolar collapse at the bedside, pointing out its regional distribution. On an experimental model in pigs, we found a good correlation between EIT and CT estimates of lung collapse during decremental PEEP trials after a maximal lung recruitment maneuver

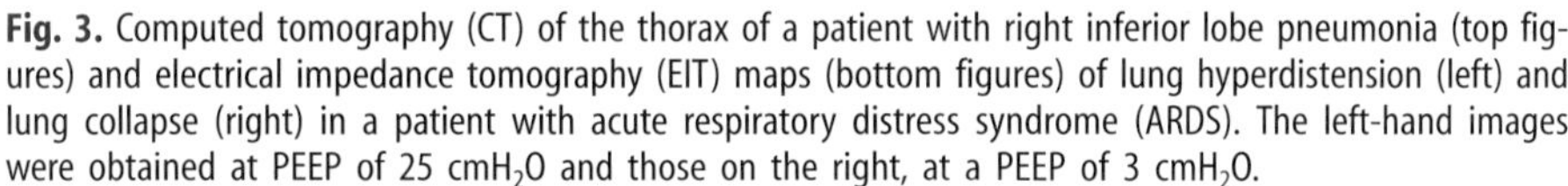

Fig. 3. Computed tomography (CT) of the thorax of a patient with right inferior lobe pneumonia (top figures) and electrical impedance tomography (EIT) maps (bottom figures) of lung hyperdistension (left) and lung collapse (right) in a patient with acute respiratory distress syndrome (ARDS). The left-hand images were obtained at PEEP of 25 cmH$_2$O and those on the right, at a PEEP of 3 cmH$_2$O.

[29]. Combining data obtained from EIT and respiratory mechanics, it is also possible to estimate the amount of overdistension during a PEEP trial, although validation of such estimates represents a challenge due to the lack of a gold standard to compare to (**Fig. 3**) [30]. Meier et al. [9] recently used EIT to monitor regional tidal volume during a PEEP titration maneuver in a model of surfactant depletion in pigs. Looking at changes in regional tidal volumes that occurred with changes in PEEP, they were able to detect the initiation of regional lung collapse and of regional lung recruitment before global changes occurred in lung mechanics. Additionally, they showed good correlation of ventilation estimated by EIT and CT, confirming the results of Victorino et al. [3]. Their results bring an exciting possibility of bedside titration of PEEP based on regional lung mechanics.

In a similar report, Luepschen et al. [31] extended the previous results by showing that the center of gravity of ventilation images moves dorsally during lung recruitment and ventrally during lung collapse. This EIT based parameter brought additional information to a fuzzy controller of ventilation that optimized lung recruitment based on oxygenation, ventilatory parameters and hemodynamics. Other authors have also used the center of ventilation to assess lung recruitment

[32]. In sixteen newborn piglets with acute lung injury (ALI) induced by whole lung lavage, Frerichs et al. showed that EIT allowed visualization of the effects of ALI, lung recruitment, surfactant administration, and subsequent mechanical ventilation strategy. They found that lung injury displaced the ventilation ventrally, and lung recruitment restored the center of ventilation to the normal position. After surfactant administration, ventilation was gradually shifted ventrally after 10 and 60 min, but remained in the pre-injury position if surfactant administration was followed by a recruitment maneuver.

Other indices to estimate lung recruitment using EIT have been proposed. In a recent report [23], the authors compared EIT measures to dynamic CT in 18 pigs divided into three groups (control, direct and indirect lung injury). EIT allowed real-time monitoring of regional ventilation distribution. During an interposed slow inflation, regional impedance time curves were used to calculate three indices: Area under the curve, slope linearity (concavity or convexity), and time delay between start of inspiration and start of regional inflation (ventilation delay index). These investigators showed that recruitment could be detected by regional EIT and was better described by the regional ventilation delay index, which also has the potential to capture intra-tidal recruitment. Unfortunately, the other two indices did not correlate with lung recruitment. Hinz et al. [33] used an index similar to the slope linearity described above and found different results. They monitored 20 mechanically ventilated patients with ALI/acute respiratory distress syndrome (ARDS) during tidal breathing and showed that the behavior of the impedance-time curve was heterogeneous within the lung suggesting the occurrence of hyperdistension and tidal recruitment in different regions of the lung. These seemingly conflicting results might be explained by simple methodological differences. First, Hinz et al. used global EIT tidal volume on the x-axis instead of time. This is important, because it eliminates the assumption that tidal volume is evenly distributed in the cephalocaudal direction. Second, performing concavity analyses on large slow inflations (maximum airway pressure of 60 cmH_2O) might be misleading because, at high lung volumes, the rib cage limits further lung expansion on the transverse plane and the additional lung inflation occurs mostly due to diaphragmatic displacement. Consequently, concavity will be biased downwards.

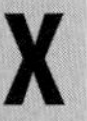

Although careful titration of PEEP is important, one should bear in mind that lung condition is constantly changing, and that a selected PEEP might not suffice to keep the lung open at all times, especially if transient depressurization of the lung takes place. Depressurization is particularly common when suctioning of the airways is required for clearance of secretions. To assess the derecruitment caused by closed-system suctioning, Wolf et al. [34] studied 6 children with ARDS on pressure controlled ventilation and continuously monitored with EIT. They showed that lung volumes decreased on average by 5.3 ml/kg after three suctioning maneuvers. Unexpectedly, they showed that the most dorsal regions of the lung were the least affected by derecruitment; since the authors used difference EIT images, they could only speculate that this region was atelectatic even before the suctioning maneuver.

Other authors have suggested that only open-system suctioning leads to significant derecruitment. In pigs monitored with EIT after surfactant depletion [8], Lindgren et al. showed that endotracheal suctioning induced collapse of the lung and decreased regional lung compliance during open-system suctioning, but not during closed-system suctioning. The collapse was predominantly in the dorsal regions, but recruitment was reestablished in less than 10 minutes by simple reconnection to the ventilator. Nevertheless, it is important to bear in mind that the model of surfactant depletion using whole lung lavage leads to lungs prone to collapse, but highly recruitable. Therefore, these results need careful scrutiny before being extrapolated to inflamed, edematous lungs of ARDS patients, on whom depressurization is best avoided.

In a different report, the same authors used EIT to assess lung collapse during bronchoscopic suctioning in mechanically ventilated patients with ALI [8]. They elegantly showed that bronchoscopy initially leads to localized auto-PEEP due to the reduced transverse area available for airflow, and that suctioning leads to a decrease in lung aeration and decrease in lung compliance even when a closed suctioning system is used. They obtained similar findings in volume-controlled and pressure-controlled ventilation. In mechanically ventilated patients being submitted to bronchoscopic procedures, EIT might prove to be a useful tool to quantify the amount of collapse and to guide post-suctioning recruitment.

Detection of Pneumothorax and Pleural Effusion

Pneumothorax is a relatively common complication in critical care patients receiving mechanical ventilation or submitted to invasive procedures such as central venous line placement or thoracocentesis. Costa et al. [10] created an algorithm for the detection of pneumothoraces using EIT. In a first set of 10 pigs, they created the algorithm which was subsequently tested in 29 pigs. EIT showed a sensitivity of 100 % (CI 93–100 %) to detect pneumothoraces as small as 20 ml (**Fig. 4.**). The major limitation of this study was the need for a baseline measurement before the occurrence of the pneumothorax, limiting the application to monitoring of situations at high risk of developing pneumothorax, such as central venous line placements or mechanical ventilation with high alveolar pressures.

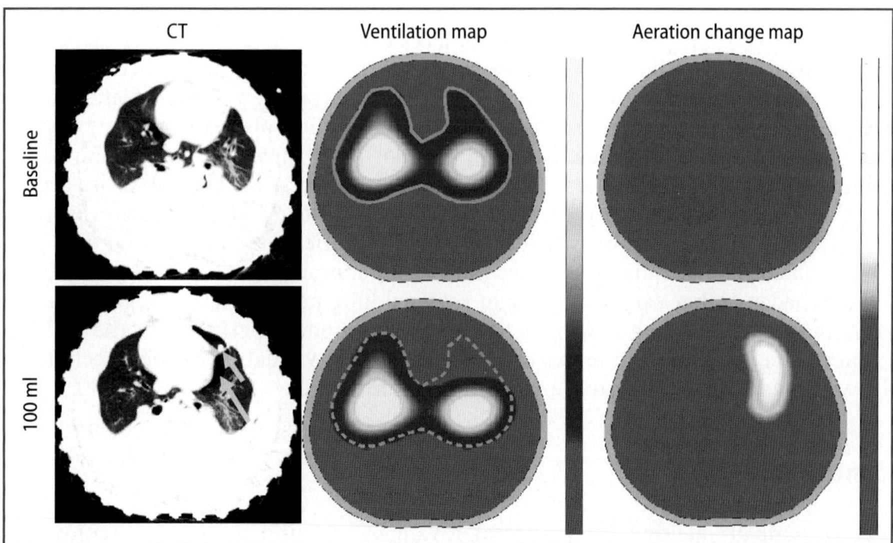

Fig. 4. Computed tomography (CT), ventilation map, and aeration change map obtained at baseline and after the induction of a 100 ml pneumothorax in a pig with partial atelectasis of the lungs. The arrows point to the accumulation of air in the pleural space. From [10] with permission

Another group of investigators [11] studied the combined use of dynamic and absolute images for the diagnosis of pneumothorax and pleural effusion. They studied five pigs and showed reproducible results with the development of pneumothorax consisting of increased impedance and decreased ventilation. Pleural effusions, being more conductive than the lung, produced a decrease in impedance associated with decreased ventilation. They further acquired images in four patients and showed that EIT absolute images were compatible with CT images.

The use of EIT as a sensitive monitoring tool for the detection of pneumothorax and pleural effusions [10, 11, 35] is appealing but probably will not be applied in clinical practice until systematic studies in patients are performed.

Correct Placement of Endotracheal Tube

Steinmann et al. [36] studied 40 patients requiring one-lung ventilation for surgical procedures. EIT monitoring started before intubation and continued throughout the protocol. All clinical decisions were based on fiberoptic bronchoscopy and EIT investigators were blinded to bronchoscopy findings. EIT reliably identified left and right one-lung ventilation, correctly diagnosing misplacement of the tube in the contralateral main bronchus. Nevertheless, using EIT parameters, they could not identify misplacement of the endobronchial cuff, suggesting that EIT cannot replace bronchoscopy as a guide to one-lung ventilation. Although not designed to address this question, this study suggests that EIT can be used to diagnose selective intubation or endotracheal tube displacement during conventional two-lung ventilation.

Potential Future Applications of Clinical Relevance

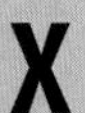

In addition to the above established applications, EIT can also be used to study lung perfusion [24, 37–39]. One of the goals of mechanical ventilation is to ensure adequate gas exchange, and the efficiency of gas exchange depends not only on ventilation, but also on pulmonary perfusion. Using dynamic filtering processes, or by means of a short period of apnea, it is possible to separate ventilation and cardiac related changes in lung impedance [24]. The amplitude of cardiac-related oscillations seen in the EIT signals, however, has not been shown to correspond to the amount of local perfusion, and further studies are necessary to explore its precise physiological meaning. A different approach to measuring lung perfusion involves the injection of small volumes (5–10 ml) of hypertonic saline in a central vein [39]. Hypertonic saline is more conductive than blood and produces regional decreases in lung impedance that vary according to regional lung perfusion. Although the above techniques offer exciting new ways to monitor pulmonary perfusion at the bedside, clinical data on these techniques are limited. Clinical validation of these techniques is warranted before they can be used in clinical practice.

Conclusion

EIT is gradually gaining acceptance as a valuable monitoring tool for critically ill patients. It is cheap, non-invasive and, up to now, has been show to reliably track changes in regional ventilation, describe regional ventilation distribution and regional lung mechanics, detect pneumothoraces, and monitor lung recruitment and derecruitment. Other applications such as monitoring of lung perfusion and of ventilation/perfusion distribution are feasible but still require further studies.

Acknowledgement: Financial support by grants from "Fundação de Amparo à Pesquisa do Estado de São Paulo (FAPESP)" and "Financiadora de Estudos e Projetos (FINEP)".

References

1. Frerichs I, Hahn G, Schiffmann H, et al (1999) Monitoring regional lung ventilation by functional electrical impedance tomography during assisted ventilation. Ann NY Acad Sci 873: 493–505
2. Barber DC, Brown BH (1984) Applied potential tomography. J Phys E Sci Instrum 17: 723–733
3. Victorino JA, Borges JB, Okamoto VN, et al (2004) Imbalances in regional lung ventilation: a validation study on electrical impedance tomography. Am J Respir Crit Care Med 169: 791–800
4. Frerichs I, Hinz J, Herrmann P, et al (2002) Detection of local lung air content by electrical impedance tomography compared with electron beam CT. J Appl Physiol 93: 660–666
5. Wolf GK Arnold JH (2005) Noninvasive assessment of lung volume: respiratory inductance plethysmography and electrical impedance tomography. Crit Care Med 33: S163–169
6. Frerichs I, Dargaville PA, Dudykevych T, et al (2003) Electrical impedance tomography: a method for monitoring regional lung aeration and tidal volume distribution? Intensive Care Med 29: 2312–2316
7. Adler A, Shinozuka N, Berthiaume Y, et al (1998) Electrical impedance tomography can monitor dynamic hyperinflation in dogs. J Appl Physiol 84: 726–732
8. Lindgren S, Odenstedt H, Olegård C, et al (2007) Regional lung derecruitment after endotracheal suction during volume- or pressure-controlled ventilation: a study using electric impedance tomography. Intensive Care Med 33: 172–180
9. Meier T, Luepschen H, Karsten J, et al (2008) Assessment of regional lung recruitment and derecruitment during a peep trial based on electrical impedance tomography. Intensive Care Med 34: 543–550
10. Costa ELV, Chaves CN, Gomes S, et al (2008) Real-time detection of pneumothorax using electrical impedance tomography. Crit Care Med 36: 1230–1238
11. Hahn G, Just A, Dudykevych T, et al (2006) Imaging pathologic pulmonary air and fluid accumulation by functional and absolute EIT. Physiol Meas 27: S187–198
12. Bayford RH (2006) Bioimpedance tomography (electrical impedance tomography). Annu Rev Biomed Eng 8: 63–91
13. Brown BH (2003) Electrical impedance tomography (EIT): a review. J Med Eng Technol 27: 97–108
14. Trigo FC, Gonzalez-Lima R Amato MBP (2004) Electrical impedance tomography using the extended kalman filter. IEEE Trans Biomed Eng 51: 72–81
15. Pai C, Mirandola L Scweder R (2005) A black-box back-projection algorithm for electrical impedance tomography. Proceedings of the 18th International Congress of Mechanical Engineering (abst)
16. Breckon WR Pidcock MK (1987) Mathematical aspects of impedance imaging. Clin Phys Physiol Meas 8 (Suppl A):77–84
17. Hua P, Woo EJ, Webster JG, et al (1993) Finite element modeling of electrode-skin contact impedance in electrical impedance tomography. IEEE Trans Biomed Eng 40: 335–343
18. Harris ND, Suggett AJ, Barber DC, et al (1987) Applications of applied potential tomography (APT) in respiratory medicine. Clin Phys Physiol Meas 8 (Suppl A):155–165
19. Adler A, Amyot R, Guardo R, et al (1997) Monitoring changes in lung air and liquid volumes with electrical impedance tomography. J Appl Physiol 83: 1762–1767
20. Gattinoni L, Pelosi P, Vitale G, et al (1991) Body position changes redistribute lung computed-tomographic density in patients with acute respiratory failure. Anesthesiology 74: 15–23

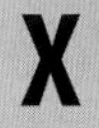

21. Borges JB, Okamoto VN, Matos GFJ, et al (2006) Reversibility of lung collapse and hypoxemia in early acute respiratory distress syndrome. Am J Respir Crit Care Med 174: 268–278.
22. Seagar AD, Barber DC, Brown BH (1987) Theoretical limits to sensitivity and resolution in impedance imaging. Clin Phys Physiol Meas 8 (Suppl A):13–31
23. Wrigge H, Zinserling J, Muders T, et al (2008) Electrical impedance tomography compared with thoracic computed tomography during a slow inflation maneuver in experimental models of lung injury. Crit Care Med 36: 903–909
24. Deibele JM, Luepschen H, Leonhardt S (2008) Dynamic separation of pulmonary and cardiac changes in electrical impedance tomography. Physiol Meas 29: S1–14
25. Villar J, Kacmarek RM, Pérez-Méndez L, et al (2006) A high positive end-expiratory pressure, low tidal volume ventilatory strategy improves outcome in persistent acute respiratory distress syndrome: a randomized, controlled trial. Crit Care Med 34: 1311–1318
26. Amato MB, Barbas CS, Medeiros DM, et al (1998) Effect of a protective-ventilation strategy on mortality in the acute respiratory distress syndrome. N Engl J Med 338: 347–354
27. Suarez-Sipmann F, Böhm SH, Tusman G, et al (2007) Use of dynamic compliance for open lung positive end-expiratory pressure titration in an experimental study. Crit Care Med 35: 214–221
28. Hinz J, Moerer O, Neumann P, et al (2006) Regional pulmonary pressure volume curves in mechanically ventilated patients with acute respiratory failure measured by electrical impedance tomography. Acta Anaesthesiol Scand 50: 331–339
29. Beraldo MA, Reske A, Borges JB, et al (2006) Peep titration by EIT (electric impedance tomography): correlation with multislice CT. Am J Respir Crit Care Med 173: A64 (abst)
30. Borges JB, Costa ELV, Beraldo MA, et al (2006) A bedside real-time monitor to detect airspace collapse in patients with ALI/ARDS. Am J Respir Crit Care Med 173: A377 (abst)
31. Luepschen H, Meier T, Grossherr M, et al (2007) Protective ventilation using electrical impedance tomography. Physiol Meas 28: S247–260
32. Frerichs I, Dargaville PA, van Genderingen H, et al (2006) Lung volume recruitment after surfactant administration modifies spatial distribution of ventilation. Am J Respir Crit Care Med 174: 772–779
33. Hinz J, Gehoff A, Moerer O, et al (2007) Regional filling characteristics of the lungs in mechanically ventilated patients with acute lung injury. Eur J Anaesthesiol 24: 414–424.
34. Wolf GK, Grychtol B, Frerichs I, et al (2007) Regional lung volume changes in children with acute respiratory distress syndrome during a derecruitment maneuver. Crit Care Med 35: 1972–1978
35. Beraldo MA, Costa ELV, Gomes S, et al (2007) Detection of pleural effusion at the bedside by EIT. Am J Respir Crit Care Med 173: A791 (abst)
36. Steinmann D, Stahl CA, Minner J, et al (2008) Electrical impedance tomography to confirm correct placement of double-lumen tube: a feasibility study. Br J Anaesth 101: 411–418
37. Smit HJ, Vonk Noordegraaf A, Marcus JT, et al (2004) Determinants of pulmonary perfusion measured by electrical impedance tomography. Eur J Appl Physiol 92: 45–49
38. Smit HJ, Handoko ML, Vonk Noordegraaf A, et al (2003) Electrical impedance tomography to measure pulmonary perfusion: is the reproducibility high enough for clinical practice? Physiol Meas 24: 491–499
39. Frerichs I, Hinz J, Herrmann P, et al (2002) Regional lung perfusion as determined by electrical impedance tomography in comparison with electron beam CT imaging. IEEE Trans Med Imaging 21: 646–652

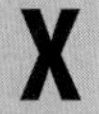

Regional Ventilation Delay Index: Detection of Tidal Recruitment using Electrical Impedance Tomography

T. Muders, H. Luepschen, and C. Putensen

Introduction

Apart from restoring adequate gas exchange, mechanical ventilation should avoid factors known to further aggravate lung injury such as inspiratory overdistension as well as cyclic opening and closing (tidal recruitment) of ventilatory units during tidal ventilation. Both are considered as major risk factors in the pathogenesis of ventilation-associated lung injury (VALI) [1–3]. The risk of inspiratory overdistension can be reduced by using small tidal volumes and by limiting inspiratory plateau pressures [4]. Low tidal volume ventilation, however, is known to promote end-expiratory alveolar collapse [5, 6], thus, potential for alveolar recruitment and risk for cyclic opening and closing of ventilatory units (tidal recruitment) is increased. To avoid end-expiratory alveolar collapse, an adequate positive end-expiratory pressure (PEEP) is needed [7, 8]. Although experimental investigations have shown that elevated PEEP levels protect from VALI [9, 10], studies comparing high-PEEP and low-PEEP strategies have failed so far to show a consistent improvement in mortality [11–13].

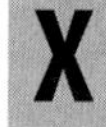

Individual PEEP Setting is Essential

Setting PEEP in order to minimize cyclic alveolar collapse (tidal recruitment) may be difficult and a strategy which considers individual differences in pulmonary responses to PEEP is required [14]. Ventilated patients with acute lung injury (ALI) often exhibit heterogeneous distribution of intrapulmonary gas and tissue due to gravity, regional surfactant dysfunction, and uneven distribution of collapsed and consolidated lung tissue. Whereas collapsed lung units can be re-opened and kept open by PEEP, consolidated lung tissue seems not to respond to increased airway pressure. Thus, the possibility of avoiding cyclic alveolar collapse and the risk of end-inspiratory overdistension by increased PEEP depends on individual potential for alveolar recruitment (collapsed lung tissue that can potentially be opened by high airway pressure) [14]. A recent multicenter computed tomography (CT) trial evaluating the amount of potentially recruitable lung in 68 patients with ALI or acute respiratory distress syndrome (ARDS) observed huge individual differences in potential for alveolar recruitment [14]. This individual potential for alveolar recruitment cannot be predicted by the origin of lung injury and correlates with poor outcome [14, 15]. Therefore, a more individual PEEP setting strategy is warranted. Individual assessment of potential for alveolar recruitment might be helpful to estimate possible effects of increased PEEP.

Global and Regional Lung Function Parameters

Although global indices of lung function, such as blood gases and respiratory mechanics, are used to optimize and monitor ventilator settings, they often provide limited or even misleading information. An increase in oxygenation does not necessarily mean lung recruitment because changes in intrathoracic pressure due to changes in ventilatory settings may affect cardiac output and regional pulmonary blood flow distribution [16]. Although theoretically based on physiological rationale, $PaCO_2$ may not be associated as expected with lung recruitment [17] since $PaCO_2$ depends on minute production of CO_2. Theoretically, the occurrence of lung recruitment with decrease of atelectasis and increase in aerated lung tissue should always lead to an improvement in respiratory mechanics. Global respiratory system compliance [18] and the profile of the global pressure–time curve (stress index) [19] have been considered for this purpose. In contrast, recent studies have shown that variations in respiratory compliance appeared to be poorly correlated with alveolar recruitment [14]. This is in part due to the fact that global lung function tests like a static pressure volume curve can only assess summarized overlapping information of several ventilatory units from different lung regions which differ in their mechanical behavior [18, 20]. The global respiratory system compliance may simultaneously determine recruitment of collapsed lung tissue (with increase in regional compliance) and overdistention of already aerated alveolar regions (with decrease in regional compliance) (**Fig. 1**). Thus, increased, decreased or unchanged global compliance will result from the balance of these two opposite regional effects. Imaging techniques such as CT that provide better insights into regional aeration heterogeneities [21, 22], however, cannot be used for bedside monitoring.

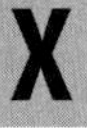

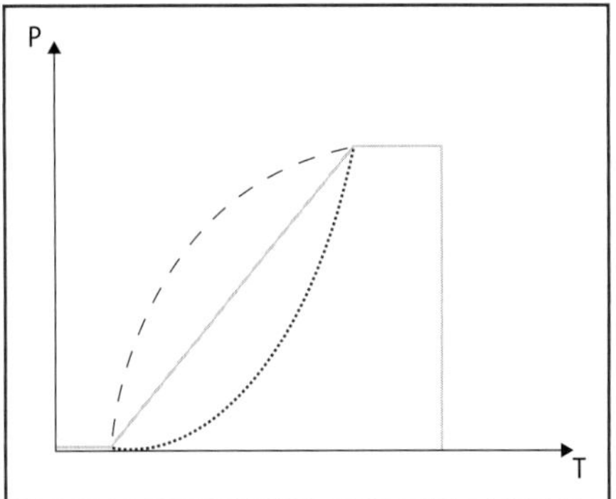

Fig. 1. Pressure-time curves during inflation with a constant flow. Dashed curve: Regional pressure-time curve during recruitment, regional compliance increases when ventilatory units are reopened. Dotted curve: Regional pressure-time curve during hyperinflation, regional compliance decreases when already opened ventilatory units are further inflated. Solid line curve: Global pressure-time curve, overlapping of opposite regional effects, global respiratory system compliance is constant during inflation.

Elecrical Impedance Tomography

Electrical impedance tomography (EIT) of the lungs is a non-invasive monitoring tool that measures relative impedance changes in lung tissue during tidal breathing and creates images of the local ventilation distribution at the bedside [23–25]. The basic principle of image generation is based on the injection of small currents of about 5 mA via surface electrodes applied circumferentially to the thorax in one plane and measurement of potential differences with pairs of passive electrodes which are not used for current injection. Hence, EIT is considered a promising tool to improve ventilatory settings by means of individualization [25–27].

However, EIT delivers complex regional information which is difficult to interpret, especially if there are no scalar parameters derived from the regional images. To overcome this difficulty, a new EIT index (regional ventilation delay index) has recently been proposed and has been shown capable of detecting recruitment during low flow inflation [25].

The Concept of the Regional Ventilation Delay Index

Similar to the global volume-time curve of the respiratory system, the global change in tissue impedance over time reflects a summation over a large number of distinct regions in the lung that may significantly differ from each other regarding their dynamic and functional behavior. Analyzing regional impedance changes over time ($\Delta Z(t)$) provides valuable information about regional lung mechanics in addition to typical parameters of global respiratory mechanics such as compliance or time constants. The concept of the regional ventilation delay index is based on these considerations and contains information about regional lung mechanics [25].

A description of the basic principles of regional ventilation delay index calculation is given in **Figure 2a**. EIT images were recorded during a slow flow inflation maneuver with a tidal volume of 1.2 l. The global impedance-time curve was then calculated as the sum over all impedance changes of the four lung regions of interest (ROI):

$$\Delta Z(t) = \sum_{ROI=1}^{4} dz_{ROI}(t).$$

Finally, the four regional ventilation delay indexes (here: four quadrants) were determined as the delay time between the start of inspiration (i.e., first increase of the global $\Delta Z(t)$ curve) and the time when the respective regional curve $dz_{ROI}(t)$ reaches a threshold of 10 % of the maximal impedance change. To address the fact that the regional ventilation delay indexes would depend on global flow rate of the low flow breath, each regional ventilation delay index was standardized by multiplication with $\Delta Z_{max\text{-}min}/\Delta t_{max\text{-}min}$ (where $\Delta Z_{max\text{-}min}$ is the maximum impedance amplitude of the global $\Delta Z(t)$ curve in arbitrary units, and $\Delta t_{max\text{-}min}$ is the time the inflation maneuver lasts [25]).

The regional ventilation delay index values showed a good correlation with the amount of recruitment of previously non-aerated lung tissue measured by CT during a inflation maneuver with a tidal volume of 1.2 l [25]. Although it seems unlikely that single recruitment maneuvers with a limited volume of 1.2 l influence pulmonary and systemic inflammation in patients with partially derecruited lungs [28], repeated maneuvers, which would be necessary during a PEEP trial in order to optimize ventilatory settings, could increase mechanical stress to the lung tissue. Thus, this original algorithm needed further improvement to integrate the promising concept of regional ventilation delay index into clinical practice.

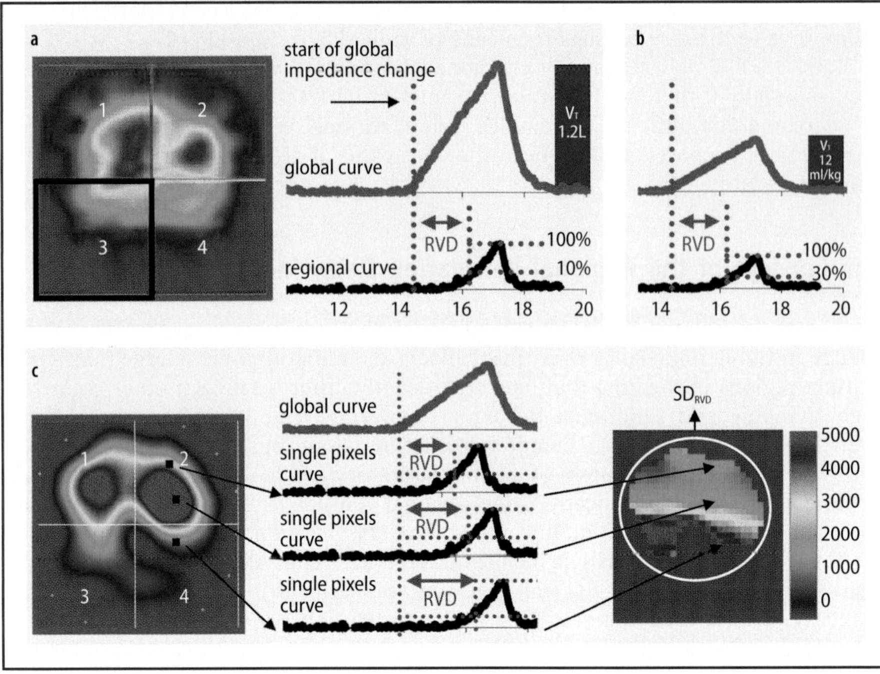

Fig. 2. a Functional image recorded by electrical impedance tomography during a slow flow inflation maneuver with a tidal volume of 1.2 l. Global (red) and regional (black) impedance/time curve. Regional ventilation delay index (RVD) of the right dorsal quadrant: Delay time from start of the global impedance change until regional curve reaches a threshold of 10% of the maximal regional impedance change. **b** to compensate for reduction of tidal volume, threshold for regional ventilation delay index calculation was increased to 30% of the regional impedance change. **c** regional ventilation delay index was calculated for any single pixel and plotted in a color coded map. Standard deviation of all single pixels' regional ventilation delay indexes was calculated to express homogeneity of regional ventilation delay.

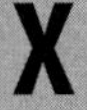

Implementing Regional Ventilation Delay Index in Clinical Practice

In an ongoing animal study, we tested whether the regional ventilation delay index could be calculated from impedance time curves obtained during a 'routinely practicable' slow flow maneuver with a tidal volume of 12 ml/kg body weight. PEEP was changed from zero end-expiratory pressure (ZEEP) to 25 cmH_2O in steps of 5 cmH_2O. Cyclic collapse and potential for alveolar recruitment were calculated from end-expiratory and end-inspiratory spiral CT scans.

The amount of cycling opening and closing lung tissue (tidal recruitment) and the potential for alveolar recruitment decreased when PEEP was increased until a PEEP of 20 cmH_2O was reached (**Fig. 3a**) (preliminary data from a single animal). Further increase in PEEP up to 25 cmH_2O did not further decrease cyclic collapse or potential for alveolar recruitment. The same was true for the amount of non-aerated lung tissue at end-expiration (**Fig. 3b**). In contrast, the end-expiratory gas volume increased whenever PEEP was increased (**Fig. 3b**).

The regional ventilation delay index was calculated from the regional impedance time curves of four equivalent quadrants as described above (**Fig. 2a**). In contrast to

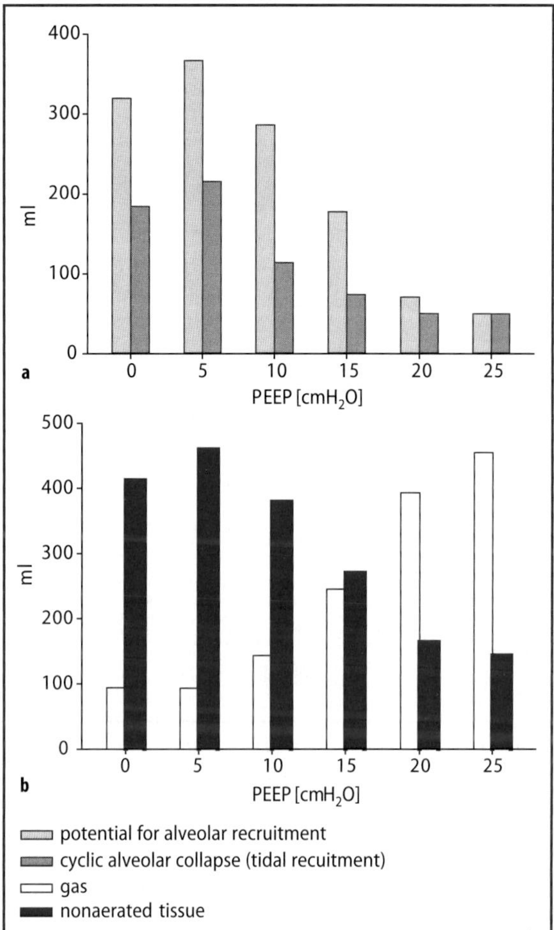

Fig. 3. a Volume of cyclic opening and closing lung tissue (cyclic collapse, tidal recruitment) and potential for alveolar recruitment. **b** volume of non-aerated lung tissue at end-expiration, and end-expiratory gas volume calculated from densitometric computed tomography analysis for any PEEP level.

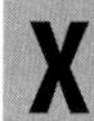

the previous validation study of regional ventilation delay index [25], the tidal volume of the slow flow inflation was reduced from 1.2 l to 360 ml (12 ml/kg body weight). To compensate for the reduction in tidal volume, the threshold for regional ventilation delay index calculation was increased from 10 % to 30 % of the maximal regional impedance change (**Fig. 2b**). Regional ventilation delay index values for all quadrants and all PEEP levels are given in **Figure 4a** (preliminary data). Regional ventilation delay index decreased in all quadrants whenever PEEP was increased without reaching a plateau. Regional ventilation delay index (measured by EIT) and cyclic collapse (obtained by CT) showed an acceptable over all correlation (**Fig. 4a**), but correlation was rather poor in single quadrants (**Fig. 4a**). A PEEP of 20 cmH_2O, which that was chosen from CT analysis to minimize the amount of cyclic collapse, could not be identified as the 'best PEEP' in this analysis of regional ventilation delay index measured in quadrants. Nevertheless, changes in regional ventilation delay index values with changes in PEEP were different in the four quadrants. Whereas the regional ventilation delay index values of the dependent quadrants were substantially different from the non-dependent, this difference was remarkably

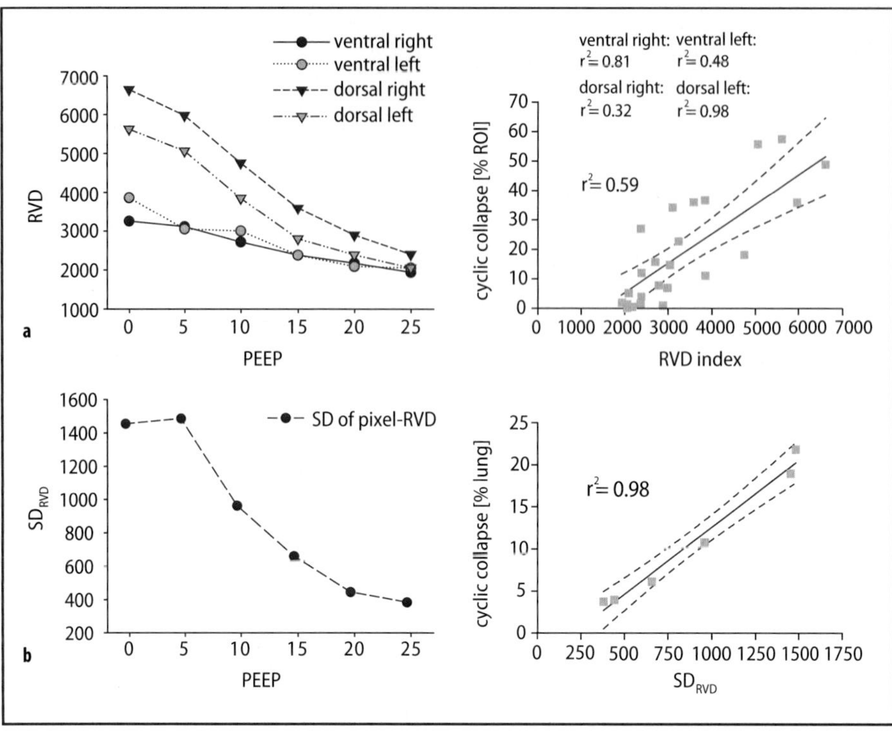

Fig. 4. a Left: Changes in regional ventilation delay index (RVD) measured in four equivalent quadrants during ventilation with PEEP from 0 to 25cm H_2O; right: Correlation between regional ventilation delay index and volume of cyclic collapse for all quadrants during ventilation with PEEP from 0 to 25 cmH_2O. **b** Left: Standard deviation of single pixels' regional ventilation delay index (SD_{RVD}) during ventilation with PEEP from 0 to 25 cmH_2O; right: Correlation between SD_{RVD} and volume of cyclic collapse during ventilation with PEEP from 0 to 25 cmH_2O.

reduced with increasing PEEP. This observation led to the assumption that homogeneity of the quadrants' regional ventilation delay index values might contain more information than the absolute values themselves.

To further improve the measure of homogeneity, a larger number of regional ventilation delay index values needed to be examined. Therefore, new regional ventilation delay index values were calculated based on the regional impedance time curves of single pixels of the dynamic EIT images (which correspond to 3D-regions of approx. $1 \times 1 \times 3$ cm^3 in the thorax). We masked out pixels that contained less than 15 % of the maximal pixel-wise ventilation signal amplitude and applied a temporal low-pass filter for each pixel with a corner frequency of 50 bpm to get rid of heart induced impedance changes. A color-coded map was then plotted to visualize the pixels' regional ventilation delay index values (**Fig. 2c**). To quantify the overall homogeneity, the standard deviation SD_{RVD} over all the single pixel regional ventilation delay index values (RVD_k) was calculated wherein k = 1...M designates all pixels of the above mentioned 15 %-threshold pixel mask and M is the number of pixels in that mask:

$$SD_{RVD} = \sqrt{\frac{\sum_{k=1}^{M} (RVD_k - RVD_{mean})^2}{M-1}} \text{ with } RVD_{mean} = \frac{\sum_{k=1}^{M} RVD_k}{M}$$

PEEP-induced changes in SD_{RVD} and correlation of SD_{RVD} with cyclic collapse are given in **Figure 4b** (preliminary data). SD_{RVD} decreased with increasing PEEP until PEEP of 20 cmH_2O was reached. Further increases in PEEP up to 25 cmH_2O did not further remarkably decrease SD_{RVD}. SD_{RVD} showed an excellent correlation with cyclic collapse ($r^2 = 0.98$, $p < 0.001$) as well as with potential for alveolar recruitment ($r^2 = 0.93$, $p > 0.001$).

Despite reduction of the tidal volume of the slow inflation maneuver from 1.2 l to 12 ml/kg body weight, the new voxel by voxel regional ventilation delay index calculation and analysis, which is independent from an exact position matching with defined CT regions such as quadrants, may provide more information on regional behavior of lung units during PEEP titration.

Conclusion

Since potential for alveolar recruitment cannot be predicted from origin of lung injury, an individual PEEP setting strategy seems to be necessary to reduce cyclic alveolar collapse and avoid end-inspiratory overdistention in mechanically ventilated patients with ALI and ARDS. Global parameters often provide limited or even misleading information. Therefore, regional information about lung function is needed. EIT imaging may be helpful for separating out different regional ventilation behaviors of the lung. This in turn may help optimize ventilator settings. The regional ventilation delay index can be calculated during a 'clinically practicable' slow flow inflation maneuver with a tidal volume of 12 ml/kg body weight. Regarding the information content of different shapes of regional impedance time curves during a slow inflation, our preliminary data suggest that using the SD_{RVD} further improved our previously described method [25] of calculating regional ventilation delay index from quadrants. SD_{RVD} reflects homogeneity of regional lung mechanics and can reliably estimate cyclic opening and closing and the potential for alveolar recruitment of previously non-aerated lung tissue. Further investigations are warranted to evaluate the value of this index for titrating PEEP during lung protective ventilation.

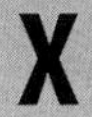

References

1. American Thoracic Society (1999) International Consensus Conferences in Intensive Care Medicine: Ventilator-associated lung injury in ARDS. Am J Respir Crit Care Med 160: 2118–2124
2. Slutsky AS (1999) Lung injury caused by mechanical ventilation. Chest 116:9S-15S
3. Uhlig S (2002) Ventilation-induced lung injury and mechanotransduction: stretching it too far? Am J Physiol Lung Cell Mol Physiol 282:L892-L896
4. The Acute Respiratory Distress Syndrome Network (2000) Ventilation with lower tidal volumes as compared with traditional tidal volumes for acute lung injury and the acute respiratory distress syndrome. N Engl J Med 342: 1301–1308
5. Chu EK, Whitehead T, Slutsky AS (2004) Effects of cyclic opening and closing at low- and high-volume ventilation on bronchoalveolar lavage cytokines. Crit Care Med 32: 168–174
6. Kallet RH, Siobal MS, Alonso JA, Warnecke EL, Katz JA, Marks JD (2001) Lung collapse during low tidal volume ventilation in acute respiratory distress syndrome. Respir Care 46: 49–52
7. Schreiter D, Reske A, Stichert B, et al (2004) Alveolar recruitment in combination with sufficient positive end-expiratory pressure increases oxygenation and lung aeration in patients with severe chest trauma. Crit Care Med 32: 968–975
8. Gattinoni L, Vagginelli F, Chiumello D, Taccone P, Carlesso E (2003) Physiologic rationale for ventilator setting in acute lung injury/acute respiratory distress syndrome patients. Crit Care Med. 31:S300-S304

9. Valenza F, Guglielmi M, Irace M, Porro GA, Sibilla S, Gattinoni L (2003) Positive end-expiratory pressure delays the progression of lung injury during ventilator strategies involving high airway pressure and lung overdistention. Crit Care Med 31: 1993 – 1998
10. Plotz FB, Slutsky AS, van Vught AJ, Heijnen CJ (2004) Ventilator-induced lung injury and multiple system organ failure: a critical review of facts and hypotheses. Intensive Care Med 30: 1865 – 1872
11. Brower RG, Lanken PN, MacIntyre N, et al (2004) Higher versus lower positive end-expiratory pressures in patients with the acute respiratory distress syndrome. N Engl J Med 351: 327 – 336
12. Meade MO, Cook DJ, Guyatt GH, et al (2008) Ventilation strategy using low tidal volumes, recruitment maneuvers, and high positive end-expiratory pressure for acute lung injury and acute respiratory distress syndrome: a randomized controlled trial. JAMA 299: 637 – 645
13. Mercat A, Richard JC, Vielle B, et al (2008) Positive end-expiratory pressure setting in adults with acute lung injury and acute respiratory distress syndrome: a randomized controlled trial. JAMA 299: 646 – 655
14. Gattinoni L, Caironi P, Cressoni M, et al (2006) Lung recruitment in patients with the acute respiratory distress syndrome. N Engl J Med 354: 1775 – 1786
15. Thille AW, Richard JC, Maggiore SM, Ranieri VM, Brochard L (2007) Alveolar recruitment in pulmonary and extrapulmonary acute respiratory distress syndrome: comparison using pressure-volume curve or static compliance. Anesthesiology 106: 212 – 217
16. Lynch JP, Mhyre JG, Dantzker DR (1979) Influence of cardiac output on intrapulmonary shunt. J Appl Physiol 46: 315 – 321
17. Henzler D, Pelosi P, Dembinski R, et al (2005) Respiratory compliance but not gas exchange correlates with changes in lung aeration after a recruitment maneuver: an experimental study in pigs with saline lavage lung injury. Crit Care 9:R471-R482
18. Jonson B, Richard JC, Straus C, Mancebo J, Lemaire F, Brochard L (1999) Pressure-volume curves and compliance in acute lung injury: evidence of recruitment above the lower inflection point. Am J Respir Crit Care Med 159: 1172 – 1178
19. Grasso S, Terragni P, Mascia L, et al (2004) Airway pressure-time curve profile (stress index) detects tidal recruitment/hyperinflation in experimental acute lung injury. Crit Care Med 32: 1018 – 1027

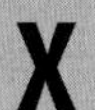

20. Hickling KG (1998) The pressure-volume curve is greatly modified by recruitment. A mathematical model of ARDS lungs. Am J Respir Crit Care Med 158: 194 – 202
21. Gattinoni L, Caironi P, Pelosi P, Goodman LR (2001) What has computed tomography taught us about the acute respiratory distress syndrome? Am J Respir Crit Care Med 164: 1701 – 1711
22. Rouby JJ, Puybasset L, Nieszkowska A, Lu Q (2003) Acute respiratory distress syndrome: lessons from computed tomography of the whole lung. Crit Care Med 31:S285-S295
23. Brown BH, Barber DC, Seagar AD (1985) Applied potential tomography: possible clinical applications. Clin Phys Physiol Meas 6: 109 – 121
24. Wolf GK, Arnold JH (2005) Noninvasive assessment of lung volume: respiratory inductance plethysmography and electrical impedance tomography. Crit Care Med 33:S163-S169
25. Wrigge H, Zinserling J, Muders T, et al (2008) Electrical impedance tomography compared with thoracic computed tomography during a slow inflation maneuver in experimental models of lung injury. Crit Care Med 36: 903 – 909
26. Luepschen H, Meier T, Grossherr M, Leibecke T, Karsten J, Leonhardt S (2007) Protective ventilation using electrical impedance tomography. Physiol Meas 28:S247-S260
27. Meier T, Luepschen H, Karsten J, et al (2008) Assessment of regional lung recruitment and derecruitment during a PEEP trial based on electrical impedance tomography. Intensive Care Med 34: 543 – 550
28. Puls A, Pollok-Kopp B, Wrigge H, Quintel M, Neumann P (2006) Effects of a single-lung recruitment maneuver on the systemic release of inflammatory mediators. Intensive Care Med 32: 1080 – 1085

Different Approaches to the Analysis of Volumetric Capnography

F. Suarez Sipmann, S.H. Böhm, and G. Tusman

Introduction

Lung mechanics and arterial blood gases are the two most common categories of variables used to assess lung function and to adjust mechanical ventilation. Analyzing the kinetics of carbon dioxide (CO_2) is another attractive approach to monitor patients receiving mechanical ventilation. CO_2 is eliminated from the blood by diffusing through the alveolar-capillary membrane. By knowing how CO_2 behaves on its way to the ambient air, physicians can obtain useful information about ventilation, perfusion, diffusion, and also convection. Despite the fact that capnography has been an essential part of monitoring during general anesthesia surprisingly it has never gained widespread use in intensive care medicine.

Capnography: Types and Applications

Time-based capnography or simply capnography represents the plot of exhaled CO_2 over time. Capnography has improved over the last few decades thanks to the development of faster infrared sensors that can measure CO_2 at the airway opening in real-time. Capnography was originally described as a means to estimate $PaCO_2$, although anesthesiologists quickly discovered its usefulness for answering many other clinical questions, such as apnea detection, esophageal intubation, or disconnection from the anesthetic circuit, to guide cardiopulmonary resuscitation (CPR) maneuvers, or to evaluate CO_2 re-absorption from capnoperitoneum to name but a few.

Another type of CO_2 monitoring is volume-based capnography, called volumetric capnography or single-breath test of CO_2 (SBT-CO_2). Volumetric capnography is the plot of expired volume of CO_2 over a single breath (**Fig. 1**).

Volumetric capnography constitutes a particularly interesting clinical tool that reflects the body's metabolism, lung perfusion, and ventilation. The rationale is that CO_2 is produced by cell metabolism, is transported to the lungs by the pulmonary blood flow, and is exclusively eliminated by the lung's ventilation. Therefore, under stable metabolic conditions, it can be assumed that volumetric capnography reflects the ventilation/perfusion relationship of the lungs.

In essence, volumetric capnography is the same as time-based capnography but enriched by specific 'volumetric' parameters like the amount of CO_2 eliminated (VCO_2), different kinds of dead spaces, and the chance to measure cardiac output using the re-breathing CO_2 technique. Volumetric capnography-derived parameters can be classified as invasive or non-invasive depending on whether a $PaCO_2$ value is needed or not.

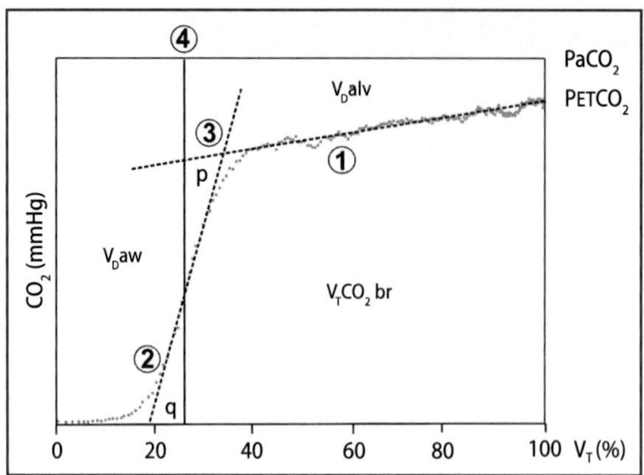

Fig. 1. Fowler's method and the Bohr-Enghoff formula applied to the volumetric capnogram. Using both these methods, a geometric representation of the dead spaces (V_D) as described by Fletcher can be drawn as shown. Fowler's method determines the position of the airway-alveolar interface as follows: (1) slope of phase III by linear regression using the data between the 40–80 % points of the expired volume; (2) the slope of phase II is calculated between the end of phase I and the 40 % tidal volume (V_T) point; (3) the intersection of lines 1 and 2 defines the limit between phase II and III; and (4) a perpendicular line is projected onto the x-axis and its position adjusted until the areas p and q on both side of it become equal.

Invasive Volumetric Capnography Variables

Dead space (V_D) describes the fraction of 'wasted' ventilation or the portion of the tidal volume (V_T) that does not participate in gas exchange. Studying this 'inefficiency' of ventilation is the best way to assess the effects of particular ventilator settings in mechanically ventilated patients. Volumetric capnography analysis by Fowler's method [1] and its modification suggested by Bohr and Enghoff [2, 3] are the standard ways to calculate dead space. The Bohr-Enghoff formula is described below:

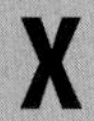

V_D/V_T = $FACO_2$ – $FeCO_2/FACO_2$ *Bohr (1891)*
V_D/V_T = $PaCO_2$ – $PeCO_2/PaCO_2$ *Enghoff (1938)*

where $FACO_2$ represents the alveolar fraction of CO_2, $FeCO_2$ the mixed concentration of CO_2 in the expired gas, and $PaCO_2$ the partial pressure of CO_2 in the arterial blood. Fraction (F) or partial pressure (P) can be used interchangeably in these formulas.

The dead space ratio (V_D/V_T) can then be separated into its subcomponents:

$V_D$phys = ($PaCO_2$ – $PeCO_2/PaCO_2$) × V_T
$V_D$alv = $V_D$phys – $V_D$aw

where $V_D$phys is the physiological dead space, which represents the total dead space within one single breath. It is constituted by the airway dead space ($V_D$aw), the gas in the main airways that is free of CO_2, and by the alveolar dead space ($V_D$alv) comprising the wasted ventilation within the alveolar compartment. The instrumental dead space represents any volumes placed between the endotracheal tube and the 'Y' piece of the ventilator's circuit and is added to the $V_D$aw naturally found within the body. This instrumental dead space becomes particularly important in small pediatric patients.

Recently, volumetric capnography and the V_D/V_T ratio have attracted increased interest in critical care medicine due to the role these parameters could play as independent prognostic factors for mortality of patients with acute respiratory distress syndrome (ARDS) [4]. Complete dead space analysis also proved useful to monitor lung recruitment maneuvers and PEEP titration in ARDS [5].

Non-invasive Volumetric Capnography Variables

It must be remembered that volumetric capnography is not centered solely on the determination of dead spaces and that non-invasive volumetric capnography derived-parameters also play an important role. In fact, most of the clinical usefulness of volumetric capnography that has been described is derived from its non-invasive parameters. The non-invasive parameters are those related to volumes or the shape of the volumetric capnography graphic, like the area under the curve (or V_TCO_2br), the slopes of phases II (S_{II}) and III (S_{III}), and the partial pressures of CO_2 at different points of the curve, like the end-tidal concentration of CO_2 ($PETCO_2$), the mean alveolar CO_2 ($PAECO_2$), or the $PeCO_2$.

Almost all the published usefulness of time and volume based capnography as clinical monitors is related to the 'shape' of these curves. For example: 1) acute arterial hypotension due to a pulmonary embolism shows a fast decrement in V_TCO_2br and $PETCO_2$ together with a leveling of S_{III} [6]; 2) a patient's inspiratory effort can be detected as a notch in the alveolar plateau phase; 3) pulmonary perfusion during weaning from extracorporeal circulation can be evaluated by the size of the area under the volumetric capnography curve [7].

Another important non-invasive calculation using volumetric capnography is the pulmonary elimination of CO_2:

$$VCO_2 = V_TCO_2br \times \text{respiratory rate (ml/minute)}$$

During steady state conditions, this variable is identical to the metabolic production of CO_2 that would be measured by a metabolic monitor provided the pulmonary perfusion and ventilation are maintained within the normal range. As CO_2 elimination depends on both lung ventilation and perfusion any decrement in these variables will decrease the VCO_2 value irrespective of the body's metabolic state.

The V_TCO_2br together with the $PETCO_2$ are used for the non-invasive calculation of cardiac output. The partial CO_2 re-breathing technique deliberately introduces changes in V_TCO_2br and $PETCO_2$ from which cardiac output can be calculated applying the Fick principle [8, 9]. However, the truth is that this method measures the non-shunted portion of cardiac output or 'effective pulmonary perfusion' since only the ventilated and perfused alveoli are able to eliminate CO_2. Therefore, this technique will show a good correlation with other cardiac output measurements only in patients with low shunt fractions.

The Bohr dead space [10] is other non-invasive volumetric capnography variable calculated as:

$$V_DBohr/V_T = PETCO_2 - PeCO_2/\ PETCO_2$$

This dead space includes only part of the V_Dalv while the shunt-related dead space (i.e., the apparent alveolar dead space effect created by shunt), is not considered by this formula. Therefore, V_DBohr does not have the same clinical value as the V_D/V_T calculated by the Bohr-Enghoff equation, although it can give a rough estimate of the efficiency of ventilation in real-time and in a non-invasive way.

S_{III} is one of the most promising non-invasive volumetric capnography derived-variables because it is mainly determined by the gas exchanging part of the lungs. The origin of this slope has been under debate for many years. Today, it is generally accepted that both ventilation and perfusion contribute to its positive slope. Ventilatory maldistribution caused by convection- and diffusion-dependent inhomogeneities in CO_2 transport, is the most important factor in the genesis of S_{III} [11–13].

X

Lung perfusion is in part also responsible for S_{III} since it continuously delivers CO_2 molecules that diffuse from the capillaries into alveoli [14]. The amount of pulmonary blood flow, but also its regional distribution within the lung, seems to play an important role, too [7]. Therefore, S_{III} has correctly been associated with the ventilation/perfusion (V/Q) relationship of the lungs.

Knowing the above concepts, S_{III} has become an attractive tool due to its non-invasiveness and ease of calculation at the bedside in real time. Increasing slopes have been related to bronchospasm [15, 16], lung destruction in chronic obstructive pulmonary disease (COPD) [17], lung growth [18], and lung perfusion [7].

It is obvious that the success of volumetric capnography as a clinical monitor depends on the quality of CO_2 and flow sensors – their time-response, resolution, accuracy, ease of the calibration procedure, and finally the synchronization between both signals. Additionally, the methodology for analyzing invasive as well as non-invasive volumetric capnography-derived parameters should be robust, reproducible, and easy to apply by computational means.

Techniques for Volumetric Capnography Analysis

There are a few different techniques for analyzing volumetric capnography. The most popular is the one proposed by Fowler in 1948 using nitrogen (N_2) instead of CO_2 [1]. Fowler developed a geometric representation of the original Bohr formula to detect the limit between conducting airways and the alveolar compartments. He determined by hand a vertical line that crossed the mid-portion of phase II thereby creating two equal areas on both sides of the expired N_2 curve. In this way, the expired tidal volume could be separated into two portions: 1) the airway dead space ($V_D$aw), i.e., the gas representing the conducting airways, and 2) the alveolar tidal volume ($V_T$alv), i.e., the part of the tidal volume that came from the alveolar compartment.

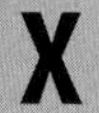

The availability of faster airflow and CO_2 sensors facilitated the application of both the Bohr-Enghoff and the Fowler concept. By combining both methods, a complete dead space calculation based on the analysis of one single breath became possible instead of having to collect expired gases in a Douglas bag for minutes (Bohr's technique). However, it was Enghoff's modification of Bohr's formula that introduced dead space measurements into the clinical arena [3]. Taking $PaCO_2$ as a surrogate for alveolar PCO_2 had practical advantages and made Bohr's concept easily applicable in patients.

Various authors [19, 20] have developed volumetric capnography as the standard for dead space analysis using the above concepts. Fletcher and Jonson's modification of Fowler's concept, in which areas of trapezoids represent dead space subdivisions, has became the most popular method for dead space analysis over the last few decades. However, for this method to become part of clinical routine, the 'manual' Fowler method must be automated by implementing it as a computational algorithm in order to suppress operator-dependent subjectivity. It is important to note that these computational 'implementations', and not Fowler's method itself, are prone to errors that might limit the clinical usefulness of volumetric capnography derived-variables. This is also true for methodologies, such as Fletcher's method, that are based on a geometrical analysis of volumetric capnography.

The key for any volumetric capnography analysis is to determine with precision the boundary between $V_T$alv and $V_D$aw or, in other words, they must be able to differentiate gas coming from the alveolar from that of the airway compartment. This boundary or stationary interface is located close to the respiratory bronchioli at the end of inspiration and moves in a mouthward direction during expiration. The interface is recovered at the airway opening by the CO_2 and flow sensors of the capnograph during expiration. By convention, the mid portion of phase II corresponds to such a limit [12, 20, 21] and thus we call it the 'airway-alveolar interface'. Any error in the assumed location of this airway-alveolar interface will affect the magnitude of most of the volumetric capnography-derived variables, such as $V_D$alv or the calculation of alveolar ventilation. To localize the interface more accurately, most of the practical implementations of Fowler's concept follow a series of sequential steps. These steps vary in different implementations and only the most common will be summarized here (**Fig. 1**):

1. S_{III} is calculated by linear regression using a fixed portion of the volumetric capnography data, commonly that between 40 and 80 % of the expired volume.
2. The maximum S_{II} is then calculated by linear regression also using a fixed portion of the volumetric capnography curve, commonly from the start of CO_2 elimination (limit between phase I and II) and 40 % of the expired volume.
3. Afterwards, lines representing phases II and III are drawn looking for their intersection, since this point represents the limit between phase II and III.
4. The position of the airway-alveolar interface is then calculated by placing a vertical line by iteratively searching between the start of phase II and its boundary to the right so that area p and area q become equal.

Two main sources of error can be observed when using this kind of interface analysis: One is the cumulative error that results from such a sequence of stepwise calculations, especially in the presence of a noisy phase III; the other is related to the analysis of volumetric capnography-derived parameters based on a fixed portion of the curve. This fact is responsible for erroneous calculations in patients with highly deformed volumetric capnography curves, such as COPD patients or when high levels of PEEP are used (see below and **Fig. 3**). X

There are other published ways of calculating the airway-alveolar interface, including the 'threshold' method described by Olsson et al. [22]. Using this technique, $V_D$aw is determined by the point at which a fixed threshold of CO_2 concentration is reached at the beginning of expiration. This method, however, systematically underestimates $V_D$aw because the calculation is based on phase I while the airway-alveolar interface belongs to phase II.

Other methods, like those suggested by Hatch et al. [23], Langley et al. [24], Cumming and Guyatt [25], and Bowes et al. [26], are based on data belonging to phase III. In contrast to the previous methods, these calculations systematically overestimate $V_D$aw because the airway-alveolar interface is erroneously displaced towards the right. However, Tang et al. [27] have elegantly demonstrated that the integration of the expired volume of CO_2 over the expired volume (Hatch-Langley method) reduces noise and make this method more precise than Fowler's technique.

Wolff et al. [28] have pointed out many of the inherent limitations of the above techniques in determining the airway-alveolar interface. These authors came up with an alternative method called the 'pre-interface expirate'. This method uses data from phase II until the point where the CO_2 concentration reaches half the $PETCO_2$ value. The first derivative of the selected raw data is calculated and plotted against the expired volume. The mean value of this distribution constitutes the pre-interface expirate. When using this method in volumetric capnograms with higher phase III slopes, unreasonably high $V_D aw$ values are obtained. This negative influence was eliminated by systematic compensation for the alveolar slope as described by the same authors and by Åström et al. [29].

Recently, Tang et al. [27] have described another modification of the 'equal area method' that fits with the results obtained by Fowler's and Fletcher's techniques. Nonetheless, even this newest modification has not overcome the intrinsic limitations that all these techniques show when confronted with deformed capnograms.

From a technical point of view, the remaining non-invasive variables like the $V_T CO_2 br$ (integration of the CO_2-flow signals) or a specific CO_2 point within the volumetric capnogram, such as the $PETCO_2$ or the $PAECO_2$, are easily calculated.

A New Algorithm for Volumetric Capnography Analysis

The volumetric capnogram is an asymmetrical sigmoid curve that can be represented by a mathematical function. Fitting an equation to measured clinical volumetric capnography data provides a systematic methodology to characterize volumetric capnography curves and to calculate the parameters derived from them in a reproducible way. We present a functional approximation of the volumetric capnography curve using acquired raw data [30]. This continuous real-valued function is obtained by non-linear least square curve fitting. Numerical algorithms are used to derive parameters from sets of non-linear data. Least squares fitting of an appropriate curve to volumetric capnography raw data can be viewed as an optimization problem; it will result in a proposed model function. This model function is based on a generalized logistic curve known as Richards' curve [31], which can be written as:

X

$$f(t,x) = f_0(t,\mathbf{x}) + f_1(t,\mathbf{x}) + f_2(t,\mathbf{x});$$

where:

$$f_0(t,\mathbf{x}) = x_1;$$

$$f_1(t,\mathbf{x}) = \frac{(x_2 - x_1)\,x_3}{(1 + e^{(-t-x_4/x_5)})};$$

$$f_2(t,\mathbf{x}) = \frac{(x_2 - x_1)(1 - x_3)}{(1 + e^{(-t-x_6/x_7)})};$$

The first term, $f_0(t,\mathbf{x})$, is the lower asymptote, the second and third terms are logistic curves, whose parameterization allows the generation of a model of the volumetric capnography curve, where t is the expired volume and f = concentration of CO_2. This model considers the well-known asymmetry of the shape of the volumetric capnography curve (**Fig. 2a**).

The parameters of the above model were found by a non-linear least square curve fitting obtained by the Levenberg-Marquardt algorithm [32, 33]. **Figure 2b** shows how volumetric capnography derived-parameters are calculated from this function. The definition of each of the parameters is based on the known physiological meaning it represents and which has been described in the literature:

- *Phase I* is the portion of the tidal volume free of CO_2 at the beginning of expiration, which belongs to the apparatus and in part to airway dead space. It is calculated from the end of inspiration (determined by the flow signal) until the

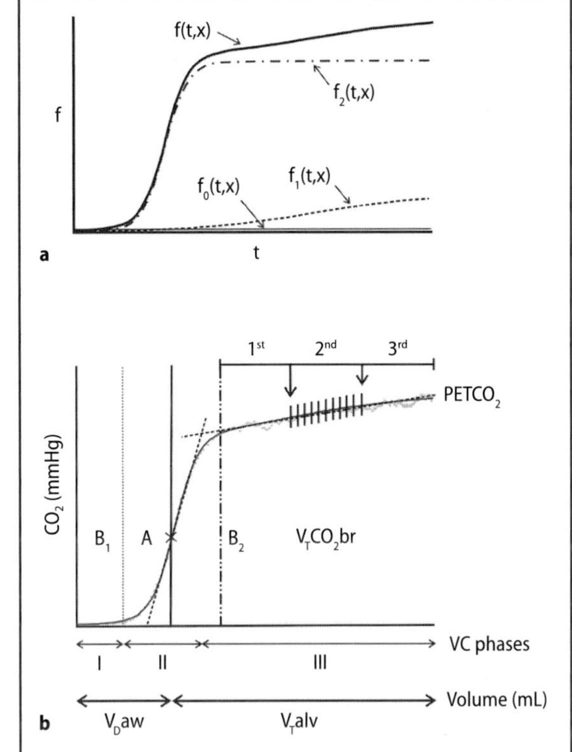

Fig. 2. a The model function where t is the expired volume and f = the concentration of CO_2. The first term $f_0(t,\mathbf{x})$ is the lower asymptote, the second $f_1(t,\mathbf{x})$ and third terms $f_2(t,\mathbf{x})$ are logistic curves, whose parameterization allows the generation of a model of the volumetric capnography (VC) curve.
b New analysis obtained by applying the Levenberg-Marquardt algorithm. The solid line represents the function [$f(t,\mathbf{x})$], which is closely fitted with the raw data (dots). The inflection point of the entire volumetric capnogram (A) defines the position of the airway-alveolar interface and thus the limit between airway dead space ($V_D$aw) and alveolar tidal volume ($V_T$alv). The limit between phases I and II is formed by the point of maximum rate of change of the 2nd derivative or left extreme of the 3rd derivative (B_1). B_2 is the right extreme of the 3rd derivative, from which the slope of phase III is calculated. The alveolar plateau ranging from line B_2 until PETCO$_2$ is divided into three equal segments. The middle third is again divided into ten equal sub-segments and their respective slopes are calculated as their 1st derivatives. The mean value of such 10 slopes constituted S_{III}. The intersection of the lines representing the slopes of phases II and III defines the limit between phases II and III. $V_TCO_2$br is the area under the curve.

start of CO_2 elimination coinciding with the point of maximum rate of change of the 2nd derivative (left extreme of the 3rd derivative – line B_1).

- *Phase II* constitutes the part of the tidal volume where a progressively increasing concentration of CO_2 is coming from lung units with different rates of ventilation and perfusion. This phase extends from the above point of maximum rate of change to the intersection of the lines representing the slopes of phases II and III.
- *Phase III* represents pure alveolar gas. It extends from the above intersection until the PETCO$_2$.
- The *airway-alveolar interface* between convective and diffusive CO_2 transport within the lungs is, by convention, placed around the midpoint of phase II [8]. This point is mathematically determined by the *inflection point* of the entire volumetric capnography curve, i.e., the point on a curve at which the curvature changed its sign.
- S_{II} is determined as the value of the 1st derivative at the inflection point (A).
- *Alpha angle* is defined by trigonometry as the angle between the regression lines representing phase II and phase III and the knowledge about their point of intersection.

- S_{III} is calculated as follows: First, B_2 is defined as the right extreme of the 3rd derivative constituting the left border of the segment, from which the slope of phase III could be calculated. Second, phase III data beyond the right of such line B_2 until the $PETCO_2$ value are divided into three equal thirds. Third, the middle third is used to calculate S_{III} because it is located safely away from any interference that the alpha angle and possible phase IV might exert on the volumetric capnogram. This middle segment is then divided into ten equidistant sections and their respective individual slopes are calculated as their 1st derivatives. The mean value of these 10 slopes finally constitutes S_{III}.
- $V_D aw$ is taken as the volume at which the vertical line running through point A crosses the x axis.
- $V_T alv$ is derived from the calculation of V_T minus $V_D$aw.
- $V_T CO_2 br$ or area under the curve of the volumetric capnogram represents the amount of CO_2 eliminated by a breath. It is calculated from the symbolic integration of the analytic function *f(t)*.
- $PETCO_2$ is the concentration or partial pressure of CO_2 at the end of expiration and is read as the value immediately before the start of inspiration.

The main advantages of the proposed method can be summarized as follows: First, the position of the airway-alveolar interface is obtained by a robust, although simple mathematical calculation from the derived function, which takes all available data points into account. It is placed at the mathematical inflection point of the entire volumetric capnography curve. Second, all volumetric capnography derived-parameters (except the limit between phases II and III) are calculated independently from each other, using the function obtained by the Levenberg-Marquardt algorithm. This approach avoids accumulative errors in the calculation of variables that are dependent on others (e.g., $V_D$aw using the Fowler's method). Third, a deformation of the volumetric capnogram caused by disease does not affect the performance of the calculations to the same extent as typically seen with other methods because their volumetric capnography analysis is mainly based on a particular and fixed portion of the curve. The new method proposed in this chapter avoids this problem because it is dynamically adapted to the shape of each individual curve.

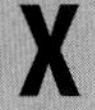

Figure 3 shows how S_{III} calculation using a fixed portion of the tidal volume is prone to error if capnograms are highly deformed as in these examples. **Figure 3a** shows a 'normal-shaped' volumetric capnogram that belongs to a patient treated with 10 cmH_2O of PEEP and adding an instrumental dead space of 25 ml that displaced the airway-alveolar interface to the right. **Figure 3b** belongs to an animal with an acute lung injury, where the limit between phases II and III is clearly blurred and S_{III} is rather high. In both these examples, the determination of S_{III} according to Fowler's traditional method would have included parts of phase II and the alpha angle within the 40–80 % region of the tidal volume, causing an erroneous overestimation of S_{III} (dotted lines A) and also a subsequent error in the $V_D$aw.

The new methodology avoids these obvious interferences because the middle third of phase III is far away from the extremes of the alveolar plateau. **Figure 3** shows how the new method, based on the Levenberg-Marquardt algorithm, is dynamically adapted to the shape of each curve. As explained above, S_{III} calculation starts safely beyond the alpha angle and ends before a possible phase IV could interfer (solid lines B).

Fourth, the new approach suggested here helps to decrease the variability in S_{III} calculation due to cardiogenic oscillations. These oscillations are produced by the

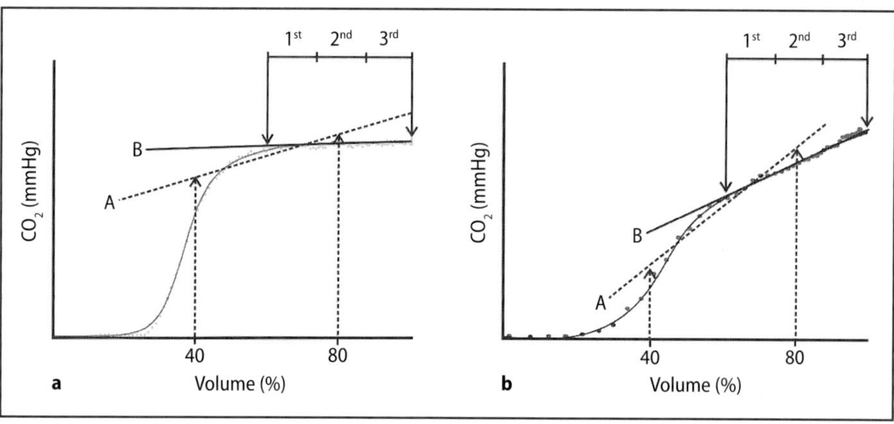

Fig. 3. Two examples (left and right panels) of phase III slopes as determined by the classical Fowler method (A, dotted lines) and by the novel method proposed in this chapter (B, closed lines). Note the erroneously high slopes of lines A that result from using a fixed portion of the expired volume in these deformed capnograms (for more details please refer to the text).

heartbeat and are a source of 'noise' in the flow and CO_2 signals. At times, large cardiogenic oscillations may affect the quality of the volumetric capnography curves considerably. Our method has the theoretical advantage of stabilizing S_{III} calculations even in the presence of cardiogenic oscillations because we are using a mean value of 10 different section measurements within the alveolar plateau.

The novel analysis of the volumetric capnography curve reduces inconsistencies in the calculations of both invasive and non-invasive parameters. This methodology has been tested and corroborated in preliminary data from patients [30]. With the rapid advances being made in sensor and computing technology, this novel method could, in the future, be implemented in real-time for clinical applications.

X

Conclusion

Volumetric capnography gives continuous and non-invasive information on the efficiency of gas exchange and the underlying processes of perfusion and ventilation in mechanically ventilated patients. Both, invasive and non-invasive volumetric capnography-derived parameters need to be determined by a method of analysis that will overcome the known limitations of current techniques. In this chapter, we propose a new methodology that is based on a mathematical function that fits all parts of the the original volumetric capnography curve and calculates parameters with robustness and accuracy. Reducing measurement-dependent variability opens new possibilities to further exploit the potential of volumetric capnography as a powerful non-invasive monitoring tool during mechanical ventilation. The future challenge will be to implement such analysis in real-time bedside monitoring.

References

1. Fowler WS (1948) Lung function studies. II. The respiratory dead space. Am J Physiol 154: 405–416
2. Bohr C (1981) Ueber die lungenathmung. Skand Archiv Physiol 2: 236–242
3. Enghoff H (1938) Volumen inefficax. Bemerkungen zur Frage des schädlichen Raumes. Uppsala Läkareforen Forhandl 44: 191–218
4. Nuckton TJ, Alonso JA, Kallet RH, et al (2002) Pulmonary dead-space fraction as a risk factor for death in the acute respiratory distress syndrome. N Engl J Med 346: 1281–1286
5. Tusman G, Suarez Sipmann F, Böhm SH, et al (2006) Monitoring dead space during recruitment and PEEP titration in an experimental model. Intensive Care Med 32: 1863–1871
6. Verschuren F, Liistro G, Coffeng R, et al (2004) Volumetric capnography as a screening test for pulmonary embolism in the emergency department. Chest 125: 841–850
7. Tusman G, Areta M, Climente C, et al (2005) Effect of pulmonary perfusion on the slopes of single-breath test of CO_2. J Appl Physiol 99: 650–655
8. Capek JM, Roy RJ (1988) Non-invasive measurements of cardiac output during partial CO_2 rebreathing. IEEE Trans Biomed Eng 35: 653–661
9. Peyton PJ, Venkatesan Y, Hood SG, Junor P, May C (2006) Noninvasive, automated and continuous cardiac output monitoring by pulmonary capnodynamics. Anesthesiology 105: 72–80
10. Rossier PH, Buhlmann A (1955) The respiratory dead space. Physiol Rev 58: 1840–1848
11. Crawford ABH, Makowska M, Paiva M, Engel LA (1985) Convection-dependent and diffusion-dependent ventilation maldistribution in normal subjects. J Appl Physiol 59: 838–846
12. Engel LA (1983) Gas mixing within acinus of the lung. J Appl Physiol 54: 609–618
13. Verbank S, Paiva M (1990) Model simulations of gas mixing and ventilation distribution in the human lung. J Appl Physiol 69: 2269–2279
14. Schwardt JF, Gobran SR, Neufeld GR, Aukburg SJ, Scherer PW (1991) Sensitivity of CO_2 washout to changes in acinar structure in a single-path model of lung airways. Ann Biomed Eng 19: 679–697
15. Blanch LL, Fernandez R, Saura P, Baigorri F, Artigas A (1999) Relationship between expired capnogram and respiratory system resistance in critically ill patients during total ventilatory support. Eur Respir J 13: 1048–1054
16. You B, Peslin R, Duvivier C, et al (1994) Expiratory capnography in asthma: evaluation of various shape indices. Eur Respir J 7: 318–323
17. Schwardt JD, Neufeld GR, Baumgardner JE, Scherer PW (1994) Noninvasive recovery of acinar anatomic information from CO_2 expirograms. Ann Biomed Eng 22: 293–306
18. Ream RS, Screiner MS, Neff JD, et al (1995) Volumetric capnography in children: influence of growth on the alveolar plateau slope. Anesthesiology 82: 64–73
19. Folkow B, Pappenheimer IR (1955) Components of the respiratory dead space and their variation with pressure breathing and with bronchoactive drugs. J Appl Physiol 8: 102–110
20. Fletcher R, Jonson B (1981) The concept of deadspace with special reference to the single breath test for carbon dioxide. Br J Anaesth 53: 77–88
21. Gomez DM (1965) A physico-mathematical study of lung function in normal subjects and in patients with obstructive pulmonary diseases. Med Thorac 22: 275–294
22. Olsson SG, Fletcher R, Jonson B, Nordstroem L, Prakash O (1980) Clinical studies of gas exchange during ventilatory support – a method using the Siemens-Elema CO2 analyzer. Br J Anaesth 52: 491–498
23. Hatch T, Cook KM, Palm PE (1953) Respiratory dead space. J Appl Physiol 5: 341–347
24. Langley F, Even P, Duroux P, Nicolas RL, Cumming G (1975) Ventilatory consequences of unilateral pulmonary artery occlusion. Les colloques de L'Institut National de la Santé et de la Recherche Medicale 51: 209–214
25. Cumming G, Guyatt AR (1982) Alveolar gas mixing efficiency in the human lung. Clin Sci (Lond) 62: 541–547
26. Bowes K. CL, Richardson JD, Cumming G, Horsfield K (1985) Effect of breathing pattern on gas mixing in a model of asymmetrical alveolar ducts. J Appl Physiol 58: 18–26
27. Tang Y, Turner MJ, Baker AB (2007) Systematic errors and susceptibility to noise of four methods for calculating anatomical dead space from the CO2 expirogram. Br J Anaesth 98: 828–834

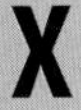

28. Wolff G, Brunner JX, Weibel W, Bowes CL, Muchenberger R, Bertschmann W (1989) Anatomical and series dead space volume: concept and measurement in clinical praxis. Appl Cardiopul Pathophysiol 2: 299–307
29. Åström E, Nicklason L, Drefeldt B, Bajc M, Jonson B (2000) Partitioning of dead space – a method of reference values in the awake human. Eur Respir J 16: 659–664
30. Scandurra AG, Maldonado EA, Dai Para AL, Tusman G, Passoni LI (2008) Modelo híbrido para la aproximación funcional de registros de capnografía volumétrica. XIV Congreso Latino Ibero Americano de Investigación de Operaciones (abst)
31. Richards FJ (1989) A flexible growth function for empirical use. J Exp Bot 10: 290–300.
32. Levenberg, K (1944) A method for the solution of certain problems in least squares. Quart Appl Math 2: 164–168.
33. Marquardt D (1963) An algorithm for least-squares estimation of nonlinear parameters. SIAM J Appl Math 11: 431–441

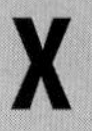

Variation in Extravascular Lung Water in ALI/ARDS Patients using Open Lung Strategy

F.J. Belda, G. Aguilar, and C. Ferrando

Introduction

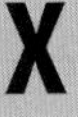

Acute lung injury (ALI) and acute respiratory distress syndrome (ARDS) are progressive forms of acute respiratory failure occurring as a result of diffuse lung inflammation. This is characterized by damage to the alveolar-capillary barrier producing alterations in permeability and pulmonary edema. The diagnosis of ALI/ARDS is based on the presence of both pulmonary and non-pulmonary risk factors and acute hypoxemia with bilateral pulmonary infiltrates on chest x-ray, not due primarily to left ventricular hypertension [1]. These current American-European Consensus Conference (AECC) definitions for ALI/ARDS, used since 1994, have been questioned over the past few years. The PaO_2/FiO_2 ratio varies with ventilator settings and should be measured by predetermined standard settings (positive end-expiratory pressure [PEEP] 10 cmH_2O and FiO_2 0.5) [2]. For the radiographic criteria, not only is there high inter-observer variability, even when used by expert investigators [3], but these criteria have also been shown to be a poor indicator of pulmonary edema. Most importantly, the use of a value for the pulmonary artery occlusion pressure (PAOP) of < 18 mmHg to exclude heart failure is of dubious value. Obviously ARDS patients can also suffer from acute heart failure, although this is not the primary cause for the pulmonary edema. In fact, more than 35 % of patients with ALI/ARDS have a PAOP > 18 mmHg. On the other hand, 21–35 % of patients with the ALI/ARDS criteria have no significant pulmonary edema [4]. Additionally, Esteban and colleagues have shown that there was not a good relationship between post-mortem findings of diffuse alveolar damage and the AECC clinical criteria of ARDS (sensitivity 75 %, specificity 84 %) [5].

For all these reasons, many authors have demanded new diagnostic criteria. For example, the proposals of Schuster in 2007 [6] and of Phua et al. in 2008 [7] indicate the need for quantification of the edema and for the use of pulmonary vascular permeability to permit clear evaluation of the magnitude and origin of the edema. Therefore, pulmonary edema (extravascular lung water, EVLW) and pulmonary vascular permeability measurements would be helpful to better characterize patients with ARDS and to follow the progress of these patients and their responses to therapeutic measures.

Measurement of EVLW at the Bedside

Quantification of edema is difficult at the bedside. Clinical examination, chest radiography, and blood gases have been proved to be of limited significance in quantifying pulmonary edema. For its part, advanced imaging techniques (quantitative computed tomography [CT], magnetic resonance imaging [MRI], positron emission tomography [PET] scan), as with the technique of pulmonary leak scans with radioactive isotopes that measures the accumulation of radioactively labeled substances (usually proteins) into the lungs, contribute valuable information, but their application in a critical care setting is difficult and makes them impractical [6].

Classically, the most commonly used method to assess EVLW at the bedside was the double (thermo-dye) indicator dilution technique. The thermal double dilution technique (COLD Z-021, Pulsion Medical Systems, Munich, Germany) was widely used in research, but had little use in clinical practice being relatively time consuming, cumbersome, and expensive. However, EVLW can now be calculated via single thermodilution, using specific analysis of the thermodilution curve (PiCCO, Pulsion Medical Systems, Munich, Germany). For the single thermodilution technique a central venous catheter is required for detection of a bolus injection of cold saline solution, and an arterial catheter with a thermistor (usually inserted into the femoral artery) is placed downstream. In fact, the easy application of this technique has renewed interest in the EVLW parameter [8].

The thermodilution curve and the formulas used to calculate EVLW by single thermodilution are shown in **Figures 1** and **2**. Briefly, cardiac output is calculated using the Stewart-Hamilton method from thermodilution curves measured in the femoral artery. The volume of distribution of the thermal indicator represents the intrathoracic thermal volume (ITTV), where ITTV (ml) = cardiac output x mean transit time of the thermal indicator. The pulmonary thermal volume (PTV) is given as PTV (ml) = cardiac output $\times\ \tau$, where τ is the exponential decay time of the thermodilution curve. Global end-diastolic volume (GEDV), the combined end-diastolic volumes of all cardiac chambers, is given as ITTV – PTV (ml). This permits calculation of intrathoracic blood volume (ITBV) from the linear relationship with GEDV: ITBV = 1.25 × GEDV – 28.4 (ml) [9]. EVLW is the difference between the thermal indicator distribution in the chest (ITTV) and the blood volume of the chest (ITBV): EVLW = ITTV – ITBV (ml).

Both the double and single thermodilution techniques have been widely evaluated in experimental and clinical studies, which have shown that EVLW assessed by double thermodilution is in close agreement with postmortem gravimetry [10–13] and with lung weight evaluated by CT scans [14]. Moreover, results from the single thermodilution technique also correlate well with gravimetry [15–17]. In an animal study of lung injury, Kuzkov et al. showed that both indicator dilution techniques

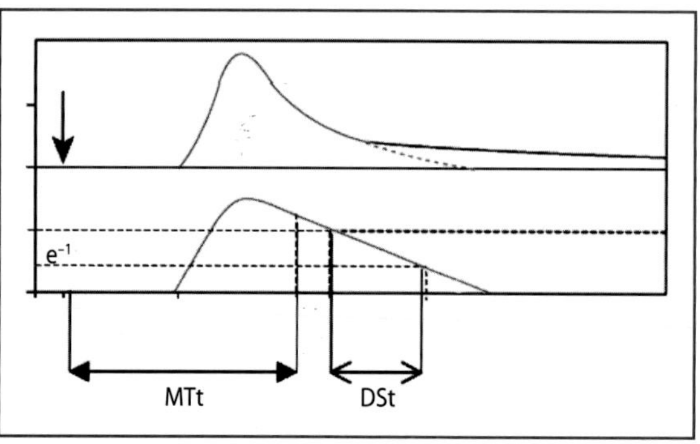

Fig. 1. Schematic description of an indicator dilution curve and the time characteristics of interest. MTt: mean transit time – represents the volume traversed by the relevant indicator, i.e., the total volume between the sites of injection and detection. This volume is often referred to as 'needle to needle volume'. DSt: downslope transit time – represents the largest individual mixing volume in a series of indicator dilution mixing chambers. (Reproduced with permission from Pulsion Medical Systems, Munich, Germany)

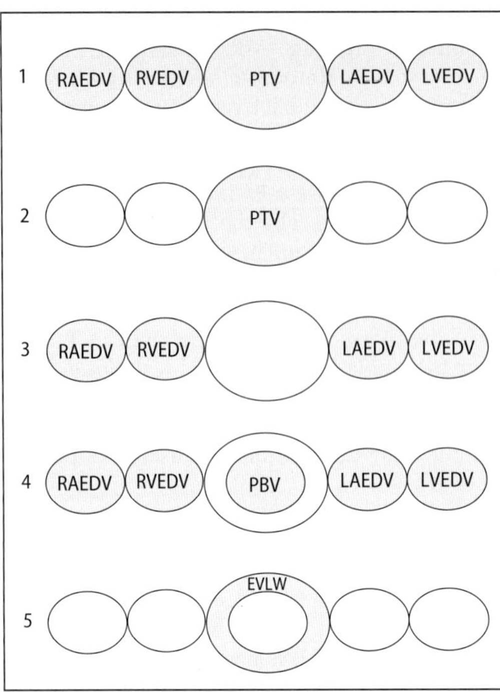

Fig. 2. Thermal volumes and extravascular lung water (EVLW) volume measurement. RAEDV: right atrial end-diastolic volume; RVEDV: right ventricular end-diastolic volume; PTV: pulmonary thermal volume; LAEDV: left atrial end-diastolic volume; LVEDV: left ventricular end-diastolic volume. **1** Multiplication of cardiac output by MTt gives the intrathoracic thermal volume (ITTV). ITTV = cardiac output × MTt. **2** Multiplication of cardiac output by downslope transit time (DSt) gives the pulmonary thermal volume (PTV). PTV = cardiac output × DSt. **3** Substraction of PTV from ITTV gives the global end-diastolic volume (GEDV), i.e., the sum of end-diastolic volume of the four cardiac chambers. **4** Assuming the correlation demonstrated by Sakka et al. [9] between GEDV and intrathoracic blood volume (ITBV): ITBV = 1.25 × GEDV – 28.4. **5** Therefore, EVLW is calculated by subtracting ITBV from ITTV: EVLW = ITTV – ITBV. (Reproduced with permission from Pulsion Medical Systems, Munich, Germany)

have a very close correlation with the gravimetric method and with CT scans [18]. Moreover, single thermodilution is highly sensitive for detecting small (10–20 %) variations in EVLW in both normal and experimental ARDS lungs [19].

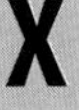

The single thermodilution technique also allows measurement of pulmonary vascular permeability. Indeed, high EVLW values along with normal pulmonary blood volume (PBV) indicate edema due to high permeability, whilst high values of both EVLW and PBV indicate hydrostatic edema. The pulmonary vascular permeability index (PVPI) is calculated by the PiCCO-technology as the ratio of EVLW/PBV with PBV derived as GEDV/4. Normal PVPI ranges between 1–3 (hydrostatic edema), with values above 3 indicating high permeability edema, distinguishing between the two types of edema with a sensitivity of 85 % and specificity of 100 % [20]. Thus, the measurement of EVLW with the single thermodilution technique has been widely used in both pediatric and adult intensive care unit (ICU) patients, including any patient who has cardiogenic and non-cardiogenic pulmonary edema, massive fluid shifts, and severe changes in microvascular permeability.

The limitations of single thermodilution have been described in detail in various reviews [8, 21]. They include the overestimation of the measurement when the technique is applied to the pediatric population or in animal experiments (pigs, sheep, dogs). This is because the software is designed for human adults (60 kg). The calculation of EVLW from single thermodilution is based on the correlation between the ITBV and the GEDV, according to the formula ITBV = 1.25 × GEDV - 28.4 ml. This correlation was established by Sakka et al. [9] in critically ill adults. In an experimental pig study, Rossi et al. [17] reduced overestimation of EVLW by applying a different equation: ITBV= 1.52 × GEDV - 49.7 ml. However this limitation only affects absolute values, since the linearity of determination is excellent at any weight [8].

Another of the limitations of intrathoracic blood volume is associated with diseases that may block the thermal indicator's passage through the lung, for example, severe pulmonary edema, massive pulmonary embolism, or hypoxic pulmonary vasoconstriction. All these situations could lead to an underestimation of EVLW. In hypoxic pulmonary vasoconstriction due to atelectasis, the application of PEEP, by lung recruitment, may induce a redistribution of pulmonary blood flow towards previously excluded areas, and hence artificially 'increase' EVLW. However, the use of high levels of PEEP producing alveolar over-distension can have the opposite effect, collapsing the lung vessels. EVLW is also underestimated in patients with lung resection. Indeed, as mentioned previously, the estimation of EVLW by single thermodilution is based on the formula, ITBV = 1.25 × GEDV – 28.4 ml. Since the difference between ITBV and GEDV is the PBV, any decrease in PBV (e.g., due to lung resection) may affect the GEDV/ITBV ratio and hence the estimation of EVLW [21].

EVLW in ALI/ARDS Patients

Amongst the advantages of measuring EVLW via the single thermodilution technique, is its good correlation with the degree of pulmonary edema, the Lung Injury Score and oxygenation [4, 8, 22]. Martin et al. [22] demonstrated in a cohort of septic patients how EVLW measured with single thermodilution could be a useful tool in the diagnosis of ARDS and may improve risk stratification and management.

The single thermodilution technique has also proved to be useful for detecting changes in EVLW, allowing proper assessment of the evolution of pulmonary edema and its treatment. Perkins et al. [23] conducted a randomized placebo-controlled clinical trial in 40 patients with ALI, treated with intravenous salbutamol or placebo. The results of this blinded trial showed that patients who were treated with intravenous salbutamol had a 40 % reduction in EVLW compared to controls. The reduction in the EVLW was matched by a reduction in the plateau airway pressure, a measure of quasi-static respiratory compliance that may reflect less pulmonary edema.

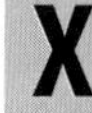

Finally, several studies have shown that monitoring EVLW may have prognostic usefulness in patients with ALI/ARDS [19, 22, 24]. Kuzkov et al. [24] studied EVLW in 38 patients with sepsis-induced ALI, and found that from the first day EVLW increased in non-survivors and decreased in the group of survivors. On the third day, this difference was statistically significant between the two groups. Recently, Phillips et al. [25] reported that the combined measurement of EVLW and pulmonary dead space in patients with ALI has a prognostic value for identifying patients at the highest risk of non-survival. In fact EVLW greater than 16 ml/kg of predicted body weight, predicted death with 100 % specificity and 86 % sensitivity.

Ventilation Strategy in ALI/ARDS and EVLW Variations

Mechanical ventilation with low tidal volume and plateau pressures reduces mortality in patients with ALI/ARDS [26]. However, ventilation with lower volumes and pressures can cause ventilator-associated lung injury (VALI) due to the loss of lung volume producing a cyclical open-closure of the alveolar atelectasis [27]. Recent publications have shown interest in new strategies of mechanical ventilation incorporating alveolar recruitment maneuvers and high levels of PEEP in order to avoid alveolar collapse [28, 29]. The aim of this open lung concept is to recruit all recruitable alveoli during an opening procedure by applying high inflation pressures and setting adequate PEEP to avoid de-recruitment. Both clinical and experimental studies have demonstrated an improvement in oxygenation and respiratory mechanics, as well as increases in lung volume [30] but no studies have been able to demonstrate that recruitment maneuvers decrease mortality in patients with ALI/ARDS [31, 32].

On the other hand, little is known thus far of side effects caused by recruitment maneuvers. Some experimental studies have concluded that lung recruitment maneuvers reduce lung injury at the histological level [33]. Another relevant experimental study [34] has shown how lung recruitment maneuvers applied to an injured lung may protect the lung endothelium, reducing EVLW but not alveolar epithelial injury.

There have been several studies looking at the effect of PEEP on EVLW in ALI/ARDS with conflicting results, some demonstrating increased EVLW [35, 36], others decreased EVLW [13, 37–39], and others no change in EVLW [40]. Maybauer et al. [35] concluded that PEEP increases EVLW because of a decrease in lung lymph flow whilst Demling and co-workers [36] reported that increasing PEEP increased EVLW when microvascular hydrostatic pressure was raised. Luecke and co-workers [37], in a surfactant-washout ARDS model, found that increased PEEP decreased EVLW and that the fall in EVLW was highly correlated to the decrease in non-aerated lung volume due to the increase in PEEP; however this decrease in EVLW did not reflect a reduction in pulmonary edema measured with CT scans. Colmenero-Ruiz et al. [13], using the same model, concluded that the early implementation of PEEP of 10 cmH_2O reduced EVLW by reducing the atelectasis produced by the oleic acid infusion, and was decreased even further by reducing the tidal volume from 12 to 6 ml/kg, avoiding over-distension of the none atelectatic lung tissue. The same group noted that PEEP reduced EVLW in a time-dependent manner [39].

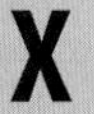

Obviously it is possible that the gradual improvement in ARDS due to PEEP may decrease edema and, therefore, the measured values of EVLW. However, it seems clear that the amount of extravascular water should not be reduced in the short term because of different PEEP settings, if the edema does not vary. It should be noted that the effect of atelectasis on EVLW assessment is still not completely understood [13, 21, 41–43]. Nevertheless, use of inappropriately high levels of PEEP producing alveolar overdistension and collapsing the lung vessels could artificially reduce EVLW values. In fact, EVLW would not be detected in low-perfused lung regions due to low cardiac output. These effects can be easily discarded when the cardiac index and other hemodynamic variables are monitored.

However, the potential impact of a standard recruitment maneuver associated with an adequate level of PEEP on pulmonary edema and EVLW measurements has not been well studied. Frank and co-workers [34] found that sustained inflation recruitment maneuvers decreased EVLW as a consequence of lung endothelium protection. Chen and co-workers [44] concluded in a study in rats with saline lavage-induced ARDS, that protective lung ventilation with an open lung strategy could reduce EVLW when compared to injurious ventilation. The two groups were ventilated with a protective strategy, with one of the groups having a sustained inflation recruitment maneuver. However, there were no significant differences in the decrease in EVLW.

We looked at the effect of recruitment maneuvers on EVLW in 18 critical care patients diagnosed with ALI/ARDS, according to the AECC definition [1]. All patients received volume control ventilation with a tidal volume of 8 ml/kg and

10–12 cmH_2O of PEEP. For the recruitment maneuver, the mode was changed to pressure assist control (A/C) with a pressure control level of 15 cmH_2O and respiratory rate of 10 breaths per minute. PEEP was increased progressively to 25 cmH_2O in order to obtain a peak inspiratory pressure (PIP) of 40 cmH_2O. After 5 breaths, pressure control was increased to 20 cmH_2O (PIP = 45 cmH_2O) and after a further 5 breaths, PEEP was increased to 30 cmH_2O (PIP = 50 cmH_2O) and continued for 20 breaths. After this period the recruitment maneuver was considered finished. A decremental PEEP trial procedure was then followed in order to determine the best compliance PEEP. For this purpose, only the PEEP setting was modified during the procedure: PEEP was reduced by steps of 2 cmH_2O every 6 breaths while dynamic compliance was measured. Following the recruitment maneuver, PEEP was adjusted to this better compliance level plus 3 cmH_2O [29].

The PiCCO was used to monitor hemodynamic measurements of EVLW and PVPI. EVLW was indexed to the predicted body weight (PBW), and PVPI was calculated as EVLW/PBV. Data were collected at time 0 (pre-recruitment maneuver), at 15 min, 1, 2, 6, and 24 hours. Arterial blood gas analyses were performed at each time point. The differences between parameters before and at different time-points after the recruitment maneuver were assessed with an analysis of variance (ANOVA) and the Bonferroni correction for multiple comparisons. The Levene test was used as a test of homogeneity.

As can be seen in **Table 1**, the lung recruitment maneuver and the establishment of the optimal PEEP produced a progressive increase in oxygenation (PaO_2/FiO_2) being significant between the control level and the value taken at 1 hour ($p = 0.014$) and in the following 24 hours ($p = 0.004$). **Table 1** also shows that the mean values of EVLW and PVPI did not change significantly after the recruitment maneuver or in the following 24 hours. **Figure 3** shows the evolution of EVLW in all patients during the study period. **Table 1** shows the hemodynamic data 15 min after the recruitment maneuver, specifically, a non-significant decrease in cardiac index and GED I. None of the hemodynamic changes during the study were significant.

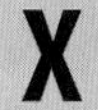

This study shows that a standard technique for lung recruitment and the adjustment of a PEEP level titrated with a decremental PEEP trial was effective in improv-

Table 1. Summary of respiratory and hemodynamic values before and after recruiting maneuver (RM).

	Pre-RM	15 min	1 h	2 h	6 h	24 h
PaO_2/FIO_2 (mmHg)	198 ± 47	220 ± 74	236 ± 69*	237 ± 71*	238 ± 82*	268 ± 74*
$PaCO_2$ (mmHg)	43 ± 7	40 ± 6	40 ± 6	40 ± 6	42 ± 7.92	43 ± 8
Pplat (cmH_2O)	26.3 ± 4.2	27.0 ± 3.4	27.3 ± 4.1	27.5 ± 4.4	26.2 ± 5.8	26.5 ± 7.6
PEEP (cmH_2O)	10.9 ± 2.5	11.7 ± 2.3	11.8 ± 2.2	11.7 ± 2.3	11.8 ± 2.9	11.7 ± 3.2
CI ($l/m/m^2$)	3.0 ± 0.9	2.9 ± 0.9	3.0 ± 0.9	2.9 ± 0.9	2.9 ± 0.9	2.8 ± 0.9
GEDVI (ml/m^2)	784 ± 216	779 ± 194	784 ± 221	794 ± 199	796 ± 197	772 ± 232
EVLWI (ml/kg/PBW)	11.5 ± 9.1	12.0 ± 9.9	10.9 ± 7.5	10.9 ± 7.1	10.9 ± 6.5	11.0 ± 5.4
PVPI	2.2 ± 1.6	2.2 ± 1.7	2.0 ± 1.2	2.0 ± 1.2	2.2 ± 1.7	2.4 ± 2.1

* indicates $p < 0.05$ when pre-RM values are compared with post-RM time points. Pplat: plateau pressure; PEEP: positive end-expiratory pressure; EVLWI: extravascular lung water index; PVPI: pulmonary vascular permeability index; PBW: predicted body weight; GEDVI: global end-diastolic volume index; CI: cardiac index

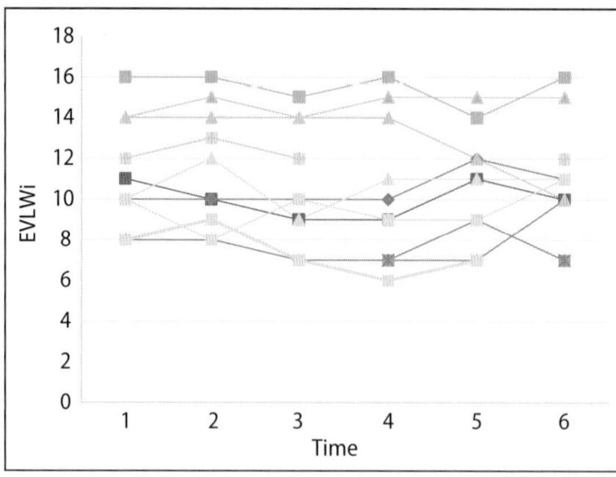

Fig. 3. Evolution of extravascular lung water index (EVLWI, indexed to predicted body weight) in all individual ALI/ARDS patients. The study period is represented by numbers: (1) Pre-recruitment maneuver; (2) 15 minutes after recruitment maneuver; (3) 1 hour after recruitment maneuver; (4) 2 hours after recruitment maneuver; (5) 6 hours after recruitment maneuver; and (6) 24 hours after recruitment maneuver.

ing the PaO_2 significantly in the subsequent hours, but that the EVLW and PVPI did not vary. These results are consistent with those obtained by Toth et al. [45]. These authors applied a recruitment maneuver (sustained inflation: 40 cmH_2O/40 sec) and a descending optimal PEEP titration in 18 ARDS patients; PaO_2 improved significantly, without any change in EVLW for up to 1 h.

From these observations, it appears that increased PEEP during recruitment maneuvers with up to 30 cmH_2O and PIP up to 50 cmH_2O is not followed by immediate changes in EVLW and PVPI, and does not support the theory that elevated PEEP causes an increase in EVLW due to increased permeability. On the contrary, increased EVLW predisposes the alveoli to atelectasis, which had to be compensated for with higher PEEP [45]. Whether there is a relationship between the evolutionary variations in the EVLW and the optimal PEEP adjusted with a decremental PEEP trial after a recruitment cannot be answered yet.

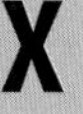

Conclusion

EVLW measured with the single thermodilution method is a very useful instrument to assess lung edema secondary to ALI/ARDS. When it is adjusted to the ideal body weight, it is a true index of the severity of edema, is useful as a prognostic factor, and also guides treatment for these patients. Lung recruitment maneuvers with high opening pressures and decremental optimal PEEP titration can be a useful therapeutic intervention in patients with ALI/ARDS and do not affect the evaluation of edema through the measurement of EVLW with single thermodilution, which may rule out any reduction or redistribution of EVLW.

References

1. Bernard GR, Artigas A, Brigham KL, et al (1994) The American-European Consensus Conference on ARDS: definitions, mechanisms, relevant outcomes. Am J Respir Crit Care Med 149: 818–824
2. Villar J, Pérez-Méndez L, López J, et al (2007) An early PEEP/FiO2 trial identifies different degrees of lung injury in patients with acute respiratory distress syndrome. Am J Respir Crit Care Med 176: 795–804

3. Rubenfeld GD, Caldwell E, Granton J, Hudson LD, Matthay MA (1999) Interobserver variability in applying a radiographic definition for ARDS. Chest 116: 1347–1353
4. Berkowitz DM, Danai PA, Eaton S, Moss M, Martin GS (2008) Accurate characterization of extravascular lung water in acute respiratory distress syndrome. Crit Care Med 36: 1803–1809
5. Esteban A, Fernandez-Segoviano P, Frutos-Vivar F, et al (2004) Comparison of clinical criteria for the acute respiratory distress syndrome with autopsy findings. Ann Intern Med 141: 440–445
6. Schuster DP (2007) The search for "objective" criteria of ARDS. Intensive Care Med 33: 400–402
7. Phua J, Stewart TE, Ferguson ND (2008) Acute respiratory distress syndrome 40 years later: time to revisit its definition. Crit Care Med 36: 2912–2921
8. Fernández-Mondejar E, Guerrero López F, Colmenero M (2007) How important is the measurement of extravascular lung water? Curr Opin Crit Care 13: 79–83
9. Sakka SG, Ruhi CC, Pfeiffer UJ, et al (2000) Assessment of cardiac preload and extravascular lung water by single transpulmonary thermodilution. Intensive Care Med 26: 180–187
10. Lewis FR, Eling VB, Hill SL, et al (1982) The measurement of extravascular lung water by thermal-green dye indicator dilution. Ann NY Acad Sci 384: 393–410.
11. Saul GM, Feeley TW, Mihn FG (1982) Effect of graded administration of PEEP on lung water in non cardiogenic pulmonary edema. Crit Care Med 10: 667–669.
12. Mihn FG, Feeley TW, Rosenthal MH, et al (1982) Measurement of extravascular lung water in dogs using the thermal-green dye indicator dilution method. Anesthesiology 57: 116–122
13. Colmenero-Ruiz M, Fernández-Mondéjar E, Fernández Sacristán MA, et al (1997) PEEP and low tidal volume reduces extravascular lung water in porcine pulmonary edema. Am J Respir Crit Care Med 155: 964–970
14. Patroniti N, Bellani G, Maggioni E, et al (2005) Measurement of pulmonary edema in patients with acute respiratory distress syndrome. Crit Care Med 33: 2547–2554
15. Katzenelson R, Perel A, Berkenstadt H, et al (2004) Accuracy of transpulmonary thermodilution versus gravimetric measurement of extravascular lung water. Crit Care Med 32: 1550–1554
16. Kirov MY, Kuzkov VV, Kuklin VN (2004) Extravascular lung water assessed by transpulmonary single thermodilution and postmortem gravimetry in sheep. Crit Care 8: R451-R458
17. Rossi P, Wanecek M, Rudehill A, et al (2006) Comparison of a single indicator and gravimetric thecnique for estimation of extravascular lung water in endotoxemic pigs. Crit Care Med 34: 1437–1443
18. Kuzkov VV, Kirov M, Waerhaug K, et al (2007) Assessment of current methods quantitating extravascular lung water and pulmonary aeration in inhomogeneus lung injury: an experimental study. Anesteziol Reanimatol 3: 4–9
19. Fernández-Mondejar E, Rivera-Fernández R, García-Delgado M, et al (2005) Small increases in extravascular lung water are accurately detected by transpulmonary thermodilution. J Trauma 59: 1420–1424
20. Monnet X, Anguel N, Osman D, Hamzaoui O, Richard C, Teboul JL (2007) Assessing pulmonary permeability by traspulmonary thermodilution allows differentiation of hydrostatic pulmonary edema from ALI/ARDS. Intensive Care Med 33: 448–453
21. Michard F (2007) Bedside assesment of extravascular lung water by dilutions methods: temptations and pitfalls. Crit Care Med 35: 1186–1192
22. Martin GS, Eaton S, Mealer M, Moss M (2005) Extravascular lung water in patients with severe sepsis: a prospective cohort study. Crit Care 9:R74–82
23. Perkins GD, McAuleyDF, Thickett DR, Gao F (2006) The beta-agonist lung injury trial (BALTI): a randomized placebo-controlled trial. Am J Respir Crit Care Med 173: 281–287
24. Kuzkov VV, Kirov MY, Sovershaev MA, et al (2006) Extravascular lung water determined with single transpulmonary thermodilution correlates with the severity of sepsis-induced acute lung injury. Crit Care Med 34: 1647–1653
25. Phillips CR, Chesnutt MS, Smith SM (2008) Extravascular lung water in sepsis-associated respiratory distress syndrome: indexing with predicted body weight improves correlation with severity of illnes and survival. Crit Care Med 36: 69–73
26. The Acute Respiratory Distress Syndrome network (2000) Ventilation with lower tidal vol-

umes as compared with traditional tidal volumes for acute lung injury and the acute respiratory distress syndrome. N Engl J Med 342: 1301–1308

27. Dreyfuss D, Saumon G (1998) Ventilator-induced lung injury: Lessons from experimental studies. Am J Respir Crit Care Med 157: 294–323
28. Brower RG, Morris A, MacIntyre N, et al (2003) Effects of recruitment maneuvers in patients with acute lung injury and acute respiratory distress syndrome ventilated with high positive end-expiratory pressure. Crit Care Med 31: 2592–2597
29. Suarez-Sipmann F, Böhm SH, Tusman G (2007) Use of dynamic compliance for open lung positive end-expiratory pressure titration in an experimental study. Crit Care Med 35: 214–221
30. Pelosi P, Goldner M, McKibben A, et al (2001) Recruitment and derecruitment during acute respiratory failure: An experimental study. Am J Respir Crit Care Med 164: 122–130
31. Meede MO, Cook DJ, Guyatt GH, et al (2008) ventilation strategy using low tidal volumes, recruitment maneuvers, and high positive end-expiratory pressure for acute lung injury and acute respiratory distress syndrome. JAMA 299(6):637–645.
32. Alain M, Jean-Christophe M.R, Bruno V, et al (2008) Positive end-expiratory setting in adults with acute lung injury and acute respiratory distress syndrome. JAMA 299: 646–655
33. Rimensberger PC, Pristine G, Mullen BM, et al (1999) Lung recruitment during small tidal volume ventilation allows minimal positive end-expiratory pressure without augmenting lung injury. Crit Care Med 27: 1940–1945
34. Frank JA, McAuley DF, Gutierrez JA, et al (2005) Differential effects of sustained inflation recruitment maneuvers on alveolar ephitelial and lung endothelial injury. Crit Care Med 33: 254–255
35. Maybauer D.M, Talke PO, Westphay M, et al (2006) Positive end-expiratory pressure ventilation increases extravascular lung water due to a decrease in lung lymph flow. Anaesth Intensive Care 34: 329–333
36. Demling RH, Staub NC, Edmunds LH Jr (1975) Effect of end-expiratory airway pressure on accumulation of extravascular lung water. J Appl Physiol 38: 907–912
37. Luecke T, Roth H, Herrmann P, et al (2003) PEEP decreases atelectasis and extravascular lung water but not lung tissue volume in surfactant-washout lung injury. Intensive Care Med 29: 2026–2033
38. Russel JA, Hoeffel J, Murray JF (1982) Effect of different levels of positive end-expiratory pressure on lung water content. J Appl Physiol 53: 9–15
39. Ruiz-Bailen M, Fernandez-Mondejar E, Hurtado-Ruiz B, et al (1999) Immediate application of positive end-expiratory pressure is more effective than delayed positive end-expiratory pressure to reduce extravascular lung water. Crit Care Med 27: 380–384
40. Myers JC, Reilley TE, Cloutier CT (1988) Effect of positive end-expiratory pressure on extravascular lung water in porcine acute respiratory failure. Crit Care Med 16: 52–54
41. Verheij J, van Lingen A, Raijmakers PG, et al (2005) Pulmonary abnormalities after cardiac surgery are better explained by atelectasis than by increased permeability oedema. Acta Anaesthesiol Scand 49: 1302–1310
42. Groeneveld AB, Verheij J, van den Berg FG, et al (2006) Increased pulmonary capillary permeability and extravascular lung water after major vascular surgery: effect on radiography and ventilatory variables. Eur J Anaesthesiol 23: 36–41
43. Szakmany T, Heigl P, Molnar Z (2004) Correlation between extravasuclar lung water and oxygenation in ALI/ARDS patients with septic shock: possible role in development of atelectasis. Anaesth Intensive Care 32: 196–201
44. Chen YM, Yang Y, Qiu HB, et al (2005) Effect of protective ventilation and open lung strategy on extravascular lung water in rabbits with acute respiratory distress syndrome. Chin J Tuberc Respir Dis 28: 615–617
45. Toth I, Leiner T, Mikor A, Szakmany T, Bogar L, Molnar Z (2007) Hemodynamic and respiratory changes during lung recruitment and descending optimal positive end-expiratory pressure titration in patients with acute respiratory distress syndome. Crit Care Med 35: 787–793

Clinical Utility of Extravascular Lung Water Measurements

X. Monnet and J.-L. Teboul

Introduction

In physiological conditions, the hydrostatic pressure of the pulmonary microvessels induces the transfer of a certain amount of fluid into the interstitial space. The lymphatic system drains this large amount of fluid toward the thoracic duct, avoiding alveolar edema. Thus, in physiology, the extravascular lung water (EVLW) is the volume of fluid that has been filtered from the vessels and that has been eliminated by lymphatic drainage. In physiological conditions, this volume is low, less than 7 ml/kg of body weight.

When the hydrostatic pressure in the pulmonary microvessels increases – for instance due to left cardiac failure – the flow of fluid transferred toward the interstitium increases. Lymphatic flow also increases. When the lymphatic drainage is overwhelmed, interstitial spaces and alveoli are flooded by edema. During cardiac failure, the increase in the pressure of the vena cava impedes lymphatic drainage and aggravates pulmonary edema formation. In case of increased permeability pulmonary edema, such as acute respiratory distress syndrome (ARDS), the transfer of fluid from the lung microvessels is due to the injury of the alveolar and capillary walls and is markedly aggravated if the hydrostatic pressure is increased.

Whatever the cause of the pulmonary leak, the accumulation of EVLW impairs gas exchange and decreases lung compliance with important clinical consequences. The EVLW can increase up to 40 or 50 ml/kg [1]. Nevertheless, neither the clinical examination, chest radiograph or gas exchange measurements allow accurate quantification of EVLW. It has been demonstrated that the level of EVLW is a prognostic factor for critically ill patients [2]. Moreover, a protocol of fluid management based upon the measurement of EVLW has been demonstrated to improve functional outcome compared to a protocol based upon the measurement of the pulmonary artery occlusion pressure (PAOP) [3]. All these factors, along with the ability of some commercial devices to measure EVLW, have led to a growing interest in this topic. In this chapter, we will detail the techniques that are available for measuring EVLW and will discuss the clinical interest of EVLW measurement at the bedside.

Measurement of EVLW

Although the clinical examination and chest radiograph are grossly able to detect the occurrence of pulmonary edema, they do not allow any accurate quantification of EVLW [4]. This measurement requires more sophisticated techniques such as gravimetry, transpulmonary dilution of markers, and pulmonary imaging techniques.

Gravimetry

Basically, gravimetry is an *ex vivo* method, which involves measuring the wet and dry weights of the lungs. The difference between the wet and dry weights corresponds to the sum of EVLW and the blood contained in the organ. The blood content is estimated from the hematocrit leaving the EVLW. Gravimetry is considered as the reference method for measuring EVLW but, obviously, can only be used for experimental purposes.

Transpulmonary Dilution Techniques

Contrary to gravimetry, these techniques can be used in the clinical setting. They are based upon the principle that the volume of dilution of a marker can be mathematically inferred from the analysis of the dilution curve. According to the Stewart-Hamilton principle, the volume (V) in which a marker injected into the circulation is diluted is proportional to the cardiac output and to the mean transit time measured on the dilution curve of the marker: V = cardiac output × mean transit time (**Fig. 1**). At a constant cardiac output, the larger the volume, the lower is the decrease in the indicator concentration at the end of the circuit.

To measure EVLW, the indicator must be injected into the vena cava, i.e., at the entrance of the thorax and the dilution must be detected at the exit of the thorax, i.e., in the aorta. Based on this principle, two techniques of transpulmonary dilution have been developed.

Double indicator dilution technique

With the double indicator technique, two different indicators are simultaneously injected into the circulation. One indicator, usually a cold fluid, diffuses into the whole thoracic volume, including intravascular and extravascular spaces. The other

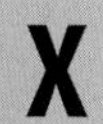

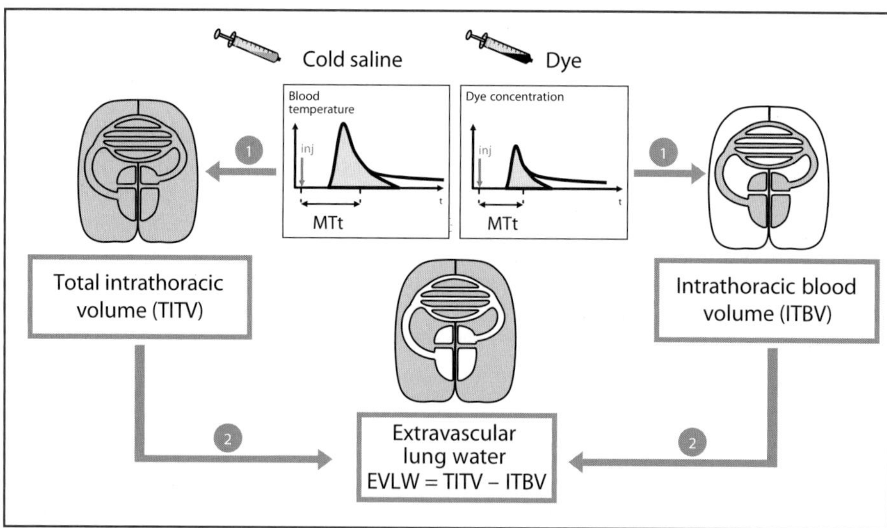

Fig. 1. Measurement of extravascular lung water (EVLW) by the double indicator dilution technique. MTt: mean transit time

indicator, usually indocyanine green (ICG), diffuses only into the vascular space. The difference between the dilution volumes of the two indicators is the thermal extravascular volume. If one considers that the volumes of the myocardium and of the thoracic vessels are negligible, this volume can be assimilated to the EVLW (**Fig. 1**).

The double indicator technique has been validated against gravimetry [5, 6]. Its reproducibility has also been well documented in some clinical studies [7, 8]. However, the cost of the ICG indicator, along with the technical difficulty of performing two injections, has led to the development of a technique using one indicator only [9].

Single indicator dilution technique

The single indicator dilution technique uses only the dilution of a cold indicator and thus allows the measurement of the global intrathoracic volume. However, the intrathoracic blood volume cannot be directly measured but only estimated from the Newman principle. According to this principle, the volume (V) of the largest chamber in which the indicator is diluting can be estimated from cardiac output and from the downslope time of the thermodilution curve after exponential transformation (**Fig. 2**): V = cardiac output/downslope time. For transpulmonary thermodilution, the larger volume in which the thermal indicator is diluting is the total pulmonary volume, corresponding to the sum of the pulmonary blood volume (PBV) and of EVLW (**Fig. 2**). By subtracting the total pulmonary volume from the total intrathoracic volume, one obtains the global end-diastolic volume (GEDV), i.e., the volume of blood contained in the four cardiac chambers at the end of diastole.

The next step is to estimate the ITBV. For this estimation, one must consider that the ITBV is proportionally linked to the GEDV [9], as demonstrated by several clinical studies [9–11]. Finally, by subtracting the estimated ITBV from the measured total intrathoracic volume, the EVLW is obtained (**Fig. 2**).

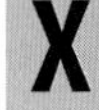

The single dilution measurement of EVLW has been validated against the double indicator transpulmonary dilution in humans [9, 12] and against the gravimetric technique in animals [13–16]. In some animal studies, a bias was sometimes observed [14], likely due to the fact that the coefficient of proportionality between the ITBV and the GEDV is different from that in humans. The reproducibility of the EVLW measurement is higher than 90 %. A commercial device (PiCCO, Pulsion Medical Systems, Germany) enables the single transpulmonary dilution technique to be performed at the bedside [9]. This device requires a central venous catheter and a femoral arterial catheter customized with a tip thermistor. It allows measurement or calculation of EVLW, cardiac output, ITBV, and GEDV.

Limitations of the Measurement of EVLW by Transpulmonary Dilution Techniques

Underestimation of EVLW during ARDS

In normal lungs, the measurement of EVLW by the transpulmonary dilution method was found to be concordant with gravimetric findings [6]. In some cases of ARDS, it has been reported that the transpulmonary dilution techniques may underestimate EVLW, especially for high values of EVLW [9, 11]. This may be due to the poor diffusion of the cold indicator in some regions of the inhomogeneous lung, leading to underestimation of the total intrathoracic volume. During ARDS, the poor diffu-

Cold saline
Blood temperature (Ts)
inj
t
MTt
ln Ts
inj
t
Dt
1
1
Total intrathoracic volume (TITV)
Total pulmonary volume (TPV)
2
2
Global end-diastolic volume
GEDV = TITV – TPV
3
Intrathoracic blood volume
ITBV = 1.25 x GEDV
4
4
Extravascular lung water
EVLW = TITV – ITBV

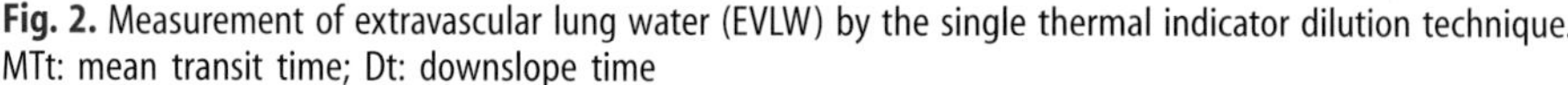

Fig. 2. Measurement of extravascular lung water (EVLW) by the single thermal indicator dilution technique. MTt: mean transit time; Dt: downslope time

X

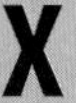

sion of the cold indicator is related to the vasoconstriction of the condensed area of the lung due to hypoxia and to the volume of the surrounding edema. Consequently, underestimation of EVLW is more pronounced when the lung injury is inhomogeneous. Accordingly, the measurement of EVLW was found to be more reliable compared to gravimetry when the ARDS was created by the instillation of oleic acid (homogeneous lesions) than when it was created by a chemical injury (heterogeneous lesions) [17, 18]. It is likely that when lung injury is heterogeneous, the indicator is redistributed toward regions with a better perfusion and with less edema. According to this hypothesis, EVLW is underestimated by the double indicator technique when one branch of the pulmonary artery is embolized [19, 20]. This also suggests that the measurement of EVLW is more reliable in extrapulmonary forms of ARDS, characterized by a homogeneous injury of the lung, than in pulmonary forms of ARDS. Nevertheless, the clinical impact of this limitation is questionable [21].

Effects of Positive End-expiratory Pressure (PEEP)

The effects of PEEP on the measurement of EVLW are controversial. On the one hand, PEEP could reduce the ITBV by squeezing the pulmonary vessels. On the other hand, PEEP could increase the ITBV [22] by recruiting some condensed regions of the lung and by reducing hypoxic vasoconstriction. Accordingly, animal studies have reported conflicting results, with PEEP leading to an overestimation [23] or to an underestimation [11, 24] of EVLW. In humans during ARDS, double dilution EVLW was reported to accurately reflect that estimated by computed tomography (CT), regardless of the level of PEEP (up to 20 cmH_2O). It is likely that PEEP has a limited clinical impact on the measurement of transpulmonary thermodilution EVLW [7].

Other limitations

One other potential source of error in the measurement of EVLW by single thermal transpulmonary dilution relates to the fact that the ITBV is not measured but is estimated from the GEDV after assuming a constant proportionality between these two variables. The coefficient of proportionality that is used in the single transpulmonary thermodilution device comes from an analysis of the whole population of a clinical study where ITBV was measured by double dilution and the GEDV measured by single thermodilution [9]. However, the coefficient of proportionality may vary from patient to patient depending on the cardio-respiratory conditions [11, 16]. In fact, the error in EVLW measurement is probably low (around 1 ml/kg) so that the impact of this limitation is small, especially when EVLW is elevated [11] or in cases of hypovolemia [16].

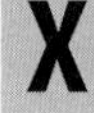

Finally, an error in the estimation of EVLW could come from indexation of EVLW to the actual patient's weight rather than to the predicted body weight, the latter being better correlated to the lungs' dimensions. Accordingly, indexing EVLW to the predicted body weight was demonstrated to reduce the number of ARDS patients with normal EVLW and to correlate better to Lung Injury Score and oxygenation [25]. In addition, the prognostic value of EVLW was found to be better in ARDS patients when the value of EVLW was indexed to the predicted rather than to the actual body weight [26].

To summarize, the transpulmonary dilution techniques enable a reliable measure of EVLW, even though the value may be underestimated in the heterogeneous forms of ARDS. In contrast to some other techniques attempting to quantify EVLW in humans, such as CT [7], lung echography [4], magnetic resonance imaging (MRI) [27], thoracic bioimpedance [28], or other isotopic techniques [29], transpulmonary thermodilution allows a measurement of EVLW that is easy, reproducible, and can be used at the bedside. The technique also provides information about cardiac output, cardiac contractility [30] and cardiac preload [31].

Clinical Utility of EVLW

Diagnosis of Pulmonary Edema

The most obvious clinical utility of measuring EVLW is to diagnose pulmonary edema in clinical situations where the diagnosis cannot be clearly established on the basis of usual criteria. This could be the case, for example, in critically ill patients receiving mechanical ventilation for several days who have already received a certain amount of fluid and who experience a worsening of gas exchange. The differential diagnosis between pulmonary edema, new episode of lung infection, atelectasis, and pleural effusion can be difficult to establish with certainty. The measurement of EVLW in such cases may be helpful in terms of diagnosis and therapeutic options.

Identification of the Mechanism of Pulmonary Edema

One of the advantages of the transpulmonary dilution technique is that it enables one to distinguish between hydrostatic and non-hydrostatic forms of pulmonary edema. Indeed, by providing the pulmonary vascular permeability index (PVPI), which is automatically calculated as the ratio between EVLW and the PBV (i.e., the ratio of the extravascular fluid to the intravascular fluid), this technique can allow bedside assessment of the pulmonary vascular permeability. This was first suggested by an animal study demonstrating that the PVPI was higher when pulmonary edema was induced by the instillation of oleic acid (increased permeability pulmonary edema) than by the inflation of a balloon in the left atrium (hydrostatic pulmonary edema) [15].

In a study conducted in 48 patients with pulmonary edema, we recently confirmed the clinical relevance of PVPI [1]. The PVPI was automatically calculated by a transpulmonary thermodilution monitor (PiCCOPlus, Pulsion Medical Systems, Germany). For each patient, the mechanism of pulmonary edema was retrospectively determined by experts who based their judgment upon the clinical history, the radiological and echocardiographic findings, the plasma B-type natriuretic peptide concentration, and the evolution of all the observed abnormalities after treatment. The PVPI was higher in patients who presented with acute lung injury (ALI) or ARDS than in patients who developed hydrostatic pulmonary edema. Moreover, a PVPI value higher than 3 enabled to discriminate between the two forms of pulmonary edema with a good diagnostic accuracy [1]. These results suggest that PVPI could be used in the clinical setting for establishing the mechanism of pulmonary edema. Furthermore, knowledge of the PVPI could be helpful in the therapeutic decision-making process, especially in patients with ALI/ARDS. For example, a very high PVPI (e.g., > 6) suggests that administration of fluid should be cautious since it has the potential to markedly increase pulmonary edema formation owing to the abnormally elevated lung permeability.

Despite the fact that ARDS is associated with an increased EVLW resulting from damage of the alveolo-capillary barrier, the consensual definition of ARDS is still based upon the presence of criteria such as hypoxemia and bilateral radiological lung infiltrates [32], which are, however, not related to the degree of EVLW elevation [33]. Another required criterion is the absence of evidence of elevated left ventricular filling pressure. Yet, the presence of a high left ventricular pressure cannot exclude that the alveolo-capillary barrier is injured and the lung microvascular permeability is abnormally increased. In this regard, in one third of patients with a diagnosis of ALI/ARDS, who by definition should, therefore, have had a

PAOP < 18 mmHg, high values of PAOP were measured during the course of their disease [34].

Interestingly, three clinical studies in patients with ARDS diagnosed by classical criteria demonstrated that EVLW was not elevated in a relatively high proportion of patients [7, 35, 36]. Even though technical limitations may have underestimated the value of EVLW, these results suggest that the conventional criteria used for diagnosing ARDS are not sufficient [37] and that EVLW may be an additional diagnostic criterion for this purpose [7]. A more complete definition of ALI/ARDS should also include a marker of increased pulmonary vascular permeability [37] such as PVPI [1].

Prognostic Evaluation of Patients with ALI/ARDS

In a study including 373 patients, among whom 13 % had ARDS, Sakka and co-workers showed that the EVLW value was higher in non-survivors than in survivors (14 ml/kg versus 10 ml/kg) [2]. Mortality was 33 % in patients with an EVLW less than 10 ml/kg and 65 % in patients with an EVLW higher than 15 ml/kg. In a more recent study in 37 patients with ALI [38], the value of EVLW obtained on Day 1 was not different between survivors and non-survivors. In contrast, the EVLW value measured on Day 3 was 60–70 % higher in non-survivors than in survivors [38]. This suggests that rather than a fixed value of EVLW, the time course of this variable should help in determining the prognosis of patients with ALI or ARDS.

Guidance of Fluid Therapy in ARDS

During recent years, a debate has emerged concerning the most appropriate fluid therapy in ALI/ARDS. On the one hand, restrictive administration of fluid in ARDS may reduce the amount of edema and improve gas exchange, but on the other hand, it could reduce cardiac preload and cardiac output and thus eventually result in organ dysfunction.

A multicenter randomized study conducted in 1000 patients with ALI/ARDS compared a liberal versus a conservative strategy of fluid administration [39]. The two strategies were based on complex algorithms including measurements of cardiac filling pressures. Although no difference in mortality was observed at 60 days, the conservative strategy was associated with a functional benefit with improved lung function, reduced duration of ventilation, and reduced length of stay in the ICU. The measurement of EVLW may be appropriately considered in this context. In line with this, a randomized study conducted years ago compared two strategies of fluid management, one based upon the measurement of the PAOP, using a pulmonary artery catheter, and the other guided by the measurement of EVLW (measured by the double indicator technique) [3]. The cumulative fluid balance was maintained stable in the group of patients in whom fluid administration was guided by EVLW while it increased in the other group. Moreover, the duration of mechanical ventilation and the length of stay in the ICU were significantly reduced in the 'EVLW-guided' group, suggesting that the measurement of EVLW could be helpful in the context of ARDS. Moreover, the transpulmonary thermodilution device also allows real-time monitoring of cardiac output and of indicators of fluid responsiveness, such as the respiratory variation of pulse pressure or of stroke volume [40]. This hemodynamic monitoring method may be particularly useful to guide fluid administration in patients with circulatory failure and lung injury since fluid responsiveness parameters help to decide when to start fluid infusion and EVLW helps to decide whether to continue or to stop fluid infusion. Knowledge of high EVLW and PVPI values may incite clinicians to restrict fluid administration in ARDS patients with severe hypoxemia, even if pulse pressure variation is high and encourage them to choose alternative interventions for restoring hemodynamic conditions.

EVLW for Guiding Ventilatory Strategy

It has been demonstrated that high frequency ventilation is more effective in patients with a very high value of EVLW. By contrast, pressure support was better tolerated in patients with a low EVLW [41]. More interestingly, the measurement of EVLW by transpulmonary thermodilution was used to demonstrate that intravenous administration of salbutamol could accelerate the resolution of alveolar edema during ALI and ARDS [33]. It can be anticipated that EVLW will be used increasingly in the near future to assess the effects of therapy on lung injury during ALI/ARDS.

Conclusion

Techniques using transpulmonary dilution of indicators enable easy and reproducible measurement of EVLW at the bedside. The reliability of these techniques has now been well demonstrated, even though some limitations may lead to the underestimation of EVLW in cases of inhomogeneous lung injury. Among the techniques available to measure EVLW, transpulmonary thermodilution has became the most utilized because of its easiness to perform. In critically ill patients, the clinical interest of measuring EVLW is now better defined. It enables a diagnosis of pulmonary edema to be established when the cause of respiratory failure is uncertain. It allows one to distinguish between hydrostatic and non-hydrostatic forms of pulmonary edema. Finally, in patients with ALI/ARDS, the measurement of EVLW may guide fluid therapy, in particular because an elevated EVLW could prompt to restrict fluid administration.

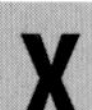

References

1. Monnet X, Anguel N, Osman D, et al (2007) Assessing pulmonary permeability by transpulmonary thermodilution allows differentiation of hydrostatic pulmonary edema from ALI/ARDS. Intensive Care Med 33: 448–453
2. Sakka SG, Klein M, Reinhart K, Meier-Hellmann A (2002) Prognostic value of extravascular lung water in critically ill patients. Chest 122: 2080–2086
3. Mitchell JP, Schuller D, Calandrino FS, Schuster DP (1992) Improved outcome based on fluid management in critically ill patients requiring pulmonary artery catheterization. Am Rev Respir Dis 145: 990–998
4. Lichtenstein D, Goldstein I, Mourgeon E, et al (2004) Comparative diagnostic performances of auscultation, chest radiography, and lung ultrasonography in acute respiratory distress syndrome. Anesthesiology 100: 9–15
5. Bock JC, Lewis FR (1990) Clinical relevance of lung water measurement with the thermal-dye dilution technique. J Surg Res 48: 254–265
6. Mihm FG, Feeley TW, Jamieson SW (1987) Thermal dye double indicator dilution measurement of lung water in man: comparison with gravimetric measurements. Thorax 42: 72–76
7. Patroniti N, Bellani G, Maggioni E, et al (2005) Measurement of pulmonary edema in patients with acute respiratory distress syndrome. Crit Care Med 33: 2547–2554
8. Godje O, Peyerl M, Seebauer T, Dewald O, Reichart B (1998) Reproducibility of double indica-

tor dilution measurements of intrathoracic blood volume compartments, extravascular lung water, and liver function. Chest 113: 1070–1077
9. Sakka SG, Ruhl CC, Pfeiffer UJ, et al (2000) Assessment of cardiac preload and extravascular lung water by single transpulmonary thermodilution. Intensive Care Med 26: 180–187
10. Reuter DA, Felbinger TW, Moerstedt K, et al (2002) Intrathoracic blood volume index measured by thermodilution for preload monitoring after cardiac surgery. J Cardiothorac Vasc Anesth 16: 191–195
11. Michard F, Schachtrupp A, Toens C (2005) Factors influencing the estimation of extravascular lung water by transpulmonary thermodilution in critically ill patients. Crit Care Med 33: 1243–1247
12. Neumann P (1999) Extravascular lung water and intrathoracic blood volume: double versus single indicator dilution technique. Intensive Care Med 25: 216–219
13. Rossi P, Wanecek M, Rudehill A, et al (2006) Comparison of a single indicator and gravimetric technique for estimation of extravascular lung water in endotoxemic pigs. Crit Care Med 34: 1437–1443
14. Kirov MY, Kuzkov VV, Kuklin VN, Waerhaug K, Bjertnaes LJ (2004) Extravascular lung water assessed by transpulmonary single thermodilution and postmortem gravimetry in sheep. Crit Care 8:R451–458
15. Katzenelson R, Perel A, Berkenstadt H, et al (2004) Accuracy of transpulmonary thermodilution versus gravimetric measurement of extravascular lung water. Crit Care Med 32: 1550–1554
16. Nirmalan M, Willard TM, Edwards DJ, Little RA, Dark PM (2005) Estimation of errors in determining intrathoracic blood volume using the single transpulmonary thermal dilution technique in hypovolemic shock. Anesthesiology 103: 805–812
17. Roch A, Michelet P, Lambert D, et al (2004) Accuracy of the double indicator method for measurement of extravascular lung water depends on the type of acute lung injury. Crit Care Med 32: 811–817
18. Carlile PV, Gray BA (1984) Type of lung injury influences the thermal-dye estimation of extravascular lung water. J Appl Physiol 57: 680–685
19. Beckett RC, Gray BA (1982) Effect of atelectasis and embolization on extravascular thermal volume of the lung. J Appl Physiol 53: 1614–1619
20. Allison RC, Parker JC, Duncan CE, Taylor AE (1983) Effect of air embolism on the measurement of extravascular lung thermal volume. J Appl Physiol 54: 943–949
21. Groeneveld AB, Verheij J (2004) Is pulmonary edema associated with a high extravascular thermal volume? Crit Care Med 32: 899–901
22. Slutsky RA (1983) Reduction in pulmonary blood volume during positive end-expiratory pressure. J Surg Res 35: 181–187
23. Carlile PV, Lowery DD, Gray BA (1986) Effect of PEEP and type of injury on thermal-dye estimation of pulmonary edema. J Appl Physiol 60: 22–31
24. Luecke T, Roth H, Herrmann P, et al (2003) PEEP decreases atelectasis and extravascular lung water but not lung tissue volume in surfactant-washout lung injury. Intensive Care Med 29: 2026–2033
25. Berkowitz DM, Danai PA, Eaton S, Moss M, Martin GS (2008) Accurate characterization of extravascular lung water in acute respiratory distress syndrome. Crit Care Med 36: 1803–1809
26. Phillips CR, Chesnutt MS, Smith SM (2008) Extravascular lung water in sepsis-associated acute respiratory distress syndrome: indexing with predicted body weight improves correlation with severity of illness and survival. Crit Care Med 36: 69–73
27. Lange NR, Schuster DP (1999) The measurement of lung water. Crit Care 3:R19-R24
28. Kunst PW, Vonk Noordegraaf A, Raaijmakers E, et al (1999) Electrical impedance tomography in the assessment of extravascular lung water in noncardiogenic acute respiratory failure. Chest 116: 1695–1702
29. Groeneveld AB, Verheij J (2006) Extravascular lung water to blood volume ratios as measures of permeability in sepsis-induced ALI/ARDS. Intensive Care Med 32: 1315–1321
30. Combes A, Berneau JB, Luyt CE, Trouillet JL (2004) Estimation of left ventricular systolic function by single transpulmonary thermodilution. Intensive Care Med 30: 1377–1383
31. Monnet X, Teboul JL (2006) Invasive measures of left ventricular preload. Curr Opin Crit Care 12: 235–240

32. Bernard GR, Artigas A, Brigham KL, et al (1994) The American-European Consensus Conference on ARDS. Definitions, mechanisms, relevant outcomes, and clinical trial coordination. Am J Respir Crit Care Med 149: 818–824
33. Perkins GD, McAuley DF, Thickett DR, Gao F (2006) The beta-agonist lung injury trial (BALTI): a randomized placebo-controlled clinical trial. Am J Respir Crit Care Med 173: 281–287
34. Ferguson ND, Meade MO, Hallett DC, Stewart TE (2002) High values of the pulmonary artery wedge pressure in patients with acute lung injury and acute respiratory distress syndrome. Intensive Care Med 28: 1073–1077
35. Martin GS, Eaton S, Mealer M, Moss M (2005) Extravascular lung water in patients with severe sepsis: a prospective cohort study. Crit Care 9:R74–82
36. Michard F, Zarka V, Alaya S (2004) Better characterization of acute lung injury/ARDS using lung water. Chest 125:1166
37. Schuster DP (2007) The search for "objective" criteria of ARDS. Intensive Care Med 33: 400–402
38. Kuzkov VV, Kirov MY, Sovershaev MA, et al (2006) Extravascular lung water determined with single transpulmonary thermodilution correlates with the severity of sepsis-induced acute lung injury. Crit Care Med 34: 1647–1653
39. Wiedemann HP, Wheeler AP, Bernard GR, et al (2006) Comparison of two fluid-management strategies in acute lung injury. N Engl J Med 354: 2564–2575
40. Monnet X, Teboul JL (2007) Volume responsiveness. Curr Opin Crit Care 13: 549–553
41. Zeravik J, Pfeiffer UJ (1989) Efficacy of high frequency ventilation combined with volume controlled ventilation in dependency of extravascular lung water. Acta Anaesthesiol Scand 33: 568–574

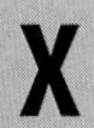

XI Perioperative Management

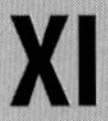

Rationalizing the Use of Surgical Critical Care: The Role of Cardiopulmonary Exercise Testing

S.J. Davies and R.J.T. Wilson

Introduction

In many hospitals, patients undergoing major elective surgery have to compete for postoperative critical care facilities with a population of unplanned emergency admissions, often resulting in delayed or cancelled procedures. Because of the competition for bed allocation in critical care, it is highly desirable that these resources are allocated to the patients that are most likely to benefit from them, and in addition it is equally desirable to identify patients that do not need to utilize these limited bed stocks after major surgery, because they have the cardiopulmonary reserve to cope with the demand that surgery entails.

A growing proportion of elderly patients with significant co-morbidities are presenting for high-risk procedures such as aortic aneurysm repair, or major cancer surgery. This surgery is associated with significant morbidity and mortality, and in the United Kingdom recently published audits have shown 30-day mortality rates of 5.6 % for elective colorectal cancer surgery [1], 19.3 % for emergency colorectal surgery, 7.3 % for elective infra-renal aortic aneurysm and aorto-iliac occlusive disease surgery [2], 9 % – 15 % for esophagectomy, and 13 % – 15 % for elective gastrectomy [3].

Heart failure has recently been shown to significantly increase the risk of death after major non-cardiac surgery [4]. In a retrospective analysis of almost 160,000 procedures, heart failure had a hazard ratio for mortality of 1.63 (95 % confidence interval 1.52 – 1.74) compared to patients without heart failure or coronary artery disease. This was in comparison to a hazard ratio of 1.08 (1.01 – 1.16) for coronary artery disease compared to patients without coronary artery disease or heart failure. In addition to this, the readmission rates to hospital were 17.1 % for patients with heart failure, 10.8 % for patients with coronary artery disease, and 8.1 % for patients with neither. In a separate study, heart failure was associated with a greater than 10-fold increase in cardiac death if present in patients at the time that they underwent major vascular surgery [5].

The hormonal and inflammatory responses that surgery generates can cause a significant increase in oxygen demand by up to 50 % that extends beyond surgery into the postoperative period [6, 7], and it has been shown that patients who have poor indices of tissue perfusion, and generate a perioperative oxygen debt due to their inability to increase cardiac output, and therefore oxygen delivery (DO_2), fare worse after major surgery [7–9]. In essence, these patients have cardiac failure defined by their inability to meet their oxygen demands.

It, therefore, seems likely that if a preoperative evaluation could identify patients with significant heart failure that limits functional capacity, it would be of use in identifying the higher-risk patient, who would gain greater benefit from postoperative critical care due to their increased risk of both mortality, morbidity, and hospital readmission.

Cardiopulmonary exercise testing is a dynamic non-invasive test that examines the ability of the patient's cardiorespiratory system to adapt to a 'stress' situation of increased oxygen demand, in effect mimicking the surgical insult. Cardiopulmonary exercise testing has been shown to identify patients at high risk of cardiorespiratory complications after major surgery through identification of their anaerobic threshold. Cardiopulmonary exercise testing allows high-risk surgical patients to be identified, and then allocated the proper resources such as enhanced perioperative hemodynamic monitoring, access to postoperative critical care services, or even, if the risk is deemed great, to explore other avenues of therapy.

In this chapter, we will explain the rationale for cardiopulmonary exercise testing, which patients should undergo cardiopulmonary exercise testing prior to surgery, the practical procedure of testing patients, and how to interpret the data into clinically useful information for perioperative management and risk stratification

Why Use Cardiopulmonary Exercise Testing as an Assessment Tool?

Why should we use cardiopulmonary exercise testing in preference to other standard preoperative tests to identify the high-risk patient? Del Guercio and Cohn [10] showed that standard preoperative assessment failed to identify physiological dysfunction in the elderly. Of the 148 patients that were cleared for surgery by standard assessment, only 13.5 % had normal physiological variables on invasive monitoring, whilst 23 % had such functional physiological derangement that it made them an unacceptable risk for surgery. In this group, which was advised against surgery, the mortality was 100 % in those who elected to proceed.

There are many tests that have been developed to look at ischemic heart disease; however, they have translated poorly into being able to stratify risk in the perioperative period. This may be because heart failure is associated with a worse outcome than coronary artery disease, as mentioned above. Transthoracic echocardiography provides excellent anatomical information; however, as a marker of cardiac function it represents a static view at a single point in time. There is poor correlation between echocardiographically assessed myocardial function and functional capacity [11]. More dynamic tests such as dobutamine stress echocardiography and dypyridamole thallium scintigraphy, have been used to try and identify high-risk patients and quantify risk. The positive predictive value of these tests for postoperative ischemic events is poor at 20 to 30 % although the negative predictive value is much higher at 95 to 100 % [12]. Importantly, these tests only evaluate the presence of myocardial ischemia and limitations on heart rate, but give little information on the extent of cardiac failure and limitations on DO_2. In addition these tests are impractical to perform as preoperative assessments.

Cardiopulmonary exercise testing has been used to stratify patients with heart failure, and the Weber Janicki classification [13] stratifies the severity of heart failure based on peak oxygen uptake and anaerobic threshold. In addition, cardiopulmonary exercise testing has been shown to be of prognostic importance in heart failure both in the short [14–18] and long term [19]. It, therefore, seems that if cardiopulmonary exercise testing can both identify and stratify patients with heart failure then it could also be used to identify patients at higher risk in terms of morbidity and mortality after surgery.

Cardiopulmonary exercise testing provides a dynamic, stressed test of cardiorespiratory reserve. Oxygen consumption (VO_2) and carbon dioxide production (VCO_2) are measured during a ramped exercise test, and as VO_2 is directly related to DO_2, and is also a linear function of cardiac output under exercise conditions, this provides an objective measurement of cardiorespiratory reserve (mainly cardiac function). The measurement of anaerobic threshold is a submaximal test that is both repeatable and relevant to perioperative risk assessment. The anaerobic threshold is the point at which DO_2 becomes inadequate to meet the energy demand of the body through pure aerobic metabolism alone, and is, therefore, supplemented by anaerobic metabolism and the consequent production of lactate. The VO_2 at which this occurs is known as the anaerobic threshold, expressed in ml/kg/min, and can be identified easily in most individuals. Older et al. measured the anaerobic threshold in 187 elderly patients before major abdominal surgery [20]: Patients who had an anaerobic threshold < 11 ml/kg/min had a mortality of 18 % compared with those who had an anaerobic threshold > 11 ml/kg/min whose mortality was 0.8 %. In patients who exhibited signs of ischemia during the testing process, mortality was 42 % for patients whose anaerobic threshold was < 11 ml/kg/min, whilst only 4 % for those whose anaerobic threshold was > 11 ml/kg/min. From these data it can be seen that poor ventricular function and, hence, poor DO_2, as measured by the anaerobic threshold, predicted a high risk for major surgery, particularly when coupled with evidence of myocardial ischemia.

Cardiopulmonary exercise testing has also been shown to be of benefit in other surgical groups. There was an inverse relationship between cardiorespiratory fitness as defined by cardiopulmonary exercise testing and major complications after bariatric surgery [21] and esophagectomy [22]. Cardiopulmonary exercise testing has also proved useful in predicting pulmonary complications after lung cancer resection surgery [23, 24]. Identification of the anaerobic threshold using cardiopulmonary exercise testing, therefore, provides a safe, objective, non-invasive, submaximal and repeatable test that is able to accurately predict those at increased risk from major abdominal surgery.

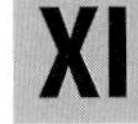

Which Patients should Undergo Cardiopulmonary Exercise Testing?

It is impractical for all surgical patients to undergo cardiopulmonary exercise testing, and indeed unnecessary as it is only the potentially at risk patient undergoing major surgery that we are interested in. In our hospital, we test all patients scheduled for aortic aneurysm repair and esophagectomy, and patients scheduled for major intra-abdominal cancer surgery who are over 55 years old, or younger if they have major co-morbidities.

Generally, there are three main reasons for surgical patients to undergo testing:

1. Surgical decision making. To aid both medical staff and patients to decide whether an operation is actually the best treatment in terms of the immediate risks of surgery balanced against the benefits that the operation may provide. In our institution, all patients with aortic aneurysms that are being considered for repair, or with esophageal tumors are treated on this basis. If patients are very high risk by virtue of their cardiopulmonary exercise test result then there are treatment alternatives that may produce equally satisfactory results. The algorithm for aortic surgical patients that will be discussed later is an example of this.

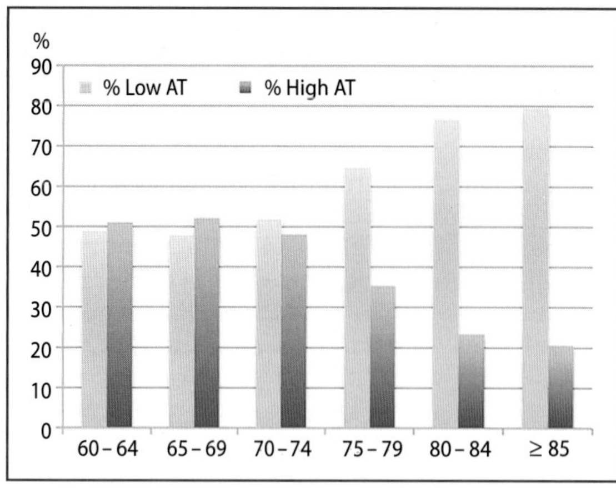

Fig. 1. Age and anaerobic threshold (AT).

2. Medical optimization. For patients where surgery is the main treatment choice, the results can be utilized to medically optimize the patient prior to surgery, usually by starting beta-blockers. This is particularly useful in view of the concerns raised in the PeriOperative ISchemic Evaluation (POISE) trial over beta-blockade of surgical patients [25], as the effect of beta-blockade can be assessed by repeat cardiopulmonary exercise testing.
3. Allocation of post-operative critical care resources. The results of cardiopulmonary exercise testing, in particular the value of the anaerobic threshold and the presence or absence of coronary artery disease, can be used in a treatment algorithm. In our hospital, the principles of the algorithm remain the same as originally published by Older et al. [20].

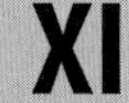

In our population of elderly patients, a significant number will have an anaerobic threshold less than 11 ml/kg/min, and therefore a high proportion of those deemed high risk can be identified (**Fig. 1**). There is no upper age limit for testing, and some form of meaningful data can be obtained from most patients. Occasionally a test is unable to be performed in patients with knee replacements, as they may not have the required degree of knee flexion to cycle effectively.

Cardiopulmonary Exercise Testing in Practice

At York, cardiopulmonary exercise testing is carried out in the general and urological surgery pre-assessment clinic as part of a routine two hour visit that covers all aspects of surgical pre-assessment. The test takes approximately 30 to 40 minutes and consists of a number of stages:

1. Preparation

Patients receive written information about the test and what to expect with their pre-assessment clinic appointment. Prior to the test, the pre-assessment nurse will take a history from the patient, measure pulse, oxygen saturations and blood pressure, and perform a resting electrocardiogram (EKG). If all is satisfactory, patients will then undergo cardiopulmonary exercise testing.

For respiratory volumes the analyzer is manually calibrated to a known volume, and for gas measurement the oxygen and carbon dioxide analyzers are calibrated to known concentrations of gas.

The patient is assisted onto a cycle ergonometer and the height of the seat is adjusted so that cycling is both comfortable and efficient. A twelve lead exercise EKG and blood pressure cuff are connected, and the patient is shown how to insert the mouthpiece for the gas analyzer. The patient is then talked through the various stages of the testing procedure and given the relevant safety information.

2. Data collection

A number of different variables are measured throughout the test including:

- 12-lead exercise EKG with ST trend analysis, with the ability to rotate through the different leads as required. This information automatically feeds to the gas analysis software to allow this to be incorporated in various measurements.
- Blood pressure is measured at the beginning and end of the test.
- For each breath the monitor measures VO_2, VCO_2, respiratory rate, respiratory exchange ratio (RER), and tidal volume.
- EKG and respiratory data collection software are interfaced, as heart rate responses to increasing work rate are useful during analysis. Gas analysis and EKG data are viewed continuously on the workstation allowing the clinician to monitor the progress of the test.

3. Unloaded Cycling

The test begins with 3 minutes of unloaded cycling. During this phase, the patient cycles without any resistance on the cycle ergonometer, at a cadence that is comfortable and sustainable for them (usually around 60 rpm). This phase is necessary as it allows the patient to get used to the cycling and to allow any anxiety based hyperventilation to settle. During this phase VO_2 usually doubles from the resting state.

4. Ramping Phase

After the 3 minutes of unloaded cycling, the resistance to cycling starts to increase. The rate of increase is determined by the patient's age and co-morbidities, and is usually an increase in work rate of 10 to 15 watts per minute. The increase in work rate is evenly distributed throughout each minute, hence the ramping effect. During this phase, the patient is encouraged to maintain a regular cadence, although the cycle ergonometer compensates for changes in cadence within limits. As the work rate increases, VO_2 will start to increase, and VCO_2 should increase in parallel whilst the patient is metabolizing aerobically. The RER during this phase should remain relatively constant, but will vary depending on diet; however it will certainly remain below 1.0. As the work rate continues to increase during the test, exercising muscle requires increasing amounts of ATP.

As ATP demand increases, a point will be reached where ATP production from anaerobic metabolic pathways starts to supplement aerobic ATP production. This is usually around 60 % of the patient's predicted maximum oxygen uptake, and the value of oxygen uptake at this point is known as the anaerobic threshold.

At the anaerobic threshold, lactate is produced from anaerobic respiration, which in turn is buffered by bicarbonate to produce carbon dioxide and water. The relative increase in carbon dioxide disrupts the usually parallel relationship between VO_2 and VCO_2, so that the two converge and eventually VCO_2 exceeds VO_2. Once this has occurred and the RER is consistently greater than 1.0 and still increasing, the test can be terminated. This type of cardiopulmonary exercise testing is submaximal, i.e., patients are not taken to their maximal VO_2, and apart from the advantage of being safe in elderly patients, it is also a point the patient is subjectively unaware of, and, therefore, it is objectively repeatable.

The test may also be prematurely terminated prior to the patient reaching anaerobic threshold if there is ST segment depression of greater than 2 mm, the patient suffers chest pain, or if they become too exhausted to continue.

5. Recovery Phase

At the termination of the test, the resistance on the cycle is removed and the patient is asked to continue cycling for approximately one minute. This is essential, as blood pressure that usually increases with exercise will decrease if there is an abrupt cessation of exercise. This recovery phase allows a gradual cessation of exercise, and avoids episode of fainting or dizziness in frail patients.

Interpretation of Cardiopulmonary Exercise Test Data

Cardiopulmonary exercise testing generates a lot of useful data, but there are specific elements that may alter clinical decision making and management:

1. The Anaerobic Threshold

XI

A graph of VO_2 against VCO_2, also known as the V-slope graph is plotted allowing the anaerobic threshold to be calculated. As discussed, at the anaerobic threshold the parallel relationship of VO_2 and VCO_2 is disrupted, with a relative increase in CO_2 production. This can be seen in the slope of the graph, and the anaerobic threshold can be calculated. The anaerobic threshold is the VO_2 in ml/kg/min when aerobic metabolism is insufficient to meet the energy demand and hence is supplemented by anaerobic metabolism. Additional information on the graph can also help to identify the anaerobic threshold, as the $PETO_2$ (end tidal oxygen tension) and V_E/VO_2 tends to rise at the anaerobic threshold while the $PETCO_2$ (end tidal CO_2) and V_E/VCO_2 remain constant for a brief period before beginning to rise due to a period of isocapnic buffering.

The anaerobic threshold value is highly significant as the work of Older et al. [20] reported that patients were at much higher risk of dying after surgery if their anaerobic threshold was < 11 ml/kg/min, with a mortality of 18 % for those with an anaerobic threshold of < 11 ml/kg/min, compared to 0.8 % with those that had an anaerobic threshold > 11 ml/kg/min; mortality was higher if patients had ischemic heart disease and a low anaerobic threshold (mortality 42 %). Our experience in York so far with over 1000 patients tested confirms Older's findings that patients with an anaerobic threshold of < 11 ml/kg/min are at the highest risk after major surgery; however our mortality figures are substantially lower.

2. Ischemic Heart Disease

It essential to identify the group of patients with ischemic heart disease as its presence confers a significant increase in peri-operative risk. At present, this group is classified as a history of myocardial infarction or angina, previous coronary artery bypass graft (CABG), or significant ST depression on exercise EKG during testing (1 mm or greater depression in two leads). However, other variables can be obtained from the cardiopulmonary exercise testing, which allow assessment of cardiac function and coronary artery disease.

a) The oxygen pulse response (VO_2/heart rate)

The oxygen pulse is calculated by dividing VO_2 by heart rate at any given point in time. It translates into the volume of oxygen taken up by the pulmonary circulation for every heart beat, and is essentially the product of stroke volume and arterial-mixed venous oxygen content difference. In health, as exercise increases the oxygen pulse should increase due to an increase in oxygen extraction and stroke volume (**Fig. 2a**). If the stroke volume is limited due to some form of myocardial dysfunction, oxygen extraction reaches its maximum early in exercise, and hence the oxygen pulse response shows little or no increase after the early stages of exercise (**Fig. 2b**).

b) Relationship of VO_2 to work rate

For each 1-watt increase in work rate, VO_2 should increase by 10 ml/min. This is a parallel relationship that remains stable across all ages in health (**Fig. 3a**). If this relationship is disrupted, i.e., the relationship is non-linear, then this may indicate ventricular dysfunction (**Fig. 3b**). Work by Belardinelli et al. [26] has suggested that the oxygen pulse response and the VO_2 work rate response are strong independent predictors of myocardial ischemia, and more accurate than standard exercise EKG stress tests.

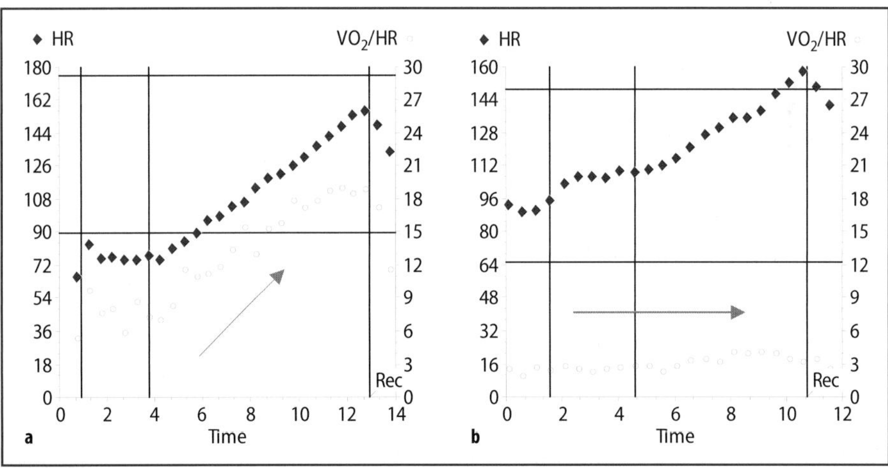

Fig. 2. Graph **a** shows a normal oxygen pulse response, with the VO_2/heart rate (HR) steadily increasing throughout exercise. The abnormal response (graph **b**) is flat, indicating that oxygen delivery is purely at the expense of heart rate, and indicates some myocardial dysfunction.

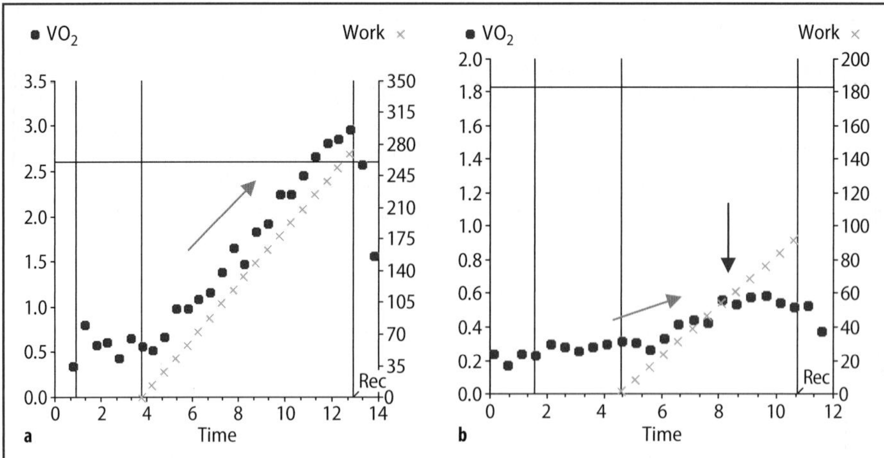

Fig. 3. Graph **a** shows the normal response of increasing VO_2 to work rate in which the two are parallel. Graph **b** shows an abnormal response, of initially a reduced gradient (pale blue arrow) indicating that VO_2 is not matching work rate increases, and then there is a flattening of the response (dark blue arrow) where the VO_2 fails to increase and indeed then starts to decrease. This is highly indicative of myocardial ischemia.

c) Ventilatory Equivalent for CO_2 (V_E/VCO_2)
This is the ratio of minute ventilation compared to the volume of CO_2 produced. The normal value is less than 34, and higher values tend to represent increased ventilation-perfusion mismatch (dead space), and in a patient with a low anaerobic threshold may indicate more severe heart failure.

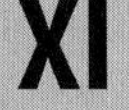

Obviously a lot of data are collected during an exercise test and its analysis may seem confusing at times. Hopefully the cases toward the end of the chapter will show what is expected on a normal and abnormal test and illustrate some of the points made above and how the data are utilized in decision making.

Risk Stratification and Management using Cardiopulmonary Exercise Testing

As stated previously, the purpose of cardiopulmonary exercise testing is to aid clinicians and patients in deciding if surgery is the most viable option, and, if it is, to plan their perioperative care and allocate appropriate resources. In a second study by Older et al. [27], over 500 patients undergoing major abdominal surgery were risk stratified by anaerobic threshold and perioperative interventions were managed on the basis of their cardiopulmonary exercise test result. The patients with an anaerobic threshold < 11 ml/kg/min (28 %) were admitted to the intensive care unit (ICU) preoperatively and had baseline hemodynamic and oxygen transport variables monitored; 115 patients (21 %) with an anaerobic threshold > 11 ml/kg/min but with evidence of myocardial ischemia on testing were admitted to the high dependency unit (HDU) postoperatively, and those with an anaerobic threshold > 11 ml/kg/min with no evidence of ischemia were cared for on a normal ward postoperatively. Of the 21 patients who died, 19 had been triaged to ICU/HDU as a result

Table 1. Odds ratios of mortality associated with anaerobic threshold values obtained by cardiopulmonary exercise testing

Cardiopulmonary exercise test result	Odds ratio (mortality)	Classification
> 11 ml/kg/min (no CAD)	1.0	Normal risk
< 11 ml/kg/min (no CAD)	2.47	Intermediate risk
11–14 ml/kg/min (+ CAD)	1.91	Intermediate risk
< 11 ml/kg/min (+ CAD)	4.42	High risk

CAD: coronary artery disease

of cardiopulmonary exercise testing and hence deemed as high risk, and the additional two deaths that were in the ward group were due to disease progression. Through cardiopulmonary exercise testing, high risk patients were suitably identified and the appropriate use of critical care beds reduced mortality in the high-risk group (low anaerobic threshold) from 18 % (original paper) to 8.9 %.

As **Table 1** shows, patient risk of mortality changes according to their anaerobic threshold and history of coronary artery disease. From our experience, not unlike that of Older et al., the high-risk patient has an anaerobic threshold < 11 ml/kg/min and coronary artery disease. This group of patients will be adequately protected with perioperative beta-blockade, will receive full invasive monitoring and intraoperative fluid optimization based on cardiac output monitoring, and will be nursed in the HDU postoperatively.

The intermediate risk group receives similar care, but can be safely managed on the nursing enhanced unit (HDU step-down care) postoperatively. The normal risk group receives no invasive monitoring unless the procedure itself demands it, and can be safely nursed postoperatively on the ward.

Utilization of these data allows effective planning of peri-operative care, rational critical care bed usage, and ultimately improved patient care and outcome. It is worth noting, however, that in some cases we would use the data to advise against surgery, even if the only alternative is palliative care, if it is deemed that the perioperative risks of surgery are too great.

Case Reports

Case 1: Normal Subject

Figure 4 shows the raw gas exchange data obtained from a fit and healthy 24-year old female and illustrates the principle features seen when conducting a cardiopulmonary exercise test. The test is commenced with 3 minutes of unloaded cycling to allow the subject to acclimatize to the test, and for any hyperventilation to settle. Data at this point show a steady VO_2 at approximately 500 ml/kg/min (unloaded cycling usually doubles VO_2 from the resting state), and VCO_2 of approximately 400 ml/kg/min, which calculates the RER at 0.8, the usual resting state for a mixed diet. When the ramping phase starts, a steady increase in VO_2 can be seen, which is mirrored by a parallel change in VCO_2. As the work rate continues to increase, the relationship between VO_2 and VCO_2 ceases to be linear and the two start to converge (and so the RER approaches 1.0) until they cross and then become divergent with VCO_2 being in excess of VO_2, and hence the RER being greater than 1.0.

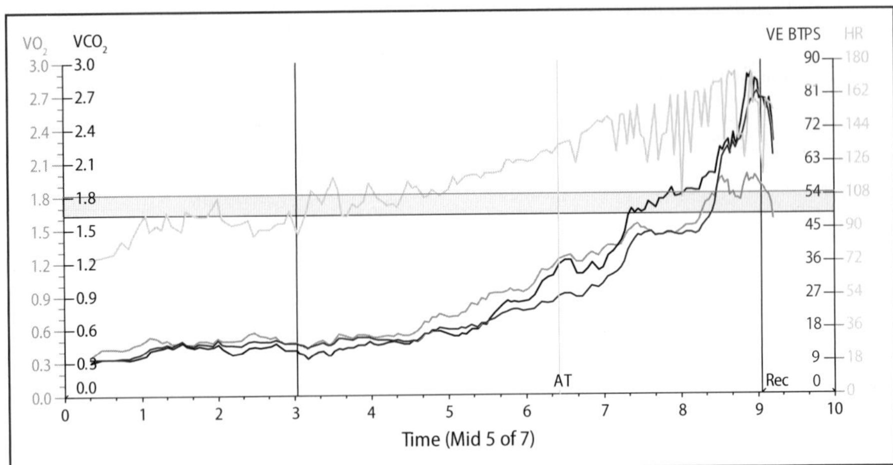

Fig. 4. Raw cardiopulmonary exercise test data from Case 1, a 'normal' subject. AT: anaerobic threshold

This convergence and subsequent relative excess of CO_2 production is due to the production of lactate from anaerobic metabolism and its subsequent buffering to CO_2. It can also be seen that there is an increase in minute ventilation at this point (brown line) due to increased respiratory drive from the increased CO_2.

Although we can estimate where we think the anaerobic threshold may be from the raw data, it must be remembered that the convergence point is not the actual anaerobic threshold, as there is a short period of isocapnic buffering. To obtain the anaerobic threshold we must look at the V-slope (**Fig. 5a**), where it can be seen there is a sudden increase in VCO_2 away from the line of intention, which also correlates to the trough of the $PETO_2$ before it rises. This is the anaerobic threshold and it can be seen that it corresponds to a VO_2 of approximately 1250 ml/min and, therefore, for a 60 kg person equates to an anaerobic threshold of 20.8 ml/kg/min.

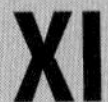

Other data can also be obtained from cardiopulmonary exercise testing as mentioned previously, and we can see data relating to cardiac function in the other panels. The oxygen pulse response shows a constant increase throughout exercise, indicating that there is appropriate inotropy and increase in stroke volume throughout exercise (**Fig. 5b**), whilst the VO_2/workrate response is normal, with a parallel increase in VO_2 to increasing work in the correct magnitude of 10 ml/min for each 1 watt increase (**Fig. 5c**). It can also be seen that the V_E/VCO_2 at the anaerobic threshold is normal at 24, indicating that there is no dead space due to cardiac failure or respiratory disease (**Fig. 5d**).

This is a perfect example of a normal exercise test, and with an anaerobic threshold of > 11 ml/kg/min would confer a normal risk for surgery.

Case 2: Resource Utilization

The data shown in **Figure 6** are from a 71-year old man scheduled for an anterior resection. He had a past medical history of hypertension but nil else of significance. He reported good exercise tolerance, and no other cardiorespiratory symptoms. His cardiopulmonary exercise test showed an anaerobic threshold of 18.1 ml/kg/min with a normal stroke volume and work rate response. Due to his 'normal' cardiopul-

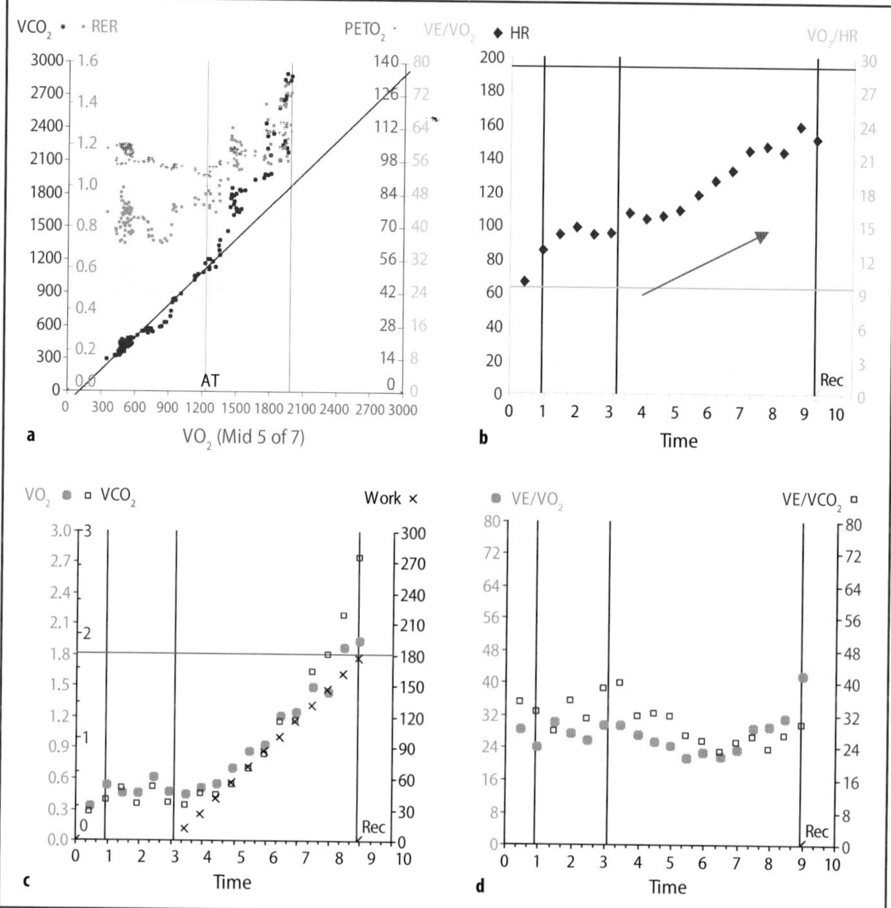

Fig. 5. V-slope **a**, oxygen pulse response **b**, VO_2/workrate response **c**, and ventilatory equivalent for CO_2 **d** from Case 1 (see text for details). AT: anaerobic threshold

monary exercise test this gentleman was deemed low risk, proceeded to surgery without invasive monitoring, was nursed uneventfully on the ward postoperatively, and was discharged on day 8.

In contrast, the cardiopulmonary exercise test data in **Figure 7** were obtained from a 67-year old male also with a history of hypertension and scheduled for elective colorectal surgery for carcinoma (left hemicolectomy). His preoperative assessment was unremarkable, and he denied any cardiac or respiratory symptoms, and claimed to have an exercise tolerance of greater than 500 m, being able to comfortably climb two flights of stairs.

It can be seen that the oxygen pulse response (**Fig. 7b**) is flat compared to case 1, suggesting that VO_2 is being predominately met by increasing heart rate, with little change in the stroke volume suggesting myocardial dysfunction. Further evidence for myocardial dysfunction is seen with a poor work rate response (**Fig. 7c**), as VO_2 changes are not parallel with work rate, and indeed there is flattening of the response at point A, which may be indicative of myocardial ischemia. An increased

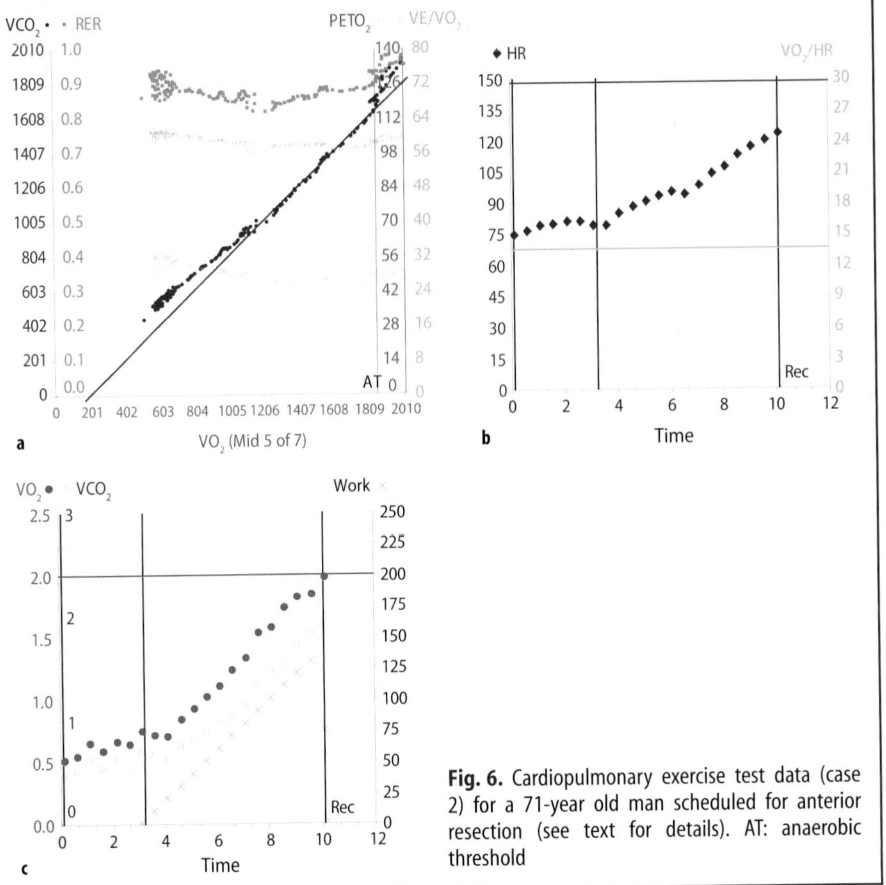

Fig. 6. Cardiopulmonary exercise test data (case 2) for a 71-year old man scheduled for anterior resection (see text for details). AT: anaerobic threshold

V_E/VCO_2 of 42 in a person with no respiratory history or symptoms also indicates increased dead space due to cardiac failure (**Fig. 7d**). The anaerobic threshold calculated by the V-slope method was 6.8 ml/kg/min.

This patient therefore has a low anaerobic threshold and signs of significant myocardial dysfunction and, therefore, has a higher risk of perioperative morbidity and mortality than the previous case; perioperative management will thus need to be modified to allow for these factors including fluid optimization, invasive monitoring, and a postoperative critical care bed.

Theses cases provide an example of how two otherwise 'fit and healthy men' of a similar age, reported exercise tolerance, and medical history have a very different objective cardiorespiratory reserve on cardiopulmonary testing. As a result, both embark on a very different perioperative course efficiently utilizing limited critical care beds.

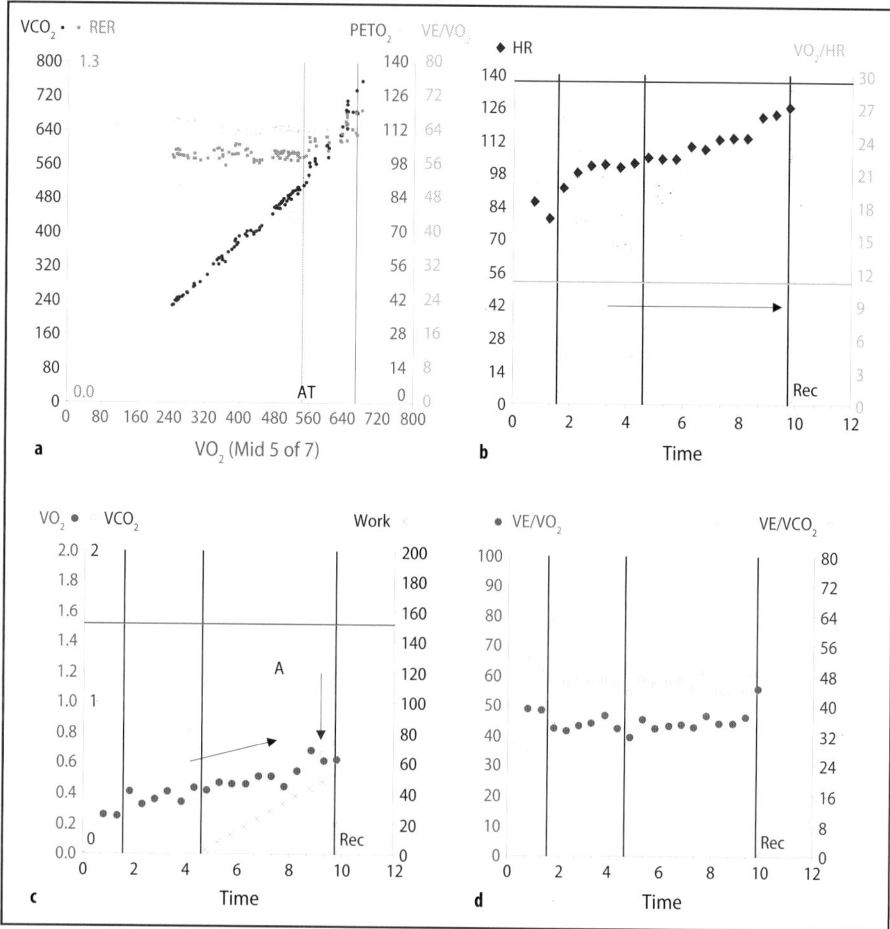

Fig. 7. Cardiopulmonary exercise test data (case 2) for a 67-year old man scheduled for elective colorectal surgery (see text for details). AT: anaerobic threshold

Case 3: Medical Perioperative Management

The data in **Figure 8** are from a 71-year old male with type 1 diabetes mellitus with no history of coronary artery disease. It can be seen from **Figure 8a** that his initial work rate response was flat suggesting coronary artery disease, but following bisoprolol 2.5 mg the work rate response improved considerably (**Fig. 8b**).

The patient's oxygen pulse response also improved, and this can be seen if we compare the initial cardiac response to exercise (**Fig. 8c**) with the response after bisoprolol 2.5 mg (**Fig. 8d**). It can be seen that the oxygen pulse is no longer flat, and the rise in the oxygen pulse during exercise following beta-blockade suggests that myocardial function has been improved.

The patient's anaerobic threshold also improved by more than 50 % from 5.7 to 9.3 ml/kg/min. This illustrates how cardiopulmonary exercise testing is able to identify myocardial impairment, and also how the effects of therapy can be evaluated by repeat testing.

XI

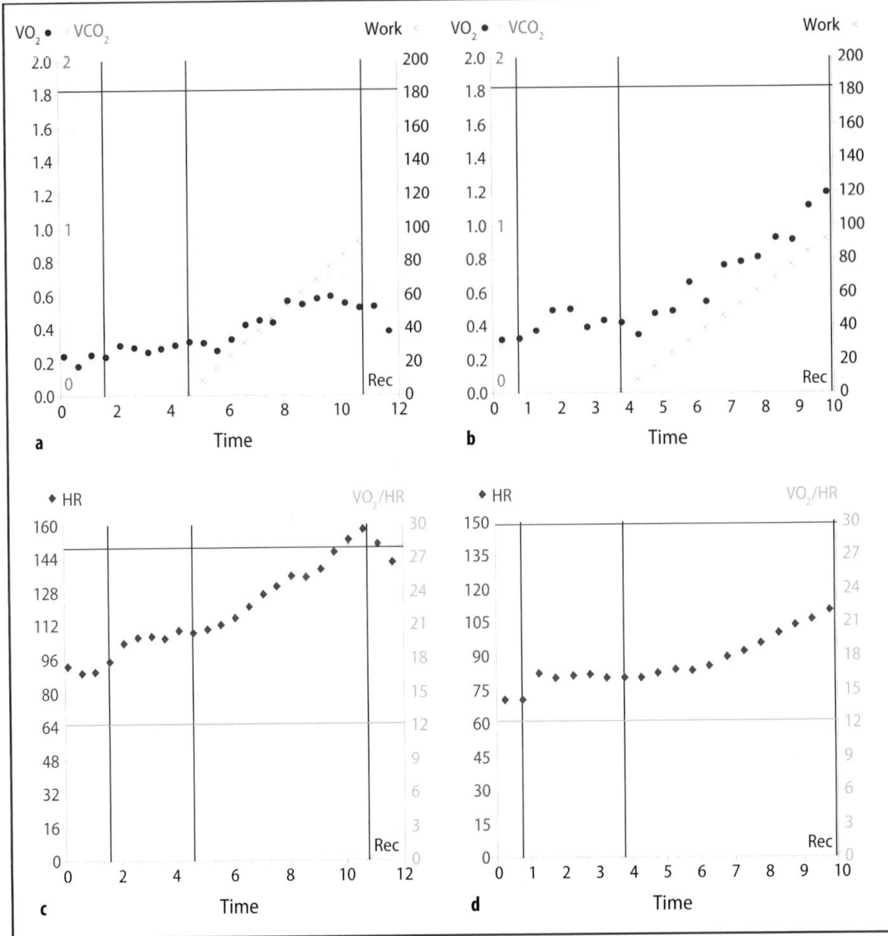

Fig. 8. VO_2/workrate response in Case 3, before **a** and after **b** bisoprolol, and oxygen-pulse response, before **c** and after **d** bisoprolol.

XI

Case 4: Surgical Decision Making

An example of how cardiopulmonary exercise testing can aid surgical decision making can be seen by looking at two patients who were scheduled for elective esophagastrectomy. The first patient was 77-years old with esophageal adenocarcinoma. The patient was an ex-smoker of greater than 40 pack years, and had a history of hypertension and angina. Cardiopulmonary exercise testing showed an anaerobic threshold of 14.1 ml/kg/min with a V_E/VCO_2 of 28. This indicated that despite multiple medical co-morbidities the patient had adequate cardiorespiratory reserve and minimal pulmonary dysfunction in order for the risk benefits of the surgery to be acceptable. The patient underwent the procedure and had an uncomplicated recovery with a 23-day hospital stay.

In contrast, a 71-year old with esophageal squamous cell carcinoma was sent for assessment by cardiopulmonary exercise testing. The patient's history was relatively unremarkable with a history of hypertension, however cardiopulmonary exercise testing showed a low anaerobic threshold of 7.7 ml/kg/min, with a significantly raised V_E/VCO_2 of 63. Due to these results and after discussion with the surgeon it was decided that surgery provided too high a risk and the patient was sent for chemo-radiotherapy. Despite this the patient remains alive and asymptomatic 37 months later.

These cases illustrate how risk can be assessed using cardiopulmonary exercise testing and the risk-benefit of treatment modalities evaluated so that the most appropriate advice and treatment option can be given to the patient.

Conclusion

Cardiopulmonary exercise testing provides objective information about cardiorespiratory reserve that allows for multidisciplinary planning of a patient's perioperative management, from preoperative interventions through to postoperative critical care utilization. This simple non-invasive test can identify not only those at high risk of perioperative complications, and hospital readmission, who will often require the services of critical care, but can also identify those patients whose physiological reserve is such that they pose a low risk for surgical intervention. It is this latter group that can safely receive their postoperative care outside of critical care facilities with a low risk of complications and unplanned emergency critical care admission.

In addition, cardiopulmonary exercise testing allows for risk stratification to enable accurate assessment of the risk-benefit ratio that surgical intervention offers the patient. Through this assessment, it can sometimes be decided that surgery provides too high a risk for an individual, and other modalities including palliation will need to be explored.

Hopefully, through the use of preoperative cardiopulmonary exercise testing, critical care utilization can be rationalized and unplanned emergency admissions to the ICU reduced.

References

1. Tekkis PP, Poloniecki JD, Thompson M, Stamatakis J (2002) ACPGBI Colorectal Cancer Study 2002. Part A: Unadjusted outcomes. Available at: http://www.nbocap.org.uk/resources/reports/ACP_report_part_A.pdf. Accessed Nov 2008
2. Bayly PJ, Matthews JN, Dobson PM, Price ML, Thomas DG (2001) In-hospital mortality from abdominal aortic surgery in Great Britain and Ireland: Vascular Anaesthesia Society audit. Br J Surg 88: 687–692
3. McCulloch P, Ward J, Tekkis PP (2003) Mortality and morbidity in gastro-oesophageal cancer surgery: initial results of ASCOT multicentre prospective cohort study. BMJ 327: 1192–1197
4. Hammill BG, Curtis LH, Bennett-Guerrero E, et al (2008) Impact of heart failure on patients undergoing major noncardiac surgery. Anesthesiology 108: 559–567
5. Sprung J, Abdelmalak B, Gottlieb A, et al (2000) Analysis of risk factors for myocardial infarction and cardiac mortality after major vascular surgery. Anesthesiology 93: 129–140
6. Older P, Smith R (1988) Experience with the preoperative invasive measurement of haemodynamic, respiratory and renal function in 100 elderly patients scheduled for major abdominal surgery. Anaesth Intensive Care 16: 389–395
7. Shoemaker WC, Appel PL, Kram HB (1992) Role of oxygen debt in the development of organ failure sepsis, and death in high-risk surgical patients. Chest 102: 208–215
8. Bland RD, Shoemaker WC, Abraham E, Cobo JC (1985) Hemodynamic and oxygen transport patterns in surviving and nonsurviving postoperative patients. Crit Care Med 13: 85–90

9. Gutierrez G, Bismar H, Dantzker DR, Silva N (1992) Comparison of gastric intramucosal pH with measures of oxygen transport and consumption in critically ill patients. Crit Care Med 20: 451–457
10. Del Guercio LR, Cohn JD (1980) Monitoring operative risk in the elderly. JAMA 243: 1350–1355
11. Halm EA, Browner WS, Tubau JF, Tateo IM, Mangano DT (1996) Echocardiography for assessing cardiac risk in patients having noncardiac surgery. Study of Perioperative Ischemia Research Group. Ann Intern Med 125: 433–441
12. Chassot PG, Delabays A, Spahn DR (2002) Preoperative evaluation of patients with, or at risk of, coronary artery disease undergoing non-cardiac surgery. Br J Anaesth 89: 747–759
13. Weber KT, Kinasewitz GT, Janicki JS, Fishman AP (1982) Oxygen utilization and ventilation during exercise in patients with chronic cardiac failure. Circulation 65: 1213–1223
14. Chua TP, Ponikowski P, Harrington D, et al (1997) Clinical correlates and prognostic significance of the ventilatory response to exercise in chronic heart failure. J Am Coll Cardiol 29: 1585–1590
15. Cohn JN, Johnson GR, Shabetai R, et al (1993) Ejection fraction, peak exercise oxygen consumption, cardiothoracic ratio, ventricular arrhythmias, and plasma norepinephrine as determinants of prognosis in heart failure. The V-HeFT VA Cooperative Studies Group. Circulation 87 (Suppl 6):VI5–16
16. Opasich C, Pinna GD, Bobbio M, et al (1998) Peak exercise oxygen consumption in chronic heart failure: toward efficient use in the individual patient. J Am Coll Cardiol 31: 766–775
17. Osada N, Chaitman BR, Miller LW, et al (1998) Cardiopulmonary exercise testing identifies low risk patients with heart failure and severely impaired exercise capacity considered for heart transplantation. J Am Coll Cardiol 31: 577–582
18. Stelken AM, Younis LT, Jennison SH, et al (1996) Prognostic value of cardiopulmonary exercise testing using percent achieved of predicted peak oxygen uptake for patients with ischemic and dilated cardiomyopathy. J Am Coll Cardiol 27: 345–352
19. Koike A, Koyama Y, Itoh H, Adachi H, Marumo F, Hiroe M (2000) Prognostic significance of cardiopulmonary exercise testing for 10-year survival in patients with mild to moderate heart failure. Jpn Circ J 64: 915–920
20. Older P, Smith R, Courtney P, Hone R (1993) Preoperative evaluation of cardiac failure and ischemia in elderly patients by cardiopulmonary exercise testing. Chest 104: 701–704
21. McCullough PA, Gallagher MJ, Dejong AT, et al (2006) Cardiorespiratory fitness and short-term complications after bariatric surgery. Chest 130: 517–525
22. Nagamatsu Y, Shima I, Yamana H, Fujita H, Shirouzu K, Ishitake T (2001) Preoperative evaluation of cardiopulmonary reserve with the use of expired gas analysis during exercise testing in patients with squamous cell carcinoma of the thoracic esophagus. J Thorac Cardiovasc Surg 121: 1064–1068
23. Bolliger CT, Jordan P, Soler M, et al (1995) Exercise capacity as a predictor of postoperative complications in lung resection candidates. Am J Respir Crit Care Med 151: 1472–1480
24. Bolliger CT, Perruchoud AP (1998) Functional evaluation of the lung resection candidate. Eur Respir J 11: 198–212
25. Devereux PJ, Yang H, Yusuf S, et al (2008) Effects of extended release metoprolol-succinate in patients undergoing non-cardiac surgery (POISE trial): a randomised controlled trial. Lancet 371: 1839–1847
26. Belardinelli R, Lacalaprice F, Carle F, et al (2003) Exercise-induced myocardial ischaemia detected by cardiopulmonary exercise testing. European heart journal 24: 1304–1313
27. Older P, Hall A, Hader R (1999) Cardiopulmonary exercise testing as a screening test for perioperative management of major surgery in the elderly. Chest 116: 355–362

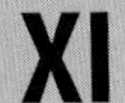

Advanced Minimally Invasive Hemodynamic Monitoring of the High-risk Major Surgery Patient

D.W. Green

Introduction

Despite major advances in monitoring technology in the last 20 years or so, perioperative management of the high-risk major surgery patient remains virtually unchanged. The vast majority of patients receive preoperative assessment which is neither designed to quantify functional capacity nor able to predict outcome. Anesthesiologists then usually monitor these patients intraoperatively using technology (e.g., oxygen saturation by pulse oximetry [SpO_2], invasive blood pressure and central venous pressure [CVP] monitoring, end-tidal carbon dioxide [$ETCO_2$], and anesthetic agent monitoring) that has not undergone major changes since the mid to late 80s. Patients are then consigned to a postoperative environment where they are managed by the most junior surgical and anesthesia staff. It is not surprising that outcome, in the UK at least, remains poor in high-risk patients [1].

I believe that there is now sufficient evidence to suggest that a combination of advanced, minimally invasive, hemodynamic assessment and monitoring markedly improves the perioperative management and outcome of high-risk surgical patients. Conventional management (as above) can lead to occult low levels of blood flow and oxygen delivery that results in complications that only occur days or weeks following surgery and give false re-assurance to the anesthesiologist that he or she is doing a 'good job'.

XI

Advanced hemodynamic management means a combined process of identification and management of the high risk surgical patient throughout the perioperative period using a set of parameters, protocols and user interfaces that facilitate assessment and optimization of anesthesia, fluids, and drugs on the major determinants of adequacy of oxygen delivery, stroke volume, and cardiac output including preload, afterload, heart rate and contractility, as well as tissue oxygenation.

In this chapter I will outline my experience with advanced haemodynamic monitoring in the perioperative period.

Definition and Role of Perioperative Optimization

Preoperative Period

Much work and energy has been expended on optimizing the high-risk patient preoperatively to usually very good effect [2]. However, it is now generally recognized that it is not cost effective to admit *all* patients pre-operatively to a high dependency environment, especially if this high quality of care is not then scrupulously maintained in the intraoperative and postoperative period [3].

Cardiopulmonary exercise testing is increasingly being used in the preoperative period to either exclude patients from major surgery if their maximum oxygen delivery does not exceed pre-defined (and arbitrary) parameters or to predict those patients who will need high dependency postoperative management and those that will not. However, despite the enthusiasm in some quarters there are relatively few data to support this form of triage in the form of randomized, controlled trials [4]. Indeed, there is little evidence to support the contention that major surgery is actually associated with or requires an increase in oxygen delivery and consumption. Such evidence is only available from randomized controlled trials in which oxygen delivery and cardiac output were not optimized *intraoperatively* [5]. Thus, the increase in oxygen delivery and consumption seen *postoperatively* probably reflect the accumulation of an *intraoperative* oxygen debt and may not be present if oxygen delivery is optimized intraoperatively. In the vast majority of trials of intraoperative optimization of fluid input (see later), measurement of stroke volume and cardiac output have only been initiated following induction of anesthesia and thus the preoperative cardiac output is not known. In the author's experience of over 150 cases of intraoperative cardiac output monitoring initiated *prior* to induction, there have been relatively few cases where cardiac output has increased substantially above preoperative levels during the procedure despite optimization of depth of anesthesia and protocol driven fluid management.

Indeed, the requirement to markedly increase cardiac output and oxygen delivery in the postoperative period may only occur in patients who are either genetically disposed to have a marked inflammatory response [6] or in those who suffer a postoperative complication and become septic.

Intraoperative Period

XI

Intraoperative fluid management regimens which result in optimization of stroke volume or other measures of fluid status have been the subject of a number of recent randomized trials. However, in most cases, fluids are administered during intra-abdominal surgery according to pre-determined 'high volume' fluid regimens (such as 5 to 15 ml/kg/h of Hartmann's/lactated Ringer's solution) based on the presumed 'third space' fluid deficit that is 'obligatory' during major intra-abdominal surgery [7]. There has thus been a presumption for nearly 50 years that patients are relatively hypovolemic during surgery unless these so called 'third space' losses are assiduously replaced. Indeed, in a recent pilot study for a major trial of fluid optimization in patients undergoing colorectal surgery using esophageal Doppler monitoring, the intervention group was scheduled to receive 1 l of Hartmann's solution per hour, i.e., approximately 15 ml/kg/h [8].

However, some trials have cast doubt on these 'high volume' fluid regimens and even suggested that fluid *restriction* may be beneficial [9], especially in thoracic and hepatic surgery. In my experience, the additional amount (i.e., excluding blood loss, urine output, and insensible loss) of crystalloid necessary to maintain pre-defined cardiovascular parameters, i.e., the average 'third space' requirement, was only 3.5 ml/kg/h with a range of 0 to 15 [10]. It is now increasingly recognized that the amount of fluid administered should be individualized to the patient's needs and not pre-determined by some liberal or restrictive regimen [11].

Unfortunately, conventional intraoperative monitoring may not accurately predict fluid requirements [12]. Since mean arterial pressure (MAP) is dependent on both cardiac output and systemic vascular resistance (SVR) it is not a good indicator of blood flow and thus oxygen delivery. Optimization of CVP has less predictive value in comparison to other measures of fluid responsiveness such as those provided by esophageal Doppler monitoring [12–14] and may be associated with more complications [15]. Recent randomized trials and meta-analyses have confirmed that intraoperative fluid optimization using esophageal Doppler monitoring improves outcome [13, 14, 16, 17].

Evidence also points to the benefits of depth of anesthesia monitoring in this context although it was not quantitatively assessed in any of the published trials of fluid optimization. It would seem futile to try and maintain 'normal' cardiovascular status using fluid administration to a patient intraoperatively when there is no quantitative estimate of how deeply (or lightly) anesthetized the patient is. Maintaining bispectral index levels between 45 and 55 will circumvent this problem while at the same time improving long term outcome [18]. However, even maintenance of seemingly adequate MAP cardiac output may still result in inadequate oxygen delivery to vital centers such as the brain. This is best demonstrated by the decreases observed in cerebral oxygen saturation in anemic elderly patients undergoing major abdominal surgery. These changes are correctable by blood transfusion [19] and there is also evidence that correction of these deficits may improve outcome in both cardiac and non cardiac surgery [20, 21]. Recent work has also demonstrated that a reduction in hemoglobin concentration, such as is found after blood donation, may significantly reduce maximum exercise capacity and thus may in itself be detrimental in the postoperative period [22].

The recent availability of equipment able to estimate beat-to-beat hemoglobin concentrations (e.g., Masimo Radical-7, Masimo Corporation, California) will allow real time assessment of oxygen delivery (see later) if used alongside continuous measurement of cardiac output. In addition, this monitor is also able to analyze beat-to-beat changes in plethysmographic variability and to produce a pleth variability index, which may prove very useful in assessing fluid status [23].

Postoperative Period

A recent study has quantified the benefit of goal-directed therapy in the immediate postoperative period using lithium indicator dilution and pulse power analysis [3]. Indeed, it is during this period that major increases in cardiac output and oxygen delivery have been observed as predictors of good outcome [5].

To be truly effective, advanced haemodynamic monitoring must be used throughout the perioperative period to maximize improvements in patient outcome.

Overview of Some Current Advanced Hemodynamic Monitors

Non- or Minimally-invasive Measurement of Cardiac Output

Esophageal Doppler monitor (ODM, Deltex Medical, Chichester)

Non-invasive measurements of cardiac output can be obtained by utilizing the principle of Doppler shift. Velocity of blood flowing in the descending aorta is obtained by measuring the Doppler shift in frequency of sound waves bounced off moving red blood cells. Thus the esophageal Doppler probe tip is positioned in the esophagus at a depth of about 35–40 cm corresponding to the anatomical level T5/T6. The sound wave frequency employed is set at 4 mHz. Cardiac output is calculated by first estimating the diameter of the descending aorta from a nomogram based on age, weight, and height and then from the distance traveled by the blood in unit time. An additional 30 % is added to this number to account for the ascending aortic blood flow. 'Peak velocity' is taken to be an indication of contractility, and the 'corrected flow time' to be an indication of preload. Fluid responsiveness is determined by assessing the effect of fluid administration on corrected flow time (ideally kept between 350 to 450 msec) and the effect of fluid challenges on increase in stroke volume [14, 24].

The basic advantage of esophageal Doppler monitoring is that it is non-invasive (although there is still the theoretical risk of esophageal trauma). Disadvantages include difficulty in positioning the probe tip, especially in the elderly patient, and shifting of the probe tip over time may lead to a sub-optimal trace.

Non-invasive cardiac output, NICO

The NICO (Philips Respironics, Amsterdam, Netherlands) apparatus calculates cardiac output using the Fick principle by a partial re-breathing technique. Although this is normally calculated using oxygen, CO_2 can also be used as in this device. Cardiac output is equal to CO_2 production (VCO_2) divided by the difference between mixed venous ($CvCO_2$) and arterial ($CaCO_2$) CO_2 content. Thus:

$$\text{Cardiac output} = VCO_2 / (CvCO_2 - CaCO_2)$$

For a non-invasive method, the need to measure $CvCO_2$ must be eliminated and this can be done by utilizing the differential Fick equation. Thus, two measurements need to be taken with different $CaCO_2$ levels in the blood (as indicated by changes in $ETCO_2$). This difference is achieved using a partial re-breathing technique by adding dead space, thereby reducing CO_2 elimination and increasing $CaCO_2$ (and its surrogate, $ETCO_2$). The increase in dead space is applied for a short enough time for there to be only a negligible change in $CvCO_2$.

The machine accurately integrates CO_2 with gas flow to obtain the volume of CO_2 passing though the airway. At 3 minute intervals it automatically introduces a loop of added dead space.

Thus, during the 3 minute cycle a baseline is first applied for 60 secs, this is then followed by rebreathing through the dead space loop for 35 sec (short enough to avoid changes in $CvCO_2$) and then stabilization for 85 sec to allow return to baseline. Cardiac output is thus proportional to the change in CO_2 elimination divided by the change in $CaCO_2$ ($ETCO_2$) during re-breathing [25].

NICO actually measures pulmonary capillary blood flow so the pulmonary shunt (using FiO_2 and SpO_2) must be calculated to obtain a true reading of cardiac output. The NICO device will not work if the $ETCO_2$ is above 10 kPa, following bicarbonate administration, if there are significant leaks in the circuit, or in other non-steady state conditions resulting in failure of the $ETCO_2$ to plateau.

The advantages of the NICO are that:

- it is totally non-invasive
- it can be applied to any patient with an endotracheal tube or supraglottic airway device
- the disposable circuit, if placed proximal to the patient airway filter, need only be changed when the circuit tubes are changed.
- there is no skill required in its use, only in the interpretation of the data.

In many studies the NICO has shown good agreement with other more invasive methods of assessing cardiac output [26]. However, it must be recognized that there may be disparity between the readings obtained from the esophageal Doppler monitor and NICO used contemporaneously and thus clinical judgment must always be used if the readings diverge [10].

The principal disadvantage is that cardiac output is only obtained at 3 minute intervals and, therefore, will not reflect sudden changes due for example to blood loss.

The LiDCO *Plus* and *Rapid*

The LiDCO system (LiDCO Ltd, Cambridge, UK) uses pulse contour power analysis to measure nominal stroke volume and thus cardiac output [27]. Lithium (c.f. dye) dilution is used to calibrate the machine so that actual cardiac outputs can be obtained. Clinical studies have been generally favorable in its ability to continuously monitor stroke volume [28–32]. However, some studies have questioned the ability of LiDCO to track rapid changes in stroke volume as a result of rapid hemorrhage in animal models or use of vasoconstrictors or dilators [33–36]. However, the limits of agreement and reproducibility are almost always within the criteria specified for such monitors [37].

Although the LiDCO*plus* has been used very widely in the intensive care environment and in the postoperative period to optimize oxygen delivery [3], the perceived difficulties encountered in calibration meant that it was little used in the operating room. Another issue related to calibration difficulties is lithium electrode drift immediately following the concomitant use of competitive neuromuscular blocking drugs; this drift does not occur with the phenylisoquinoline neuromuscular blocking drugs, atracurium and cisatracurium.

However, in most cases the anesthesiologist is (or should be) concerned with maintenance of pre-operative values rather than needing to know the actual values in the vast majority of patients. This can best be obtained by placement of the radial arterial line prior to induction of anesthesia to obtain key baseline hemodynamic parameters.

Facilitation of the use of LiDCO technology in the operating room, based on the issues raised above, has led to the development of the LiDCO*rapid*. This has a much simpler interface and display which focuses on the cardiovascular parameters essential for patient optimization (**Fig. 1**), including nominal cardiac output and stroke volume and stroke volume variation (SVV) as well as screens to follow the effects of fluid administration. Nominal cardiac output and nominal stroke volume are determined by estimating aortic capacitance from nomograms using the patient's age, weight, and height [38]. Unlike the LiDCO*plus*, there is no inbuilt calibration system but one can enter externally validated cardiac outputs such as that obtained by the NICO or indeed esophageal Doppler monitoring. However, in my opinion, it is change, displayed by trends over time, which is much more important.

Recent work has demonstrated that the displayed preload parameters (SVV trend over 10 mins and change in stroke volume per beat) are useful indicators of fluid status and fluid responsiveness and are superior to left ventricular end-diastolic volume and CVP [27, 29, 39, 40]. It is this ability to measure SVV that makes this device such a useful intraoperative monitor in the absence of significant dysrhythmia. The ease of use and relevance of displayed data make the new LiDCO*rapid* an excellent addition to our armamentarium of minimally invasive intraoperative monitors.

Future developments should include the ability to incorporate continuous oxygen content and thus oxygen delivery and also the ability to transfer intraoperative data to the postoperative high dependency environment where high quality monitoring can then continue.

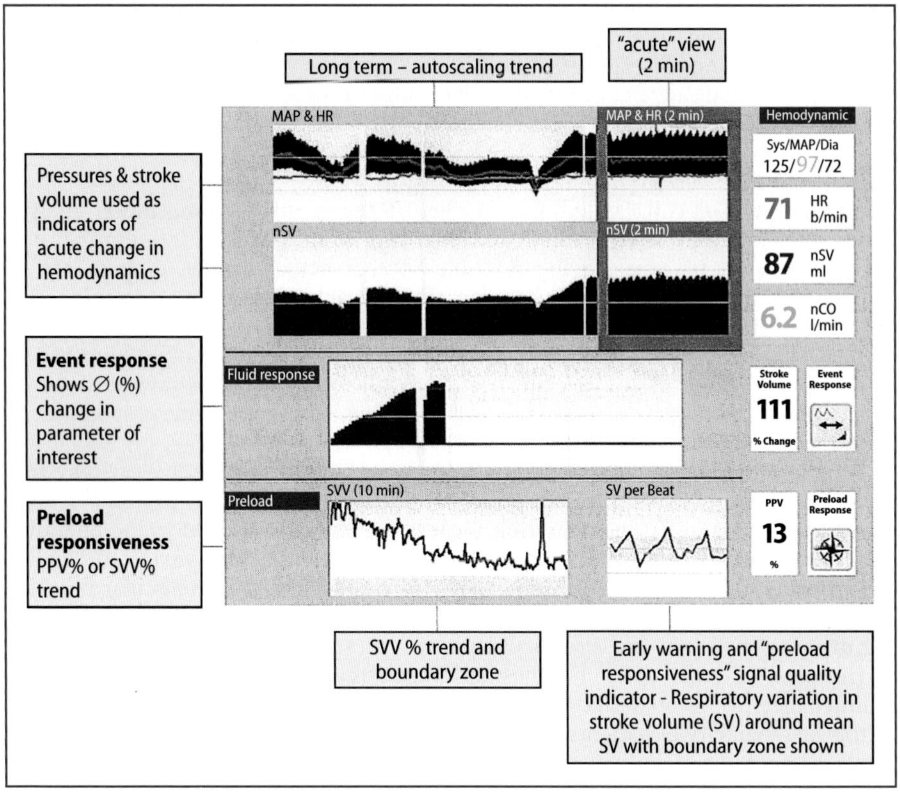

Long term – autoscaling trend

"acute" view (2 min)

Pressures & stroke volume used as indicators of acute change in hemodynamics

MAP & HR

MAP & HR (2 min)

Hemodynamic

Sys/MAP/Dia 125/97/72

71 HR b/min

nSV

nSV (2 min)

87 nSV ml

6.2 nCO l/min

Event response Shows ∅ (%) change in parameter of interest

Fluid response

Stroke Volume 111 % Change

Event Response

Preload responsiveness PPV% or SVV% trend

Preload

SVV (10 min)

SV per Beat

PPV 13 %

Preload Response

SVV % trend and boundary zone

Early warning and "preload responsiveness" signal quality indicator - Respiratory variation in stroke volume (SV) around mean SV with boundary zone shown

Fig. 1. The LiDCO*rapid* display (for full explanation of the displayed parameters see text). PPV: pulse pressure variation; SVV: stroke volume variation

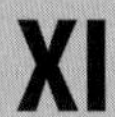

Comparison of cardiac outputs from monitors used contemporaneously in the operating room

A number of studies have been performed recently comparing the results obtained from one monitor versus another [34, 41–46]. However, it is outside the scope of this chapter to review these in detail. I will thus concentrate on studies that I have performed.

In a study of 12 patients undergoing major abdominal surgery, cardiac outputs obtained from the ODM and NICO were compared. **Figure 2** demonstrates that the limits of agreement are quite large and casts some doubt on the accuracy of either method in this context. However, in most cases there was good trend agreement as is shown in the sequential chart, **Figure 3** [10].

A recent study in foals showed good agreement between the NICO and a calibrated LiDCO*plus* [41]. Are the readings obtained from these monitors consistent and comparable in daily clinical practice in humans with the LiDCO*rapid*? The LiDCO*rapid* and NICO were used contemporaneously in 20 patients. However, the NICO could not be expected to respond as quickly as the *LiDCOrapid* to the dynamic changes that occur during surgery and anesthesia. Taking all 20 patients studied together there appears to be reasonable correlation between the readings ($p < 0.0001$, $r = 0.34$), suggesting that they both seem to track changes in a similar

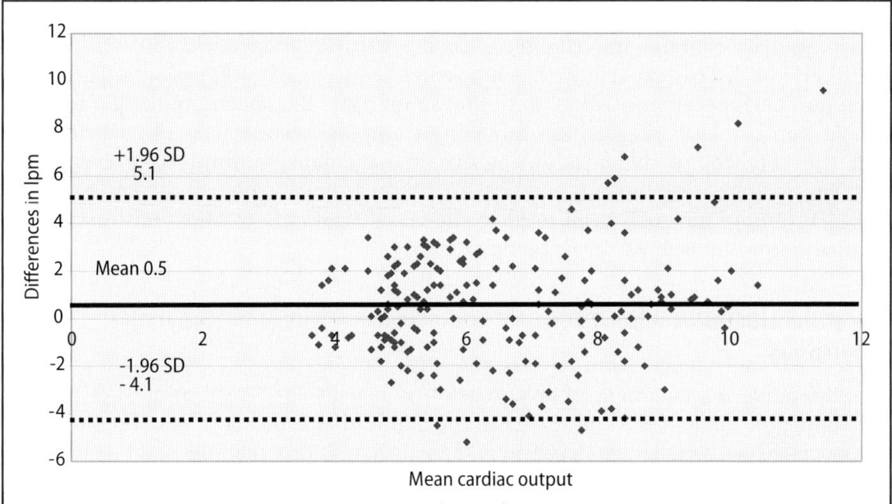

Fig. 2. Bland Altman plot showing the differences between the cardiac outputs obtained by the NICO (Respironics) and the esophageal Doppler monitor (ODM, Deltex). The x axis is the mean cardiac output from paired readings and the y axis is the difference in lpm between paired readings. The bias is 0.5 lpm and the limits of agreement are +5.1 to −4.1 (± 1.96 SD). For full details see text. From [10] with permission.

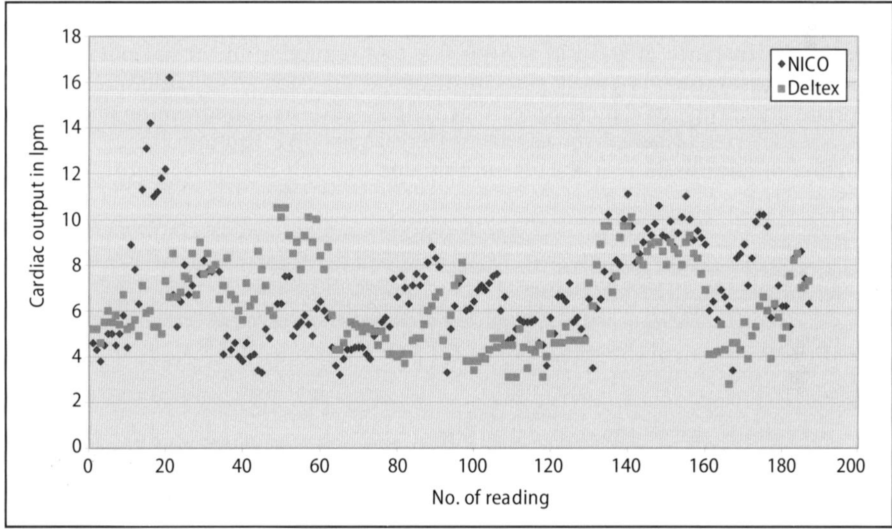

Fig. 3. A sequential plot of all readings obtained by the NICO (Respironics) and the Esophageal Doppler monitor (ODM, Deltex). Although there is general agreement in the plot between the two, significant outliers exist. From [10] with permission.

fashion. However, since the LiDCO*rapid* was mainly used in its normal uncalibrated mode, Bland Altman analysis was not used.

Our initial experience with the cerebral oximeter (Invos®, Somanetics, Troy) demonstrated the superiority of this device over transcranial Doppler measurement and conscious state assessment for demonstrating adequacy of cerebral perfusion and oxygenation following clamping during carotid endarterectomy under local anesthesia [47]. This experience has now extended to nearly 100 patients. There have been no perioperative strokes and the shunt rate has been markedly reduced. Changes in cerebral oxygenation following clamping precede loss of consciousness and the cerebral oximeter allows active management to limit or prevent such changes by increasing mean blood pressure and cardiac output. In the latter context, the LiDCO*rapid* has also been used in the last 40 patients to allow optimization of cardiac output as well as mean blood pressure.

Use of the LiDCO*plus* and LiDCO*rapid* in the management of intraoperative hypotension

Intraoperative management of hypotension is usually empirical and takes place in the context of inadequate knowledge of the depth of anesthesia. Thus, if hypotension is associated with excessive depth (e.g., a bispectral index reading of 30 or below) it would surely be more appropriate to reduce the concentration of anesthetic agents in the first instance rather than use other methods such as fluids and vasoactive agents to increase blood pressure. However, in many elderly patients, depth of anesthesia may already be excessively light and reducing the concentration of anesthetic agents still further may lead to awareness. In the absence of depth of anesthesia monitoring, fluid administration and vasoactive agents are commonly used to correct hypotension. Use of the LiDCO*rapid* enables the effects of fluid administration on stroke volume to be quantified and the appropriate vasoactive drug to be selected. For instance, if a fall in MAP is due to a reduction in cardiac output (as is usually the case) use of a purely vasoconstrictor drug, such as metaraminol, is inappropriate and drugs that increase cardiac output, such as ephedrine or phenylephrine, are preferred. **Figure 4** shows that a decrease in MAP (bottom trace) following induction of anesthesia (mark 2) is entirely due to a fall in cardiac output as there

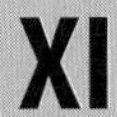

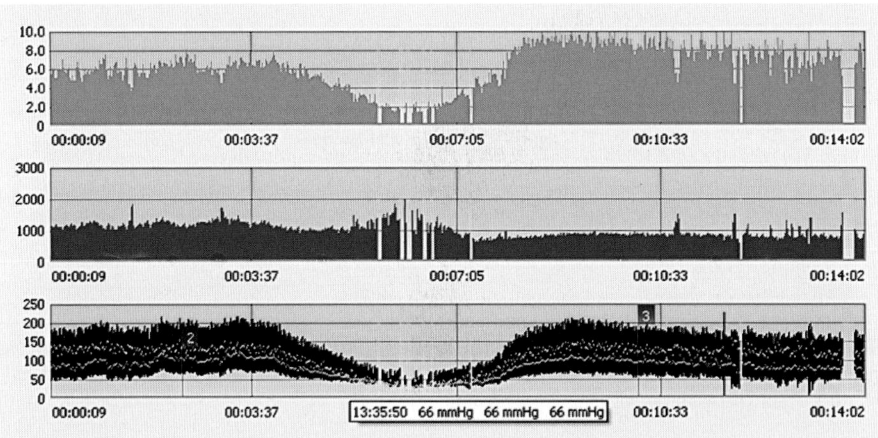

Fig. 4. The LiDCO display shows that the fall in blood pressure (lower trace) at induction of anesthesia (2) is entirely due to a proportional fall in cardiac output (top trace, y axis in lpm). The middle trace shows a slight increase in systemic vascular resistance (SVR). This case was successfully treated with phenylephrine infusion (3). A pure vasoconstrictor, such as metaraminol, would have been inappropriate. (Display obtained after downloading the data using LiDCO *Analysis Plus* software).

is no decrease in SVR. Treatment is by phenylephrine bolus and infusion (mark 3). This restores both MAP and cardiac output.

Figure 5 shows the effect of two vasoactive drugs, metaraminol (mark 2) and ephedrine (mark 4) on MAP and cardiac output during anesthesia. It can be seen that metaraminol produces a short lived increase in MAP which is purely due to an increased SVR and is associated with a slight decline in cardiac output, whereas ephedrine has a beneficial effect on both MAP and cardiac output with no change in SVR.

In other situations, as in **Figure 6**, the decrease in MAP (bottom trace) from 100 mmHg to 60 mmHg after induction (mark 2) may be due entirely to a decrease

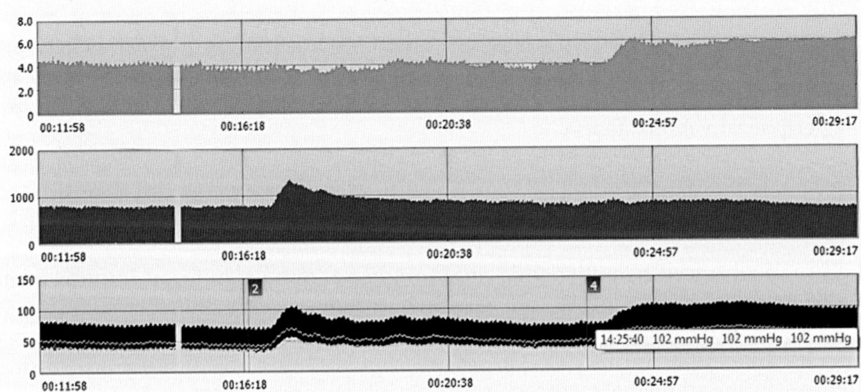

Fig. 5. The effect of two vasoactive drugs, metaraminol (2) and ephedrine (4) on mean blood pressure (MAP bottom trace) and cardiac output (top trace) during anesthesia. It can be seen that metaraminol produces a short lived increase in MAP which is purely due to an increased systemic vascular resistance (SVR, middle trace) and is associated with a slight decline in cardiac output, whereas ephedrine has a beneficial effect on both MAP and cardiac output with no change in SVR. (Display obtained after downloading the data using LiDCO *Analysis Plus* software).

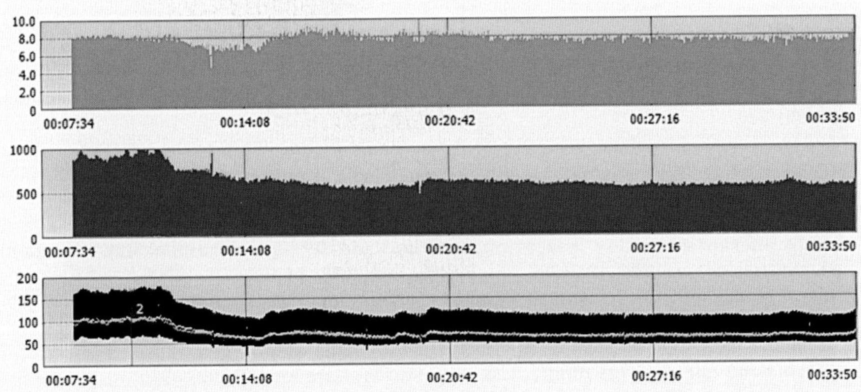

Fig. 6. The LiDCO display shows the fall in mean arterial pressure (MAP, bottom trace) from 100 mmHg to 60 mmHg after induction (2) is due almost entirely to a fall in systemic vascular resistance (SVR, middle trace) with no change in cardiac output (top trace). Here either metaraminol or ephedrine, if deemed necessary, may be appropriate. (Display obtained after downloading the data using LiDCO *Analysis Plus* software).

in SVR (middle trace) with no change in cardiac output (top trace). Here, either metaraminol or ephedrine, if deemed necessary, may be appropriate.

Decline in Use of Central Venous Catheterization for Major Surgery

Use of non-invasive monitoring devices, such as LiDCO*rapid* and ODM, has resulted in a dramatic reduction in the use of centrally placed venous catheters in high-risk patients undergoing major peripheral vascular and abdominal surgery. This reduces the risk of complications associated with the use of these devices [15, 48, 49]. Since CVP is no longer seen to be a satisfactory measure to optimize fluid administration, its use can now be questioned intraoperatively except perhaps in cases of hepatic resection where it is also desirable to keep the CVP low [50]. In my own experience, the use of triple lumen central lines in major abdominal and vascular surgery has decreased from 85 to 10 %, now being reserved solely for those patients with difficult peripheral venous access..

Conclusion

The use of advanced hemodynamic monitors has allowed significant improvements in perioperative management and patient outcome. However, further benefit may only be seen if these monitors are used in combination (e.g., LiDCO, NICO, cerebral oximeter and bispectral index). The use of this intraoperative technology must be extended to the immediate postoperative period and funding must be identified to allow this to happen. The requirement now is for the development of more highly evolved and integrated monitors with smart screens where the data captured are presented as organized and meaningful information to the end user, whether anesthesiologist, surgeon or nurse, to inform appropriate interventions. This new generation of monitors must also allow for the data to be archived and used for informing further high quality clinical trials using this technology.

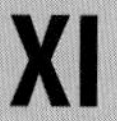

References

1. Jhanji S, Thomas B, Ely A, Watson D, Hinds CJ, Pearse RM (2008) Mortality and utilisation of critical care resources amongst high-risk surgical patients in a large NHS trust. Anaesthesia 63: 695–700
2. Boyd O, Grounds RM, Bennett ED (1993) A randomized clinical trial of the effect of deliberate perioperative increase of oxygen delivery on mortality in high-risk surgical patients. JAMA 270: 2699–2707
3. Pearse R, Dawson D, Fawcett J, Rhodes A, Grounds RM, Bennett ED (2005) Early goal-directed therapy after major surgery reduces complications and duration of hospital stay. A randomised, controlled trial [ISRCTN38797445]. Crit Care 9:R687–693
4. Older P, Hall A (2004) Clinical review: how to identify high-risk surgical patients. Crit Care 8: 369–372
5. Shoemaker WC, Appel PL, Kram HB (1993) Hemodynamic and oxygen transport responses in survivors and nonsurvivors of high-risk surgery. Crit Care Med 21: 977–990
6. Lee JT, Chaloner EJ, Hollingsworth SJ (2006) The role of cardiopulmonary fitness and its genetic influences on surgical outcomes. Br J Surg 93: 147–157
7. Shires T, Williams J, Brown F (1961) Acute change in extracellular fluids associated with major surgical procedures. Ann Surg 154: 803–810
8. McFall MR, Woods WG, Wakeling HG (2004) The use of oesophageal Doppler cardiac output

measurement to optimize fluid management during colorectal surgery. Eur J Anaesthesiol 21: 581–583

9. Brandstrup B, Tonnesen H, Beier-Holgersen R, et al (2003) Effects of intravenous fluid restriction on postoperative complications: comparison of two perioperative fluid regimens: a randomized assessor-blinded multicenter trial. Ann Surg 238: 641–648
10. Green DW (2007) Comparison of cardiac outputs during major surgery using the Deltex CardioQ oesophageal Doppler monitor and the Novametrix-Respironics NICO: a prospective observational study. Int J Surg 5: 176–182
11. Holte K, Foss NB, Andersen J, et al (2007) Liberal or restrictive fluid administration in fast-track colonic surgery: a randomized, double-blind study. Br J Anaesth 99: 500–508
12. Junghans T, Neuss H, Strohauer M, et al (2006) Hypovolemia after traditional preoperative care in patients undergoing colonic surgery is underrepresented in conventional hemodynamic monitoring. Int J Colorectal Dis 21: 693–697
13. Lee JH, Kim JT, Yoon SZ, et al (2007) Evaluation of corrected flow time in oesophageal Doppler as a predictor of fluid responsiveness. Br J Anaesth 99: 343–348
14. Wakeling HG, McFall MR, Jenkins CS, et al (2005) Intraoperative oesophageal Doppler guided fluid management shortens postoperative hospital stay after major bowel surgery. Br J Anaesth 95: 634–642
15. Venn R, Steele A, Richardson P, Poloniecki J, Grounds M, Newman P (2002) Randomized controlled trial to investigate influence of the fluid challenge on duration of hospital stay and perioperative morbidity in patients with hip fractures. Br J Anaesth 88: 65–71
16. Abbas SM, Hill AG (2008) Systematic review of the literature for the use of oesophageal Doppler monitor for fluid replacement in major abdominal surgery. Anaesthesia 63: 44–51
17. Noblett SE, Snowden CP, Shenton BK, Horgan AF (2006) Randomized clinical trial assessing the effect of Doppler-optimized fluid management on outcome after elective colorectal resection. Br J Surg 93: 1069–1076
18. Monk TG, Saini V, Weldon BC, Sigl JC (2005) Anesthetic management and one-year mortality after noncardiac surgery. Anesth Analg 100: 4–10
19. Green DW (2007) A retrospective study of changes in cerebral oxygenation using a cerebral oximeter in older patients undergoing prolonged major abdominal surgery. Eur J Anaesthesiol 24: 230–234
20. Casati A, Fanelli G, Pietropaoli P, et al (2005) Continuous monitoring of cerebral oxygen saturation in elderly patients undergoing major abdominal surgery minimizes brain exposure to potential hypoxia. Anesth Analg 101: 740–747
21. Murkin JM, Adams SJ, Novick RJ, et al (2007) Monitoring brain oxygen saturation during coronary bypass surgery: a randomized, prospective study. Anesth Analg 104: 51–58
22. Dellweg D, Siemon K, Mahler F, Appelhans P, Klauke M, Kohler D (2008) [Cardiopulmonary exercise testing before and after blood donation]. Pneumologie 62: 372–377
23. Cannesson M, Desebbe O, Rosamel P, et al (2008) Pleth variability index to monitor the respiratory variations in the pulse oximeter plethysmographic waveform amplitude and predict fluid responsiveness in the operating theatre. Br J Anaesth 101: 200–206
24. Gan TJ, Soppitt A, Maroof M, et al (2002) Goal-directed intraoperative fluid administration reduces length of hospital stay after major surgery. Anesthesiology 97: 820–826
25. Jaffe MB (1999) Partial CO2 rebreathing cardiac output--operating principles of the NICO system. J Clin Monit Comput 15: 387–401
26. Cholley BP, Payen D (2005) Noninvasive techniques for measurements of cardiac output. Curr Opin Crit Care 11: 424–429
27. Jonas MM, Tanser SJ (2002) Lithium dilution measurement of cardiac output and arterial pulse waveform analysis: an indicator dilution calibrated beat-by-beat system for continuous estimation of cardiac output. Curr Opin Crit Care 8: 257–261
28. Dyer RA, Piercy JL, Reed AR, Lombard CJ, Schoeman LK, James MF (2008) Hemodynamic changes associated with spinal anesthesia for cesarean delivery in severe preeclampsia. Anesthesiology 108: 802–811
29. Belloni L, Pisano A, Natale A, et al (2008) Assessment of fluid-responsiveness parameters for off-pump coronary artery bypass surgery: A comparison among LiDCO, transesophageal echochardiography, and pulmonary artery catheter. J Cardiothorac Vasc Anesth 22: 243–248

30. Pearse RM, Ikram K, Barry J (2004) Equipment review: an appraisal of the LiDCO plus method of measuring cardiac output. Crit Care 8: 190–195
31. Pittman J, Bar-Yosef S, SumPing J, Sherwood M, Mark J (2005) Continuous cardiac output monitoring with pulse contour analysis: a comparison with lithium indicator dilution cardiac output measurement. Crit Care Med 33: 2015–2021
32. Costa MG, Della Rocca G, Chiarandini P, et al (2008) Continuous and intermittent cardiac output measurement in hyperdynamic conditions: pulmonary artery catheter vs. lithium dilution technique. Intensive Care Med 34: 257–263
33. Yamashita K, Nishiyama T, Yokoyama T, Abe H, Manabe M (2007) Effects of vasodilation on cardiac output measured by PulseCO. J Clin Monit Comput 21: 335–339
34. de Wilde RB, Schreuder JJ, van den Berg PC, Jansen JR (2007) An evaluation of cardiac output by five arterial pulse contour techniques during cardiac surgery. Anaesthesia 62: 760–768
35. Cooper ES, Muir WW (2007) Continuous cardiac output monitoring via arterial pressure waveform analysis following severe hemorrhagic shock in dogs. Crit Care Med 35: 1724–1729
36. Berberian G, Quinn TA, Vigilance DW, et al (2005) Validation study of PulseCO system for continuous cardiac output measurement. Asaio J 51: 37–40
37. Critchley LA, Critchley JA (1999) A meta-analysis of studies using bias and precision statistics to compare cardiac output measurement techniques. J Clin Monit Comput 15: 85–91
38. Langewouters GJ, Wesseling KH, Goedhard WJ (1985) The pressure dependent dynamic elasticity of 35 thoracic and 16 abdominal human aortas in vitro described by a five component model. J Biomech 18: 613–20
39. Preisman S, Kogan S, Berkenstadt H, Perel A (2005) Predicting fluid responsiveness in patients undergoing cardiac surgery: functional haemodynamic parameters including the Respiratory Systolic Variation Test and static preload indicators. Br J Anaesth 95: 746–755
40. Berkenstadt H, Margalit N, Hadani M, et al (2001) Stroke volume variation as a predictor of fluid responsiveness in patients undergoing brain surgery. Anesth Analg 92: 984–989
41. Valverde A, Giguere S, Morey TE, Sanchez LC, Shih A (2007) Comparison of noninvasive cardiac output measured by use of partial carbon dioxide rebreathing or the lithium dilution method in anesthetized foals. Am J Vet Res 68: 141–147
42. Opdam HI, Wan L, Bellomo R (2007) A pilot assessment of the FloTrac(TM) cardiac output monitoring system. Intensive Care Med 33: 344–349
43. Manecke GR Jr, Auger WR (2007) Cardiac output determination from the arterial pressure wave: clinical testing of a novel algorithm that does not require calibration. J Cardiothorac Vasc Anesth 21: 3–7
44. Gueret G, Kiss G, Khaldi S, et al (2007) Comparison of cardiac output measurements between NICO and the pulmonary artery catheter during repeat surgery for total hip replacement. Eur J Anaesthesiol 24: 1028–1033
45. Baylor P (2006) Lack of agreement between thermodilution and fick methods in the measurement of cardiac output. J Intensive Care Med 21: 93–98
46. Hallowell GD, Corley KT (2005) Use of lithium dilution and pulse contour analysis cardiac output determination in anaesthetized horses: a clinical evaluation. Vet Anaesth Analg 32: 201–211
47. Fassiadis N, Zayed H, Rashid H, Green DW (2006) Invos(R) Cerebral Oximeter compared with the transcranial Doppler for monitoring adequacy of cerebral perfusion in patients undergoing carotid endarterectomy. Int Angiol 25: 401–406
48. Orme RM, McSwiney MM, Chamberlain-Webber RF (2007) Fatal cardiac tamponade as a result of a peripherally inserted central venous catheter: a case report and review of the literature. Br J Anaesth 99: 384–388
49. Wigmore TJ, Smythe JF, Hacking MB, Raobaikady R, MacCallum NS (2007) Effect of the implementation of NICE guidelines for ultrasound guidance on the complication rates associated with central venous catheter placement in patients presenting for routine surgery in a tertiary referral centre. Br J Anaesth 99: 662–665
50. Wang WD, Liang LJ, Huang XQ, Yin XY (2006) Low central venous pressure reduces blood loss in hepatectomy. World J Gastroenterol 12: 935–939

Post-pneumonectomy Pulmonary Edema

D. Cook, E. Powell, and F. Gao-Smith

Introduction

The first successful pneumonectomy was performed as a two step procedure by Rudolf Nissen in 1930. Although lesser resections are now performed when possible, in certain cases of non-small cell lung cancer, pneumonectomy provides the only potentially curative option. However, it is a procedure associated with a high mortality (3.3–9.3 %) and morbidity (30.6–59 %) [1–5]. Post-pneumonectomy pulmonary edema is not an infrequent complication of pneumonectomy (incidence 4–7 %) [6] and one that is associated with a mortality of at least 50 % [7]. Post-pneumonectomy pulmonary edema is often called post-lung resection acute lung injury, firstly due to its pathophysiological and clinical similarities to acute lung injury (ALI) and acute respiratory distress syndrome (ARDS), and secondly because it occurs following lobectomy as well as pneumonectomy. This chapter outlines the diagnosis and prevalence of this condition and then discusses the potential etiological factors.

Diagnostic Criteria

In the early years of its recognition, post-pneumonectomy pulmonary edema was a diagnosis based on a clinical picture of postoperative respiratory failure associated with diffuse radiographic changes. It was often termed non-cardiogenic pulmonary edema [8, 9]. As time progressed, different authors used slightly different definitions, although the common theme remained the presence of diffuse radiographic infiltrates with respiratory distress/hypoxia following lung resection, as previously, but increasingly with the active exclusion of other potential causes, e.g., infection, thromboembolism, and cardiac failure. Post-pneumonectomy pulmonary edema has been used to describe lung injury following both lobectomy and pneumonectomy and pneumonectomy alone. In 1993, Turnage and Lunn [8] demonstrated that cases of post-pneumonectomy pulmonary edema had post-mortem features identical to classical ARDS raising the possibility of using the American-European Consensus Guidelines for ARDS to diagnose post-pneumonectomy pulmonary edema [10].

Prevalence

In 1995, Hayes et al. [11] used these guidelines in the diagnosis of ALI/ARDS in 469 patients after lung resection, including pneumonectomy, lobectomy and wedge resection. These authors reported an overall incidence of ALI/ARDS of 5.1 %, which is similar to other published incidences of between 2 -7 % [7–9, 12–14]. Several studies have demonstrated a higher prevalence of, and mortality from, post-pneumonectomy pulmonary edema following pneumonectomy than following lesser resections [7, 12, 13]. A recent study by Tang et al. [15] compared the incidence and mortality of ARDS after pulmonary resection between two study periods (1991–1997 and 2000–2005). These authors reported that the incidence and mortality had fallen significantly between these study periods (incidence from 3.2 % to 1.6 % and mortality from 72 % to 45 %) and concluded that this was partly explained by more aggressive strategies to avoid pneumonectomy in the latter study period.

Pathology

As mentioned previously, post-mortem studies following post-pneumonectomy pulmonary edema have found the classical features of ARDS seen from other causes, e.g., sepsis. These features included hyaline membrane formation and pulmonary vascular thrombosis [8]. ARDS in its initial phase is characterized by an exudative alveolar edema containing plasma proteins, various mediators/cytokines and inflammatory cells (predominantly neutrophils) [16]. This increase in alveolar permeability is thought to be due to a breakdown in the integrity of the alveolar-capillary barrier. Overall, this initial ARDS phase is exactly the same process seen following lung resection [14]. The increased permeability seen in post-pneumonectomy pulmonary edema has also been found using radionucleotide studies and is consistent with the changes seen in the well-recognized early exudative phase of classical ARDS [9, 14, 17–19].

Following this initial exudative phase, post-pneumonectomy pulmonary edema and ARDS both follow the same path consisting of hyaline membrane formation, type I pneumocyte necrosis, extensive microthrombosis [20] and a predominant neutrophil cell profile in the alveolar fluid [16, 20]. A proliferative and regenerative phase then occurs with proliferation of type II pneumocytes and fibroblasts. The type II pneumocytes then differentiate into type I pneumocytes, many of which were lost in the exudative phase. During this phase, fibrosis and remodeling takes place, sometimes resulting in extensive remodeling of the pulmonary vascular bed and scarred damaged lungs [6, 16, 20]. This, however, is not inevitable and both the pathological and functional outcomes of ARDS are variable.

Etiology

The definitive etiology of post-pneumonectomy pulmonary edema has not been determined as yet, although several factors associated with the development of post-pneumonectomy pulmonary edema have been suggested. These include right pneumonectomy, excessive fluid administration, ventilation with large tidal volumes, and transfusion of blood products. Cerfolio et al. demonstrated that perioperative steroid administration reduces the incidence of post-pneumonectomy pulmonary edema, which suggests that the pathogenesis of post-pneumonectomy pulmonary edema involves inflammation, similarly to ARDS [21].

Discussed below are some of the factors thought to be of significance in the etiology of ARDS and post-pneumonectomy pulmonary edema (**Table 1**).

Table 1. Possible factors involved in the etiology of post-pneumonectomy pulmonary edema

Primary Insults
Oxidative damage/ischemia–reperfusion injury
Ventilation with large volumes/pressures
Surgical trauma
Pathogenesis
Inflammation
Oxidative damage and ischemia-reperfusion injury
Exacerbating factors
Over-zealous fluid administration
Increased pulmonary capillary pressure
Disrupted lymphatic drainage
Chronic alcohol consumption
Transfusion of blood products
Unbalanced chest drainage

Inflammation

It is well known that during ALI/ARDS there is a proliferation of inflammatory cells and mediators that can be detected in both bronchoalveolar lavage (BAL) fluid and plasma [22, 23].

1. Eicosanoids

Eicosanoids are compounds derived from arachidonic acid metabolism (prostanoids and leukotrienes) that act as mediators in several physiological pathways including inflammation and hemostasis. Increased levels of prostanoids have been detected following pulmonary resection [24] and increased levels of leukotrienes have been reported in ARDS. In fact, there is a suggestion that leukotriene B4 (LTB4) levels may be an early predictor of the development of ARDS in groups at risk [25]. The known physiological effects of the leukotrienes and prostanoids would be consistent with them having a role. LTB4 is one of the most powerful neutrophil chemotactic agents known [26], as well as promoting neutrophil adhesion to the vascular endothelium and transendothelial migration. The cysteinyl leukotrienes (LTC4, LTD4, LTE4) cause increased vascular permeability (1000 times more potent than histamine), which is a recognized component of ARDS and post-pneumonectomy pulmonary edema.

2. Vascular endothelial growth factor (VEGF)

VEGF has also been linked with the early phase of, and recovery from, ARDS. Thikkett et al. [27] demonstrated that VEGF levels were increased in plasma from ARDS patients compared to controls. They demonstrated that recombinant VEGF and ARDS patients' plasma increased the flux of albumin across epithelial cell monolayers more than controls and VEGF inhibitors decreased this flux by 48 %. More recently, the same group demonstrated that levels of alveolar VEGF were lower in patients with ARDS than those at risk and that alveolar levels increased during recovery from ARDS [28]. The conclusion from these observations is that VEGF may play an important role in the increased permeability state that exists in early ARDS and that increased alveolar levels are associated with resolution of ARDS. Whether this is applicable to post-pneumonectomy pulmonary edema is unknown.

3. Tumor necrosis factor (TNF)-α and the interleukins (IL)
IL-8 is a potent neutrophil chemotactic agent. Donnelly et al. [29] reported increased IL-8 levels in patients at risk of ARDS who subsequently developed ARDS compared to those who did not. This difference was only significant in BAL fluid and not in the plasma samples. Amat et al. [25] found increased plasma levels of IL-8 in patients who already had ARDS compared to at risk patients. IL-1 and TNF-α are pro-inflammatory cytokines involved in the early phase of inflammation being released within the first 30–90 minutes after exposure to endotoxin (lipopolysaccharide, LPS). Both can induce a septic shock like pattern on infusion in animals [30] and IL-1 in particular is potent in the activation of neutrophils and the up-regulation of adhesion molecules essential for the progression of ARDS [31]. These cytokines also stimulate the release of further inflammatory cytokines, e.g., IL-6. Increased levels of IL-1 and TNF-α have been identified in the BAL fluid of patients with ARDS in comparison to those with cardiogenic pulmonary edema [23].

In summary there seems to be a fair amount of evidence that activation of the inflammatory cascade and release of certain inflammatory mediators is associated with the development of ARDS. There is much less work concerning the influence of inflammatory mediators in post-pneumonectomy pulmonary edema. However, considering the potential stimuli for inflammation during lung resection (surgical stimulus, ischemia-reperfusion injury, oxidative damage) and the similarities in pathology between ARDS and post-pneumonectomy pulmonary edema, it is likely that inflammation is integral to the pathogenesis of post-pneumonectomy pulmonary edema.

Fluid Therapy and Reduction in Volume of the Pulmonary Vascular Bed

Over-zealous fluid therapy was first considered a potential etiological factor in post-pneumonectomy pulmonary edema by Zeldin et al. in 1984 [32]. These authors reported on 10 cases of post-pneumonectomy pulmonary edema and found that these patients had significantly higher fluid inputs than those who did not develop post-pneumonectomy pulmonary edema. Several other studies have since demonstrated an association between fluid therapy and post-pneumonectomy pulmonary edema [12, 13], but others have not [8, 9, 33]. Mathru et al. [14] studied five patients with post-pneumonectomy pulmonary edema and measured the pulmonary capillary pressure and protein content of the edema fluid. These investigators found that pulmonary capillary pressures were raised due to a reduction in the volume of the pulmonary vascular bed. They also found the edema fluid protein to serum protein ratio was 0.6 or greater suggesting permeability pulmonary edema [14]. Waller et al. [19] also demonstrated that the permeability of the non-operated lung in pneumonectomy patients increases, which is consistent with Mathru's findings [14]. Groeneveld [18] looked at the relationship between extravascular lung water (EVLW) and pulmonary capillary filtration pressure in normal and increased permeability states. He reported a significant relationship between pulmonary capillary filtration pressure (which is related to the fluid load) and EVLW in increased permeability states only.

In summary, excessive fluid therapy has often been associated with but not been proved to cause post-pneumonectomy pulmonary edema/ARDS. However, as pneumonectomy is associated with increased endothelial permeability [19], and fluid loading can cause a significant increase in EVLW in increased permeability states [18], it seems logical that cautious perioperative fluid therapy is important. It also seems logical that measures are taken to prevent, as far as possible, increases in pulmonary capillary pressure.

Disrupted Lymphatic Drainage

Altered lymphatic drainage from the lungs has been suggested to be a contributing factor in the development of post-pneumonectomy pulmonary edema by the mechanism of slowing the clearing of excessive fluid administration from the lungs. Lymphatic vessels are unavoidably damaged during pulmonary resections and nodal dissection and sampling will clearly add to this. Anatomical studies have suggested that the left lung relies far more on contralateral lymphatic drainage than the right lung raising a theoretical reason for the quoted excess number of cases of post-pneumonectomy pulmonary edema in right sided pneumonectomies [6, 34, 35].

The effect of lymphatic disruption on extravascular fluid accumulation is difficult to estimate in real life situations although common sense would indicate that decreasing the ability of the lymphatic system to clear fluid is likely to impair the ability of the thorax as a whole to clear fluids. This would have the effect of increased hydrostatic pressure in favor of edema formation. This mechanism, however, does not explain the exudative nature of the edema and the high levels of cytokines in that fluid. Therefore, lymphatic disruption is at most likely to exacerbate rather than cause post-pneumonectomy pulmonary edema.

Oxidative Damage and Ischemia-Reperfusion Injury

Oxygen free radicals (reactive oxygen species, ROS) have been shown to be important in the pathogenesis of ARDS [36]. Several pathways for generation of oxygen free radicals are known, including the mitochondrial metabolic pathways, the enzyme, xanthine oxidase, arachidonic acid metabolism, and direct production by neutrophils and macrophages [37]. In normal conditions, circulating and local antioxidants, such as vitamins A, C, and E, and antioxidant enzymes, such as superoxide dismutase, prevent significant oxidant damage [37]. In ARDS there is evidence of increased oxidative damage associated with decreased levels of antioxidants [38].

Williams et al. [39] studied oxidative damage in patients undergoing thoracic surgery. They found a significant perioperative fall in plasma thiol levels (due to oxidation) with a significant perioperative rise in plasma carbonyl levels, all consistent with oxidative protein damage. This significant difference was only present in patients undergoing a pneumonectomy or lobectomy and was not present in patients undergoing a biopsy or wedge resection. The overall conclusion of the study was that, as in ARDS, there is evidence for oxidative damage in pulmonary resection patients.

Ischemia, followed by reperfusion (ischemia-reperfusion injury) has been reported to be the primary cause of graft failure in lung transplant patients. The damage in ischemia-reperfusion injury is thought to occur through the production of ROS [40]. Williams et al. [41] postulated that oxidant generation secondary to ischemia-reperfusion injury may occur during pulmonary resection. They looked at this in isolated rat lungs comparing controls to a group undergoing one lung ventilation followed by a pneumonectomy compared to another group undergoing one lung ventilation followed by re-inflation of the collapsed lung without resection. In both groups, the authors found evidence of oxidant damage associated with a fall in oxygenation. They reported that these changes were attenuated following treatment with superoxide dismutase, the conclusion being that ischemia-reperfusion injury may be important in thoracic surgery and a potential source of ROS [41].

In summary there is evidence for oxidative damage in both ARDS and post-pneumonectomy pulmonary edema. However, the significance of oxidative damage in terms of the development of, and morbidity and mortality associated with, ARDS and post-pneumonectomy pulmonary edema is presently undetermined.

Ventilation

Ventilation with high volumes and pressures during pneumonectomy is likely to be a contributing factor in the development of post-pneumonectomy pulmonary edema. In ARDS patients, Brower et al. clearly showed a 22 % relative risk reduction with a low tidal volume ventilation strategy compared to a high tidal volume strategy, demonstrating a clear link with ARDS and ventilator strategy [42]. In 1997, van der Werff et al. [33] reported that higher ventilation pressures were significantly associated with the development of post-pneumonectomy pulmonary edema, with a relative risk of 3.0 (95 % CI 1.2–7.3). In 2003, Licker et al. [13] found that the plateau inspiratory pressure and the ventilatory hyperpressure index (a value taking into account plateau inspiratory pressure and the duration of one lung ventilation) were significantly associated with the development of ALI following lung resection, with an odds ratio of 3.53 (CI 1.7–8.5) for the ventilation hyperpressure index. In 2006, Fernández-Pérez et al. [43] demonstrated an increased risk of post-pneumonectomy pulmonary edema with large tidal volume ventilation. It is thought that ventilation with higher volumes and pressures results in amplification of the inflammatory cascade. This is supported by a study showing that a 'lung-protective' ventilation strategy was associated with decreased bronchoalveolar and plasma cytokine levels compared to conventional ventilation [44].

Comorbidities

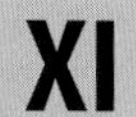

A number of studies have looked at possible risk factors for post-pneumonectomy pulmonary edema including co-morbidities [8, 12, 13, 33]. Licker et al. [13] studied many comorbidities, including coronary artery disease, hypertension, diabetes, alcohol consumption, and chronic obstructive pulmonary disease (COPD). The authors found that chronic alcohol consumption was a significant risk factor for the development of post-pneumonectomy pulmonary edema in multivariate analysis. Interestingly, Moss et al. [45] showed that chronic alcohol consumption increased the risk of ARDS and Guidot and Roman [46] studied the role of alcohol in the pathogenesis of ALI and suggested it may increase oxidative stress, impair alveolar liquid clearance, and alter epithelial cell permeability. There is also evidence suggesting that patients undergoing lung resection who have a raised preoperative C-reactive protein (CRP), are more at risk of postoperative complications [47] and that CRP is raised in patients who abuse alcohol [48].

Chest Drains

Acute mediastinal shift secondary to the negative pressure generated by the underwater seal in a chest drain has been postulated to be a contributing factor for the development of post-pneumonectomy pulmonary edema. Animal studies have suggested that negative pressure in the mediastinum compared to normal pressure increases the likelihood of ARDS developing [49]. Alvarez et al. [50] performed a retrospective analysis of practice in their institution following a change from underwater seals to a balanced drainage system, to maintain mediastinal pressure within normal limits. These authors found a significant reduction in the incidence of post-pneumonectomy pulmonary edema, from 14.3 to 0 %. These data seem compelling in themselves, but the obvious problem exists in that the underwater seal group acted as historical controls for the balanced seal group and the problems of interpreting results from historical controls are well known. Nevertheless, this study raises the potential that a fairly simple intervention may have a large influence on post-pneumonectomy pulmonary edema and certainly warrants a larger prospective trial.

Transfusion of Blood Products

An association between transfusion of fresh frozen plasma (FFP) and post-pneumonectomy pulmonary edema was described by van der Werff et al. in 1997 [33]. These authors postulated an immune reaction as the cause for the increase in cases of post-pneumonectomy pulmonary edema in the FFP group speculating a similar pathology to transfusion related acute lung injury (TRALI), with activated leukocytes and granulocytes migrating into the pulmonary interstitium. A more recent retrospective analysis by Thomas et al. [51] found blood transfusion to be the strongest predictor of post-pneumonectomy respiratory distress. They also found that among the twelve patients who received plasma, nine developed postoperative respiratory failure [51]. However, Licker et al. [13] found no association between blood transfusion and post-pneumonectomy pulmonary edema. It must also be remembered that patients receiving blood transfusions, especially FFP, are more likely to have had a greater surgical insult, a greater duration of ventilation, increased fluid infusion, and possibly a greater risk of oxidative damage.

Conclusion

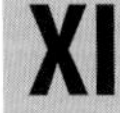

Post-pneumonectomy pulmonary edema is a not infrequent complication of lung resection and carries a high mortality. Evidence suggests that the incidence of post-pneumonectomy pulmonary edema is decreasing which may be due to a reduction in the number of pneumonectomies being performed and also a greater application of careful fluid balance and ventilation strategies [15]. It is likely that inflammation plays an integral part in the pathogenesis of post-pneumonectomy pulmonary edema and that several factors may initiate the inflammatory cascade (ventilation with high volumes/pressures, ischemia-reperfusion injury and oxidative damage, surgical insult) while other factors increase susceptibility to post-pneumonectomy pulmonary edema (chronic alcohol consumption) and still others contribute to the severity of the edema (fluid loading, increased pulmonary capillary pressures, chest drains, lymphatic disruption).

There are limited treatment options for post-pneumonectomy pulmonary edema once it occurs. Assuming that post-pneumonectomy pulmonary edema is a post pneumonectomy version of ALI/ARDS then standard ALI/ARDS treatment is logical. There are measures that can be taken in order to try and prevent cases of post-pneumonectomy pulmonary edema: Limiting surgical resection as far as possible, careful fluid balance, avoiding high inspired oxygen, minimizing pulmonary capillary pressures, and avoiding ventilation with large volumes. However, these measures are not always possible, especially in the more borderline cases of lung resection. Perhaps future research could be directed at the role of anti-inflammatory drugs or anti-oxidants in the prevention and treatment of post-pneumonectomy pulmonary edema.

References

1. Alexiou C, Beggs D, Rogers ML, Beggs L, Asopa S, Salama FD (2001) Pneumonectomy for non-small cell lung cancer: predictors of operative mortality and survival. Eur J Cardiothorac Surg 20: 476–480
2. Algar FJ, Alvarez A, Salvatierra A, Baamonde C, Aranda JL, Lopez-Pujol FJ (2003) Predicting pulmonary complications after pneumonectomy for lung cancer. Eur J Cardiothorac Surg 23: 201–208
3. Bernard A, Deschamps C, Allen MS, et al (2001) Pneumonectomy for malignant disease: factors affecting early morbidity and mortality. J Thorac Cardiovasc Surg 121: 1076–1082
4. Dancewicz M, Kowalewski J, Peplinski J (2006) Factors associated with perioperative complications after pneumonectomy for primary carcinoma of the lung. Interact Cardiovasc Thorac Surg 5: 97–100
5. Licker M, Spiliopoulos A, Frey JG, et al (2002) Risk factors for early mortality and major complications following pneumonectomy for non-small cell carcinoma of the lung. Chest 121: 1890–1897
6. Jordan S, Mitchell JA, Quinlan GJ, Goldstraw P, Evans TW (2000) The pathogenesis of lung injury following pulmonary resection. Eur Respir J 15: 790–799
7. Dulu A, Pastores SM, Park B, Riedel E, Rusch V, Halpern NA (2006) Prevalence and mortality of acute lung injury and ARDS after lung resection. Chest 130: 73–78
8. Turnage WS, Lunn JJ (1993) Postpneumonectomy pulmonary edema. A retrospective analysis of associated variables. Chest 103: 1646–1650
9. Waller DA, Gebitekin C, Saunders NR, Walker DR (1993) Noncardiogenic pulmonary edema complicating lung resection. Ann Thorac Surg 55: 140–143
10. Bernard GR, Artigas A, Brigham KL, et al (1994) The American-European Consensus Conference on ARDS. Definitions, mechanisms, relevant outcomes, and clinical trial coordination. Am J Respir Crit Care Med 149: 818–824
11. Hayes JP, Williams EA, Goldstraw P, Evans TW (1995) Lung injury in patients following thoracotomy. Thorax 50: 990–991
12. Alam N, Park BJ, Wilton A, et al (2007) Incidence and risk factors for lung injury after lung cancer resection. Ann Thorac Surg 84: 1085–1091
13. Licker M, de Perrot M, Spiliopoulos A, et al (2003) Risk factors for acute lung injury after thoracic surgery for lung cancer. Anesth Analg 97: 1558–1565
14. Mathru M, Blakeman B, Dries DJ, Kleinman B, Kumar P (1990) Permeability pulmonary edema following lung resection. Chest 98: 1216–1218
15. Tang SS, Redmond K, Griffiths M, Ladas G, Goldstraw P, Dusmet M (2008) The mortality from acute respiratory distress syndrome after pulmonary resection is reducing: a 10-year single institutional experience. Eur J Cardiothorac Surg 34: 898–902
16. Bellingan GJ (2002) The pulmonary physician in critical care * 6: The pathogenesis of ALI/ARDS. Thorax 57: 540–546
17. Groeneveld AB (1997) Radionuclide assessment of pulmonary microvascular permeability. Eur J Nucl Med 24: 449–461
18. Groeneveld AB (2002) Vascular pharmacology of acute lung injury and acute respiratory distress syndrome. Vascul Pharmacol 39: 247–256
19. Waller DA, Keavey P, Woodfine L, Dark JH (1996) Pulmonary endothelial permeability changes after major lung resection. Ann Thorac Surg 61: 1435–1440
20. Baudouin SV (2003) Lung injury after thoracotomy. Br J Anaesth 91: 132–142
21. Cerfolio RJ, Bryant AS, Thurber JS, Bass CS, Lell WA, Bartolucci AA (2003) Intraoperative solumedrol helps prevent postpneumonectomy pulmonary edema. Ann Thorac Surg 76: 1029–1033
22. Park WY, Goodman RB, Steinberg KP, et al (2001) Cytokine balance in the lungs of patients with acute respiratory distress syndrome. Am J Respir Crit Care Med 164: 1896–1903

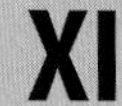

23. Schutte H, Lohmeyer J, Rosseau S, et al (1996) Bronchoalveolar and systemic cytokine profiles in patients with ARDS, severe pneumonia and cardiogenic pulmonary oedema. Eur Respir J 9: 1858–1867
24. Gebhard F, Marzinzig M, Hartel W, Bruckner UB (1997) [Systemic release of prostanoids after surgically-induced injury of lung tissue]. Langenbecks Arch Chir 382: 243–251
25. Amat M, Barcons M, Mancebo J, et al (2000) Evolution of leukotriene B4, peptide leukotrienes, and interleukin-8 plasma concentrations in patients at risk of acute respiratory distress syndrome and with acute respiratory distress syndrome: mortality prognostic study. Crit Care Med 28: 57–62
26. Sampson SE, Costello JF, Sampson AP (1997) The effect of inhaled leukotriene B4 in normal and in asthmatic subjects. Am J Respir Crit Care Med 155: 1789–1792
27. Thickett DR, Armstrong L, Christie SJ, Millar AB (2001) Vascular endothelial growth factor may contribute to increased vascular permeability in acute respiratory distress syndrome. Am J Respir Crit Care Med 164: 1601–1605
28. Thickett DR, Armstrong L, Millar AB (2002) A role for vascular endothelial growth factor in acute and resolving lung injury. Am J Respir Crit Care Med 166: 1332–1337
29. Donnelly SC, Strieter RM, Kunkel SL, et al (1993) Interleukin-8 and development of adult respiratory distress syndrome in at-risk patient groups. Lancet 341: 643–647
30. Okusawa S, Gelfand JA, Ikejima T, Connolly RJ, Dinarello CA (1988) Interleukin 1 induces a shock-like state in rabbits. Synergism with tumor necrosis factor and the effect of cyclooxygenase inhibition. J Clin Invest 81: 1162–1172
31. Bhatia M, Moochhala S (2004) Role of inflammatory mediators in the pathophysiology of acute respiratory distress syndrome. J Pathol 202: 145–156
32. Zeldin RA, Normandin D, Landtwing D, Peters RM (1984) Postpneumonectomy pulmonary edema. J Thorac Cardiovasc Surg 87: 359–365
33. van der Werff YD, van der Houwen HK, Heijmans PJ, et al (1997) Postpneumonectomy pulmonary edema. A retrospective analysis of incidence and possible risk factors. Chest 111: 1278–1284
34. Baker NH, Hill L, Ewy HG, Marable S (1967) Pulmonary lymphatic drainage. J Thorac Cardiovasc Surg 54: 695–696
35. Nohl-Oser HC (1972) An investigation of the anatomy of the lymphatic drainage of the lungs as shown by the lymphatic spread of bronchial carcinoma. Ann R Coll Surg Engl 51: 157–176
36. Lang JD, McArdle PJ, O'Reilly PJ, Matalon S (2002) Oxidant-antioxidant balance in acute lung injury. Chest 122:314S-320S
37. Zhang H, Slutsky AS, Vincent JL (2000) Oxygen free radicals in ARDS, septic shock and organ dysfunction. Intensive Care Med 26: 474–476
38. Metnitz PG, Bartens C, Fischer M, Fridrich P, Steltzer H, Druml W (1999) Antioxidant status in patients with acute respiratory distress syndrome. Intensive Care Med 25: 180–185
39. Williams EA, Quinlan GJ, Goldstraw P, Gothard JW, Evans TW (1998) Postoperative lung injury and oxidative damage in patients undergoing pulmonary resection. Eur Respir J 11: 1028–1034
40. de Perrot M, Liu M, Waddell TK, Keshavjee S (2003) Ischemia-reperfusion-induced lung injury. Am J Respir Crit Care Med 167: 490–511
41. Williams EA, Quinlan GJ, Anning PB, Goldstraw P, Evans TW (1999) Lung injury following pulmonary resection in the isolated, blood-perfused rat lung. Eur Respir J 14: 745–750
42. The Acute Respiratory Distress Syndrome Network. (2000) Ventilation with lower tidal volumes as compared with traditional tidal volumes for acute lung injury and the acute respiratory distress syndrome. N Engl J Med 342: 1301–1308
43. Fernandez-Perez ER, Keegan MT, Brown DR, Hubmayr RD, Gajic O (2006) Intraoperative tidal volume as a risk factor for respiratory failure after pneumonectomy. Anesthesiology 105: 14–18
44. Ranieri VM, Suter PM, Tortorella C, et al (1999) Effect of mechanical ventilation on inflammatory mediators in patients with acute respiratory distress syndrome: a randomized controlled trial. JAMA 282: 54–61
45. Moss M, Parsons PE, Steinberg KP, et al (2003) Chronic alcohol abuse is associated with an increased incidence of acute respiratory distress syndrome and severity of multiple organ dysfunction in patients with septic shock. Crit Care Med 31: 869–877

46. Guidot DM, Roman J (2002) Chronic ethanol ingestion increases susceptibility to acute lung injury: role of oxidative stress and tissue remodeling. Chest 122:309S-314S
47. Amar D, Zhang H, Park B, Heerdt PM, Fleisher M, Thaler HT (2007) Inflammation and outcome after general thoracic surgery. Eur J Cardiothorac Surg 32: 431–434
48. Alho H, Sillanaukee P, Kalela A, Jaakkola O, Laine S, Nikkari ST (2004) Alcohol misuse increases serum antibodies to oxidized LDL and C-reactive protein. Alcohol Alcohol 39: 312–315
49. Ramenofsky ML (1979) The effects of intrapleural pressure on respiratory insufficiency. J Pediatr Surg 14: 750–756
50. Alvarez JM, Panda RK, Newman MA, Slinger P, Deslauriers J, Ferguson M (2003) Postpneumonectomy pulmonary edema. J Cardiothorac Vasc Anesth 17: 388–395
51. Thomas P, Michelet P, Barlesi F, et al (2007) Impact of blood transfusions on outcome after pneumonectomy for thoracic malignancies. Eur Respir J 29: 565–570

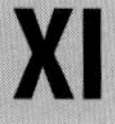

The Role of Phenylephrine in Perioperative Medicine

C. Ertmer, A. Morelli, and M. Westphal

Introduction

Phenylephrine is a synthetic, direct sympathomimetic agent that is mainly used to induce locoregional vasoconstriction. For this purpose, phenylephrine is contained in several decongestant nasal sprays [1] and mydriatics [2] in doses usually not exerting significant systemic cardiovascular effects. In 1976, oral phenylephrine was approved for non-prescription use as a decongestant by the Food and Drug Administration (FDA) [3]. In addition, local phenylephrine injection may be considered to treat regional hyperemia, e.g., in patients with priapism [4]. Intravenous phenylephrine represents an effective vasopressor in a variety of clinical indications, particularly including Cesarean section and cardiovascular surgery. This chapter summarizes the pharmacology of intravenous phenylephrine and clinical studies investigating its use in the perioperative setting and provides recommendations for perioperative use.

Pharmacological Characteristics of Phenylephrine

Phenylephrine (chemical name: 3-[(1R)-1-hydroxy-2-methylaminoethyl]phenol) is closely related to epinephrine but lacks the hydroxyl group in position 4 of the latter molecule. Because of the absence of the typical catechol (benzene-1,2-diol) structure (**Fig. 1**), from a chemical point of view phenylephrine does not belong to the group of catecholamines.

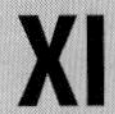

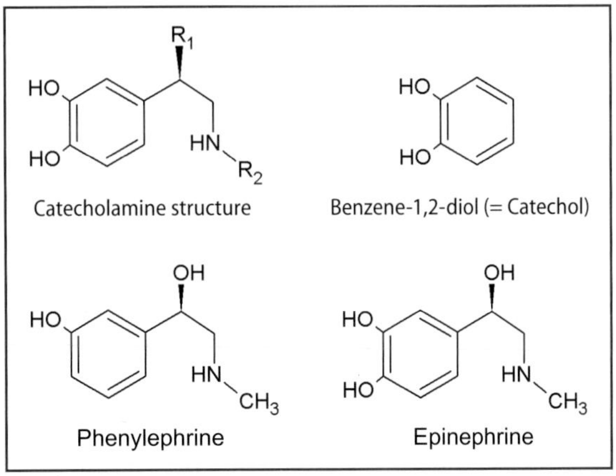

Catecholamine structure

Benzene-1,2-diol (= Catechol)

Phenylephrine

Epinephrine

Fig. 1. Chemical structures of catechol, epinephrine and phenylephrine.

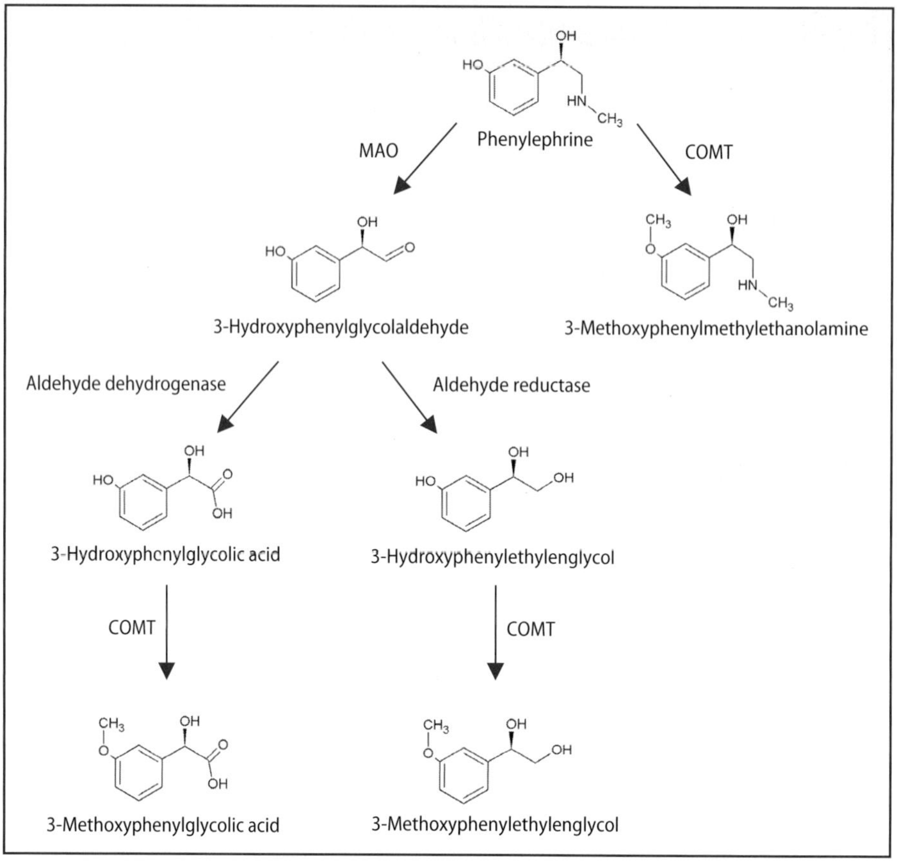

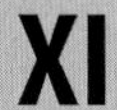

Fig. 2. Endogenous metabolism of phenylephrine. MAO: monoamine oxidase; COMT: catechol-O-methyl transferase

Orally ingested phenylephrine is subjected to a marked first-pass mechanism with a bioavailability of about 38 % [5]. Following hepatic metabolism by monoamine oxidase and to a lesser extent by the catechol-O-methyl transferases (**Fig. 2**), 80 % of orally and 86 % of intravenously administered phenylephrine are excreted via the urine [5]. This, in turn, suggests complete uptake of the drug following oral ingestion. In contrast, as a result of the reduced bioavailability, the fraction of free plasma phenylephrine is largely reduced following oral uptake (2.6 %) as compared to intravenous infusion (16 %) [5]. In addition, no relevant changes in blood pressure or heart rate were observed following intranasal installation of up to 15 mg phenylephrine [1]. Pharmacokinetic variables, such as biological half-life (2.1 – 3.4 h), total clearance (~35 ml/min), and volume of distribution (340 l) are comparable to those of structurally related amines [5].

Phenylephrine binds to adrenergic α_1 receptors and induces contraction of vascular smooth muscle cells. The subsequent vasoconstriction lasts up to 20 minutes following intravenous bolus infusion and up to 1 hour after intramuscular injection [6]. Phenylephrine is currently available for intravenous infusion in 1 ml vials containing 10 mg of the drug. Prior to infusion, the vial content should be diluted with

99 ml of the vehicle fluid to achieve a concentration of 100 μg/ml. Doses for intravenous bolus injection average between 50 and 200 μg. For continuous infusion, doses range between 0.05 and 5 μg/kg/min, depending on the severity of arterial hypotension. When high doses are required, solutions with higher phenylephrine concentrations (up to 1 mg/ml) may be prepared.

Due to the increase in total peripheral resistance, reflex bradycardia may ensue following injection of phenylephrine, which can be explained by the activation of baroreceptors [7]. While this effect may potentially be advantageous in vasoplegic patients with tachycardia, it could also be detrimental in patients with symptomatic bradycardia or aortic or mitral valve regurgitation. Thus, whenever phenylephrine is used, inotropic drugs should be available to counteract potential myocardial depression. On the other hand, due to the high selectivity of phenylephrine at the α_1 receptor, combination with β-adrenergic drugs may be ideal in titrating vasoconstrictive and inotropic effects in critically ill patients.

Contraindications for the Use of Phenylephrine

As with all vasoconstrictors, phenylephrine should not be infused in hypertensive or hypovolemic patients. Hypovolemia should be counteracted by goal-directed fluid therapy prior to phenylephrine infusion to prevent vasopressor-masked hypovolemia, which may foster the pathogenesis of multiple organ failure [8]. In addition, phenylephrine should be avoided or used with great caution in patients not able to cope with sudden increases in myocardial afterload or reductions in heart rate. Such conditions include congestive heart failure, aortic or mitral valve insufficiency, as well as ventricular wall aneurysm. To date, no data are available for patients with vasospastic diathesis, such as patients with Raynaud's syndrome or recent subarachnoid hemorrhage.

Use of Phenylephrine to Treat Perioperative Arterial Hypotension

General and Regional Anesthesia

General and neuroaxial anesthesia are commonly related to relevant arterial hypotension according to reductions in sympathetic tone, myocardial inotropy, and vascular resistance. Infusion of 100 μg phenylephrine proved effective in preventing arterial hypotension following induction of anesthesia with propofol in 135 patients (American Society of Anesthesiologists [ASA] physical status I or II) [9]. In 16 healthy patients undergoing general anesthesia, phenylephrine increased mean arterial pressure (MAP) as effectively as norepinephrine, but reduced stroke volume and the velocity of myocardial fiber shortening [10]. In addition, it has been reported that phenylephrine infusion (0.5 μg/kg/min) reduced the magnitude of redistribution hypothermia as compared to a control group by maintaining precapillary vasoconstriction of cutaneous arterioles [11]. Furthermore, in patients with chronic pulmonary hypertension undergoing general anesthesia complicated by systemic hypotension, norepinephrine appears preferable over phenylephrine, since only norepinephrine decreased the pulmonary to systemic arterial pressure ratio [12].

Depending on their specific lipid solubility, vasopressor agents may even exert distinct effects on anesthesia depth. In this context, it has been demonstrated that ephedrine (high lipid solubility due to the lack of hydroxyl residues bonded to the phenyl ring) increases bispectral index values (i.e., lowers anesthesia depth), whereas the hydrophilic phenylephrine (**Fig. 1**) does not [13]. A Japanese study group confirmed these findings and provided evidence that the differences in anesthesia depth were not related to changes in anesthetic concentrations [14].

Apart from general anesthesia, several studies have investigated the effects of phenylephrine when used to treat arterial hypotension associated with neuroaxial blockade. In 30 patients undergoing total hip athroplasty under epidural anesthesia, Sharrock and co-workers reported the effects of intravenous phenylephrine (10.6 ± 6.2 μg/min ≈ 0.15 μg/kg/min) versus epinephrine (2.6 ± 1.02 μg/min ≈ 0.03 μg/kg/min) on intraoperative hemodynamics [15]. Notably, this relatively low phenylephrine dose stabilized MAP at ≈ 60 mmHg and heart rate between 50 and 60 bpm, whereas epinephrine was associated with heart rates around 80 bpm at an even lower level of MAP (≈ 50 mmHg). However, due to the occurrence of reflex bradycardia in the phenylephrine group and epinephrine-mediated stimulation of β-receptors, cardiac output was higher in the epinephrine group. In a subsequent study, the same research group did not notice any differences between the vasopressors on coagulation variables or thrombembolic events that may have potentially resulted from differences in venous blood flow [16]. In addition, the same authors reported that the lower cardiac output with phenylephrine was not associated with lower intraoperative blood loss [17]. However, total blood loss was very low in both groups (≈ 250 ml). Therefore, it remains unclear whether in cases of severe bleeding during hip athroplasty (such as intraoperative laceration of the superficial femoral artery), epinephrine infusion may increase blood loss as compared to phenylephrine due to higher femoral arterial blood flow.

In patients with spinal anesthesia undergoing elective surgery, phenylephrine better maintained mean and diastolic blood pressure as compared to epinephrine, thereby lowering heart rate and cardiac output [18].

From the above studies investigating the use of phenylephrine in general and regional anesthesia, it can be concluded that phenylephrine effectively increases blood pressure and decreases heart rate without relevant adverse effects. From a pragmatic approach, it may be suggested that phenylephrine is the optimal vasopressor in normovolemic, hypotensive patients, whose heart rate is judged as 'too high'. Comparable effects can be attained with the combination of norepinephrine and beta-blockers. This combination, however, has not yet been compared to phenylephrine. In hypotensive bradycardic patients, phenylephrine should be avoided, since it may further decrease heart rate.

Cardiac Surgery

Arterial hypotension is a common complication in patients undergoing cardiac surgery and may result from myocardial insufficiency, hypovolemia, and/or vasodilation associated with anesthesia and cardiopulmonary bypass (CPB). The ideal vasoactive drug to increase MAP in this setting is still unclear. In patients with coronary artery disease scheduled for coronary artery bypass grafting, phenylephrine (100 μg i.v. bolus) exerts similar effects to norepinephrine (10 μg i.v. bolus) by increasing MAP and systemic vascular resistance (SVR) without affecting cardiac output [19]. Phenylephrine is thus suitable for increasing coronary perfusion pressure in patients with coronary artery disease. Even direct infusion of phenylephrine into the coronary arteries of healthy patients and patients with coronary spastic angina did not induce coronary vasospasm [20]. Furthermore, phenylephrine does not exert significant vasoconstrictive effects on radial artery grafts when used to increase coronary perfusion pressure [21]. However, in coronary artery disease, bolus infusion of phenylephrine (1 µg/kg) is associated with transient impairment of systolic left ventricular function, as assessed by transesophageal echocardiography (TEE) [22]. It may be relevant that the latter adverse effect has not been observed following bolus infusion of norepinephrine (0.05 µg/kg). However, it remains elusive whether the absence of myocardial depression following norepinephrine bolus infusion was dose-related. In contrast, in patients with valvular aortic stenosis, systolic left ventricular function is well maintained following phenylephrine infusion to restore MAP [22]. In addition, phenylephrine has been reported to impair diastolic left ventricular function in patients with and without coronary artery disease [23]. In patients with valvular aortic stenosis, diastolic function of the left ventricle remained unchanged. Phenylephrine may, therefore, be preferable to norepinephrine in these patients due to unwanted β-adrenergic effects of the latter drug. Phenylephrine infusion may furthermore be beneficial to increase pulmonary blood flow and oxygenation in patients with right ventricular outflow tract obstruction and pulmo-systemic shunt (e.g., tetralogy of Fallot) [24]. In this condition, phenylephrine increases SVR and, therefore, ameliorates the shunt fraction from the right to the left ventricle.

Non-cardiac Vascular Surgery

Patients with significant stenosis of arterial vessels are particularly susceptible to sudden decreases in arterial pressure. Especially in patients with carotid stenosis undergoing endarterectomy, sustained arterial hypotension may result in severe postoperative neurologic deficits [25, 26]. In this context, Mutch and co-workers reported on the feasibility and safety of phenylephrine to titrate MAP to 110 ± 10 % of baseline values during carotid endarterectomy [27]. Borum et al. demonstrated that the mean phenylephrine dosage needed to titrate MAP to baseline values during carotid endarterectomy under general anesthesia was ~0.5 µg/kg/min [28]. Interestingly, vasopressor doses may be reduced by ~40 % with concomitant transesophageal atrial pacing aimed at increasing cardiac output. Notably, phenylephrine should not be used routinely to counteract decreases in blood pressure secondary to anesthesia that is too deep. In this regard, Smith and co-workers found that patients anesthetized with ~1 minimal alveolar concentration (MAC) of isoflurane were less likely to suffer from myocardial ischemia or new onset segmental wall motion abnormalities than those anesthetized with 1.5 MAC of isoflurane during carotid surgery [29]. The latter group needed phenylephrine to compensate for the arterial hypotension induced by deep anesthesia. However, it appears that the adverse events observed in this study [29] were due to overdosage of anesthetic drugs rather than to phenylephrine infusion *per se*. In view of the current evidence, phenylephrine appears to be a safe vasopressor during carotid surgery. Unfortunately, there are no studies comparing phenylephrine with other vasopressors in this situation.

Cesarean Section

General anesthesia is awkward in females undergoing Cesarean section because of the risks of pulmonary aspiration, intubation problems, maternal hypotension, and anesthetic exposure to the fetus, possibly resulting in fetal hypoxemia and acidosis. Thus, except for emergency cases or severe contraindications, spinal anesthesia currently represents the anesthetic technique of choice in this indication. Although modern techniques using combinations of intrathecal opiates and low-dose local anesthetics largely reduce the incidence of arterial hypotension, the high anesthetic level targeted (mostly 4th thoracic dermatome) often requires the use of vasoactive drugs. Whereas the Anglo-American literature reports on the widespread use of ephedrine [30], combinations of theodrenaline and cafedrine (Akrinor®) are often applied in Germany and Austria [31]. These compounds have been shown to increase maternal blood pressure without impairing uteroplacental perfusion [30, 32]. However, in women treated with β-agonists for tocolysis or patients with coronary artery disease, inotropic drugs may further increase heart rate and myocardial oxygen demand and should, therefore, be avoided. A multitude of clinical studies has investigated the use of phenylephrine to treat arterial hypotension in this setting. As an example, a German group [33] reported on the successful treatment of arterial hypotension with phenylephrine in a female with hypertrophic, obstructive cardiomyopathy (HOCM) undergoing Cesarean section, where β-adrenergic treatment or excessive increases in endogenous catecholamine concentrations are known to be deleterious.

Moran and co-workers were the first to compare the efficacy and safety of ephedrine (initial dose 10 mg, repetitive doses 5–10 mg) and phenylephrine (initial dose 80 μg, repetitive doses 40–80 μg) in 60 females undergoing spinal anesthesia for Cesarean section [34]. In both groups, umbilical pH, partial pressure of carbon dioxide (PCO_2), and base deficit were maintained in the normal range, with significant group differences in favor of phenylephrine. There were no differences in neonatal Apgar (Appearance, Pulse, Grimace, Activity, Respiration) scores or maternal nausea and vomiting. LaPorta et al. confirmed these findings using a similar study design, and reported that maternal and fetal norepinephrine concentrations were considerably lower with phenylephrine treatment [35]. This may well be explained by the indirect sympathomimetic effects of ephedrine. Moreover, Pierce et al. demonstrated equality of ephedrine and phenylephrine in terms of umbilical natriuretic peptide concentrations, which have been shown to affect feto-placental circulatory homeostasis [36]. In contrast, Hall and colleagues reported that considerably lower doses of phenylephrine (continuous infusion of 10 μg/min, supplemented by bolus infusions of 20 μg) were significantly less effective in terms of increasing maternal blood pressure as compared to ephedrine (continuous infusion of 1–2 mg/min, supplemented by bolus infusions of 6 mg) [37]. Higher bolus doses (100 μg of phenylephrine), on the other hand, may be associated with relevant bradycardia requiring infusion of atropine [38]. Notably, in the latter study, fetal acid-base characteristics were even better maintained with the high phenylephrine dose as compared to ephedrine (5 mg bolus infusions), despite intermittent bradycardia. Using continuous intravenous infusions, Cooper et al. compared phenylephrine (100 μg/ml), ephedrine (3 mg/ml) and a combination of both drugs (50 μg phenylephrine plus 1.5 mg ephedrine per ml), and reported a lower incidence of arterial hypotension, tachycardia, and fetal acidosis in both phenylephrine groups [39]. The rate of nausea and vomiting was higher with the combination therapy as compared to sole phenylephrine. The authors therefore concluded that a combination therapy with ephedrine and phenylephrine had no advantage over sole phenylephrine in their study. In a large study including 125 parturients, Ngan Kee and co-workers randomly compared the effects of different combinations of phenylephrine and ephedrine (ranging from 0 % phenylephrine plus 100 % ephedrine to 100 % phenylephrine plus 0 % ephedrine) to maintain systolic blood pressure at baseline [40]. Notably, as the proportion of phenylephrine decreased and the proportion of ephedrine increased among groups, the incidences of hypotension and nausea/vomiting increased. In addition, the magnitude of deviations of blood pressure above or below baseline values increased, maternal heart rate was faster, and fetal pH, base excess, and umbilical arterial oxygen content decreased. The authors concluded that combinations of phenylephrine and ephedrine appear to have no advantage compared with phenylephrine alone. In contrast, Loughrey and co-workers reported that a combination of phenylephrine and ephedrine (40 μg phenylephrine plus 10 mg ephedrine as initial bolus; 20 μg plus 5 mg for subsequent bolus infusions) had no superior effects over sole ephedrine (10 mg for initial, 5 mg for subsequent bolus infusions) [41]. However, considering the very high incidence of arterial hypotension in that study (80 % and 95 % in the sole ephedrine and combination groups, respectively), which is substantially higher than in previous studies, these results should be judged with extreme caution.

In addition to correction of arterial hypotension, several studies investigated the efficacy and safety of phenylephrine administered to prevent reductions in blood pressure. Ayorinde et al. demonstrated that an intramuscular injection of 4 mg phenylephrine given immediately after induction of spinal anesthesia effectively maintained MAP in two thirds of study patients (n = 108) and reduced total rescue intravenous ephedrine requirements as compared to placebo or only 2 mg phenylephrine [42]. Notably, the incidence of arterial hypotension was 48 % in patients treated with 45 mg intramuscular ephedrine (compared to 33 % with 4 mg phenylephrine). The relatively high rate of arterial hypotension may partly be explained by the high dose of intrathecal anesthetic used in the study (2.2 ml hyperbaric bupivacaine 0.5 % plus fentanyl 20 μg). In a French study, the combination of pre-emptive intravenous ephedrine (2 mg/min) plus phenylephrine (10 mg/min) reduced the incidence of arterial hypotension to 37 % as compared to 75 % with sole ephedrine [42]. Apgar scores were equally good in both groups with significantly higher umbilical artery pH with the combination therapy. Again, high doses of local anesthetics (2.2 ml hyperbaric bupivacaine 0.5 %) combined with opioids were injected and may thus explain the high rate of arterial hypotension.

Regarding the goal blood pressure values during Cesarean section, a Chinese research group compared different phenylephrine infusion regimens aimed at preserving systolic blood pressure at 100 %, 90 %, or 80 % of baseline values [43]. Notably, the 100 % group received more phenylephrine but had fewer episodes of severe hypotension (systolic blood pressure below 80 % of baseline value), less nausea and vomiting, and higher umbilical arterial pH as compared to the other two groups. In similar studies, the same authors confirmed their beneficial findings associated with liberal phenylephrine infusion [40, 44–46]. It appears, therefore, that systolic blood pressure should be titrated to establish baseline values in normotensive women undergoing Cesarean section in spinal anesthesia.

Prevention and treatment of arterial hypotension in patients undergoing Cesarean section in spinal anesthesia includes a multifactorial approach consisting of avoidance of aortocaval compression, compression of the lower extremities, prehydration with colloids, low-dose spinal anesthesia, and goal-directed infusion of vasoactive drugs [47]. Thus, at our institution, patients are prehydrated with 500 ml of 6 % hydroxyethyl starch (HES) 130/0.4, receive low-dose spinal anesthesia in the right lateral position (1.6 ml hyperbaric bupivacaine 0.5 %, 5 μg sufentanil, 100 μg morphine), and immediately thereafter are turned to the Trendelenburg position with inclination to the left side. Only if necessary, is 50 μg phenylephrine repeatedly infused to maintain systolic blood pressure at baseline values. In view of the current literature, it appears that phenylephrine (administered in single intravenous doses ≤ 100 μg) is at least as safe and effective as ephedrine, and may be particularly beneficial in patients presenting with contraindications to inotropic drugs.

Use of Phenylephrine in Postoperative Intensive Care Medicine

Despite widespread use of phenylephrine to treat arterial hypotension in the perioperative setting, its clinical efficacy in postoperative intensive care unit (ICU) patients remains to be further investigated. Due to its pharmacological features (i.e., α-adrenergic activity and minimal affinity for β-adrenergic receptors) phenylephrine is commonly used as a bolus infusion to immediately counteract sudden severe arterial hypotension. However, ICU patients often require hemodynamic support over a long time period, and continuous infusion may, therefore, be preferable over bolus infusion. The following paragraphs specifically focus on the efficacy of phenylephrine relevant to the treatment of cardiovascular diseases in ICU patients. Specifically, the role of phenylephrine in the treatment of the two most common causes of arterial hypotension is discussed, i.e., vasodilatory shock after CPB and septic shock.

Vasodilatory Shock after Cardiac Surgery and Cardiopulmonary Bypass

Vasodilatory shock after CPB is characterized by profound arteriolar vasodilation resulting in low SVR and arterial hypotension. Norepinephrine is commonly used for the treatment of hypotension in this setting [48]. Data on the use of phenylephrine to treat arterial hypotension after postcardiotomy shock are scarce. However, Nygren and colleagues [49] recently compared the effects of phenylephrine and norepinephrine on systemic and regional hemodynamics in a series of uncomplicated, normotensive, postcardiac surgery patients. The authors reported that low doses of norepinephrine (0.052 ± 0.009 μg/kg/min) and phenylephrine (0.50 ± 0.22 μg/kg/min) induced a 30 % increase in MAP. Nevertheless, for the same MAP and cardiac output, phenylephrine caused a more pronounced increase in splanchnic oxygen extraction and mixed venous-hepatic vein oxygen saturation gradient compared to norepinephrine. These findings suggest that phenylephrine induces more pronounced splanchnic vasoconstriction compared with norepinephrine [49]. Notably, a decrease in splanchnic blood flow was previously observed in pigs treated with phenylephrine at a dose of 2.4 ± 0.6 μg/kg/min during CPB [50]. In contrast to the impairment in the splanchnic oxygen demand-supply relationship, however, phenylephrine did not affect the gastric-arterial PCO_2 gradient, suggesting that phenylephrine did not alter the regional gastric-mucosal relationship between blood flow and metabolism [49]. Taking into account the limitations related to the protocol design as well as the baseline hemodynamics and the low-doses of catecholamines administered to the enrolled patients, the study by Nygren et al. [49] strengthens the notion that norepinephrine may be safer than phenylephrine to counteract arterial hypotension in postcardiac surgery patients. In view of the current literature on this topic, although limited in extent, it appears reasonable to use phenylephrine only with great caution in patients with vasodilatory shock after cardiac surgery.

Use of Phenylephrine in Sepsis-related Arterial Hypotension

Current guidelines on the management of septic shock recommend norepinephrine or dopamine as first-line agents to increase peripheral vascular resistance and preserve organ perfusion following adequate volume therapy [51]. Moreover, the Surviving Sepsis Campaign recommends that phenylephrine should not be used as the initial vasopressor in septic shock [51], since phenylephrine may reduce splanchnic blood flow and oxygen delivery in septic shock patients [52, 53]. Nevertheless, it is important to note that these recommendations are based on a limited number of studies that have evaluated the clinical use of phenylephrine in septic shock [52, 54, 55]. More importantly, a direct comparison between phenylephrine and norepinephrine or dopamine in human septic shock has not yet been performed.

Phenylephrine increases SVR by selectively stimulating α_1-adrenoceptors without a compensatory increase in myocardial contractility and thus in cardiac output [56]. This may be especially problematic in conditions of increased oxygen demand, such as early sepsis [57–59]. From a hemodynamic point of view, it could be argued that in volume-resuscitated patients, norepinephrine may potentially be advantageous over phenylephrine since it simultaneously stimulates α_1-, β_1- and β_2-receptors, thereby counteracting arterial hypotension by increasing SVR and myocardial inotropy [56]. On the other hand, phenylephrine could be preferable to norepinephrine, since β_1 stimulation may increase heart rate and myocardial oxygen demand. In this regard, Sander et al. [60] reported that prolonged tachycardia may increase the incidence of major cardiac events in critically ill patients.

Our research group reported that in a series of septic shock patients, systemic hemodynamics and global oxygen transport remained unchanged after replacing norepinephrine by phenylephrine except for a significant decrease in heart rate [61]. However, the different severities of cardiovascular dysfunction among the studied patients could have affected the results of this study [61]. In addition, the studied patients were already treated with high norepinephrine dosages (0.8 ± 0.7 μg/kg/min) at study entry. Finally, the protocol design (lack of a control group) did not allow a direct time-dependent effect unrelated to the specific agent to be identified [61]. In order to overcome these crucial weaknesses, we recently performed a direct comparison aimed at investigating the effects of first-line therapy with either phenylephrine or norepinephrine on systemic and regional hemodynamics in patients with early, volume-resuscitated septic shock. Interestingly, we did not find any differences between the groups treated with norepinephrine or phenylephrine in terms of systemic hemodynamics (unpublished data). It is, therefore, conceivable that compared to delayed treatment, early administration of phenylephrine in these hypotensive septic patients could have played a pivotal role in this regard [57–59]. Taken together, our observations suggest that there are no apparent advantages in terms of cardiopulmonary performance and global oxygen transport, when one catecholamine is administered instead of another in the initial hemodynamic support of septic shock.

Pulmonary hypertension occurs frequently in critically ill patients with acute respiratory distress syndrome (ARDS) or chronic obstructive pulmonary disease (COPD). In this context, it may be important to consider that phenylephrine increases mean pulmonary arterial pressure and pulmonary vascular resistance and may decrease cardiac output, thus worsening right ventricular pressure overload [12, 62]. Therefore, phenylephrine should not be used in septic patients with significant pulmonary hypertension [63].

Few clinical studies have been performed on phenylephrine in septic shock, but several experimental studies have evaluated the impact of phenylephrine on splanchnic perfusion. Breslow at al. reported no differences between phenylephrine (5.9 ± 2.7 μg/kg/min) and norepinephrine (3.0 ± 1.6 μg/kg/min) in terms of splanchnic oxygen supply [64]. These findings were confirmed by Schwarz et al. [65], who reported that progressively increasing doses of phenylephrine (from 0.1 to 10 μg/kg/min) did not decrease jejunal tissue oxygen supply as compared to norepinephrine (from 0.01 to 2 μg/kg/min). Nevertheless, in the study by Schwarz et al. [65] increasing doses of norepinephrine increased cardiac output and led to significant tachycardia as compared to phenylephrine. In endotoxemic dogs, Zhang et al. [66] demonstrated that 1 μg/kg/min of phenylephrine did not influence hepatosplanchnic blood flow or global and liver oxygen extraction capabilities. Most recently, Krejci et al. [67] reported that norepinephrine distributes blood flow away from the splanchnic circulation (e.g., small intestine) to other regions of the body by β-adrenergic stimulation. Notably, whereas norepinephrine reduced blood flow in both the jejunal mucosa and in the jejunal muscularis, phenylephrine at doses of 3.1 ± 1.0 μg/kg/min did not affect blood flow in the jejunal mucosa and even increased blood flow in the jejunal muscularis.

Compared to the experimental setting, the effects of phenylephrine on gastric-arterial PCO_2 gradients or jejunal mucosal perfusion in patients with septic shock are still not fully understood. We recently reported for the first time that phenylephrine did not impair gastrointestinal mucosal perfusion, as measured by gastric-arterial PCO_2 gap, in a series of 15 septic shock patients [61]. Nevertheless, in striking contrast to the finding of preserved gastrointestinal mucosal perfusion, we found that phenylephrine impaired hepatosplanchnic blood flow [61]. Notably, our findings were in harmony with the results from a study by Reinelt et al. [52], who showed that hepatosplanchnic oxygen delivery and blood flow in six patients suffering from septic shock decreased when norepinephrine was gradually replaced by phenylephrine at identical levels of MAP and cardiac index.

XI

In contrast, we observed that early administration of phenylephrine to counteract arterial hypotension did not impair hepatosplanchnic blood flow or increase arterial lactate concentrations (unpublished data). It appears, therefore, that a different hemodynamic condition at baseline (i.e., arterial hypotension) and, more importantly, administration of phenylephrine as a first-line agent could have played a pivotal role in this regard [59]. However, it should be stressed that previous studies [68] demonstrated that the β-adrenergic response may become predominant in endotoxic animals because of a progressive reduction in the number of α-adrenergic receptors and thus a relative increase in β-receptors. It is, therefore, plausible that early administration of phenylephrine may be more effective than delayed treatment.

The effects of phenylephrine on renal function have not yet been fully elucidated. In the current literature there are no direct comparative studies of phenylephrine and norepinephrine on renal function in septic shock. We recently reported that delayed administration of phenylephrine replacing norepinephrine (i.e., cross-over protocol design) in a series of septic shock patients negatively affected renal function, as indicated by a decrease in creatinine clearance, compared to norepinephrine [61]. Nevertheless, early administration of phenylephrine did not decrease creatinine clearance even though we observed a tendency towards an increase in the number of patients who required renal replacement therapy at the end of the observational period (unpublished data). Although speculative, this finding supports the notion that mixed α- and β-adrenergic agents may preserve renal function when given to increase or maintain MAP, even in critically ill patients with acute kidney injury [69].

The different impact on hepatosplanchnic perfusion and renal function of early compared to delayed administration of phenylephrine [61], strengthens the assumption that the efficacy of hemodynamic optimization by fluids and vasopressor agents critically depends on the urgency of the therapy and not only on the type of vasopressor used [59]. At present, in view of the available literature, adrenergic agents with both α- and β-adrenergic properties, such as norepinephrine, appear to be safer than phenylephrine in the hemodynamic support of septic patients.

Use of Phenylephrine in Cardiopulmonary Resuscitation

The rationale of therapy with vasoactive drugs in the setting of cardiopulmonary resuscitation (CPR) is to induce maximal vasoconstriction in non-vital organs to increase the proportion of blood delivered to vital organs, i.e., the heart and brain. Ideally, such drugs should not increase myocardial oxygen demand. Thus, from a theoretical point of view, selective α_1 agonists, such as phenylephrine, would represent suitable substances in this setting. In 1985, Silfvast and colleagues investigated the effects of 1 mg of phenylephrine compared to 0.5 mg of epinephrine in 65 patients with out-of-hospital cardiac arrest [70]. Interestingly, the authors noticed no significant differences in return of spontaneous circulation between the groups (31 vs. 28 % in patients treated with phenylephrine or epinephrine, respectively) [70]. However, given the marked changes in performance of CPR over the last few decades [71], the small sample size of the latter study and the relatively small phenylephrine dose (intrinsic sympathomimetic activity of phenylephrine vs. epinephrine ~1:5 to 1:10), it is unclear whether these results would hold true at present. Thus, future studies are warranted to compare phenylephrine with currently used vasopressors in the setting of CPR (i.e., epinephrine and/or vasopressin), before final conclusions can be drawn.

Summary and Conclusion

Phenylephrine represents an effective and safe vasopressor agent to treat arterial hypotension in the setting of general and regional anesthesia. The reflex reduction in heart rate may potentially be desirable in certain patients with tachycardia. In specific cardiac diseases associated with impaired myocardial oxygen delivery or obstruction of the left ventricular outflow tract (e.g., valvular aortic stenosis or HOCM), phenylephrine appears to be the ideal vasoactive agent, since it increases coronary perfusion pressure without exerting inotropic effects. In women undergoing Cesarean section under spinal anesthesia, phenylephrine is the vasopressor of choice, as it is at least as safe and effective as ephedrine and reduces the rate of nausea and vomiting. Despite its pure α-agonistic effect, uteroplacental hemodynamics and fetal oxygenation are well maintained when phenylephrine is used to maintain systolic arterial pressure at baseline. In patients with bradycardia or patients in whom a decrease in heart rate might be detrimental (e.g., mitral valve regurgitation), phenylephrine should be avoided. The available data on the role of phenylephrine in postoperative intensive care medicine do not support its use for hemodynamic support, since mixed α- and β-agonistic catecholamines, such as norepinephrine, appear to be safer and more effective.

References

1. Myers MG, Iazzetta JJ (1982) Intranasally administered phenylephrine and blood pressure. Can Med Assoc J 127: 365–368
2. Tanner V, Casswell AG (1996) A comparative study of the efficacy of 2.5 % phenylephrine and 10 % phenylephrine in pre-operative mydriasis for routine cataract surgery. Eye 10: 95–98
3. Department of Health, Education, and Welfare, Food and Drug Administration (1976) Establishment of a monograph for OTC cold, cough, allergy, bronchodilator, and antiasthmatic products. Fed Regist 41: 38399–38400
4. Azocar Hidalgo G, Van Cauwelaert R, Castillo Cadiz O, Aguirre Aguirre C, Wohler Campos C (1994) [Treatment of priapism with phenylephrine]. Arch Esp Urol 47: 785–787
5. Hengstmann JH, Goronzy J (1982) Pharmacokinetics of 3H-phenylephrine in man. Eur J Clin Pharmacol 21: 335–341
6. Plumb DC (2002) Veterinary Drug Handbook, 4th edn. PharmaVet Publishing, White Bear Lake
7. La Rovere MT, Pinna GD, Raczak G (2008) Baroreflex sensitivity: measurement and clinical implications. Ann Noninvasive Electrocardiol 13: 191–207
8. Hinder F, Stubbe HD, Van Aken H, et al (2003) Early multiple organ failure after recurrent endotoxemia in the presence of vasoconstrictor-masked hypovolemia. Crit Care Med 31: 903–909
9. Imran M, Khan FH, Khan MA (2007) Attenuation of hypotension using phenylephrine during induction of anaesthesia with propofol. J Pak Med Assoc 57: 543–547
10. Goertz AW, Schmidt M, Seefelder C, Lindner KH, Georgieff M (1993) The effect of phenylephrine bolus administration on left ventricular function during isoflurane-induced hypotension. Anesth Analg 77: 227–231
11. Ikeda T, Ozaki M, Sessler DI, Kazama T, Ikeda K, Sato S (1999) Intraoperative phenylephrine infusion decreases the magnitude of redistribution hypothermia. Anesth Analg 89: 462–465
12. Kwak YL, Lee CS, Park YH, Hong YW (2002) The effect of phenylephrine and norepinephrine in patients with chronic pulmonary hypertension. Anaesthesia 57: 9–14
13. Ishiyama T, Oguchi T, Iijima T, Matsukawa T, Kashimoto S, Kumazawa T (2003) Ephedrine, but not phenylephrine, increases bispectral index values during combined general and epidural anesthesia. Anesth Analg 97: 780–784
14. Takizawa D, Takizawa E, Miyoshi S, et al (2006) The effect of ephedrine and phenylephrine on BIS values during propofol anaesthesia. Eur J Anaesthesiol 23: 654–657
15. Sharrock NE, Go G, Mineo R (1991) Effect of i.v. low-dose adrenaline and phenylephrine infusions on plasma concentrations of bupivacaine after lumbar extradural anaesthesia in elderly patients. Br J Anaesth 67: 694–698
16. Sharrock NE, Go G, Mineo R, Harpel PC (1992) The hemodynamic and fibrinolytic response to low dose epinephrine and phenylephrine infusions during total hip replacement under epidural anesthesia. Thromb Haemost 68: 436–441
17. Sharrock NE, Mineo R, Go G (1993) The effect of cardiac output on intraoperative blood loss during total hip arthroplasty. Reg Anesth 18: 24–29
18. Brooker RF, Butterworth JF, Kitzman DW, Berman JM, Kashtan HI, McKinley AC (1997) Treatment of hypotension after hyperbaric tetracaine spinal anesthesia. A randomized, double-blind, cross-over comparison of phenylephrine and epinephrine. Anesthesiology 86: 797–805
19. Baraka A, Haroun S, Baroody MA, et al (1991) The hemodynamic effects of intravenous norepinephrine versus epinephrine and phenylephrine in patients with ischemic heart disease. Middle East J Anesthesiol 11: 53–62
20. Kugiyama K, Ohgushi M, Motoyama T, et al (1999) Enhancement of constrictor response of spastic coronary arteries to acetylcholine but not to phenylephrine in patients with coronary spastic angina. J Cardiovasc Pharmacol 33: 414–419
21. Skubas N, Barner HB, Apostolidou I, Lappas DG (2005) Phenylephrine to increase blood flow in the radial artery used as a coronary bypass conduit. J Thorac Cardiovasc Surg 130: 687–692
22. Goertz AW, Lindner KH, Seefelder C, Schirmer U, Beyer M, Georgieff M (1993) Effect of phenylephrine bolus administration on global left ventricular function in patients with coronary artery disease and patients with valvular aortic stenosis. Anesthesiology 78: 834–841

23. Goertz AW, Lindner KH, Schutz W, Schirmer U, Beyer M, Georgieff M (1994) Influence of phenylephrine bolus administration on left ventricular filling dynamics in patients with coronary artery disease and patients with valvular aortic stenosis. Anesthesiology 81: 49–58
24. Tanaka K, Kitahata H, Kawahito S, Nozaki J, Tomiyama Y, Oshita S (2003) Phenylephrine increases pulmonary blood flow in children with tetralogy of Fallot. Can J Anaesth 50: 926–929
25. Howell SJ (2007) Carotid endarterectomy. Br J Anaesth 99: 119–131
26. Ghogawala Z, Westerveld M, Amin-Hanjani S (2008) Cognitive outcomes after carotid revascularization: the role of cerebral emboli and hypoperfusion. Neurosurgery 62: 385–395
27. Mutch WA, White IW, Donen N, et al (1995) Haemodynamic instability and myocardial ischaemia during carotid endarterectomy: a comparison of propofol and isoflurane. Can J Anaesth 42: 577–587
28. Borum SE, Bittenbinder TM, Buckley CJ (2000) Transesophageal atrial pacing reduces phenylephrine needed for blood pressure support during carotid endarterectomy. J Cardiothorac Vasc Anesth 14: 277–280
29. Smith JS, Roizen MF, Cahalan MK, et al (1988) Does anesthetic technique make a difference? Augmentation of systolic blood pressure during carotid endarterectomy: effects of phenylephrine versus light anesthesia and of isoflurane versus halothane on the incidence of myocardial ischemia. Anesthesiology 69: 846–853
30. Turkoz A, Togal T, Gokdeniz R, Toprak HI, Ersoy O (2002) Effectiveness of intravenous ephedrine infusion during spinal anaesthesia for caesarean section based on maternal hypotension, neonatal acid-base status and lactate levels. Anaesth Intensive Care 30: 316–320
31. Aniset L, Konrad C, Schley M (2006) [Ephedrine as alternative to Akrinor in regional obstetric anesthesia]. Anaesthesist 55: 784–790
32. James FM 3rd, Greiss FC, Jr., Kemp RA (1970) An evaluation of vasopressor therapy for maternal hypotension during spinal anesthesia. Anesthesiology 33: 25–34
33. Deiml R, Hess W, Bahlmann E (2000) [Primary cesarean section. Use of phenylephrine during anesthesia in a patient with hypertrophic obstructive cardiomyopathy]. Anaesthesist 49: 527–531
34. Moran DH, Perillo M, LaPorta RF, Bader AM, Datta S (1991) Phenylephrine in the prevention of hypotension following spinal anesthesia for cesarean delivery. J Clin Anesth 3: 301–305
35. LaPorta RF, Arthur GR, Datta S (1995) Phenylephrine in treating maternal hypotension due to spinal anaesthesia for caesarean delivery: effects on neonatal catecholamine concentrations, acid base status and Apgar scores. Acta Anaesthesiol Scand 39: 901–905
36. Pierce ET, Carr DB, Datta S (1994) Effects of ephedrine and phenylephrine on maternal and fetal atrial natriuretic peptide levels during elective cesarean section. Acta Anaesthesiol Scand 38: 48–51
37. Hall PA, Bennett A, Wilkes MP, Lewis M (1994) Spinal anaesthesia for caesarean section: comparison of infusions of phenylephrine and ephedrine. Br J Anaesth 73: 471–474
38. Thomas DG, Robson SC, Redfern N, Hughes D, Boys RJ (1996) Randomized trial of bolus phenylephrine or ephedrine for maintenance of arterial pressure during spinal anaesthesia for Caesarean section. Br J Anaesth 76: 61–65
39. Cooper DW, Carpenter M, Mowbray P, Desira WR, Ryall DM, Kokri MS (2002) Fetal and maternal effects of phenylephrine and ephedrine during spinal anesthesia for cesarean delivery. Anesthesiology 97: 1582–1590
40. Ngan Kee WD, Lee A, Khaw KS, Ng FF, Karmakar MK, Gin T (2008) A randomized double-blinded comparison of phenylephrine and ephedrine infusion combinations to maintain blood pressure during spinal anesthesia for cesarean delivery: the effects on fetal acid-base status and hemodynamic control. Anesth Analg 107: 1295–1302
41. Loughrey JP, Yao N, Datta S, Segal S, Pian-Smith M, Tsen LC (2005) Hemodynamic effects of spinal anesthesia and simultaneous intravenous bolus of combined phenylephrine and ephedrine versus ephedrine for cesarean delivery. Int J Obstet Anesth 14: 43–47
42. Ayorinde BT, Buczkowski P, Brown J, Shah J, Buggy DJ (2001) Evaluation of pre-emptive intramuscular phenylephrine and ephedrine for reduction of spinal anaesthesia-induced hypotension during Caesarean section. Br J Anaesth 86: 372–376
43. Ngan Kee WD, Khaw KS, Ng FF (2004) Comparison of phenylephrine infusion regimens for maintaining maternal blood pressure during spinal anaesthesia for Caesarean section. Br J Anaesth 92: 469–474

44. Ngan Kee WD, Khaw KS, Ng FF, Lee BB (2004) Prophylactic phenylephrine infusion for preventing hypotension during spinal anesthesia for cesarean delivery. Anesth Analg 98: 815–821
45. Ngan Kee WD, Khaw KS, Ng FF (2005) Prevention of hypotension during spinal anesthesia for cesarean delivery: an effective technique using combination phenylephrine infusion and crystalloid cohydration. Anesthesiology 103: 744–750
46. Ngan Kee WD, Tam YH, Khaw KS, Ng FF, Critchley LA, Karmakar MK (2007) Closed-loop feedback computer-controlled infusion of phenylephrine for maintaining blood pressure during spinal anaesthesia for caesarean section: a preliminary descriptive study. Anaesthesia 62: 1251–1256
47. Erler I, Gogarten W (2007) [Prevention and treatment of hypotension during Caesarean delivery]. Anasthesiol Intensivmed Notfallmed Schmerzther 42: 208–213
48. Dunser MW, Mayr AJ, Ulmer H, et al (2001) The effects of vasopressin on systemic hemodynamics in catecholamine-resistant septic and postcardiotomy shock: a retrospective analysis. Anesth Analg 93: 7–13
49. Nygren A, Thoren A, Ricksten SE (2006) Vasopressors and intestinal mucosal perfusion after cardiac surgery: Norepinephrine vs. phenylephrine. Crit Care Med 34: 722–729
50. O'Dwyer C, Woodson LC, Conroy BP, et al (1997) Regional perfusion abnormalities with phenylephrine during normothermic bypass. Ann Thorac Surg 63: 728–735
51. Dellinger RP, Levy MM, Carlet JM, et al (2008) Surviving Sepsis Campaign: International guidelines for management of severe sepsis and septic shock: 2008. Intensive Care Med 34: 17–60
52. Reinelt H, Radermacher P, Kiefer P, et al (1999) Impact of exogenous beta-adrenergic receptor stimulation on hepatosplanchnic oxygen kinetics and metabolic activity in septic shock. Crit Care Med 27: 325–331
53. Beale RJ, Hollenberg SM, Vincent JL, Parrillo JE (2004) Vasopressor and inotropic support in septic shock: an evidence-based review. Crit Care Med 32 (Suppl 11):S455–465
54. Gregory JS, Bonfiglio MF, Dasta JF, Reilley TE, Townsend MC, Flancbaum L (1991) Experience with phenylephrine as a component of the pharmacologic support of septic shock. Crit Care Med 19: 1395–1400
55. Flancbaum L, Dick M, Dasta J, Sinha R, Choban P (1997) A dose-response study of phenylephrine in critically ill, septic surgical patients. Eur J Clin Pharmacol 51: 461–465
56. Hofmann BB, Lefkowitz RJ (1990) Catecholamines and sympathomimetic drugs. In: Gilman AG, Rail TW, Nies AS, Taylor P (eds) Goodman and Gilman's The Pharmacological Basis of Therapeutics. Pergamon, New York, pp 187–220

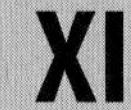

57. Rivers E, Nguyen B, Havstad S, et al (2001) Early goal-directed therapy in the treatment of severe sepsis and septic shock. N Engl J Med 345: 1368–1377
58. Rivers E, Coba V, Whitmill M (2008) Early goal directed therapy in severe sepsis and septic shock: A Contemporary review of the literature. Curr Opin Anesthesiol 21: 128–140
59. Parrillo JE (2008) Septic shock--vasopressin, norepinephrine, and urgency. N Engl J Med 358: 954–956
60. Sander O, Welters ID, Foex P, Sear JW (2005) Impact of prolonged elevated heart rate on incidence of major cardiac events in critically ill patients with a high risk of cardiac complications. Crit Care Med 33: 81–88
61. Morelli A, Lange M, Ertmer C, et al (2008) Short-term effects of phenylephrine on systemic and regional hemodynamics in patients with septic shock: A crossover pilot study. Shock 29: 446–451
62. Rich S, Gubin S, Hart K (1990) The effects of phenylephrine on right ventricular performance in patients with pulmonary hypertension. Chest 98: 1102–1106
63. Zamanian RT, Haddad F, Doyle RL, Weinacker AB (2007) Management strategies for patients with pulmonary hypertension in the intensive care unit. Crit Care Med 35: 2037–2050
64. Breslow MJ, Miller CF, Parker SD, Walman AT, Traystman RJ (1987) Effect of vasopressors on organ blood flow during endotoxin shock in pigs. Am J Physiol 252:H291–300
65. Schwarz B, Hofstotter H, Salak N, et al (2001) Effects of norepinephrine and phenylephrine on intestinal oxygen supply and mucosal tissue oxygen tension. Intensive Care Med 27: 593–601
66. Zhang H, De Jongh R, De Backer D, Cherkaoui S, Vray B, Vincent JL (2001) Effects of alpha

– and beta -adrenergic stimulation on hepatosplanchnic perfusion and oxygen extraction in endotoxic shock. Crit Care Med 29: 581 – 588
67. Krejci V, Hiltebrand LB, Sigurdsson GH (2006) Effects of epinephrine, norepinephrine, and phenylephrine on microcirculatory blood flow in the gastrointestinal tract in sepsis. Crit Care Med 34: 1456 – 1463
68. Pittner RA, Spitzer JA (1993) Shift from alpha- to beta-type adrenergic receptor-mediated responses in chronically endotoxemic rats. Am J Physiol 264:E650 – 654
69. Bellomo R, Wan L, May C (2008) Vasoactive drugs and acute kidney injury. Crit Care Med 36 (Suppl 4):S179 – 186
70. Silfvast T, Saarnivaara L, Kinnunen A, et al (1985) Comparison of adrenaline and phenylephrine in out-of-hospital cardiopulmonary resuscitation. A double-blind study. Acta Anaesthesiol Scand 29: 610 – 613
71. American Heart Association (2005) Guidelines for Cardiopulmonary Resuscitation and Emergency Cardiovascular Care. Circulation 112 (Suppl 24):IV1 – 203

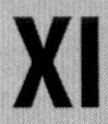

Role of the Calcium Sensitizer, Levosimendan, in Perioperative Intensive Care Medicine

S. Rehberg, P. Enkhbaatar, and D.L. Traber

Introduction

The calcium (Ca^{2+})-sensitizer, levosimendan, is recommended by the European Heart Association and the European Society of Intensive Care Medicine for the treatment of low output heart failure, when standard treatment is insufficient [1]. Despite encouraging results from experimental and randomized clinical studies, a recent large randomized, double-blind, multicenter trial in patients with acute decompensated heart failure (Survival Of Patients With Acute Heart Failure In Need Of Intravenous Inotropic Support, SURVIVE study), did not reveal any significant reduction in 31- or 180-day mortality with levosimendan compared to dobutamine [2]. The elementary question that needs to be addressed and was recently elegantly worded by Dr. Butler and colleagues, is whether "to abandon or not to abandon levosimendan?" [3].

The opposing party may indicate that classic inotropic agents, such as β_1-adrenoceptor agonists and phosphodiesterase-III (PDE-III) inhibitors, have a well established record of clinical efficiency and there is no need for a new compound that is 'only' as effective. In addition, the drug-related costs of dobutamine, for example, are less than half those of levosimendan [4]. However, supporters of levosimendan have strong arguments, too. First of all, there are some details about the SURVIVE study that need to be discussed. In this context, a subgroup analysis of patients receiving β_1-adrenergic antagonists showed reduced mortality in patients treated with levosimendan [5]. In addition, several aspects of the study design are controversial and may have influenced the results, such as the dosing of the two treatment drugs, the exclusion of patients in need of catecholamines, and the absence of continuous hemodynamic monitoring potentially resulting in undetected hypovolemic patients [6]. Last but not least, we have to ask ourselves, whether we can really expect a substantial effect on 6-month mortality of a drug that is administered for only 24 hours (even though the effects of levosimendan may last for a minimum of 2 days)? In this regard, a tendency towards a progressive amelioration of a potential mortality benefit with levosimendan over time was seen in the SURVIVE study [3].

Second, against the background of the current literature, the therapeutic potential of levosimendan does not seem to be limited to low output heart failure. The purpose of this chapter, therefore, is to review recent experimental and clinical trials to present new insights into the effects of and possible indications for levosimendan in perioperative intensive care medicine. For more extensive information about the current role of levosimendan in the treatment of heart failure, we recommend, among others, the recent meta-analysis by Dr. Delaney and colleagues [7], the review article by Dr. Lehtonen and Dr. Poder [8], and the study by Dr. Parissis and colleagues [9].

Mode of Action

The effects of levosimendan mainly depend on two predominant mechanisms: Ca^{2+} sensitization of contractile myofilaments and activation of adenosine triphosphate (ATP) dependent potassium (K^+) channels in vascular smooth muscle cells and the mitochondria. The inhibition of PDE-III is of minor importance, because it only occurs at doses higher than those clinically recommended. However, PDE-III inhibition may potentially contribute to the positive lusitropic effect of levosimendan [6, 10, 11].

The positive inotropic effect of levosimendan is linked to selective binding to the N-domain of Ca^{2+} binding cardiac troponin C (cTnC) and stabilizing of the interaction between cTnC and cTnI. Since levosimendan dissociates from cTnC when Ca^{2+} levels decrease, it only acts during systole and does not impair diastolic relaxation [12]. Another advantage over 'classic' inotropes, such as β_1-adrenoreceptor agonists or PDE-III inhibitors, is that levosimendan does not increase intracellular Ca^{2+} concentration or myocardial oxygen consumption [13].

Activation of K^+ channels in vascular smooth muscle cells is responsible for the vasodilation associated with levosimendan in the systemic and pulmonary vasculature. Although the channel distribution and physiologic regulation of vascular tone may differ between the individual vascular beds, it is currently accepted that levosimendan opens large conductance Ca^{2+} activated and voltage-gated K^+ channels in large conductance vessels and ATP dependent K^+ channels in small resistance vessels (**Fig. 1**) [14]. The vasodilation caused by levosimendan may potentially be a double-edged sword. On the one hand, the decrease in left and right ventricular afterload might be beneficial. On the other hand, a decrease in mean arterial pressure (MAP) in intensive care patients may be associated with detrimental consequences, if not treated properly.

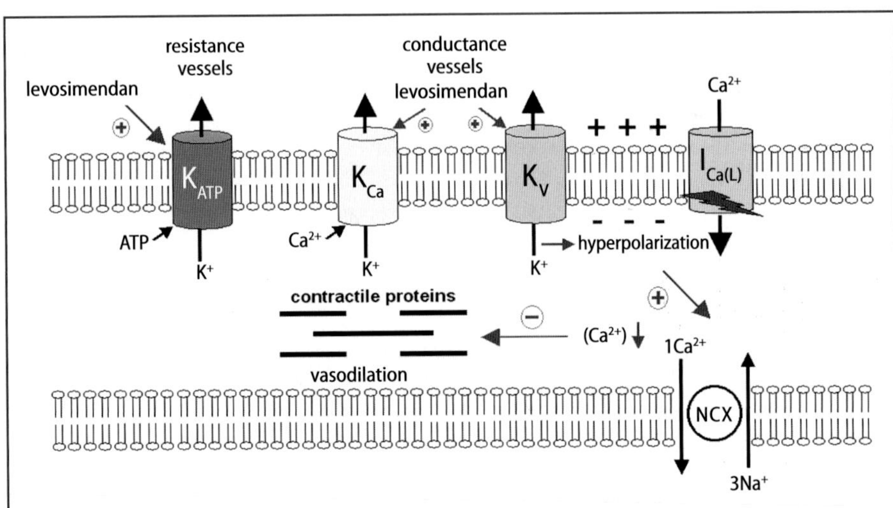

Fig. 1. Cellular mechanisms of vasodilation caused by levosimendan. ATP: adenosine triphosphate; Ca^{2+}: calcium ion; $I_{Ca(L)}$: calcium ion transporter; Na^+: sodium ion; NCX: sodium-calcium-exchanger; K_{xxx}: xxx-dependent potassium channel

XI

In addition, levosimendan activates ATP-sensitive K^+ channels in the mitochondria, thereby possibly maintaining mitochondrial volume, ameliorating Ca^{2+} overload, and preserving mitochondrial function during ischemia [15]. These mechanisms seem to be responsible for myocardial protection during ischemia-reperfusion injury [16] and improved myocardial function of stunned myocardium in response to levosimendan administration [17]. However, mitochondrial dysfunction is not limited to the myocardium. It also plays a pivotal role in multiple organ failure [18], possibly turning levosimendan into a therapeutic approach for a larger number of critically ill patients.

Over the last few years there is growing evidence for immunomodulatory and anti-apoptotic effects of levosimendan. These properties may represent an additional biologic mechanism that prevents further cytotoxic and hemodynamic consequences of abnormal immune and neurohormonal responses in critically ill patients, leading to organ protection, and beneficially intervening in the progression of the disease. Experimental results suggest that levosimendan exerts cardioprotective effects through its antioxidant properties and seems to be a potent inhibitor of hydrogen peroxide (H_2O_2)-induced cardiomyocyte apoptotic cell death [19]. Clinical data demonstrate that levosimendan prevents the increase in markers of oxidative and nitrosative stress seen in advanced chronic heart failure patients [20]. In addition, the reduction of pro-inflammatory markers, like interleukin (IL)-6, tumor necrosis factor (TNF)-α, intercellular and vascular adhesion molecules as well as endothelin-1, has been described in chronic heart failure patients [21–23]. **Figure 2** gives an overview of the main effects of levosimendan.

Recently, Kaptan and colleagues described a significant inhibitory effect of clinically relevant doses of levosimendan on platelet aggregation of healthy volunteers *in vitro* [24]. The clinical implications of this result remain to be clarified in future studies.

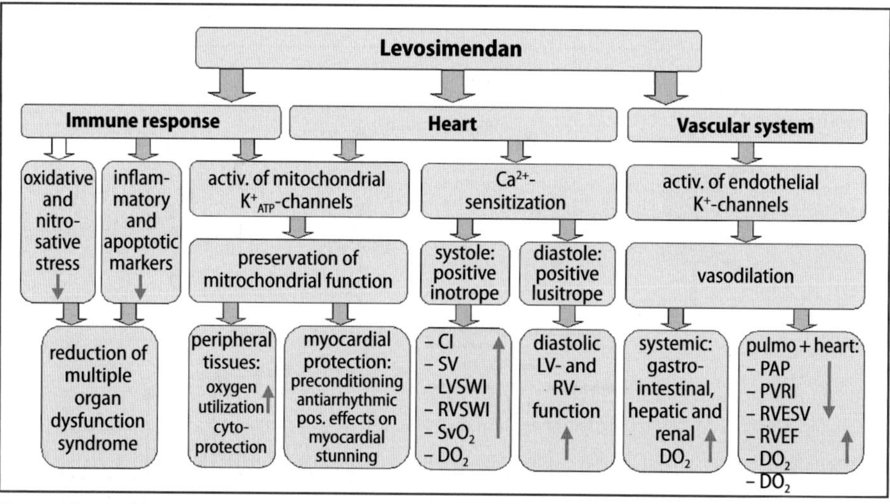

Fig. 2. Effects of levosimendan. activ.: activation; Ca^{2+}: calcium ion; CI, cardiac index; DO_2: oxygen delivery; K^+_{ATP}-channels: adenosine triphosphate sensitive potassium channels; LV: left ventricular; PAP: pulmonary artery pressure; PVRI: pulmonary vascular resistance index; RV, right ventricular; RVEF; right ventricular ejection fraction; RVESV: right ventricular endsystolic volume; SV: stroke volume; SvO_2: mixed venous oxygen saturation; ↑: increased values; ↓: decreased values

Dosage and Pharmacokinetics

Levosimendan (Simdax™, Abbott, Illonois, USA) is the (-) enantiomer of {[4-(1,4,5,6-tetrahydro-4-methyl-6-oxo-3-pyridazinyl)phenyl]hydrazono} propanedinitrile and is commercially available as a powder to be dissolved in a solution of glucose 5 % in water [11]. Recommendations for the treatment of low output heart failure suggest an initial bolus of 6–12 (-24) μg/kg followed by a continuous infusion of 0.05–0.2 μg/kg/min [25]. However, based on the results of recent clinical trials it may be advantageous to restrict the treatment to a continuous infusion in order to reduce potential side effects in hypovolemic patients, like a decrease in MAP and an increase in heart rate. This is even more important in situations when vasodilation is already present, like in septic shock [2, 26, 27]. Notably, levosimendan has also been shown to be effective when administered by nebulization [28]. In a rat model of ventilator-induced lung injury (VILI), administration of prophylactic nebulized levosimendan reduced the amount of inflammatory markers, like IL-1β, and prolonged survival as compared to placebo. However, the dose needed was more than ten times higher than for intravenous administration.

While no dose adaptation is necessary in patients with impaired hepatic function [29], the dose should be reduced in patients with severe renal insufficiency because of a 1.5-fold prolonged half-life of levosimendan metabolites [30]. Pharmacokinetic properties are not influenced by age, race, gender, or the different physiology in heart failure patients. In addition, levosimendan seems to be as effective in fast as in slow acetylators, despite the fact that the enzyme N-acetyltransferase-2, which is responsible for the metabolism of OR-1855 to OR-1896, is polymorphically distributed in the population [31].

Clinically Relevant Side Effects

Levosimendan is generally well tolerated in patients with severe heart failure. Common side effects, like arterial hypotension, headache, dizziness and nausea, seem to primarily relate to vasodilation. The incidence of cardiac arrhythmias is not increased as compared to placebo and is even lower than with dobutamine [32]. Bolus administration and high doses of levosimendan are especially associated with these unwanted effects. In addition, the majority of clinical trials report no serious interaction with routine drugs used in heart failure, such as β-adrenoceptor inhibitors, digoxin, or furosemide [2].

Metabolism

Levosimendan has a short half-life (approximately 1 h) and is characterized by a fast onset of drug action. Although levosimendan is administered intravenously, it is excreted into the small intestine and reduced by intestinal bacteria to an amino phenolpyridazinone metabolite (OR-1855). This metabolite is further metabolized by acetylation to an N-acetylated conjugate (OR-1896). OR-1896 has a similar pharmacological profile to levosimendan. Because of its half-life of 75–80 h, OR-1896 is responsible for the persistence of hemodynamic and neurohumeral effects after the termination of a 24 hour infusion of levosimendan for at least one week. In fact, peak concentrations of OR-1896 are reached after 2 days [13, 31].

Severe Sepsis and Septic Shock

Severe sepsis and septic shock are among the leading causes of death in non-coronary intensive care units (ICUs) [11]. Despite recent improvements in the treatment of these patients [33], in the presence of septic shock mortality increases up to 70 % and higher [34]. Because of its vasodilating properties, levosimendan should be used with adequate precautions in patients with septic shock, including continuous hemodynamic monitoring and ensuring sufficient volume status of the patient. An experimental study in endotoxemic pigs revealed an aggravation of tachycardia and arterial hypotension under levosimendan treatment associated with decreased coronary perfusion pressures and a mortality rate of 5 out of 6 animals versus 2 out of 6 in the placebo group [35]. A closer look at the study design teaches us three important pitfalls regarding the use of levosimendan in septic shock: First, the dosage of levosimendan was more than 4 times higher than clinically recommended; second, no additional vasopressor was administered; and last, but not least, volume resuscitation was probably insufficient.

Comparing the different pathomechanisms in sepsis with recent insights into the effects of levosimendan (as described above), levosimendan provides a huge potential in septic shock and might not even be restricted to patients with left ventricular failure [36]. Myocardial dysfunction in sepsis, also called septic cardiomyopathy, is characterized by desensitization of myocardial myofilaments to Ca^{2+}, impaired β-adrenergic signaling and the combination of systolic and diastolic dysfunction of both ventricles [37]. Levosimendan increases the sensitivity of contractile myofilaments to Ca^{2+} in both ventricles without impairment of diastolic function and independent of β-adrenergic signaling [10]. Several experimental studies reported an increased biventricular contractility and improvements in ventriculo-vascular coupling and systolic as well as diastolic function [38–40]. The decrease in MAP was small and seemed to be beneficial, due to the decrease in left ventricular afterload, rather than harmful. In an ovine model of fecal peritonitis-induced septic shock, the combination therapy of levosimendan and arginine-vasopressin improved not only myocardial but also pulmonary function as reflected in lower pulmonary vascular resistance indices (PVRI) and improved PaO_2/FiO_2 ratio as compared to single arginine-vasopressin or placebo treatment [38].

XI

Splanchnic vasoconstriction and impaired microcirculation in the gut play a pivotal role in the pathophysiology of sepsis-associated organ failure [41]. In experimental ovine endotoxemic shock, levosimendan (in contrast to dobutamine) increased superior mesenteric arterial blood flow, splanchnic oxygen delivery (DO_2) and mucosal oxygen saturation [42]. Accordingly, the beneficial effects of levosimendan on renal function in endotoxemic rats may be related to the increased renal blood flow due to K^+ channel activation [43]. Recently, Dr. Fries and colleagues made a very interesting finding. In a rat model of endotoxemic shock, the administration of 0.3 μg/kg/min levosimendan improved microvascular oxygenation but not perfusion [44]. The authors concluded that a mechanism relatively independent of macrocirculatory hemodynamics and overall microvascular perfusion (protection of mitochondrial function?) may account for these observations. The improved oxygenation of the gastrointestinal mucosa combined with the reduced endothelial dysfunction resulting from the inhibition of intercellular adhesion molecule (ICAM)-1 and vascular cell adhesion molecule (VCAM)-1 [21] may be very useful to preserve splanchnic barrier function with a subsequent attenuation of sepsis-related organ failure.

Mitochondrial dysfunction and over-activation of inflammatory cascades are critically involved in the pathogenesis of sepsis [18]. Given its anti-inflammatory properties and the beneficial effects on mitochondrial function (as described above), levosimendan represents a more than interesting therapeutic approach in septic shock. In fact, but this is only speculative at this point in time, these effects could be an explanation for the increased tissue oxygenation without improved microvascular perfusion reported by Fries et al. [44].

Morelli and colleagues published the first randomized, controlled clinical trial evaluating the effects of levosimendan in patients suffering from septic shock with persistent left ventricular ejection fraction (LVEF) below 45 % after 2 days of standard treatment (volume substitution, norepinephrine and dobutamine) [27]. The continuous infusion of 0.2 μg/kg/min levosimendan over 24 hours improved left ventricular stroke work index (LVSWI), end-systolic and end-diastolic volume index, increased oxygen consumption and delivery index and urinary output, and reduced arterial lactate levels and gastric mucosal hypoxia compared to dobutamine. No increase in norepinephrine requirements to keep MAP between 70 and 80 mmHg was seen in these patients, suggesting compensation of levosimendan-related vasodilation.

A subsequent randomized controlled study by the same group investigated the effects of levosimendan in septic shock patients with acute respiratory distress syndrome (ARDS) and right ventricular failure [26]. A 24 hour infusion of 0.2 μg/kg/min levosimendan reduced PVRI and increased right ventricular function as reflected by increases in right ventricular ejection fraction (RVEF) and decreases in right ventricular end-systolic volume index (RVESVI). As in the previous study, levosimendan led to improved mixed venous oxygen saturation (SvO_2) and DO_2.

Summarizing the current literature, levosimendan may be a promising therapeutic approach in the treatment of severe sepsis and septic shock not only restricted to patients with impaired myocardial function. However, sufficient fluid resuscitation, combination with a vasopressor agent, and continuous hemodynamic monitoring must be ensured to prevent side effects. Especially if a bolus administration is necessary, the dose chosen should be as low as possible and precautions should be taken to avoid a sudden decrease in MAP. The first results of an ongoing prospective, randomized, placebo-controlled trial investigating the use of levosimendan as a rescue therapy in refractory septic shock are impatiently awaited [36].

Perioperative Administration

Clinical experience with perioperative use of levosimendan almost exclusively comes from cardiac surgery. Tritapepe et al. reported an increased cardiac index and lower troponin I concentrations 48 hours after coronary artery bypass grafting (CABG) compared to placebo in patients who received a levosimendan bolus (24 μg/kg) just before placement on cardiopulmonary bypass (CPB) [45]. In patients with a preoperative ejection fraction ≤ 30 % scheduled for CABG, the intraoperative combination of dobutamine and levosimendan was associated with lower norepinephrine doses and a shorter duration of inotropic drug administration and tracheal intubation compared to combined milrinone and dobutamine. In addition, the stroke volume was better maintained in patients treated with levosimendan [46]. In a very interesting study, Dr. Tasouli and colleagues investigated the influence of different time points for the infusion start on intra- and postoperative outcome parameters in patients undergoing open-heart surgery. Patients were randomized to receive a continuous infusion of levosimendan (0.1 μg/kg/min) either started intra- or postoperatively on the ICU. Both treatment strategies were safe and efficacious in increasing cardiac index, SvO_2 and LVEF. Notably, the earlier (intraoperative) start of levosimendan infusion was associated with a shorter length of ICU and hospital stay [47].

Given that levosimendan is mostly used as a last resort therapy, the prophylactic administration of levosimendan in patients with preoperative low output syndrome appears to be almost revolutionary. However, first results from small clinical trials seem promising. Bolus administration of 12–24 μg/kg levosimendan combined with 500 ml hydroxyethyl starch (HES) 6 % 20 min before coronary surgery improved left ventricular function without any decrease in MAP or tachycardia compared to placebo [48]. Even more interesting, because not limited to cardiac surgery, two studies recently reported the use of preoperative levosimendan infusion in heart failure patients undergoing non-cardiac surgery [49, 50]. Twelve patients with preoperative LVEF < 30 % received a loading dose (24 μg/kg) followed by a 24 hour continuous infusion (0.1 μg/kg/min) levosimendan one day before the surgery under continuous hemodynamic monitoring on the ICU. While no adverse reactions, complications, or mortality occurred during the 30-day follow-up, treated patients had a significantly increased LVEF and a reduced ejection time 7 days after levosimendan infusion than before [49]. Ponschab et al. administered a total dose of 12.5 mg levosimendan with an infusion rate of 0.1 μg/kg/min started at least 2 hours before urgent hip fracture surgery in 10 patients with symptomatic heart failure and a LVEF of less than 35 %. Levosimendan increased intra- and postoperative cardiac and stroke volume indices and decreased SVRI and plasma levels of B-type natriuretic peptide up to 48 hours [50]. In their review article, Drs Archan and Toller state that in their department high-risk patients for cardiac surgery are routinely transferred to the ICU to receive a continuous infusion of levosimendan (0.1 μg/kg/min) 4–12 hours before surgery under continuous hemodynamic monitoring [6]. According to the authors, so far no serious adverse events have occurred.

If the positive results for the early or prophylactic use of levosimendan are verified in larger, randomized trials, the discussion about initially increased costs compared to standard treatment would certainly change significantly.

Right Ventricular Dysfunction

Because of its thinner wall in comparison to the left ventricle and the usually low pulmonary resistance, the right ventricle is very sensitive to any increases in afterload. In this case, the right ventricle generates pressure at the expense of volume and a mismatch between pulmonary vascular load and right ventricular contractile reserve occurs resulting in ventriculo-vascular uncoupling and finally dilatation of the ventricle.

While this pathomechanism of right ventricular failure may be adaptive in case of pulmonary fibrosis, for example, it develops very fast when acute increases in pulmonary resistance occur. Therefore, there is an urgent need for drugs that support the failing right ventricle for the time necessary to treat the causative pulmonary obstruction.

Since levosimendan increases myocardial contractility and in parallel reduces right ventricular afterload by pulmonary vasodilation, its use in patients with right ventricular dysfunction seems to be more than reasonable. In two porcine models of right ventricular dysfunction, the administration of levosimendan (single 20 μg/kg bolus or 20 μg/kg bolus followed by a continuous infusion of 1 μg/kg/min for 45 min) increased right ventricular contractility, improved right ventriculo-vascular coupling and reduced right ventricular afterload compared to placebo [51, 52]. Kerbaul and colleagues showed that levosimendan was superior to dobutamine in pressure load-induced right ventricular failure in dogs because of its additional pulmonary vasodilatory effects [53]. These positive effects of levosimendan on right ventricular function have also been verified in small clinical trials. In patients with sepsis and ARDS, levosimendan (continuous infusion of 0.2 μg/kg/min) decreased mean pulmonary artery pressures and improved right ventricular performance [26]. Poelzl et al. recently reported that levosimendan therapy was feasible and improved hemodynamics in patients with acute predominantly right heart failure. The authors further proposed the increase in right ventricular contractility, rather than a reduction in afterload, as the possible pathophysiological mechanism [54]. In agreement with effects on the left ventricle, levosimendan seems to improve systolic as well as diastolic right ventricular function in patients with advanced heart failure [55] and acute decompensated heart failure with ischemic cardiomyopathy [56].

Cardiogenic Shock

There are two main theories that justify the use of levosimendan in cardiogenic shock. First, alternatives to the standard inotropic drug, dobutamine, are warranted since its use may be associated with an increased myocardial infarction size, an increased risk of arrhythmias, and a loss of hemodynamic effects with prolonged infusion [57]. Second, systemic inflammation and secondary multiple organ dysfunction are the leading causes of death in patients with cardiogenic shock [58]. Levosimendan seems to provide an answer to these problems, because it is known to increase myocardial contractility independent of the β-adrenergic system at low energy costs [10, 13] and provides anti-inflammatory and cyto-protective effects [19–23, 28].

The administration of levosimendan (0.1 μg/kg/min for 24 hours) combined with norepinephrine and sufficient volume therapy in ten patients with cardiogenic shock refractory to standard treatment increased cardiac index and decreased SVRI, without lowering MAP. Four of these patients were still alive after 6 months [59]. In patients with persisting cardiogenic shock 24 hours after revascularization, the addition of levosimendan (bolus of 12 μg/kg followed by a 24 hour infusion of 0.05–0.2 μg/kg/min) to conventional therapy (norepinephrine and dobutamine) led to sustained improvements in cardiovascular hemodynamics (increased cardiac and cardiac power index, decreased SVRI) as compared to continued standard treatment without significant changes in MAP [60]. A recently published prospective, randomized, controlled single-center trial investigated the effects of levosimendan (12 μg/kg bolus over 10 min followed by a 50 min infusion of 0.1 μg/kg/min and a 23 hour infusion of 0.2 μg/kg/min) compared with the PDE-III inhibitor, enoximone (fractional loading dose of 0.5 mg/kg followed by 2–10 μg/kg/min continuously), in refractory cardiogenic shock complicating acute myocardial infarction, on top of current therapy [61]. Levosimendan significantly increased 30-day survival compared to enoximone and was associated with lower cumulative doses of catecholamines after 72 hours. In addition, multiple organ failure leading to death occurred exclusively in the enoximone group.

Although these results are encouraging, and the disappointing results of the SURVIVE-trial [2] do not apply to patients suffering from cardiogenic shock (these patients were excluded from the study), so far there is no large randomized study proving the benefit of levosimendan treatment in cardiogenic shock. Therefore, levosimendan should be used with care and cannot be recommended as therapy of choice yet.

Cardiopulmonary Resuscitation

Data regarding the use of levosimendan during cardiopulmonary resuscitation (CPR) are scarce and restricted to experimental studies and single case reports. Dr. Koudouna and colleagues reported increased coronary perfusion pressures and an improved initial resuscitation success rate when epinephrine was combined with a bolus of 12 μg/kg levosimendan instead of placebo in pigs after 8 min of untreated ventricular fibrillation [62]. Levosimendan treatment after successful resuscitation led to greater LVEF and fractional area changes as compared to dobutamine in pigs [63]. However, the dose of levosimendan in this study was twice as high as recommended. In addition to its positive inotropic effects during CPR and related ischemia-reperfusion injury, the myocardial protection of levosimendan due to ATP dependent K^+ channel activation may be the cause of its beneficial effects. In a rat model of ventricular fibrillation, the positive results after levosimendan treatment (fewer electrical shocks, lower ST-elevations, and prolonged survival) were abolished by prophylactic administration of the non-selective K^+ channel inhibitor, glibenclamide [64].

Two recently published case reports suggest beneficial effects of levosimendan during CPR. In a woman suffering from prostaglandin-induced cardiac arrest and fulminant pulmonary failure after postpartum atonic uterine bleeding, the addition of levosimendan (bolus of 12 μg/kg and subsequent continuous infusion of 0.2 μg/kg/min) to standard medication following recovery of spontaneous circulation after 90 min resulted in hemodynamic stabilization within 30 min [65]. A 32-year old man with idiopathic cardiomyopathy and electromechanical dissociation completely recovered from 2.5 hours of CPR using an additional infusion of 0.3 μg/kg/min levosimendan [66].

Although it is too soon to draw any conclusions based on these references, the results encourage further investigation. So far, levosimendan represents at least a final option for CPR after failure of standard treatment.

Conclusion

The Ca^{2+}-sensitizer, levosimendan, is the best investigated inotropic drug with more controlled clinical data than any other. In view of the current literature, levosimendan seems to be more than just a drug with positive inotropic effects. Due to its vasodilatory, but even more important anti-inflammatory and cyto-protective properties, the number of indications in perioperative intensive care may soon be larger than just the treatment of low output heart failure. However, sufficient volume status, combination with a vasopressor agent, and continuous hemodynamic monitoring must be guaranteed. Bolus administration of levosimendan should be restricted to emergency situations and precautions should be taken to avoid a sudden decrease in MAP. Importantly, early administration seems to be more efficient than the often applied 'last resort' therapy. If verified in large randomized trials, the reduced ICU and hospital stays after prophylactic preoperative treatment of high risk patients for cardiac as well as non-cardiac surgery may influence considerably the discussion about the high therapy costs associated with levosimendan. In summary, the current indication of levosimendan for the treatment of low-output heart failure may only represent the famous 'tip of the iceberg'. Future studies are warranted regarding patient selection and the optimum regimen and dosing of levosimendan for each of the potential indications to support and complete these initial results.

References

1. Nieminen MS, Böhm M, Cowie MR, et al (2005) Executive summary of the guidelines on the diagnosis and treatment of acute heart failure: the Task Force on Acute Herat Failure of the European Society of Cardiology. Eur Heart J 26: 384–416
2. Mebazaa A, Nieminen MS, Packer M, et al (2007) Levosimendan vs dobutamine for patients with acute decompensated heart failure: the SURVIVE Randomized Trial. JAMA 297: 1883–1891
3. Butler J, Giamouzis G, Giannakoulas G (2007) A struggle to SURVIVE: to abandon or not to abandon levosimendan? Cardiovasc Drugs Ther 21: 401–402
4. Oliveira MTJ, Follador W, Martins ML, et al (2005) Cost analysis of the treatment of acute decompensated heart failure. Levosimendan versus dobutamine. Arq Bras Cardiol 85: 9–14
5. Mebazaa A, Cohan-Solal A, Kleber FX, et al (2007) Levosimendan reduces mortality, when compared with dobutamine in patients receiving beta blockers. Eur J Heart Fail 6:109 (abst)
6. Archan S, Toller W (2008) Levosimendan: current status and future prospects. Curr Opin Anaesthesiol 21: 78–84
7. Delaney A, Bradford C, McCaffrey J, Bagshaw SM, Lee R (2009) Levosimendan for the treatment of acute severe heart failure: A meta-analysis of randomised controlled trials. Int J Cardiol (in press)
8. Lehtonen L, Poder P (2007) The utility of levosimendan in the treatment of heart failure. Ann Med 39: 2–17
9. Parissis JT, Papadopoulos C, Nikolaou M, et al (2007) Effects of levosimendan on quality of life and emotional stress in advanced heart failure patients. Cardiovasc Drugs Ther 21: 263–268
10. Rehberg S, Ertmer C, Van Aken H, et al (2007) Role of Levosimendan in intensive care treatment of myocardial insufficiency. Anaesthesist 56: 30–43
11. Pinto BB, Rehberg S, Ertmer C, Westphal M (2008) Role of levosimendan in sepsis and septic shock. Curr Opin Anaesthesiol 21: 168–177
12. Sorsa T, Pollesello P, Solaro RJ (2004) The contractile apparatus as a target for drugs against heart failure: interaction of levosimendan, a calcium sensitiser, with cardiac troponin c. Mol Cell Biochem 266: 87–107
13. Toller WG, Stranz C (2006) Levosimendan, a new inotropic and vasodilator agent. Anesthesiology 104: 556–569
14. Yildiz O (2007) Vasodilating mechanisms of levosimendan: involvement of K+ channels. J Pharmacol Sci 104: 1–5
15. Kopustinskiene DM, Pollesello P, Saris NE (2001) Levosimendan is a mitochondrial K(ATP) channel opener. Eur J Pharmacol 428: 311–314
16. Moiseyev VS, Poder P, Andrejevs N, et al (2002) Safety and efficacy of a novel calcium sensitizer, levosimendan, in patients with left ventricular failure due to an acute myocardial infarction. A randomized, placebo-controlled, double-blind study (RUSSLAN). Eur Heart J 23: 1422–1432
17. Sonntag S, Sundberg S, Lehtonen LA, Kleber FX (2004) The calcium sensitizer levosimendan improves the function of stunned myocardium after percutaneous transluminal coronary angioplasty in acute myocardial ischemia. J Am Coll Cardiol 43: 2177–2182
18. Singer M (2007) Mitochondrial function in sepsis: acute phase versus multiple organ failure. Crit Care Med 35:S441–448

19. Sahin AS, Gormus N, Duman A (2007) Preconditioning with levosimendan prevents contractile dysfunction due to H2O2-induced oxidative stress in human myocardium. J Cardiovasc Pharmacol 50: 419–423
20. Parissis JT, Andreadou I, Markantonis SL, et al (2007) Effects of Levosimendan on circulating markers of oxidative and nitrosative stress in patients with advanced heart failure. Atherosclerosis 195:e210–215
21. Parissis JT, Karavidas A, Bistola V, et al (2008) Effects of levosimendan on flow-mediated vasodilation and soluble adhesion molecules in patients with advanced chronic heart failure. Atherosclerosis 197: 278–282
22. Adamopoulos S, Parissis JT, Iliodromitis EK, et al (2006) Effects of levosimendan versus dobutamine on inflammatory and apoptotic pathways in acutely decompensated chronic heart failure. Am J Cardiol 98: 102–106
23. Parissis JT, Adamopoulos S, Farmakis D, et al (2006) Effects of serial levosimendan infusions on left ventricular performance and plasma biomarkers of myocardial injury and neurohormonal and immune activation in patients with advanced heart failure. Heart 92: 1768–1772
24. Kaptan K, Erinc K, Ifran A, et al (2008) Levosimendan has an inhibitory effect on platelet function. Am J Hematol 83: 46–49
25. Nieminen MS, Akkila J, Hasenfuss G, et al (2000) Hemodynamic and neurohumeral effects of continuous infusion of levosimendan in patients with congestive heart failure. J Am Coll Cardiol 36: 1903–1912
26. Morelli A, Teboul JL, Maggiore SM, et al (2006) Effects of levosimendan on right ventricular afterload in patients with acute respiratory distress syndrome: a pilot study. Crit Care Med 34: 2287–2293
27. Morelli A, De Castro S, Teboul JL, et al (2005) Effects of levosimendan on systemic and regional hemodynamics in septic myocardial depression. Intensive Care Med 31: 638–644
28. Boost KA, Hoegl S, Dolfen A, et al (2008) Inhaled levosimendan reduces mortality and release of proinflammatory mediators in a rat model of experimental ventilator-induced lung injury. Crit Care Med 36: 1873–1879
29. Puttonen J, Kantele S, Ruck A, et al (2008) Pharmacokinetics of intravenous levosimendan and its metabolites in subjects with hepatic impairment. J Clin Pharmacol 48: 445–454
30. Puttonen J, Kantele S, Kivikko M, et al (2007) Effect of severe renal failure and haemodialysis on the pharmacokinetics of levosimendan and its metabolites. Clin Pharmacokinet 46: 235–246
31. Antila S, Sundberg S, Lehtonen LA (2007) Clinical pharmacology of levosimendan. Clin Pharmacokinet 46: 535–552
32. Follath F, Cleland JG, Just H, et al (2002) Efficacy and safety of intravenous levosimendan compared with dobutamine in severe low-output heart failure (the LIDO study): a randomised double-blind trial. Lancet 360: 196–202
33. Dellinger RP, Levy MM, Carlet JM, et al (2008) Surviving Sepsis Campaign: international guidelines for management of severe sepsis and septic shock: 2008. Crit Care Med 36: 296–327
34. Russell JA (2006) Management of sepsis. N Engl J Med 355: 1699–1713
35. Cunha-Goncalves D, Perez-de-Sa V, Dahm P, Grins E, Thorne J, Blomquist S (2007) Cardiovascular effects of levosimendan in the early stages of endotoxemia. Shock 28: 71–77
36. Powell BP, De Keulenaer BL (2007) Levosimendan in septic shock: a case series. Br J Anaesth 99: 447–448
37. Muller-Werdan U, Buerke M, Ebelt H, et al (2006) Septic cardiomyopathy – A not yet discovered cardiomyopathy? Exp Clin Cardiol 11: 226–236
38. Rehberg S, Ertmer C, Lange M, Morelli A, Van Aken H, Westphal M (2007) Combined levosimendan and vasopressin prolong survival in ovine septic shock. Crit Care Med 35 (Suppl 12): A61 (abst)
39. Oldner A, Konrad D, Weitzberg E, Rudehill A, Rossi P, Wanecek M (2001) Effects of levosimendan, a novel inotropic calcium-sensitizing drug, in experimental septic shock. Crit Care Med 29: 2185–2193
40. Barraud D, Faivre V, Damy T, et al (2007) Levosimendan restores both systolic and diastolic cardiac performance in lipopolysaccharide-treated rabbits: comparison with dobutamine and milrinone. Crit Care Med 35: 1376–1382

41. Hotchkiss RS, Karl IE (2003) The pathophysiology and treatment of sepsis. N Engl J Med 348: 138–150
42. Dubin A, Murias G, Sottile JP, et al (2007) Effects of levosimendan and dobutamine in experimental acute endotoxemia: a preliminary controlled study. Intensive Care Med 33: 485–494
43. Zager RA, Johnson AC, Lund S, Hanson SY, Abrass CK (2006) Levosimendan protects against experimental endotoxemic acute renal failure. Am J Physiol Renal Physiol 290:F1453–1462
44. Fries M, Ince C, Rossaint R, et al (2008) Levosimendan but not norepinephrine improves microvascular oxygenation during experimental septic shock. Crit Care Med 36: 1886–1891
45. Tritapepe L, De Santis V, Vitale D, et al (2006) Preconditioning effects of levosimendan in coronary artery bypass grafting--a pilot study. Br J Anaesth 96: 694–700
46. De Hert SG, Lorsomradee S, Cromheecke S, Van der Linden PJ (2007) The effects of levosimendan in cardiac surgery patients with poor left ventricular function. Anesth Analg 104: 766–773
47. Tasouli A, Papadopoulos K, Antoniou T, et al (2007) Efficacy and safety of perioperative infusion of levosimendan in patients with compromised cardiac function undergoing open-heart surgery: importance of early use. Eur J Cardiothorac Surg 32: 629–633
48. Barisin S, Husedzinovic I, Sonicki Z, Bradic N, Barisin A, Tonkovic D (2004) Levosimendan in off-pump coronary artery bypass: a four-times masked controlled study. J Cardiovasc Pharmacol 44: 703–708
49. Katsaragakis S, Kapralou A, Markogiannakis H, et al (2008) Preoperative levosimendan in heart failure patients undergoing noncardiac surgery. Neth J Med 66: 154–159
50. Ponschab M, Hochmair N, Ghazwinian N, Mueller T, Plochl W (2008) Levosimendan infusion improves haemodynamics in elderly heart failure patients undergoing urgent hip fracture repair. Eur J Anaesthesiol 25: 627–633
51. Missant C, Rex S, Segers P, Wouters PF (2007) Levosimendan improves right ventriculovascular coupling in a porcine model of right ventricular dysfunction. Crit Care Med 35: 707–715
52. Kerbaul F, Gariboldi V, Giorgi R, et al (2007) Effects of levosimendan on acute pulmonary embolism-induced right ventricular failure. Crit Care Med 35: 1948–1954
53. Kerbaul F, Rondelet B, Demester JP, et al (2006) Effects of levosimendan versus dobutamine on pressure load-induced right ventricular failure. Crit Care Med 34: 2814–2819
54. Poelzl G, Zwick RH, Grander W, et al (2008) Safety and Effectiveness of Levosimendan in Patients with Predominant Right Heart Failure. Herz 33: 368–373
55. Parissis JT, Paraskevaidis I, Bistola V, et al (2006) Effects of levosimendan on right ventricular function in patients with advanced heart failure. Am J Cardiol 98: 1489–1492
56. Duygu H, Ozerkan F, Zoghi M, et al (2008) Effect of levosimendan on right ventricular systolic and diastolic functions in patients with ischaemic heart failure. Int J Clin Pract 62: 228–233
57. Schulz R, Rose J, Martin C, Brodde OE, Heusch G (1993) Development of short-term myocardial hibernation. Its limitation by the severity of ischemia and inotropic stimulation. Circulation 88: 684–695
58. Buerke M, Prondzinsky R (2008) Levosimendan in cardiogenic shock: better than enoximone! Crit Care Med 36: 2450–2451
59. Delle Karth G, Buberl A, Geppert A, et al (2003) Hemodynamic effects of a continuous infusion of levosimendan in critically ill patients with cardiogenic shock requiring catecholamines. Acta Anaesthesiol Scand 47: 1251–1256
60. Russ MA, Prondzinsky R, Christoph A, et al (2007) Hemodynamic improvement following levosimendan treatment in patients with acute myocardial infarction and cardiogenic shock. Crit Care Med 35: 2732–2739
61. Fuhrmann JT, Schmeisser A, Schulze MR, et al (2008) Levosimendan is superior to enoximone in refractory cardiogenic shock complicating acute myocardial infarction. Crit Care Med 36: 2257–2266
62. Koudouna E, Xanthos T, Bassiakou E, et al (2007) Levosimendan improves the initial outcome of cardiopulmonary resuscitation in a swine model of cardiac arrest. Acta Anaesthesiol Scand 51: 1123–1129
63. Huang L, Weil MH, Tang W, Sun S, Wang J (2005) Comparison between dobutamine and levosimendan for management of postresuscitation myocardial dysfunction. Crit Care Med 33: 487–491

64. Cammarata GA, Weil MH, Sun S, Huang L, Fang X, Tang W (2006) Levosimendan improves cardiopulmonary resuscitation and survival by K(ATP) channel activation. J Am Coll Cardiol 47: 1083–1085
65. Krumnikl JJ, Toller WG, Prenner G, Metzler H (2006) Beneficial outcome after prostaglandin-induced post-partum cardiac arrest using levosimendan and extracorporeal membrane oxygenation. Acta Anaesthesiol Scand 50: 768–770
66. Tsagalou EP, Nanas JN (2006) Resuscitation from adrenaline resistant electro-mechanical dissociation facilitated by levosimendan in a young man with idiopathic dilated cardiomyopathy. Resuscitation 68: 147–149

Inhaled Nitric Oxide Therapy in Adult Cardiac Surgery

B.C. Creagh-Brown and T.W. Evans

Introduction

Nitric oxide (NO) is a naturally-occurring free radical that exists as a colorless and odorless gas. In biological solutions, NO is highly diffusible both in water and through biological membranes, with a half-life measured in seconds. Prior to the recognition that NO was the same molecule as an endothelium-derived relaxing factor some 20 years ago [1] it was considered to be mainly an environmental pollutant. However, NO is now recognized as an endogenously produced vasodilator that modulates vascular tone and, thereby, regulates systemic and pulmonary blood flow. It has also been found to have diverse roles throughout mammalian physiology, including neurotransmission and host defense.

Generation and Metabolism

NO is formed via the action of nitric oxide synthase (NOS) on the semi-essential amino acid, L-arginine, in the presence of molecular oxygen. The neuronal isoform (nNOS) was the first to be identified, followed by inducible (iNOS or NOS2), and endothelial (eNOS or NOS3) isoforms. iNOS is calcium-independent and generates higher concentrations of NO [2] than the calcium-dependent nNOS and eNOS; excessive iNOS activity is implicated in the pathogenesis of septic shock. There is controversy over the nature of a mitochondrial NOS and whether it represents a specific isotype [3]. In addition to *de novo* synthesis, the supposedly inert anions nitrate (NO_3^-) and nitrite (NO_2^-) can be recycled to form NO, particularly in hypoxic states [4]. Exogenous NO may be administered via controlled inhalation of the gas or through administration of pharmacological donors such as sodium nitroprusside or nitroglycerine (glyceryl trinitrate, GTN).

Traditionally, NO was thought to be rapidly inactivated by hemoglobin, such that when inhaled its actions would be confined to ventilated alveolar units without remote effects. However, it is now postulated that remote signaling can be achieved through redox-related NO adducts. These include the S-nitrosothiols (SNOs) which are formed through NO binding to cysteine residues in proteins or peptides, albumin (to form S-nitrosoalbumin) and hemoglobin. Interactions between NO and hemoglobin are highly complex, and are governed not only by hemoglobin oxygen saturation but also by local redox conditions. Classically, NO reacts with oxyhemoglobin to form methemoglobin and nitrate or heme-iron nitrosyl hemoglobin; however SNO-Hb is also formed. As such, circulating erythrocytes may effectively store and release NO peripherally in areas of low oxygen tension [5]. Thus, in isolation

NO can act as an autocrine or paracrine mediator, but when stabilized may exert endocrine influences [6].

When inhaled with high concentrations of oxygen, gaseous NO slowly forms the toxic product nitrogen dioxide (NO_2). Other potential reactions include nitration (addition of NO^{2+}), nitrosation (addition of NO^+) or nitrosylation (addition of NO). Furthermore, NO may react with reactive oxygen species (ROS), such as superoxide, to form reactive nitrogen species (RNS) such as peroxynitrite ($ONOO^-$), a powerful oxidant that can decompose further to yield NO_2 and hydroxyl radicals. Therefore, NO is potentially cytotoxic, and covalent nitration of tyrosine in proteins by reactive nitrogen species has been used as a marker of oxidative stress. Almost 70 % of inhaled NO is excreted within 48 hours as nitrate in the urine [7].

Local Cardiopulmonary Effects

NO-mediated activation of soluble guanylyl cyclase leads to cyclic guanosine 3' 5'-monophosphate (cGMP) formation which activates its associated protein kinase. This decreases the sensitivity of myosin to calcium-induced contraction and lowers the intracellular calcium concentration by activating calcium-sensitive potassium channels and inhibiting the release of calcium from the sarcoplasmic reticulum. When administered by inhalation, pulmonary vascular resistance (PVR) decreases. Consequently, pulmonary arterial pressure and right ventricular afterload fall. Where right ventricular function is impaired, the decrease in afterload can improve cardiac output. By contrast, in patients with left ventricular impairment, increased right ventricular output can cause left atrial pressure to increase excessively leading to, or exacerbating, pulmonary edema. Similarly, pulmonary hydrostatic pressure may be adversely affected by a greater degree of dilatation of the pre-capillary than post-capillary vasculature. NO may also influence the development or resolution of pulmonary edema through non-hydrostatic mechanisms. These include alterations in pulmonary vascular permeability through limiting inflammation, or improving the integrity of the alveolar-capillary membrane [8].

Inhaled NO improves ventilation-perfusion matching and systemic oxygenation. However, the beneficial effects of inhaled NO on oxygenation are limited if hypoxemia is not consequent upon ventilation-perfusion mismatch and hypoxic pulmonary vasoconstriction (HPV). Thus, experimental data confirm that intravenously administered vasodilators may worsen oxygenation, presumably by counteracting HPV [9].

Non-cardiovascular Effects

The increasingly recognized peripheral effects of inhaled NO are dose-dependent and can take place in the absence of any change in systemic hemodynamics. Cell-specific effects go beyond relaxation of vascular smooth muscle, and include inhibition of platelet aggregation and leukocyte adhesion and migration [5]. In the peripheral vasculature there is altered regional blood flow. In the kidneys there is increased renal blood flow, glomerular filtration rate, and urine output. Improved tissue oxygenation can be detected in the liver. NO has multiple immunoregulatory and antimicrobial functions. Its precise effects on host defense are likely to be concentration-, redox environment-, and pathogen-dependent [10].

Pulmonary Hypertension and Right Ventricular Failure after Cardiac Surgery

Pulmonary Hypertension

The pathogenesis of pulmonary hypertension after surgery necessitating cardiopulmonary bypass (CPB) is multi-factorial. Importantly, CPB *per se* causes diminished endogenous NO production [11] which may be alleviated by inhaled NO [12]. Inhaled NO has also been proposed to lessen the systemic inflammatory response syndrome (SIRS) associated with CPB [13]. Post-CPB, pulmonary hypertension has more severe consequences in the presence of cardiopulmonary pathology such as pre-existing right ventricular impairment. Indeed, in patients with impaired left ventricular function undergoing elective coronary artery bypass grafting (CABG), those with concomitant right ventricular impairment had significantly worse outcomes [14]. Despite surgical correction of valvular defects and/or reduced left atrial pressure there may be residual pulmonary hypertension due to remodeling of the pulmonary vasculature resultant upon chronic left atrial hypertension.

Right Ventricular Failure

Right ventricular performance depends upon right coronary artery perfusion or blood flow, which is determined by the difference between aortic and right ventricular pressures. In contrast to the left ventricle, right coronary arterial blood flow can occur during both systole and diastole as the tissue pressure in the right ventricle does not usually exceed aortic pressure. However, as right ventricular systolic pressure increases, the dynamics change with a decline in coronary perfusion during systole. Impaired perfusion causes impaired contractility. Right ventricular dysfunction may therefore result from ischemia when right ventricular pressures are high and/or systemic pressures are low, or when there is any limitation of flow within the right coronary artery or its grafts [15] (**Fig. 1**). The geometry of the right ventricle permits relatively constant cardiac output in the face of variable venous return but this adaptation is at the expense of the ability to generate high pressures. Under pathological circumstances the functions of the right and left ventricle become more directly linked (ventricular interdependence) and the contribution of left ventricular contraction to right ventricular function becomes more important [16]. The pericardium limits total cardiac volume, such that when the right ventricle increases in size, there is a corresponding fall in left ventricular volume. The slope of the Frank-Starling curve is flatter for the right ventricle and the overall effect is decreased cardiac output.

Diagnosis

Measurements of peri-operative pulmonary hypertension and right ventricular ejection fraction (RVEF) can be made using a pulmonary artery catheter (PAC), and estimations made using echocardiography (transthoracic or transesophageal) [17]. Left atrial pressure (LAP) is usually higher than RAP because the right ventricle has greater compliance than the left ventricle. An early indication of right ventricular impairment may be when RAP starts to approximate to LAP [15].

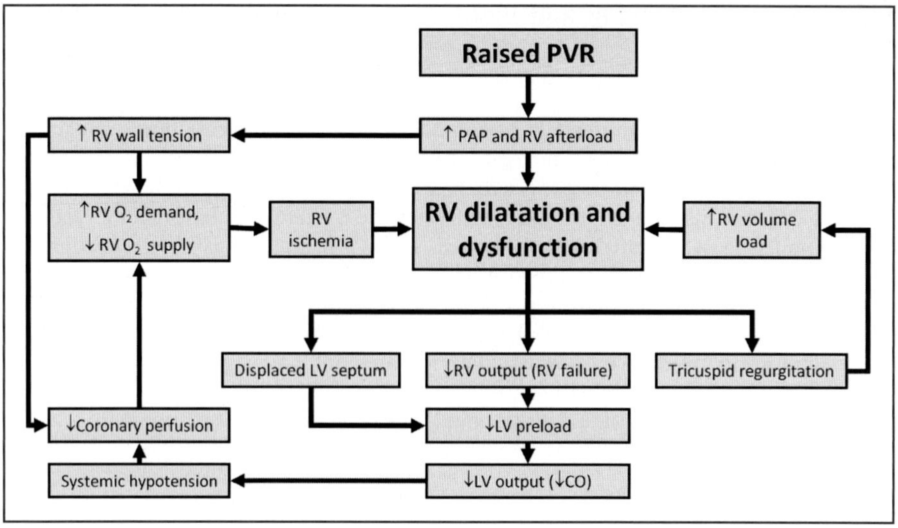

Raised PVR
↑ PAP and RV afterload
↑ RV wall tension
↑RV O_2 demand,
↓ RV O_2 supply
RV ischemia
RV dilatation and dysfunction
↑RV volume load
Displaced LV septum
↓RV output (RV failure)
Tricuspid regurgitation
↓Coronary perfusion
↓LV preload
Systemic hypotension
↓LV output (↓CO)

Fig. 1. Downward spiral of right ventricular (RV) dysfunction after cardiopulmonary bypass. PVR: pulmonary vascular resistance; PAP: pulmonary artery pressure; LV: left ventricular; CO: cardiac output

Administration of Nitric Oxide

Internationally, the licensed indication for inhaled NO therapy is restricted to persistent pulmonary hypertension in neonates. However, the majority (~70 %) of usage is outside this arena (personal communication, Peter Rothery, iNO Therpeutics). An advisory board under the auspices of the European Society of Intensive Care Medicine and European Association of Cardiothoracic Anaesthesiologists published guidelines for the use of NO in 2005 [18]. Inhaled NO is usually administered via a ventilator circuit protected by a cuffed endotracheal tube. To minimize admixture of high concentrations of oxygen with NO (risk of NO_2 formation) the NO/nitrogen mixture is introduced into the inspiratory limb of the circuit as near to the patient as possible. It is obligatory to monitor NO and NO_2 concentrations and although concentrations of inhaled NO administered clinically should not cause methemoglobinemia, guidelines recommend regular measurement of methemoglobin. Inhaled NO administration reduces endogenous NO production and rapid withdrawal can cause significant rebound pulmonary hypertension. In clinical practice, this can be avoided by gradual withdrawal of therapy [8].

There is marked variation in response to inhaled NO between patients [8] and in the same patient at different times. After prolonged use there is a leftward shift in the dose-response curve such that without regular titration against a relevant physiological index there is a risk of excessive inhaled NO administration. Such excessive dosing can lead to worsening oxygenation [19].

A survey of therapeutic use of inhaled NO in adult patients from a single US center (2000–2003) demonstrated that the commonest indication was to treat pulmonary and right ventricular failure in patients after cardiac surgery, followed by (in decreasing order) orthotopic heart transplantation, ventricular assist device placement, medical patients, orthotopic lung transplantation and for hypoxemia in other surgery. Overall mortality was lower when inhaled NO was used after orthotopic heart transplantation (25.4 %) and orthotopic lung transplantation (37.8 %) than following cardiac surgery (61 %), insertion of ventricular assist device (62 %), or other surgery (75 %); and was highest among medical patients (90 %), possibly due to its use as a therapy of last resort [20].

Cardiac Surgery

Studies in patients undergoing cardiac surgery confirm that inhaled NO acts as a selective pulmonary vasodilator irrespective of the presence of a ventricular assist device, or infusion of nitrates and is as effective after CPB as before. Administration at 20 or 40 parts per million (ppm) [21, 22] decreases PVR without altering systemic hemodynamics [23]. PVR is diminished to a greater extent in patients with higher baseline resistance [24, 25]. Importantly, inhaled NO's unique virtue of selective pulmonary vasodilation is invaluable when the right ventricle may benefit from reduction in afterload, but there is a relative contraindication to the use of a non-specific vasodilator. This is usually because vasopressors are already required to maintain adequate systemic pressure. A non-blinded study comparing inhaled NO to the non-selective vasodilator, milrinone, in 45 adult cardiac surgical patients with pulmonary hypertension confirmed that inhaled NO use was associated with a higher RVEF and lower requirements for vasopressor agents [26]. Similarly, a trial comparing inhaled NO either with inhaled prostacyclin (prostaglandin PGI2: epoprostanol) or intravenous vasodilators in 58 patients undergoing surgery for severe mitral stenosis with pulmonary hypertension showed that both inhaled agents were superior to intravenous vasodilatators at preserving systemic pressures [27].

The European inhaled NO guidelines suggest that optimization of right ventricular function should be achieved through all available means prior to starting inhaled NO. It is of course reasonable to ensure that ventilation, preload, and coronary perfusion are optimal, and to employ other measures to lower PVR and reduce myocardial oxygen consumption. However, it is debatable whether thoracic decompression (prolonged open sternotomy) with its attendant risks [28, 29] should be obligatory prior to the use of inhaled NO.

Valve Operations

Measures of right ventricular function are predictive of mortality in patients undergoing aortic or mitral valve replacement [30]. Pulmonary hypertension associated with mitral valve disease can significantly complicate repair or replacement and inhaled NO has been used with good result in this context [31, 32]. In 27 patients with mitral and/or aortic valve disease with post-operative pulmonary hypertension, hemodynamics and markers of oxygen delivery improved significantly [33]. Similarly, in 34 patients with complex cardiac surgery inhaled NO improved hemodynamics (mean pulmonary artery pressure, cardiac index and mean systemic pressure) and was important for weaning from CPB and later for continued right ventricular support [34].

Adult Congenital Heart Disease

In adult patients with congenital heart disease who have cardiac surgery, inhaled NO is a valuable adjuvant therapy [35] as both pulmonary hypertension and impaired right ventricular function are common.

Ventricular Assist Device

When a left ventricular assist device (LVAD) is used to support left ventricular function, the loss of contribution that left ventricular contraction makes to right ventricular function may be significant. Although the LVAD reduces left atrial pressures and, therefore, right ventricular afterload, the decrease in right ventricular function may be critical, particularly when it was already impaired [15, 36]. Inhaled NO has been used to alleviate right ventricular failure in this context [37].

Heart Transplantation

Donor organ ischemia and pre-existent or perioperative pulmonary hypertension contribute to the development of right ventricular failure [38] in orthotopic heart transplantation patients. Pulmonary hypertension in a recipient is associated with adverse outcome as it can cause right ventricular failure in the immediate postoperative period. Increased PVR is therefore a relative contraindication to heart transplantation in some centers. Inhaled NO is an effective therapy for right ventricular failure after heart transplantation, which may be associated with a reduction in mortality [39]. Some centers advocate use of inhaled NO preoperatively when there is pre-existent pulmonary hyperension [40].

Lung Transplantation

Early ischemia/reperfusion injury after orthotopic lung transplantation manifests clinically as pulmonary edema and is a cause of significant morbidity and mortality [41, 42]. Endogenous NO activity is decreased after orthotopic lung transplantation despite increased eNOS expression. Although inhaled NO has been shown to be a useful therapy in this circumstance [43] it has not been shown to prevent ischemia-reperfusion injury in clinical lung transplantation.

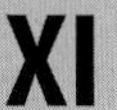

Trial Data Relating to Outcome

There are no published randomized controlled trials of inhaled NO against placebo or an alternative vasodilator in adult cardiac surgery with patient outcome as an endpoint. In children, a study of pulmonary hypertensive crises after cardiac surgery for correction of congenital heart disease demonstrated a trend towards a reduction in mortality with inhaled NO but this was not statistically significant [44]. Pulmonary hypertensive crises were defined as episodes where the pulmonary/systemic artery pressure ratio increased unacceptably (more than 0.75).

Conclusion

There is a strong physiological rationale supporting the use of inhaled NO in the context of right ventricular dysfunction complicating cardiac surgery. Given the immediate and beneficial effects that are often seen after commencement, and considering the limitations of alternatives [45], it may prove impossible to identify investigators with sufficient equipoise to enrol patients in a comparative trial of outcome with inhaled NO and placebo. Comparing clinical outcomes with inhaled NO versus other inhaled or intravenous vasodilators would be preferable. Further problems in designing and conducting randomized controlled trials on the efficacy of inhaled NO in the context of adult cardiac surgery include difficulty with blinding as the effects of inhaled NO are immediately apparent, and recruitment may be limited as the onset of acute pulmonary hypertension/right ventricular failure can be rapidly life-threatening with little time for consent/assent or randomization.

References

1. Palmer RM, Ferrige AG, Moncada S (1987) Nitric oxide release accounts for the biological activity of endothelium-derived relaxing factor. Nature 327: 524–526
2. McCarthy HO, Coulter JA, Robson T, Hirst DG (2008) Gene therapy via inducible nitric oxide synthase: a tool for the treatment of a diverse range of pathological conditions. J Pharm Pharmacol 60: 999–1017
3. Davidson SM, Duchen MR (2006) Effects of NO on mitochondrial function in cardiomyocytes: Pathophysiological relevance. Cardiovasc Res 71: 10–21
4. Lundberg JO, Weitzberg E, Gladwin MT (2008) The nitrate-nitrite-nitric oxide pathway in physiology and therapeutics. Nat Rev Drug Discov 7: 156–167
5. McMahon TJ, Doctor A (2006) Extrapulmonary effects of inhaled nitric oxide: role of reversible S-nitrosylation of erythrocytic hemoglobin. Proc Am Thorac Soc 3: 153–160
6. Cokic VP, Schechter AN (2008) Effects of nitric oxide on red blood cell development and phenotype. Curr Top Dev Biol 82169–215
7. Young JD, Sear JW, Valvini EM (1996) Kinetics of methaemoglobin and serum nitrogen oxide production during inhalation of nitric oxide in volunteers. Br J Anaesth 76: 652–656
8. Griffiths MJ, Evans TW (2005) Inhaled nitric oxide therapy in adults. N Engl J Med 353: 2683–2695
9. Rossaint R, Falke KJ, Lopez F, Slama K, Pison U, Zapol WM (1993) Inhaled nitric oxide for the adult respiratory distress syndrome. N Engl J Med 328: 399–405
10. Mannick JB (2006) Immunoregulatory and antimicrobial effects of nitrogen oxides. Proc Am Thorac Soc 3: 161–165
11. Morita K, Ihnken K, Buckberg GD, Sherman MP, Ignarro LJ (1996) Pulmonary vasoconstriction due to impaired nitric oxide production after cardiopulmonary bypass. Ann Thorac Surg 61: 1775–1780
12. Wessel DL, Adatia I, Giglia TM, Thompson JE, Kulik TJ (1993) Use of inhaled nitric oxide and acetylcholine in the evaluation of pulmonary hypertension and endothelial function after cardiopulmonary bypass. Circulation 88: 2128–2138
13. Gianetti J, Del Sarto P, Bevilacqua S, et al (2004) Supplemental nitric oxide and its effect on myocardial injury and function in patients undergoing cardiac surgery with extracorporeal circulation. J Thorac Cardiovasc Surg 127: 44–50
14. Maslow AD, Regan MM, Panzica P, Heindel S, Mashikian J, Comunale ME (2002) Precardiopulmonary bypass right ventricular function is associated with poor outcome after coronary artery bypass grafting in patients with severe left ventricular systolic dysfunction. Anesth Analg 95: 1507–1518
15. Vlahakes GJ (2005) Right ventricular failure following cardiac surgery. Coron Artery Dis 16: 27–30
16. Klima U, Guerrero JL, Vlahakes GJ (1998) Contribution of the interventricular septum to maximal right ventricular function. Eur J Cardiothorac Surg 14: 250–255
17. De Simone R, Wolf I, Mottl-Link S, et al (2005) Intraoperative assessment of right ventricular volume and function. Eur J Cardiothorac Surg 27: 988–993
18. Germann P, Braschi A, Della Rocca G, et al (2005) Inhaled nitric oxide therapy in adults: European expert recommendations. Intensive Care Med 31: 1029–1041
19. Gerlach H, Keh D, Semmerow A, et al (2003) Dose-response characteristics during long-term inhalation of nitric oxide in patients with severe acute respiratory distress syndrome: a prospective, randomized, controlled study. Am J Respir Crit Care Med 167: 1008–1015
20. George I, Xydas S, Topkara VK, et al (2006) Clinical indication for use and outcomes after inhaled nitric oxide therapy. Ann Thorac Surg 82: 2161–2169

21. Rich GF, Murphy GD Jr, Roos CM, Johns RA (1993) Inhaled nitric oxide. Selective pulmonary vasodilation in cardiac surgical patients. Anesthesiology 78: 1028–1035
22. Snow DJ, Gray SJ, Ghosh S, et al (1994) Inhaled nitric oxide in patients with normal and increased pulmonary vascular resistance after cardiac surgery. Br J Anaesth 72: 185–189
23. Hare JM, Shernan SK, Body SC, Graydon E, Colucci WS, Couper GS (1997) Influence of inhaled nitric oxide on systemic flow and ventricular filling pressure in patients receiving mechanical circulatory assistance. Circulation 95: 2250–2253
24. Della Rocca G, Pugliese F, Antonini M, et al (1997) Hemodynamics during inhaled nitric oxide in lung transplant candidates. Transplant Proc 29: 3367–3370
25. Solina AR, Ginsberg SH, Papp D, et al (2002) Response to nitric oxide during adult cardiac surgery. J Invest Surg 15: 5–14
26. Solina A, Papp D, Ginsberg S, et al (2000) A comparison of inhaled nitric oxide and milrinone for the treatment of pulmonary hypertension in adult cardiac surgery patients. J Cardiothorac Vasc Anesth 14: 12–17
27. Fattouch K, Sbraga F, Sampognaro R, et al (2006) Treatment of pulmonary hypertension in patients undergoing cardiac surgery with cardiopulmonary bypass: a randomized, prospective, double-blind study. J Cardiovasc Med 7: 119–123
28. Anderson CA, Filsoufi F, Aklog L, Farivar RS, Byrne JG, Adams DH (2002) Liberal use of delayed sternal closure for postcardiotomy hemodynamic instability. Ann Thorac Surg 73: 1484–1488
29. Christenson JT, Maurice J, Simonet F, Velebit V, Schmuziger M (1996) Open chest and delayed sternal closure after cardiac surgery. Eur J Cardiothorac Surg 10: 305–311
30. Haddad F, Denault AY, Couture P, et al (2007) Right ventricular myocardial performance index predicts perioperative mortality or circulatory failure in high-risk valvular surgery. J Am Soc Echocardiogr 20: 1065–1072.
31. Healy DG, Veerasingam D, McHale J, Luke D (2006) Successful perioperative utilisation of inhaled nitric oxide in mitral valve surgery. J Cardiovasc Surg (Torino) 47: 217–220
32. Girard C, Lehot JJ, Pannetier JC, Filley S, Ffrench P, Estanove S (1992) Inhaled nitric oxide after mitral valve replacement in patients with chronic pulmonary artery hypertension. Anesthesiology 77: 880–883
33. Santini F, Casali G, Franchi G, et al (2005) Hemodynamic effects of inhaled nitric oxide and phosphodiesterase inhibitor (dipyridamole) on secondary pulmonary hypertension following heart valve surgery in adults. Int J Cardiol 103: 156–163
34. Beck JR, Mongero LB, Kroslowitz RM, et al (1999) Inhaled nitric oxide improves hemodynamics in patients with acute pulmonary hypertension after high-risk cardiac surgery. Perfusion 14: 37–42
35. Price S, Jaggar SI, Jordan S, et al (2007) Adult congenital heart disease: intensive care management and outcome prediction. Intensive Care Med 33: 652–659
36. Ochiai Y, McCarthy PM, Smedira NG, et al (2002) Predictors of severe right ventricular failure after implantable left ventricular assist device insertion: analysis of 245 patients. Circulation 106 (Suppl 1):I198–202
37. Wagner F, Dandel M, Gunther G, et al (1997) Nitric oxide inhalation in the treatment of right ventricular dysfunction following left ventricular assist device implantation. Circulation 96 (Suppl 9):II-291–296
38. Kaul TK, Fields BL (2000) Postoperative acute refractory right ventricular failure: incidence, pathogenesis, management and prognosis. Cardiovasc Surg 8: 1–9
39. Mosquera I, Crespo-Leiro MG, Tabuyo T, et al (2002) Pulmonary hypertension and right ventricular failure after heart transplantation: usefulness of nitric oxide. Transplant Proc 34: 166–167
40. Stobierska-Dzierzek B, Awad H, Michler RE (2001) The evolving management of acute right-sided heart failure in cardiac transplant recipients. J Am Coll Cardiol 38: 923–931
41. King RC, Binns OA, Rodriguez F, et al (2000) Reperfusion injury significantly impacts clinical outcome after pulmonary transplantation. Ann Thorac Surg 69: 1681–1685
42. de Perrot M, Liu M, Waddell TK, Keshavjee S (2003) Ischemia-reperfusion-induced lung injury. Am J Respir Crit Care Med 167: 490–511
43. Kemming GI (1998) Inhaled nitric oxide (NO) for the treatment of early allograft failure after lung transplantation. Munich Lung Transplant Group. Intensive Care Med 24: 1173–1180

44. Miller OI, Tang SF, Keech A, Pigott NB, Beller E, Celermajer DS (2000) Inhaled nitric oxide and prevention of pulmonary hypertension after congenital heart surgery: a randomised double-blind study. Lancet 356: 1464–1469
45. Dickstein ML (2005) Con: inhaled prostaglandin as a pulmonary vasodilator instead of nitric oxide. J Cardiothorac Vasc Anesth 19: 403–405

XI

XII Cardiac Function

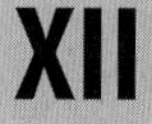

Use of Natriuretic Peptides in the Emergency Department and the ICU

T. Reichlin, M. Noveanu, and C. Mueller

Introduction

The clinical importance of a specific disease marker is related to the overall importance of the disease or biological signal it quantifies, the availability of alternative methods to reliably diagnose the disease and quantify disease severity, and, of course, the performance of the marker. Natriuretic peptides, as quantitative markers of cardiac stress and heart failure, owe their clinical importance to the fact that heart failure is a major public health problem, the uncertainty in the clinical diagnosis and management of heart failure, and to their excellent diagnostic and prognostic utility [1–5].

Natriuretic Peptides are Quantitative Markers of Cardiac Stress and Heart Failure

Most clinical data on natriuretic peptides have been obtained with assays measuring either B-type natriuretic peptide (BNP) or N-terminal pro BNP (NT-proBNP). Preliminary data suggest that other members of the natriuretic peptide family, including midregional proANP and proANP, may have comparable clinical utility at least in some indications [6–8].

Natriuretic peptides can be seen as quantitative markers of cardiac stress and heart failure summarizing the extent of systolic and diastolic left ventricular dysfunction, valvular dysfunction, and right ventricular dysfunction (**Fig. 1**). In general, levels of BNP and NT-proBNP are directly related to the severity of heart failure symptoms and to the severity of the cardiac abnormality. BNP is a 32-amino acid peptide that is secreted with the inactive aminoterminal proBNP (NT-proBNP) and intact proBNP from the left and the right cardiac atria and ventricles in response to ventricular volume expansion and pressure overload [9–15]. Recent data suggest that left ventricular end-diastolic wall stress and wall stiffness may be the predominate triggers of BNP release [13, 14].

Two important principles should underlie the clinical use of natriuretic peptides. First, a natriuretic peptide level is not a stand-alone test. It is always of greatest value when it complements the physician's clinical skills along with other available diagnostic tools. Second, natriuretic peptide levels should be interpreted and used as continuous variables in order to make full use of the biological information provided by the measurement (like, e.g., calculated glomerular filtration rate).

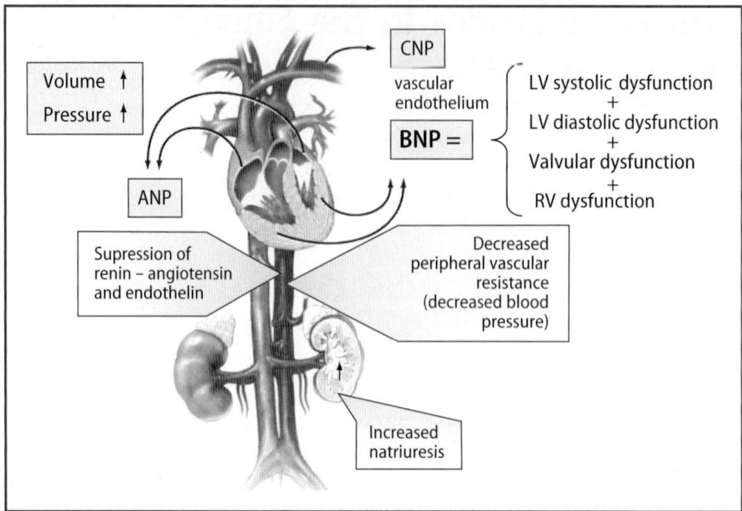

Fig. 1. Natriuretic peptides are quantitative markers of cardiac stress and heart failure. RV: right ventricular; LV: left ventricular; BNP: B-type natriuretic peptide; ANP: A-type natriuretic peptide; CNP: C-type natriuretic peptide

Clinical Indications: Patients with Acute Dyspnea

Current evidence is sufficient to recommend the routine clinical use of natriuretic peptides in only one situation: The diagnosis and management of patients presenting with acute dyspnea. Although other indications in the emergency department (ED) are the subject of intensive investigation and natriuretic peptides have been shown to be powerful tools for risk stratification also, e.g., in patients with acute coronary syndromes, pulmonary embolism, and pneumonia, further research is needed to justify routine clinical use [3].

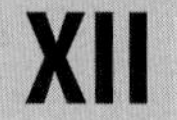

The rapid and accurate differentiation of heart failure from other causes of acute dyspnea remains a clinical challenge, both in the ED and in the intensive care unit (ICU). After evaluating a patient's symptoms, conducting a physical examination, and performing electrocardiography (EKG) and chest radiography, the clinician is often left with considerable diagnostic uncertainty, which can result in misdiagnosis and delay the initiation of appropriate therapy [1–5].

Diagnostic Value of Natriuretic Peptides in Patients with Acute Dyspnea

Numerous observational studies including patients presenting with acute dyspnea have validated natriuretic peptides against a gold standard diagnosis of heart failure and shown convincingly that natriuretic peptides have a very high diagnostic accuracy [6, 8, 16–24]. The higher the natriuretic peptide level the higher the probability that acute dyspnea is caused by heart failure. The largest validating study included more than 1500 patients and found that adding BNP to clinical judgment would have enhanced diagnostic accuracy from 74 % to 81 %. The areas under the receiver operating characteristic (ROC) curve were 0.86, 0.90, and 0.93 for clinical judgment, for BNP, and for the two in combination, respectively ($p < 0.0001$ for all pair-wise comparisons) [4, 5].

Prognostic Value of Natriuretic Peptides in Patients with Acute Dyspnea

Natriuretic peptides predict prognosis and help risk stratify patients with dyspnea irrespective of the cause of dyspnea (heart failure or non-cardiac) [20, 25–28]. The natriuretic peptide level quantifies cardiac stress and accurately predicts the risk of death, both in-hospital and long-term. The areas under the ROC curve for the ability of natriuretic peptide to predict death were 0.70 to 0.75. For example, a NT-proBNP value of 5180 pg/ml or higher at presentation to the ED predicted death within 76 days with a sensitivity of 68 %, a specificity of 72 %, and a negative predictive value of 96 % in patients with acute heart failure [20].

Impact of Natriuretic Peptide on the Management of Patients with Acute Dyspnea

Easily applicable algorithms for the interpretation of BNP and NT-proBNP using specific cut-off levels have been developed. In order to make best use of the diagnostic and prognostic information from natriuretic peptide levels, the clinician needs to understand that natriuretic peptides are quantitative markers of cardiac stress and heart failure. The higher the natriuretic peptide level, the higher the likelihood that the dyspnea in the individual patient is caused by heart failure. It has become common to use two cut-off values: A lower one with a high negative predictive value to reliably exclude heart failure as the cause of acute dyspnea, and a second, higher cut-off with a high positive predictive value to 'rule in' heart failure as the cause of dyspnea. For BNP, the two cut-off levels 100 pg/ml and 400 pg/ml should be used. These cut-off values apply irrespective of age and sex [29, 30]. However, these cut-offs do need to be adjusted in the presence of two clinical conditions: Kidney disease and obesity. In patients with kidney disease and an estimated glomerular filtration rate of less than 60 ml/min, 200–225 pg/ml rather than 100 pg/ml is the most appropriate cut-off value to rule out heart failure [31, 32]. In contrast, the presence of obesity requires the use of lower cut-off values. In patients with severe obesity and a body mass index (BMI) above 35, we recommend a BNP cut-off value of 60 pg/ml to rule out and 200 pg/ml to rule in heart failure as the cause of acute dyspnea [33,34].

The International Collaborative for NT-proBNP Study defined the most appropriate cut-off values for NT-proBNP [19, 20]: 300 pg/ml should be used to 'rule out' heart failure. Depending on age (< 50, 50–75, and > 75 years), 450 pg/ml, 900 pg/ml, or 1800 pg/ml should be used to 'rule in' heart failure. As renal function in this population was closely related to age, no further adjustment for renal function was necessary. Obesity is also associated with lower NT-proBNP levels [35]. It is a matter of debate whether NT-proBNP levels should be adjusted for obesity.

Added Value of Using Natriuretic Peptide in the Management of Patients with Acute Dyspnea

The added value of natriuretic peptide in the management of patients with acute dyspnea was examined in two randomized controlled trials including patients presenting to the ED [36, 37] Together, these randomized studies provide a clear answer to the remaining key question: Does the increase in diagnostic accuracy associated with the use of natriuretic peptide translate into improved patient management when used in clinical practice?

The BNP for Acute Shortness of Breath Evaluation (BASEL) study randomized 452 consecutive patients presenting with dyspnea to the ED to either BNP-guided management or standard management without the use of BNP [36]. The use of BNP resulted in a reduction in the time from presentation at the ED to the initiation of the appropriate therapy according to the final discharge, a reduction in hospital admission rate, a reduction in the need for intensive care, and a reduction in the time to discharge. The total cost of treatment was $5,410 in the BNP group compared with $7,264 in the control group, a significant reduction of 26 %. These data support the conclusion that, when used in conjunction with other clinical information, rapid measurement of BNP in the ED improves medical and economic outcome. These findings were recently confirmed by a Canadian multicenter study (IMPROVE-CHF) using NT-proBNP [37]. Five hundred patients presenting with dyspnea to seven EDs were studied. Knowledge of NT-proBNP results reduced the duration of ED visit by 21 %, the number of patients rehospitalized over 60 days by 35 %, and direct medical costs of all ED visits, hospitalizations, and subsequent outpatient services (US $6129 to US $5180 per patient; $p = 0.023$) over 60 days from enrolment. Adding NT-proBNP to clinical judgment enhanced the accuracy of a diagnosis; the area under the ROC curve increased from 0.83 to 0.90 ($p < 0.00001$).

The BASEL study also assessed the cost-effectiveness of BNP testing during long-term follow-up [38, 39]. To address the fact that tailoring of resources may well be cost-effective initially, but may result in large secondary costs due to recurrent symptoms, cost-effectiveness analyses were performed at 180 and 360 days follow-up. BNP testing was found to be cost-effective also at these time points. The use of BNP levels significantly reduced total treatment cost. This reduction was driven by significantly fewer days spent in-hospital in the BNP group. A large part of this reduction occurred during the initial presentation and was fully maintained throughout 360 days.

The importance of obtaining the natriuretic peptide level immediately at presentation to the ED was further highlighted by a recent analysis from a large registry indicating that delayed measurement of natriuretic peptide levels and delay in treatment for acute heart failure were strongly associated. These delays were linked with modestly increased in-hospital mortality, independent of other prognostic variables. The adverse impact of delay was most notable in patients with greater natriuretic peptide levels [40].

Based on these data it seems appropriate to recommend the measurement of natriuretic peptides at presentation in all patients presenting with acute dyspnea as their main complaint.

ICU Perspective

As diagnostic dilemmas in the ICU are often as challenging as in the ED, recent studies have begun to evaluate whether the use of natriuretic peptides may also be helpful in the ICU. The value of a biomarker to detect heart failure in the ICU is based on the observation that heart failure is common in the ICU and on the assumption that the detection of heart failure in the ICU allows the early initiation of specific heart failure therapy in order to improve morbidity and mortality. However, there are major differences in patient characteristics, disease severity, co-morbidity, resources available for the individual patient, and therapies between the ICU and the ED, so that the role of natriuretic peptides should be specifically assessed in critically ill patients.

The number of patients included in recent ICU studies has been small. Therefore, most recent studies may be considered hypothesis generating rather than confirmatory. Overall, current evidence does not seem strong enough to recommend the routine clinical use of natriuretic peptides in the ICU. However, in some situations, very exciting initial data have recently been reported [41]. As one example, the diagnostic use of natriuretic peptide in patients with hypoxemic respiratory failure and bilateral infiltrates on chest radiograph has been briefly described. This setting often requires the evaluation of cardiac function using pulmonary artery catheterization or echocardiography. These techniques help to differentiate between cardiogenic pulmonary edema from an acute lung injury (ALI). Natriuretic peptides have also been proposed to help in the differentiation between cardiogenic and non-cardiogenic pulmonary edema. Jefic et al. [42] performed a prospective study on 41 consecutive patients with hypoxic respiratory failure undergoing pulmonary artery catheterization to evaluate whether BNP or NT-proBNP or both could be used to differentiate high pulmonary artery occlusion pressure (PAOP) versus low PAOP pulmonary edema. In this study, BNP and NT-proBNP failed to reliably differentiate between patients with high and low PAOP. Additional work by Bal et al. [43] and Forfia et al. [44] underlines the recognition that natriuretic peptide and PAOP provide different windows on the heart. More recently, Karmpaliotis et al. [45] reported data from 81 ICU patients suffering from acute pulmonary edema. BNP offered good discriminatory performance for the final diagnosis established by two independent intensivists. In this study, the median BNP was 1260 pg/ml in patients with heart failure (cardiogenic pulmonary edema) and 325 pg/ml in those with acute respiratory distress syndrome (ARDS). A BNP level below 200 pg/ml offered a specificity of 91 % for the final diagnosis of ARDS, whereas a BNP of at least 1200 pg/ml offered a specificity of 92 % for the final diagnosis of cardiogenic pulmonary edema. Obviously, further evidence from larger studies is needed to appropriately define the potential clinical use of natriuretic peptide for differentiating cardiogenic pulmonary edema from ALI.

Conclusion

Natriuretic peptides have been shown to be very helpful in the diagnosis and management of patients presenting with acute dyspnea. Natriuretic peptides can be seen as quantitative markers of cardiac stress and heart failure, summarizing the extent of systolic and diastolic left ventricular dysfunction, valvular dysfunction, and right ventricular dysfunction. Current evidence supports the routine use of natriuretic peptides in patients with acute dyspnea. As cardiac stress also determines prognosis in other common cardiac and non-cardiac disorders in the ED and in the ICU, the use of natriuretic peptide may also be helpful in many additional disorders including patients with acute coronary syndromes, pulmonary embolism, severe sepsis and septic shock [46].

Acknowledgement: Dr. Mueller was supported by research grants from the Swiss National Science Foundation, the Swiss Heart Foundation, the Novartis Foundation, the Krokus Foundation, Abbott, Biosite, Brahms, Roche, Siemens, and the University of Basel.

References

1. Nieminen MS, Böhm M, Cowie MR, et al (2005) Executive summary of the guidelines on the diagnosis and treatment of acute heart failure. Eur Heart J 26: 384–416
2. Cowie MR, Struthers AD, Wood DA, et al (1997) Value of natriuretic peptides in assessment of patients with possible new heart failure in primary care. Lancet 350: 1349–1353
3. Mueller C, Breidthardt T, Laule-Kilian K, Christ M, Perruchoud AP (2007) The integration of BNP and NT-proBNP into clinical medicine. Swiss Med Wkly 137: 4–12
4. Maisel AS, Krishnaswamy P, Nowak RM, et al (2002) Rapid measurement of B-type natriuretic peptide in the emergency diagnosis of heart failure. N Engl J Med 347: 161–167
5. McCullough PA, Nowak RM, McCord J, et al (2002) B-type natriuretic peptide and clinical judgement in emergency diagnosis of heart failure. Analysis from Breathing Not Properly (BNP) Multinational Study. Circulation 106: 416–422
6. Gegenhuber A, Struck J, Poelz W, et al (2006) Midregional pro-A-type natriuretic peptide measurements for diagnosis of acute destabilized heart failure in short-of-breath patients: comparison with B-type natriuretic peptide (BNP) and amino-terminal proBNP. Clin Chem 52: 827–831
7. Gegenhuber A, Struck J, Dieplinger B, et al (2007) Comparative evaluation of B-type natriuretic peptide, mid-regional pro-A-type natriuretic peptide, mid-regional pro-adrenomedullin, and Copeptin to predict 1-year mortality in patients with acute destabilized heart failure. J Card Fail 13: 42–49
8. Potocki M, Breidthardt T, Reichlin T, et al (2008) Comparison of midregional pro-atrial natriuretic peptide with N-terminal pro-B-type natriuretic peptide in the diagnosis of heart failure. Eur Heart J 29:180a (abst)
9. Mukoyama M, Nakao K, Hosoda K, et al (1991) Brain natriuretic peptide as a novel cardiac hormone in humans. Evidence for an exquisite dual natriuretic peptide system, atrial natriuretic peptide and brain natriuretic peptide. J Clin Invest 87: 1402–1412
10. Yasue H, Yoshimura M, Sumida H, et al (1994) Localization and mechanism of secretion of B-type natriuretic peptide in comparison with those of A-type natriuretic peptide in normal subjects and patients with heart failure. Circulation 90: 195–203
11. Davis M, Espiner E, Richards G, et al (1994) Plasma brain natriuretic peptide in assessment of acute dyspnea. Lancet 343: 440–444
12. McDonagh TA, Robb SD, Murdoch DR, et al (1998) Biochemical detection of left-ventricular systolic dysfunction. Lancet 351: 9–13
13. Iwanaga Y, Nishi I, Furuichi S, et al (2006) B-type natriuretic peptide strongly reflects diastolic wall stress in patients with chronic heart failure. Comparison between systolic and diastolic heart failure. J Am Coll Cardiol 47: 742–748
14. Watanabe S, Shite J, Takaoka H, et al (2006) myocardial stiffness is an important determinant of the plasma brain natriuretic peptide concentration in patients with both diastolic and systolic heart failure. Eur Heart J 27: 832–838
15. Troughton RW, Prior DL, Pereira JJ, et al (2004) Plasma B-type natriuretic peptide levels in systolic heart failure. Importance of left ventricular diastolic function and right ventricular systolic function. J Am Coll Cardiol 43: 416–422
16. Lainchbury JG, Campbell E, Frampton CM, et al (2003) Brain natriuretic peptide and N-terminal brain natriuretic peptide in the diagnosis of heart failure in patients with acute shortness of breath. J Am Coll Cardiol 42: 728–735
17. Svendstrup Nielsen L, Svanegaard J, Klitgaard NA, Egeblad H (2004) N-terminal pro-brain natriuretic peptide for discriminating between cardiac and non-cardiac dyspnoea. Eur J Heart Fail 6: 63–70
18. Dao Q, Krishnaswamy P, Kazanegra R, et al (2001) Utility of B-type natriuretic peptide in the diagnosis of congestive heart failure in an urgent-care setting. J Am Coll Cardiol 37: 379–385
19. Januzzi JL, Camargo CA, Anwaruddin S, et al (2005) The N-terminal pro-BNP investigation of dyspnea in the emergency department (PRIDE) study. Am J Cardiol 95: 948–954
20. Januzzi JL, van Rimmenade R, Lainchbury J, et al (2006) NT-proBNP testing for diagnosis and short-term prognosis in acute destabilized heart failure: an international pooled analysis of 1256 patients. The International Collaborative of NT-proBNP Study. Eur Heart J 27: 330–337

21. Wright SP, Doughty RN, Pearl A, et al (2003) Plasma amino-terminal pro-brain natriuretic peptide and accuracy of heart-failure diagnosis in primary care. A randomized, controlled trial. J Am Coll Cardiol 42: 1793–1800
22. Zaphiriou A, Robb S, Murray-Thomas T, et al (2005) The diagnostic accuracy of plasma BNP and NTproBNP in patients referred from primary care with suspected heart failure: results of the UK natriuretic peptide study. Eur J Heart Fail 7: 537–541
23. Ray P, Arthaud M, Birolleau S, et al (2005) Comparison of brain natriuretic peptide and pro-brain natriuretic peptide in the diagnosis of cardiogenic pulmonary edema in patients aged 65 and older. J Am Geriatr Soc 53: 643–648
24. Mueller T, Gegenhuber A, Poelz W, Haltmayer M (2005) Diagnostic accuracy of b-type natriuretic peptide and amino terminal proBNP in the emergency diagnosis of heart failure. Heart 91: 606–612
25. Fonarow GC, Peacock WF, Phillips CO, et al (2007) Admission B-type natriuretic peptide levels and in-hospital mortality in acute decompensated heart failure ADHERE Scientific Advisory Committee and Investigators. J Am Coll Cardiol 49: 1943–1950
26. Januzzi JL, Sakhuja R, O'Donoghue M, et al (2006) Utility of amino-terminal pro-brain natriuretic peptide testing for the prediction of 1-year mortality in patients with dyspnea treated in the emergency department. Arch Intern Med 166: 315–320
27. Christ M, Laule-Kilian K, Hochholzer W, et al (2006) Gender-specific risk stratification using B-type natriuretic peptide levels in patients with acute dyspnea: Insights from the BASEL study. J Am Coll Cardiol 48: 1808–1812
28. Christ M, Thuerlimann A, Laule K, et al (2007) Long-term prognostic value of B-type natriuretic peptide level in cardiac and non-cardiac causes of acute dyspnea. Eur J Clin Invest 37: 834–841
29. Maisel AS, Clopton P, Krishnaswamy P, et al (2004) Impact of age, race, and sex on the ability of B-type natriuretic peptide to aid in the emergency diagnosis of heart failure: results from Breathing Not Properly (BNP) Multinational Study. Am Heart J 147: 1078–1084
30. Mueller C, Laule-Kilian K, Scholer A, et al (2004) Use of B-type natriuretic peptide for the management of women with dyspnea. Am J Cardiol 94: 1510–1514
31. McCullough PA, Duc P, Omland T, et al (2003) B-type natriuretic peptide and renal function in the diagnosis of heart failure: An Analysis from the breathing not properly multinational study. Am J Kidney Dis 41: 571–575
32. Mueller C, Laule Kilian K, Scholer A, et al (2005) B-type natriuretic peptide for acute dyspnea in patients with kidney disease: insights from a randomized comparison. Kidney Int 67: 278–284.
33. Wang TJ, Larson MG, Levy D, et al (2004) Impact of obesity on plasma natriuretic peptide levels. Circulation 109: 594–600
34. McCord J, Mundy BJ, Hudson MP, et al (2004) Relationship between obesity and B-type natriuretic peptide levels. Arch Intern Med 164: 2247–2252
35. Krauser DG, Llyod-Jones DM, Chae CU, et al (2005) Effect of body mass index on natriuretic peptide levels in patients with acute congestive heart failure: A proBNP Investigation of dyspnea in the emergency department (PRIDE) substudy. Am Heart J 149: 744–750
36. Mueller C, Scholer A, Laule-Kilian K, et al (2004) Use of B-type natriuretic peptide in the evaluation and management of acute dyspnea. N Engl J Med 350: 647–654
37. Moe GW, Howlett J, Januzzi JL, et al (2007) N-terminal pro-B-type natriuretic peptide testing improves the management of patients with suspected acute heart failure: primary results of the Canadian prospective randomized multicenter IMPROVE-CHF study. Circulation 115: 3103–3110
38. Mueller C, Laule-Kilian K, Schindler C, et al (2006) Cost-effectiveness of B-type natriuretic peptide testing in patients with acute dyspnea. Arch Intern Med 166: 1081–1087
39. Breidthardt T, Laule K, Strohmeyer AH, et al (2007) Medical and economic long-term effects of B-type natriuretic peptide testing in patients with acute dyspnea. Clin Chem 53: 1415–1422
40. Maisel AS, Peacock WF, McMullin N, Jessie R, Fonarow GC, Wynne J, Mills RM (2008) Timing of immunoreactive B-type natriuretic peptide levels and treatment delay in acute decompensated heart failure: an ADHERE (Acute Decompensated Heart Failure National Registry) analysis. J Am Coll Cardiol 52: 534–540

41. Mueller C (2007) The use of B-type natriuretic peptides in the intensive care unit. Crit Care Med 35: 2438–2439
42. Jefic D, Lee JW, Jefic D, et al (2005) Utility of B-type natriuretic peptide and N-terminal pro B-type natriuretic peptide in evaluation of respiratory failure in critically ill patients. Chest 128: 288–295
43. Bal L, Thierry S, Brocas E, et al (2006) B-type natriuretic peptide (BNP) and N-terminal-proBNP for heart failure diagnosis in shock or acute respiratory distress. Acta Anaesthesiol Scand 50: 340–347
44. Forfia PR, Watkins SP, Rame JE, et al (2005) Relationship between B-type natriuretic peptides and pulmonary capillary wedge pressure in the intensive care unit. J Am Coll Cardiol 45: 1667–1671
45. Karmpaliotis D, Kirtane AJ, Ruisi CP, et al (2007) Diagnostic and prognostic utility of brain natriuretic Peptide in subjects admitted to the ICU with hypoxic respiratory failure due to noncardiogenic and cardiogenic pulmonary edema. Chest 131: 964–971
46. Maisel AS, Mueller C, Adams K, et al (2008) State of the art: Using natriuretic peptide levels in clinical practice. Eur J Heart Fail 10: 824–839

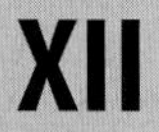

Abnormalities of the ST Segment

D. Gallo, J.M. Pines, and W. Brady

Introduction

The ST segment represents the period between depolarization and repolarization of the left ventricle. In the normal state, the ST segment is isoelectric, meaning that it is neither elevated nor depressed relative to the TP segment. Abnormalities of the ST segment of clinical import include ST segment elevation and ST segment depression. The electrocardiographic (EKG) differential diagnosis of abnormalities of the ST segment is broad, containing ominous and benign entities, including ST elevation myocardial infarction (STEMI), bundle branch block (BBB), acute pericarditis, benign early repolarization, left ventricular hypertrophy, ventricular paced rhythm, digoxin effect, myocarditis, cardiomyopathy, etc [1–3].

Electrocardiographic Evaluation

EKG features to consider in the differential diagnosis of ST abnormalities include the type of segment deviation (i.e., elevation vs. depression); the magnitude, morphology, and distribution of the ST segment abnormality; the width and size of the accompanying QRS complex; and associated T wave anomalies [2, 4, 5]. Over-reliance on any single feature of the EKG, however, is not encouraged. Each piece of the diagnostic puzzle must be viewed as a part of the entire picture – the history, examination, EKG, and other investigations. In addition, the 12-lead EKG, once ST segment elevation is noted, should be scrutinized in a systematic fashion – such an approach allows for a more reasoned review of the EKG and reduces the chance of missed features (**Fig. 1**).

Thus, the presence of an ST segment abnormality on the EKG itself in no way confirms the diagnosis of acute coronary syndrome (ACS). ST segment elevation is seen in approximately 20 % of chest pain patients in the emergency department while ST segment depression is more frequent. A significant minority of these chest pain patients with ST segment abnormality will be diagnosed with ACS; in fact, the most common cause of ST segment elevation among chest pain patients in the emergency department is a non-infarction diagnosis (**Fig. 2**) [1–3].

ST segment elevation results from a number of EKG syndromes, such as STEMI, left ventricular hypertrophy, BBB, and benign early repolarization. For instance, in a study of prehospital chest pain patients, the investigators demonstrated that the majority of patients manifesting ST segment elevation on the EKG did not have STEMI as the final diagnosis; left ventricular hypertrophy and left BBB (LBBB) accounted for the majority of these cases of ST segment elevation [6]. In the emer-

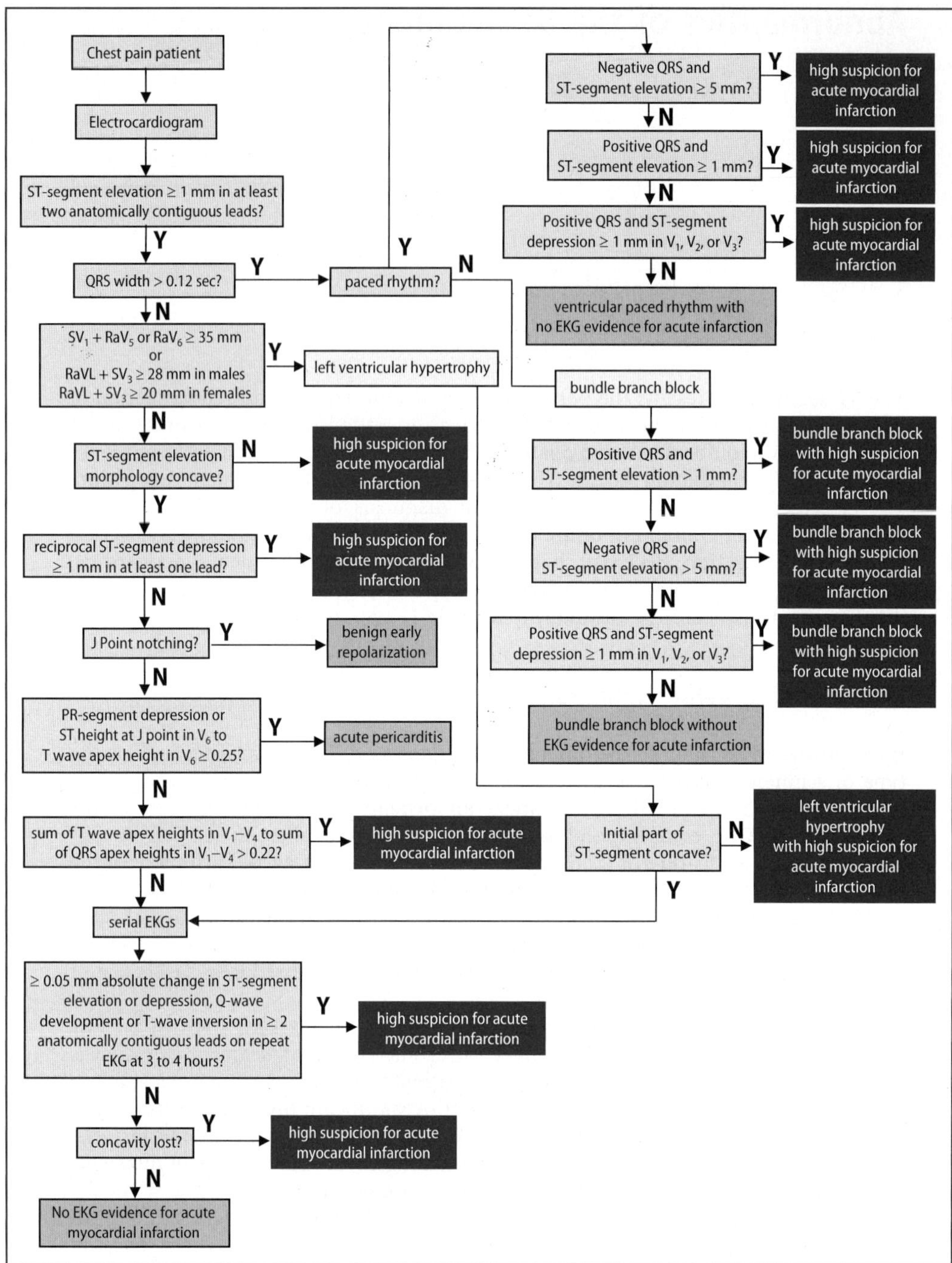

Fig. 1. An algorithmic approach to the interpretation of ST segment elevation in patients with chest pain.

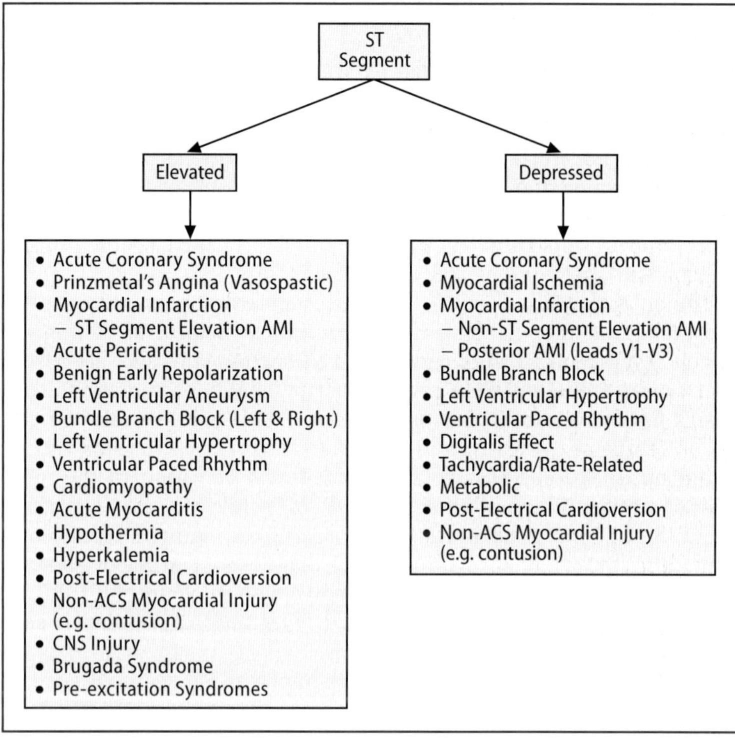

Fig. 2. Causes of ST segment abnormality encountered in patients with chest pain. AMI: acute myocardial infarction; ACS: acute coronary syndrome

gency department chest pain population, left ventricular hypertrophy is the most frequent cause of ST segment elevation encountered; LBBB and STEMI are the next most common causes of elevation followed by right BBB (RBBB), benign early repolarization, pericarditis, ventricular paced rhythm, left ventricular aneurysm, and other miscellaneous syndromes [1, 2]. In the coronary care unit, it has been shown that in patients with ST segment elevation and suspected acute myocardial infarction (AMI), the ST segment abnormality was actually diagnostic for STEMI in only half of the patients; as with the prehospital and emergency department populations, the range of etiologies responsible for the ST segment elevation was very broad.

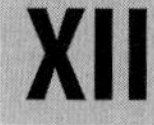

While ST segment elevation is not significantly predictive of STEMI in all chest pain patients, ST segment depression is more often associated with an ACS diagnosis in this population [3]. For example, in a study of chest pain patients in the emergency department, investigators noted that approximately 30 % of these individuals had ST segment depression on the EKG. Of those patients with ST segment depression, approximately 70 % had an ACS diagnosis. Considering all patients with ST segment depression in this group, the following EKG diagnoses were encountered: STEMI (with associated reciprocal ST segment depression), left ventricular hypertrophy, BBB, and ventricular paced rhythm [3].

Considering the magnitude of ST segment changes, the total amount of ST segment elevation is greater in the AMI patient compared to the non-infarction patient [4]. The total amount of ST segment elevation is defined as the milli-volt summation of elevation in all involved EKG leads. This observation is noted from numerous perspectives, including the single lead as well as the entire 12-lead EKG. For instance, the magnitude of individual lead ST segment elevation in AMI patterns averages 4.4 mV while, in non-AMI syndromes, 1.8 mV is found. From the perspective of the 12-lead EKG, the total summation of ST segment elevation remains greater in AMI (15.3 mV) versus non-AMI (7.4 mV) presentations. Furthermore, in the STEMI patient, the total amount of ST segment deviation (the sum of elevation and depression) is significantly greater in the STEMI patient (17.8 mV versus 10.5 mV); this later observation results from the presence of reciprocal ST segment depression in many inferior and anterior AMI presentations [4–6].

The anatomic distribution of the ST segment abnormality can be considered in this evaluation though this information is less helpful in distinguishing ACS from non-ACS syndromes. More widespread ST segment changes are associated with non-AMI causes while localized changes occur in ACS presentations though this difference is not significant in most situations. STEMI demonstrates ST segment elevation in an average of 3.4 leads; non-AMI patterns display 4.1 leads with ST segment elevation on a typical EKG. Isolated ST segment elevation in the inferior and lateral leads, however, frequently suggests STEMI while anterior elevation most often is found in non-AMI syndromes [4]. Regarding ST segment depression, a specific anatomic distribution is not helpful in the diagnosis of ACS. An anatomic distribution, however, is significant in the left ventricular hypertrophy, BBB, and ventricular paced patterns – in these syndromes, ST segment depression is seen in leads with predominantly positive QRS complexes.

An analysis of the contour of the abnormal ST segment may be of assistance (**Fig. 3**); this observation is true for both ST segment elevation and ST segment depression. In the consideration of ST segment elevation, this technique uses the morphology of the initial portion of the elevated ST-segment/T-wave – defined as beginning at the J point and ending at the apex of the T-wave. Patients with non-infarctional ST segment elevation (i.e., with benign early repolarization- or left ventricular hypertrophy-related changes) tend to have a concave morphology of the waveform. Conversely, patients with ST segment elevation due to AMI have either obliquely flat or convex waveforms (grouped together as non-concave). The use of this ST segment elevation waveform analysis in emergency department chest pain patients is a very specific clinical tool – meaning that it should be employed in the second tier of medical decision-making with respect to the EKG (**Fig. 1**) allowing the clinician to *rule-in* STEMI. Atypical patterns of STEMI can present with a concave pattern while non-infarction causes of ST segment elevation can manifest a non-concave morphology of the elevated segment. Furthermore, anterior wall STEMI, early in the course of the illness, can manifest concave forms of ST segment elevation [2, 7].

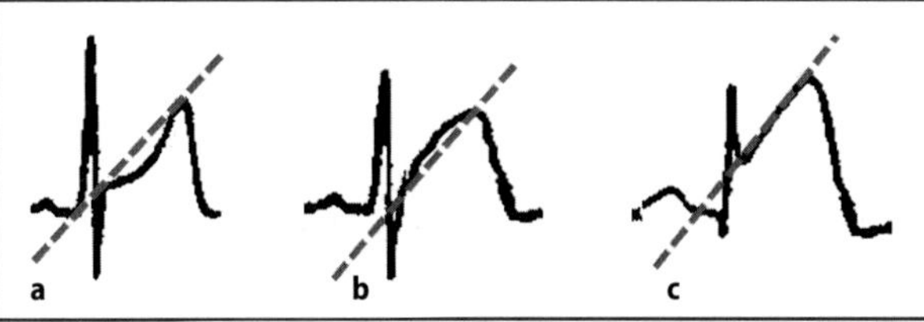

Fig. 3. Morphologic analysis of the elevated ST segment. **a** Concave ST segment elevation (likely non-acute myocardial infarction [AMI]); **b** Convex ST segment elevation (likely AMI); **c** Obliquely straight ST segment elevation (likely AMI).

The shape of the depressed ST segment can also assist in the EKG diagnosis of ACS. ST segment depression is divided into three morphologic classifications: Downsloping, horizontal (flat), and upsloping. Considering the EKG ST depression morphology as a criterion for the diagnosis of ACS, the non-downsloping pattern (horizontal and upsloping) demonstrates reasonably good specificity (91 %) yet a poor sensitivity (35 %) for an ACS diagnosis. Certain patterns with abnormal intraventricular conduction – BBB, ventricular paced rhythm, and left ventricular hypertrophy – will present with ST segment depression as a result of abnormal repolarization. If these patterns are removed, the characteristics of this test are more impressive, with an increased specificity (97 %) for ACS – in other words, the presence of either the flat or upsloping ST depression morphology in chest pain patients with normal intraventricular conduction strongly supports an ACS diagnosis [3].

As seen in BBB, ventricular paced rhythm, and left ventricular hypertrophy patterns, abnormal QRS complex presentations – both increased width and amplitude – can produce ST segment and T wave abnormalities which both mimic and confound the evaluation of potential ACS (**Fig. 4**). A widened complex is one criterion for BBB and/or ventricular-paced rhythm which may cause ST segment/T wave abnormalities. In BBB, the EKG demonstrates a broad QRS complex with a width greater than 0.12 seconds. The LBBB pattern is characterized by a primarily negative QRS complex in lead V1 – usually a QS or rS complex. In leads V5 and V6, a large, positive R wave is seen with similar structures found in leads I and aVl. Poor R wave progression or QS complexes are noted in the right to mid precordial leads, rarely

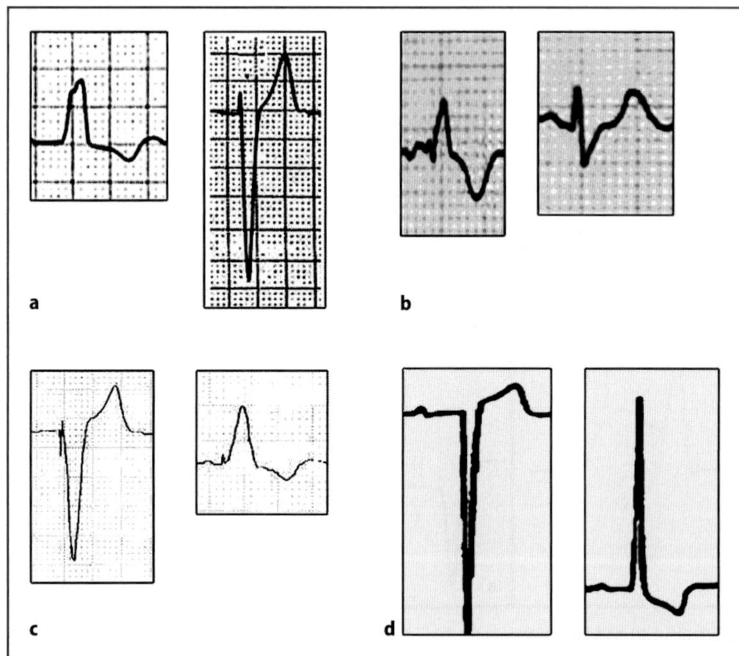

Fig. 4. ST segment and T wave abnormalities associated with left bundle branch block (**a**), right bundle branch block (**b**), right ventricular paced rhythm (**c**), and left ventricular hypertrophy (by voltage criteria) with strain pattern (**d**).

XII

extending beyond leads V4 or V5. QS complexes may also be encountered in leads III and aVF. RBBB most often presents with a wide R wave in lead V1 with a range of specific morphologies, including monophasic R, biphasic RSR', or qR configurations. In lead V6, a wide S or RS wave is seen. QS complexes are encountered in the inferior leads. In the ventricular-paced electrocardiographic pattern, a primarily negative QRS complex is seen in the precordial leads, characterized by either a QS or rS configuration complex. A large monophasic R wave is noted in leads I and aVL and, on occasion, in leads V5 and V6. QS complexes may also be encountered in leads II, III and aVF.

In patients with either BBB or a ventricular-paced EKG pattern, the anticipated or expected ST segment-T wave configurations are discordant, directed opposite from the terminal portion of the QRS complex. This QRS complex-T wave axis discordance is best described using the rule of appropriate discordance (**Fig. 5**). According to this rule, leads with either QS or rS complexes (i.e., complexes which are partially or entirely negative in deflection) may have markedly elevated ST segments while leads with large monophasic R waves (i.e., positive QRS complexes) demonstrate ST segment depression. The T wave, in leads with a negative or primarily negative QRS complex, is prominent with a convex upward shape or a tall, vaulting appearance. The T waves in leads with positive QRS complexes are frequently inverted. Thus, the ST segments and, to a lesser extent, the T waves must be interpreted in a different fashion (**Fig. 6**) if the QRS complex is abnormally large (i.e., left ventricular hypertrophy) or abnormally wide (BBB or ventricular paced rhythm).

As described above, BBB and ventricular-paced rhythms alter the expected ST segment and T wave configurations; the left ventricular hypertrophy pattern also changes the anticipated ST segment and T wave appearances. Large amplitude QRS complexes are a potential clue to EKG left ventricular hypertrophy which, if present, may cause ST segment/T waves changes; in fact, ST segment/T wave changes resulting from altered repolarization of the hypertrophied myocardium, the so-called "strain" pattern, are noted in approximately 70 % of patients with the left ventricular hypertrophy pattern [8]. The left ventricular hypertrophy pattern is identified on the EKG by voltage criteria, including cumulative voltage of the S wave in lead V1 and the R wave in lead V5 or V6, totaling more than 35 millimeters.

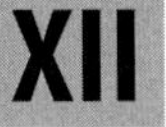

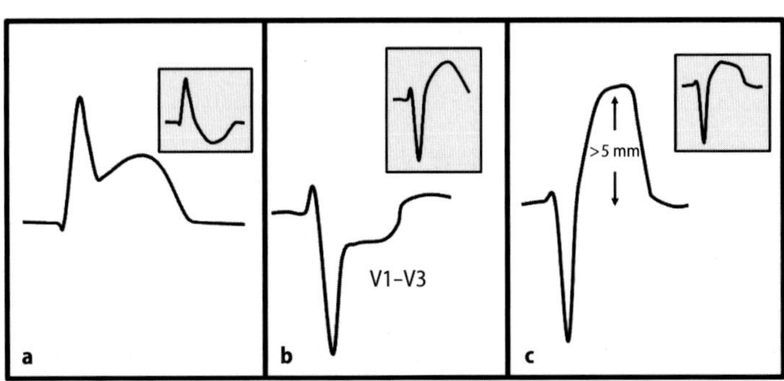

Fig. 5. The concept of appropriate discordance in patients with abnormal intraventricular conduction (bundle branch block and ventricular paced rhythm. **a** Concordant ST segment elevation (normal discordant ST segment depression in box); **b** Concordant ST segment depression in leads V1 to V3 (normal discordant ST segment elevation in box); **c** Excessive (> 5 mm) discordant ST segment elevation (normal [< 5 mm] discordant ST segment elevation in box).

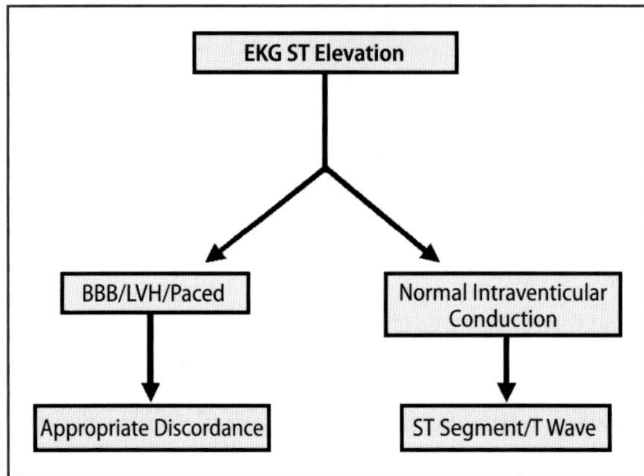

Fig. 6. The impact of abnormal QRS complex configurations on interpretation of ST segment abnormalities.

The EKG consequences of the left ventricular hypertrophy pattern are significant (**Fig. 4**). Left ventricular hypertrophy is associated with poor R wave progression in the right to mid-precordial leads, producing a QS pattern in leads V1, V2, and V3. As predicted by the rule of appropriate discordance, ST segment elevation is encountered in this distribution along with prominent T waves. ST segment depression, characterized by downsloping ST segment depression with asymmetric, biphasic, or inverted T waves in leads with prominent R waves, is seen in the lateral leads.

The presence of T wave abnormality can also assist in establishing the EKG diagnosis. Prominent, upright T waves can suggest early STEMI; the differential diagnosis for the prominent, 'hyperacute' T wave is broad, including early STEMI, hyperkalemia, left ventricular hypertrophy, BBB, benign early repolarization, and acute myopericarditis. Inverted T waves, while not specific for ACS, are associated with acute coronary presentations as well as the sequelae of myocardial infarction; these inverted T waves range in amplitude from minimal to maximal. Other EKG features to consider include PR segment changes (depression and elevation) which is highly associated with acute pericarditis and irregularity of the J point which suggests benign early repolarization.

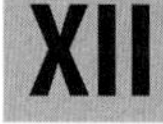

Electrocardiographic Differential Diagnosis – ST Segment Abnormalities[1]

Acute Coronary Syndrome

Acute coronary events can present with a range of ST segment abnormalities, including elevation and depression as well as other changes. Unstable angina, Prinzmetal's (vasospastic or variant) angina, non-ST segment elevation AMI (NSTEMI), and STEMI can demonstrate ST segment abnormalities on the 12-lead EKG. Both unstable angina and NSTEMI have variable EKG presentations with the ultimate distinction between the two diagnoses made by serum marker analysis. A combination of two diagnostic criteria has typically been required in at least one EKG lead to

1 Note the discussion of BBB, ventricular paced rhythm, and left ventricular hypertrophy is found in the *Electrocardiographic Evaluation* section

diagnose a non-STEMI ACS: 1) at least 1.0 mm (0.10 mV) depression at the J point, or 2) either horizontal or downsloping ST segment depression. ST segment depression due to ACS is usually diffuse though it can be located in a specific anatomic distribution (e.g., anterior, lateral, or inferior leads).

One particular ST segment depression presentation is highly associated with STEMI; this form of ST segment depression is termed reciprocal ST segment depression or reciprocal change. This type of ST segment depression occurs in the setting of simultaneous ST segment elevation. The presence of reciprocal change increases the positive predictive value for a diagnosis of AMI to greater than 90 % – i.e., ST segment depression on the EKG in the setting of anatomically arrayed ST segment elevation greatly increases the chance that the ST segment elevation results from AMI. Importantly, ST segment depression seen in EKG situations involving left ventricular hypertrophy, BBB, and/or ventricular-paced patterns is not considered reciprocal ST segment depression.

Within the realm of ACS, ST segment elevation represents either Prinzmetal's angina or STEMI. Prinzmetal's angina will demonstrate ST segment elevation which is obliquely straight or convex; this finding is impossible to distinguish from STEMI without serial measurement of the 12-lead EKG and serum marker analysis. The ST segment elevation related to AMI must be present in at least two anatomically contiguous EKG leads. The magnitude of the elevation ranges from minimal to maximal; at least 1.0 mV of such elevation is necessary.

A subset of the STEMI presentation concerns the isolated posterior wall AMI. From the perspective of the 12-lead EKG, ST segment depression with prominent R wave and upright T wave is seen in the right precordial leads (V1 to V3, **Fig. 7**). When viewed from the posterior perspective (i.e., leads V8 and V9), however, the posterior wall AMI will demonstrate ST segment elevation. EKG abnormalities suggestive of a posterior wall AMI include the following (in leads V1, V2, or V3): Horizontal ST segment depression with tall, upright T waves; a tall, wide R wave; and an R/S wave ratio greater than 1.0 mV in lead V2.

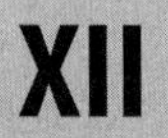

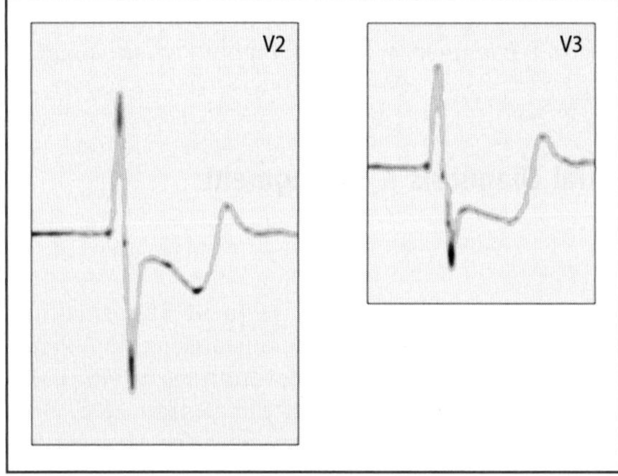

Fig. 7. ST segment depression in the right precordial leads (V2 and V3) suggestive of posterior wall acute myocardial infarction: Prominent R wave, ST segment depression, and upright T wave.

Benign Early Repolarization

Benign early repolarization describes a pattern of ST segment elevation with prominent T waves most often seen in young, apparently healthy male patients; this pattern is a normal variant without known association with cardiac illness. Benign early repolarization occurs in up to one-third of young adult, active patients; the mean age is approximately 40 years with a range of mid teenage to the advanced elderly stages of life. Most patients with benign early repolarization are less than 50 years of age and it is rarely seen in individuals over age 70.

On the EKG, benign early repolarization is diagnosed using the following criteria (**Fig. 8**): ST segment elevation; concavity of the initial, upsloping portion of the ST segment; notching or slurring of the J point; symmetric, concordant, prominent T waves; widespread distribution of the EKG abnormalities on the EKG; and temporal stability. The ST segment is elevated in the benign early repolarization pattern, usually in the 1 to 2 mm range but it may approach 5 mm; the contour of the elevated segment is concave – the ST segment appears to have been lifted off the baseline starting at the J point. In the benign early repolarization pattern, the J point itself is frequently notched or irregular – a highly characteristic finding. Prominent T waves are encountered with a large amplitude and slightly asymmetric morphology. The amplitude of the T wave is greatest in the precordial leads with heights of approximately 6 to 8 mm; T waves in the limb leads are usually 4 to 6 mm in height. The T waves are concordant with the QRS complex (i.e., oriented in the same direction as the major portion of the QRS complex) and are usually found in leads V1 to V4.

Benign early repolarization most often will demonstrate ST segment elevation in the precordial leads followed by a combination of the precordial and limb leads. Importantly, the limb leads less often manifest ST segment elevation – in other words, ST segment elevation in the limb leads without similar findings in the precordial leads is rare and should prompt consideration of another diagnosis, such as AMI.

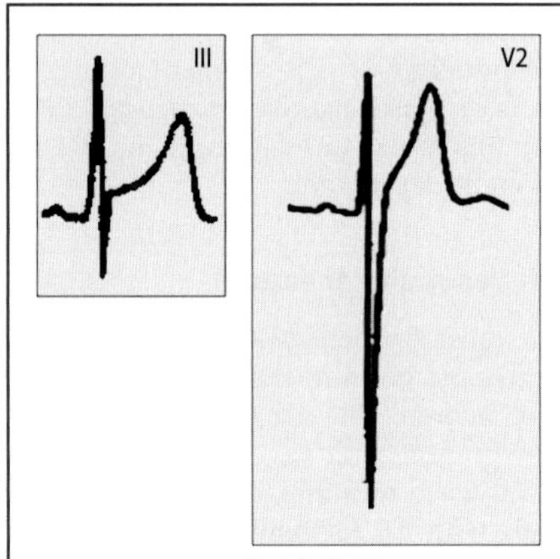

Fig. 8. ST segment elevation as seen in benign early repolarization.

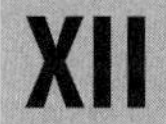

Acute Myopericarditis

Acute myopericarditis presents across a variable range of EKG abnormalities. These abnormalities result from epicardial inflammation; note that the pericardial membrane is electrically silent. The EKG abnormalities evolve through four classic stages. Stage I is characterized by ST segment elevation, prominent T wave, and PR segment depression (**Fig. 9**). Stage II is distinguished by a normalization of the initial abnormalities while stage III involves T wave inversion in the anatomic segments previously affected with the ST segment elevation. Stage IV is characterized by a normalization of all changes with a return to the baseline. The evolution of these EKG stages occurs in a very unpredictable manner with stages I through III developing over several hours to several days; stage IV then occurs over a generally longer period of time.

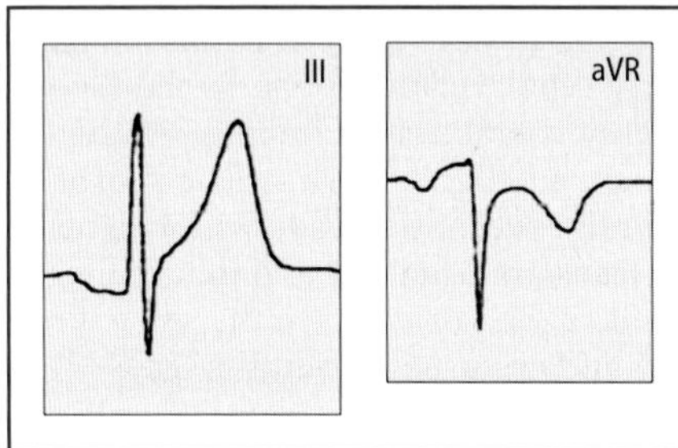

Fig. 9. ST segment elevation as seen in acute myopericarditis (lead III); also note the ST segment depression with PR segment elevation in lead aVR.

Stage I abnormality, namely ST segment elevation, is usually electrocardiographically obvious. The ST segment elevation is usually less than 5 mm in magnitude, concave in morphology, and widespread in distribution. Reciprocal ST segment depression is seen in lead aVR and occasionally in lead V1. The ST segment elevation is most often seen in many leads simultaneously though it may be limited to a specific anatomic segment if the process is focal. PR segment abnormality, resulting from atrial epicardial inflammation, is a highly suggestive EKG feature of stage I myopericarditis. PR segment depression is described as "almost diagnostic" for acute myopericarditis; "reciprocal" PR segment elevation is seen in lead aVR (**Fig. 9**); in many cases, this finding is in fact more obvious to the clinician compared to PR segment depression.

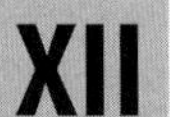

Left Ventricular Aneurysm

The most frequent EKG manifestation of ventricular aneurysm is ST segment elevation, most often in the anterior distribution; inferior and lateral aneurysms are also encountered. The actual ST segment abnormality due to the ventricular aneurysm may present with varying morphologies, ranging from obvious, convex ST segment elevation to minimal, concave elevations. Pathologic Q waves are usually observed in leads with ST segment elevation. A calculation of the ratio of the amplitude of the T wave to the QRS complex may help distinguish anterior STEMI from ventricular aneurysm. If the ratio of the amplitude of the T wave to the QRS complex exceeds 0.36 in any single lead, the EKG likely reflects AMI. If this ratio is less than 0.36 in all leads, however, the findings likely result from ventricular aneurysm [9].

Other Patterns with ST Segment Abnormality

Certain intracranial events, such as subarachnoid hemorrhage and intracerebral bleeds, may produce ST segment/T wave changes. Most often, these alterations involve the T wave with deep inversions in the right to mid precordial leads. Relatively minor degrees of ST segment elevation are also encountered in leads with obviously abnormal T waves.

The hypothermic EKG triad includes the Osborne (or J) wave, bradycardia, and tremor artifact. The Osborne wave is formed at the juncture between the terminal portion of the QRS complex and the initial ST segment – the J point. The J point itself and the immediately adjacent ST segment appears to have lifted unevenly off the baseline.

The EKG manifestations of digitalis – the digoxin effect – include a 'scooped' form of ST segment depression, most prominent in the inferior and anterior leads. The ST segment morphology is characterized by a gradual, downsloping initial limb and an abrupt return to the baseline. Note that this form of ST segment depression is not indicative of digoxin toxicity.

Cardiomyopathy may produce EKG patterns such as ST segment changes, T wave abnormalities, widened QRS complexes, and pathologic Q waves. Cardiomyopathy may produce significant Q waves in the inferior and anterior leads. These leads can also demonstrate ST segment elevation with prominent T waves.

The Brugada syndrome is characterized by a RBBB pattern with ST segment elevation in the right precordial leads; these patients have a tendency for sudden cardiac death resulting from polymorphic ventricular tachycardia [10]. EKG abnormalities that suggest the diagnosis include RBBB (complete and incomplete) and ST segment elevation in leads V1, V2, and/or V3.

Takastubo cardiomyopathy (also known as the left ventricular apical ballooning syndrome) is a recently described disorder in which patients develop anginal symptoms with acute congestive heart failure during times of stress; on occasion, serum markers can be abnormal yet, at cardiac catheterization, abnormal left ventricular function and normal coronary arteries are noted [11]. EKG findings seen include ST segment elevation (90 % of patients), T wave inversion (50 %), and abnormal Q waves (25 %). These findings are most often transient, presenting only when the patient is symptomatic and resolving during physiologically normal periods [12].

Numerous other clinical scenarios and events will manifest ST segment abnormality, including post-electrical cardioversion, non-ACS myocardial injury (e.g., traumatic contusion), and rate-related (non-ACS) changes seen in tachycardic patients.

References

1. Brady WJ, Perron AD, Martin ML, Beagle C, Aufderheide TP (2001) Electrocardiographic ST segment elevation in emergency department chest pain center patients: Etiology responsible for the ST segment abnormality. Am J Emerg Med 19: 25–28
2. Brady WJ, Syverud SA, Beagle C, et al (2001) Electrocardiographic ST segment elevation: The diagnosis of AMI by morphologic analysis of the ST segment. Acad Emerg Med 8: 961–967
3. Brady WJ, Dobson T, Holstege C, et al (2004): Electrocardiographic ST segment depression: Association with ACS. Acad Emerg Med 11: 419 (abst)
4. Brady WJ, Perron AD, Ullman EA (2002) ST segment elevation: A comparison of electrocardiographic features of AMI and non-AMI ECG syndromes. Am J Emerg Med 20: 609–612
5. Brady WJ, Perron AD, Syverud SA, et al (2002) Reciprocal ST segment depression: Impact on

the electrocardiographic diagnosis of ST segment elevation acute myocardial infarction. Am J Emerg Med 20: 35–38

6. Otto LA, Aufderheide TP (1994) Evaluation of ST segment elevation criteria for the prehospital electrocardiographic diagnosis of acute myocardial infarction. Ann Emerg Med 23: 17–24
7. Kosuge M, Kimura K, Ishikawa T, et al (1999) Value of ST-segment elevation pattern in predicting infarct size and left ventricular function at discharge in patients with reperfused acute anterior myocardial infarction. Am Heart J 137: 522–527
8. Huwez FU, Pringle SD, Macfarlane PW (1992) Variable patterns of ST-T abnormalities in patients with left ventricular hypertrophy and normal coronary arteries. Br Heart J 67: 304–307
9. Smith S, Nolan M (2003) Ratio of T amplitude to QRS amplitude best distinguishes acute anterior MI from anterior left ventricular aneurysm. Acad Emerg Med 10: 516 (abst)
10. Brugada P, Brugada J (1992) Right bundle branch block, persistent ST segment elevation and sudden cardiac death: A distinct clinical and electrocardiographic syndrome. J Am Coll Cardiol 20: 1391–1396
11. Akashi YJ, Nakazawa K, Sakakibara M, Miyake F, Koike H, Sasaka K (2003) The clinical features of takotsubo cardiomyopathy. QJM 96: 563–573
12. Tsuchihashi K, Ueshima K, Uchida T, et al (2001) Transient left ventricular apical ballooning without coronary artery stenosis: A novel heart syndrome mimicking AMI. J Am Col Cardiol 38: 11–18

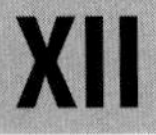

Functional Mitral Regurgitation in the Critically Ill

J. Poelaert

Introduction

Functional mitral regurgitation is the consequence of left ventricular systolic dysfunction in the presence of an anatomically normal mitral valve. Systolic left ventricular failure is often the cause of congestive heart failure, which is a frequent reason for admission to the intensive care unit (ICU). The most frequent cause of left ventricular dysfunction is ischemic heart disease. Both the ventricle and the mitral valve apparatus are involved in the pathogenesis of functional mitral regurgitation. The mitral valve is a complex apparatus, composed of the mitral valve leaflets, the chordae tendineae, papillary muscles, and the related regional area of the ventricular wall (**Fig. 1**). Malfunction of one or more components of this apparatus engenders improper functioning of the mitral valve.

Pathological mitral regurgitation, although heterogeneous in etiology, is a common corollary of ischemic cardiomyopathy, with great impact on mortality and morbidity, and its prevalence increases with age. Other causes of mitral regurgitation are related to myxomatous degeneration, endocarditis, and rheumatic disease [1]. The clinical outcome of this disease in the critically ill is scantily defined. The frequency of mitral regurgitation within society is difficult to estimate, but its causes are easier

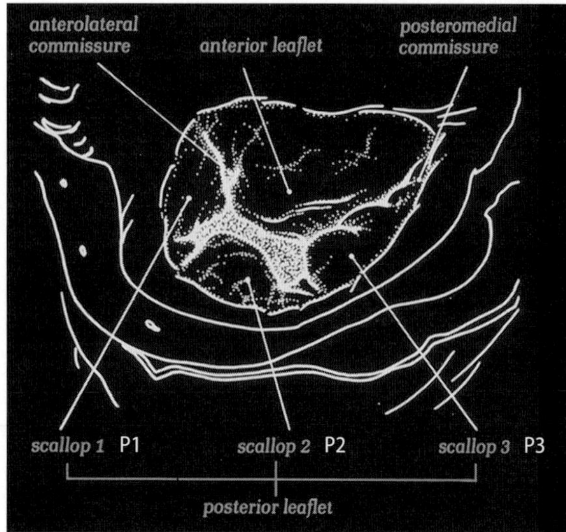

Fig. 1. The anatomy of the normal mitral valve. The different segments as used by cardiac surgeons, have been indicated.

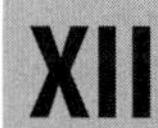

to assess. Ischemic heart disease is the most frequent cause of death with great impact on quality of life for survivors. Ischemic mitral regurgitation doubles late mortality [2, 3]. Optimal care must include estimation of ventricular contractile reserve with respect to estimation of function and prognosis [4]. Furthermore, high-risk subgroups must be defined. To improve outcomes, these high-risk patients, even with asymptomatic mitral regurgitation, may benefit from surgical treatment [5]. The presence of mitral regurgitation after myocardial infarction should thus be taken into account in post-myocardial infarction risk stratification [6].

In this chapter, we will summarize the pathophysiological mechanisms, the diagnostic features, and the subsequent therapeutic management of functional mitral regurgitation.

Definition

Functional mitral regurgitation is the insufficiency occurring as a consequence of left ventricular dysfunction. The valve leaflets are completely normal and the regurgitant jet is straight into the left atrium, underlining the absence of any pathologic feature of the valve leaflets. Characteristic to functional mitral regurgitation is the abnormal and increased tension on the leaflets (tethering force), in conjunction with a sometimes severely (although potentially intermittent) decreased left ventricular function. **Table 1** summarizes the different causes of acute mitral regurgitation.

Mitral regurgitation is not always pathological. In a transesophageal echocardiographic (TEE) study, mitral regurgitation was shown to be present in 36 % of healthy volunteers [7]. Pathological mitral regurgitation flows are characterized by broad (> 10 mm) regurgitant jets with a long duration (> 30 ms) (**Fig. 2**). Further-

Table 1. Causes of acute mitral regurgitation in the critically ill.

Leaflet disorders
Myxomatous degeneration with acute deterioration of function
Rheumatic valve disease
Infective endocarditis
Trauma: penetrating or iatrogenic
Annular disorders
Dilation, concomitant with LV dilatation
Calcification
Chordae tendineae
Rupture (ischemic heart disease, calcification, trauma)
Lengthening
Retraction: rheumatic valve disease
Papillary muscles
Displacement, secondary to left ventricular remodeling
Infarction
Trauma
Regional wall motion abnormalities: Ischemic heart disease
Invading disorders
Infiltrative disorders: Amyloidosis, sarcoidosis
Tumors: atrial myxoma

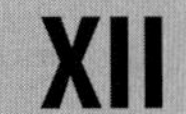

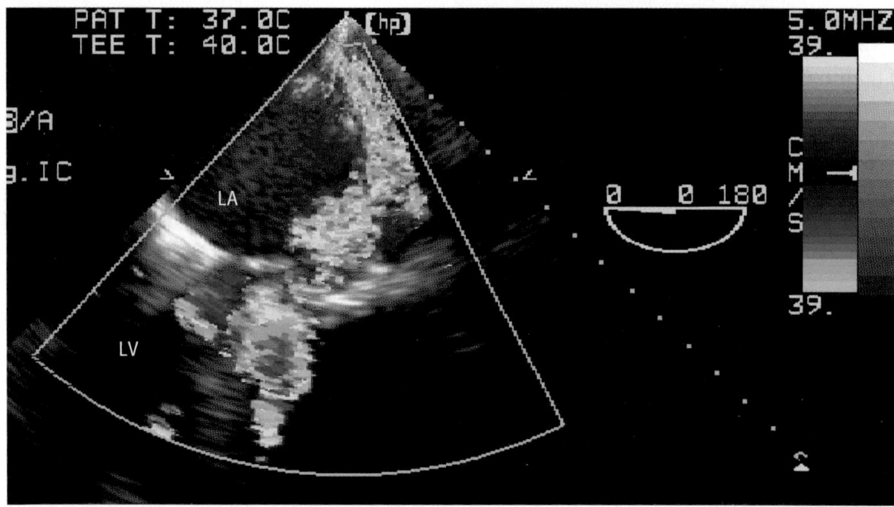

Fig. 2. Color Doppler evaluation is the mainstay for grading the severity of mitral regurgitation. Both the width and the length of the regurgitant jet in the left atrium (LA) should be assessed. LV: left ventricle

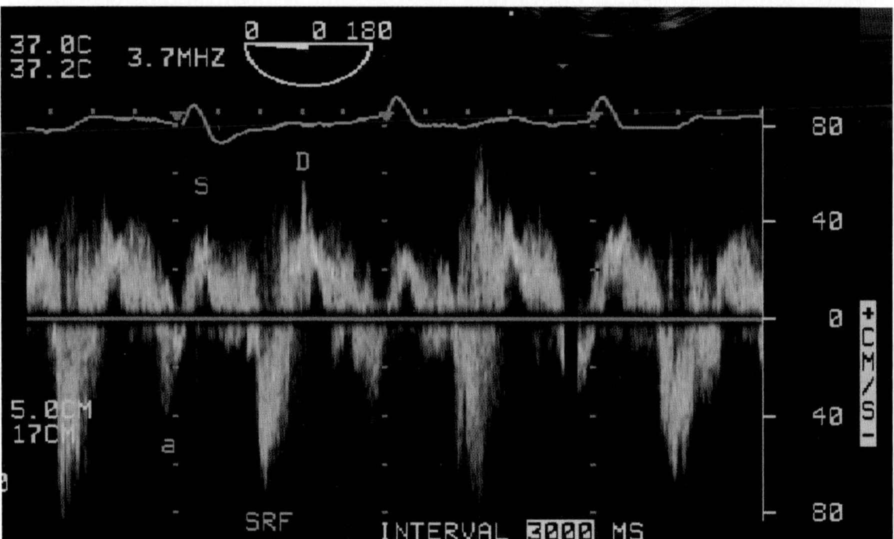

Fig. 3. Characteristic pattern of a pulmonary venous Doppler signal, with a large systolic reverse flow wave (SRF) and an enlarged reverse atrial contraction wave (a).

more, a characteristic pattern in the pulmonary veins is obtained with pulsed wave Doppler: the regurgitant flow is so high that it is deviated towards the right and/or left pulmonary veins (**Fig. 3**), inducing a backward directed increased atrial contraction flow wave due to the high residual volume in the left atrium, a blunted systolic forward flow wave, mainly due to a major systolic reverse flow wave, and finally a delayed filling of the left atrium with an increased diastolic flow wave. Other diagnostic features will be discussed below.

Pathophysiology

Opening of the mitral valve depends completely on the pressure gradient created throughout diastole; filling of the left ventricle starts with the energy consuming left ventricular relaxation and concomitant descent of left ventricular pressure below left atrial pressure. Proper closure of the mitral valve depends on the balance between the closing force, generated by the contraction of the left ventricle, and the tethering forces, built up between the anterolateral and posteromedial papillary muscles and the mitral annulus. Coaptation time and length are two features of the closure of the mitral valve. Functional mitral regurgitation is characterized by an imbalance between the tethering forces, inducing tenting of the mitral valve, and the closing force of the left ventricle. Coaptation time will be reduced when tethering forces are inadequately opposed by, e.g., decreased systolic left ventricular function, inhibiting the leaflets from reaching their proper closing point in time, at the level of the annulus. Coaptation length is reduced by tethering of the papillary muscles and the annular dilatation. The pathophysiological triad of mitral regurgitation was originally described by Carpentier et al., identifying three distinct classes of mitral valve disease [8]. These are summarized in **Table 2**. Functional mitral regurgitation is the first class. In contrast to the other classes described by Carpentier et al., a completely normal mitral valve is found in functional mitral regurgitation.

At the level of the leaking mitral valve, the regurgitant blood volume depends on the afterload characteristics of the left ventricle. Increased afterload (arterial hypertension, aortic stenosis) will increase, and low blood pressure and shock will decrease the regurgitant volume. In addition, whenever the tethering forces decrease, e.g., with akinesia or dyskinesia of the zone of a papillary muscle, mitral regurgitation may decrease or vanish completely, even with diminished closing force of the left ventricle.

Analysis of the acute effects of mitral regurgitation in comparison with aortic regurgitation on the left ventricle show a lesser increase in left ventricular end-diastolic pressure and volume following acute mitral regurgitation. In comparison with acute aortic regurgitation, acute mitral regurgitation reduces intraventricular pressure and left ventricular radius more, decreasing left ventricular wall tension. Hence, the ratio of left ventricular end-systolic wall thickness to radius is lower with acute mitral regurgitation than with acute aortic regurgitation [9].

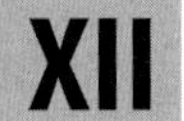

Functional mitral regurgitation is rather the consequence of dilation of the left ventricle, decreased closing force, and systolic mitral valve tenting and, hence,

Table 2. Different characteristics of the mitral valve apparatus with respect to the various types of mitral regurgitation, as described by Carpentier et al. [8].

type	leaflets	leaflet motion	coaptation annulus	annulus	papillary muscles
I	Normal	normal	below	dilation	perforation possible
II	Thickening possible	Increased (prolapse)	above		(chordal) rupture/elongation
IIIa	Thickening	Systole, diastole restricted	below	thickening	
IIIb	Thickening	Systole restricted	below	thickening	apical displacement

incomplete closure of the mitral leaflets [10]. Dilation of the left ventricle alone already induces incomplete closure of the leaflets and production of a systolic mitral regurgitation flow. Characteristically, this jet is directed towards the roof of the left atrium [11]. After a myocardial infarction, the left ventricle undergoes secondary remodeling, explaining why recurrent leakage of the mitral valve may occur after initial correction of the mitral leakage by mitral annuloplasty [12].

Whenever regional wall motion abnormalities (severe hypokinesia, akinesia or dyskinesia) are present in the region of the papillary muscles, displacement of the papillary muscles as a consequence of left ventricular remodeling may occur. Traction occurs on the leaflets, displacing the coaptation point apically, finally resulting in a tented mitral valve (**Table 2**). In contrast, leaflet movement above the level of the annulus is either the consequence of rupture of chordae at the tip of or in the middle of the leaflet, resulting in prolapse or bulging of the leaflet, respectively (**Table 2**).

Diagnosis

Echocardiographic evaluation of a mitral valve should include the following aspects:

1. assessment of closure of the leaflets at the annular level
2. appropriateness of the closure (coaptation)
3. completeness of the valvular apparatus (i.e., chordae tendineae, papillary muscles, regional function of the ventricular wall)
4. color Doppler of the mitral valve, including estimation of the effective regurgitant orifice, the width and length of the jet, Doppler flow assessment of both transmitral and pulmonary veins (left and right)
5. assessment of right ventricular function and pulmonary hypertension
6. exclusion of aortic regurgitation/stenosis.

It cannot be stressed sufficiently that in acute circumstances an echocardiographic investigation should start with a short axis view of the left and right ventricle [13, 14], providing direct insight into important features, such as global systolic function, including presence of dilatation, (static) preload, and presence of regional wall motion abnormalities. The importance of obtaining all this information by eye-balling one view is immense; both exclusion of the heart as a cause of shock in a newly admitted ICU patient, and immediate (although rough) diagnosis of ventricular failure may be addressed with one view [14].

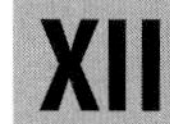

Estimation of the severity of functional mitral regurgitation is summarized in **Table 3**. Assessment of closure of the leaflets should encompass the level of closure. Closure above the annular plane indicates billowing (fixed tips of the leaflets and thus, intact chordae tendineae at this level, although ruptured chordae or part of a papillary muscle attached in the middle of the leaflet), prolapse (ruptured chordae, connected to the tips of the leaflets), or both. Closure below the annular level suggests increased tethering forces of the chordae resulting in tenting of the mitral valve leaflets. All these features can be elegantly seen with 3D-echocardiography [15].

It is essential to assess left ventricular size and function. A left ventricular end-systolic diameter above 45 mm is an important sign of dilatation, resulting in inadequate coaptation of the leaflets, even hampering closure at the level of the mitral annulus. Patients with an effective regurgitant orifice of 40 mm^2 minimally, have been shown to be at higher risk of death and complications than those with a smaller effective regurgitant orifice [5]. In addition to simple eye-balling, left ven-

Table 3. Estimation of the severity of functional mitral regurgitation, characterized by a central regurgitant jet.

Technique	mild	severe
Color Doppler jet length	not to LA roof	to LA roof
Vena contracta width	< 0.3 cm	> 0.6 cm
Filling LA by color jet	< 20 %	> 40 %
Flow convergence	absent or minimal	large
Pulmonary venous Doppler	$S > D$	$S < D$
LV end-systolic diameter	< 45 mm	> 45 mm
EROA	< 0.2 cm^2	≥ 0.4 cm^2

D, diastolic flow wave velocity, obtained at the level of one of the entries of the pulmonary veins; EROA, effective regurgitant orifice area (cm^2); LA, left atrium; LV, left ventricle; S, systolic flow wave velocity, obtained at the level of one of the entries of the pulmonary veins.

tricular systolic function can now be assessed easily using myocardial Doppler imaging at the level of the mitral annulus [16]. Systolic tissue velocities below 8 cm/s suggest decreased left ventricular systolic function. Care should be taken to interpret these data in view of preload conditions, as the systolic tissue velocity at the mitral annulus is preload dependent [17].

Furthermore, the completeness of the mitral valvular apparatus and its function must be checked, including chordae, papillary muscles, and the function of the ventricular wall.

Echocardiographic estimation of the presence of increased pulmonary artery pressures is best obtained from a continuous wave Doppler signal across the tricuspid valve [18, 19].

Associated pathology may have considerable impact on prognosis and outcome determination. Decreased right ventricular systolic function in conjunction with functional mitral regurgitation was reported to have a mortality rate of 28 % [20]. Survivors had a prolonged stay in the hospital because of heart failure. In this respect, it is important to evaluate both left and right ventricular function and estimate right ventricular systolic pressure from a trans-tricuspid flow pattern [18]. Knowledge of pulmonary artery hypertension is important in view of optimal support of right ventricular function.

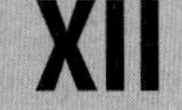

Finally, the difference between acute and chronic mitral regurgitation should be discussed (**Table 4**). In chronic mitral regurgitation, onset is most often insidious and gradual, with symptomatology (dyspnea) rather moderate. The left heart bears the stigmata of chronic disease: A dilated left atrium with decreased compliance, emptying into a dilated and sometimes hypertrophic left ventricle with decreased

Table 4. Differences between acute and chronic severe mitral regurgitation, with respect to functional mitral regurgitation.

Symptomatology	Acute	Chronic
Onset	Acute	Insidious, gradual
Clinical picture	Severely ill	Moderate dyspnea
Echo LV size	Normal	Dilation, LVH
Echo LV function	Hyperkinesia	Normal-reduced
Echo LA size/compliance	Normal/normal-reduced	Dilation/reduced
Etiology	AMI, trauma, ...	IHD, endocarditis, ...

AMI, acute myocardial infarction; IHD, ischemic heart disease; LA, left atrium; LVH, left ventricular hypertrophy.

function. In contrast, acute mitral regurgitation is often combined with a hyperkinetic left ventricle.

Therapeutic Management

Medical

Medical treatment alone is indicated whenever asymptomatic mitral regurgitation is present and the effective regurgitant orifice is < 40 mm^2, as explained above. All measures valid for the support of heart failure should be included in the treatment of functional mitral regurgitation. In this respect, vasodilator therapy is the mainstay to unload the left ventricle and to reduce regurgitation into the left atrium as much as possible. In acute mitral regurgitation, nitroprusside, a mixed venous and arterial vasodilator, is the drug of choice. Endocarditis prophylaxis should be started concomitantly. Measures should be undertaken to also support right and left ventricular function and to reduce pulmonary hypertension.

Surgical

Surgery should be considered in symptomatic patients with important mitral regurgitation. Coronary artery bypass grafting (CABG) alone, without concomitant mitral annuloplasty appears to have little benefit on outcome [21], suggesting that preoperative evaluation to guide intraoperative therapy is warranted. Intraoperative TEE consistently underestimates preoperative findings [21–23]. Several therapeutic options have been introduced over the years. Mitral annuloplasty seems a logical approach, to compensate for the dilation of the left ventricle [8]. Introduction of an undersized annuloplasty ring leads to reduction of end-diastolic left ventricular volume, improvement of ejection fraction, and diminished regurgitant volumes [24]. Care should be taken of residual mitral regurgitation, which could be related to inadequate downsizing of the annular ring, resulting in inadequate coaptation. A new development results in improved coaptation due to a reduced anteroposterior dimension allowing the often tethered P2-P3 segments to coapt more appropriately. Three-dimensional echocardiography may help to improve the choice of the annular ring, in particular when considering imitating the saddle shape of the native mitral annulus [15]. Recurrent mitral regurgitation is often related to continued remodeling of the left ventricle.

More than the surgical procedure itself, it is important for intensivists to know when patients with acute mitral regurgitation should be scheduled for surgery. It is now general policy to present patients in cardiac failure class II (dyspnea on heavy exertion) with an end-systolic left ventricular diameter > 45 mm and an end-systolic volume of > 50 ml/m^2 body surface area. Less symptomatic patients should be carefully followed even after discharge from the ICU.

Conclusion

Full understanding of the nature of functional mitral regurgitation should help in correctly detecting this disease with all its pitfalls and consequences in the critically ill. Diagnosis starts with awareness of its potential presence and a subsequent pathophysiological approach to the mechanisms of this mitral regurgitation. Assessment should encompass all facets of Doppler-echocardiography, including Doppler, myocardial Doppler imaging, and 3D-echocardiography, if available, to assess left and right ventricular function, and the respective preloads and afterloads. All facets of the mitral valve apparatus should be examined in this respect. Only these measures, followed by appropriate management will improve survival of patients with functional mitral regurgitation.

References

1. Cohn LH, Kowalker W, Bhatia S, et al (1988) Comparative morbidity of mitral valve repair versus replacement for mitral regurgitation with and without coronary artery disease. Ann Thorac Surg 45: 284–290
2. Gomez-Doblas JJ, Schor J, Vignola P, et al (2001) Left ventricular geometry and operative mortality in patients undergoing mitral valve replacement. Clin Cardiol 24: 717–722
3. Lamas GA, Mitchell GF, Flaker GC, et al (1997) Clinical significance of mitral regurgitation after acute myocardial infarction. Survival and Ventricular Enlargement Investigators. Circulation 96: 827–833
4. Lee R, Haluska B, Leung DY, Case C, Mundy J, Marwick TH (2005) Functional and prognostic implications of left ventricular contractile reserve in patients with asymptomatic severe mitral regurgitation. Heart 91: 1407–1412
5. Enriquez-Sarano M, Avierinos JF, Messika-Zeitoun D, et al (2005) Quantitative determinants of the outcome of asymptomatic mitral regurgitation. N Engl J Med 352: 875–883
6. Bursi F, Enriquez-Sarano M, Nkomo VT, et al (2005) Heart failure and death after myocardial infarction in the community: the emerging role of mitral regurgitation. Circulation 111: 295–301
7. Taams MA, Gussenhoven EJ, Cahalan MK, et al (1989) Transesophageal Doppler color flow imaging in the detection of native and Bjork-Shiley mitral valve regurgitation. J Am Coll Cardiol 13: 95–99
8. Carpentier A, Chauvaud S, Fabiani JN, et al (1980) Reconstructive surgery of mitral valve incompetence: ten-year appraisal. J Thorac Cardiovasc Surg 79: 338–348
9. Nwasokwa O, Camesas A, Weg I, Bodenheimer MM (1989) Differences in left ventricular adaptation to chronic mitral and aortic regurgitation. Chest 95: 106–110
10. Yiu SF, Enriquez-Sarano M, Tribouilloy C, Seward JB, Tajik AJ (2000) Determinants of the degree of functional mitral regurgitation in patients with systolic left ventricular dysfunction: A quantitative clinical study. Circulation 102: 1400–1406
11. Yoshida K, Yoshikawa J, Yamaura Y, et al (1990) Value of acceleration flows and regurgitant jet direction by color Doppler flow mapping in the evaluation of mitral valve prolapse. Circulation 81: 879–885
12. Hung J, Papakostas L, Tahta SA, et al (2004) Mechanism of recurrent ischemic mitral regurgitation after annuloplasty: continued LV remodeling as a moving target. Circulation 110: II85–90
13. Poelaert J, Schmidt C, Colardyn F (1998) Transoesophageal echocardiography in the critically ill. Anaesthesia 53: 55–68
14. Poelaert JI, Schupfer G (2005) Hemodynamic monitoring utilizing transesophageal echocardiography: The relationships among pressure, flow, and function. Chest 127: 379–390
15. Otsuji Y, Handschumacher MD, Schwammenthal E, et al (1997) Insights from three-dimensional echocardiography into the mechanism of functional mitral regurgitation: direct in vivo demonstration of altered leaflet tethering geometry. Circulation 96: 1999–2008
16. Edvardsen T, Urheim S, Skulstad H, Steine K, Ihlen H, Smiseth OA (2002) Quantification of left ventricular systolic function by tissue doppler echocardiography: Added value of measuring pre- and postejection velocities in ischemic myocardium. Circulation 105: 2071–2077
17. Amà R, Segers P, Roosens C, Claessens T, Verdonck P, Poelaert J (2004) Effects of load on systolic mitral annular velocity by tissue Doppler imaging. Anesth Analg 99: 332–338
18. Berger M, Haimowitz A, Van Tosh A, Berdoff R, Goldberg E (1985) Quantitative assessment of pulmonary hypertension in patients with tricuspid regurgitation using continuous wave Doppler ultrasound. J Am Coll Cardiol 6: 359–365

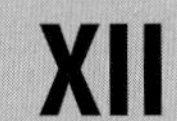

19. Quiles J, Garcia-Fernandez MA, Almeida PB, et al (2003) Portable spectral Doppler echocardiographic device: overcoming limitations. Heart 89: 1014–1018
20. Dini FL, Conti U, Fontanive P, et al (2007) Right ventricular dysfunction is a major predictor of outcome in patients with moderate to severe mitral regurgitation and left ventricular dysfunction. Am Heart J 154: 172–179
21. Aklog L, Filsoufi F, Flores KQ, et al (2001) Does coronary artery bypass grafting alone correct moderate ischemic mitral regurgitation? Circulation 104:I68–75
22. Czer LS, Maurer G, Bolger AF, DeRobertis M, Chaux A, Matloff JM (1996) Revascularization alone or combined with suture annuloplasty for ischemic mitral regurgitation. Evaluation by color Doppler echocardiography. Tex Heart Inst J 23: 270–278
23. Bach D, Deeb M, Bolling S (1995) Accuracy of intraoperative transesophageal echocardiography for estimating the severity of functional mitral regurgitation. Am J Cardiol 76: 508–512
24. Bolling SF (2002) Mitral reconstruction in cardiomyopathy. J Heart Valve Dis 11 (Suppl 1):S26–31

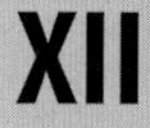

XIII Cardiopulmonary Resuscitation

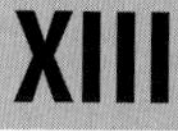

Feedback to Improve the Quality of CPR

J. Yeung, J. Soar, and G.D. Perkins

Introduction

Ischemic heart disease is a leading cause of death in the world and many people die prematurely from sudden cardiac arrest. It is estimated that 40–46,0000 people in the USA and 700,000 people in Europe experience sudden cardiac arrest each year [1]. Cardiopulmonary resuscitation (CPR) is the attempt to restore spontaneous circulation by performing chest compressions with or without ventilations [2]. Early and effective CPR, prompt defibrillation, early advanced life support, and post-resuscitation care are key components in the 'Chain of Survival' [3]. Standardized resuscitation guidelines and training courses in CPR and advanced life support have been developed in order to improve outcomes from cardiac arrest. These have been implemented through most of Europe, the USA and many other developed countries. Despite this, observational studies report that the quality of CPR in both the out-of-hospital and in-hospital setting is often poor and that survival rates remain low despite significant advances in the science of resuscitation [4–6]. Technological advances mean that it is now possible to measure the quality of CPR during actual resuscitation attempts. Feedback techniques for both individuals and teams are now being developed to improve the quality of CPR during both training and actual resuscitation attempts.

The Importance of Quality CPR

Studies from the early 1990s were among the first to start to make the link between the quality of CPR and patient outcome. Wik and colleagues observed that the quality of CPR by bystanders was associated with outcome [4]. Good quality CPR was defined in this study as the presence of a palpable pulse upon arrival of the paramedic. The investigators found improved survival to hospital discharge rates among patients who received good quality bystander CPR (23 % survival) as opposed to poor quality CPR (1 % survival) or no CPR (6 % survival) prior to the arrival of the emergency medical service (EMS). Similar findings were also observed at the same time by Gallagher et al. [5] and Van Hoeyweghen et al. [6] in 2071 and 3306 consecutive out-of-hospital cardiac arrests in New York and Belgium, respectively.

Chest Compressions

Effective chest compressions are essential to promote forward blood flow and maintain heart and brain perfusion. However, even optimal chest compressions only deliver 20–25 % of normal organ blood flow [7]. Chest compression depth, rate, and interruptions in chest compressions have been shown to have a direct influence on patient outcome [7, 8].

Animal studies show a linear relationship between chest compression depth and coronary perfusion pressure and that the 'effectiveness' of CPR is sensitive to small changes in compression depth [9, 10]. These findings were confirmed in humans in the late 1980s by Ornato et al. who demonstrated a linear relationship between compression force delivered by a Thumper™ device and systolic blood pressure and end-tidal CO_2 [11]. Based on these data the International Liaison Committee for Resuscitation recommended that chest compression depth should be between 40–50 mm in adults [12]. This corresponds to approximately 20 % of the anteroposterior diameter of an adult chest [13].

Recent studies have shown that chest compression depth does influence patient survival. Using an accelerometer device placed on the chest to measure sternal movement, Edelson et al. [7] found an association between chest compression depth and the probability of shock success in a mixed population of in- and out-of-hospital patients in ventricular fibrillation. A higher mean compression depth during the 30 seconds of CPR preceding a defibrillation attempt was associated with an increased chance of shock success (adjusted odds ratio 1.99 for every 5 mm increase; 95 % confidence interval 1.08–3.66). In this study, all five patients with a mean compression depth of 50 mm had successful defibrillation. Using the same device, Kramer-Johansen et al. [8] showed in a logistic regression analysis of 208 out-of-hospital resuscitation attempts that an increase in compression depth was associated with a better chance of admission to hospital alive (odds ratio 1.05 (95 % CI; 1.01, 1.09) per mm increase in compression depth).

The International Liaison Committee for Resuscitation recommends that chest compressions are performed at a rate of 100 per minute. Animal models of cardiac arrest [14–16] show a constant stroke volume and improved hemodynamics by increasing compression rate up to 130 to 150/min, with the duty cycle maintained at 50 % (time in compression versus decompression). Abella et al. examined chest compressions in 97 in-hospital resuscitation attempts and found a greater return of spontaneous circulation in patients receiving chest compressions at rates above 87 per minute compared to those with a compression rate below 72 per minute (75 % versus 43 %) [17].

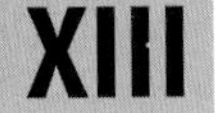

Interruptions in Chest Compressions

Interruptions in chest compressions (also referred to as no-flow time or hands-off time) are common during resuscitation [18, 19]. Whilst some interruptions are necessary such as during defibrillation or pulse/rhythm checks, many of the interruptions observed in practice are avoidable. Two specific contributors to no-flow time are the period between cessation of chest compression prior to a defibrillation shock (known as the pre-shock pause) and the time following the shock to resumption of chest compression (post-shock pause) [8]. Prolonged pre- and post-shock pauses are associated with a reduced chance of successful defibrillation.

Yu et al. were one of first groups to demonstrate the adverse effects of prolonged pre-shock pauses [20]. Using a porcine model of prolonged (7 min) ventricular fibrillation the effect of increasing pre-shock pauses on return of spontaneous circulation rates and post resuscitation hemodynamic function was evaluated. The durations of pre-shock pauses were modeled on the time taken for commercially available automated external defibrillators to analyze the rhythm, charge the capacitor, and deliver a shock (range 10 to 19.5 seconds). The study showed that return of spontaneous circulation rates were significantly higher in animals treated with minimal (3 second) pre-shock pause as opposed to those treated with a 15 or 20 second pre-shock pause (100 % survival versus 20 % and 0 % respectively). Prolonged pre-shock pauses were associated with more marked myocardial dysfunction in the 24 hours after return of spontaneous circulation.

Two physiological explanations have been suggested for how interruptions in chest compressions reduce shock success. The traditional explanation is that interruptions in chest compressions reduce coronary perfusion pressure [20], which decreases the probability of return of spontaneous circulation after attempted defibrillation [21]. Alternatively, Chamberlain et al. suggest that chest compressions empty the right ventricle and thus reduce ventricular interaction in the arrested heart. Reducing ventricular interaction will increase left ventricular volume and hence myocyte stretch. Therefore, when defibrillation takes place and coordinated electrical activity is restored, the heart is able to generate an effective contraction [22].

The findings by Yu et al. [20] were subsequently confirmed in observational studies in humans which showed that an increase in the duration of the pre-shock pause was associated with a reduction in the likelihood of shock success. Eftestol et al. used ventricular fibrillation waveform prediction models on electrocardiogram (EKG) outputs from humans in cardiac arrest to show that increasing pre-shock pauses (as brief as 5 seconds) were associated with a 50 % relative reduction in the calculated probability of return of spontaneous circulation [23]. Edelson et al. demonstrated that first shock success (defined as removal of ventricular fibrillation for at least 5 seconds following defibrillation) was associated with shorter pre-shock pauses (adjusted odds ratio of 1.86 for every 5 second decrease in pre-shock pause) [7]. Berg and colleagues used a pig model of prolonged ventricular fibrillation to show that a delay in resuming chest compressions after defibrillation was associated with reduced return of spontaneous circulation and neurologically intact survival at 48 hours [24]. These data provide a clear rationale for reducing the duration of pre-shock and post-shock pauses.

Ventilation Rate and Hyperventilation

Resuscitation guidelines in 2005 recommended a ventilation rate of 8–10 breaths per minute during CPR [2]. In practice, most rescuers ventilate at much higher rates leading to hyperventilation and hypocarbia [25]. Ventilations can interrupt chest compression and reduce vital organ perfusion. Positive pressure ventilation increases intrathoracic pressure and decreases venous return to the heart, rendering CPR less effective. Aufderheide et al. [26] reproduced ventilation rates seen in an observational study during actual resuscitation attempts in a pig model of ventricular fibrillation cardiac arrest. The study showed that an excessive ventilation rate (30/min) increased intrathoracic pressure, reduced coronary perfusion pressure and lowered survival compared to a slower ventilation rate (12/min). The addition of supplemental CO_2 to the inspired gas in the hyperventilation group to correct for hypocarbia failed to correct these harmful effects. This implies that raised intrathoracic pressure is the predominant harmful mechanism when high ventilation rates are used during CPR.

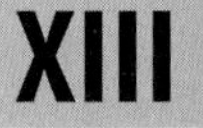

The Quality of CPR is often Sub-optimal during Clinical Resuscitation Attempts

A number of prospective observational studies have demonstrated that the quality of CPR during in-hospital and out-of--hospital resuscitation attempts is frequently sub-optimal. Abella et al. [18] studied 67 patients who suffered in hospital cardiac arrests and analyzed parameters of CPR quality. Chest compression rates were too slow (< 90/min) 28.1 % of the time and 37.4 % of chest compressions were of inadequate depth (< 38 mm). Ventilation rates were excessive nearly two thirds of the time. Chest compressions were only performed for 76 % of the resuscitation attempts [18]. The findings were similar in the study by Wik et al. of 176 out-of-hospital resuscitation attempts [19]. In this study, chest compressions were not given during 48 % (95 % CI, 45 – 51 %) of the resuscitation attempts. Chest compression depth averaged 34 mm (95 % CI, 33 – 35 mm) with 72 % of compressions below 38 mm [19]. Poor quality CPR is not limited to clinical resuscitation attempts. In an observational study of clinicians under direct supervision during advanced resuscitation simulation training, we found that chest compressions were almost always too shallow (97 %) and no compressions were performed for 37 % of the resuscitation attempts [27].

Losert et al. reported that it is possible to perform high quality CPR with a motivated and experienced team [28]. Data from 80 patients with non-traumatic cardiac arrest admitted to the emergency department showed that the highly trained emergency department staff performed good quality chest compressions (rate 96/min) with only 7 % of chest compressions being too shallow and that no-flow durations (without chest compressions) were similarly low (12.7 %). However, there was scope for improvement as 32 % of patients were hyperventilated.

Technologies introduced to facilitate early defibrillation such as the automated external defibrillator (AED or shock advisory defibrillator) may not be achieving their full potential due to the delays imposed by the device between cessation of chest compression and shock delivery. Pauses ranging from 5.2 to 28.4 seconds [29] have been reported during which the defibrillators analyzed the underlying heart rhythm and charged the capacitor in preparation for shock delivery. A direct comparison between AEDs and manual defibrillation showed that the pre- and post-shock pauses were longer in patients receiving shocks from AEDs than from manual defibrillators (22 vs 15 s and 20 vs 9 s, respectively). However, 26 % of shocks given via the manual defibrillator were given inappropriately (when the adjudication panel defined the rhythm as non-shockable) compared to only 6 % in the AED group [30].

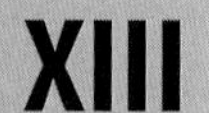

Strategies for Improving the Quality of CPR

Real-time Feedback during CPR Training and Actual Resuscitation

Subjective evaluation of resuscitation performance by CPR instructors is limited by the difficulty of assessing the adequacy of performance by observation alone, particularly the adequacy of ventilation and chest compression [31]. Audio (e.g., metronome for compression rate or audible click when adequate compression depth is achieved) and visual feedback (e.g., lights illuminating when adequate compression depth is achieved) have been incorporated into resuscitation training manikins for a number of years. The use of these devices during training has a positive effect on both initial skill acquisition and retention of skills several weeks after initial training [32].

More sophisticated devices have been developed recently that convert objective measures of CPR performance (e.g., compression depth) into spoken instructions on how performance can be improved (e.g., shallow chest compressions prompt the instruction "press a little harder"). The audible instructions can be combined with visual displays to further enhance performance. Wik et al. showed that the use of one of these devices during basic life support training improved the proportion of correctly performed compressions from a mean of 33 to 77 % and correct inflations from a mean of 9 to 58 % [33]. The improved performance was maintained both 6 and 12 months after initial training [34, 35]. Sutton et al. also found similar improvements in skill acquisition in providers of pediatric basic life support using this technology compared to one-on-one instructor led training. In addition to better CPR parameters, volunteers also had lower error rates in chest compressions and ventilations, resulting in higher pass rates in skills testing [36].

Technological advances have allowed the integration of performance feedback into portable devices which can be used during actual resuscitation attempts. **Figure 1** shows an example of two such devices where feedback from an accelerometer placed on the victim's chest (to measure compression parameters) and transthoracic impedance measurements (to detect ventilation) are used to provide audio and visual feedback on performance during actual resuscitation attempts.

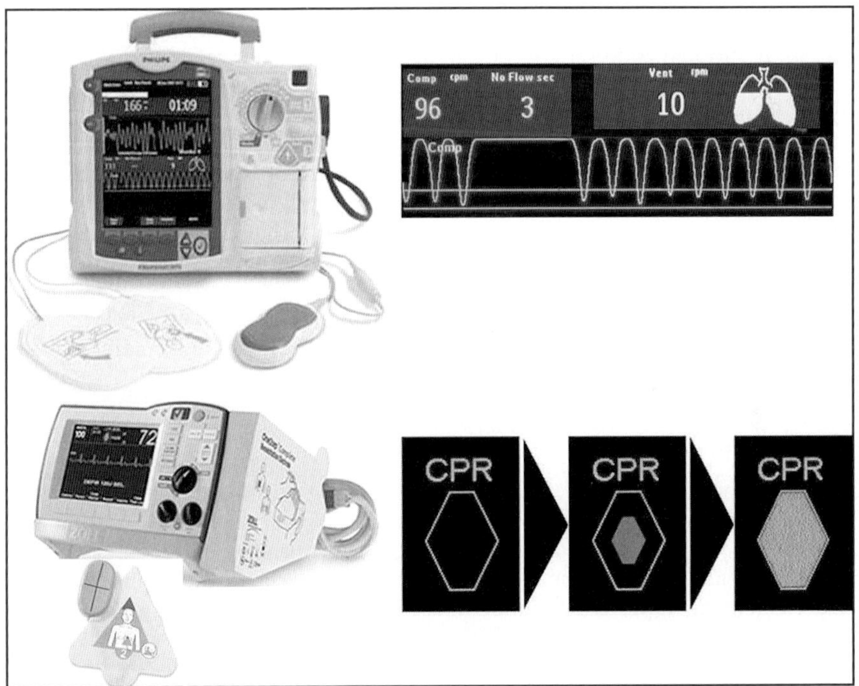

Fig. 1. Examples of commercially available cardiopulmonary resuscitation (CPR) feedback devices. The small rectangular box (accelerometer) is placed on the patient's sternum and used to measure sternal movement and compression rate. Changes in transthoracic impedance or end-tidal CO_2 are used to monitor ventilation rates. Displays on the defibrillator monitor provide visual feedback on compression +/- ventilation performance. The visual feedback may be supplemented by audible prompts such as "compress the chest deeper".

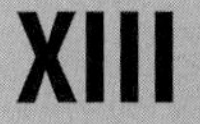

The impact of introducing this technology into clinical practice has been evaluated in three prospective before-after cohort studies. Kramer-Johansen et al. [8] reported improved CPR quality with real time automated feedback in pre-hospital cardiac arrests when the technology was introduced across three European ambulance services. Resuscitation attempts after introduction of the device had significantly greater compression depth (38 versus 34 mm), percentage of correct compression depth (53 versus 24 %) and compression rate (109 versus 121/min). The importance of introducing the technology in a coordinated and structured manner with supporting education and training was highlighted when the same team introduced it into a fourth ambulance service [37]. On this occasion the feedback technology failed to lead to any improvement in CPR quality. This was ascribed to a lack of supporting infrastructure and training for those using the device. A similarly disappointing result was found when the device was introduced into a hospital based resuscitation system. Despite showing less variation in CPR quality measures between resuscitation attempts in the feedback group there were no significant differences in the quality of CPR after the introduction of the feedback technology [38].

The use of these devices is not without potential limitations. The accuracy of the devices for measuring chest compression depth may be influenced by the surface the victim is positioned on. If the victim is situated on a compressible surface such as a bed and mattress then most devices are unable to take account of the degree of compression of the underlying mattress. Thus compressions registering on the device as being of adequate depth may in fact still be too shallow due to a failure to compensate for additional compression of the mattress [39]. We investigated this phenomenon using a commercially available accelerometer device and found that CPR guided by the feedback device led to significant under compression of the chest as 35–40 % of the total compression depth measured was attributable to compression of the underlying mattress [40]. Using a backboard to increase the stiffness of the bed/mattress had little effect on improving compression depth in this model. Other potential limitations to feedback devices include increased mechanical work required to perform chest compressions [41] and the potential for injury to rescuers associated with moving parts in certain devices [42]. To date, no randomized controlled clinical trials have been conducted to investigate the clinical benefits or otherwise of these devices, so the clinical impact of introducing these technologies remains to be determined.

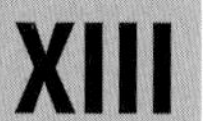

Post-event Debriefing

The use of post event debriefing in simulator based training has been shown to significantly improve team performance [43] and is widely used by the military and in aviation for improving future performance particularly in the context of rare or stressful events. Participation as a member of a cardiac arrest team can be a stressful and challenging experience. Junior doctors have reported feeling un-prepared and concerned about managing cardiac arrest and have called for more feedback on their performance [44]. In addition to potentially being able to improve the quality of CPR, post-event debriefing may have a part to play in reducing stress amongst members of the resuscitation team.

Dine et al. investigated a strategy of post-event debriefing among nurses during advanced resuscitation training [45]. Following a simulated cardiac arrest, participants received a 5-min structured program of post-arrest debriefing in which the participants were shown the actual transcript of their own CPR efforts and briefly counseled on how to improve their CPR to comply with consensus resuscitation guidelines. Post-event debriefing in this format led to significant improvements in the quality of CPR. These improvements were further augmented when real-time audiovisual feedback was available during the resuscitation attempt. The combination of feedback and debriefing improved compression rate compliance from 45 to 84 % ($p = 0.001$) and doubled the number of compressions of adequate rate and depth (29 versus 64 %, $p = 0.005$).

Post-event debriefing of medical residents after in-hospital resuscitation attempts was studied in a before-after cohort study by investigators from the University of Chicago [46]. A unique debriefing program (Resuscitation with Actual Performance Integrated Debriefing, RAPID) was introduced to allow discussion of cases during a 45 minute session each week. Cardiac arrest data transcripts detailing the quality of CPR, EKG traces, and problems with specific resuscitation attempts were converted into presentation slides. These were used to provide feedback on performance and to reinforce the scientific evidence behind resuscitation techniques. Compared to the historical control group (who received real time audiovisual feedback on CPR performance only) the RAPID cohort delivered improved ventilation rates (13 vs 18/min, $p < 0.001$) and increased compression depth (50 vs 44 mm, $p = 0.001$) compared with the control group. Knowledge about resuscitation among the members of the cardiac arrest team also improved significantly. There were also improved patient outcomes (increase in return of spontaneous circulation rate from 44.6 to 59.4 %, $p = 0.03$). This is the best real patient study to date supporting the use of debriefings for resuscitation teams. The study used a historical control group and spanned the change in resuscitation guidelines in 2005. This is a potential confounding factor as the new guidelines emphasized the importance of CPR quality and of minimizing interruptions in chest compression.

Future Developments in Technology

Remote guidance and feedback to lay rescuers who witness a collapse may be possible with new mobile cellular phone technology in the future. In a manikin study, untrained individuals given audiovisual prompts sent by an ambulance dispatch center to a cellular phone were more likely to deliver chest compressions than those who received telephone instructions alone [47]. The use of new video phones to guide and provide feedback during a resuscitation attempt is also being studied.

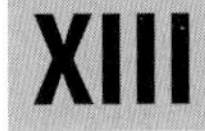

Strategies to reduce the pre-shock pause imposed by AEDs are also being investigated. These may include reducing the number of voice prompts, pre-charging the capacitor during CPR, and new diagnostic algorithms to reduce the time taken for rhythm analysis. Filtering technology to remove the artefacts created by CPR has also now been developed. This would allow rhythm analysis to take place during ongoing CPR. This approach was investigated using a databank of EKG traces from 229 patients in cardiac arrest [48]. The algorithm was able to identify a shockable rhythm with a sensitivity of 93 % and a specificity of 89 %, yielding a positive predictive value of 91 %. A non-shockable rhythm was identified with a sensitivity of 89 %, a specificity of 93 %, and a positive predictive value of 91 % during uninterrupted chest compression.

Utilization of signals frequently collected by defibrillators, such as transthoracic impedance and EKG signals, may also play a role in providing feedback on the quality of CPR. Transthoracic impedance measurements through defibrillator pads are already used in some defibrillators to monitor ventilation rate. In an experimental study in humans, investigators found that monitoring transthoracic impedance could also reliably detect esophageal intubation [49]. Analysis of the EKG signal, particularly the characteristics of the ventricular fibrillation waveform is able to predict the likelihood of shock success. Using this technology Li et al. were able to differentiate between good and poor quality CPR in a pig model of cardiac arrest [50]. The development of these and related technologies is likely to play an increasing role in providing feedback to aid the delivery of optimal CPR to patients in the future.

Conclusion

Good quality CPR improves survival from cardiac arrest. Numerous studies show that the quality of CPR is poor during training and real resuscitation attempts. Feedback devices that measure CPR quality during actual skill performance and provide prompts to correct any deficiencies can improve skill performance. Feedback devices may reduce rescuer fatigue and improve willingness to perform CPR in lay people. Real time audio feedback during CPR has been called 'The Guardian Angel of CPR' [51]. It has also been suggested that audio feedback on AEDs will enable 'the untrained layperson to become the next critical care practitioner' [52]. There is good evidence to support the regular use of feedback devices during training and whenever available in cardiac arrest situations. The use of feedback devices during actual CPR followed by a post-event briefing may further improve skill performance during subsequent resuscitation attempts.

References

1. International Liaison Committee for Resuscitation (2005) International Consensus on Cardiopulmonary Resuscitation and Emergency Cardiovascular Care Science with Treatment Recommendations. Part 1: introduction. Resuscitation 67: 181–186
2. Jacobs I, Nadkarni V, Bahr J, et al (2004) Cardiac arrest and cardiopulmonary resuscitation outcome reports: update and simplification of the Utstein templates for resuscitation registries. A statement for healthcare professionals from a task force of the international liaison committee on resuscitation. Resuscitation 63: 233–249
3. Perkins GD, Soar J (2005) In hospital cardiac arrest: missing links in the chain of survival. Resuscitation 66: 253–255
4. Wik L, Steen PA, Bircher NG (1994) Quality of bystander cardiopulmonary resuscitation influences outcome after prehospital cardiac arrest. Resuscitation 28: 195–203
5. Gallagher EJ, Lombardi G, Gennis P (1995) Effectiveness of bystander cardiopulmonary resuscitation and survival following out-of-hospital cardiac arrest. JAMA 274: 1922–1925
6. Van Hoeyweghen RJ, Bossaert LL, Mullie A, et al (1993) Quality and efficiency of bystander CPR. Belgian Cerebral Resuscitation Study Group. Resuscitation 26: 47–52
7. Edelson DP, Abella BS, Kramer-Johansen J, et al (2006) Effects of compression depth and preshock pauses predict defibrillation failure during cardiac arrest. Resuscitation 71: 137–145
8. Kramer-Johansen J, Myklebust H, Wik L, et al (2006) Quality of out-of-hospital cardiopulmonary resuscitation with real time automated feedback: a prospective interventional study. Resuscitation 71: 283–292
9. Babbs CF, Voorhees WD, Fitzgerald KR, Holmes HR, Geddes LA (1983) Relationship of blood pressure and flow during CPR to chest compression amplitude: evidence for an effective compression threshold. Ann Emerg Med 12: 527–532
10. Bellamy RF, DeGuzman LR, Pedersen DC (1984) Coronary blood flow during cardiopulmonary resuscitation in swine. Circulation 69: 174–180

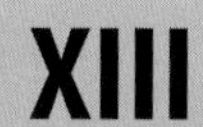

11. Ornato JP, Levine RL, Young DS, Racht EM, Garnett AR, Gonzalez ER (1989) The effect of applied chest compression force on systemic arterial pressure and end-tidal carbon dioxide concentration during CPR in human beings. Ann Emerg Med 18: 732–737
12. International Liaison Committee for Resuscitation (2005) International Consensus on Cardiopulmonary Resuscitation and Emergency Cardiovascular Care Science with Treatment Recommendations. Part 2: Adult basic life support. Resuscitation 67: 187–201
13. Pickard A, Darby M, Soar J (2006) Radiological assessment of the adult chest: implications for chest compressions. Resuscitation 71: 387–390
14. Maier GW, Tyson GS Jr, Olsen CO, et al (1984) The physiology of external cardiac massage: high-impulse cardiopulmonary resuscitation. Circulation 70: 86–101
15. Halperin HR, Tsitlik JE, Guerci AD, et al (1986) Determinants of blood flow to vital organs during cardiopulmonary resuscitation in dogs. Circulation 73: 539–550
16. Feneley MP, Maier GW, Kern KB, et al (1988) Influence of compression rate on initial success of resuscitation and 24 hour survival after prolonged manual cardiopulmonary resuscitation in dogs. Circulation 77: 240–250
17. Abella BS, Sandbo N, Vassilatos P, et al (2005) Chest compression rates during cardiopulmonary resuscitation are suboptimal: a prospective study during in-hospital cardiac arrest. Circulation 111: 428–434
18. Abella BS, Alvarado JP, Myklebust H, et al (2005) Quality of cardiopulmonary resuscitation during in-hospital cardiac arrest. JAMA 293: 305–310
19. Wik L, Kramer-Johansen J, Myklebust H, et al (2005) Quality of cardiopulmonary resuscitation during out-of-hospital cardiac arrest. JAMA 293: 299–304
20. Yu T, Weil MH, Tang W, et al (2002) Adverse outcomes of interrupted precordial compression during automated defibrillation. Circulation 106: 368–372
21. Paradis NA, Martin GB, Rivers EP, et al (1990) Coronary perfusion pressure and the return of spontaneous circulation in human cardiopulmonary resuscitation. JAMA 263: 1106–1113
22. Chamberlain D, Frenneaux M, Steen S, Smith A (2008) Why do chest compressions aid delayed defibrillation? Resuscitation 77: 10–15
23. Eftestol T, Sunde K, Steen PA (2002) Effects of interrupting precordial compressions on the calculated probability of defibrillation success during out-of-hospital cardiac arrest. Circulation 105: 2270–2273
24. Berg RA, Hilwig RW, Berg MD, et al (2008) Immediate post-shock chest compressions improve outcome from prolonged ventricular fibrillation. Resuscitation 78: 71–76
25. O'Neill JF, Deakin CD (2007) Do we hyperventilate cardiac arrest patients? Resuscitation 73: 82–85
26. Aufderheide TP, Sigurdsson G, Pirrallo RG, et al (2004) Hyperventilation-induced hypotension during cardiopulmonary resuscitation. Circulation 109: 1960–1965
27. Perkins GD, Boyle W, Bridgestock H, et al (2008) Quality of CPR during advanced resuscitation training. Resuscitation 77: 69–74
28. Losert H, Sterz F, Kohler K, et al (2006) Quality of cardiopulmonary resuscitation among highly trained staff in an emergency department setting. Arch Intern Med 166: 2375–2380
29. Snyder D, Morgan C (2004) Wide variation in cardiopulmonary resuscitation interruption intervals among commercially available automated external defibrillators may affect survival despite high defibrillation efficacy. Crit Care Med 32:S421–424
30. Kramer-Johansen J, Edelson DP, Abella BS, et al (2007) Pauses in chest compression and inappropriate shocks: A comparison of manual and semi-automatic defibrillation attempts. Resuscitation 73: 212–220
31. Lynch B, Einspruch EL, Nichol G, Aufderheide TP (2008) Assessment of BLS skills: Optimizing use of instructor and manikin measures. Resuscitation 76: 233–243
32. Spooner BB, Fallaha JF, Kocierz L, et al (2007) An evaluation of objective feedback in basic life support (BLS) training. Resuscitation 73: 417–424
33. Wik L, Thowsen J, Steen PA (2001) An automated voice advisory manikin system for training in basic life support without an instructor. A novel approach to CPR training. Resuscitation 50: 167–172
34. Wik L, Myklebust H, Auestad BH, Steen PA (2002) Retention of basic life support skills 6 months after training with an automated voice advisory manikin system without instructor involvement. Resuscitation 52: 273–279

35. Wik L, Myklebust H, Auestad BH, Steen PA (2005) Twelve-month retention of CPR skills with automatic correcting verbal feedback. Resuscitation 66: 27–30
36. Sutton RM, Donoghue A, Myklebust H, et al (2007) The voice advisory manikin (VAM): an innovative approach to pediatric lay provider basic life support skill education. Resuscitation 75: 161–168
37. Olasveengen TM, Tomlinson AE, Wik L, et al (2007) A failed attempt to improve quality of out-of-hospital CPR through performance evaluation. Prehosp Emerg Care 11: 427–433
38. Abella BS, Edelson DP, Kim S, et al (2007) CPR quality improvement during in-hospital cardiac arrest using a real-time audiovisual feedback system. Resuscitation 73: 54–61
39. Perkins GD, Smith CM, Augre C, et al (2006) Effects of a backboard, bed height, and operator position on compression depth during simulated resuscitation. Intensive Care Med 32: 1632–1635
40. Perkins GD, Kocierz L, Smith SCL, McCulloch R, Davies RP (2009) Compression feedback devices over estimate chest compression depth when performed on a bed. Resuscitation 80: 79–82
41. van Berkom PF, Noordergraaf GJ, Scheffer GJ, Noordergraaf A (2008) Does use of the CPREzy involve more work than CPR without feedback? Resuscitation 78: 66–70
42. Perkins GD, Augre C, Rogers H, Allan M, Thickett DR (2005) CPREzy: an evaluation during simulated cardiac arrest on a hospital bed. Resuscitation 64: 103–108
43. Townsend RN, Clark R, Ramenofsky ML, Diamond DL (1993) ATLS-based videotape trauma resuscitation review: education and outcome. J Trauma 34: 133–138
44. Hayes CW, Rhee A, Detsky ME, Leblanc VR, Wax RS (2007) Residents feel unprepared and unsupervised as leaders of cardiac arrest teams in teaching hospitals: a survey of internal medicine residents. Crit Care Med 35: 1668–1672
45. Dine CJ, Gersh RE, Leary M, et al (2008) Improving cardiopulmonary resuscitation quality and resuscitation training by combining audiovisual feedback and debriefing. Crit Care Med 36: 2817–2822
46. Edelson DP, Litzinger B, Arora V, et al (2008) Resuscitation with actual performance integrated debriefing (RAPID) improves CPR quality and initial patient survival. Resuscitation Science Symposium A61:29 (abst)
47. Choa M, Park I, Chung HS, et al (2008) The effectiveness of cardiopulmonary resuscitation instruction: animation versus dispatcher through a cellular phone. Resuscitation 77: 87–94
48. Li Y, Bisera J, Geheb F, Tang W, Weil MH (2008) Identifying potentially shockable rhythms without interrupting cardiopulmonary resuscitation. Crit Care Med 36: 198–203
49. Kohler KW, Losert H, Myklebust H, et al (2008) Detection of malintubation via defibrillator pads. Resuscitation 77: 339–344
50. Li Y, Ristagno G, Bisera J, et al (2008) Electrocardiogram waveforms for monitoring effectiveness of chest compression during cardiopulmonary resuscitation. Crit Care Med 36: 211–215
51. Heightman AJ (2005) The guardian angel of CPR. JEMS 30:4
52. Pepe PE, Wigginton JG (2006) Key advances in critical care in the out-of-hospital setting: the evolving role of laypersons and technology. Crit Care 10:119

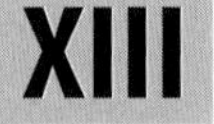

The Post-cardiac Arrest Syndrome

J.P. Nolan and R.W. Neumar

Introduction

Survival rates following in- and out-of-hospital cardiac arrest remain disappointingly low [1–3] but there is good evidence that interventions applied after return of spontaneous circulation influence significantly the chances of survival with good neurological outcome [4]. Among those patients admitted to an intensive care unit (ICU) after cardiac arrest, approximately two thirds will not survive to be discharged from hospital [5, 6], but there is considerable variation in post-cardiac arrest treatment and patient outcome between institutions [6, 7]. The prolonged period of systemic ischemia during cardiac arrest and the subsequent reperfusion response that occurs after return of spontaneous circulation results in a complex combination of pathophysiological processes that have been termed recently the post-cardiac arrest syndrome [8]. The components of post-cardiac arrest syndrome comprise post-cardiac arrest brain injury, post-cardiac arrest myocardial dysfunction, systemic ischemia/reperfusion response, and persistent precipitating pathology. A recent scientific statement from the International Liaison Committee on Resuscitation (ILCOR) and several other organizations provides comprehensive information about the epidemiology, pathophysiology, treatment, and prognostication of the post-cardiac arrest syndrome [8]. This chapter will highlight the main messages to come from this scientific statement.

Phases of the Post-cardiac Arrest Syndrome

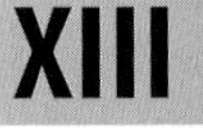

The post-cardiac arrest period can be divided into four phases (**Fig. 1**) [8]. The immediate post-arrest phase is defined as the first 20 minutes after return of spontaneous circulation. This phase will be influenced by interventions that are typically applied at the site of the initial collapse. The early post-arrest phase is between 20 minutes and 6 to 12 hours after return of spontaneous circulation; early interventions applied during transport, in the emergency department and in the ICU will impact this phase. The intermediate phase is between 6 to 12 hours and 72 hours when injury pathways are still active and may be influenced by further treatment in the ICU. Finally, the recovery phase is the period beyond 3 days – this is when prognostication becomes more reliable.

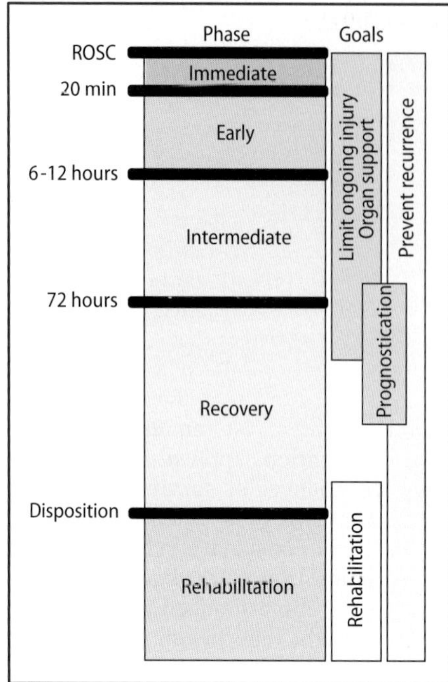

Fig. 1. Phases of post-cardiac arrest syndrome. ROSC = return of spontaneous circulation. From [8] with permission.

Pathophysiology of Post-cardiac Arrest Syndrome

The severity of the post-cardiac arrest syndrome will vary depending on the severity of the ischemic insult, the cause of cardiac arrest, and the patient's pre-arrest state of health. The post–cardiac arrest syndrome is unlikely to occur if return of spontaneous circulation is achieved rapidly.

Post-cardiac Arrest Brain Injury

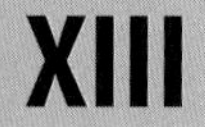

Of those patients who survive to ICU admission but who die later in hospital, brain injury is the cause of death in approximately two thirds of cases after out-of hospital cardiac arrest and in about a quarter of cases after in-hospital cardiac arrest [9]. The pathophysiological processes leading to brain injury in these circumstances are complex and include excitotoxicity, disrupted calcium homeostasis, free radical formation, pathological protease cascades, and activation of cell death signaling pathways [10]. Many of these processes occur over hours to days after return of spontaneous circulation, which provides a reasonable window for potential treatment. Intravascular thrombosis may occur during prolonged cardiac arrest and, after return of spontaneous circulation, can impair cerebral microcirculatory reperfusion despite adequate cerebral perfusion pressure (CPP) [11]. This provides part of the rationale for the use of thrombolytic therapy during cardiac arrest [12]. Although there is cerebral microcirculatory failure, elevated CPP and impaired cerebrovascular autoregulation may result in high cerebral blood flow (CBF) soon after return of spontaneous circulation [13]; this may result in transient brain edema, especially after asphyxial cardiac arrest, but it is rarely associated with clinically relevant increases in intracranial pressure (ICP). The CPP necessary to maintain optimal cerebral perfusion will vary among individual post-cardiac arrest patients and with the interval after return of spontaneous circulation.

Pyrexia [14], seizures [15], and hyperglycemia [16] are all associated with worse neurological outcome among post-cardiac arrest patients.

Post-cardiac Arrest Myocardial Dysfunction

Post–cardiac arrest global myocardial dysfunction is common but is often responsive to therapy and reversible [17]. In one series of 148 patients who survived out-of-hospital cardiac arrest, cardiac index was lowest at 8 hours after resuscitation and returned to normal by 72 hours [17].

Systemic Ischemia/reperfusion Response

With the onset of cardiac arrest, the delivery of oxygen and metabolic substrates and the removal of metabolites cease. Cardiopulmonary resuscitation (CPR) only partially reverses this process, achieving cardiac output and oxygen delivery that is much less than normal. The whole body ischemia/reperfusion of cardiac arrest followed by return of spontaneous circulation activates immunological and coagulation pathways causing a systemic inflammatory response syndrome (SIRS) that resembles sepsis [18, 19]. Activation of blood coagulation without adequate activation of endogenous fibrinolysis causes widespread microvascular thrombosis [20].

Persistent Precipitating Pathology

The pathophysiology of the post–cardiac arrest syndrome may be complicated by the presence of precipitating pathologies such as acute coronary syndrome (ACS), pulmonary diseases, hemorrhage and sepsis. Acute myocardial infarction is documented in approximately 50 % of adult out-of-hospital cardiac arrest patients and in many cases there is no history of chest pain and ST-segment elevation is absent [4, 21]. Pulmonary emboli have been reported in 2 % to 10 % of sudden deaths [3, 22]. The incidence of pulmonary embolism among patients who achieve return of spontaneous circulation after cardiac arrest is unknown. Multiple organ failure is a more common cause of death in the ICU after initial resuscitation from in-hospital cardiac arrest than after out-of-hospital cardiac arrest. This may reflect the greater contribution of infections to cardiac arrest in the hospital [9].

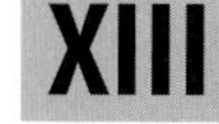

Treatment of the Post-cardiac Arrest Syndrome

Treatment of the post–cardiac arrest patient will involve several specialties. Some of these patients will have a prolonged ICU stay and require multiple organ support. There is some evidence that a coordinated multimodal approach improves outcome when compared with historical controls [4]. A post-cardiac arrest ICU care bundle has been proposed and comprises: Early coronary reperfusion and hemodynamic optimization; control of ventilation; blood glucose control; temperature control; and treatment of seizures [23].

Airway and Ventilation

There are no data supporting precise indications for intubation, ventilation, and sedation after cardiac arrest. Although cerebral autoregulation is either absent or altered in most patients in the acute phase after cardiac arrest [13], cerebrovascular reactivity to changes in arterial carbon dioxide tension is preserved [24]. Extrapolation from studies of brain-injured patients indicating that hyperventilation induces cerebral ischemia implies that ventilation to normocarbia is probably optimal.

Adequate oxygen delivery is essential, but animal data indicate that too much oxygen during the initial stages of reperfusion can exacerbate neuronal damage through production of free radicals and mitochondrial injury [25]. Animal studies have demonstrated neurological benefits of controlled reoxygenation during the initial phases of resuscitation by ventilating with the minimum FiO_2 required to maintain adequate oxygen saturation of arterial blood (SaO_2 94–96 %) [26]. Based on these data, avoid unnecessary arterial hyperoxia, particularly during the initial post-cardiac arrest period. This can be achieved by adjusting the FiO_2 to produce an SaO_2 of 94–96 %. Controlled reoxygenation has yet to be studied in randomized prospective clinical trials. The British Thoracic Society has recently published guidelines for emergency oxygen use in adult patients [27]. These recommend a target SaO_2 of 94–98 % for those critically ill patients not at risk of hypercapnic respiratory failure.

Circulation

In one review, acute changes in coronary plaque morphology were found in 40 to 86 % of cardiac arrest survivors and in 15 to 64 % of autopsy studies [28]. Several case series and studies with historical controls document the feasibility and success of early percutaneous coronary intervention (PCI) after out-of-hospital cardiac arrest [4, 21, 29]. Patients resuscitated from cardiac arrest and who have electrocardiogram (EKG) criteria for ST-segment elevation myocardial infarction (STEMI) should undergo immediate coronary angiography with subsequent PCI if indicated. Given the high incidence of ACS in patients with out-of-hospital cardiac arrest and limitations of EKG-based diagnosis, it is appropriate to consider immediate coronary angiography in all post–cardiac arrest patients in whom ACS is suspected. In the absence of a PCI facility, thrombolytic therapy is an appropriate alternative for post-cardiac arrest management of STEMI.

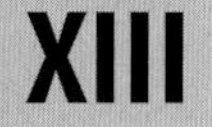

Following return of spontaneous circulation, myocardial dysfunction, hypovolemia and impaired vasoregulation commonly result in hemodynamic instability in the form of dysrhythmias, hypotension, and low cardiac index [17]. These patients will frequently require surprisingly large volumes of fluid (e.g., 3.5 – 6.5 l of crystalloid) to maintain adequate right-heart filling pressures [4, 17]. Myocardial dysfunction after return of spontaneous circulation is common but is generally reversible and responsive to inotropes [17, 18]. Early echocardiography will enable the extent of myocardial dysfunction to be quantified and may guide therapy. Impaired vasoregulation may occur for up to 72 hours after cardiac arrest [17]. Treatment with an inotrope and/or vasopressor may be guided by blood pressure, heart rate, plasma lactate concentration, urine output and central venous oxygen saturation ($ScvO_2$). Although a pulmonary artery catheter (PAC) or non-invasive cardiac output monitoring will enable treatment to be guided by cardiac index and systemic vascular resistance there is no evidence that use of these monitors improves outcome after cardiac arrest. If fluid resuscitation combined with inotropes and/or vasopressors does not restore adequate organ perfusion, insertion of an intra-aortic balloon pump (IABP) may be beneficial [4].

Relative adrenal insufficiency occurs frequently after successful resuscitation of out-of-hospital cardiac arrest and is associated with increased mortality [30] but there is no evidence that treatment with steroids in the post-cardiac arrest phase improves long-term outcomes.

Early goal-directed therapy is established for sepsis [31], but there are few data to support this strategy in post-cardiac arrest syndrome. The optimal mean arterial pressure (MAP) for post-cardiac arrest patients is unknown. Loss of cerebral autoregulation implies the need for an adequate perfusion pressure to ensure optimal cerebral blood flow but a high MAP will increase myocardial afterload. On the basis of the limited available evidence, reasonable goals for post-cardiac arrest syndrome include a MAP of 65–100 mm Hg (taking into consideration the patient's normal blood pressure, cause of arrest, and severity of any myocardial dysfunction), central venous pressure (CVP) 8–12 mm Hg, $ScvO_2 > 70$ %, urine output > 1 ml/kg/h and a normal or decreasing serum or blood lactate value. The optimum hemoglobin concentration during post-cardiac arrest has not been defined.

Disability (optimizing neurological recovery)

Interventions in the post-cardiac arrest period that may determine the final neurological outcome include control of cerebral perfusion, control of seizures, control of plasma glucose concentration, and control of temperature. Maintenance of an adequate CPP has been discussed above.

Control of seizures

Seizures and/or myoclonus occur in 5 to 15 % of adult patients who achieve return of spontaneous circulation and 10 to 40 % of those who remain comatose [15, 32]. Seizures increase cerebral metabolism by up to 3-fold and should be treated promptly and effectively with benzodiazepines, phenytoin, sodium valproate, propofol, or a barbiturate. Clonazepam is the drug of choice for the treatment of myoclonus, but sodium valproate and levetiracetam may also be effective.

Glucose Control

Hyperglycemia is common after cardiac arrest. Although one study has shown that tight control of blood glucose (4.4 to 6.1 mmol/l or 80 to 110 mg/dl) with insulin reduced hospital mortality rates in a surgical ICU [33], recent studies indicate that post-cardiac arrest patients may be treated optimally with a slightly higher target range for blood glucose concentration of up to 8 mmol/l (144 mg/dl) [4, 34, 35]. The lower value of 6.1 mmol/l may not reduce mortality any further but instead may expose patients to the potentially harmful effects of hypoglycemia. Glucose control may be particularly beneficial for those patients staying in the ICU for at least 3 days [36]; the median length of ICU stay for post-cardiac arrest patients is approximately 3.4 days [4, 5]. Regardless of the chosen glucose target range, blood glucose must be measured frequently [4, 34], especially when insulin is started and during cooling and rewarming periods.

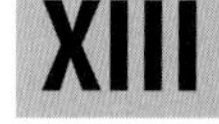

Temperature control

Therapeutic hypothermia is considered widely as part of a standardized treatment strategy for comatose survivors of cardiac arrest [4, 37, 38]. Two randomized clinical trials showed improved outcome in adults who remained comatose after initial resuscitation from out-of-hospital ventricular fibrillation (VF) cardiac arrest and who were cooled within minutes to hours after return of spontaneous circulation [39, 40]. Patients in these studies were cooled to 33 °C or the range of 32 °C to 34 °C for 12 to 24 hours. Four studies with historical control groups reported benefit after therapeutic hypothermia in comatose survivors of out-of-hospital non-VF arrest and all rhythm arrests [8]. Other observational studies provide evidence for possible benefit after cardiac arrest from other initial rhythms and in other settings [41]. Which patients may benefit most from mild hypothermia has not been fully elucidated, and the ideal induction technique, target temperature, duration, and rewarming rate have not been determined. There is some clinical evidence that a shorter time to achieve target temperature is associated with a better neurological outcome [42].

Hypothermia can be induced easily with intravenous ice-cold fluids (30 ml/kg of 0.9 % saline or Ringer's lactate) [43] or placing ice packs on the groin and armpits and around the neck and head. Initial cooling is facilitated by concomitant neuromuscular blockade with sedation to prevent shivering. Magnesium sulfate reduces shivering threshold and can be given (5 g infused over 5 h) to reduce shivering during cooling. As it is a vasodilator, magnesium sulfate increases cooling and has antiarrhythmic properties. Patients can be transferred to the angiography laboratory while being cooled [4]. Hypothermia is best maintained with external or internal cooling devices that include continuous temperature feedback to achieve a target temperature. External devices include cooling blankets or pads with water-filled circulating systems or more advanced systems in which cold air is circulated through a tent. Intravascular cooling catheters are usually inserted into a femoral or subclavian vein. Less sophisticated methods, such as cold wet blankets and ice packs can also be used to maintain hypothermia but these methods may be more time consuming for nursing staff, result in greater temperature fluctuations, and do not enable controlled rewarming [44]. The optimal rate of rewarming is not known, but current consensus is to rewarm at about 0.25 °C to 0.5 °C per hour [41]. Therapeutic hypothermia is associated with several complications (**Table 1**); metabolic rate,

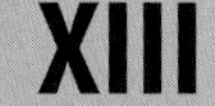

Table 1. Complications associated with therapeutic hypothermia

Shivering – particularly during the induction phase	
Increased systemic vascular resistance	
Dysrhythmias – bradycardia is the most common	
Diuresis – may cause hypovolemia and electrolyte abnormalities	
Electrolyte abnormalities:	hypophosphatemia hypokalemia hypomagnesemia hypocalcemia
Decreased insulin sensitivity and insulin secretion – hyperglycemia	
Impaired coagulation and increased bleeding	
Impairment of the immune system – increased infection rates, e.g., pneumonia	
Hyperamylasemia	
Reduced drug clearance	e.g., clearance of sedative drugs and neuromuscular blockers is reduced by up to 30 % at a temperature of 34°C

plasma electrolyte concentrations, and hemodynamic conditions may change rapidly during both the cooling and rewarming phases.

If therapeutic hypothermia is not indicated, prevention of pyrexia is critically important. Pyrexia is common in the first 48 hours after cardiac arrest [45] and the risk of a poor neurological outcome increases for each degree of body temperature > 37 °C [14].

Post-cardiac Arrest Prognostication

Although several recent systematic reviews have evaluated predictors of poor outcome in those remaining comatose after cardiac arrest [46–48] prognostication of futility remains controversial. The situation has been compounded by the introduction of therapeutic hypothermia – there are few data on its impact on the accuracy of prognostication. The ILCOR Scientific Statement on the Post-Cardiac Arrest Syndrome summarizes most of the available data on prognostication but some of the salient points on this topic are:

- Prognosis cannot be based on the circumstances surrounding cardiac arrest and CPR.
- The reliability of all prognosticating tools is dependent on when they are applied after cardiac arrest
- Neurologic exam does not reliably prognosticate futility in the first 24 hours after return of spontaneous circulation.
- Absence of pupillary light response, corneal reflex, or motor response to painful stimuli at day 3 after return of spontaneous circulation provide the most reliable predictors of poor outcome (vegetative state or death) [32, 46, 48].
- In the comatose patient after a primary cardiac arrest, myoclonic status epilepticus reliably predicts a poor outcome [46], but it may be misdiagnosed by non-neurologists.
- Burst suppression or generalized epileptiform discharges on the electroencephalogram (EEG) predict poor outcome but this is too imprecise for use in individual cases.
- Bilateral absence of the N20 component of the somatosensory evoked potential with median nerve stimulation recorded on days 1–3 or later accurately predicts a poor outcome [46–48].
- There are too few data to determine the value of radiological investigations in predicting outcome in comatose post-cardiac arrest patients.
- Until more is known about the impact of therapeutic hypothermia, prognostication should probably be delayed but the optimal time for this has yet to be determined.

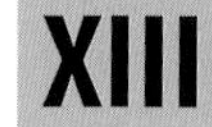

Organ Donation

The reported incidence of patients with clinical brain death following sustained return of spontaneous circulation after cardiac arrest ranges from 8 to 16 % [49, 50]. These patients can be considered for organ donation. A number of studies have reported no difference in transplant outcomes when the organs were obtained from appropriately selected post–cardiac arrest patients or from other brain-dead donors [50]. The proportion of cardiac arrest patients dying in the critical care unit and who might be suitable non-heart-beating donors has not been documented.

Conclusion

A recent scientific statement has outlined the pathophysiology, treatment, and prognosis of patients who regain spontaneous circulation after cardiac arrest. The components of post-cardiac arrest syndrome comprise post-cardiac arrest brain injury, post-cardiac arrest myocardial dysfunction, systemic ischemia/reperfusion response, and persistent precipitating pathology. Treatment may include prolonged multiple-organ support as well as time-critical input from specialists from several disciplines. Historically, about one third of post-cardiac arrest patients admitted to the ICU survive to be discharged from hospital. Studies utilizing therapeutic hypothermia and optimized post-cardiac arrest care suggest that 50 % survival with good neurologic outcome is an achievable goal.

References

1. Nichol G, Thomas E, Callaway CW, et al (2008) Regional variation in out-of-hospital cardiac arrest incidence and outcome. JAMA 300: 1423–1431
2. Sandroni C, Nolan J, Cavallaro F, Antonelli M (2007) In-hospital cardiac arrest: incidence, prognosis and possible measures to improve survival. Intensive Care Med 33: 237–245
3. Nadkarni VM, Larkin GL, Peberdy MA, et al (2006) First documented rhythm and clinical outcome from in-hospital cardiac arrest among children and adults. JAMA 295: 50–57
4. Sunde K, Pytte M, Jacobsen D, et al (2007) Implementation of a standardised treatment protocol for post resuscitation care after out-of-hospital cardiac arrest. Resuscitation 73: 29–39
5. Nolan JP, Laver SR, Welch CA, Harrison DA, Gupta V, Rowan K (2007) Outcome following admission to UK intensive care units after cardiac arrest: a secondary analysis of the ICNARC Case Mix Programme Database. Anaesthesia 62: 1207–1216
6. Carr BG, Kahn JM, Merchant RM, Kramer AA, Neumar RW (2009) Inter-hospital variability in post-cardiac arrest mortality. Resuscitation 80: 30–34
7. Langhelle A, Tyvold SS, Lexow K, Hapnes SA, Sunde K, Steen PA (2003) In-hospital factors associated with improved outcome after out-of-hospital cardiac arrest. A comparison between four regions in Norway. Resuscitation 56: 247–263
8. Neumar R, Nolan JP, Adrie C, et al (2008) Post-Cardiac Arrest Syndrome: Epidemiology, pathophysiology, treatment and prognostication. Circulation 118: 2452–2483
9. Laver S, Farrow C, Turner D, Nolan J (2004) Mode of death after admission to an intensive care unit following cardiac arrest. Intensive Care Med 30: 2126–2128
10. Neumar RW (2000) Molecular mechanisms of ischemic neuronal injury. Ann Emerg Med 36: 483–506
11. Wolfson SK Jr, Safar P, Reich H, et al (1992) Dynamic heterogeneity of cerebral hypoperfusion after prolonged cardiac arrest in dogs measured by the stable xenon/CT technique: a preliminary study. Resuscitation 23: 1–20
12. Bottiger BW, Krumnikl JJ, Gass P, Schmitz B, Motsch J, Martin E (1997) The cerebral 'no-reflow' phenomenon after cardiac arrest in rats – influence of low-flow reperfusion. Resuscitation 34: 79–87
13. Sundgreen C, Larsen FS, Herzog TM, Knudsen GM, Boesgaard S, Aldershvile J (2001) Autoregulation of cerebral blood flow in patients resuscitated from cardiac arrest. Stroke 32: 128–132
14. Zeiner A, Holzer M, Sterz F, et al (2001) Hyperthermia after cardiac arrest is associated with an unfavorable neurologic outcome. Arch Intern Med 161: 2007–2012
15. Krumholz A, Stern BJ, Weiss HD, (1988) Outcome from coma after cardiopulmonary resuscitation: relation to seizures and myoclonus. Neurology 38: 401–405
16. Mullner M, Sterz F, Binder M, Schreiber W, Deimel A, Laggner AN (1997) Blood glucose concentration after cardiopulmonary resuscitation influences functional neurological recovery in human cardiac arrest survivors. J Cereb Blood Flow Metab 17: 430–436
17. Laurent I, Monchi M, Chiche JD, et al (2002) Reversible myocardial dysfunction in survivors of out-of-hospital cardiac arrest. J Am Coll Cardiol 40: 2110–2116

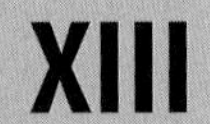

18. Adrie C, Adib-Conquy M, Laurent I, et al (2002) Successful cardiopulmonary resuscitation after cardiac arrest as a "sepsis-like" syndrome. Circulation 106: 562–568
19. Adrie C, Laurent I, Monchi M, Cariou A, Dhainaou JF, Spaulding C (2004) Postresuscitation disease after cardiac arrest: a sepsis-like syndrome? Curr Opin Crit Care 10: 208–212
20. Adrie C, Monchi M, Laurent I, et al (2005) Coagulopathy after successful cardiopulmonary resuscitation following cardiac arrest: implication of the protein C anticoagulant pathway. J Am Coll Cardiol 46: 21–28
21. Spaulding CM, Joly LM, Rosenberg A, et al (1997) Immediate coronary angiography in survivors of out-of-hospital cardiac arrest. N Engl J Med 336: 1629–1633
22. Kurkciyan I, Meron G, Sterz F, et al (2000) Pulmonary embolism as a cause of cardiac arrest: presentation and outcome. Arch Intern Med 160: 1529–1535
23. Nolan JP, Soar J (2008) Post resuscitation care – time for a care bundle? Resuscitation 76: 161–162
24. Buunk G, van der Hoeven JG, Meinders AE (1997) Cerebrovascular reactivity in comatose patients resuscitated from a cardiac arrest. Stroke 28: 1569–1573
25. Liu Y, Rosenthal RE, Haywood Y, Miljkovic-Lolic M, Vanderhoek JY, Fiskum G (1998) Normoxic ventilation after cardiac arrest reduces oxidation of brain lipids and improves neurological outcome. Stroke 29: 1679–1686
26. Balan IS, Fiskum G, Hazelton J, Cotto-Cumba C, Rosenthal RE, (2006) Oximetry-guided reoxygenation improves neurological outcome after experimental cardiac arrest. Stroke 37: 3008–3013
27. O'Driscoll BR, Howard LS, Davison AG (2008) Guideline for emergency oxygen use in adult patients. Thorax 63: vi1-vi73
28. Zipes DP, Wellens HJ (1998) Sudden cardiac death. Circulation 98: 2334–2351
29. Garot P, Lefevre T, Eltchaninoff H, et al (2007) Six-month outcome of emergency percutaneous coronary intervention in resuscitated patients after cardiac arrest complicating ST-elevation myocardial infarction. Circulation 115: 1354–1362
30. Pene F, Hyvernat H, Mallet V, et al (2005) Prognostic value of relative adrenal insufficiency after out-of-hospital cardiac arrest. Intensive Care Med 31: 627–633
31. Rivers E, Nguyen B, Havstad S, et al (2001) Early goal-directed therapy in the treatment of severe sepsis and septic shock. N Engl J Med 345: 1368–1377
32. Zandbergen EG, Hijdra A, Koelman JH, et al (2006) Prediction of poor outcome within the first 3 days of postanoxic coma. Neurology 66: 62–68
33. van den Berghe G, Wouters P, Weekers F, et al (2001) Intensive insulin therapy in the critically ill patients. N Engl J Med 345: 1359–1367
34. Oksanen T, Skrifvars MB, Varpula T, et al (2007) Strict versus moderate glucose control after resuscitation from ventricular fibrillation. Intensive Care Med 33: 2093–2100
35. Losert H, Sterz F, Roine RO, et al (2008) Strict normoglycaemic blood glucose levels in the therapeutic management of patients within 12h after cardiac arrest might not be necessary. Resuscitation 76: 214–220
36. Van den Berghe G, Wilmer A, Hermans G, et al (2006) Intensive insulin therapy in the medical ICU. N Engl J Med 354: 449–461
37. Nolan JP, Morley PT, Vanden Hoek TL, Hickey RW (2003) Therapeutic hypothermia after cardiac arrest. An advisory statement by the Advancement Life support Task Force of the International Liaison committee on Resuscitation. Resuscitation 57: 231–235
38. Soar J, Nolan JP (2007) Mild hypothermia for post cardiac arrest syndrome. BMJ 335: 459–460
39. Hypothermia After Cardiac Arrest Study Group (2002) Mild therapeutic hypothermia to improve the neurologic outcome after cardiac arrest. N Engl J Med 346: 549–556
40. Bernard SA, Gray TW, Buist MD, et al (2002) Treatment of comatose survivors of out-of-hospital cardiac arrest with induced hypothermia. N Engl J Med 346: 557–563
41. Arrich J (2007) Clinical application of mild therapeutic hypothermia after cardiac arrest. Crit Care Med 35: 1041–1047
42. Wolff B, Machill K, Schumacher D, Schulzki I, Werner D (2009) Early achievement of mild therapeutic hypothermia and the neurologic outcome after cardiac arrest. Int J Cardiol (in press)
43. Kim F, Olsufka M, Longstreth WT Jr, et al (2007) Pilot randomized clinical trial of prehospi-

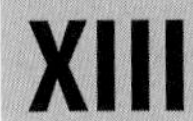

tal induction of mild hypothermia in out-of-hospital cardiac arrest patients with a rapid infusion of 4 degrees C normal saline. Circulation 115: 3064–3070

44. Merchant RM, Abella BS, Peberdy MA, et al (2006) Therapeutic hypothermia after cardiac arrest: Unintentional overcooling is common using ice packs and conventional cooling blankets. Crit Care Med 34: S490-S494
45. Hickey RW, Kochanek PM, Ferimer H, Alexander HL, Garman RH, Graham SH, (2003) Induced hyperthermia exacerbates neurologic neuronal histologic damage after asphyxial cardiac arrest in rats. Crit Care Med 31: 531–535
46. Wijdicks EF, Hijdra A, Young GB, Bassetti CL, Wiebe S (2006) Practice parameter: prediction of outcome in comatose survivors after cardiopulmonary resuscitation (an evidence-based review): report of the Quality Standards Subcommittee of the American Academy of Neurology. Neurology 67: 203–210
47. Booth CM, Boone RH, Tomlinson G, Detsky AS (2004) Is this patient dead, vegetative, or severely neurologically impaired? Assessing outcome for comatose survivors of cardiac arrest. JAMA 291: 870–879
48. Zandbergen EG, de Haan RJ, Stoutenbeek CP, Koelman JH, Hijdra A (1998) Systematic review of early prediction of poor outcome in anoxic-ischaemic coma. Lancet 352: 1808–1812
49. Peberdy MA, Kaye W, Ornato JP, et al (2003) Cardiopulmonary resuscitation of adults in the hospital: a report of 14720 cardiac arrests from the National Registry of Cardiopulmonary Resuscitation. Resuscitation 58: 297–308
50. Adrie C, Haouache H, Saleh M, et al (2008) An underrecognized source of organ donors: patients with brain death after successfully resuscitated cardiac arrest. Intensive Care Med 34: 132–137

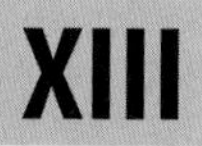

Use of a Standardized Treatment Protocol for Post-cardiac Resuscitation Care

M.A. Kuiper, P.E. Spronk, and M.J. Schultz

Introduction

For a long time, the outcome of patients after out-of-hospital cardiac arrest has been extremely poor, with only 5–10 % of survivors having a good neurological outcome. In recent years, several studies have demonstrated an increase in survival of cardiac arrest patients admitted to the intensive care unit (ICU), often with more than 60 % having good neurological outcome [1–6]. Since the introduction of cardiopulmonary resuscitation (CPR) in the early 1960s by Safar and McMahon (mouth-to-mouth respiration) [7] and Kouwenhoven et al. (closed chest-compression) [8], the emphasis in resuscitation medicine has been on the treatment of cardiac arrest until return of spontaneous circulation, with manual CPR and early defibrillation of convertible cardiac rhythms being the two most important items. The general consensus was that improvement of outcome of cardiac arrest patients would solely lie in shortening the period of circulatory standstill, thus minimizing the, mainly neurological, damage. Having restored the circulation, treating physicians "could only wait and see what the outcome would be". However, alongside the processes of recovery and compensation, a pathological state may develop with associated organ failure – the so-called post-resuscitation syndrome. Physicians should be aware of this condition and actively treat its complications to improve the condition of the patient and to increase the chance of a good neurological outcome after cardiac arrest. Induced mild hypothermia is an important factor in this aspect and has become an established treatment for the post-resuscitation patient. However, induced mild hypothermia is not the sole treatment modality that should be used.

Indeed, Sunde et al. [4] reported on the use of a standardized treatment protocol and showed improved outcomes of patients treated with a bundle of strategies compared with historic controls. This chapter discusses the role of several strategies in patients after cardiac arrest and details of post-resuscitation care. It provides a rationale for the different treatment steps of a standardized treatment protocol for the post-resuscitation patient (**Table 1**).

Chain of Survival

The chain of survival as advocated by the various societies of resuscitation, promotes getting help, basic life support with manual CPR to buy time, early defibrillation to restart the circulation, and advanced life support by professionals. In the past, the emphasis in resuscitation medicine has mainly been on the first three steps of resuscitation: Getting help, early and good quality CPR, and early defibrillation.

Table 1. Proposed model for standardized post-resuscitation treatment. Treatment protocol based on Sunde et al. [4], Polderman [19] and Arawwawala and Brett [50]

- After return of spontaneous circulation: Control hemodynamics and oxygenation; diagnose and treat the cause of arrest; reperfusion (PCI; thrombolysis) after STEMI
- Therapeutic hypothermia (32–34 °C in comatose patients for 24 h) should be initiated as quickly as possible. Try to reach temperatures below 34°C and then achieve target temperature as rapidly as possible. Initially 2–3 l of ice-cold (4 °C) Ringer's lactate or 0.9 % NaCl intravenously and as soon as possible start endovascular or surface cooling for maintenance, striving for minimal fluctuations of temperature.
- Blood pressure: MAP > 75 mmHg
  Cardiac output during hypothermia may be 20–30 %. Use SvO_2 to monitor oxygen balance; SvO_2 > 70 %
  Use volume, inotropes and/or vasopressors to reach these goals
  Consider IABP in cardiogenic shock
  Heart rate: 60–100/min – use volume, sedation, beta-blocker (normally not indicated when using therapeutic hypothermia because of relative bradycardia)
  Temperature 32–34 °C for 24 h
  SpO_2 95–98 – using controlled ventilation, not support ventilation; tidal volumes of 6 ml/kg/ideal body weight
  PCO_2 5–6 kPa (avoid hyperventilation/hypocapnia)
  Blood glucose 4.4–6.1 mmol/l actrapid-infusion (insulin resistance; avoid hypoglycemia/hypokalemia)
  Electrolytes: Aim for normal values
  Hemoglobin 5.5–6.0 mmol/l (9–10 g/dl) – transfusion if necessary
  Diuresis > 0.5 ml/kg/h – use volume, inotropes, and/or vasopressors. Start renal replacement therapy early in acute kidney failure.
  pH > 7.20, base excess > –10. When indicated use sodium bicarbonate or start CVVH
  Seizures: Prevent/treat seizures using sedation, and/or specific anticonvulsive medication
  EEG when indicated
  Sedation and analgesia: Morphine or fentanyl and midazolam
  Treat shivering with magnesium, meperidine (pethidine); paralysis only when necessary. Use strategies to prevent complications, such as (ventilator associated) pneumonia, wound infections, and bedsores.
  Use of other evidenced based critical care strategies, such as thrombo-prophylaxis and early enteral feeding
- Monitoring:
  Continuous EKG
  Arterial catheter
  SpO_2
  $ScvO_2$ or SvO_2
  Cardiac output
  Central venous line with central venous pressure
  Core temperature
  Arterial blood gases (pH, BE, PCO_2, PO_2; lactate)
  Blood glucose and electrolytes
  Echocardiography, chest X-ray
  EEG and SEP
- After 24 h of cooling, patients should be slowly re-warmed in a controlled fashion (0.2–0.5 °C /h). Sedation may be stopped after the body temperature has reached 36.0 °C.
- Use only established predictors of death and/or unfavorable outcome in patients remaining unconscious after cardiac arrest. Indicators of poor outcome after CPR are absent pupillary light response or corneal reflexes, and extensor or no motor response to pain after 3 days of observation; myoclonus status epilepticus; and bilateral absent cortical responses on somatosensory evoked potential studies recorded 3 days after CPR.

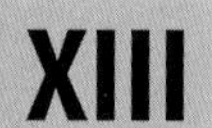

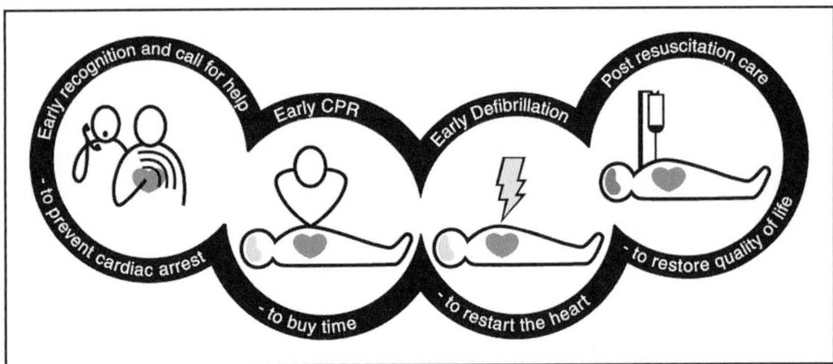

Fig. 1. European Resuscitation Council Chain of survival

The 4th step of the chain of survival, advanced life support, was probably never as well defined as the earlier steps. As early defibrillation is likely the most crucial step in the early phase of cardiac arrest, the use of automated external defibrillators (AEDs) has most probably led to a better neurological outcome in cardiac arrest patients. Also early coronary interventions have improved outcome.

The two landmark studies by the Hypothermia after Cardiac Arrest (HACA) group [9] and by Bernard et al. [10] showing benefit of induced mild hypothermia after cardiac arrest have shifted the focus and there is now an increasing interest in post-resuscitation treatment. However, it was not until 2005, that the 4th ring of the chain of survival was updated to reflect the importance of post resuscitation care in determining the ultimate outcome following cardiac arrest [12] (**Fig. 1**).

The Post-resuscitation Syndrome

The post-resuscitation syndrome is defined as a condition after resuscitation following (prolonged) cardiac arrest and, therefore, whole body ischemia and reperfusion with multiple-organ dysfunction, most notably of, but not limited to, the brain. Negovsky, one pioneer of "reanimatology" and therapeutic hypothermia, was probably the first to introduce the concept of the post-resuscitation syndrome [12]. Negovsky found pathophysiological changes after resuscitation that differed substantially from those caused by ischemia and hypoxia. In the brain, redistribution of Ca^{2+}, together with the formation of free radicals was observed, causing damage to DNA and organelle membranes, followed by development of progressive autoimmune pathology, reflecting the damage to the blood-brain barrier [12, 13]. The post-resuscitation or post-cardiac arrest syndrome is at present believed to be a form of systemic inflammatory response syndrome (SIRS), caused by ischemia-reperfusion. As this 'sepsis–like syndrome' [14] may precede the development to multiple-organ dysfunction syndrome, even after successful and swift restoration of the circulation, a patient after cardiac arrest may ultimately die of the consequences of post-resuscitation syndrome. On the other hand, this syndrome gives physicians the opportunity to intervene and strive to improve outcome by supporting the function of failing organs with ventilation, hemodynamic support, or renal replacement therapy.

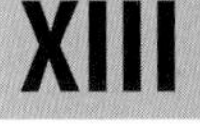

Early Coronary Intervention

Early revascularization after myocardial infarction improves outcome. Compared with thrombolytic therapy, percutaneous coronary intervention (PCI) results in a higher rate of patency of the infarct-related coronary artery, lower rates of stroke and re-infarction, and higher long-term survival rates [15]. Induced mild hypothermia in combination with PCI is feasible and safe in patients resuscitated after cardiac arrest due to acute myocardial infarction (AMI) [16]. In patients with cardiac arrest due to ST-segment elevation myocardial infarction (STEMI), it may be acceptable to use thrombolytic therapy as the reperfusion strategy of first choice. This applies especially in hospitals where immediate PCI is not available [17]. The diagnosis of STEMI can be established in the field immediately after return of spontantous circulation in most patients. This may enable an early decision about reperfusion therapy, i.e., immediate out-of-hospital thrombolytic therapy or targeted transfer for PCI [18]. In view of the existing evidence, PCI after cardiac arrest due to STEMI should be the preferred mode of treatment in regions and situations where this is possible.

Induced Mild Hypothermia

Since the landmark publications by the HACA group [9] and Bernard et al. [10], many studies have been published using a non-randomized design or matched historical controls, all showing a profound improvement of outcome since therapeutic hypothermia has been implemented (**Fig. 2**). The two original studies provided us with the evidence for treating patients with mild hypothermia if they fulfilled the criteria for inclusion (HACA study: witnessed cardiac arrest, ventricular fibrillation, or ventricular tachycardia as the initial cardiac rhythm, presumed cardiac origin of the arrest, age between 18–75 years, estimated interval of 5–15 minutes from the patient's collapse to the first attempt at resuscitation by emergency medical personnel, and an interval of no more than 60 minutes from collapse to restoration of spontaneous circulation). These inclusion criteria must have led to exclusion of many cardiac arrest patients. Indeed, out of 3551 patients assessed for eligibility in the HACA study, 3246 did not meet these inclusion criteria. There is accumulating evidence, however, that induced mild hypothermia is probably also valuable for patients not strictly fulfilling these criteria, such as patients with asystole or pulseless electrical activity [19, 20] or patients above 75 years of age [21]. It seems reasonable to consider induced mild hypothermia for all patients admitted to the ICU after cardiac arrest, which is supported by the ILCOR statement on therapeutic hypothermia [22].

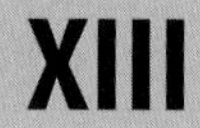

Why should all patients after circulatory arrest and return of spontaneous circulation receive induced hypothermia? Therapeutic hypothermia affects brain metabolism, lowering the metabolism by 40–50 % when temperature decreases from 38 °C to 32 °C, thereby decreasing oxygen demand. Moreover, the level of inflammation is attenuated and intracranial pressure (ICP) decreases [19]. However, we may view mild hypothermia not so much as a neuro-protective strategy alone, but as an active treatment strategy to improve the function of the brain as well as other organs. Apart from improving brain function, therapeutic hypothermia may (or can) improve function of other organs: Studies suggest positive effects in cardiogenic shock, seizures, acute respiratory distress syndrome (ARDS), nephropathy, hepatic

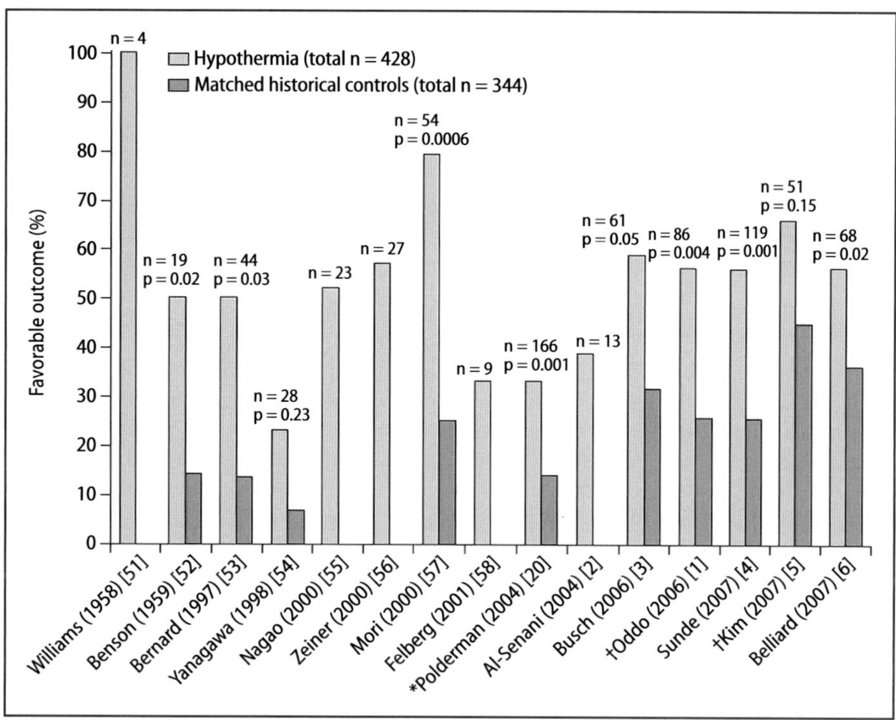

Fig. 2. Use of hypothermia in cardiac arrest, non-randomized studies. *Patients with witnessed arrest and initial rhythm of asystole or pulseless electrical activity; †Studies enrolling several categories of patients, only patients with initial rhythm of ventricular tachycardia/fibrillation shown. Modified from [19] with permission

failure, or arrhythmias [20]. These strategies remain to be proven, however. A non-significant reduction in infarct size in myocardial infarction has also been reported [23].

Data from surveys in Europe and the United States suggest that rates of use of induced mild hypothermia in post-cardiac arrest patients may be as low as 30–40 % among physicians [24]. A recent e-mail invitation anonymous web-based survey was held among ICUs in the Netherlands: 37 of the participating ICUs (50 %) said they always treated these patients with therapeutic hypothermia; 42 % only treated patients with therapeutic hypothermia when CPR fulfilled several criteria, such as ventricular fibrillation as the presenting cardiac rhythm at arrival of ambulance (82 %) and duration of time to return of spontaneous circulation (55 %); 6 ICUs (8 %) never induced hypothermia. The most important reason for not inducing hypothermia was lack of equipment. Surface cooling (86 %) and cold intravenous fluids (71 %) were most frequently used to reach the target temperature. Hemodynamic instability was most often cited as a reason to discontinue treatment with therapeutic hypothermia. Thus, in the Netherlands, therapeutic hypothermia after CPR is implemented in almost all ICUs, which is, compared to previous reports from other countries, exceedingly high (unpublished data). Despite varying acceptance and implementation across the world, lack of scientific evidence for the use of induced mild hypothermia after cardiac arrest may no longer be used as an argument for not implementing this treatment.

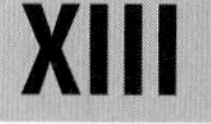

Cerebral Blood Flow and Mean Arterial Blood Pressure

Initially, shortly after return of spontaneous circulation, there is a change in cerebral blood flow (CBF), which normalizes later (after 72 hours) [25]. The mean flow velocities, as assessed using transcranial Doppler are lowered, while oxygen extraction is initially normal but decreases with time. This latter effect is significantly more pronounced in non-survivors.

After cardiac arrest, cerebral autoregulation is disturbed, but not completely absent [26]. As this mechanism regulates the CBF to maintain steady oxygen delivery to the brain during changes in blood pressure, this means that CBF is highly pressure dependent during impairment of the autoregulation and therefore a high mean arterial blood pressure (MAP) is most probably needed. There is no clinical evidence for a specific limit for the MAP, but as the ICP following CPR is not necessarily elevated, and in general remains below 15 mmHg [27], maintaining the MAP > 75 mmHg and thus a cerebral perfusion pressure (CPP) of > 60 mmHg, is justifiable. The optimal MAP for post-cardiac arrest patients may even be higher [28]. Of note, the MAP in the study by Bernard et al. [10] was approximately 90 mmHg in both the hypothermia and normothermia groups. In patients with severe myocardial dysfunction after cardiac arrest, these values may be difficult to obtain, and a balance needs to be found between the optimal blood pressure for CBF and the burden for the myocardium to meet this demand.

Hemodynamic Support and Monitoring

Hemodynamic monitoring is warranted to optimize circulation and balance oxygen supply to demand. Heart rate, blood pressure, cardiac output, mixed (SvO_2) or central ($ScvO_2$) venous oxygen saturation, lactate, and arterial blood gases need to be monitored. While all of these methods of monitoring the circulation have their own obvious limitations, monitoring may prevent severe misbalances between oxygen delivery and oxygen consumption. Cardiac output during hypothermia may be 20–30 % lower and, therefore, be accepted below normal limits. The use of $ScvO_2$ or SvO_2 measurements to monitor oxygen balance and maintaining $Scv0_2$ > 70 % is probably a reasonable approach. Volume, inotropes and/or vasopressors will often be necessary to reach these goals. We may need to consider the use of an intra-aortic balloon pump (IABP) in patients with (refractory) cardiogenic shock due to myocardial infarction or myocardial stunning.

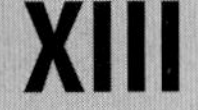

In line with guidelines for pharmacological prevention of perioperative cardiac complications in high risk patients undergoing non-cardiac surgery aimed at maintaining adequate oxygen delivery while preventing myocardial ischemia, the heart rate needs to be maintained between 60–100/minute, using volume, sedation, beta-blockers or a pacemaker to obtain this. As hypothermia often leads to relative bradycardia, beta-blockers are rarely needed, however. Anti-arrhythmic drugs may be needed to maintain sinus rhythm. In patients who survive but are prone to arrhythmias, implantable cardiac defibrillators can be considered. Close monitoring of the circulation is warranted in order to balance oxygen demand and supply while at the same time taking care to relieve the myocardial burden and prevent secondary myocardial ischemia.

Ventilation

In post-resuscitation patients, the use of controlled ventilation as opposed to a support mode of ventilation is rational, as in most cases this decreases oxygen consumption [29]. The use of tidal volumes of 6 ml/kg predicted or ideal bodyweight is advocated to diminish the occurrence of acute lung injury (ALI) as there is accumulating and convincing clinical and preclinical evidence that ventilation with tidal volumes of 6 ml/kg predicted or ideal bodyweight prevents the development of ALI [30].

As the metabolic rate decreases 5–8 % per each °C, there is a concomitant decrease in oxygen consumption and carbon dioxide production. Ventilator settings need to be adjusted accordingly to prevent hyperventilation and thus hypocapnia. Hypocapnia leads to cerebral vasoconstriction and diminished CBF and oxygen delivery. Blood gases need to be repeatedly checked to be able to maintain normoventilation.

While there is no discussion about the need to treat and prevent hypoxia, this invariably leads to hyperoxia, which may be detrimental in itself, especially after a period of hypoxia. While there is preclinical evidence to promote the use of a limited fraction of inspired oxygen (FiO_2), there is no evidence for limiting FiO_2 in humans. Striving for a peripheral oxygen saturation (SpO_2) of 95–98 % would seem reasonable to prevent hypoxemia and hyperoxemia, but while hyperoxemia is potentially detrimental after ischemia, especially beyond 5 minutes, hypoxemia is obviously worse.

Blood Glucose and Electrolyte Monitoring

As hypothermia can decrease insulin sensitivity as well as reduce insulin secretion by pancreatic islet cells, patients who are cooled have a high risk of developing hyperglycemia. Control of blood glucose using insulin therapy is, therefore, necessary. While there is no clinical outcome study showing benefit in a strictly defined subgroup of post-cardiac arrest patients, there is sufficient evidence for controlling blood glucose using insulin from the Van den Berghe studies [31, 32] to include this strategy in post-resuscitation treatment.

Electrolyte disturbances are to be expected in patients treated with hypothermia because of changes in renal function, combined with electrolyte shifts to the intracellular compartment. Hypomagnesemia in particular can easily occur and is associated with increased risks of adverse outcome. As magnesium has a pivotal role in many central nervous and cardiovascular processes, it is advisable to start magnesium supplementation early. Administering magnesium helps prevent hypokalemia, hypophosphatemia, hypocalcemia, and hyponatremia, so controlling magnesium facilitates the control of other electrolytes. During hypothermia, hypokalemia may also occur, especially in patients with increased urine production. It is beyond the scope of this paper to discuss all possible effects of electrolyte disturbances during induced mild hypothermia. It is generally advised that magnesium, potassium and phosphate should be kept in the normal to high-normal range, and sodium be kept in the normal range. [33]

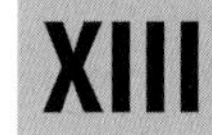

Patients after cardiac arrest will have a lowered pH, due to increases in PCO_2 and lactate. As the patient is mechanically ventilated, the PCO_2 will often not pose a problem and will normalize, and restoration of the circulation will most often lead to clearance of lactate, reducing these levels and normalizing the pH. As a low pH induces a pro-inflammatory state, and because many enzyme mediated processes are compromised at a pH lower than 7.20–7.25, measures need to be taken to maintain pH > 7.20. Sunde et al. showed that using a goal directed, standardized approach in the treatment of post-resuscitation patients leads to a significantly less negative base excess, and therefore a higher pH, without changes in PCO_2 [4].

In patients with electrolyte disturbances, low pH and/or acute kidney failure, one might consider using a form of continuous renal replacement therapy (CRRT), such as continuous veno-venous hemofiltration (CVVH). CVVH may aid in maintaining a normal acid-base and electrolyte balance.

Thrombolytic Therapy Aimed at Improving Brain Perfusion

Fischer et al. showed in a cat model that thrombolytic therapy with recombinant tissue type plasminogen activator (rtPA) and heparin after cardiac arrest and successful CPR reduced non-perfused brain areas and improved microcirculatory reperfusion [34]. In a retrospective study, Richling et al. reported a trend towards better neurological outcome using thrombolytic therapy compared to PCI in patients with cardiac arrest due to STEMI [17]. At the moment however, there are insufficient clinical data to support this strategy.

Brain Monitoring

Monitoring of the brain can be achieved using a (continuous) electroencephalogram (EEG). A study evaluating the use of continuous EEG monitoring after cardiac arrest showed development of EEG status epilepticus during therapeutic hypothermia in 26 out of 94 evaluated cardiac arrest patients, and this status epilepticus correlated with poor outcome [35]. Continuous EEG monitoring provides an opportunity of treating EEG status epilepticus in the absence of clinical signs (non-convulsive status epilepticus) in patients treated with hypothermia, sedation and paralyzing agents, which prevent clinical signs and symptoms from becoming overt. As EEG status epilepticus is known to increase oxygen consumption of the brain, it seems reasonable to try to terminate it. Anti-convulsant drugs and sedatives can be used to prevent and/or treat this status epilepticus. Although this may seem a reasonable approach, there are as yet no convincing data on outcome to support this strategy.

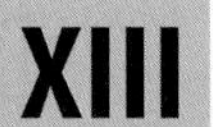

Prevention of Infection

Therapeutic hypothermia increases the risk of infections due to immune suppression. A retrospective cohort study of patients after cardiac arrest reported an increased incidence of lower respiratory tract infections in patients treated with mild hypothermia [36]. Sunde et al. compared a prospective cohort treated with hypothermia with a retrospective cohort before the use of therapeutic hypothermia [4]. These authors found no increase in the rate of pneumonia as a result of hypothermia, but their reported percentage of pneumonia was also high: 57 % in the cardiac arrest patient cohort before implementing therapeutic hypothermia compared with 48 % in the cohort treated with therapeutic hypothermia. This is most likely a detrimental factor as ventilator-associated pneumonia (VAP) is known to increase mortality and also because infections may cause fever, which is harmful for the compromised nervous system. There are various options to decrease the possibility of infection, one being the use of selective decontamination of the digestive tract, which is a well-proven strategy to prevent VAP and mortality in ICU patients [37, 38].

Use of Sedation, Analgesia and Paralyzing Agents

Use of sedation in comatose post-cardiac arrest patients is rational, as it not only facilitates the use of hypothermia and controlled ventilation, but also reduces oxygen consumption. The use of analgesics is rational as well: A state of post-anoxic coma does not eliminate the need for anesthesia and/or analgesia [13]. Patients with an AMI may experience pain, which may even be aggravated by prolonged periods of chest compressions, necessitating the use of analgesic agents, which on their own can reduce oxygen consumption. Sedation and analgesia are also used to avoid shivering during hypothermia. Shivering greatly increases oxygen demand and needs to be diagnosed and treated. If sedation and analgesia are not sufficient to abolish shivering, magnesium may be used, as well as meperidine (pethidine®). If the patient still shows signs of shivering, a paralyzing agent needs to be added.

The choice of sedatives is not always considered crucial. It needs to be mentioned that the protocol of the Bernard study [10] demanded the use of midazolam, while in the HACA study [9] the combination of midazolam and fentanyl was used. If other sedatives or analgesics are preferred, potential drawbacks of the drugs need to be considered. Propofol, for instance, often used as a sedative for patients with neurological critical care disorders, has a more profound negative inotropic effect than midazolam, thereby possibly compromising the circulation and negatively affecting the prognosis. Shivering was treated with the paralyzing agents vecuronium in the Bernard study [10] and pancuronium in the HACA trial [9].

Slow, Passive or Active Re-warming and the Prevention of Fever

Re-warming after therapeutic hypothermia needs to be slow and controlled (0.2-0-5 °C/h). Rapid re-warming in patients with traumatic brain injury (TBI) and in the peri-operative setting has resulted in worse outcomes than slow re-warming [19]. Animal studies have shown that rapid re-warming can adversely affect outcome and that slow re-warming preserves the benefits of cooling [39]. Rapid re-warming may cause regional or general imbalances between CBF and oxygen consumption and, thus, cause hypoxia, leading to additional ischemic neuronal damage [19]. In clinical studies, rapid re-warming also increases the risk of electrolyte shifts and especially of hyperkalemia. Re-warming also affects the sensitivity of the cell to insulin; so during re-warming blood glucose should be closely monitored.

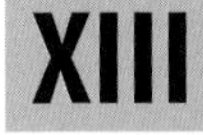

Increasing evidence suggests that fever is harmful to the injured brain, and it seems reasonable to maintain normothermia in most patients with neurological injuries who have decreased consciousness (especially in those previously treated with hypothermia) for at least 72 hours after injury [19].

Passive re-warming cannot be strictly controlled; as slow re-warming and prevention of fever are of the utmost importance, it is reasonable to choose slow, active and controlled re-warming.

Prognostication

Unpublished data from the PROPAC study [40] by Zandbergen et al. on differences in outcome of patients after cardiac arrest related to early do-not-resuscitate (DNR) orders after admittance suggest that installing treatment limitations within the first 24 hours leads to a decreased chance of survival.

Pupillary light response, corneal reflexes, motor responses to pain, myoclonus status epilepticus, and somatosensory evoked potential (SEP) studies can reliably assist in accurately predicting poor outcome in comatose patients after CPR for cardiac arrest [41]. Myoclonus status epilepticus is, however, rare and should not be confused with myclonus, which in itself does not reliably predict poor outcome or death. As mild hypothermia mandates the use of analgesics, sedatives, and sometimes paralytic agents, and as the pharmacokinetics of these drugs are changed, resulting in a reduced clearance, utmost care needs to be taken when performing a neurological assessment of these patients. While an absent cortical response (N20) of the SEP has been demonstrated to have a positive predictive value of 100 %, the presence of a N20 does not in any way predict good outcome.

Serum neuron-specific enolase (NSE) has also been suggested as a predictable parameter in establishing prognosis after cardiac arrest, but recent studies in patients treated with hypothermia show higher serum NSE values than previously reported in patients surviving with good neurological outcome [42]. This probably limits the usefulness of NSE in establishing a reliable prognosis.

Prognosis cannot be based on the circumstances of CPR *per se*. Witnessed or not witnessed, basic life support or not, and time to return of spontaneous circulation do not reliably predict outcome in an individual patient. For prognostication we should only use established predictors. Poor outcome in post-anoxic coma can be reliably predicted with good neurological assessment after three days and with SEPs in a substantial number of patients. Establishing DNR orders within the first 24 hours after cardiac arrest leads to a decreased chance of survival of the post-resuscitation patient.

Future Perspectives

We are now witnessing a great leap forward in the treatment of post-cardiac arrest patients, and many possible treatment modes are under investigation to further improve outcome.

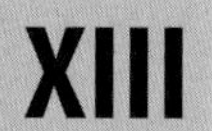

1) During advanced life support, a device for automated chest compressions is potentially useful in assisting and improving CPR. We await convincing clinical data before widespread use can be advocated. Impedance threshold devices to produce negative intrathoracic pressure during ventilation in CPR can be used to improve preload and thereby hemodynamics and CBF during CPR [43]. On-site cooling after out-of-hospital cardiac arrest has been shown to be feasible [44]; no clinical data are yet available to show survival benefit.

2) Cardio-cerebral or chest compression-only resuscitation has been advocated by Ewy who claims substantial outcome benefit with this approach after cardiac arrest [45]. On March 31, 2008, the American Heart Association issued a statement that recommended performing chest-compression-only CPR if the rescuer is a bystander without CPR training or "previously trained in CPR but not confident in his or her ability to provide conventional CPR, including high-quality chest compressions (i.e.,

compressions of adequate rate and depth with minimal interruptions) with rescue breath." [46]. This recommendation has not been adopted by the European Resuscitation Council.

3) Coenzyme Q10 (CoQ10) is an essential mitochondrial cofactor that has been shown to possess neuroprotective qualities in neurodegenerative disorders and may also have a cardioprotective effect in cardiosurgery. Combining CoQ10 with mild hypothermia immediately after CPR may improve survival and may improve neurological outcome in survivors [47].

4) Erythropoietin (EPO) may also have neuroprotective properties. A small clinical study using EPO in out-of-hospital cardiac arrest patients failed, however, to show significant survival benefit [48].

5) Will applying rules for pre-hospital termination of resuscitation in out-of-hospital cardiac arrest affect outcomes of patients surviving to the emergency room or the ICU? In a recent retrospective validation study, Sasson et al. found that basic and advanced life support termination-of-resuscitation rules performed well in identifying out-of-hospital cardiac arrest patients who have little or no chance of survival [49]. Strict stopping rules for basic and advanced life support were defined. For basic life support the rules were "Event not witnessed by emergency medical services personnel; no automated external defibrillator used or manual shock applied in out of-hospital setting; no return of spontaneous circulation in out-of-hospital setting". Additional rules for advanced life support were: "Arrest not witnessed by bystander; no bystander-administered CPR". A patient must meet all of the criteria in either category to warrant termination of resuscitation in the out-of-hospital setting. Pre-hospital selection of post-cardiac arrest patients who will invariably die will increase the likelihood of survival for the remaining cohort, and probably change the attitude of the treating physicians towards these patients, theoretically resulting in more aggressive treatment and better outcome [49].

Conclusion

After cardiac arrest, immediate restoration of the circulation is of the utmost importance. Good quality basic life support and early defibrillation are crucial steps in this phase of CPR. After return of spontaneous circulation, considerable improvement in outcome of the post-resuscitation patient can be achieved by actively treating many complications of the ischemia-reperfusion phenomena known as the post-resuscitation syndrome. The most important treatment modality in this situation is induced mild hypothermia. Other important treatment modalities include early coronary reperfusion, controlled ventilation to achieve normal arterial blood PO_2 and PCO_2, hemodynamic optimization, judicious use of sedatives and analgesics and prevention of shivering to reduce oxygen consumption, tight control of electrolytes and glucose, prevention and treatment of seizures, prevention of complications such as infections, and the use of validated predictors for prognosis.

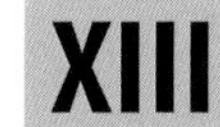

Presently, there is accumulating evidence to support the view that a standardized protocol should be used to optimize the treatment of the post-resuscitation patient admitted to the ICU.

References

1. Oddo M, Schaller MD, Feihl F, Ribordy V, Liaudet L (2006) From evidence to clinical practice: effective implementation of therapeutic hypothermia to improve patient outcome after cardiac arrest. Crit Care Med 34: 1865–1873
2. Al-Senani FM, Graffagnino C, Grotta JC, et al (2004) A prospective, multicenter pilot study to evaluate the feasibility and safety of using the CoolGard System and Icy catheter following cardiac arrest. Resuscitation 62: 143–150
3. Busch M, Soreide E, Lossius HM, Lexow K, Dickstein K (2006) Rapid implementation of therapeutic hypothermia in comatose out-of-hospital cardiac arrest survivors. Acta Anaesthesiol Scand 50: 1277–1283
4. Sunde K, Pytte M, Jacobsen D, et al (2007) Implementation of a standardised treatment protocol for post resuscitation care after out-of-hospital cardiac arrest. Resuscitation 73: 29–39
5. Kim F, Olsufka M, Longstreth WT Jr, et al (2007) Pilot randomized clinical trial of prehospital induction of mild hypothermia in out-of-hospital cardiac arrest patients with a rapid infusion of 4 degrees C normal saline. Circulation 115: 3064–3070
6. Belliard G, Catez E, Charron C, et al (2007) Efficacy of therapeutic hypothermia after out-of-hospital cardiac arrest due to ventricular fibrillation. Resuscitation 75: 252–259
7. Safar P, McMahon M (1958) Mouth-to-airway emergency artificial respiration. JAMA 166: 1459–1460
8. Kouwenhoven WB, Jude JR, Knickerbocker GG (1960) Closed chest cardiac massage. JAMA 173: 1064–1067
9. The HACA Study Group (2002) Mild therapeutic hypothermia to improve the neurologic outcome after cardiac arrest. N Engl J Med 346: 549–556
10. Bernard S, Gray TW, Buist MD, et al (2002) Treatment of comatose survivors of out-of-hospital cardiac arrest with induced hypothermia. N Engl J Med 346: 557–563
11. Nolan J, Soar J, Eikeland H (2006) The chain of survival. Resuscitation 71: 270–271
12. Negovsky VA (1972) The second step in resuscitation--the treatment of the 'post-resuscitation disease'. Resuscitation 1: 1–7
13. Negovsky VA, Gurvitch AM (1995) Post-resuscitation disease--a new nosological entity. Its reality and significance. Resuscitation 30: 23–27
14. Adrie C, Adib-Conquy M, Laurent I, et al (2002) Successful cardiopulmonary resuscitation after cardiac arrest as a "sepsis-like"syndrome. Circulation 106: 562–568
15. Zijlstra F, Hoorntje JC, de Boer MJ, et al (1999) Long-term benefit of primary angioplasty as compared with thrombolytic therapy for acute myocardial infarction. N Engl J Med 341: 1413–1419
16. Wolfrum S, Pierau C, Radke PW, Schunkert H, Kurowski V (2008) Mild therapeutic hypothermia in patients after out-of-hospital cardiac arrest due to acute ST-segment elevation myocardial infarction undergoing immediate percutaneous coronary intervention. Crit Care Med 36: 1780–1786
17. Richling N, Herkner H, Holzer M, Riedmueller E, Sterz F, Schreiber W (2007) Thrombolytic therapy vs primary percutaneous intervention after ventricular fibrillation cardiac arrest due to acute ST-segment elevation myocardial infarction and its effect on outcome. Am J Emerg Med 25: 545–550
18. Müller D, Schnitzer L, Brandt J. Arntz HR (2008) The accuracy of an out-of-hospital 12-lead ECG for the detection of ST-elevation myocardial infarction immediately after resuscitation. Ann Emerg Med 52: 658–664
19. Polderman KH (2008) Induced hypothermia and fever control for prevention and treatment of neurological injuries. Lancet 371: 1955–1969
20. Polderman KH, Sterz F, van Zanten ARH, et al (2003) Induced hypothermia improves neurological outcome in asystolic patients with out-of hospital cardiac arrest. Circulation 108:IV–581 (abst)
21. Van Lelyveld LE, Tjan DH, van Zanten AR (2008) Mild therapeutic hypothermia after cardiopulmonary resuscitation; patients over the age of 75. Intensive Care Med 34:S212 (abst)
22. Nolan JP, Morley PT, Hoek TL, Hickey RW (2003) Therapeutic hypothermia after cardiac arrest. An advisory statement by the Advancement Life support Task Force of the International Liaison committee on Resuscitation. Resuscitation 57: 231–235

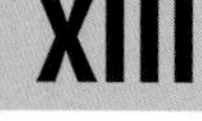

23. Dixon SR, Whitbourn RJ, Dae MW, et al (2002) Induction of mild systemic hypothermia with endovascular cooling during primary percutaneous coronary intervention for acute myocardial infarction. J Am Coll Cardiol 40: 1928–1934
24. Brooks SC, Morrison LJ (2008) Implementation of therapeutic hypothermia guidelines for post-cardiac arrest syndrome at a glacial pace: Seeking guidance from the knowledge translation literature. Resuscitation 77: 286–292
25. Lemiale V, Huet O, Vigué B, et al (2008) in cerebral blood flow and oxygen extraction during post-resuscitation syndrome. Resuscitation 76: 17–24
26. Nishizawa H, Kudoh I (1996) Cerebral autoregulation is impaired in patients resuscitated form cardiac arrest. Acta Anaesthesiol Scand 40: 1149–1153
27. Sakabe T, Tateishi A, Miyauchi Y, et al (1987) Intracranial pressure following cardiopulmonary resuscitation. Intensive Care Med 13: 256–259
28. Leonov Y, Sterz F, Safar P, Johnson DW, Tisherman SA, Oku K (1992) Hypertension with hemodilution prevents multifocal cerebral hypoperfusion after cardiac arrest in dogs. Stroke 23: 45–53
29. Lewis WD, Chwals W, Benotti PN, et al (1988) Bedside assessment of the work of breathing. Crit Care Med 16: 117–122
30. Schultz MJ, Determann RM, Wolthuis EK (2008)Ventilation with lower tidal volumes as compared with normal tidal volumes for patients without acute lung injury – a preventive randomized controlled trial. Intensive Care Med 34:S10 (abst)
31. Van den Berghe G, Wouters P, Weekers F, et al (2001) Intensive insulin therapy in the critically ill patients. N Engl J Med 345: 1359–1367
32. Van den Berghe G, Wilmer A, Hermans G, et al (2006) Intensive insulin therapy in the medical ICU. N Engl J Med 354: 449–461
33. Behringer W, Bernard S, Holzer M, Polderman K, Tiainen M, Roine RO (2007) Prevention of post-resuscitation neurologic dysfunction and injury by the use of therapeutic hypothermia. In: Paradis NA, Halperin HR, Kern KB, Wenzel V, Chamberlain DA (eds) Cardiac Arrest. The Science and Practice of Resuscitation Medicine. 2nd edn. Cambridge University Press, Cambridge, pp 848–884
34. Fischer M, Böttiger BW, Popov-Cenic S, Hossmann KA (1996) Thrombolysis using plasminogen activator and heparin reduces cerebral no-reflow after resuscitation from cardiac arrest: an experimental study in the cat. Intensive Care Med 22: 1214–1223
35. Rundgren M, Westhall E, Cronberg T, Rosén I, H. Friberg H (2008) Amplitude integrated EEG (AEEG) predicts outcome in hypothermia treated cardiac arrest patients. Intensive Care Med 34:S102 (abst)
36. Nieuwendijk R, Struys AA, Gommers D, Simoons ML, Bakker J (2008) Treatment with induced hypothermia after out-of-hospital cardiac arrest has a high incidence of lower respiratory infections. Intensive Care Med 34:S211 (abst)
37. Stoutenbeek CP, van Saene HFK, Miranda DR, Zandstra DF (1984) The effect of selective decontamination of the digestive tract on colonisation and infection rate in multiple trauma patients. Intensive Care Medicine 10: 185–192
38. de Jonge E, Schultz MJ, Spanjaard L, et al (2003) Effects of selective decontamination of digestive tract on mortality and acquisition of resistant bacteria in intensive care: a randomised controlled trial. Lancet 362: 1011–1016
39. Alam HB, Rhee P, Honma K, et al (2006) Does the rate of rewarming from profound hypothermic arrest influence the outcome in a swine model of lethal hemorrhage? J Trauma 60: 134–146
40. Zandbergen EG, Hijdra A, Koelman JH, et al (2006) Prediction of poor outcome within the first 3 days of postanoxic coma. Neurology 66: 62–68
41. Wijdicks EF, Hijdra A, Young GB, Bassetti CL, Wiebe S, Quality Standards Subcommittee of the American Academy of Neurology (2006) Practice parameter: prediction of outcome in comatose survivors after cardiopulmonary resuscitation (an evidence-based review): report of the Quality Standards Subcommittee of the American Academy of Neurology. Neurology 67: 203–210
42. Reisinger J, Höllinger K, Lang W (2007) Prediction of neurological outcome after cardiopulmonary resuscitation by serial determination of serum neuron-specific enolase. Eur Heart J 28: 52–58

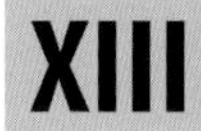

43. Aufderheide TP, Lurie KG (2006) Vital organ blood flow with the impedance threshold device. Crit Care Med 34:S466–473
44. Busch H, Brunner M, Schwab H, Inderbitzen B, Barbut D, Schwab T (2008) Pre-treatment with trans-nasal cooling for the induction of therapeutic hypothermia in patients with cardiac arrest leads to a significant faster achievement of target temperature during systemic cooling. Intensive Care Med 34:S250 (abst)
45. Ewy GA (2007) Cardiac arrest--guideline changes urgently needed. Lancet 369: 882–884
46. Sayre MR, Berg RA, Cave DM, et al (2008) Hands-only (compression-only) cardiopulmonary resuscitation: a call to action for bystander response to adults who experience out-of-hospital sudden cardiac arrest: a science advisory for the public from the American Heart Association Emergency Cardiovascular Care Committee. Circulation 117: 2162–2167
47. Damian MS, Ellenberg D, Gildemeister R, et al (2004) Coenzyme Q10 combined with mild hypothermia after cardiac arrest: a preliminary study. Circulation 110: 3011–3016
48. Cariou A, Claessens YE, Pène F, et al (2008) Early high-dose erythropoietin therapy and hypothermia after out-of-hospital cardiac arrest: a matched control study. Resuscitation 76: 397–404
49. Sasson C, Hegg AJ, Macy M, Park A, Kellermann A, McNally B, CARES Surveillance Group (2008) Prehospital termination of resuscitation in cases of refractory out-of-hospital cardiac arrest. JAMA 300: 1432–1438
50. Arawwawala D, Brett SJ (2007) Clinical review: beyond immediate survival from resuscitation-long-term outcome considerations after cardiac arrest. Crit Care 11:235
51. Williams GR, Spencer FC (1958) The clinical use of hypothermia following cardiac arrest. Ann Surg 148: 462–468
52. Benson DW, Williams GR, Spencer FC, Yates AT (1959) The use of hypothermia after cardiac arrest. Anesth Analg 38: 423–428
53. Bernard SA, Jones BM, Horne MK (1997) Clinical trial of induced hypothermia in comatose survivors of out-of-hospital cardiac arrest. Ann Emerg Med 30: 146–153
54. Yanagawa Y, Ishihara S, Norio H, et al (1998) Preliminary clinical outcome study of mild resuscitative hypothermia after out-of-hospital cardiopulmonary arrest. Resuscitation 39: 61–66
55. Nagao K, Hayashi N, Kanmatsuse K, et al (2000) Cardiopulmonary cerebral resuscitation using emergency cardiopulmonary bypass, coronary reperfusion therapy and mild hypothermia in patients with cardiac arrest outside the hospital. J Am Coll Cardiol 36: 776–783
56. Zeiner A, Holzer M, Sterz F, et al (2000) Mild resuscitative hypothermia to improve neurological outcome after cardiac arrest. A clinical feasibility trial. Stroke 31: 86–94
57. Mori K, Takeyama Y, Itoh Y, et al (2000) A multivariate analysis of prognostic factors in survivors of out-of-hospital cardiac arrest with brain hypothermia therapy. Crit Care Med 28 (12 suppl):A168 (abst)
58. Felberg RA, Krieger DW, Chuang R, et al (2001) Hypothermia after cardiac arrest: feasibility and safety of an external cooling protocol. Circulation 104: 1799–1804

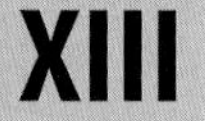

Therapeutic Hypothermia after Cardiac Arrest

G. Ristagno and W. Tang

Introduction

Patients who are successfully resuscitated following cardiac arrest often present with what is now termed 'post-resuscitation disease' [1]. Most prominent, are post-resuscitation myocardial failure and ischemic brain damage. Although post-resuscitation myocardial dysfunction has been implicated as an important mechanism accounting for fatal outcomes after cardiac resuscitation [2–4], morbidity and mortality after successful cardiopulmonary resuscitation (CPR) largely also depends on recovery of neurologic function. As many as 30 % of survivors of cardiac arrest in fact manifest permanent brain damage [5–7]. The greatest post-resuscitation emphasis has been on long-term neurologically intact survival [8]. Evidence favoring correction of electrolyte and glucose abnormalities, control of post-resuscitation cardiac rate, rhythm, systemic blood pressure, and intravascular volumes are cited but objective proof of these interventions is still anedoctal. Of all interventions, the most persuasive benefits have followed the use of hypothermia [8].

Therapeutic hypothermia following return of spontaneous circulation was advocated for decades prior to its clinical acceptance [9]. More than a decade ago, it was reported that young and healthy people who underwent accidental deep hypothermia with cardiac arrest were able to survive with no or minimal cerebral impairment even after prolonged cardiac arrest [10]. The concept of hypothermia for reducing either or both ischemic and reperfusion injury of the brain represents a pioneering contribution of the late Professor Peter Safar and the persistence of his efforts through his students, and especially Professor Fritz Sterz [9, 11]. In 1996, Professor Safar and colleagues induced hypothermia by instilling Ringer's solution maintained at a temperature of 4 °C into the abdominal cavity of dogs after resuscitation from cardiac arrest. Cooling was maintained for 12 hours. Functional recovery was associated with minimal histological brain damage [9]. Two of the largest randomized clinical trials on systemic hypothermia published in 2002 [11, 12] objectively demonstrated improvements in neurological outcomes and, within a short 5 years, this therapeutic intervention has finally proved to be neuroprotective [8, 11, 12].

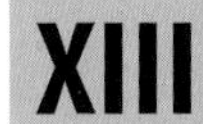

At present, therapeutic hypothermia has become a well-recognized useful tool in the physician's armamentarium for providing neuroprotection following cerebral ischemic events, including global cerebral ischemia following cardiac arrest. The International Liaison Committee and the American Heart Association (AHA) recommend post-resuscitation hypothermia in the range of 32°C to 34°C for between 12 and 24 hours in adult victims who are comatose following return of spontaneous circulation [8].

Effects of Hypothermia on Neurological Function Following Cardiac Arrest

Post-resuscitation neurological function largely depends on the duration of the arrest time, with no blood flow and development of ischemic injury. The severity of neurologic dysfunction after circulatory arrest also relates to the cerebral reperfusion disturbances observed during and after reperfusion following resuscitation. During ischemic episodes, there is increased blood viscosity and blood consequently stagnates within the microcirculation facilitating red cell aggregation. Constriction of blood vessels and perivascular edema have also been frequently observed [13, 14]. All these mechanisms may be implicated in increasing cerebral vascular resistance which culminates in marked impairment of reflow after return of spontaneous circulation and cerebral hypoperfusion, especially in the forebrain and cerebellar regions. Severe hypoperfusion to as low as 6 to 20 % of the normal level that developed in the first 10 to 20 minutes of reperfusion has been reported to last for at least 2 hours [15]. In a recent investigation performed in our laboratories [16], of special interest was the relationship between macro- and microvascular flows and the severity of brain tissue ischemia during and following cardiac arrest and return of spontaneous circulation. We reported that increases in cerebral cortical tissue PCO_2, a useful quantitative measurement of the metabolic severity of low flow states, were observed after onset of cardiac arrest and were progressive during (CPR). After return of spontaneous circulation, although macro- and microvascular flows were restored quite promptly, cerebral cortical ischemia was more slowly reversed. Hence, these studies pinpointed delays in reversal of brain ischemia after resuscitation with early brain protection such as initiating hypothermia during CPR rather than after resuscitation.

Hypothermia slows down most of the cerebral metabolic processes and, therefore, may inhibit deleterious biochemical or cerebrovascular events during reperfusion [17, 18]. Hypothermia also decreases damaging free radical production [18] and excitatory amino acid release [19] and instead promotes neuronal recovery after both focal and global brain ischemia.

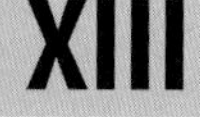

Cerebral blood flow modifications in response to cooling are not as yet clearly understood. Previous studies have shown local or global decreases in blood reperfusion in the brain during whole body or selective brain cooling [20, 21]. This was explained as a direct result of the coupling between the local blood reperfusion and local metabolism that usually decreases when temperature drops. However, this coupling might be disrupted during ischemia [22]. In experimental models, Kuluz et al. [23] described increases in cerebral large vessel blood flow following selective brain cooling. In different settings, cooling of carotid artery preparations induced a reversible graded vasodilation and decreased or abolished the effect of vasocontractile neurotransmitters. Isometric tensions in rodent carotid artery strips were further assessed during stepwise cooling [24]. Lowering of the temperature, from 37 °C to 4 °C, induced a rapid and reproducible stepwise decrease in the arterial wall tone and when the temperature was reset to 37 °C, the tone rapidly returned to the basal level. Cooling also significantly reduced or totally abolished norepinephrine-induced contractions of the large cerebral vessels. In organs other than brain, hypothermia instead induced a clear-cut increase in basal tone of the smooth muscles of the blood vessels. Therefore, the basic mechanisms underlying hypothermic reactions of smooth muscle in blood vessels and other conduits of the body are regionally different and adjusted to serve the functional requirements of the organism when exposed to hypothermia. In different settings, when cerebral perfusion was measured during hyperthermia, defined as increases of 4 °C from the basal temperature, carotid artery contraction and decreases in cerebral blood flow were observed [25].

Additional benefits of brain hypothermia are also identified in the ability of hypothermia to significantly reduce intracranial pressure (ICP) after restoration of flow and this might account for greater perfusion [26]. When ICP increases due to brain edema, neurons may be damaged thus jeopardizing cerebral perfusion. Induced hypothermia might, therefore, be considered to control increases in ICP, without compromising cerebral autoregulation [26, 27].

Effects of Hypothermia on Myocardial Function after Cardiac Arrest

More than 50 % of all patients initially resuscitated from cardiac arrest subsequently die before leaving the hospital. Studies in animals and in human patients support the notion that the majority of these deaths are due to impaired myocardial function primarily due to heart failure and/or recurrent ventricular fibrillation [28]. This high incidence of fatal outcomes related to post-resuscitation myocardial dysfunction has prompted research on options for myocardial preservation during cardiac arrest and resuscitation. In addition to neuroprotection [11, 12], hypothermia has also appeared to be an important intervention to protect the heart after cardiac arrest.

Hypothermia, in fact, has been shown to protect from ischemia-reperfusion injury [29], and to aid in diminishing myocardial infarct size in animal models of coronary artery occlusion [30, 31]. Such protection seemed to be mediated by increased nitric oxide (NO) generation via activation of protein kinase C-epsilon (PKCε) [29]. Hypothermia also reduced metabolic demand and high energy phosphate utilization in the myocardium [32], as well as oxygen utilization [33] with consequent reductions in ATP depletion [34]. In models of ischemia-reperfusion in cardiomyocytes, cooling prior to reperfusion conferred improved cell viability and attenuated a number of intracellular injury pathway mechanisms, including apoptotic enzymes, in comparison to reperfusion without cooling [29]. In settings of cardiac arrest, temperature preconditioning induced by short-term hypothermic perfusion and rewarming, protected hearts au pair to ischemic preconditioning [35]. Prior to inducing ischemia, hearts underwent cycles of hypothermic perfusion at 26°C interspersed with intervals of normothermic perfusion. During reperfusion following ischemia, hypothermia improved hemodynamic recovery, decreased arrhythmias, and reduced necrotic damage.

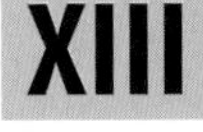

Moreover, rapid cooling has also been previously reported to lead to increases in mammalian cardiac muscle twitch force, probably related to increases in the calcium sensitivity of the myofilaments [36]. When we investigated the effects of a range of temperatures on ventricular myocyte contractility, we observed that decreases in perfusion temperatures were highly related to significant increases in myocyte contractility (unpublished data). Reductions in perfusion temperature were accompanied by corresponding increases in cell shortening percentage (**Fig. 1**).

All these effects of hypothermia may contribute to the explanation of more recent observations of increased myocardial contractility following cooling treatment after cardiac arrest. In isolated hearts perfused and exposed to mild or moderate hypothermia during 120 minutes of ischemia, moderate hypothermia suppressed anaerobic metabolism during ischemia and significantly diminished left ventricular end-

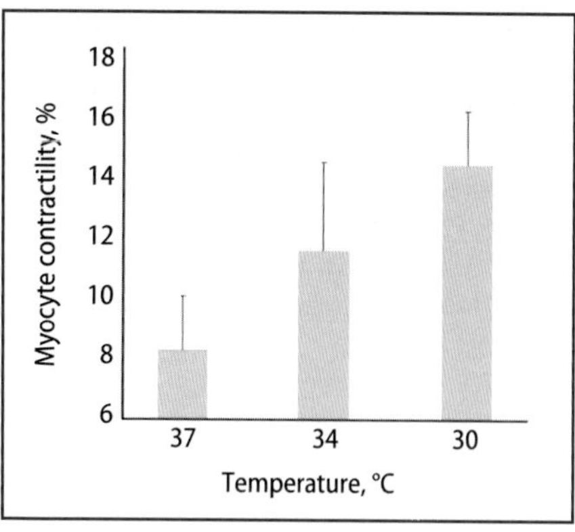

Fig. 1. Myocyte contractility expressed in % of baseline length during different perfusion temperatures.

diastolic pressure at the end of ischemia. Hypothermia therefore contributed to the preservation of myocardial function, coronary flow, and oxygen consumption compared with normal control hearts [37]. Interesting data, highlighting improvements of myocardial contractility in animals that received hypothermia treatment following cardiac arrest, have been recently published by Zhao et al [38]. In these experiments, hypothermic cardiovascular reperfusion resulted in considerably greater cardiac output with concomitant lesser systolic and diastolic myocardial dysfunction during the post-arrest period. Accordingly, we have recently confirmed, employing a different method of cooling to provide rapid selective head cooling initiated during CPR, improvements not only on post-resuscitation neurological outcome but also increases in coronary perfusion pressure during chest compressions, with consequent greater success of resuscitation and better post-resuscitation myocardial function and survival [39–41].

Finally, hypothermia has been reported to reduce the defibrillation threshold to terminate ventricular fibrillation [42]. Boddicker et al. [32] demonstrated that moderate or severe systemic hypothermia, induced by surrounding the head, thorax, and abdomen with ice, prior to resuscitation, improved the success of defibrillation and return of spontaneous circulation in a prolonged porcine model of cardiac arrest. Severe surface hypothermia facilitated transthoracic defibrillation through modifications in mechanical and electrophysiological myocardium properties, shown by increases in thoracic impedance with a decrease in current.

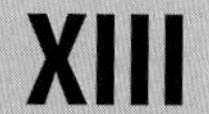

Timing and Methods for Inducing Hypothermia

Currently, hypothermic treatment is initiated during the post-resuscitation period in order to minimize reperfusion injury following ischemia. However, several experimental investigations have raised the importance of starting hypothermia as soon as possible and have also suggested that intra-arrest hypothermia may provide additional survival benefits [38–41, 43, 44]. The theoretical advantages of earlier cooling include decreasing reperfusion related injury mechanisms, attenuation of the oxidant burst seen within minutes of normothermic reperfusion, and inhibition of reperfusion related apoptosis [45].

When mild cerebral hypothermia was induced in pigs immediately after return of spontaneous circulation, improved cerebral functional and morphologic outcomes were observed in contrast to animals not subjected to cooling, whereas a delay of as little as 15 minutes in initiation of cooling after reperfusion slightly decreased tissue damage but did not improve functional outcome [46]. Subsequently, when hypothermia was initiated during cardiac arrest, early cooling not only improved neurological outcome but also yielded better 72-hour survival, in contrast to delayed hypothermia and normothermic resuscitation [44]. Even when resuscitative efforts were delayed in order to facilitate external surface cooling before initiation of CPR, better hemodynamics, survival and neurological function have been reported [38].

These findings support the concept that post-resuscitation injury processes begin immediately after return of spontaneous circulation, and that intra-arrest cooling might serve as a useful therapeutic approach to improve both cerebral outcome and finally survival. The beneficial effects of early initiation of hypothermia on survival and outcomes of CPR have been further confirmed in the clinical scenario. The institution of hypothermic treatment based on a 'control of the time to target temperature', so as to achieve mild hypothermic temperature as fast as possible, was associated with reduced hypoxic brain injury and favored better neurologic outcome in resuscitated victims of cardiac arrest [47]. Therefore, although delayed hospital cooling has been demonstrated to improve outcomes after cardiac arrest, in-field cooling started immediately after return of spontaneous circulation has the potential to be more beneficial. When victims of out of hospital cardiac arrest were randomized to receive intravenous infusion of up to 2 l of 4 °C normal saline in the field, mean temperature decreased over 1.24 °C reaching an average temperature of 34.7 °C prior to hospital arrival. This in-field cooling was not associated with adverse consequences in terms of blood pressure, heart rate, arterial oxygenation, or evidence of pulmonary edema, and instead was associated with improvement regarding awakening and survival to hospital discharge [48].

Traditionally, hypothermia has been accomplished by two methods. The first is 'external cooling', which employs cold packs or cooling blankets and sophisticated machines with automatic feedback control; the second is 'internal cooling', which uses cold intravenous infusions, intravascular cooling catheters, body cavity lavage, extra-corporeal circuits, and, more recently, selective brain cooling. Other non-invasive methods include drugs and cold liquid ventilation. Improved cooling technologies have resulted in earlier attainment of target temperature and even more robust clinical benefits in the management of the survivors of cardiac arrest. Most of these methods are quite invasive and are still at an experimental stage. The optimal timing and technique for the induction of hypothermia after cardiac arrest have not as yet been defined, and are currently a major topic of ongoing research. External methods cool first the skin and peripheral compartments of the body and internal methods cool the blood, thus directly cooling the core compartment of the body. These methods are, however, slow to achieve significant cooling of the brain because they are targeted at cooling the entire body, rather than the injured cerebral area. A reduction in brain temperature of as little as 2 °C has been shown to reduce ischemic damage and significantly improves outcomes in patients with stroke, head injuries or after cardiac arrest. The major challenge facing clinicians is represented by the need to maximize the protective effects of brain hypothermia and thereby the time to delivery of this type of treatment. Cooling the entire body or the total arterial blood to achieve a temperature reduction in the brain may not be necessary, since the brain receives only 20 % of the resting cardiac output. The long cooling period may be reduced if only the head is cooled. Selective brain hypothermia using different devices has, therefore, been proposed [22, 39]. In our recent experience, we uti-

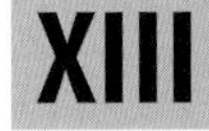

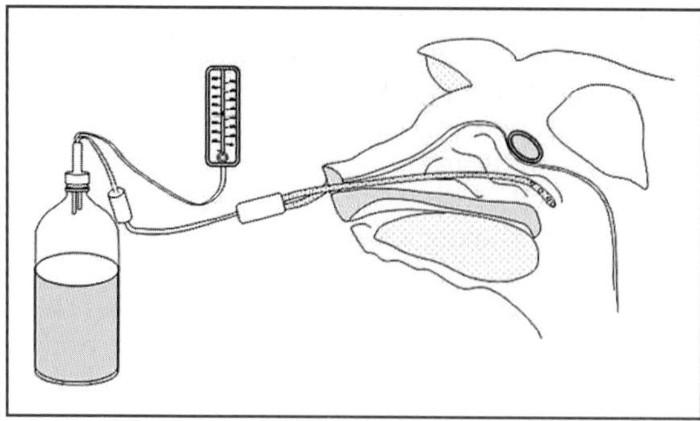

Fig. 2. Schematic representation of the system for head cooling (Bene-Chill Inc., San Diego, CA) applied in a pig.

lize the nasopharynx cavity to induce hypothermia. A chemically and biologically inert volatile fluorocarbon is vaporized and propelled into the nasopharynx by oxygen where it produces evaporative cooling. This natural cavity into the head takes advantage of overcoming the obstacle of cooling the brain through the skull. This approach can, therefore, significantly cool the nasopharynx cavity and offers the ability to cool the brain more quickly via direct conductive mechanisms and indirect hematogenous mechanisms (**Fig. 2**).

Preliminary Experience with Selective Brain Cooling: Effects on Neurological and Myocardial Functions

When pigs were cooled coincident with onset of CPR, the jugular venous temperature was reduced from 38 °C to 34 °C over 5 minutes. The likelihood of successful defibrillation after 10 minutes of untreated cardiac arrest and 5 minutes of CPR was significantly increased with head cooling. Eight cooled animals survived for 96 hours with full neurological recovery. Only 2 of 8 normothermic controls survived and both had persistent neurological deficits. Quite unexpectedly and in the absence of more than a 1.3 °C decrease in body temperature over the ensuing hour, left ventricular systolic function, reflected by ejection fraction and fractional area change together with left ventricular diastolic function, represented by isovolumic relaxation time and E/E' ratio, were significantly better in head cooled animals (**Fig. 3**) [39, 40]. Several mechanisms may have contributed to the observed improvement in myocardial performance. The cooled animals had a higher defibrillation success rate ($p = 0.034$), required a shorter duration of CPR ($p = 0.01$) and a lesser total dose of epinephrine ($p = 0.009$), in comparison to the control group. Greater post-resuscitation hemodynamic stability was also observed in cooled animals. Immediately post-return of spontaneous circulation, arterial pressures and coronary perfusion pressures, in fact, increased in cooled animals and were significantly greater compared to control animals, in which pressures decreased. Brain cooling during CPR therefore improved myocardial perfusion and this was reflected in less recurrent ventricular fibrillation and ultimately in improvements in myocardial performance (**Table 1**).

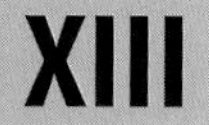

These beneficial effects on ease of defibrillation and a more benign post-resuscitation course were subsequently confirmed in animals in which the duration of untreated cardiac arrest was extended to 15 minutes [41]. Also unexpectedly there

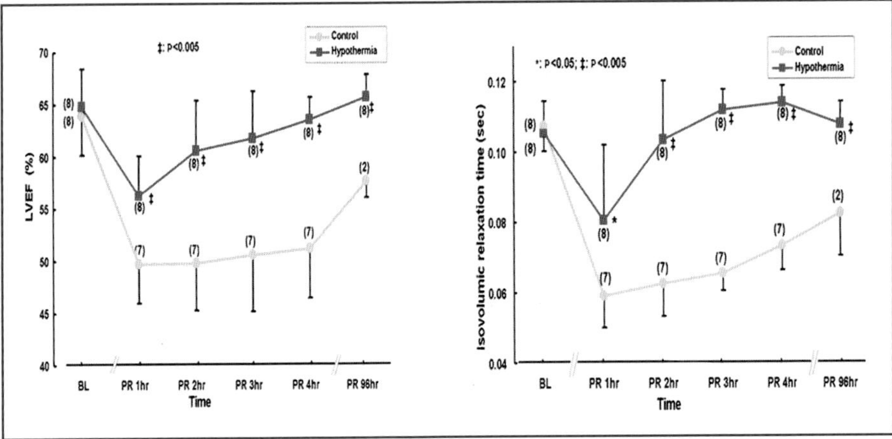

Fig. 3. Post-resuscitation left ventricular ejection fraction (LVEF) and isovolumic relaxation time. BL: baseline; PR: post-resuscitation.

Table 1. Effects of head cooling on post-resuscitation hemodynamics.

	Control (8)	Head Cooled (8)	p value
Brain temperature, °C			
Baseline	38 ± 0.3	38.01 ± 0.3	NS
Post-resuscitation	38.3 ± 0.2	35.8 ± 2.3	0.016
Core temperature, °C			
Baseline	37.9 ± 0.1	38 ± 0.3	NS
Post-resuscitation	38.1 ± 0.3	38 ± 0.3	NS
Number of recurrent VF	12 ± 7	6 ± 4	0.05
Coronary perfusion pressure, mmHg			
Baseline	73 ± 11	73 ± 14	NS
Post-resuscitation	30 ± 17	61 ± 25	0.009
Mean arterial pressure, mmHg			
Baseline	119 ± 12	119 ± 11	NS
Post-resuscitation	71 ± 23	130 ± 6	< 0.001

VF: ventricular fibrillation

was a remarkably higher coronary perfusion pressure in head cooled animals and this was consistent with greater success of defibrillation ($p < 0.01$).

The mechanism by which selective brain cooling improved the likelihood of return of spontaneous circulation is not fully understood. It is conceivable that targeted cooling of the underside of the brain using nasopharyngeal cooling alters the firing rates of efferent autonomic nerves in the cervical chain. Inhibition of sympathetic firing during systemic hypothermia has been reported previously as temperature was reduced from 38°C to 31°C [49]. Experimental studies in healthy volunteers demonstrated that plasma norepinephrine and total peripheral resistances were reduced during moderately cold head immersion for 20 minutes. Moreover, hypothermia has been reported to attenuate ischemia-induced release of norepinephrine and acetylcholine [50]. The paraventricular nucleus of the hypothalamus is a focal point in the complex of interacting systems regulating stress response and, in our model, those brain regions were close to the source of cooling. When we measured plasma norepinephrine concentration during CPR prior to return of spontaneous circulation, it was lower in the cooled animals than in the control animals.

In assessing the critical perfusion condition during and after resuscitation from cardiac arrest, both investigators and clinicians have focused on pressure and blood flow through large vessels and specifically arterial and large venous vessels and cardiac output. CPR interventions and especially chest compressions focused on increasing and maintaining optimal pressures so as to favor large vessel supplies to the brain and the heart. With the advent of methods by which microvessels and especially capillaries are visualized, it has become apparent that large vessel pressures and flows alone may not be predictive of the extent to which microvessels and, therefore, tissues are perfused. Yet, it is the microvessels and specifically the capillaries, which serve as the ultimate exchange sites for vital metabolites. In a preliminary study in pigs, we have addressed effects of selective head cooling on cerebral microcirculatory flows in relation to carotid blood flows. After 4 minutes of untreated ventricular fibrillation and 4 minutes of CPR, carotid artery diameters and flows increased during selective head cooling, even though cardiac output was not changed in comparison to controls at that time point. The increases in carotid blood flows were associated with concurrent increases in the numbers of perfused capillaries visualized in the cerebral cortex (**Fig. 4**).

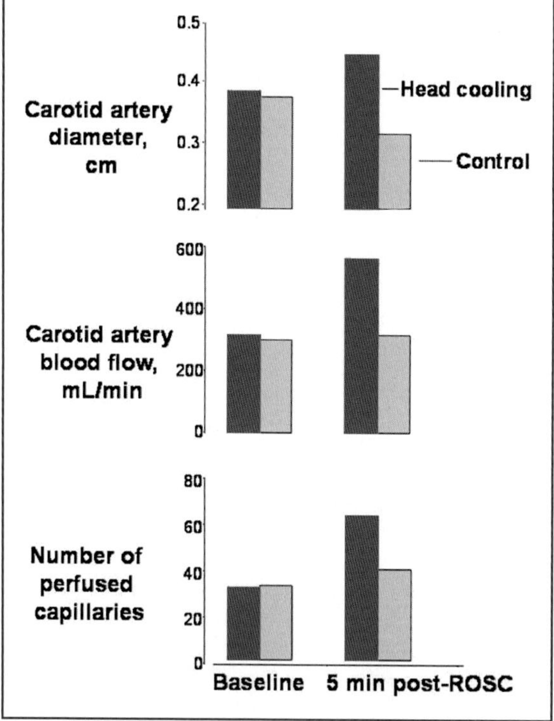

Fig. 4. Carotid artery diameter and flow and number of perfused cerebral cortical microvessels in animals resuscitated from cardiac arrest and subjected to head cooling or control. ROSC: return of spontaneous circulation

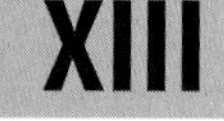

Conclusion

Over the past few years, the implementation of therapeutic hypothermia has provided an exciting opportunity toward improving neurological outcome from out-of-hospital cardiac arrest. The pioneering approaches of Doctor Safar, more than a decade ago, to introduce hypothermia as a valid treatment to reduce ischemic brain injury following cardiac arrest, represented the initial steps toward its affirmation as useful neuroprotective treatment. The need to initiate hypothermia as soon as possible following resuscitation has now been clearly recognized. However, there are compelling data suggesting the importance to begin hypothermia during the intra-arrest period and resuscitative maneuvers. This approach may provide significant additional survival benefits. Early initiation of therapeutic hypothermia is, in fact, emerging as a method able to preserve not only cerebral function but also myocardial function and, therefore, improve survival after resuscitation from cardiac arrest.

References

1. Adrie C, Laurent I, Monchi M, et al (2004) Postresuscitation disease after cardiac arrest: a sepsis-like syndrome? Curr Opin Crit Care 10: 208-212
2. Tang W, Weil MH, Sun S, et al (1993) Progressive myocardial dysfunction after cardiac resuscitation. Crit Care Med 21: 1046-1050
3. Peatfield RC, Sillett RW, Taylor D, McNicol MW (1977) Survival after cardiac arrest in the hospital. Lancet 1: 1223-1225
4. DeBard ML (1981) Cardiopulmonary resuscitation: analysis of six years' experience and review of the literature. Ann Emerg Med 10: 408-416
5. Safar P (1993) Cerebral resuscitation after cardiac arrest: research initiatives and future directions. Ann Emerg Med 22: 324-349
6. Brain Resuscitation Clinical Trial II Study Group (1991) A randomized clinical study of a calcium-entry blocker (lidoflazine) in the treatment of comatose survivors of cardiac arrest. N Engl J Med 324: 1225-1231
7. Eisenberg MS, Horwood BT, Cummins RO, Reynolds-Haertle R, Hearne TR (1990) Cardiac arrest and resuscitation: a tale of 29 cities. Ann Emerg Med 19: 179-186
8. American Heart Association (2005) Guidelines for Cardiopulmonary Resuscitation and Emergency Cardiovascular Care Part 7.5: Postresuscitation support. Circulation 112: IV-84-IV-88
9. Safar P, Xiao F, Radovsky A, et al (1996) Improved cerebral resuscitation from cardiac arrest in dogs with mild hypothermia plus blood flow promotion. Stroke 27: 105-113
10. Walpoth BH, Walpoth-Aslan BN, Mattle HP, et al (1997) Outcome of survivors of accidental deep hypothermia and circulatory arrest treated with extracorporeal blood warming. N Engl J Med 337: 1500-1505
11. The Hypothermia After Cardiac Arrest Study Group (2002) Mild therapeutic hypothermia to improve the neurologic outcome after cardiac arrest. N Engl J Med 346: 549-556
12. Bernard SA, Gray TW, Buist MD, et al (2002) Treatment of comatose survivors of out-of-hospital cardiac arrest with induced hypothermia. N Engl J Med 346: 557-563
13. Shaffner DH, Eleff SM, Koehler RC, Traystman RJ (1998) Effect of the no-flow interval and hypothermia on cerebral blood flow and metabolism during cardiopulmonary resuscitation in dogs. Stroke 29: 2607-2615
14. Fischer M, Hossmann KA (1995) No-reflow after cardiac arrest. Intensive Care Med 21: 132-141
15. Liachenko S, Tang P, Hamilton RL, Xu Y (2001) Regional dependence of cerebral reperfusion after circulatory arrest in rats. J Cereb Blood Flow Metab 21: 1320-1329
16. Ristagno G, Tang W, Sun S, Weil MH (2008) Cerebral cortical microvascular flow during and following cardiopulmonary resuscitation after short duration of cardiac arrest. Resuscitation 77: 229-234

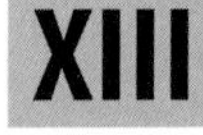

17. D'Cruz BJ, Fertig KC, Filiano AJ, Hicks SD, DeFranco DB, Callaway CW (2002) Hypothermic reperfusion after cardiac arrest augments brain-derived neurotrophic factor activation. J Cereb Blood Flow Metab 22: 843–851
18. Dietrich WD, Busto R, Alonso O, Globus MY-T, Ginsberg MD (1993) Intraischemic but not postischemic brain hypothermia protects chronically following global forebrain ischemia in rats. J Cereb Blood Flow Metab 14: 541-549
19. Ooboshi H, Ibayashi S, Takano K, et al (2000) Hypothermia inhibits ischemia-induced efflux of amino acids and neuronal damage in the hippocampus of aged rats. Brain Res 884: 23-30
20. Busijia DW, Leffler CW (1987) Hypothermia reduces cerebral metabolic rate and cerebral blood flow in newborn pigs. Am J Physiol 253: H869-H873
21. Okubo K, Itoh S, Isobe K (2001) Cerebral metabolism and regional blood flow during moderate systemic cooling in newborn piglets. Pediatr Int 43: 496–501
22. Wang Y, Zhu L (2007) Targeted brain hypothermia induced by an interstitial cooling device in human neck: theoretical analyses. Eur J Appl Physiol 101: 31–40
23. Kuluz JW, Prado R, Chang J, et al (1993) Selective brain cooling increases cortical cerebral blood flow in rats. Am J Physiol 265: H824-H827
24. Mustafa S, Thulesius O (2002) Cooling-induced carotid artery dilatation: an experimental study in isolated vessels. Stroke 33: 256–260
25. Mustafa S, Elgazzar AH, Ismael HN (2007) Influence of hyperthermia on carotid blood flow using 99mTc-HMPAO. Eur J Appl Physiol 101: 257–262
26. Strauch JT, Spielvogel D, Haldenwang PL, et al (2003) Cerebral physiology and outcome after hypothermic circulatory arrest followed by selective cerebral perfusion. Ann Thorac Surg 76: 1972–1981
27. Lavinio A, Timofeev I, Nortje J, et al (2007) Carebrovascular reactivity during hypothermia and rewarming. Br J Anaesth 99: 237–244
28. Tang W, Weil MH, Sun S, Pernat A, Mason E (2000) K(ATP) channel activation reduces the severity of postresuscitation myocardial dysfunction. Am J Physiol Heart Circ Physiol 279: H1609-H1615
29. Shao ZH, Chang WT, Chan KC, et al (2007) Hypothermia-induced cardioprotection using extended ischemia and early reperfusion cooling. Am J Physiol Heart Circ Physiol 292: H1995-H2003
30. Dave RH, Hale SL, Kloner RA (1998) Hypothermic, closed circuit pericardioperfusion: a potential cardioprotective technique in acute regional ischemia. J Am Coll Cardiol 31: 1667–1671
31. Tissier R, Hamanaka K, Kuno A, Parker JC, Cohen MV, Downey JM (2007) Total liquid ventilation provides ultra-fast cardioprotective cooling. J Am Coll Cardiol 49: 601–605
32. Boddicker KA, Zhang Y, Zimmerman MB, Davies LR, Kerber RE (2005) Hypothermia improved defibrillation success and resuscitation outcomes from ventricular fibrillation. Circulation 111: 3195–3201
33. Buckberg GD, Brazier JR, Nelson RL, et al (1977) Studies of the effects of hypothermia on regional myocardial blood flow and metabolism during cardiopulmonary bypass. I. The adequately perfused beating, fibrillating, and arrested heart. J Thorac Cardiovasc Surg 73: 87–94
34. Ning XH, Xu CS, Portman MA (1999) Mitochondrial protein and HSP70 signaling after ischemia in hypothermic-adapted hearts augmented with glucose. Am J Physiol 277: R11-R17
35. Khaliulin I, Clarke SJ, Lin H, Parker J, Suleiman MS, Halestrap AP (2007) Temperature preconditioning of isolated rat hearts--a potent cardioprotective mechanism involving a reduction in oxidative stress and inhibition of the mitochondrial permeability transition pore. J Physiol 581: 1147–1161
36. Harrison SM, Bers DM (1989) Influence of temperature on the calcium sensitivity of the myofilaments of skinned ventricular muscle from the rabbit. J Gen Physiol 93: 411–428
37. Ning XH, Chi EY, Buroker NE, et al (2007) Moderate hypothermia (30 degrees C) maintains myocardial integrity and modifies response of cell survival proteins after reperfusion. Am J Physiol Heart Circ Physiol 293: H2119-H2128
38. Zhao D, Abella BS, Beiser DG, et al (2008) Intra-arrest cooling with delayed reperfusion yields higher survival than earlier normothermic resuscitation in a mouse model of cardiac arrest. Resuscitation 77: 242–249
39. Tsai MS, Barbut D, Tang W, et al (2008) Rapid head cooling initiated coincident with cardio-

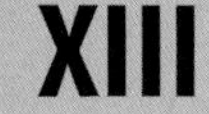

pulmonary resuscitation improves success of defibrillation and post-resuscitation myocardial function in a porcine model of prolonged cardiac arrest. J Am Coll Cardiol 51: 1988–1990
40. Guan J, Tang W, Wang H, et al (2007) Early head cooling during resuscitation culminating in systemic hypothermia results in better neurological outcome than delayed systemic hypothermia in pigs. Crit Care Med 35: A95 (abst)
41. Wang H, Tsai MS, Guan J, Tang W, Sun S, Weil MH (2007) Intra-arrest rapid head cooling improves success of resuscitation in a porcine model of prolonged cardiac arrest. Crit Care Med 35: A94 (abst)
42. Rhee BJ, Zhang Y, Boddicker KA, et al (2005) Effect of hypothermia on transthoracic defibrillation in a swine model. Resuscitation 65: 79–85
43. Leonov Y, Sterz F, Safar P, et al (1990) Mild cerebral hypothermia during and after cardiac arrest improves neurologic outcome in dogs. J Cereb Blood Flow Metab 10: 57–70
44. Abella BS, Zhao D, Alvarado J, Hamann K, Vanden Hoek TL, Becker LB (2004) Intra-arrest cooling improves outcomes in a murine cardiac arrest model. Circulation 09: 2786–2791
45. Maier CM, Abern K, Cheng ML, et al (1998) Optimal depth and duration of mild hypothermia in a focal model of transient cerebral ischemia: effects on neurologic outcome, infarct size, apoptosis, and inflammation. Stroke 29: 2171–2180
46. Kuboyama K, Safar P, Radovsky A, Tisherman SA, Stezoski SW, Alexander H (1993) Delay in cooling negates the beneficial effect of mild resuscitative cerebral hypothermia after cardiac arrest in dogs: a prospective, randomized study. Crit Care Med 21: 1348–1358
47. Wolff B, Machill K, Schumacher D, Schulzki I, Werner D (2009) Early achievement of mild therapeutic hypothermia and the neurologic outcome after cardiac arrest. Int J Cardiol (in press)
48. Kim F, Olsufka M, Longstreth WT Jr, et al (2007) Pilot randomized clinical trial of prehospital induction of mild hypothermia in out-of-hospital cardiac arrest patients with a rapid infusion of 4 degrees C normal saline. Circulation 115: 3064–3070
49. Frank SM, Cattaneo CG, Wieneke-Brady MB, et al (2002) Threshold for adrenomedullary activation and increased cardiac work during mild core hypothermia. Clin Sci (Lond) 102: 119–125
50. Kawada T, Kitagawa H, Yamazaki T, et al (2007) Hypothermia reduces ischemia- and stimulation-induced myocardial interstitial norepinephrine and acetylcholine releases. J Appl Physiol 102: 622–627

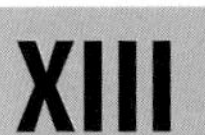

XIV Renal Function

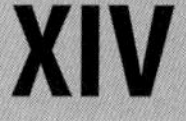

Biomarkers of Acute Kidney Injury in Critical Illness

F. Adams and B. Venkatesh

Introduction

In the last decade, epidemiological studies worldwide have shown an increase in the incidence of acute renal failure in critically ill patients [1–3]. The consequences of renal failure in the critically ill are well recognized. Despite recent advances in renal replacement therapy, the mortality rate from acute renal failure remains high, ranging from 20–50 %. The increased incidence may be due in part to the changing demographic of the critically ill patient. The increasing age of the population, as well as increased co-morbidities, such as hypertension and diabetes mellitus, increase the susceptibility to renal injury. Increasing incidence of sepsis, use of nephrotoxic drugs, and the use of radio contrast media all contribute to the increased likelihood of acute kidney injury (AKI).

Delays, both in the diagnosis of AKI and in initiation of renal supportive therapy, will contribute to a failure to reduce the morbidity and mortality associated with AKI in this high-risk group. In view of the magnitude of the problem, early detection seems mandatory to facilitate therapeutic measures to prevent established acute renal failure and the resultant need for dialytic therapy. Experimentally, it has been shown that earlier intervention in AKI results in an improved outcome [4]. The search has, therefore, been on for an early biomarker of AKI rather than acute renal failure. Consequently, the analogy that these biomarkers represent the 'troponins of the kidney' has been applied. The American Society of Nephrology has designated the development of biomarkers for AKI as an area of top research priority. The properties of an ideal biomarker of AKI are listed in **Table 1**.

The question, however, is which is the most reliable biomarker for diagnosis and prognostication of renal injury? Several contenders for the ideal AKI biomarker have emerged in the last decade (**Table 2**). Whilst their diagnostic potential has been examined in both experimental and clinical acute renal failure, limited data exist on

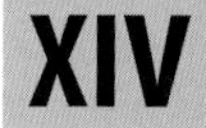

Table 1. Properties of the ideal biomarker

Properties
Detectable early in course of disease
High sensitivity
High specificity
Biological stability
Easily and rapidly performed
Reproducible
Wide biological range allowing risk stratification
Able to be detected on readily accessible body fluids such as serum or urine

Table 2. Biomarkers of acute kidney injury

Biomarker	Site of detection
N-acetyl-β-D-glucosaminidase, NAG	urine
Cystatin C	urine/plasma
Kidney injury molecule-1, KIM 1	urine
Neutrophil gelatinase-associated lipocalin, NGAL	urine/plasma
Cysteine-rich protein, CYR61	urine
Interleukin-18, IL-18	urine
Sodium hydrogen exchanger 3, NHE3	urine
Tubular enzymes	urine
Fetuin A	urine

their utility in the intensive care setting. In comparison to the patient with stable chronic kidney disease or in the general medical ward, the milieu of the critically ill patient is complicated by the presence of systemic inflammatory response syndrome (SIRS), cytokinemia and multi-organ dysfunction, which may affect biomarker generation, turnover, and clearance. In this commentary, we examine the published data on biomarkers of AKI in the intensive care setting and discuss their potential role in the evaluation and management of acute renal injury in the critically ill patient.

Conventionally used Indices of Renal Injury

Historically, renal function has been monitored by using estimations of the serum creatinine (formed by muscle breakdown) and creatinine clearance as surrogates for the glomerular filtration rate (GFR). As dynamic markers of renal function and AKI, serum creatinine and creatinine clearance are less than ideal. Serum creatinine can be affected by age, sex, muscle mass, drugs and diet; ingestion of meat can increase the serum creatinine by as much as 30 % 7 hours after a meal. Creatinine is a relatively insensitive indicator of GFR; GFR has to be reduced by 40–50 % before the serum creatinine begins to increase. An isolated serum creatinine value is unable to differentiate between acute and chronic renal disease.

Other indices, such as creatinine clearance (affected by inaccurate body weight estimations, edema), urine output (affected by solute load, drugs, renal obstruction, and errors in data collection), and urinary electrolytes (affected by diuretics), as indicators of AKI are neither sensitive nor specific.

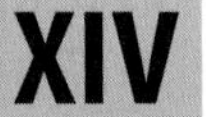

Biomarkers of Renal Injury

A biomarker is "a biological characteristic that is objectively measured and evaluated as an indicator of normal biological process, pathogenic process or pharmacological response to a therapeutic intervention" [5]. The ideal biomarker of AKI would have a high sensitivity and specificity, biological stability, and be easily and rapidly performed. A single biomarker may fail if its level is influenced by several diseases. It needs to be detectable early enough so that therapeutic intervention to halt/reverse the disease process is possible. A wide biological range allowing risk stratification would enable selected targeting of therapy. It should also be readily

Table 3. Temporal characteristics of biomarkers

Biomarker	Time to earliest detection from initial insult	Time to peak level
NGAL (urine)	< 2 hours	4–6 hours
IL-18 (urine)	2–4 hours	12 hours
KIM 1 (urine)	4–6 hours	24 hours
CYR61	3–6 hours	6–9 hours

NGAL: neutrophil gelatinase-associated lipocalin; IL: interleukin; KIM: kidney injury molecule; CYR: cysteine-rich protein

assayed on easily accessible body fluids such as serum and urine. The ideal biomarker would allow discrimination between various types of AKI, and between AKI and other causes of acute renal disease [6].

In AKI, advantage is taken of the biological response of the renal tissue to ischemic and toxic injury. The biological response results in several cellular and enzyme changes, which can be readily measured using genomic, proteomic, and microarray technologies. Some of the novel biomarkers of AKI, with special reference to critical illness are described below. The temporal relationship from insult to detection for some of the biomarkers is described in **Table 3**.

Serum Markers

The novel serum markers under investigation include human neutrophil gelatinase-associated lipocalin (NGAL), and cystatin C.

Neutrophil gelatinase-associated lipocalin

NGAL is a 25 kDa protein which belongs to the lipocalin superfamily. It is covalently bound to gelatinase from human neutrophils and expressed at low levels in several tissues, including kidney, trachea, lungs, stomach, and colon. It is one of the most upregulated genes and over-expressed proteins following renal ischemia. Its expression is also increased in bacterial infections due to the secondary inflammatory activation of leukocytes. Following injury, NGAL induction is a rapid event detectable within a few hours, characterizing NGAL as one of the immediate early genes or acute phase reactants, such as interleukin (IL)-6 and C-reactive protein (CRP).

NGAL concentrations have been demonstrated to increase rapidly in serum and/or urine in response to ischemic renal injury in a number of studies. In a study of 71 children undergoing cardiopulmonary bypass (CPB) of whom 20 developed acute renal failure, the urinary concentration of NGAL at two hours after bypass was the most significant indicator for renal injury in multivariate analysis [7]. Similar results have been reported among adults undergoing cardiac surgery [8] and percutaneous coronary intervention. In ischemia-reperfusion injuries and cisplatin nephropathy [9], NGAL induction precedes the elevation of classical markers for kidney damage: Serum creatinine, urinary N-acetyl-β-D-glucosaminidase, β 2-microglobulin levels. Furthermore, Mori et al. [10] and other groups have reported that NGAL protein accumulates abundantly in the blood, urine, and renal proximal and distal tubules in acute renal failure, in cases associated with renal ischemia (sepsis, hypovolemia, and heart failure) [11], nephrotoxin (antibiotics, cisplatin, bisphosphonate non-steroidal anti-inflammatory drugs [9], radiocontrast, and hemoglobinuria), kidney-parenchymal damage (glomerulonephrits, minimal change disease, focal segmental glomeru-

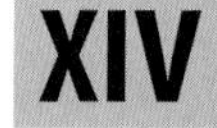

losclerosis, and diabetic nephropathy) [12], hemolytic-uremic syndrome, and post-transplant rejection [13].

There are few published data on NGAL in critically ill patients. The published literature is largely confined to the post-CPB population, where elevated NGAL has been shown to be a highly predictive early biomarker of AKI after cardiac surgery [7]. Other limitations include the fact that there are non-renal sources of NGAL, thus elevated serum concentrations may be found in conditions other than in renal failure.

Cystatin C

Cystatin C is a cationic cysteine protease inhibitor which is synthesized by all nucleated cells. It is freely filtered at the glomerulus and completely reabsorbed at the proximal tubule. It is thought that blood concentrations of cystatin C are unaffected by age and muscle mass, although the latter point has been disputed [14]. A reduction in GFR is associated with an increase in serum cystatin C concentrations. Urinary levels increase in the context of acute tubular injury. The role of cystatin C as a biomarker was substantiated in a prospective study of 85 intensive care unit (ICU) patients at high risk of developing AKI: 44 patients developed AKI and 41 patients acted as controls [15]. All patients had a normal GFR, defined by a serum creatinine less than 110 μmol/l. Increases in cystatin C levels of 50 % or more occurred 1.5 ± 0.6 days earlier than a comparable rise in serum creatinine. Sensitivity and specificity of cystatin C two days prior to D0, were 0.53 and 0.82, respectively, with a positive predictive value of 0.45 [15]. A sensitivity of this level is unlikely to be helpful to the intensive care physician with regard to whether or not to institute renal support. Prospective, albeit small, studies [16, 17] would support this view.

Urine Markers of AKI

Several novel urine markers of AKI have been investigated and are summarized in **Table 4**. Other urinary markers evaluated as potential biomarkers of AKI include urinary endothelin [18], cysteine rich protein 61 [19], perforin and granzyme B [20]. While elevated urinary concentrations of these markers have been reported in experimental renal failure, human studies on their clinical utility are minimal.

Data on Biomarkers of AKI in Critical Illness

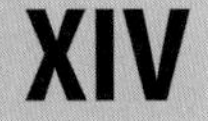

In **Table 5**, we provide a summary of the clinical studies examining the utility of biomarkers in critical illness As seen above, several studies on biomarkers of AKI have been performed in critically ill patients, The level of accuracy for the prediction of AKI noted in non-critically ill patients has not been achieved in the intensive care population. Several explanations for this finding can be proposed. First, not all of these biomarkers are renally generated; for example there are non-renal sources of NGAL [21, 22]. Therefore, non-renal diseases can increase biomarker concentrations. In this context, it is important to note that kidney injury molecule (KIM)-1 is a marker of renal cancer [23] and cystatin C can also be elevated in malignancy [24]. Second, an important factor which predisposes to elevation of these biomarkers is the inflammatory response and cytokinemia. Therefore, conditions which induce a marked inflammatory response, such as sepsis [25], vascular injury, and use of certain types of colloids [26] can result in elevations in the concentrations of these markers independent of renal injury. Third, diuretics such as furosemide and dopa-

Table 4. Urinary biomarkers of acute kidney injury (AKI)

Biomarker	Biological basis	Clinical value/limitations	Sensitivity	Specificity	AUC
Urinary enzymes: Alkaline phosphatase,	Apical surface of proximal tubular epithelial cells contain several enzymes, released into the urine either by leakage or by exocytosis	– Earlier marker as compared to serum creatinine, but limited sensitivity and specificity – Cut-off points vary in different diseases – Even mild reversible injury of the kidney not progressing to acute renal failure also results in enzymuria	50 %	95 %	0.863
n-acetyl β-D glucosaminidase [NAG]			100 %	81 %	0.845
α-glutathione S-transferase (GST)			75 %	90 %	0.893
π-GST			100 %	90 %	0.929
gamma glutamyl transpeptidase (GGT)			100 %	90 %	0.95
Sodium hydrogen exchanger 3 (NHE3)	Major sodium transporter along the proximal tubule, with excretion increased in AKI	– Increased urinary levels in both pre-renal and renal failure – Dopamine also increases urinary excretion even in the absence of renal dysfunction thus limiting its utility.			
Urinary interleukin (IL)-18, 300 pg/mg	A pro-inflammatory cytokine that is induced and cleaved in the proximal tubule by the action of capsase 1 on pro-IL-18	Significantly increased in ischemic acute tubular necrosis compared with other renal diseases. Precise timing of the appearance in urine merits additional studies	95 %	82 %	0.95
Kidney injury molecule (KIM)-1,7 ng/mg	A transmembrane protein with extracellular immunoglobulin and mucin domains, expressed in very low levels in the normal kidney. Potential role in cell-cell and cell-matrix interactions in the normal kidney. In AKI, the ectodomain of KIM-1 is shed from the tubular cells into the urine and these can be detected by ELISA	Urinary marker. Precise timing of the appearance in urine merits additional studies			
6 hours post-injury			85 %	21 %	0.52
12 hours post-injury			32 %	90 %	0.83
Urinary neutrophil gelatinase-associated lipocalin (NGAL) 85 µg/g			93 %	98 %	0.948
Urinary cystatin C	Normally cystatin C is freely filtered and fully reabsorbed in the renal tubules. Tubular injury results in reduced tubular reabsorption and increased urinary excretion.		92 %	83 %	0.92

Urinary enzyme indices from [30], IL-18 indices from [31], KIM-1 indices from [32], NGAL indices from [33], cystatin C indices from [15]. AUC: area under the curve

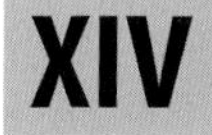

Table 5. Clincial data on biomarkers of acute kidney injury (AKI) in critical illness

First author [ref]	Biomarker	Patient population	Key findings
Westhuyzen [30]	Urinary enzymes	26 critically ill patients – medical/surgical ICU	GGT and GST appeared to have the highest sensitivity and AUC as compared to other urinary enzymes.
Herget-Rosenthal [15]	Serum cystatin C	85 critically ill patients at risk of developing acute renal failure	Cystatin C an earlier predictor of AKI and also reliably predicted the need for RRT.
Ahlstrom [34]	Serum cystatin C	202 critically ill patients	Serum cystatin C was as good as plasma creatinine in detecting acute renal failure in intensive care patients. Neither marker was clinically useful in predicting mortality.
Parikh [35]	Urine IL-18	A nested case-control study was performed within the ARDS Network trial (52 patients and 86 controls)	Urine IL-18 $>$ 100 pg/ml was highly predictive of AKI in the next 24 h. Urine IL-18 values were independent predictors of mortality.
Wheeler [36]	Serum NGAL	145 critically ill children with SIRS or septic shock and 25 healthy controls	Serum NGAL was significantly increased in critically ill children with SIRS and septic shock. Serum NGAL is a highly sensitive but nonspecific predictor of AKI in critically ill children with septic shock.
Washburn [37]	Urine IL-18	137 critically ill children	Urinary IL-18 concentration $\geq$ 100 pg/ml and $>$ 200 pg/ml had a specificity to predict AKI development within 24 h and to predict the AKI duration $>$ or $=$ 48 h respectively. Urinary IL-18 was also associated with mortality (odds ratio = 1.29, $p < 0.05$), independent of the PRISM II score.
Zappitelli [38]	Urine NGAL	140 critically ill children	Urinary NGAL was found to be a useful early AKI marker that predicted development of severe AKI in a heterogeneous group of patients with unknown timing of kidney injury.
Herrero-Morin [39]	Serum cystatin C	25 critically ill children	Serum cystatin C was found to be better than serum creatinine, in detecting AKI in critically ill children.
du Cheyron [40]	Urine NHE3	68 critically ill patients	Urine NHE3 levels were elevated in pre-renal azotemia and in patients with tubular necrosis suggesting that it is a marker of tubular damage.

NGAL: neutrophil gelatinase-associated lipocalin; IL: interleukin; NHE3: Sodium hydrogen exchanger 3; AUC: area under the curve; ARDS: acute respiratory distress syndrome; SIRS: systemic inflammatory response syndrome, GGT: gamma glutamyl transpeptidase; GST: glutathione S-transferase; PRISM: Pediatric Risk of Mortality; RRT: renal replacement therapy

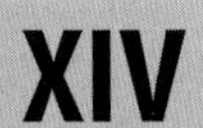

mine may result in increased urinary excretion of certain markers. Finally, there has been a lack of consensus regarding the diagnosis and severity stratification of AKI among the published studies resulting in varied levels of reported accuracies for the various markers. However, the advent of the Risk, Injury, Failure, Loss of Kidney Function, End-stage Kidney Disease (RIFLE) criteria and greater adherence to the Standards for Reporting Diagnostic Accuracy (STARD) protocols may help minimize the effect of this confounding variable

Biomarkers on the Horizon

Two new biomarkers of AKI have been described. These are exosomal fetuin A and netrin I. Exosomal fetuin A is an exosomal protein and, in a study by Zhou et al. [27], urinary fetuin A was markedly increased in response to nephrotoxins and ischemia in a rat model. Urinary levels were not elevated in prerenal azotemia.

Netrin 1 is a laminin-like molecule expressed in the kidney and in preliminary murine models and in patients with acute renal failure, has shown promise as an emerging marker of early renal injury [28].

What should an Intensivist do When Faced with an Abnormal Biomarker Result?

As with any investigation, the result should be viewed in a clinical context – treat the patient not the result. The presence of an elevated biomarker in a critically ill patient should make the clinician wary to the fact that there is an increased risk of onset of AKI. Clinical stratagems to retard or reverse (further) renal deterioration are based on an understanding of renal pathophysiology. Such measures include the restoration of intravascular volume and maintenance of an adequate renal perfusion pressure. Avoidance of nephrotoxic drugs (non-steroidal anti-inflammatory drugs, aminoglycosides), minimizing the use of contrast studies, and aggressive treatment of sepsis are also of paramount importance. There may be a role for pre-emptive renal replacement therapy, although this needs to be validated in clinical trials.

Conclusion

The morbidity and mortality associated with AKI make it an imperative that progress is made in the effective management of this condition. This laudable ideal is fraught with difficulty. The disease may be asymptomatic for much of its course, meaning the clinician has to have a high index of suspicion. Significant increases in morbidity and mortality are associated with modest increase in serum creatinine [29]. In the research setting, the myriad end-points, as well as the various pathophysiological aspects of AKI, make comparing interventions and outcomes complex. This is compounded by the fact that it may be incorrect to extrapolate between clinical models; the mechanisms of AKI in sepsis may not be the same as in ischemia. The varying time course of the putative biomarkers may produce difficulties when comparing clinical efficacy. It is likely that no one biomarker will be used to detect AKI; more likely they will be used as part of a 'biomarker panel' to delineate the path of AKI and help the clinician act in a timely fashion to improve outcome.

References

1. Waikar SS, Curhan GC, Wald R , McCarthy F.P Chertow GM (2006) Declining mortality of patients with acute renal failure,1998 to 2002. J Am Soc Nephrol 17: 1143–1150
2. Cole L, Bellomo R, Silvester W, Reeves JH (2000) A prospective, multicenter study of the epidemiology, management, and outcome of severe acute renal failure in a "closed" ICU. Am J Respir Crit Care Med 162: 191–196
3. Uchino S, Kellum JA, Bellomo R, et al (2005) Acute renal failure in critically ill patients; a multinational, multicentre study JAMA 294: 813–818
4. Jo S-K, Xuzhen H, Yuen P, Aslamkhan A, Pritchard J, Dear J, Star R (2004) Delayed DMSO administration protects the kidney from mercuric chloride injury. J Am Soc Nephrol 15: 2648–2654
5. Hewitt SM, Dear J, Star R (2004) Discovery of protein biomarkers for renal disease. J Am Soc Nephrol 15: 1677–1689
6. Deverajan P, Williams LM (2007) Proteomics for biomarker discovery in acute kidney injury. Semin Nephrol 27: 637–651
7. Mishra J, Dent C, Tarabishi R, et al (2005) Neutrophil gelatinase associated lipocalin (NGAL) as a biomarker for acute renal injury after cardiac surgery. Lancet 365: 1231–1238
8. Wagener G, Jan M, Kim M, et al (2006) Association between increase in urinary neutrophil gelatinase associated lipocalin and acute renal dysfunction after adult cardiac surgery. Anaesthesiology 105: 485–491
9. Mishra J, Mori K, Ma Q, Kelly C, Barasch J, Devarajn P (2004) Neutrophil gelatinase associated lipocalin:a novel early urinary biomarker for cisplatin nephropathy. Am J Nephrol 24: 307–315
10. Mori K, Lee T, Rapoport D, et al (2005) Endocyte delivery of lipocalin-siderophore-iron complex rescues the kidney from ischaemia reperfusion injury. J Clin Invest 115: 610–621
11. Mishra J, Ma Q, Prada A, et al (2003) Identification of neutrophil gelatinase-associated lipocalin as a novel early urinary biomarker for ischaemic renal injury. J Am Soc Nephrol 14: 2534–2543
12. Ding H, He Y, Li K, et al (2007) Urinary Neutrophil gelatinase associated lipocalin (NGAL) is an early biomarker for renal tubulointerstitial injury in IgA nephropathy. Clin Immunol 123: 227–234
13. Mishra J, Ma Q, Kelly C, et al (2006) Kidney NGAL is a novel early biomarker of acute injury following transplantation. Pediatr Nephrol 21: 856–863
14. Macdonald J, Marcora S, Jibani M, et al (2006) GFR estimation using cystatin C is not independent of body composition Am J Kidney Dis 48: 712–719
15. Herget-Rosenthal S, Marggraf G, Husing J, et al (2004) Early detection of renal failure by cystatin C. Kidney Int 66: 1115–1122
16. Delanaye P, Lambermont B, Chapelle J-P, Gielen J, Gerard P, Rorive G. (2004) Plasmatic cystatin c for estimation of glomerular filtration rates in intensive care units. Intensive Care Med 30: 980–983
17. Herrero-Morin JD, Malaga S, Fernandez N,et al. (2007) Cystatin C and beta 2 microglobulin: markers of glomerular filtration in critically ill children. Crit Care 11:R59
18. Wilhelm SM, Stowe NT, Robinson AV, Schulak JK (2001) The use of the endothelial antagonist lezosentan before or after renal ischaemia protects renal function. Transplantation 71: 211–216
19. Muramatsu Y, Tsujie M, Kodha Y, et al (2002) Early detection of cysteine rich protein 61-(CYR61,CCN1) in urine following renal ischaemic reperfusion injury. Kidney Int 62: 1601–1610
20. Li B, Hartono C, Ding R, et al (2001) Non invasive diagnosis of renal allograft rejection by measurement of messenger RNA for perforin and granzyme B in urine N Engl J Med 344: 947–954
21. Moniaux M, Chakraborty S, Yalniz M, et al (2008) Early diagnosis of pancreatic cancer: neutrophil gelatinase associated lipocalin as a marker of pancreatic intra epithelial neoplasia. Br J Cancer 98 1540–1547
22. Lim R, Ahmed N, Borregard V (2007) Neutrophil gelatinase associated lipocalin (NGAL) an early screening biomarker for ovarian cancer: NGAL is associated with epidermal growth factor inducedepithelio-mesenchymal transition. Int J Cancer 120: 2426–2434

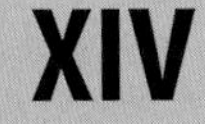

23. Han WK, Alinain A, Wu C-L, et al (2005) Human kidney injury molecule 1 is a tissue and urinary tumour marker of renal cell carcinoma. J Am Soc Nephrol 16: 1126–1134
24. Nakai K, Kikuchi M, Fujimoto K, et al (2008) Serum levels of cystatin C in patients with malignancy. Clin Exp Nephrol 12: 132–139
25. Tschoeke SK, Oberholzer A, Moldawer L (2006) Interleukin 18:A novel prognostic cytokine in bacteria induced sepsis. Crit Care Med 34: 1225–1233
26. Boldt J, Brosch C, Rohn K, Papsdorf M, Mengistu A (2008) Comparison of the effects of gelatin and a modern hydroxyethyl starch on renal function and inflammatory response in elderly cardiac surgical patients. Br J Anaesth 100: 457–464
27. Zhou H, Pisitkun T, Aponte A, et al (2006) Exosomal fetuin A identified by proteomics: A novel urinary biomarker for detecting acute kidney injury. Kidney Int 70: 1847–1857
28. Reeves B, Kwon W, Ramesh G (2008) Netrin 1 and kidney injury. II Netrin I is an early biomarker of acute kidney injury Am J Physiol Renal Physiol 294:F371–378
29. Coca SG, Peixoto AJ, Garg AV, Krunholz HM, Parikh CR (2007) The prognostic importance of a small acute decrement in kidney function in hospitalised patients: a systematic review and meta analysis. Am J Kidney Dis 50: 712–720
30. Westhuyzen J, Endre Z, Reece G, Reith D, Saltissi D, Morgan TJ (2003) Measurement of tubular enzymuria facilitates early detection of acute renal impairment in the intensive care unit. Nephrol Dial Transplant 18: 534–551
31. Parikh CR, Mishra J, Thiessen-Philbrook, et al (2006) Urinary IL 18 is an early predictive biomarker of acute kidney injury after cardiac surgery Kidney Int 70: 199–203
32. Han WK, Waikar SS, Johnson A, et al (2008) Urinary biomarkers in the early diagnosis of acute kidney injury. Kidney Int 73: 863–969
33. Nickolas TL, O'Rourke MJ, Yang J, et al (2008) Sensitivity and specificity of a single emergency department measurement of urinary Neutrophil Gelatinase Associated Lipocalin for diagnosing acute kidney injury. Ann Intern Med 148: 810–819
34. Ahlstrom A, Tallgren M, Pellonen S, Pettila V (2004) Evolution and predictive power of serum Cystatin C in acute renal failure. Clinical Nephrol 62: 344–350
35. Parikh CR, Abraham E, Ancukiewicz M, Edelstein CL (2005) Urine ILl8 is an early diagnostic marker for acute kidney injury and predicts mortality in the intensive care unit. J Am Soc Nephrol 16: 3046–3052
36. Wheeler DS, Devarajan P, Ma Q, et al (2008) serum neutrophil gelatinase associated lipocalin (NGAL) as a marker of acute kidney injury in critically ill children with septic shock. Crit Care Med 36: 1297–1303
37. Washburn KK, Zappitelli M, Arikan AA, et al (2008) Urinary IL18 is an acute kidney injury biomarker in critically ill children. Nephrol Dial Transplant 23: 566–572
38. Zappitelli M, Washburn KK, Arikan AA, et al (2007) Urine neutrophil gelatinase associated lipocalin is an early marker of acute kidney injury in critically ill children: a prospective cohort study. Crit Care 11:R84
39. Herrero-Morin JD, Malaga S, Fernandez N, et al (2007) Cystatin C and beta 2 microglobulin: marker of glomerular filtration in critically ill children. Crit Care 11:R59
40. du Cheyron D, Daubin C, Poggioli J, et al (2003) Urinary measurement of Na+/H+ exchange isoform 3 (NHE3) protein as a new marker of tubule injury in critically ill patients in acute renal failure. Am J Kidney Dis 42: 497–506

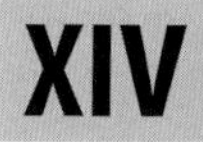

The Role of Biomarkers in Cardiac Surgery-associated Acute Kidney Injury

A. Shaw, M. Stafford-Smith, and M. Swaminathan

Introduction

Cardiac surgery associated-acute kidney injury (AKI) is common, affecting up to 40 % of heart surgery patients (depending on the definition used) [1]. Five to ten percent of these patients will require new renal replacement therapy, and this carries a high price in terms of morbidity, mortality and resource utilization [2]. Despite decades of successful animal research, there have been remarkably few positive human clinical trials of cardiac surgery associated-AKI prevention and treatment, and no treatment has been confirmed effective in large, multicenter randomized clinical trials [3]. Much of the problem has been attributed to delayed diagnosis – serum creatinine does not rise until 48 hours after surgery – such that by the time the diagnosis is made, it is too late to intervene. In prevention trials, lack of a clear consensus definition of AKI has hampered endpoint adjudication such that it still remains unclear which therapies may be effective, in which patient subtypes they should be used, and what is the correct time to begin and end them. The advent of a new generation of biomarkers coming hot on the heels of a consensus definition system for AKI [4] means that we may be poised to make significant advances in this area. This chapter reviews the place of existing and novel biomarkers in the diagnosis, risk stratification and prognosis of cardiac surgery associated-AKI.

What are the Characteristics of an Ideal Biomarker of Cardiac Surgery-associated-AKI?

The ideal biomarker should provide quick, reliable, and inexpensive measurement of a biological process that is inextricably linked to cardiac surgery associated-AKI. It should be readily quantifiable in accessible clinical samples (e.g., plasma or urine), with levels greatly increased specifically in cardiac surgery associated-AKI. There should be minimal to no overlap in biomarker levels between cases and control subjects, nor should levels be subject to wide variation in the general heart surgery population. Biomarker levels should correlate with the total burden of disease, but be unaffected by unrelated conditions and associated comorbid factors, and should correlate closely with the established parameters of disease that are known to influence quality of life and survival. They should vary rapidly in response to specific treatments, and large deviations of the biomarker from the reference values in the control population should have predictive power for disease severity and prognosis. Such a biomarker does not exist, nor is it likely to, and it is more probable that panels of biomarkers assessing different aspects of renal function and damage will be most useful in the management of patients with cardiac surgery associated-AKI [5].

Diagnostic Performance: How Good is a Test?

Before attempting to understand how good any particular biomarker is for the diagnosis of cardiac surgery associated-AKI, it is important to understand the terms commonly used to describe the measures of accuracy of any diagnostic test, such that meaningful interpretation of the results of studies evaluating novel biomarkers may be made.

Diagnostic tests may return values that are categorical (has AKI/does not have AKI), that are ordinal (has stage 1, 2 or 3 AKI) or that are continuous (quantitative measurement of functional defect). In general, categorical tests may be assessed in terms of sensitivity, specificity, positive predictive value, negative value, and receiver operating characteristic (ROC) curve analysis. For diagnostic purposes, continuous tests are usually dichotomized into yes/no categories and sometimes also into bins of severity to permit simpler interpretation. Although this makes them easier to understand, in general continuous variables are more powerful descriptors of physiological aberration and thus many biomarker discovery studies have used this approach instead of straightforward categorical descriptions. Below we outline what is meant by the commonly used descriptors of diagnostic test performance.

- Sensitivity (true positive rate): This is the probability that a test will make a diagnosis of AKI in a patient who really does have AKI. It is the true positive rate, and is given by the fraction of all AKI patients who have a positive test.
- Specificity (true negative rate): This is the probability that a test will make a diagnosis of no AKI in a patient who really does not have AKI. It is the true negative rate, and is given by the fraction of patients without AKI who have a negative test.
- Positive predictive value (precision rate): This is the proportion of patients with positive test results who are correctly diagnosed. It is given by the fraction of positive test results that actually have AKI. It is dependent on the prevalence of the disease however, increasing in direct proportion with disease prevalence.
- Negative predictive value: This is the probability that a patient with a negative test does not have AKI. It is given by the fraction of patients with negative test results that indeed truly do not have AKI. The various operating characteristics of diagnostic tests are summarized in **Table 1**.

One of the problems commonly facing diagnostic tests is that the operating characteristics (sensitivity and specificity) may change across the potential range of cut-off

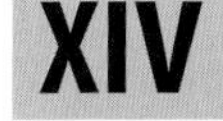

Table 1. Features of a diagnostic test

	Acute kidney injury	No acute kidney injury	Utility
Positive test	True positive	False positive (Type 1 error)	Positive predictive value
Negative test	False negative (Type 2 error)	True negative	Negative predictive value
Test characteristic	Sensitivity	Specificity	

values for a 'positive' diagnosis. A test that is 100 % sensitive but 10 % specific will not retain much clinical utility, particularly if the consequences of an erroneous diagnosis are not trivial. In practice, the operating characteristics of a test across different cut off values may be assessed using a ROC curve [6]. This curve plots the true positive rate (sensitivity) against the false positive rate (1-specificity), and the area under the curve (AUC) provides a single estimate of how 'good' the test is for the diagnosis of a disease. Generally, values of 0.8 and higher are accepted as being clinically useful. A perfect classifier would lead to a curve where the elbow of the curve lay on the upper left corner of the plot, and would have an AUC of 1.0.

What Biomarkers are Needed?

Given the limitations of using serum creatinine and urine output for detecting AKI, there is a need for better biomarkers that can more reliably help refine the diagnosis of AKI [7]. Potentially, these novel biomarkers may allow subcategorization of this disease in a manner analogous to the way hematological malignancies have been subcategorized, now that information about their molecular subtypes is available. It is probable that cardiac surgery associated-AKI is not a single disease, rather a panoply of illnesses that appear similar from a functional deficit perspective, but that are mediated by different pathological processes. This may also explain why we have failed to translate therapies that are effective in (single mechanism) animal models of AKI into the human domain.

If a panel of biomarkers could be developed such that the diagnosis of AKI could be made soon after the injury (i.e., within hours), then the window of opportunity for effective therapies may be advanced earlier in the disease process, and potentially even during the initiation or propagation phase. In addition, an earlier and more reliable diagnosis of AKI would facilitate better risk stratification. Examples of outcomes that could be predicted might include AKI patients who subsequently require renal replacement therapy, duration of AKI, development of subsequent chronic kidney disease, and all cause mortality. Analogous to the cardiology composite of MACE (Major Adverse Cardiac Events), these outcomes may collectively be considered as a composite renal variable known as Major Adverse Kidney Events (MAKE).

What Biomarkers are Currently Available and How Good are They?

The biomarkers currently available to us for the diagnosis of cardiac surgery associated-AKI are unsatisfactory [8]. This is somewhat surprising since AKI is diagnosed exclusively on changes in laboratory parameters (serum creatinine, blood urea nitrogen). Once renal dysfunction develops it can be defined in a number of ways. The variables traditionally used to characterize postoperative renal dysfunction include peak postoperative serum creatinine, absolute and/or percentage change in serum creatinine, postoperative estimated creatinine clearance, absolute and/or percentage change in creatinine clearance, and need for renal replacement therapy [5]. All have previously been shown to be predictive of adverse postoperative outcomes.

Until the advent of cystatin C (see below), there had been no new tests of renal function in widespread use for more than 50 years. Increasingly, laboratories are beginning to offer cystatin C as a test of renal function, in the belief that it is a better indicator of renal filtration function than estimates of serum creatinine. Whether this is actually true or not is unknown.

The most important reason to find a replacement for serum creatinine for the diagnosis and prognosis of AKI in general, and cardiac surgery associated-AKI in particular, is that there is a delay of at least 48 hours after an insult before the serum creatinine rises. This means we cannot currently intervene until it is too late; indeed, it is like providing coronary revascularization two days after a myocardial infarction. Novel tests of actual kidney damage (urinary neutrophil gelatinase-associated lipocalin [NGAL], kidney injury molecule [KIM]-1) may allow earlier diagnosis of tubular damage, rather than declining function, which in turn may allow much earlier interventions to be tested.

What Biomarkers are Under Development?

Prompted by these potential benefits of an improved biomarker for detecting AKI, several new biomarkers have been identified while some previously identified ones have been more intensely studied [9]. Although there have been over 20 unique biomarkers of AKI identified or under investigation, most of the current interest has focused on a handful of promising biomarkers: NGAL, cystatin C, interleukin (IL)-18, and KIM-1 [10].

Neutrophil Gelatinase-associated Lipocalin

NGAL is an immunological protein that is covalently bound to gelatinase from neutrophils and expressed at low levels by various human tissues including the kidneys. In the setting of cardiac surgery, NGAL has been demonstrated to be a highly sensitive and specific biomarker of postoperative AKI. Its gene is one of the earliest and the most upregulated in the kidney after ischemic injury. In one study of 71 children undergoing cardiopulmonary bypass (CPB), the incidence of AKI was found to be 28 %. Both urine and serum NGAL increased 2 hours after CPB and were found to be the most powerful independent predictors of AKI in this population. Two additional studies have demonstrated that both urine NGAL (at 2 hours) and plasma NGAL (at 12 hours) strongly correlate with mortality in children [11, 12]. Similar results have been observed in the adult cardiac surgical population [13]. In a study of 81 adult cardiac patients, 20 % of the patients developed postoperative AKI: NGAL was higher in patients with AKI at 1 hour, 3 hours, and 18 hours post-CPB when compared with their non-AKI counterparts.

A more recent study found that the use of aprotinin versus epsilon amino-caproic acid in patients undergoing cardiac surgery resulted in a twofold incidence of AKI in the aprotinin group. Urinary NGAL was significantly higher at both 0 and 3 hours post-CPB in patients receiving aprotinin [14]. Whether urinary NGAL may turn out to be a better predictor of cardiac surgery-associated-AKI than plasma NGAL remains to be demonstrated conclusively. One recent study found this to be the case [15], suggesting that plasma NGAL elevations may be more indicative of a global inflammatory insult induced by the CPB machine rather than a specific kidney insult. If this is the case, then the combination of plasma and urinary NGAL data may allow a more temporal approach to AKI diagnosis than has been possible previously.

Interleukin-18

IL-18, a pro-inflammatory cytokine that belongs to the IL-1 superfamily, has been shown to be both a mediator and biomarker of ischemic AKI. In a study of 55 children following CPB, urinary IL-18 was detectable at 4–6 hours, peaked at 12 hours, and remained elevated for over 48 hours [16]. Further multivariate analysis suggested that urine IL-18 may also be a marker of AKI severity. Similar results have been also been observed in non-cardiac populations with AKI [17–19].

Kidney Injury Molecule-1

KIM-1 is an immunoglobulin superfamily transmembrane protein normally present at low levels in proximal renal tubular cells that dramatically increases in expression following acute ischemic or nephrotoxic insult [20]. Recent findings in cell cultures also demonstrate that it transforms renal epithelial cells into 'semiprofessional' phagocytes that may assist with clearance of the apoptotic and necrotic cells that result from AKI [21]. Several studies in non-cardiac patients have demonstrated that KIM-1 is a very sensitive indicator of AKI [20–22]. However, fewer studies exist specifically in the cardiac surgery literature. In a cohort study of 103 adult patients undergoing CPB, KIM-1 levels increased significantly at both 2 hours and 24 hours postoperatively in patients with AKI [22].

Cystatin C

Cystatin C is a protein that is produced by all nucleated cells [23]. It has been suggested that cystatin C is an ideal molecule for measuring glomerular filtration rate (GFR) because it is freely filtered by the glomerulus, completely reabsorbed by the proximal convoluted tubules, and is not secreted [23, 24]. Unlike creatinine, it is not affected by age, gender, sex, or body mass [24]. There have only been a few studies to date that have explored cystatin C as a biomarker for AKI post-cardiac surgery [15]. In this prospective study, cystatin C and NGAL were measured in serum and urine samples of 72 adults who underwent cardiac surgery. Within the first 6 hours, serum values for cystatin C and NGAL were not predictive of AKI while urinary values were elevated. These findings suggest that urinary biomarkers may be superior to serum values for early detection of AKI.

Limitations of New Biomarkers

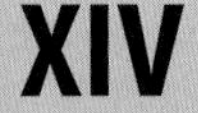

Despite the promise of earlier detection of AKI, and with greater sensitivity, each biomarker has its limitations. NGAL may be influenced by pre-existing renal disease as well as infections [25]. KIM-1 is more specific for ischemic and nephrotoxic AKI and may not be useful in detecting other types of renal injury [20]. IL-18 peaks later than many other leading biomarkers, and is more specific for ischemic AKI [16]. Finally, cystatin C is not specific for ischemic AKI and its serum level rises much later than NGAL, KIM-1, and IL-18. In addition to their individual limitations, a variety of statistical and methodologic issues must be appropriately considered when determining the overall diagnostic performance of biomarkers. First, odds ratios or relative risks alone are inadequate to discriminate between individuals who may or may not have AKI. Rather, the accuracy and validity of biomarkers are better summarized using ROC curves as discussed earlier [8]. Next, errors in the reference standard may threaten the validity of biomarker studies, but may be addressed by using hard outcomes (e.g., renal replacement therapy-requiring AKI, death) that are not subject to the same potential for misclassification that is inherent in diagnosing AKI. Additionally, risk prediction in individual patients requires that the biomarker have strong discriminatory characteristics that include a large difference in risk between low versus high values of the biomarker. Finally, the diagnostic characteristics of biomarkers will need to be evaluated with a consistent gold standard at well-defined time points.

Although determining their individual test characteristics will represent a significant advance in this field, combinations of biomarkers in multi-marker panels may provide a leap forward with the ability to differentiate between various AKI phenotypes and detect ischemic AKI earlier with greater precision and prognostic capacity.

One further limitation of the use of urinary protein levels for detection of cardiac surgery-associated-AKI is the fact that antifibrinolytic agents such as aminocaproic acid and tranexamic acid are both known to induce a temporary proteinuria during their administration [26]. Although this phenomenon is temporary and self limiting, it is important to consider when interpreting urinary protein data in patients who have received these drugs.

How will New Biomarkers Change the Diagnosis and Treatment of AKI?

As mentioned above, novel biomarkers of acute kidney damage and acute deteriorations of renal function will allow earlier diagnosis of a defect, and potentially may allow us to refine the diagnostic approach to AKI by pointing to disease mechanisms. This in turn may allow more targeted application of salvage therapies, and even preventive therapies if there are common pathophysiological pathways involved [8].

Second, new biomarkers of prognosis are required in order that we may predict who will require renal replacement therapy and who will not [27]. If a person will ultimately require renal replacement therapy then there is little to be gained by delaying its initiation, since all that will generally occur is the development of fluid and electrolyte abnormalities that will take longer to correct once renal replacement therapy is finally begun. Biomarkers of disease progression, then, will also be important to identify.

Third, new biomarkers of outcome will greatly assist with individual patient prognostication. If it could be shown that certain patterns in relevant biomarkers are associated with consistent outcomes, then this will assist physicians as they make difficult decisions about ongoing treatment in advanced multiorgan disease. Acute renal failure is almost always a feature of multiple organ failure, and if it is known that permanent renal replacement therapy will be required because the kidneys have failed to a point where they will never recover then this information will be important to integrate into the overall clinical decision making process.

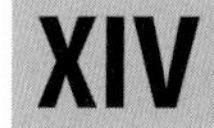

Conclusion

In summary, there has been a lack of new biomarkers for more than half a century. Accompanying the recent consensus on diagnosis of AKI (albeit one which uses serum creatinine which itself may one day be replaced) has been the discovery and initial validation of new biomarkers of both renal function and kidney damage. This will hopefully allow more focused investigation of their role in disease diagnosis, prognosis and classification such that we do not have to face a further 30 years of failed translational research. Indeed, it may be the case that we should re-explore some therapies that have been consigned to the pharmacological trash can, in the light of new information about disease mechanisms in different clinical settings. Lastly, cardiac surgery associated-AKI represents a prime arena for such investigation, since we know precisely when the insult occurs, and are ideally poised to intervene.

References

1. Shaw A, Swaminathan M, Stafford-Smith M (2008) Cardiac surgery-associated acute kidney injury: putting together the pieces of the puzzle. Nephron Physiol 109: 55–60
2. Thakar CV, Worley S, Arrigain S, et al (2005) Influence of renal dysfunction on mortality after cardiac surgery: modifying effect of preoperative renal function. Kidney Int 67: 1112–1119
3. Schetz M, Bove T, Morelli A, et al (2008) Prevention of cardiac surgery-associated acute kidney injury. Int J Artif Organs 31: 179–189
4. Mehta RL, Kellum JA, Shah SV, et al (2007) Acute Kidney Injury Network: report of an initiative to improve outcomes in acute kidney injury. Crit Care 11:R31.
5. Dennen P, Parikh CR (2007) Biomarkers of acute kidney injury: can we replace serum creatinine? Clin Nephrol 68: 269–278
6. Zweig MH, Campbell G (1993) Receiver-operating characteristic (ROC) plots: a fundamental evaluation tool in clinical medicine. Clin Chem 39: 561–577
7. Molitoris BA, Melnikov VY, Okusa MD, et al (2008) Technology Insight: biomarker development in acute kidney injury--what can we anticipate? Nat Clin Pract Nephrol 4: 154–165
8. Coca SG, Yalavarthy R, Concato J, Parikh CR (2008) Biomarkers for the diagnosis and risk stratification of acute kidney injury: a systematic review. Kidney Int 73: 1008–1016
9. Thurman JM, Parikh CR (2008) Peeking into the black box: new biomarkers for acute kidney injury. Kidney Int 73: 379–381
10. Edelstein CL (2008) Biomarkers of acute kidney injury. Adv Chronic Kidney Dis 15: 222–234
11. Dent CL, Ma Q, Dastrala S, et al (2007) Plasma neutrophil gelatinase-associated lipocalin predicts acute kidney injury, morbidity and mortality after pediatric cardiac surgery: a prospective uncontrolled cohort study. Crit Care 11:R127.
12. Bennett M, Dent CL, Ma Q, et al (2008) Urine NGAL predicts severity of acute kidney injury after cardiac surgery: a prospective study. Clin J Am Soc Nephrol 3: 665–673
13. Wagener G, Jan M, Kim M, et al (2006) Association between increases in urinary neutrophil gelatinase-associated lipocalin and acute renal dysfunction after adult cardiac surgery. Anesthesiology 105: 485–491
14. Wagener G, Gubitosa G, Wang S, et al (2008) Increased incidence of acute kidney injury with aprotinin use during cardiac surgery detected with urinary NGAL. Am J Nephrol 28: 576–582
15. Koyner JL, Bennett MR, Worcester EM, et al (2008) Urinary cystatin C as an early biomarker of acute kidney injury following adult cardiothoracic surgery. Kidney Int 74: 1059–1069
16. Parikh CR, Mishra J, Thiessen-Philbrook H, et al (2006) Urinary IL-18 is an early predictive biomarker of acute kidney injury after cardiac surgery. Kidney Int 70: 199–203
17. Mehta RL (2006) Urine IL-18 levels as a predictor of acute kidney injury in intensive care patients. Nat Clin Pract Nephrol 2: 252–253
18. Parikh CR, Abraham E, Ancukiewicz M, Edelstein CL (2005) Urine IL-18 is an early diagnostic marker for acute kidney injury and predicts mortality in the intensive care unit. J Am Soc Nephrol 16: 3046–3052
19. Parikh C R, Jani A, Melnikov VY, Faubel S, Edelstein CL (2004) Urinary interleukin-18 is a marker of human acute tubular necrosis. Am J Kidney Dis 43: 405–414
20. Han WK, Bailly V, Abichandani R, et al (2002) Kidney Injury Molecule-1 (KIM-1): a novel biomarker for human renal proximal tubule injury. Kidney Int 62: 237–244

21. Ichimura T, Asseldonk EJ, Humphreys BD, Gunaratnam L, Duffield JS, Bonventre JV (2008) Kidney injury molecule-1 is a phosphatidylserine receptor that confers a phagocytic phenotype on epithelial cells. J Clin Invest 118: 1657–1668
22. Liangos O, Perianayagam MC, Vaidya VS, et al (2007) Urinary N-acetyl-beta-(D)-glucosaminidase activity and kidney injury molecule-1 level are associated with adverse outcomes in acute renal failure. J Am Soc Nephrol 18: 904–912
23. Herget-Rosenthal S, Marggraf G, Husing J, et al (2004) Early detection of acute renal failure by serum cystatin C. Kidney Int 66: 1115–1122
24. Dharnidharka VR, Kwon C, Stevens G (2002) Serum cystatin C is superior to serum creatinine as a marker of kidney function: a meta-analysis. Am J Kidney Dis 40: 221–226
25. Mitsnefes MM, Kathman TS, Mishra J, et al (2007) Serum neutrophil gelatinase-associated lipocalin as a marker of renal function in children with chronic kidney disease. Pediatr Nephrol 22: 101–108
26. Stafford Smith M (1999) Antifibrinolytic agents make alpha1- and beta2-microglobulinuria poor markers of post cardiac surgery renal dysfunction. Anesthesiology 90: 928–929
27. Arthur JM, Janech MG, Varghese SA, Almeida JS, Powell TB (2008) Diagnostic and prognostic biomarkers in acute renal failure. Contrib Nephrol 160: 53–64

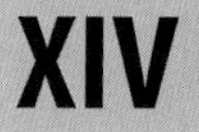

Neutrophil Gelatinase-associated Lipocalin: An Emerging Biomarker for Angina Renalis

P. Devarajan

Introduction

Angina pectoris is symptomatic, and sensitive biomarkers such as troponin that are released from affected myocytes have revolutionized the early diagnosis and successful treatment of ischemic myocardial injury. In contrast, ischemic acute kidney injury (AKI), analogously referred to as *angina renalis*, is largely devoid of symptoms. Although common and serious (about one-third of intensive care patients develop AKI), the diagnosis using conventional biomarkers such as serum creatinine is unreliable and delayed [1]. Therefore, potentially effective interventions are delayed, and AKI remains an important contributor to the high mortality rate in affected critically ill subjects [2, 3]. Fortunately, recent advances have unraveled the early stress response of kidney tubule cells to ischemic injury, and have provided several novel biomarkers for AKI [4–6]. The current status of neutrophil gelatinase-associated lipocalin (NGAL), possibly the most promising AKI biomarker in intensive care and emergency medicine settings, is outlined below.

Discovery of NGAL as an AKI Biomarker

Preclinical high-throughput gene expression experiments identified *Ngal* (also known as lipocalin 2 or *lcn2*) to be one of the most upregulated genes in the kidney very early after acute injury in animal models [7]. NGAL was also found to be one of the most highly induced proteins in the kidney after ischemic or nephrotoxic AKI, and the NGAL protein was easily detected in the urine and blood in animal models [8–10]. In a translational human cross-sectional study, patients in the intensive care unit (ICU) with established AKI (doubling of serum creatinine) displayed a marked increase in urine and serum NGAL by Western blotting [11]. Urine and serum NGAL levels correlated with serum creatinine, and kidney biopsies in subjects with AKI showed intense accumulation of immunoreactive NGAL in cortical tubules, confirming NGAL as a sensitive index of established AKI in humans.

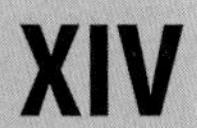

NGAL for the Early Diagnosis of AKI

An increasing number of human studies have now identified NGAL as an early non-invasive diagnostic biomarker of AKI in common intensive care and emergency department settings, preceding a rise in serum creatinine by several hours to days (**Table 1**). In prospective studies of children with normal kidney function and no co-

Table 1. NGAL for the early prediction of acute kidney injury (AKI) and its clinical outcomes

Biomarker property	Cardiopulmonary bypass (CPB)	Contrast-induced nephropathy	Kidney transplantation	Critical care or emergency setting
Time post-event	2 h post-CPB	2 h post-contrast	2–12 h post-transplant	At presentation
Time preceding AKI	2 days pre-AKI	1–2 days pre AKI	2–3 days pre-DGF	2 days pre-AKI
ROC AUC	0.61–0.99	0.91–0.92	0.90	0.78–0.95
AKI outcomes predicted	Duration, severity, death	No data available	Duration, severity	Duration, severity, death
References	[12–18, 30–35]	[22–26]	[19–21]	[27–29]

AKI, defined as a 50 % or greater increase in serum creatinine from baseline. DGF: delayed graft function, defined as dialysis requirement within the first week after transplant. ROC AUC, area under the receiver operating characteristic curve. Times shown are the earliest time points when the biomarker becomes significantly increased from baseline.

morbid conditions who underwent cardiopulmonary bypass (CPB) surgery, AKI (defined as a 50 % increase in serum creatinine) occurred 2–3 days postoperatively [12–14]. In contrast, NGAL measurements by ELISA revealed a dramatic increase in the urine and plasma, within 2–6 hours of cardiac surgery in those who subsequently developed AKI. Both urine and plasma NGAL were excellent independent predictors of AKI, with an area under the curve (AUC) of > 0.9 for the 2–6 hour urine and plasma NGAL measurements [12–14]. These findings have now been confirmed in prospective studies of adults who developed AKI after CPB surgery, in whom urinary NGAL was significantly elevated by 1–3 hours after the operation [15–17]. These early urinary NGAL measurements correlated well with bypass time and aortic cross-clamp time, whereas neither peak serum creatinine nor relative changes in serum creatinine correlated with these well known indices of intraoperative renal hypoperfusion [17]. The AUCs for the prediction of AKI were in the 0.61–0.80 range, the somewhat inferior performance perhaps reflective of confounding variables (such as old age, pre-existing kidney disease, prolonged bypass times, chronic illness, and diabetes), variations in the definition of AKI, and technical issues with the NGAL measurements [3]. A recent prospective study in adult cardiac surgical patients has also revealed a good predictive value of plasma NGAL measurements obtained on arrival in the ICU, with an AUC of 0.80 for the prediction of AKI (> 50 % increase in serum creatinine) which occurred 1–2 days later [18].

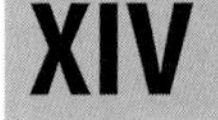

NGAL has been evaluated as a biomarker of AKI in kidney transplantation. Protocol biopsies of kidneys obtained 1 hour after vascular anastomosis revealed a significant correlation between NGAL staining intensity and the subsequent development of delayed graft function [19]. In a prospective multicenter study, NGAL levels in urine samples collected on the day of transplant identified those who subsequently developed delayed graft function (which typically occurred 2–4 days later), with an AUC of 0.9 [20]. Plasma NGAL measurements have also been correlated with delayed graft function following kidney transplantation from donors after cardiac death [21].

Several investigators have examined the role of NGAL as a predictive biomarker of nephrotoxicity following contrast administration [22–26]. In a prospective study of children undergoing elective cardiac catheterization with contrast administration, both urine and plasma NGAL predicted contrast-induced nephropathy (defined as a 50 % increase in serum creatinine from baseline) within 2 hours after contrast administration, with an AUC of 0.91–0.92 [26]. In studies of adults administered contrast, an early rise in both urine (4 hours) and plasma (2 hours) NGAL were documented, in comparison with a much later increase in plasma cystatin C levels (8–24 hours after contrast administration), providing further support for NGAL as an early biomarker of contrast nephropathy [23, 24].

Urine and plasma NGAL measurements represent early biomarkers of AKI in the pediatric intensive care setting, being able to predict this complication about 2 days prior to the rise in serum creatinine, with high sensitivity and AUCs of 0.68–0.78 [27, 28]. In patients seen in the emergency department for a myriad of reasons, a single measurement of urine NGAL at the time of initial presentation predicted AKI with an outstanding AUC of 0.95 [29]. Thus, NGAL is a useful early AKI marker that predicts development of AKI even in heterogeneous groups of patients with multiple co-morbidities and with unknown timing of kidney injury.

The results described thus far have been obtained using research-based assays, which are not practical in the clinical setting. In this regard, a major advance has been the development of a standardized point-of-care kit for the clinical measurement of plasma NGAL (Triage® NGAL Device, Biosite Incorporated). In children undergoing cardiac surgery, the 2-hour plasma NGAL measurement measured by the Triage® Device showed an AUC of 0.96, sensitivity of 0.84, and specificity of 0.94 for prediction of AKI using a cut-off value of 150 ng/ml [30]. The assay is facile with quantitative results available in 15 minutes, and requires only microliter quantities of whole blood or plasma. In addition, a urine NGAL immunoassay has been developed for a standardized clinical platform (Architect® analyzer, Abbott Diagnostics). In children undergoing cardiac surgery, the 2-hour urine NGAL measurement by Architect® analyzer showed an AUC of 0.95, sensitivity of 0.79, and specificity of 0.92 for prediction of AKI using a cut-off value of 150 mg/ml [31]. This assay is also easy to perform with no manual pretreatment steps, a first result available within 35 minutes, and requires only 150 microliters of urine. Both assays are currently undergoing multicenter validation in adult populations.

NGAL for Monitoring the Response to AKI Therapy

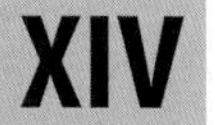

Because of its high predictive properties for AKI, NGAL is also emerging as an early biomarker in interventional trials. For example, a reduction in urine NGAL has been employed as an outcome variable in clinical trials demonstrating the improved efficacy of a modern hydroxyethyl starch (HES) preparation over albumin or gelatin in maintaining renal function in elderly cardiac surgery patients [32, 33]. Similarly, the response of urine NGAL was attenuated in adult cardiac surgery patients who experienced a lower incidence of AKI after sodium bicarbonate therapy when compared to sodium chloride [34]. In addition, adults who developed AKI after aprotinin use during cardiac surgery displayed a dramatic rise in urine NGAL in the immediate postoperative period, attesting to the potential use of NGAL for the prediction of nephrotoxic AKI [35]. The use of NGAL as a trigger to initiate and monitor novel therapies, and as a safety biomarker when using potentially nephrotoxic agents, is expected to increase in the near future.

NGAL for the Prediction of AKI Outcomes

Recent studies have demonstrated the utility of early NGAL measurements for predicting clinical outcomes of AKI in various common clinical settings (**Table 1**). In children undergoing cardiac surgery, the 2 hour post-operative plasma NGAL levels measured by the Triage® device strongly correlated with duration and severity of AKI, and length of hospital stay. In addition, the 12 hour plasma NGAL strongly correlated with mortality [30]. Similarly, the 2 hour urine NGAL levels measured by the Architect® analyzer highly correlated with duration and severity of AKI, length of hospital stay, dialysis requirement, and death [31]. In a multicenter study of children with diarrhea-associated hemolytic uremic syndrome, urine NGAL obtained early during the hospitalization predicted the severity of AKI and dialysis requirement with high sensitivity [36]. Early urine NGAL levels were also predictive of duration of AKI (AUC 0.79) in a heterogeneous cohort of critically ill subjects [27]. In adults undergoing CPB, those who subsequently required renal replacement therapy were found to have the highest urine NGAL values upon arrival in the ICU [16]. In adult kidney transplant patients undergoing either protocol biopsies or clinically indicated biopsies, urine NGAL measurements were found to be predictive of tubulitis or other tubular pathologies [37], raising the possibility of NGAL representing a non-invasive screening tool for the detection of tubulo-interstitial disease in the early months following kidney transplantation.

Limitations of NGAL as an AKI Biomarker

Clearly, NGAL represents a novel predictive biomarker for AKI and its outcomes. However, the majority of studies published thus far have involved relatively small numbers of subjects from single centers, in which NGAL appears to be most sensitive and specific in homogeneous patient populations with predictable forms of AKI. Plasma NGAL measurements may be influenced by a number of coexisting variables such as chronic kidney disease, chronic hypertension, systemic infections, inflammatory conditions, and malignancies [38–43]. In the chronic kidney disease population, plasma NGAL levels correlate with the severity of renal impairment [38, 42, 43]. However, the increase in plasma NGAL in these situations is generally much less than that typically encountered in AKI.

There is an emerging literature suggesting that urine NGAL is also a marker of chronic kidney disease and its severity [44]. In subjects with chronic kidney disease due to glomerulonephritides, urine NGAL levels were elevated and significantly correlated with serum creatinine, glomerular filtration rate (GFR) and proteinuria [45]. In patients with autosomal dominant polycystic kidney disease, urine NGAL measurements correlated with residual GFR and severity of cystic disease [40]. Urine NGAL has also been shown to represent an early biomarker for the degree of chronic injury in patients with IgA nephropathy [46], lupus nephritis [47, 48], and congestive heart failure [49], and may be increased in urinary tract infections. However, the levels of urine NGAL in these situations are significantly blunted compared to those typically measured in intrinsic AKI. This was most recently demonstrated in a study examining unselected patients presenting to an emergency room, in whom a single measurement of urine NGAL at the time of initial presentation reliably distinguished intrinsic AKI from prerenal azotemia and from chronic kidney disease [29].

Conclusion

NGAL as an AKI biomarker appears to have successfully passed through the preclinical, assay development, and initial clinical testing stages of the biomarker development process. It has now entered the prospective screening stage, facilitated by the development of commercial tools for the measurement of NGAL on large populations across different laboratories. The current status of NGAL as an AKI biomarker is shown in **Table 1**. But will any single biomarker such as NGAL suffice in AKI? In addition to early diagnosis and prediction, it would be desirable to identify biomarkers capable of discerning AKI subtypes, identifying etiologies, predicting clinical outcomes, allowing for risk stratification, and monitoring the response to interventions. In order to obtain all of this desired information, a panel of validated biomarkers may be needed. Other AKI panel candidates may include interleukin-18 (IL-18), kidney injury molecule-1 (KIM-1), cystatin C, and liver-type fatty acid binding protein (L-FABP), to name a few [1–6].

The availability of such a panel of AKI biomarkers could revolutionize renal and critical care. However, we must remain cognizant of the technical and fiscal issues surrounding the identification, validation, commercial development, and acceptance of multi-marker panels. Deriving from the recent cardiology literature, a clinically useful biomarker should (a) be easily measurable at a reasonable cost with short turnaround times; (b) provide information that is not already available from clinical assessment; and (c) aid in medical decision making [50]. In this respect, troponin as a stand-alone biomarker provides excellent diagnostic and prognostic information in acute coronary syndromes and acute decompensated heart failure. If the current prospective multicenter studies of NGAL measurements with standardized laboratory platforms provide promising results, we may already have a troponin-like biomarker for *angina renalis*.

Acknowledgements: Studies cited in this review that were performed by the author's laboratory were supported by grants from the NIH (R01 DK53289, RO1 DK069749 and R21 DK070163).

References

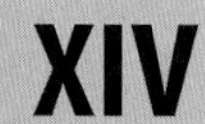

1. Parikh CR, Devarajan P (2008) New biomarkers of acute kidney injury. Crit Care Med 36 (Suppl): S159-S165
2. Devarajan P (2008) Neutrophil gelatinase-associated lipocalin – an emerging troponin for kidney injury. Nephrol Dial Transplant 23: 3737–3743
3. Devarajan P (2008) NGAL in acute kidney injury: from serendipity to utility. Am J Kidney Dis 52: 395–399
4. Devarajan P (2006) Update on mechanisms of ischemic acute kidney injury. J Am Soc Nephrol 17: 1503–1520
5. Devarajan P (2008) Proteomics for the investigation of acute kidney injury. Contrib Nephrol 160: 1–16
6. Devarajan P, Parikh C, Barasch J (2008) Case 31–2007: a man with abdominal pain and elevated creatinine. N Engl J Med 358:312
7. Supavekin S, Zhang W, Kucherlapati R, et al (2003) Differential gene expression following early renal ischemia-reperfusion. Kidney Int 63: 1714–1724
8. Mishra J, Ma Q, Prada A, et al (2003) Identification of neutrophil gelatinase-associated lipocalin as a novel urinary biomarker for ischemic injury. J Am Soc Nephrol 4: 2534–2543
9. Mishra J, Mori K, Ma Q, et al (2004) Neutrophil gelatinase-associated lipocalin (NGAL): a novel urinary biomarker for cisplatin nephrotoxicity. Am J Nephrol 24: 307–315

10. Mishra J, Mori K, Ma Q, et al (2004) Amelioration of ischemic acute renal injury by neutrophil gelatinase-associated lipocalin. J Am Soc Nephrol 15: 3073–3082
11. Mori K, Lee HT, Rapoport D, et al (2005) Endocytic delivery of lipocalin-siderophore-iron complex rescues the kidney from ischemia-reperfusion injury. J Clin Invest 115: 610–621
12. Mishra J, Dent C, Tarabishi R, et al (2005) Neutrophil gelatinase-associated lipocalin (NGAL) as a biomarker for acute renal injury following cardiac surgery. Lancet 365: 1231–1238
13. Parikh CR, Mishra J, Thiessen-Philbrook H, et al (2006) Urinary IL-18 is an early predictive biomarker of acute kidney injury after cardiac surgery. Kidney Int 70: 199–203
14. Portilla D, Dent C, Sugaya T, et al (2008) Liver Fatty Acid-Binding Protein as a biomarker of acute kidney injury after cardiac surgery. Kidney Int 73: 465–472
15. Wagener G, Jan M, Kim M, et al (2006) Association between increases in urinary neutrophil-associated lipocalin and acute renal dysfunction after adult cardiac surgery. Anesthesiology 105: 485–491
16. Koyner J, Bennett M, Worcester E, et al (2008) Urinary cystatin C: A novel early biomarker of AKI development and severity after adult cardiothoracic surgery. Kidney Int 74: 1059–1069
17. Wagener G, Gubitosa G, Wang S, Borregaard N, Kim M, Lee HT (2008) Urinary neutrophil gelatinase-associated lipocalin and acute kidney injury after cardiac surgery. Am J Kidney Dis 52: 425–433
18. Haase-Fielitz A, Bellomo R, Devarajan P, et al (2009) Novel and conventional biomarkers predicting acute kidney injury in adult cardiac surgery – a prospective cohort study. Crit Care Med (in press)
19. Mishra J, Ma Q, Kelly C, et al (2006) Kidney NGAL is a novel early marker of acute injury following transplantation. Pediatr Nephrol 21: 856–863
20. Parikh CR, Jani A, Mishra J, et al (2006) Urine NGAL and IL-18 are predictive biomarkers for delayed graft function following kidney transplantation. Am J Transplant 6: 1639–1645
21. Kusaka M, Kuroyanagi Y, Mori T, et al (2008) Serum neutrophil gelatinase-associated lipocalin as a predictor of organ recovery from delayed graft function after kidney transplantation from donors after cardiac death. Cell Transplant 17: 129–134
22. Bachorzewska-Gajewska H, Malyszko J, Sitniewska E, et al (2006) Neutrophil-gelatinase-associated lipocalin and renal function after percutaneous coronary interventions. Am J Nephrol 26: 287–292
23. Bachorzewska-Gajewska H, Malyszko J, Sitniewska E, et al (2007) Neutrophil gelatinase-associated lipocalin (NGAL) correlations with cystatin C, serum creatinine and eGFR in patients with normal serum creatinine undergoing coronary angiography. Nephrol Dial Transplant 22: 295–296
24. Bachorzewska-Gajewska H, Malyszko J, Sitniewska E, et al (2007) Could neutrophil-gelatinase-associated lipocalin and cystatin C predict the development of contrast-induced nephropathy after percutaneous coronary interventions in patients with stable angina and normal serum creatinine values? Kidney Blood Press Res 30: 408–415
25. Ling W, Zhaohui N, Ben H, et al (2008) Urinary IL-18 and NGAL as early predictive biomarkers in contrast-induced nephropathy after coronary angiography. Nephron Clin Pract 108: c176-c181
26. Hirsch R, Dent C, Pfriem H, et al (2007) NGAL is an early predictive biomarker of contrast-induced nephropathy in children. Pediatr Nephrol 22: 2089–2095
27. Zappitelli M, Washburn KM, Arikan AA, et al (2007) Urine NGAL is an early marker of acute kidney injury in critically ill children. Crit Care 11: R84
28. Wheeler DS, Devarajan P, Ma Q, et al (2008) Serum neutrophil gelatinase-associated lipocalin (NGAL) as a marker of acute kidney injury in critically ill children with septic shock. Crit Care Med 36: 1297–1303
29. Nickolas TL, O'Rourke MJ, Yang J, et al (2008) Sensitivity and specificity of a single emergency department measurement of urinary neutrophil gelatinase-associated lipocalin for diagnosing acute kidney injury. Ann Intern Med 148: 810–819
30. Dent CL, Ma Q, Dastrala S, et al (2007) Plasma NGAL predicts acute kidney injury, morbidity and mortality after pediatric cardiac surgery: a prospective uncontrolled cohort study. Crit Care 11: R127
31. Bennett M, Dent CL, Ma Q, et al (2008) Urine NGAL predicts severity of acute kidney injury after cardiac surgery: A prospective study. Clin J Am Soc Nephrol 3: 665–673

32. Boldt J, Brosch C, Ducke M, et al (2007) Influence of volume therapy with a modern hydroxyethylstarch preparation on kidney function in cardiac surgery patients with compromised renal function: a comparison with human albumin. Crit Care Med 35: 2740–2746
33. Boldt J, Brosch Ch, Rohm K, et al (2008) Comparison of the effects of gelatin and a modern hydroxyethylstarch solution on renal function and inflammatory response in elderly cardiac surgery patients. Br J Anaesth 100: 457–464
34. Haase M, Fielitz-Haase A, Bellomo R, et al (2008) Sodium bicarbonate to prevent acute kidney injury after cardiac surgery: a pilot double-blind, randomised controlled trial. Nephrol Dial Transplant 1 (Suppl 2): ii212 (abst)
35. Wagener G, Gubitosa G, Wang S, et al (2008) Increased incidence of acute kidney injury with aprotinin use during cardiac surgery detected with urinary NGAL. Am J Nephrol 28: 576–582
36. Trachtman H, Christen E, Cnaan A, et al (2006) Urinary neutrophil gelatinase-associated lipocalcin in D+HUS: a novel marker of renal injury. Pediatr Nephrol 21: 989–994
37. Schaub S, Mayr M, Hönger G, et al (2007) Detection of subclinical tubular injury after renal transplantation: comparison of urine protein analysis with allograft histopathology. Transplantation 84: 104–112
38. Mitsnefes M, Kathman T, Mishra J, et al (2007) Serum NGAL as a marker of renal function in children with chronic kidney disease. Pediatr Nephrol 22: 101–108
39. Devarajan P (2007) Neutrophil gelatinase-associated lipocalin: new paths for an old shuttle. Cancer Therapy 5: 463–470
40. Bolignano D, Coppolino G, Campo S, et al (2007) Neutrophil gelatinase-associated lipocalin in patients with autosomal-dominant polycystic kidney disease. Am J Nephrol 27: 373–378
41. Malyszko J, Bachorzewska-Gajewska H, Malyszko JS, et al (2008) Serum neutrophil gelatinase-associated lipocalin as a marker of renal function in hypertensive and normotensive patents with coronary artery disease. Nephrology (Carlton) 13: 153–156
42. Malyszko J, Bachorzewska-Gajewska H, Sitniewska E, et al (2008) Serum neutrophil gelatinase-associated lipocalin as a marker of renal function in non-diabetic patients with stage 2–4 chronic kidney disease. Renal Failure 30: 1–4
43. Bolignano D, Lacquaniti A, Coppolino G, et al (2008) Neutrophil gelatinase-associated lipocalin reflects the severity of renal impairment in subjects affected by chronic kidney disease. Kidney Blood Press Res 31: 255–258
44. Nickolas TL, Barasch J, Devarajan P (2008) Biomarkers in acute and chronic kidney disease. Curr Opin Nephrol Hypertens 17: 127–132
45. Bolignano D, Coppolino G, Campo S, et al (2008) Urinary neutrophil gelatinase-associated lipocalin (NGAL) is associated with severity of renal disease in proteinuric patients. Nephrol Dial Transplant 23: 414–416
46. Ding H, He Y, Li K, et al (2007) Urinary neutrophil gelatinase-associated lipocalin (NGAL) is an early biomarker for renal tubulointerstitial injury in IgA nephropathy. Clin Immunol 123: 227–234
47. Brunner HI, Mueller M, Rutherford C, et al (2006) Urinary NGAL as a biomarker of nephritis in childhood-onset SLE. Arthritis Rheum 54: 2577–2584
48. Suzuki M, Wiers KM, Klein-Gitelman MS, et al (2008) Neutrophil gelatinase-associated lipocalin as a biomarker of disease activity in pediatric lupus nephritis. Pediatr Nephrol 23: 403–412
49. Damman K, van Veldhuisen DJ, Navis G, Voors AA, Hillege HL (2008) Urinary neutrophil gelatinase associated lipocalin (NGAL), a marker of tubular damage, is increased in patients with chronic heart failure. Eur J Heart Fail 10: 997–1000
50. Braunwald E (2008) Biomarkers in heart disease. N Engl J Med 358: 2148–2159

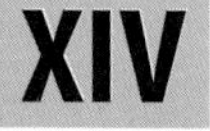

XV Hepatosplanchnic Function

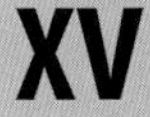

How does Intra-abdominal Pressure Affect the Daily Management of My Patients?

I.E. De laet, J.J. De Waele, and M.L.N.G. Malbrain

Introduction

A compartment syndrome exists when increased pressure in a closed anatomic space threatens the viability of the enclosed tissue. When this occurs in the abdominal cavity the impact on end-organ function within and outside the cavity can be devastating. The abdominal compartment syndrome (ACS) is not a disease; as such it can have many causes and it can develop within many disease processes. Unlike many commonly encountered disease processes which remain within the purview of a given discipline, intra-abdominal hypertension (IAH) and the ACS readily cross the usual barriers and may occur in any patient population regardless of age, illness, or injury. In an attempt to bring together all physicians and other health care workers who are confronted on a regular basis with the adverse effects of IAH, the World Society of the Abdominal Compartment Syndrome (WSACS, www.wsacs.org) was founded.

Recent animal and human data suggest that the adverse effects of elevated intra-abdominal pressure (IAP) can already occur at lower levels than previously thought and even before the development of clinically overt ACS. Therefore, clinicians should be aware of all the different effects of IAH on organ function and incorporate the concept of IAH into their everyday clinical management. This chapter will give a brief overview of definitions, etiology, and epidemiology of IAH/ACS and focus on the influence of IAH on the general ICU management of the critically ill patient and how IAP can be used in daily practice irrespective of interventions specifically aimed at reducing IAP, which will not be discussed here.

Definitions

The results of the 2004 consensus conference of the WSACS held in Noosa, Australia were published in 2006 and contain a set of definitions related to IAH and ACS [1] (**Table 1**). These definitions are based on the best available scientific data today, but are likely to undergo some minor changes in the future.

IAH is defined by a sustained or repeated pathologic elevation of IAP ≥ 12 mmHg and ACS is defined as a sustained IAP ≥ 20 mmHg that is associated with new organ dysfunction/failure. ACS can be classified into primary, secondary, and recurrent ACS.

Table 1. Consensus definitions for intra-abdominal hypertension (IAH) and abdominal compartment syndrome (ACS) (adapted from [1])

Definition 1	IAP is the steady-state pressure concealed within the abdominal cavity.
Definition 2	APP = MAP – IAP
Definition 3	FG = GFP – PTP = MAP – 2 x IAP
Definition 4	IAP should be expressed in mmHg and measured at end-expiration in the complete supine position after ensuring that abdominal muscle contractions are absent and with the transducer zeroed at the level of the mid-axillary line.
Definition 5	The reference standard for intermittent IAP measurement is via the bladder with a maximal instillation volume of 25 ml of sterile saline.
Definition 6	Normal IAP is approximately 5–7 mmHg in critically ill adults.
Definition 7	IAH is defined by a sustained or repeated pathological elevation of IAP ≥ 12 mmHg.
Definition 8	IAH is graded as follows: • Grade I: IAP 12–15 mmHg • Grade II: IAP 16–20 mmHg • Grade III: IAP 21–25 mmHg • Grade IV: IAP > 25 mmHg
Definition 9	ACS is defined as a sustained IAP > 20 mmHg (with or without an APP < 60 mmHg) that is associated with new organ dysfunction/failure.
Definition 10	Primary ACS is a condition associated with injury or disease in the abdomino-pelvic region that frequently requires early surgical or interventional radiological intervention.
Definition 11	Secondary ACS refers to conditions that do not originate from the abdomino-pelvic region.
Definition 12	Recurrent ACS refers to the condition in which ACS redevelops following previous surgical or medical treatment of primary or secondary ACS.

APP: abdominal perfusion pressure; FG: filtration gradient; GFP: glomerular filtration pressure; IAP: intra-abdominal pressure; MAP: mean arterial pressure; PTP: proximal tubular pressure

Epidemiology and Etiology

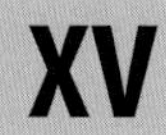

IAP may increase most obviously because of increased intra-abdominal volume in the abdominal cavity (consisting of both the retroperitoneal space and the peritoneal cavity), but the compliance of the abdominal wall is equally important. Similar to the situation in the brain, there are essentially two parts to the abdominal pressure-volume curve. When the abdominal wall is very compliant and at low intra-abdominal volumes, relatively large increases in volume will lead to minor changes in IAP only [2]. However, at higher volumes the abdominal wall compliance may decrease and small volume changes can lead to important increases in IAP. This means that a small increase in intra-abdominal volume can lead to clinically important effects on organ function, but also that relatively small decreases in volume can lower IAP substantially, which offers options for treatment. This abdominal pressure-volume curve is shifted to the left in situations where the abdominal wall compliance is decreased due to hematoma, voluntary muscle activity, edema, or other factors. The occurrence of IAH is usually associated with a situation that causes increased abdominal volume or decreased abdominal compliance but often a combination of both these factors. The WSACS published a list of risk factors associated with these situations [1]. They are summarized in **Table 2**.

Techniques for IAP Measurement

Surveys among clinicians show that many of them use clinical examination for the diagnosis of ACS, a practice which has repeatedly been shown to be unreliable with a sensitivity and positive predictive value of around 40–60 % [3, 4]. The use of abdominal perimeter is equally inaccurate. Radiologic investigation, with plain radiography of the chest or abdomen, abdominal ultrasound, or computed tomography (CT)-scan are also insensitive to the presence of increased IAP. However, they can be indicated to illustrate the cause of IAH (e.g., bleeding, hematoma, ascites, abscess) and may offer clues for management (e.g., paracentesis, drainage of collections).

The most important tool in establishing the diagnosis of IAH or ACS is IAP measurement [2]. Since the abdominal contents are primarily non-compressive in nature and predominantly fluid-based, they can be assumed to behave according to Pascal's law. Therefore, the IAP measured at one point can be assumed to be the pressure throughout the abdominal cavity. IAP increases with inspiration (due to downward displacement of the diaphragm) and decreases with expiration (due to diaphragmatic relaxation).

'Normal' IAP is variable. In the strict sense it is less than 5 mmHg in adults under resting conditions. However, in obese persons, in pregnant women or in patients with chronic ascites, it can be higher, up to 10 or even 15 mmHg, without causing significant adverse effects, probably due to the chronic nature of the IAP increase with adaptation of the individual's physiology. In children, the normal IAP is generally lower. In general, IAP readings must be interpreted relative to the individual patient's physiologic state.

IAP can be measured directly or indirectly, intermittently or continuously.

Transvesical IAP Measurement

The bladder has been studied and used most extensively to measure IAP. The technique described by Kron et al. [5] has been adapted over the years by Cheatham and Safcsak [6] and served as a model for commercially available devices such as the Abvisor (WolfeTory Medical, Salt Lake City, USA) [2].

A manometer technique can also be used, which was first described by Harrahill in 1998 [7]. The patient's own urine is used as a transducing medium, and the height of the fluid column in the catheter reflects the IAP. Based on this technique, a commercially available device has been developed (FoleyManometer, Holtech Medical, Copenhagen, Denmark) [2]. Using this technique, an IAP can be obtained at regular intervals, but it remains labor intensive, especially when hourly IAP measurements are needed.

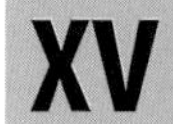

Continuous IAP measurement techniques have, therefore, been investigated. Balogh et al. [8, 9] introduced a method for continuous IAP measurement using a three way Foley catheter, which was found to perform excellently in ICU patients [2].

Transgastric IAP Measurement

Transgastric measurement of IAP has been reported, but is not used frequently in clinical practice. Collee et al. [10] used a fluid column in the nasogastric tube to measure IAP, but this technique has been replaced by the use of a balloon tipped catheter [2, 11], which can be used in a continuous or semi-continuous fashion. However, experience in critically ill patients is limited, and the influence of intestinal peristalsis and enteral nutrition, to name just two possible interfering factors, has not been studied so far.

Recommendations for IAP Measurement

Should I Measure IAP in all Patients?

Although the incidence of IAH in critically ill patients is considerable [12], routine IAP measurement in all patients admitted to the ICU is currently rarely performed, and probably not indicated. The WSACS has provided a list of risk factors associated with IAH and ACS (**Table 2**) [1]; in patients with two or more risk factors routine IAP monitoring is advised.

What Technique should I Use?

According to the WSACS consensus guidelines, IAP should be measured transvesically at end-expiration in the complete supine position after ensuring that abdominal muscle contractions are absent and with the transducer zeroed at the mid-axillary line at the level of the iliac crest. The technique used should be determined based on the indication and the condition of the patient, the available monitoring equipment, and the experience of the nursing staff with regards to possible pitfalls related to the technique used.

In some patients, a continuous technique may be preferable, e.g., when the abdominal perfusion pressure (APP) is used as a resuscitation endpoint, or in patients with impending ACS requiring urgent abdominal decompression. For most patients however, an intermittent technique may be adequate.

The manometer techniques can be used without the need for additional electronic equipment, which also allows for IAP measurement in the general ward when IAH or ACS is suspected.

Ideally, a protocol describing the preferred method of IAP measurement with details regarding the conditions in which it should be obtained should be available in every ICU.

What Frequency?

When an intermittent method is used, measurements should be obtained at least every 4 hours, and in patients with evolving organ dysfunction, this frequency should be increased up to hourly measurements.

When Should I Stop IAP Measurement?

IAP measurement can be discontinued when the patient has no signs of acute organ dysfunction, and IAP values have been below 10 mmHg for 24–48 hours. In case of recurrent organ dysfunction, IAP measurement should be reconsidered.

Table 2. Risk factors for the development of intra-abdominal hypertension (IAH) and abdominal compartment syndrome (ACS) [1]

A. Related to diminished abdominal wall compliance
- Mechanical ventilation, especially fighting with the ventilator and the use of accessory muscles
- Use of positive end-expiratory pressure (PEEP) or the presence of auto-PEEP
- Basal pleuropneumonia
- High body mass index
- Pneumoperitoneum
- Abdominal (vascular) surgery, especially with tight abdominal closures
- Pneumatic anti-shock garments
- Prone and other body positioning
- Abdominal wall bleeding or rectus sheath hematomas
- Correction of large hernias, gastroschisis or omphalocele
- Burns with abdominal eschars

B. Related to increased intra-abdominal contents
- Gastroparesis
- Gastric distension
- Ileus
- Volvulus
- Colonic pseudo-obstruction
- Abdominal tumor
- Retroperitoneal/abdominal wall hematoma
- Enteral feeding
- Intra-abdominal or retroperitoneal tumor
- Damage control laparotomy

C. Related to abdominal collections of fluid, air or blood
- Liver dysfunction with ascites
- Abdominal infection (pancreatitis, peritonitis, abscess,...)
- Hemoperitoneum
- Pneumoperitoneum
- Laparoscopy with excessive inflation pressures
- Major trauma
- Peritoneal dialysis

D. Related to capillary leak and fluid resuscitation
- Acidosis* (pH below 7.2)
- Hypothermia* (core temperature below 33 °C)
- Coagulopathy* (platelet count below 50000/mm^3 OR an activated partial thromboplastin time (aPTT) more than 2 times normal OR a prothrombin time (PT) below 50 % OR an international standardized ratio (INR) more than 1.5)
- Polytransfusion/trauma (> 10 units of packed red cells/24 hours)
- Sepsis (as defined by the American–European Consensus Conference definitions)
- Severe sepsis or bacteremia
- Septic shock
- Massive fluid resuscitation (> 5 l of colloid or > 10 l of crystalloid/24 hours with capillary leak and positive fluid balance)
- Major burns

* The combination of acidosis, hypothermia, and coagulopathy has been put forward in the literature as the deadly triad.

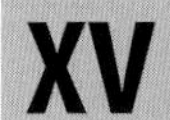

The Impact of IAH on Organ Function Management

ACS is diagnosed when the IAH is above 20 mmHg and there is evidence of new end-organ dysfunction [13]. IAH is diagnosed at lower levels of IAP when the patient is at risk, but there is no evidence of organ dysfunction, although subtle forms of organ dysfunction may be present at levels of IAP previously deemed to be safe [1]. There probably is a 'dose-dependent' association between IAP and organ dysfunction. Therefore, lowering IAP should have a beneficial effect on organ function and, indeed, decompressive laparotomy has been shown to improve organ function. However, at lower levels of IAH where decompressive laparotomy is not indicated, the increased IAP still has an impact on organ function, either as a causal agent or as an aggravating factor for other causes of organ dysfunction. IAH also has an impact on the parameters we use to monitor organ function as will be shown below. Therefore, whatever contribution IAH may have on organ dysfunction, IAP should be taken into account when assessing and managing IAH. We will provide an overview of the impact of IAH on monitoring and management of the different organ systems.

Effect on Cardiovascular Management

IAH is associated with a number of effects on the cardiovascular system that are caused by multiple factors [14]. First, due to the cranial movement of the diaphragm during IAH, the intrathoracic pressure will rise during IAH. Animal and human experiments have shown that 20–80 % of the IAP is transmitted to the thorax. This leads to compression of the heart and reduction of end-diastolic volume. Second, cardiac preload decreases due to decreased venous return from the abdomen and the systemic afterload is initially increased due to direct compression of vascular beds and activation of the renin-angiotensin-aldosterone pathway [15–18]. This leads to decreased cardiac output. Mean arterial blood pressure (MAP) may initially increase due to shunting of blood away from the abdominal cavity but, thereafter, normalizes or decreases [14, 19]. The cardiovascular effects are aggravated by hypovolemia and the application of positive end-expiratory pressure (PEEP) [20–24], whereas hypervolemia has a temporary protective effect [25].

IAH also has a marked effect on the reliability of hemodynamic monitoring. Preload estimation is most profoundly affected.

Preload estimation

Due to the abdomino-thoracic transmission of pressure, traditional filling pressures (central venous pressure [CVP] and pulmonary artery occlusion pressure [PAOP]) are falsely elevated in the presence of IAH, and do not reflect true cardiac filling. Due to the physiologic complexity of patients with IAH/ACS, resuscitation to arbitrary, absolute PAOP or CVP values should, therefore, be avoided as such a practice can lead to inappropriate therapeutic decisions, under-resuscitation, and organ failure. This must especially be kept in mind given the recent renewed interest in CVP as a resuscitation endpoint during early-goal directed therapy for severe sepsis and the propensity for sepsis and its treatment to result in subsequent IAH/ACS. Recognizing the impact of elevated IAP and intrathoracic pressure on the validity of intracardiac filling pressure measurements, some authors have suggested calculating the transmural PAOP ($PAOP_{tm}$) or CVP (CVP_{tm}) in an attempt to improve the accuracy of PAOP and CVP as resuscitation endpoints. Assuming proper placement of a pul-

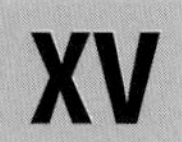

monary artery catheter (PAC) and the absence of other confounding factors, $PAOP_{tm}$ may be calculated as end-expiratory PAOP ($PAOP_{ee}$) minus pleural pressure (Ppl) with CVP_{tm} calculated as CVP_{ee} – Ppl · Ppl is typically determined by measuring lower esophageal pressure using a balloon catheter. Kallet et al. calculated $PAOP_{tm}$ using esophageal pressure for Ppl, and reported that this improved the ability of $PAOP_{ee}$ alone to predict fluid responsiveness, i.e., preload recruitable increases in cardiac output [26]. Other authors have advocated the practice of measuring PAOP during disconnection of the patient's airway (the so-called "pop-off" PAOP) to minimize the effect of Ppl. Such a practice would not be valid in the patient with elevated IAP, however, as this does not reduce the contribution of IAP to the patient's Ppl. Moreover, such maneuvers may be harmful in that they result in temporary loss of PEEP and derecruitment, which is to be avoided in patients with acute respiratory distress syndrome (ARDS, which is often associated with ACS). We recently evaluated several equations for calculating $PAOP_{tm}$ in patients with IAH and PEEP levels from 0 to 20 cmH_2O [18]. Confirming the findings of previous authors, a significant correlation was found between IAP and Ppl with approximately 80 % of the IAP being transmitted to the intrathoracic compartment ($Ppl = 0.8 \times IAP + 1.6$ ($r^2 = 0.8$, $p < 0.0001$)). Of the four equations evaluated, all were equivalent in predicting preload-recruitable increases in cardiac output. As a result, we concluded that the simple calculation of subtracting half the IAP from $PAOP_{ee}$ or CVP_{ee} may provide a rapid bedside estimate of true transmural filling pressure. This finding has important implications. The Surviving Sepsis Campaign guidelines, targeting initial and ongoing resuscitation towards a CVP of 8 to 12 mmHg [27], and other studies, targeting a MAP of 65 mmHg [28], should be interpreted and adjusted according to these findings.

Due to the problems in using cardiac filling pressures in the presence of IAH, it may be more useful to use volumetric monitoring parameters such as right ventricular end diastolic volume index (RVEDVI) or global end-diastolic volume index (GEDVI). These parameters are particularly useful because of the changing ventricular compliance and elevated intrathoracic pressure [18, 29–32]. Cheatham et al. [33] and Chang et al. [34] independently compared PAOP, CVP, and RVEDVI as estimates of preload status in patients with elevated IAP before and after abdominal decompression. In both studies, cardiac index (CI) was noted to correlate significantly with RVEDVI and inversely with PAOP and CVP. While some have raised concern that mathematical coupling, the interdependence of two variables when one is used to calculate the other, may explain the significant correlation between RVEDVI and CI, three separate studies have confirmed the validity of RVEDVI as a predictor of preload recruitable increases in CI [18].

Brienza et al. [35] and Malbrain et al. [36] have both demonstrated that elevated intrathoracic pressure and IAP result in significant decreases in GEDVI despite paradoxical increases in measured PAOP and CVP. As with RVEDVI, GEDVI appears to be superior to PAOP and CVP in predicting preload status, especially in patients with elevated intrathoracic pressure or IAP where transmission of these pressures to the pulmonary capillaries can erroneously increase measured PAOP and CVP values.

Assessing fluid responsiveness

It is clear from the discussion above that preload measurement or estimation is a complex issue. This complexity is increased further by the fact that volume status alone does not completely predict the effect of volume administration on cardiovascular function. Fluid responsiveness, i.e., increase in CI after administration of fluids, is an even more elusive concept than preload as such. Apart from crude clinical tests, such as the passive leg raising test or a limited fluid bolus test, fluid responsiveness has been shown to correlate best with stroke volume variation (SVV) and pulse pressure variation (PPV), parameters which can be derived from the arterial waveform, e.g., using the PiCCO device (Pulsion Medical Systems, Munich. Germany). However, there are some pitfalls [37]. SVV and PPV are only reliable predictors of fluid responsiveness in the absence of spontaneous breathing movements and in regular sinus rhythm, since stroke volume exhibits beat-to-beat variations in the presence of irregular cardiac rhythms or due to the pressure swings associated with spontaneous breathing. Furthermore, Duperret et al. showed in a pig model that SVV and PPV are increased when experimental IAH is induced [38]. However, since the pigs were not subjected to a fluid bolus, it is impossible to determine whether this was due to real hypovolemia induced by the decreased venous return in IAH, or a 'false' increase in SVV and PPV due to erroneous measurement.

Abdominal perfusion pressure

During the early evolution of IAH and ACS, attempts were made to identify a single 'critical' IAP that could be used to guide decision making in patients with IAH. This oversimplifies what is actually a highly complex and variable physiologic process. While IAP is a major determinant of patient outcome during critical illness, the IAP that defines both IAH and ACS clearly varies from patient to patient and even within the same patient as their disease process evolves. As a result, a single threshold value of IAP cannot be globally applied to decision making in all critically ill patients.

One approach to improving the sensitivity of IAP for decision making is to incorporate it into an assessment of abdominal perfusion as a resuscitation endpoint. Cheatham and colleagues first proposed the concept of APP as a predictor of survival in patients with IAH or ACS [39]. APP assesses not only the severity of IAH present, but also the adequacy of the patient's systemic perfusion. Analogous to the widely accepted and utilized concept of cerebral perfusion pressure (CPP), calculated as MAP minus intracranial pressure (ICP), APP, calculated as MAP minus IAP, has been proposed as a more accurate marker of critical illness and endpoint for resuscitation in patients with IAH [40].

APP provides an easily calculated measure that has been demonstrated to be superior to the clinical prediction of IAP alone. Cheatham et al. [39] in a retrospective trial of surgical/trauma patients with IAH (mean IAP 22 ± 8 mmHg) concluded that an APP ≥ 50 mmHg optimized survival. APP was also found to be statistically superior to arterial pH, base deficit, arterial lactate, and hourly urinary output in its ability to predict patient outcome. Malbrain [40] in three subsequent trials in mixed medical-surgical patients (mean IAP 10 ± 4 mmHg) suggested that an APP ≥ 60 mmHg represented an appropriate resuscitation goal. Persistence of IAH and failure to maintain an APP ≥ 60 mmHg by day 3 was found to discriminate between survivors and non-survivors.

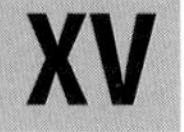

As a resuscitation endpoint, APP has yet to be subjected to a prospective, randomized clinical trial (although such a study is currently being prepared by the WSACS). Further, the therapeutic threshold above which raising MAP to achieve a particular APP becomes futile or even detrimental remains unknown. Indiscriminate fluid administration places the patient at risk for secondary ACS and should be avoided. Target APP values may be achieved through a balance of judicious fluid resuscitation and application of vasoactive medications. Notwithstanding these concerns, maintaining an APP of 50–60 mmHg appears to predict improved survival from IAH/ACS that is not identified by IAP alone.

Effects of IAH on Respiratory Management

The transmission of IAP to the thorax also has an impact on the respiratory system. Patients with primary ACS will often develop secondary ARDS and may require a different ventilatory strategy and more specific treatment than a patient with primary ARDS [41, 42]. The major problem lies in the reduction of the functional residual capacity (FRC). Together with the alterations caused by secondary ARDS this will lead to the so-called 'baby-lung'. IAH decreases total respiratory system compliance by a decrease in chest wall compliance, while lung compliance remains virtually unchanged [43, 44]. Theoretically, the compliance of the thoracic and abdominal wall can be improved by the use of neuromuscular blockers. Several authors have looked at the effect of neuromuscular blockers on IAP and found that bolus injections do have a temporary lowering effect on the IAP [45]. Although there are no data on the effect on respiratory system compliance in the presence of IAH, it is safe to assume that the decreased IAP in itself has a beneficial effect. Therefore, the use of neuromuscular blockers can be considered, but the expected benefit has to be balanced against known complications of neuromuscular blockers such as increased incidence of dorsobasal atelectasis, ventilator-associated pneumonia (VAP), critical illness polyneuropathy, and ICU-related muscular weakness.

Quintel et al. [46] studied the effect of instillation of oleic acid into the lungs of dogs to induce acute lung injury (ALI), followed by an increase in IAP (by instillation of fluid into the abdominal cavity). This study demonstrated that the ALI and lung edema induced by oleic acid were aggravated in the presence of IAH.

Some recommendations can be made in terms of ventilation strategy for patients with IAH:

- Patients with IAH should be ventilated according to low tidal volume strategies as put forward in the ARDS Network Guidelines [47].
- Best PEEP should be set to counteract IAP while at the same time avoiding over-inflation of already well-aerated lung regions
  - Best PEEP = IAP
- During lung protective ventilation, the plateau pressures (Pplat) should be limited to transmural plateau pressures below 35 cmH_2O
  - $Pplat_{tm} = Pplat - IAP / 2$
- Monitoring of extravascular lung water index (EVLWI) seems warranted in at risk patients since IAH is associated with increased risk of lung edema [46]
- In patients with decreased thoracic wall compliance, the use of neuromuscular blockers can be considered.

The Effect of IAH on Renal Function Management

Renal dysfunction is one of the most consistently described organ dysfunctions associated with IAH [48–52]. The etiology is multifactorial and offers a unique insight into the deleterious and sometimes cumulative effects of IAH on organ function.

XV

The most important effect of IAH on the kidney is related to renal blood flow [53]. IAH has been shown to lead to renal venous compression and increased renal venous pressure. Renal arterial blood flow and microcirculatory flow in the renal cortex are also decreased. Direct compression of the renal cortex may be a contributing factor. The changes in renal blood flow lead to activation of the renin-angiotensin-aldosterone pathway and anti-diuretic hormone (ADH) secretion is also increased in IAH. The clinical importance of these changes is still unclear.

The management of renal function is one of the areas in which the presence of IAH markedly affects clinical management. Impairment of kidney function has been seen at relatively low levels of IAH previously deemed to be safe. In many instances, the first action taken when renal function starts to deteriorate is administration of fluids and, as explained before, fluid resuscitation indeed has a temporary protective effect from the deleterious effects of IAH in the early stages. However, fluid resuscitation will also lead to increased edema formation, third spacing and possibly to a vicious cycle of ongoing IAH. In fact, fluid loading is one of the major risk factors for the development of IAH and the major contributor to secondary ACS, the morbidity and mortality of which is even higher than for primary ACS. Therefore, although an initial fluid challenge at the first sign of kidney failure can be considered (especially at lower IAP values when the etiology of the kidney dysfunction is uncertain), we recommend that great care be taken to avoid fluid overload. In this light, colloid resuscitation may be preferable to crystalloids and mobilization of edema by administration of albumin (to increase colloid osmotic pressure) and diuretics can be attempted. As IAH-induced kidney function progresses, patients often do not respond to diuretic therapy. Fluid removal by means of ultrafiltration has been shown to have a beneficial effect on IAP and possibly on organ function [54]. The institution of renal replacement therapy with fluid removal, if hemodynamically tolerated, should not be delayed. There are no reliable data on the preferred method of renal replacement therapy.

The Effect of IAH on the Management of the Patient with Intracranial Hypertension

A direct relationship between IAP and ICP has been observed in animal and human studies [25, 55–59]. Several authors hypothesized that the increase in ICP secondary to IAH was caused by increased intrathoracic pressure, leading to increased CVP and decreased venous return from the brain and, thus, venous congestion and brain edema. This hypothesis gained acceptance when Bloomfield et al. [25] demonstrated that the association between IAP and ICP could be abolished by performing a sternotomy and bilateral pleuropericardiotomy in pigs. The reduced systemic blood pressure associated with decreased cardiac preload and the increase in ICP will lead to a decrease in CPP. Some authors have even demonstrated successful treatment of refractory intracranial hypertension with abdominal decompression or curarization [56, 59].

Some recommendations:

- IAP monitoring is essential for all trauma or non-trauma patients at risk of intracranial hypertension or IAH (according to the risk factors published by the WSACS)
- In all patients with intracranial hypertension, preventive measures should be undertaken to avoid increase in IAP
- Neurologic status should be frequently monitored in patients with IAH
- Avoid hypervolemia in patients with IAH to prevent further increase in ICP.
- Provide adequate treatment for IAH, especially if intracranial hypertension is also present
- Avoid laparoscopy in patients at risk for intracranial hypertension. The pneumoperitoneum used for laparoscopy creates a situation analogous to experimental settings of IAH and intracranial hypertension in which detrimental effects on ICP have been observed. This is especially important in trauma patients with associated brain and abdominal injuries.

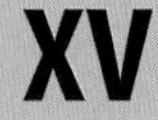

The Influence of IAH on the Management of Specific Patient Groups

IAH and Patients with Severe Sepsis

Sepsis-induced IAH is probably due to a 'first hit', the systemic infection, followed by a 'second hit' characterized by a massive inflammatory reaction and capillary leak syndrome. In this acute phase, patients receive large amounts of fluids which leads to edema formation and IAH [60]. Where the digestive tract is concerned, IAH causes diminished perfusion, mucosal acidosis, and sets the stage for multiple organ failure. The pathological changes are more pronounced after sequential insults of ischemia-reperfusion and IAH. It appears that IAH and ACS may serve as the second insult in the two-hit phenomenon of the causation of multiple-organ dysfunction syndrome. Recent clinical studies have demonstrated a temporal relationship between ACS and subsequent multiple organ dysfunction syndrome.

Understanding this pathologic string of events, it is important to adjust sepsis treatment to the presence of IAH. In septic shock, fluid resuscitation is the first therapeutic action recommended in the Surviving Sepsis Campaign Guidelines [27]. Traditionally, fluid resuscitation protocols are aimed at correction of 'basic' physiological parameters such as blood pressure, CVP, and urine output. However, as we have described before, all these physiologic parameters can be affected by the presence of IAH. Abdominothoracic pressure transmission can lead to overestimation of the actual filling pressures and underresusctiation of the patient, while IAH-induced kidney injury can decrease urine output and lead to overresuscitation which is equally detrimental. There is increasing evidence that IAH may be the missing link between overresuscitation, multiple organ failure, and death.

Daugherty et al. recently conducted a prospective cohort study of 468 medical ICU patients [61]. Forty patients (8.5 %) had a net positive fluid balance of more than 5 l after 24 hours (all risk factors for primary ACS served as exclusion criteria). The incidence of IAH in this group was a staggering 85 % and 25 % developed secondary ACS. The study was not powered to detect differences in mortality and outcome parameters were not statistically different between patients with or without IAH and ACS. Nevertheless, there was a trend towards higher mortality in the IAH groups and mortality figures reached 80 % in the ACS group. Although epidemiologic research regarding this subject is virtually non-existent, the increase in reported series seems to indicate an increasing incidence of this highly lethal complication.

In light of this increasing body of evidence regarding the association between massive fluid resuscitation, IAH, organ dysfunction, and mortality, it seems wise to at least incorporate IAP as a parameter in all future studies regarding fluid management, and to put into question current clinical practice guidelines, not in terms of whether to administer fluids at all, but in terms of the parameters we use to guide our treatment.

IAH and the Burn Patient

Another population where fluid resuscitation has been a cornerstone of therapy for decades is burn patients. Undoubtedly, fluid resuscitation protocols have saved countless lives in burn patients. However, increasing numbers of reports in recent years have highlighted the association between administration of large amounts of fluids in the first 24 h after burn injury and the development of secondary ACS. This can be avoided by using adjusted fluid resuscitation protocols. Oda et al. [62]

reported a reduced risk of ACS (as well as lower fluid requirements during the first 24 hours and lower peak inspiratory pressures after 24 hours) when using hypertonic lactated saline for burn resuscitation, and O'Mara et al. [63] reported lower fluid requirements and lower IAP using colloids.

IAH and the Hematology Patient

Recent studies have alluded to the increased incidence and consequences of IAH in hematological patients [64]. The causes for this finding are multifactorial:

- Growth factor-induced capillary leak syndrome with concomitant large volume fluid resuscitation and third space sequestration
- Chemotherapy-induced ileus, colonic pseudo-obstruction (Ogilvie's syndrome), mucositis or gastroenteritis
- Sepsis and infectious complications aggravating intestinal and capillary permeability
- Extramedullary hematopoiesis as seen with chronic myeloid leukemia resulting in hepatosplenomegaly, chronic IAH, and chronic (irreversible) pulmonary hypertension
- The mechanisms of veno-occlusive disease seen after stem cell transplantation may be triggered by or related to increased IAP

Therefore, critically ill hematological patients should be managed according to the principles described above.

IAH in Morbidly Obese Patients

Recent studies show that obese patients have higher baseline IAP values [65]. As with IAH in the critically ill, elevated IAP in the morbidly obese patient can have far reaching effects on end organ function. Disease processes common in morbidly obese patients, such as obesity hypoventilation syndrome, pseudotumor cerebri, gastroesophageal reflux and stress urinary incontinence are now being recognized as being caused by the increased IAP occurring with an elevated body mass index [66–68]. Furthermore the increased incidence of poor fascial healing and higher incisional hernia rates have been related to IAH-induced reductions in rectus sheath and abdominal wall blood flow.

A New Concept: Acute Bowel Injury and Acute Intestinal Distress Syndrome

Although few epidemiologic data are available to confirm this observation, it is our impression that the incidence of primary IAH/ACS is decreasing due to increased awareness of the problem among surgeons, who are more likely to leave the abdomen open in high risk surgery cases. This observation was also mentioned by Kimball et al. [69] in a review of patients with ruptured aortic aneurysm.

The focus of attention is shifting to secondary ACS and rightfully so. This syndrome is highly prevalent in critically ill patients and leads to even higher mortality than primary IAH. As described by Kimball [70] and Kirkpatrick et al. [71], a variety of noxious stimuli (such as infection, trauma, burns, sepsis) can lead to activation of the innate immune system and neutrophil activation. This systemic immune response causes release of cytokines into the circulation leading to systemic inflammatory response syndrome (SIRS) and capillary leak. Apart from a direct negative impact on cellular organ function, this syndrome also exerts its deleterious effect through accumulation of extravascular fluids in the tissues and local ischemia. This mechanism of injury is widely recognized and accepted in the lung, where it is classified as ALI or ARDS. However, the same pathological process occurs in the gut, but recognition of this concept is taking much slower to seep through into general ICU practice.

Why is this the case? It is undoubtedly true that bowel function is much harder to quantify than, e.g., lung function. PaO_2/FiO_2 ratios are very easy to calculate at the bedside and monitoring parameters such as EVLWI have been demonstrated to be accurate prognostic predictors. The same goes for the kidney. Urinary output and serum creatinine levels as crude indicators of kidney function are readily available and the acute kidney injury (AKI) RIFLE (Risk of kidney dysfunction, Injury to kidney, Failure of kidney function, Loss of kidney function, End-Stage kidney disease) classification has been linked with mortality. However, the role of the gut as the motor of organ dysfunction syndrome may be equally important and difficulties in assessing gut function should not deter us from recognizing that concept. In fact, in analogy to ALI and AKI, we propose the introduction of a concept named Acute Bowel Injury (ABI) which is manifest through bowel edema and the ensuing IAH. Even more than for other organ dysfunction syndromes, ABI has a negative impact on distant organ systems through the development of IAH, and can contribute to the development of AKI and ALI.

No specific markers of bowel function have been identified, apart from the very crude on/off parameter of enteral feeding tolerance. However, since capillary leak and bowel edema are cornerstones of this syndrome, ABI can probably best be defined, at least partially, in terms of IAP levels. Another plus for IAP is that it has already been linked to prognosis in several epidemiologic studies. One might argue then that the ABI concept is just another word for IAH. However, ABI reflects a more basic concept of complex bowel injury caused by a first hit (either directly, such as in abdominal sepsis or trauma, or indirectly such as in ischemia due to hypovolemic or distributive shock), followed by a second hit in the form of capillary leak, bowel edema, and local ischemia, of which (secondary) IAH is the result (**Fig. 1**). If the vicious cycle is not stopped this will eventually lead to acute intestinal distress syndrome and ACS. This definition set can evolve to a more intuitive understanding of the complexity of the pathologic process instead of a purely mechanical viewpoint of increased pressure in a confined anatomical space. Another viable option for definition of ABI and acute intestinal distress syndrome may be to use a gastrointestinal failure score based on both IAP values and enteral feeding tolerance such as proposed by Reintam et al. [72].

Conclusion

IAH and ACS occur frequently in ICU patients and are independently associated with mortality. The presence of IAH also has a profound effect on monitoring and support of almost all organ functions within the human body. Apart from specific strategies aimed at decreasing IAP and improving organ function, the IAP should be integrated in the supportive management of the various organ systems. This chapter has provided an overview of the different effects of IAH on organ function and its

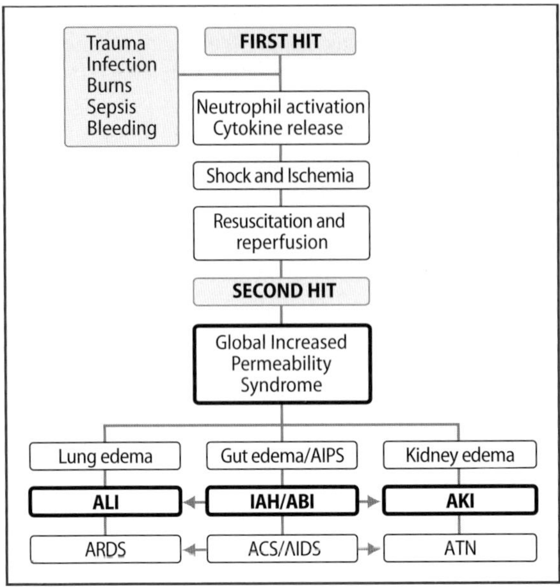

Fig. 1. The two hit model leading to intra-abdominal hypertension (adapted from [60] with permission). ABI: acute bowel injury; ACS: abdominal compartment syndrome; AIDS: acute intestinal distress syndrome; AIPS: acute intestinal permeability syndrome; AKI: acute kidney injury; ALI: acute lung injury; ARDS: acute respiratory distress syndrome; ATN: acute tubular necrosis; IAH: intra-abdominal hypertension

implications for management, and highlighted some patient populations in which these concepts are especially important.

References

1. Malbrain ML, Cheatham ML, Kirkpatrick A, et al (2006) Results from the International Conference of Experts on Intra-abdominal Hypertension and Abdominal Compartment Syndrome. I. Definitions. Intensive Care Med 32: 1722–1732
2. Malbrain ML (2004) Different techniques to measure intra-abdominal pressure (IAP): time for a critical re-appraisal. Intensive Care Med 30: 357–371
3. Kirkpatrick AW, Brenneman FD, McLean RF, Rapanos T, Boulanger BR (2000) Is clinical examination an accurate indicator of raised intra-abdominal pressure in critically injured patients? Can J Surg 43: 207–211
4. Sugrue M, Bauman A, Jones F, et al (2002) Clinical examination is an inaccurate predictor of intraabdominal pressure. World J Surg 26: 1428–1431
5. Kron IL, Harman PK, Nolan SP (1984) The measurement of intra-abdominal pressure as a criterion for abdominal re-exploration. Ann Surg 199: 28–30
6. Cheatham ML, Safcsak K (1998) Intraabdominal pressure: a revised method for measurement. J Am Coll Surg 186: 594–595
7. Harrahill M (1998) Intra-abdominal pressure monitoring. J Emerg Nurs 24: 465–466
8. Balogh Z, De Waele JJ, Malbrain ML (2007) Continuous intra-abdominal pressure monitoring. Acta Clin Belg Suppl 62: 26–32
9. Balogh Z, Jones F, D'Amours S, Parr M, Sugrue M (2004) Continuous intra-abdominal pressure measurement technique. Am J Surg 188: 679–684
10. Collee GG, Lomax DM, Ferguson C, Hanson GC (1993) Bedside measurement of intra-abdominal pressure (IAP) via an indwelling naso-gastric tube: clinical validation of the technique. Intensive Care Med 19: 478–480
11. Malbrain ML, De Laet I, Viaene D, Schoonheydt K, Dits H (2008) In vitro validation of a novel method for continuous intra-abdominal pressure monitoring. Intensive Care Med 34: 740–745
12. Malbrain ML, Chiumello D, Pelosi P, et al (2005) Incidence and prognosis of intraabdominal

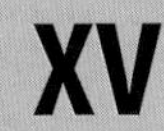

hypertension in a mixed population of critically ill patients: A multiple-center epidemiological study. Crit Care Med 33: 315–322
13. Malbrain ML, Deeren D, De Potter TJ (2005) Intra-abdominal hypertension in the critically ill: it is time to pay attention. Curr Opin Crit Care 11: 156–171
14. Cheatham M, Malbrain M (2006) Cardiovascular implications of elevated intra-abdominal pressure. In: Ivatury R, Cheatham M, Malbrain M, Sugrue M (eds) Abdominal compartment syndrome. Landes Bioscience, Georgetown, pp 89–104.
15. Kashtan J, Green JF, Parsons EQ, Holcroft JW (1981) Hemodynamic effect of increased abdominal pressure. J Surg Res 30: 249–255
16. Ridings PC, Bloomfield GL, Blocher CR, Sugerman HJ (1995) Cardiopulmonary effects of raised intra-abdominal pressure before and after intravascular volume expansion. J Trauma 39: 1071–1075
17. Richardson JD, Trinkle JK (1976) Hemodynamic and respiratory alterations with increased intra-abdominal pressure. J Surg Res 20: 401–404
18. Malbrain ML, Cheatham ML (2004) Cardiovascular effects and optimal preload markers in intra-abdominal hypertension. In: Vincent JL (ed) Yearbook of Intensive Care and Emergency Medicine. Springer-Verlag, Heidelberg, pp 519–543
19. Cheatham M, Malbrain M (2006) Abdominal perfusion pressure. In: Ivatury R, Cheatham M, Malbrain M, Sugrue M (eds) Abdominal Compartment Syndrome. Landes Bioscience, Georgetown 69–81
20. Simon RJ, Friedlander MH, Ivatury RR, DiRaimo R, Machiedo GW (1997) Hemorrhage lowers the threshold for intra-abdominal hypertension-induced pulmonary dysfunction. J Trauma 42: 398–403
21. Burchard KW, Ciombor DM, McLeod MK, Slothman GJ, Gann DS (1985) Positive end expiratory pressure with increased intra-abdominal pressure. Surg Gynecol Obstet 161: 313–318
22. Pelosi P, Ravagnan I, Giurati G, et al (1999) Positive end-expiratory pressure improves respiratory function in obese but not in normal subjects during anesthesia and paralysis. Anesthesiology 91: 1221–1231
23. Sugrue M, D'Amours S (2001) The problems with positive end expiratory pressure (PEEP) in association with abdominal compartment syndrome (ACS). J Trauma 51: 419–420
24. Sussman AM, Boyd CR, Williams JS, DiBenedetto RJ (1991) Effect of positive end-expiratory pressure on intra-abdominal pressure. South Med J 84: 697–700
25. Bloomfield GL, Ridings PC, Blocher CR, Marmarou A, Sugerman HJ (1997) A proposed relationship between increased intra-abdominal, intrathoracic, and intracranial pressure. Crit Care Med 25: 496–503
26. Kallet RH, Katz JA, Pittet JF, et al (2000) Measuring intra-esophageal pressure to assess transmural pulmonary arterial occlusion pressure in patients with acute lung injury: a case series and review. Respir Care 45: 1072–1084
27. Dellinger RP, Carlet JM, Masur H, et al (2004) Surviving Sepsis Campaign guidelines for management of severe sepsis and septic shock. Intensive Care Med 30: 536–555
28. Rivers E, Nguyen B, Havstad S, et al (2001) Early goal-directed therapy in the treatment of severe sepsis and septic shock. N Engl J Med 345: 1368–1377
29. Cheatham ML, Block EF, Nelson LD, Safcsak K (1998) Superior predictor of the hemodynamic response to fluid challenge in critically ill patients. Chest 114: 1226–1227
30. Cheatham ML, Nelson LD, Chang MC, Safcsak K (1998) Right ventricular end-diastolic volume index as a predictor of preload status in patients on positive end-expiratory pressure. Crit Care Med 26: 1801–1806
31. Schachtrupp A, Graf J, Tons C, Hoer J, Fackeldey V, Schumpelick V (2003) Intravascular volume depletion in a 24-hour porcine model of intra-abdominal hypertension. J Trauma 55: 734–740
32. Michard F, Alaya S, Zarka V, Bahloul M, Richard C, Teboul JL (2003) Global end-diastolic volume as an indicator of cardiac preload in patients with septic shock. Chest 124: 1900–1908
33. Cheatham ML, Safcsak K, Block EF, Nelson LD (1999) Preload assessment in patients with an open abdomen. J Trauma 46: 16–22
34. Chang MC, Miller PR, D'Agostino R Jr, Meredith JW (1998) Effects of abdominal decompression on cardiopulmonary function and visceral perfusion in patients with intra-abdominal hypertension. J Trauma 44: 440–445

35. Brienza N, Dambrosio M, Cinnella G, Conte M, Puntillo N, Bruno F (1996) [Effects of PEEP on intrathoracic and extrathoracic blood volumes evaluated with the COLD system in patients with acute respiratory failure. Preliminary study]. Minerva Anestesiol 62: 235–242
36. Malbrain M, Debaveye Y, Bertieaux S (2000) Effect of abdominal compression and decompression on cardiorespiratory function and regional perfusion. Intensive Care Med 26:S264 (abst)
37. Malbrain ML, De Laet I (2008) Functional haemodynamics during intra-abdominal hypertension: what to use and what not. Acta Anaesthesiol Scand 52: 576–577
38. Duperret S, Lhuillier F, Piriou V, et al (2007) Increased intra-abdominal pressure affects respiratory variations in arterial pressure in normovolaemic and hypovolaemic mechanically ventilated healthy pigs. Intensive Care Med 33: 163–171
39. Cheatham ML, White MW, Sagraves SG, Johnson JL, Block EF (2000) Abdominal perfusion pressure: a superior parameter in the assessment of intra-abdominal hypertension. J Trauma 49: 621–626
40. Malbrain ML (2002) Abdominal perfusion pressure as a prognostic marker in intra-abdominal hypertension. In: Vincent JL (ed) Yearbook of Intensive Care and Emergency Medicine. Springer-Verlag, Heidelberg, pp 792–814
41. Ranieri VM, Brienza N, Santostasi S, et al (1997) Impairment of lung and chest wall mechanics in patients with acute respiratory distress syndrome: role of abdominal distension. Am J Respir Crit Care Med 156: 1082–1091
42. Gattinoni L, Pelosi P, Suter PM, Pedoto A, Vercesi P, Lissoni A (1998) Acute respiratory distress syndrome caused by pulmonary and extrapulmonary disease. Different syndromes? Am J Respir Crit Care Med 158: 3–11
43. Mutoh T, Lamm WJ, Embree LJ, Hildebrandt J, Albert RK (1991) Abdominal distension alters regional pleural pressures and chest wall mechanics in pigs in vivo. J Appl Physiol 70: 2611–2618
44. Mutoh T, Lamm WJ, Embree LJ, Hildebrandt J, Albert RK (1992) Volume infusion produces abdominal distension, lung compression, and chest wall stiffening in pigs. J Appl Physiol 72: 575–582
45. De laet I, Malbrain ML (2007) ICU management of the patient with intra-abdominal hypertension: what to do, when and to whom? Acta Clin Belg Suppl 62: 190–199
46. Quintel M, Pelosi P, Caironi P, et al (2004) An increase of abdominal pressure increases pulmonary edema in oleic acid-induced lung injury. Am J Respir Crit Care Med 169: 534–541
47. Slutsky AS, Ranieri VM (2000) Mechanical ventilation: lessons from the ARDSNet trial. Respir Res 1: 73–77
48. Biancofiore G, Bindi L, Romanelli AM, et al (2002) Renal failure and abdominal hypertension after liver transplantation: determination of critical intra-abdominal pressure. Liver Transpl 8: 1175–1181
49. Biancofiore G, Bindi ML, Romanelli AM, et al (2003) Postoperative intra-abdominal pressure and renal function after liver transplantation. Arch Surg 138: 703–706
50. Sugrue M, Buist MD, Hourihan F, Deane S, Bauman A, Hillman K (1995) Prospective study of intra-abdominal hypertension and renal function after laparotomy. Br J Surg 82: 235–238
51. Sugrue M, Hallal A, D'Amours S (2006) Intra-abdominal pressure hypertension and the kidney. In: Ivatury R, Cheatham M, Malbrain M, Sugrue M (eds) Abdominal Compartment Syndrome. Landes Bioscience, Georgetown, pp 119–128
52. Sugrue M, Jones F, Deane SA, Bishop G, Bauman A, Hillman K (1999) Intra-abdominal hypertension is an independent cause of postoperative renal impairment. Arch Surg 134: 1082–1085
53. De laet I, Malbrain ML, Jadoul JL, Rogiers P, Sugrue M (2007) Renal implications of increased intra-abdominal pressure: are the kidneys the canary for abdominal hypertension? Acta Clin Belg Suppl 62: 119–130
54. Kula R, Szturz P, Sklienka P, Neiser J, Jahoda J (2004) A role for negative fluid balance in septic patients with abdominal compartment syndrome? Intensive Care Med 30: 2138–2139
55. De laet I, Citerio G, Malbrain ML (2007) The influence of intraabdominal hypertension on the central nervous system: current insights and clinical recommendations, is it all in the head? Acta Clin Belg Suppl 62: 89–97
56. Josephs LG, Este-McDonald JR, Birkett DH, Hirsch EF (1994) Diagnostic laparoscopy increases intracranial pressure. J Trauma 36: 815–818

57. Bloomfield GL, Ridings PC, Blocher CR, Marmarou A, Sugerman HJ (1996) Effects of increased intra-abdominal pressure upon intracranial and cerebral perfusion pressure before and after volume expansion. J Trauma 40: 936–941
58. Citerio G, Vascotto E, Villa F, Celotti S, Pesenti A (2001) Induced abdominal compartment syndrome increases intracranial pressure in neurotrauma patients: a prospective study. Crit Care Med 29: 1466–1471
59. Deeren D, Dits H, Malbrain MLNG (2005) Correlation between intra-abdominal and intracranial pressure in nontraumatic brain injury. Intensive Care Med 31: 1577–1581
60. Malbrain ML, De laet I (2008) AIDS is coming to your ICU: be prepared for acute bowel injury and acute intestinal distress syndrome. Intensive Care Med 34: 1565–1569
61. Daugherty EL, Hongyan L, Taichman D, Hansen-Flaschen J, Fuchs BD (2007) Abdominal compartment syndrome is common in medical intensive care unit patients receiving large-volume resuscitation. J Intensive Care Med 22: 294–299
62. Oda J, Ueyama M, Yamashita K, et al (2006) Hypertonic lactated saline resuscitation reduces the risk of abdominal compartment syndrome in severely burned patients. J Trauma 60: 64–71
63. O'Mara MS, Slater H, Goldfarb IW, Caushaj PF (2005) A prospective, randomized evaluation of intra-abdominal pressures with crystalloid and colloid resuscitation in burn patients. J Trauma 58: 1011–1018
64. Ziakas PD, Voulgarelis M, Felekouras E, Anagnostou D, Tzelepis GE (2005) Myelofibrosis-associated massive splenomegaly: a cause of increased intra-abdominal pressure, pulmonary hypertension, and positional dyspnea. Am J Hematol 80: 128–132
65. Hamad GG, Peitzman AB (2006) Morbid obesity and chronic intra-abdominal hypertension. In: Ivatury R, Cheatham M, Malbrain M, Sugrue M (eds) Abdominal Compartment Syndrome. Landes Bioscience, Georgetown, pp 187–194
66. Sugerman HJ (2001) Effects of increased intra-abdominal pressure in severe obesity. Surg Clin North Am 81: 1063–1075
67. Sugerman HJ (1998) Increased intra-abdominal pressure in obesity. Int J Obes Relat Metab Disord 22:1138
68. Sugerman HJ, DeMaria EJ, Felton WL III, Nakatsuka M, Sismanis A (1997) Increased intra-abdominal pressure and cardiac filling pressures in obesity-associated pseudotumor cerebri. Neurology 49: 507–511
69. Kimball EJ, Kinikini DV, Mone MC, et al (2006) Delayed abdominal closure in the management of ruptured abdominal aortic aneurysm. Crit Care Med 33 (suppl 12):A38 (abst)
70. Kimball EJ (2006) Intra-abdominal hypertension and the abdominal compartment syndrome: 'ARDS' of the gut. Int J Intensive Care Spring:1–7
71. Kirkpatrick AW, Balogh Z, Ball CG, et al (2006) The secondary abdominal compartment syndrome: iatrogenic or unavoidable? J Am Coll Surg 202: 668–679
72. Reintam A, Parm P, Kitus R, Starkopf J, Kern H (2008) Gastrointestinal Failure Score in critically ill patients: a prospective observational study. Crit Care 12:R90

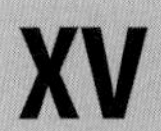

ICG Clearance Monitoring in ICU Patients

E. Levesque and F. Saliba

Introduction

Indocyanine green (ICG) clearance has been used, since the 1950s, as an indicator of dynamic liver function. The emergence of static liver function tests together with imaging and histology, has reduced the use of ICG measurements in the clinical setting. During the last two decades, methods to assess the hepatosplanchnic circulation and liver function have been the focus of intense investigation. The monitoring of this regional circulation has been shown to be the best predictor of outcome in critically ill patients [1]. As technologies advance, two mains goals can be identified concerning hemodynamic monitoring: The first is to make measurements using non-invasive tools in order to eliminate the risks associated with invasive monitoring; the second is to find a single measurement that could predict patient status. The same points are currently needed in regional hemodynamic monitoring. This chapter briefly considers ICG clearance physiology and its various methods of measurement, reviews the indications for ICG clearance measurement, and defines the current interests and limits of this technique with regard to hepatic functional impairment in critically ill patients with sepsis, liver disease, or after major hepatic surgery and liver transplantation.

Physiology of Indocyanine Green

ICG is a water-soluble, nontoxic tricarbocyanine dye. The active substance or dyestuff, ICG, is the mono-sodium salt of 1-[sulfobutyl] 3.3 dimethyl 2 {7 [(4 sulfo butyl) 3.3 dimethyl 4.5 benzoindoliny liden (2)] heptatrien(1.3.5) yl} 4.5. benzoindolium iodide. Its molecular formula is $C_{43}H_{47}N_2NaO_6S_2$, and its molecular weight is 774.97 Da.

The principal characteristic of ICG is that it is extracted nearly exclusively by the hepatic parenchymal cells and excreted almost entirely into the bile without enterohepatic circulation [2]. Indeed, after injection, ICG binds almost completely, within 1–2 seconds, to plasma proteins (globulin, α_1-lipoproteins) without extravascular distribution. It is taken up by the parenchymal cells of the liver, bound by acceptor proteins, and then, through the hepatic cells, excreted via the canalicular membrane and eliminated with the bile in unchanged form. ICG is detectable 15 minutes after injection into the bile, with a maximum concentration from 1/2 to 2 hours after injection, depending on the amount injected. The kinetic of ICG plasma disappearance has been thoroughly described in previous articles [3, 4]. Because of its metabolism, the ICG elimination rate, a dynamic test, has been largely used to assess liver function, hepatic blood flow, and hepatosplanchnic hemodynamics [5–7].

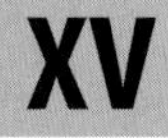

ICG is, in general, very well tolerated and safe. In all of the reported studies using ICG, no side-effect has been related to its use. However, in patients with an iodine allergy or thyrotoxicosis, use of ICG is not advised, since it contains iodine. ICG injection can, in extremely rare cases, cause nausea and an anaphylactic reaction (incidence of approximately 1:40000) with the main manifestations being pruritus, urticaria, tachycardia, hypotension, dyspnea, and shortness of breath.

Principles of Measurement

Various techniques (invasive and non-invasive) are available to evaluate ICG elimination after an intravenous injection. These methods give us various derived values that quantify ICG elimination: the clearance (Cl-ICG), the plasma disappearance rate (PDR-ICG), which is the percentage of ICG eliminated in 1 minute after an ICG bolus, and the retention rate at 15 minutes (R15) (**Table 1**).

Invasive Methods

Spectrophotometric concentration analysis at regular time intervals on serial blood samples was the first method described and remains the gold standard. To decrease the number of blood samplings, which are cost- and time-consuming, the insertion of a fiber-optic aortic catheter into the femoral artery has been proposed (COLD-System Z_{021}, Pulsion Medical Systems, Munich, Germany). Currently, because of its invasiveness, its use is limited to experimental settings.

Non-Invasive Methods

For 10 years now, ICG elimination can also be determined non-invasively by a measure based on spectrophotometry. The patient is monitored with an ICG finger clip, which is connected to a liver function monitor (LiMON®, Pulsion Medical System, Munich, Germany) via an optical probe. After injection, ICG is detected from fractional pulsatile changes in optical absorption. The optical peak absorptions of 805 nm and 890 nm allow continuous measurements of PDR-ICG. For each measure, a 0.25 to 0.5 mg/kg bolus of ICG is injected through a peripheral or central venous catheter and immediately flushed with 10 ml of normal saline. Administration is always performed after dilution of the lyophilisate in 10 ml of accompanying solvent or ice-cold 5 % dextrose, in order to obtain a concentration of 2.5 mg/ml. The dose administered per patient is calculated from the weight of the patient on the basis of 0.25 to 0.5 mg/kg. Sakka et al. showed that a dosage of ICG of 0.25 mg/kg appeared to be more accurate for transcutaneous measures of PDR-ICG than a 0.5 mg/kg bolus in critically ill patients ($r = 0.95$, $p < 0.0001$, with a mean bias 1.0 ± 2.5 %/min) [8]. The monitor

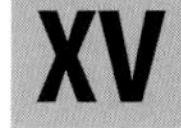

Table 1. Parameters that quantify indocyanine green (ICG) elimination

Parameter	Calculation	Normal range	Unit
Plasma disappearance rate of ICG (PDR-ICG)	$\ln 2/t_{1/2} \times 100$	18–25	%/min
ICG clearance	$Vd_{circ} \times PDR$	500–750	ml/min
ICG retention rate after 15 min	$[ICG_{t=15}] / [ICG_{t=0}] \times 100$	0–10	%

Vd_{circ}: volume of distribution of the dye

then determines automatically the PDR-ICG by a mono-exponential transformation of the original ICG concentration curve and backward extrapolation to the time point 'zero' (100 %), describing the decay as the percentage of change per time.

With this non-invasive monitoring, the ICG elimination is determined without any time delay, (the results being obtained within a few minutes, depending on the circulation time). This can be done at the bedside and reduces the number of blood samples. Recently, several studies have reported a good correlation between invasive and non-invasive methods [9–14]. A good correlation between invasive and non-invasive techniques (r^2: 0.81 to 0.97) has been reported in different clinical settings, i.e., critically ill patients [13], patients awaiting liver transplantation, liver transplanted patients [10, 12, 14], and patients being assessed for suitability of hepatic resection [9]. However, von Spiegel et al. [12], in 9 patients undergoing liver transplantation, observed that the PDR-ICG values measured by the non-invasive method tended to be relatively lower than the invasive Cl-ICG. This difference is linked, in these patients, to an increase in the volume of distribution (Vd_{circ}) of ICG just after the surgery. The pulse dye densitometry method for assessing liver function and hepatic blood flow can be used in hemodynamically stable and unstable patients [11]. However, the PDR-ICG value should be interpreted with caution in some situations.

Limits of ICG Pharmacokinetics Interpretation

The moment in the course of the day when ICG measurements are obtained is important. Indeed, circadian variations in hepatic blood flow and in ICG kinetics have been observed in healthy male volunteers [15]. The plasma clearance of ICG was lowest at 14:00 and highest during the night. Two previous studies have shown that several factors (postural change and exercise [16], food [17], drugs, such as angiotensin converting enzyme inhibitors [18] or N-acetylcysteine [19]) modify liver blood flow and ICG clearance. Physiologically, it has been shown that the volume of distribution of ICG is distributed in the vascular bed and is equal to the plasma volume assessed by [^{131}I]-labeled albumin [6].

The Current Place of ICG in Clinical Practice (Table 2)

Prognostic Marker in the Intensive Care Unit

Several prognostic scores have been tested and validated in intensive care patients. In many of these (Simplified Acute Physiology Score [SAPS] II, Sequential Organ Failure Assessment [SOFA]...], bilirubin is the only variable used to assess liver function and hepatosplanchnic blood flow. Yet, Sakka et al. have shown that the ICG-PDR on admission to the intensive care unit (ICU) was as sensible as other scores, such as APACHE II or SAPS II [20]. In their study, in 336 patients admitted to the ICU, PDR-ICG was as sensible as and more specific than bilirubin (area under the curve [AUC] 0.831 for PDR-ICG, with a cut-off point ≤ 10.3 %/min versus AUC 0.782 for bilirubin ($p < 0.06$), using receiver operating characteristic [ROC] curves) [21]. Gottlieb et al. [22] also observed, in seven injured patients with hepatic venous catheters, an earlier decrease in ICG clearance compared to bilirubin in cases of liver dysfunction. They concluded that ICG clearance was more sensitive than bilirubin for detecting liver dysfunction [22]. Similar results have been obtained in subgroups

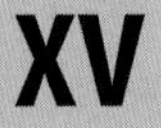

Table 2. Current use of indocyanine green clearance (ICG) monitoring

In the intensive care unit	• Prognostic markers (in critically ill patients, in septic shock) • Assessment of hepato-splanchnic hemodynamics
In hepatology	• Assessment of liver functional reserve in cirrhosis • Prognostic value in cirrhosis
In surgery	• Evaluate hepatic functional reserve before liver resection • Predict mortality and morbidity after surgery (liver resection, thoracic surgery, cardiac surgery) • To use in decision trees to select the surgical procedures in patients with impaired liver functional reserve
In liver transplantation (LT)	• Before LT: for selection of the graft • During LT: inform about the graft reperfusion • After LT: evaluate graft function and identify early graft dysfunction, predict graft and patient outcome, help to diagnose hepatic artery thrombosis and acute rejection.

of critically ill patients. In surgical critically ill patients, the plasma clearance rate of ICG was higher in survivors compared to non-survivors (11.1 ± 7.1 % versus 4.8 ± 4.3 %) [23]. In another study in 42 patients with trauma or shock, PDR-ICG predicted survival (15.0 ± 6.9 %/min in the survivors vs. 6.6 ± 5.0 %/min in non-survivors) whereas total bilirubin, alkaline phosphatase, and serum glutamic-oxalacetic transaminase, were identical in the two groups [24].

In patients with septic shock, the ICG elimination rate is an indicator of hepatocellular dysfunction; indeed, in a recent article, Kimura et al. reported an association between hepatocellular injury and a reduction in hepatic ICG clearance [25]. Moreover, in patients with septic shock, Kimura et al. showed that sequential changes in the elimination rate of ICG could predict survival. When the Cl-ICG increased, from 24 to 120 hours after the onset of the septic shock, it was associated with a good outcome; however, when the Cl-ICG remained stable or decreased, the patients died [25]. Knowing that regional variables are more important predictors of mortality compared with global volume-related hemodynamic [1], the PDR-ICG appears to be a very useful tool in the ICU. It is an excellent test to estimate hepatosplanchnic blood flow in patients with hemodynamic shock, and can be used as a prognostic factor on admission to the ICU.

Hepatosplanchnic Hemodynamics In Different Clinical Settings

Multiple organ failure syndrome is a major cause of death in patients in the ICU. It is associated with hepatosplanchnic hypoperfusion leading to an inadequate perfusion of the gut and damage to the mucosa of the intestine. This could result in a loss of its barrier function and lead to translocation of bacteria or endothelin into the circulation. After surgical interventions, the incidence of hepatosplanchnic hypoperfusion ranges from 1 to 2 %, depending on hemodynamic disturbances, with the same consequences as in septic shock.

The PDR-ICG (non-invasive method) has been validated as a marker of hepatosplanchnic perfusion [20, 26]. Several authors have used the PDR-ICG to evaluate the effects of treatments on the hepatosplanchnic circulation. After surgery, the PDR-ICG has been used to select patients at risk of hepatosplanchnic hypoperfusion and to guide therapy or to decide when to use more invasive devices to monitor this perfusion [27]. For example, in patients with septic shock, in whom the ICG clearance is predictive of survival, Lehmann et al. showed an increase in PDR-ICG after prostaglandin (PGI2 analog – Iloprost) administration and a protective effect of this drug on the hepatosplanchnic circulation [26]. The same results were observed with dopexamine with a positive effect on the PDR-ICG [27].

In another setting, the PDR-ICG has been largely used to evaluate the ventilator effect of positive end-expiratory pressure (PEEP) on venous return, thus altering systemic hemodynamic patterns and hepatosplanchnic blood flow. It was shown that PEEP decreased venous return and modified splanchnic hemodynamics in an experimental setting. However, in patients after orthotopic liver transplantation, in spite of the increase in the PEEP (from 0 to 10 cmH_2O) and deterioration of cardiac flow in half the patients, the PDR-ICG remained normal and stable [29]. After cardiac surgery, with the same PEEP level, the PDR-ICG remained unchanged [30].

In chronic intestinal ischemia [31] and during abdominal compartment syndrome [32, 33], ICG clearance was used to evaluate the effect on hepatosplanchnic hemodynamics of increasing cardiac output by fluid loading. The limitation of these studies is the lack of evaluation of the ICG distribution volume.

Cirrhosis

ICG clearance is thought to be adequate as an estimate of liver functional reserve in patients with cirrhosis and to reflect the degree of sinusoidal capillarization, portovenous shunt, and modifications in liver blood flow [4]. In cirrhotic patients, ICG clearance is significantly lower than in healthy patients, mainly with an intrinsic decrease of ICG hepatic uptake [34]. Indeed, the liver parenchymal cell volume in cirrhotic patients (874 ± 161 ml) was significantly smaller that in patients without cirrhosis (1284 ± 352 ml) [35]; the parenchymal cell volume per body weight was significantly correlated to ICG clearance.

Few data are available on ICG clearance and its prognostic value in cirrhotic patients. In a series of 102 cirrhotic patients (cirrhosis of various etiologies), the PDR-ICG was correlated with the Child-Pugh score [36]. Similarly, Herold et al., in patients with hepatitis C virus cirrhosis, reported an inverse correlation between several quantitative tests of liver function with ICG clearance and the Child-Pugh score [37]. In this study, patients with Child-Pugh A had an ICG clearance (0.15 ± 0.05 l/min) at the lower limit of normal; in patients with Child-Pugh B and Child Pugh C, the ICG clearance was significantly lower (0.07 ± 0.04 l/min and 0.03 ± 0.02 l/min, respectively).

During the follow-up of cirrhotic patients, ICG has been used as a predictor of survival [38]. In this study, 105 cirrhotic patients were followed for an average of 31 months, with 38 deaths over this period. The probability of survival was lower in patients with an ICG clearance less than 300 ml/min (70 %), than in patients with an ICG clearance greater than 1000 ml/min (80 %). However, among the covariates, ICG clearance was not independently associated with survival [38].

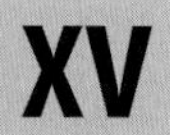

In a prospective study, Oellerich et al. [39] suggested that dynamic liver function tests such as Cl-ICG were superior to conventional liver function tests in assessing short-term prognosis in cirrhotic patients [39]. In this study, 107 adult candidates for liver transplantation were included; 18 died in the 120 days following inclusion. The patients who survived for at least 120 days showed a significantly lower ICG half-life compared to non-survivors (24.5 vs 12.3 min).

Major Hepatic Surgery

Post-operative hepatic failure is a life threatening complication that occurs in 1 to 5 % of hepatic resections. Evaluating the hepatic functional reserve is essential before surgery in order to limit the risk of post-operative hepatic failure. Thus, to predict mortality and morbidity after liver resection, several authors have used ICG clearance in addition to imaging and volumetric assessment [40, 41].

Nonami et al. [42] examined various predictive factors in 315 patients over 11 years. In this study, there were 291 survivors and 24 patients with post-operative liver failure. Among the factors studied, ICG clearance and blood loss during surgery were the only factors independently correlated to survival. Similarly, Lau et al. [43], in a series of 127 patients, reported cut-off values for ICG retention rate at 15 minutes of 14 % for major hepatectomy and 23 % for minor hepatectomy. The relative risk of death for major hepatectomy was 3 if the ICG retention rate at 15 min exceeded the cut-off [43]. For Hemming et al. [44], neither age nor standard liver function tests were useful as preoperative prognostic indicators of survival; only ICG clearance was a significant marker in determining outcome. According to the authors [44], below the cut-off point of 5.2 ml/min/kg, liver resection should not be attempted. Moreover, after liver resection in patients with hepatocellular carcinoma, a higher value of ICG retention rate at 15 minutes seemed linked to a higher recurrence rate [45]. It should be noted that all these studies included patients undergoing liver resection for hepatocellular carcinoma with cirrhosis. However, Yamanaka et al. [46] reported the same result in a study of 434 patients with a subgroup of 58 patients with liver metastases. According to these results, scoring systems and decision trees have been established using ICG clearance to estimate post-operative hepatic reserve prior to liver resection. Hence, Nagashima et al. [47] proposed the chronic liver dysfunction score that included five parameters, including the ICG retention rate (with the most important weight); this score provides a reliable assessment of the risk of partial liver resection. Decision trees have also been established to select the surgical procedures in patients with impaired liver functional reserve. Imamura el al. [4], using such a decision tree, observed a mortality rate of less than 1 % in patients with Child-Turcotte-Pugh A, undergoing liver resection for hepatocellular carcinoma. In their decision tree, the possible operative procedure (enucleation, limited resection, segmentectomy, mono- to bisectoriectomy, and trisectriectomy) depended on the total bilirubin level, the presence of ascites, and the ICG retention rate at 15 minutes. ICG clearance has also been used after thoracic surgery in cirrhotic patients [48]. Iwata et al. showed, as for preoperative serum alpha-fetoprotein or total bilirubin, that the ICG retention rate at 15 minutes was a predictive factor for postoperative liver failure after lung cancer surgery in patients with liver cirrhosis. Indeed, in the liver failure group, the preoperative value of the ICG retention rate at 15 minutes was significantly higher than in the non-liver failure group [48].

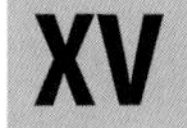

Liver Transplantation

Before Liver Transplantation

Successful liver transplantation depends on numerous factors that affect either the donor or the recipient. Assessing liver function in donors remains a major problem. With this aim, Wesslau et al. [49] studied several characteristics in 41 liver graft donors, 21 of whom were accepted for transplantation. The authors observed that a

PDR-ICG value of less than 15 %/min was associated with primary non-function of the graft [49]. On the other hand, 19 livers were found unsuitable for transplantation (based on the subjective decision of the surgeon). Only three of these had a PDR-ICG value greater than 15 %/min. Thus, the ICG clearance could be used as a prognostic index prior to organ explantation.

During liver transplantation

To identify graft dysfunction, von Spiegel et al. [12] analyzed the time course of ICG elimination from before surgery until 24 h post-surgery in 9 patients (12). The authors observed that during the anhepatic phase, the Cl-ICG or PDR-ICG remained low. Immediately after reperfusion of the graft, the PDR-ICG and Cl-ICG increased to supranormal values, before decreasing during the first 24 postoperative hours. The absence, after reperfusion, of an increase in ICG elimination could, therefore, provide information on graft function. In a case report, Mandell et al. [50] suspected graft dysfunction because the ICG elimination value was similar before and after reperfusion. The intra-operative ultrasound showed a reduction in portal venous blood flow. After reconstruction, ICG elimination was normal.

After liver transplantation

The ICG elimination rate, measured either by an invasive method (Cl-ICG) or a non-invasive method (PDR-ICG or retention rate), has been widely used to evaluate graft function [14, 51–54]. These various studies showed that ICG elimination, measured on the day of liver transplantation, reflected graft function and could be used to predict graft viability and patient survival. In these studies, the authors showed a good correlation between Cl-ICG and outcome. For Jalan et al. [51] and Plevris et al. [54], a Cl-ICG cut-off of 200 ml/min predicted survival. In a recent investigation in a cohort of 72 transplant recipients, we observed that a low PDR-ICG (< 12.85 %/min) was significantly associated with postoperative complications (primary non-function, hemorrhagic or septic shock, acute rejection, hepatic artery thrombosis) (**Fig. 1**) [55]. In all the studies, the ICG elimination rate was highly sensitive of liver dysfunction but not specific for the reason of the dysfunction. Analyzing the sequential changes in our series, we showed that the PDR-ICG can be used to help identify early graft dysfunction. Indeed, among patients with a complication after liver transplantation, a persistently low PDR-ICG (< 12.85 %/min) between day 0 and day 5 was associated with septic shock, prolonged liver dysfunction or hepatic artery thrombosis (**Fig. 2**), and these patients required retransplantation or prolonged

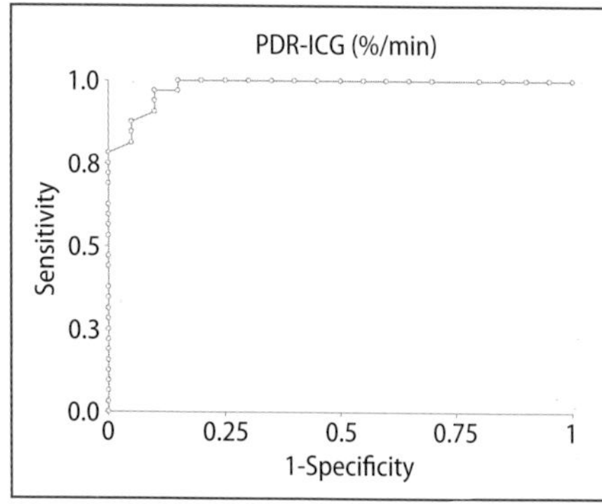

Fig. 1. Sensitivity and specificity of lowest value of plasma disappearance rate of indocyanine green (PDR-ICG) with respect to outcome according to receiver operating characteristic (ROC) curves in 72 transplant patients [55]. A PDR-ICG value, between day 0 and day 5 post-transplantation, less than 12.85 %/min is predictive of post-operative complications, with 90 % specificity and 97 % sensitivity. The area under the curve was 0.983.

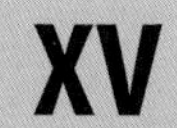

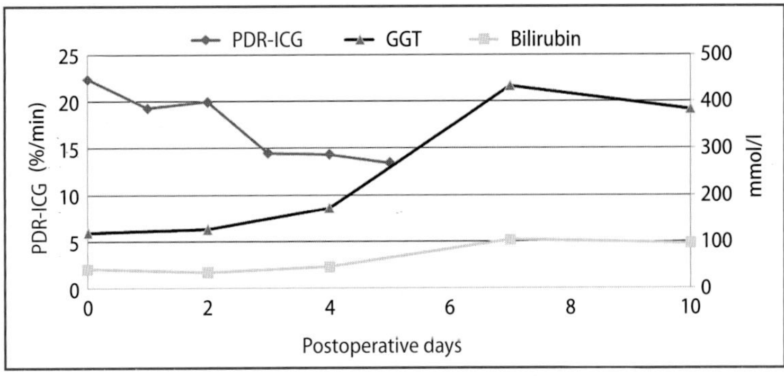

Fig. 2. Sequential changes of plasma disappearance rate of indocyanine green (PDR-ICG), bilirubin and gamma glutamyl transpeptidase, between day 0 and day 10 post-transplantation [55].

intensive medical support. Patients with a normal PDR-ICG on day 1 and day 2 after transplantation who had a secondary decrease in PDR-ICG during their ICU stay, developed acute rejection [55]. Previous studies demonstrated that acute rejection was associated with a reduction in ICG clearance due to a fall in liver blood flow [56]. We observed, only in patients with acute rejection, significant sequential changes in PDR-ICG after liver transplantation. The decrease in PDR-ICG, between the third and fifth days post-transplantation, was an early marker of acute rejection, earlier than the increase in liver enzymes.

A low PDR-ICG value after liver transplantation indicates the need for more invasive exams and should influence treatment decisions. A Doppler-ultrasound or angiography must be scheduled to look for hepatic artery thrombosis, the frequency of which ranges from 2 to 12 % after liver transplantation [57, 58]. Indeed, in our study evaluating ICG after liver transplantation, we observed four patients who had low PDR-ICG values and completely stopped blood flow in the hepatic artery [55]. In these four patients, the presence of hepatic artery thrombosis (early post-orthotopic liver transplantation), was confirmed by angiography. Moreover, treatment of the hepatic artery thrombosis (surgical repair or retransplantation) was followed by an increase in PDR-ICG. In one patient who developed hepatic artery thrombosis 13 years after orthotopic liver transplantation, the same result was obtained. Similarly, Krenn et al. [59] observed a decrease in PDR-ICG from 24.8 % (post-reperfusion) to 0 % (10 hours after admission to the ICU). Angiography showed a complete stop of blood flow in the hepatic artery, as well as in the portal vein. In this case, retransplantation was carried out as an emergency. In three other patients with normal PDR-ICG and no blood flow in the hepatic artery on Doppler-ultrasound, the diagnosis of hepatic artery thrombosis was eliminated either by angiography or computed tomography angio-scan. In these three cases, the PDR-ICG remained normal. Thus, we suggest that ICG elimination reflected by the PDR-ICG may be of considerable help in the diagnosis of hepatic artery thrombosis when the Doppler-ultrasound is difficult to interpret.

ICG clearance can be used to evaluate, as a meaningful liver function parameter, different treatments for early allograft dysfunction after liver transplantation. In primary dysfunction of the graft after liver transplantation, albumin dialysis with the molecular adsorbents recirculating system (MARS®) provides a safe approach [60, 61]. In a pilot study, evaluating the effects of MARS therapy in this situation, the authors observed a significant increase in PDR-ICG after the treatment [60]. This PDR-ICG change before the first and the last sessions of MARS therapy was observed only among survivors. It is to be noted that, when the laboratory data on inclusion into this study were compared, only total bilirubin and PDR-ICG (4.65 %/min vs 15.8 %/min) were significantly different between the MARS treated group and the control group. Moreover, the monitoring of PDR-ICG was superior to bilirubin and prothrombin time measurements for determining graft function, especially in patients with primary non-function and graft dysfunction undergoing MARS therapy [62].

The PDR-ICG has also been used to achieve adequate blood levels of tacrolimus following liver transplantation to optimize rejection prophylaxis [63]. In this study, without finding an association between PDR-ICG and acute rejection, a mixed model analysis of variance revealed an interaction between post-operative day 1 (18 hours post-reperfusion) PDR-ICG value, and the linear increase in the blood level of tacrolimus.

Conclusion

Currently, few tests are available to evaluate liver function. Apart from static markers, such as bilirubin (the only parameter include in major prognostic scores or organ dysfunction scores), serum activities of liver enzymes or liver proteins (prothrombin time, albumin, fibrinogen), ICG clearance is the only dynamic test that can be used in clinical practice.

Over the last decade, ICG elimination, known for nearly half a century, has been used to quantify liver function and to evaluate hepatosplanchnic hemodynamics. Its prognostic value in critically ill patients and in hepatic surgery patients (hepatectomy or liver transplantation) has been demonstrated. With the use of a finger clip sensor connected to an ambulant monitor and any peripheral or central venous access (for injection of the ICG), this measure is now non-invasive, safe, and quick. A low PDR-ICG value should alert the clinician. An urgent investigation is then needed to check the patency of hepatic blood vessels and regional hemodynamics. ICG monitoring can also help guide treatment.

References

1. Poeze M, Solberg BC, Greve JW, Ramsay G (2005) Monitoring global volume-related hemodynamic or regional variables after initial resuscitation: What is a better predictor of outcome in critically ill septic patients? Crit Care Med 33: 2494–2500
2. Wheeler HO, Cranston WI, Meltzer JI (1958) Hepatic uptake and biliary excretion of indocyanine green in the dog. Proc Soc Exp Biol Med 99: 11–14
3. Ott P (1998) Hepatic elimination of indocyanine green with special reference to distribution kinetics and the influence of plasma protein binding. Pharmacol Toxicol 83 Suppl 2: 1–48
4. Imamura H, Sano K, Sugawara Y, Kokudo N, Makuuchi M (2005) Assessment of hepatic reserve for indication of hepatic resection: decision tree incorporating indocyanine green test. J Hepatobiliary Pancreat Surg 12: 16–22
5. Hunton DB, Bollman JL, Hoffman HN (1960) Studies of hepatic function with indocyanine green. Gastroenterology 39: 713–724
6. Caesar J, Shaldon S, Chiandussi L, Guevara L, Sherlock S (1961) The use of indocyanine green in the measurement of hepatic blood flow and as a test of hepatic function. Clin Sci 21: 43–57
7. Sakka SG (2007) Assessing liver function. Curr Opin Crit Care 13: 207–214
8. Sakka SG, Koeck H, Meier-Hellmann A (2004) Measurement of indocyanine green plasma disappearance rate by two different dosages. Intensive Care Med 30: 506–509

9. Purcell R, Kruger P, Jones M (2006) Indocyanine green elimination: a comparison of the LiMON and serial blood sampling methods. ANZ J Surg 76: 75–77
10. Hsieh CB, Chen CJ, Chen TW, et al (2004) Accuracy of indocyanine green pulse spectrophotometry clearance test for liver function prediction in transplanted patients. World J Gastroenterol 10: 2394–2396
11. Faybik P, Krenn CG, Baker A, et al (2004) Comparison of invasive and noninvasive measurement of plasma disappearance rate of indocyanine green in patients undergoing liver transplantation: a prospective investigator-blinded study. Liver Transpl 10: 1060–1064
12. von Spiegel T, Scholz M, Wietasch G, et al (2002) Perioperative monitoring of indocyanine green clearance and plasma disappearance rate in patients undergoing liver transplantation. Anaesthesist 51: 359–366
13. Sakka SG, Reinhart K, Meier-Hellmann A (2000) Comparison of invasive and noninvasive measurements of indocyanine green plasma disappearance rate in critically ill patients with mechanical ventilation and stable hemodynamics. Intensive Care Med 26: 1553–1556
14. Tsubono T, Todo S, Jabbour N, et al (1996) Indocyanine green elimination test in orthotopic liver recipients. Hepatology 24: 1165–1171
15. Lemmer B, Nold G (1991) Circadian changes in estimated hepatic blood flow in healthy subjects. Br J Clin Pharmacol 32: 627–629
16. Daneshmend TK, Jackson L, Roberts CJ (1981) Physiological and pharmacological variability in estimated hepatic blood flow in man. Br J Clin Pharmacol 11: 491–496
17. Svensson CK, Edwards DJ, Mauriello PM, et al (1983). Effect of food on hepatic blood flow: implications in the "food effect" phenomenon. Clin Pharmacol Ther 34: 316–323
18. Geneve J, Le Dinh T, Brouard A, Bails M, Segrestaa JM, Caulin C (1990) Changes in indocyanine green kinetics after the administration of enalapril to healthy subjects. Br J Clin Pharmacol 30: 297–300
19. Devlin J, Ellis AE, McPeake J, et al (1997) N-acetylcysteine improves indocyanine green extraction and oxygen transport during hepatic dysfunction. Crit Care Med 25: 236–242
20. Sakka SG, Meier-Hellmann A (2001) Indocyanine green for the assessment of liver function in critically ill patients. In: Vincent JL (ed) Yearbook of Intensive Care and Emergency Medicine. Springer-Verlag, Heidelberg, pp 611–618
21. Sakka SG, Reinhart K, Meier-Hellmann A (2002) Prognostic value of indocyanine green plasma disappearance rate in critically ill patients. Chest 122: 1715–1720
22. Gottlieb ME, Stratton HH, Newell JC, Shah DM (1984) Indocyanine green. Its use as an early indicator of hepatic dysfunction following injury in man. Arch Surg 119: 264–268
23. Kholoussy AM, Pollack D, Matsumoto T (1984) Prognostic significance of indocyanine green clearance in critically ill surgical patients. Crit Care Med 12: 115–116
24. Pollack DS, Sufian S, Matsumoto T (1979) Indocyanine green clearance in critically ill patients. Surg Gynecol Obstet 149: 852–854
25. Kimura S, Yoshioka T, Shibuya M, et al (2001) Indocyanine green elimination rate detects hepatocellular dysfunction early in septic shock and correlates with survival. Crit Care Med 29: 1159–1163
26. Lehmann C, Taymoorian K, Wauer H, et al (2000) Effects of the stable prostacyclin analogue iloprost on the plasma disappearance rate of indocyanine green in human septic shock. Intensive Care Med 26: 1557–1560
27. Sander M, Spies CD, Foer A, Syn DY, Grubitzsch H, Von Heymann C (2007) Peri-operative plasma disappearance rate of indocyanine green after coronary artery bypass surgery. Cardiovasc J Afr 18: 375–379
28. Birnbaum J, Lehmann C, Taymoorian K, et al (2003) The effect of dopexamine and iloprost on plasma disappearance rate of indocyanine green in patients in septic shock. Anaesthesist 52: 1014–1019
29. Krenn CG, Krafft P, Schaefer B, et al (2000) Effects of positive end-expiratory pressure on hemodynamics and indocyanine green kinetics in patients after orthotopic liver transplantation. Crit Care Med 28: 1760–1765
30. Holland A, Thuemer O, Schelenz C, van Hout N, Sakka SG (2007) Positive end-expiratory pressure does not affect indocyanine green plasma disappearance rate or gastric mucosal perfusion after cardiac surgery. Eur J Anaesthesiol 24: 141–147
31. Henriksen JH, Winkler K (1987) Hepatic blood flow determination. A comparison of 99mTc-

diethyl-IDA and indocyanine green as hepatic blood flow indicators in man. J Hepatol 4: 66–70

32. Sakka SG (2007) Indocyanine green plasma disappearance rate as an indicator of hepato-splanchnic ischemia during abdominal compartment syndrome. Anesth Analg 104: 1003–1004
33. Hofmann D, Thuemer O, Schelenz C, van Hout N, Sakka SG (2005) Increasing cardiac output by fluid loading: effects on indocyanine green plasma disappearance rate and splanchnic microcirculation. Acta Anaesthesiol Scand 49: 1280–1286
34. Kawasaki S, Sugiyama Y, Iga T, et al (1985) Pharmacokinetic study on the hepatic uptake of indocyanine green in cirrhotic patients. Am J Gastroenterol 80: 801–806
35. Hashimoto M, Watanabe G (2000) Hepatic parenchymal cell volume and the indocyanine green tolerance test. J Surg Res 92: 222–227
36. Mukherjee S, Rogers MA, Buniak B (2006) Comparison of indocyanine green clearance with Child's-Pugh score and hepatic histology: a multivariate analysis. Hepatogastroenterology 53: 120–123
37. Herold C, Heinz R, Radespiel-Tröger M, Schneider HT, Schuppan D, Hahn EG (2001) Quantitative testing of liver function in patients with cirrhosis due to chronic hepatitis C to assess disease severity. Liver 21: 26–30
38. Merkel C, Bolognesi M, Finucci GF, et al (1989) Indocyanine green intrinsic hepatic clearance as a prognostic index of survival in patients with cirrhosis. J Hepatol 9: 16–22
39. Oellerich M, Burdelski M, Lautz HU, et al (1991) Assessment of pretransplant prognosis in patients with cirrhosis. Transplantation 51: 801–806
40. Hsia CY, Lui WY, Chau GY, King KL, Loong CC, Wu CW (2000) Perioperative safety and prognosis in hepatocellular carcinoma patients with impaired liver function. J Am Coll Surg 190: 574–579
41. Fan ST, Lai EC, Lo CM, Ng IO, Wong J (1995) Hospital mortality of major hepatectomy for hepatocellular carcinoma associated with cirrhosis. Arch Surg 130: 198–203
42. Nonami T, Nakao A, Kurokawa T, et al (1999) Blood loss and ICG clearance as best prognostic markers of posthepatectomy liver failure. Hepatogastroenterology 46: 1669–1672
43. Lau H, Man K, Fan ST, et al (1997) Evaluation of preoperative hepatic function in patients with hepatocellular carcinoma undergoing hepatectomy. Br J Surg 84: 1255–1259
44. Hemming AW, Scudamore CH, Shackleton CR, et al (1992) Indocyanine green clearance as a predictor of successful hepatic resection in cirrhotic patients. Am J Surg 163: 515–518
45. Hanazaki K, Kajikawa S, Shimozawa N, et al (2000) Survival and recurrence after hepatic resection of 386 consecutive patients with hepatocellular carcinoma. J Am Coll Surg 191: 381–388
46. Yamanaka N, Okamoto E, Oriyama T, et al (1994) A prediction scoring system to select the surgical treatment of liver cancer. Further refinement based on 10 years of use. Ann Surg 219: 342–346
47. Nagashima I, Takada T, Okinaga K, Nagawa H (2005) A scoring system for the assessment of the risk of mortality after partial hepatectomy in patients with chronic liver dysfunction. J Hepatobiliary Pancreat Surg 12: 44–8
48. Iwata T, Inoue K, Nishiyama N, et al (2007) Factors predicting early postoperative liver cirrhosis-related complications after lung cancer surgery in patients with liver cirrhosis. Interact Cardiovasc Thorac Surg 6: 720–730
49. Wesslau C, Kruger R, May G (1994) Clinical investigations using indocyanine green clearance for evaluation of liver function in organ donors. Transplantology 5: 7–9
50. Mandell MS, Wachs M, Niemann CU, Henthorn TK (2002) Elimination of indocyanine green in the perioperative evaluation of donor liver function. Anesth Analg 95: 1182–1184
51. Jalan R, Plevris JN, Jalan AR, et al (1994) A pilot study of indocyanine green clearance as an early predictor of graft function. Transplantation 58: 196–200
52. Yamanaka N, Okamoto E, Kato T, et al (1992) Usefulness of monitoring the ICG retention rate as an early indicator of allograft function in liver transplantation. Transplant Proc 24: 1614–1617
53. Hori T, Iida T, Yagi S, et al (2006) K(ICG) value, a reliable real-time estimator of graft function, accurately predicts outcomes in adult living-donor liver transplantation. Liver Transpl 12: 605–613

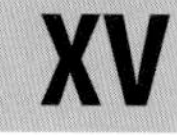

54. Plevris JN, Jalan R, Bzeizi KI, et al (1999) Indocyanine green clearance reflects reperfusion injury following liver transplantation and is an early predictor of graft function. J Hepatol 30: 142–148
55. Levesque E, Saliba F, Benhamida S, et al (2009) Plasma disappearance rate of indocyanine green: a tool to evaluate early graft outcome after liver transplantation. Liver Transpl (in press)
56. Clements D, McMaster P, Elias E (1988) Indocyanine green clearance in acute rejection after liver transplantation. Transplantation 4: 383–385
57. Stange BJ, Glanemann M, Nuessler NC, Settmacher U, Steinmüller T, Neuhaus P (2003) Hepatic artery thrombosis after adult liver transplantation. Liver Transpl 9: 612–620
58. Sánchez-Bueno F, Robles R, Acosta F, et al (2000) Hepatic artery complications in a series of 300 orthotopic liver transplants. Transplant Proc 32: 2669–2670
59. Krenn CG, Schafer B, Berlakovich GA, Steininger R, Steltzer H, Spiss CK (1998) Detection of graft nonfunction after liver transplantation by assessment of indocyanine green kinetics. Anesth Analg 87: 34–36
60. Hetz H, Faybik P, Berlakovich G, et al (2006) Molecular adsorbent recirculating system in patients with early allograft dysfunction after liver transplantation: a pilot study. Liver Transpl 12: 1357–1364
61. Saliba F, Ichaï P, Samuel D (2008) Artificial liver Support: Current status. In: Vincent JL (ed) Yearbook of Intensive Care and Emergency Medicine. Springer-Verlag, Heidelberg, pp 785–798
62. Scheingraber S, Richter S, Igna D, et al (2007) Indocyanine green elimination but not bilirubin indicates improvement of graft function during MARS therapy. Clin Transplant 21: 689–695
63. Parker BM, Cywinski JB, Alster JM, et al (2008) Predicting immunosuppressant dosing in the early postoperative period with noninvasive indocyanine green elimination following orthotopic liver transplantation. Liver Transpl 14: 46–52

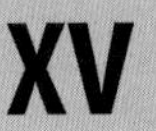

Acute-on-Chronic Liver Failure in Cirrhosis: Defining and Managing Organ Dysfunction

D. Shawcross and J. Wendon

Introduction

The term 'acute-on-chronic liver failure' was first used in the 1960s mainly in relation to flares of viral hepatitis. It was not until the turn of the millennium, however, that the term entered the everyday vocabulary of hepatologists when it was used to describe the pathophysiological deterioration in patients with cirrhosis mainly in the context of trials utilizing liver support devices [1]. Since then, a consensus definition of acute-on-chronic liver failure has been fiercely debated. The terms 'compensated' and 'decompensated' liver disease are rarely used in the critical care arena with patients being defined with regard to the degree of organ dysfunction rather than by quantifying liver synthetic function *per se*. Moreover, it has been shown that the prognosis in patients with cirrhosis is strongly correlated with the number of failing organs [2–4] and that certain cohorts of patients with severe hepatic encephalopathy, acute variceal bleeding, and organ failure benefit from admission to a critical care environment [5].

In this chapter, we define acute-on-chronic liver failure as it is normally used and suggest an alternative definition of liver failure requiring critical care and organ support. Furthermore, we will describe the common precipitants and therapeutic modalities, concentrating on critically ill patients with cirrhosis.

Defining Acute-on-Chronic Liver Failure

To hepatologists, acute-on-chronic liver failure encompasses patients with cirrhosis in whom a precipitating factor or triggering event such as infection or acute variceal bleeding results in an acute pathophysiologic deterioration with progressive organ dysfunction. In some patients the precipitant is overt, while in others it remains elusive. The acute deterioration is typically characterized by a hyperdynamic circulation, low systemic vascular resistance, renal dysfunction, worsening portal hypertension and hepatic encephalopathy. These patients have striking similarities with other critically ill patient groups [6] and early aggressive management and organ-targeted goal-directed therapies may prevent progression to irreversible organ failure and death [7].

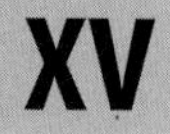

Quantifying Organ Dysfunction in Cirrhosis

Figure 1 encapsulates the major organ systems which are affected to one degree or another in patients with cirrhosis. It is particularly important to factor in the significant effects of liver dysfunction on the immune system, adrenals, gut, and portal circulation. Although it has not been examined in depth it is likely that 'septic liver dysfunction' will have many of the phenotypical characteristics that are seen in 'decompensated' chronic liver disease. It may indeed be that low-grade portal hypertension and its complications may be present and relevant to the patient with 'septic' liver dysfunction.

The admission to an intensive care unit (ICU) environment will encompass patients with recognized chronic liver disease and its associated complications. In addition however, we must consider those with disease processes who are not normally considered to have pre-existing liver disease. One of the largest such groups are those with non-alcoholic fatty liver disease, a rapidly growing cohort of patients in the general population. These individuals will not be recognized as having 'preceding liver disease'. This is a group of patients whose livers are highly susceptible to oxidative stress, have pre-existing insulin resistance, and who will develop 'stiff' livers with early development of cholestasis and ascites.

Another cohort of patients who frequently develop liver dysfunction are those undergoing liver resection. Many of these patients will have received preoperative chemotherapy and will have significant fatty livers. Removal of a significant amount

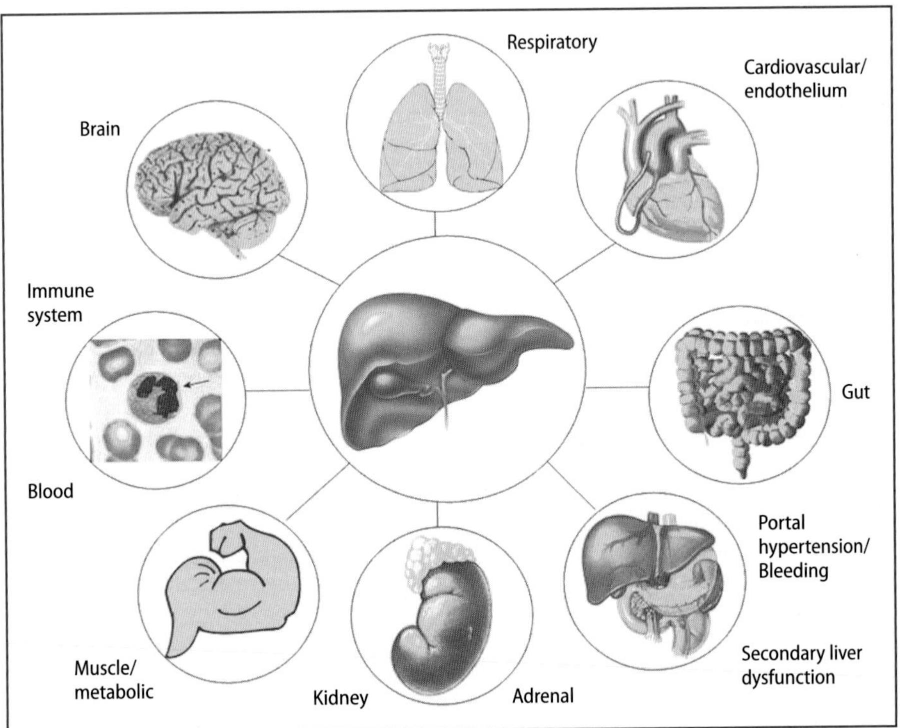

Fig. 1. A pictorial representation of the major organ systems that are affected in patients with cirrhosis.

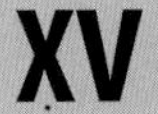

of liver with a fatty baseline will result in a markedly reduced 'functional' residual volume. Such patients will then develop many of the features of 'small for size' syndrome with cholestasis and portal hypertension. It may be that many of the features of end organ dysfunction such as portal hypertension, gut edema and congestion, renal vasoconstriction, portal shunting and hepatic encephalopathy may be seen at 'low titer' in those with so called 'septic liver cholestasis'.

Physiological derangement can be numerically quantified using a variety of scoring tools including the Acute Physiology and Chronic Health Evaluation (APACHE) [2, 8] and Sequential Organ Failure Assessment Score (SOFA) [9]. These scores have been validated to predict survival in general ICU populations but have been examined to a lesser extent in patients with cirrhosis (reviewed in [10]). Specific scoring systems for cirrhosis, such as the Child-Pugh-Turcotte system [11] and Model of End-stage Liver Disease (MELD) [12] have not been examined to any significant degree in critical care environments. More recently the RIFLE (Risk of renal failure, Injury to the kidney, Failure of kidney function and End-stage renal failure) classification was shown to demonstrate high discriminative power as an independent variable along with a SOFA score of ≥ 9 in predicting hospital mortality in critically ill patients with cirrhosis [13]. The outcome of patients with cirrhosis admitted to ICU and the utility of the various organ scoring systems in relation to predicting survival is reviewed in [10] and will not be the subject of this chapter. Instead we will focus on an evidence-based approach to the management of organ dysfunction in cirrhosis.

It should perhaps be considered that the definitions of acute-on-chronic liver failure (**Table 1**) may require adaptation for patients with liver disease in the critical environ. There already exists in the hepatology world considerable discussion as to the definition and distinction of 'decompensated' liver disease and acute-on-chronic liver failure. Many of the patients described with these syndromes are managed in a ward or even outpatient environment. The more severe end of the spectrum of organ dysfunction, with associated liver failure is not adequately described by the existing definitions. We would suggest that the term 'liver failure requiring critical care and organ support' (**Table 1**) could be adopted to encompass a number of subgroups, which would envelop the disease spectra that are encountered on a daily basis in the ICU. The subgroups and suggested features are summarized in **Table 1**.

Pathogenesis

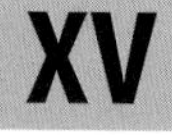

It is generally well recognized that the development of organ dysfunction in cirrhosis can be triggered in several different ways characterized by a 'second hit' in a patient with pre-existing chronic liver disease. Of all of these precipitants, infection, and the resultant systemic inflammatory response syndrome (SIRS), is perhaps the most important and most prevalent within this population. Patients with cirrhosis are functionally immunosuppressed and prone to infection [14]. Sepsis and/or SIRS occur in approximately 40 % of hospitalized patients with cirrhosis and the resultant organ failure is a major cause of death [15]. Specifically, the interplay between infection/inflammation and the development of hepatic encephalopathy has become well recognized and one of the ongoing challenges will be the separation of inflammation from infection. Similar functional immunosuppression can be seen in patients with acute liver function [16].

An ammonia load resulting from upper gastrointestinal bleeding or following the formation of a portocaval shunt or TIPS (transjugular intrahepatic portosystemic

Table 1. Definitions

1. Liver failure not requiring organ support (incorporating acute-on-chronic liver failure/ 'decompensated' cirrhosis) The development of ascites, hyperbilirubinemia, renal dysfunction, grade 1/2 hepatic encephalopathy in a patient with pre-existing cirrhosis
2. Liver failure requiring critical care and organ support The term encompasses the following 3 groups: 1. The critically ill patient with cirrhosis [Point 3] 2. Liver dysfunction in association with critical illness [Point 4] 3. Acute liver failure [Point 5]
3. The critically ill patient with cirrhosis Pre-existing cirrhosis in association with one of more of the following: • Major variceal hemorrhage requiring airway management • Severe hepatic encephalopathy (grade 3/4) • Acute renal dysfunction requiring renal replacement therapy • Hypotension (requiring fluids and vasopressors) • Intra-abdominal hypertension with end-organ dysfunction • Metabolic acidosis
4. Acute liver dysfunction in association with critical illness The term encompasses the following 3 groups: 1. Septic cholestasis 2. 'Small for size' syndrome post-liver resection (ascites, portal hypertension, cholestasis +/− hepatic encephalopathy) 3. Liver trauma
5. Acute liver failure with organ dysfunction Acute liver dysfunction (with no pre-exisiting liver disease) in association with any of the following: • Coagulopathy • Hepatic encephalopathy • Metabolic acidosis • Renal dysfunction • Cardiovascular failure • Respiratory failure

shunt) can lead to the development of hepatic encephalopathy [17] or the resultant change in systemic and splanchnic hemodynamics can precipitate right heart dysfunction [18].

It is important to recognize that the development of organ dysfunction is likely to be observed as a down-stream occurrence following an inflammatory event, with patients moving from a chronic stable phenotype to that of organ dysfunction and critical illness (**Fig. 2**). Other precipitants resulting in clinical deterioration, such as new onset portal vein thrombosis, hepatocellular carcinoma, use of non steroidal anti-inflammatory drugs, over use of diuretics, and use of sedatives should also be considered. One of the major challenges in the management of this cohort of critically ill patients with cirrhosis is the separation of those with reversible organ dysfunction in association with a precipitant and those where the deterioration is that of inexorable decline in association with end-stage liver disease.

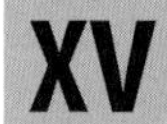

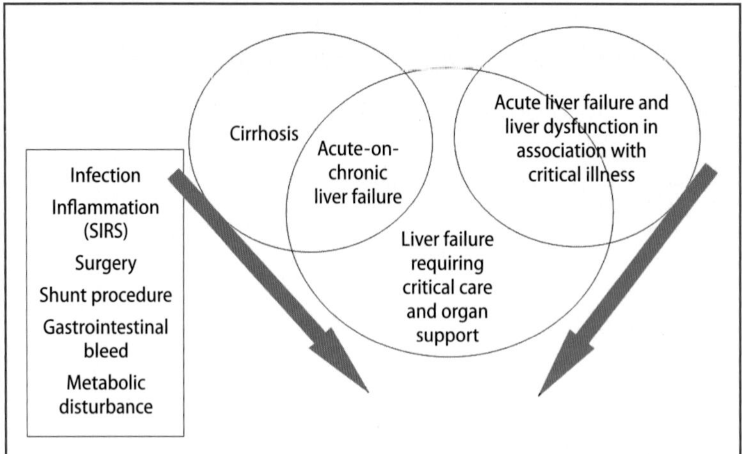

Fig. 2. A diagrammatic representation of the relationship between acute liver failure, liver dysfunction in association with critical illness and the patient with cirrhosis, and the development of liver failure requiring critical care and organ support. Factors such as infection and inflammation (systemic inflammatory response syndrome [SIRS]) can precipitate the development of multiorgan dysfunction.

Associated Organ Dysfunction

Adrenal

A number of studies have shown that relative adrenal insufficiency (defined as an impaired adrenal response to adrenocorticotropic hormone (ACTH) is common in critically ill patients with cirrhosis and its incidence correlates with the severity of liver disease (Child-Pugh and MELD scores) in addition to physiological derangements (APACHE II and SOFA scores) [19]. These authors [19] also noted a significantly increased mortality in patients with impaired adrenal response compared to those without. This phenomenon can exist in the absence of sepsis and led one group to propose the term 'hepatoadrenal syndrome'; this group also noted a relationship with cholesterol levels [20]. The effect of treating patients with cirrhosis and septic shock with low dose hydrocortisone has been evaluated prospectively in a small study [21]. Relative adrenal insufficiency was diagnosed in 68 % of patients and this group was treated with hydrocortisone. Treated patients had a quicker resolution of shock and an apparent survival benefit compared to historical controls that had not undergone adrenal function testing. A similar incidence is seen in patients with acute liver failure [19].

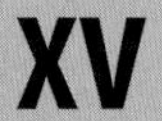

Brain

Hepatic encephalopathy remains a major clinical problem in patients with cirrhosis and when hepatic encephaolopathy is severe in cirrhosis, patients may develop varying degrees of confusion and coma [22]. In patients with severe liver dysfunction and, therefore, impaired urea synthesis, glutamine is synthesized from ammonia and glutamate and acts as a major alternative ammonia detoxification pathway. Glutamine synthesis occurs within astrocytes and may be one of the main causes of brain swelling. Clinically significant brain swelling and increased intracranial pressure (ICP) are effectively only seen in acute liver failure. More recent studies have suggested that intracranial hypertension is less frequent than previously described, being seen in 25 % of acute and hyperacute etiologies but in only 9 % of those with subacute liver failure. Magnetic resonance imaging (MRI) studies in liver cirrhosis have shown evidence of astrocyte swelling in patients with cirrhosis, with the degree of abnormality correlating with neuropsychological function and normalizing after liver transplantation [23]. In rare circumstances, clinically significant brain swelling may be seen; this should be considered especially when patients are exposed to a TIPS shunt without prior exposure to hyperammonemia [17].

To date, current therapies for hepatic encephalopathy have been based upon ammonia lowering strategies based on the hypothesis that the colon is the primary organ responsible for the generation of ammonia. Therefore, the mainstay of current therapy of hepatic encephalopathy has been the administration of non-absorbable antibiotics, lactulose, and protein restricted diets. However, the results of two recently published studies [24, 25] suggest that the colon may not be the only focus for ammonia reduction suggesting that the role of other organs in ammonia metabolism needs to be explored. In a recently published systematic review of 22 randomized trials using lactulose/lactitol and non-absorbable antibiotics for hepatic encephalopathy, it was concluded that there is 'insufficient' evidence at present to recommend or refute their use in hepatic encephalopathy [24]. Compared with placebo or no intervention, lactulose/lactitol had no significant effect on mortality.

Historically, protein restriction for the treatment of hepatic encephalopathy has been advocated based on anecdotal observations. This is in direct opposition to the fact that in cirrhosis, higher protein intakes are required to maintain a positive nitrogen balance. A recent small randomized study in cirrhotic patients with hepatic encephalopathy demonstrated that diets with a normal protein content can be administered safely and without detrimental effect on resolution of encephalopathy [25].

The most important management principal in patients with grade 3/4 hepatic encephalopathy is care of the airway. Patients with cirrhosis and hepatic encephalopathy alone should have a good prognosis providing the airway is protected against aspiration and that secondary chest sepsis is avoided.

Although we know that ammonia is important in the pathogenesis of hepatic encephalopathy, clinical observations do not always show a consistent correlation between the concentration of ammonia in the blood and the symptoms of hepatic encephalopathy. Therefore, it is probable that other factors, in addition to hyperammonemia, are important in modulating the effects of hyperammonemia. Recently the role of inflammation on the development of hepatic encephalopathy has been highlighted. Sepsis/inflammation is a frequent precipitant of hepatic encephalopathy and studies have suggested rapid progression in the severity of hepatic encephalopathy in those patients with acute liver failure who have more marked inflammation [26]. These observations have been confirmed in cirrhotic patients [27]. Altering the gut flora and gut permeability may justify the use of probiotic therapy, however, further work is required before this can be considered as standard therapy [28]. The role of beta-blockers, well recognized in the stable patient to decrease portal hypertensive enteropathy and thus 'gut leak', should be considered in the critical care setting if hemodynamics allow.

The use of a 'detoxification device' in liver failure might lead to a temporary improvement in the patient's condition, allowing the liver to recover spontaneously. Liver support systems, such as MARS (molecular adsorbents recirculating system), may have a role and has been found to be of benefit in improving hepatic encephalopathy grade in patients with acute-on-chronic liver failure independently of changes in ammonia and cytokines. A recent study looking at MARS showed improved resolution of hepatic encephalopathy but did not demonstrate any survival benefit; although the study was not powered for survival [29]. In the meantime, current guidelines will need to be revised with strict attention being paid to treating the precipitating factors, correction of dehydration, electrolyte and acid-base imbalance, constipation, and infection.

The management of hepatic encephalopathy in association with acute liver failure requires a different management protocol. The development of grade 3/4 hepatic encephalopathy is associated with a worse prognosis and more importantly may be complicated by the development of cerebral edema and raised ICP. Management is similar to that of neurocritical care although these cohorts of patients frequently do not autoregulate to pressure and increasing blood pressure without access to ICP monitoring is inadvisable. Fever and a SIRS-type response are associated with increased risk of elevated ICP and should be avoided. The use of hypothermia is being examined in a randomized controlled trial. The ICU management of acute liver failure requires a multidisciplinary approach in a center offering emergency liver transplantation [30].

Blood (Coagulopathy)

Patients with cirrhosis are invariably coagulopathic, resulting from a combination of poor liver synthetic function impairing the ability to produce clotting factors and fibrinogen, and thrombocytopenia. Platelets, fresh frozen plasma, and cryoprecipitate frequently need to be infused in the context of invasive procedures and variceal bleeding. It is also important to consider immune mediated thrombocytopenia and heparin-induced thrombocytopenia in addition to hypersplenism in those patients with thrombocytopenia. Standard measures of coagulation may be inadequate and the role of thromboelastography in the monitoring and management of patients with cirrhosis in the ICU can be invaluable [31, 32]. Thromboelastography provides a global assessment of hemostatic function from initial clot formation to clot dissolution. Prothrombotic states are not uncommon in liver disease and may not be adequately recognized using standard clotting profiles but can be characterized by thromboelastography. Such patients may be at increased risk of venous thrombosis (including portal vein) and embolic disease.

Cardiovascular

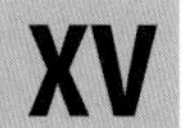

Cardiac and vascular dysfunction is common in cirrhosis but often underestimated. The presence of a hyperdynamic circulation in patients with cirrhosis and portal hypertension is well established, manifesting as high cardiac output, a hyporesponsive peripheral circulation, low systemic vascular resistance, and increased portosystemic shunting [33]. These phenomena may be secondary to a reduction in vascular responsiveness and desensitization to vasoconstrictors (endothelin I, angiotensin II and sympathomimetics) or to the effects of vasodilators (nitric oxide and prostacyclins) with resultant vasodilatation. These hemodynamic changes are responsible for many of the complications of cirrhosis we see including variceal bleeding, recurrent ascites and hepatorenal syndrome. Despite having an increased circulating blood volume, patients with cirrhosis are centrally volume deplete prior to the development of an acute insult. As such, they have limited reserve to accommodate further vasodilatation and hypotension and are inevitably profoundly volume depleted with the additional insult of sepsis or variceal hemorrhage. The cornerstone of management is thus early and aggressive volume repletion despite the presence of peripheral edema and ascites. Salt restriction in critically ill patients with cirrhosis is not required. The presence of cirrhotic cardiomyopathy and diastolic dysfunction may further complicate matters [34] and thus optimal volume repletion may be difficult to ascertain. Invasive monitoring is, therefore, frequently indicated. Dynamic hemodynamic monitoring as opposed to static cardiac measurements may be a better indication of volume responsiveness particularly in the context of diastolic dysfunction.

Portopulmonary syndrome (the development of pulmonary hypertension in a patient with portal hypertension resulting from intense vasoconstriction of pulmonary capillaries and pulmonary vascular remodeling) should always be considered and may be screened for using echocardiography. If present, a pulmonary flotation catheter may be placed in order to monitor therapies administered to decrease pulmonary hypertension such as sidenafil or prostacyclin.

If volume repletion is inadequate as a first line therapy then vasopressors should be instituted using norepinephrine in the first instance. Recently there has been a vogue for introduction of low dose vasopressin as an adjunct to catecholamines in refractory septic shock. A recent multicenter randomized double blind trial did not show a survival benefit [35] but this does not rule out a role for vasopressin in those patients who have high requirements for catecholamines. In patients with sepsis and vasopressor-dependent shock, international guidelines recommend the use of steroids although this remains an area of controversy. Initial studies were very positive with improved outcome [36] whilst a recent large multicenter study could not demonstrate any survival benefit.

Gut/nutrition

The gastrointestinal tract is often a neglected organ in patients with cirrhosis. It is important to remember that the small intestine provides a significant contribution to ammonia generation (along with the kidney), that it contributes significantly to endotoxemia through decreased integrity of the bowel wall leading to bacterial translocation, that portal hypertensive enteropathy causes malabsorption and chronic blood loss, and the implications of significantly raised intra-abdominal pressure from the accumulation of ascites. Moreover, adequate nutrition with appropriate supplementation of vitamins and trace elements is perhaps one of the most important therapies that can be given to patients with alcoholic hepatitis and acute-on-chronic liver failure who are invariably malnourished with little muscle mass and are in a catabolic state. The most appropriate type and nature of nutrition has yet to be established in prospective trials.

Intra-abdominal pressure can be measured through a nasogastric tube or via the urinary catheter. Intra-abdominal hypertension is deleterious to cardiovascular, respiratory and renal function [37] and can be reduced effectively by judicious low volume (4–6 liters) paracentesis.

Immune System

Patients with cirrhosis are particularly prone to infection which is frequently a precipitant of hepatic encephalopathy, renal failure, and circulatory collapse. Bacterial infections are of particular concern in patients with cirrhosis because they are poorly tolerated [15]. The increased risk of infection is secondary to impairment of several host defense mechanisms including impaired neutrophil function [38]. The hemodynamic derangement of cirrhosis resembles that produced by endotoxin, and bacteremia can greatly exacerbate this state, producing hypotension, hepatorenal syndrome, deterioration in mental status, and increased portal hypertension with risk of variceal bleeding. Factors that predispose to bacterial infection include malnutrition with impaired cell-mediated immunity, decreased integrity of the bowel wall leading to bacterial translocation, and impaired phagocytic activity of the hepatic and splenic reticuloendothelial system resulting from portal hypertension. Tuftsin, a natural tetrapeptide known to stimulate phagocytosis by neutrophils, has also been shown to be reduced in cirrhosis [39]. Neutrophils from patients with superimposed acute alcoholic hepatitis have depressed phagocytosis, intracellular killing and metabolic activity, although they have a greater capacity for ingestion and killing of bacteria than neutrophils of patients with cirrhosis alone [38]. Neutrophil dysfunction with high resting oxidative burst and reduced phagocytic capacity is present in patients with cirrhosis and alcoholic hepatitis and has been associated with a significantly greater risk of infection, organ failure and mortality [40]. Neutrophil phagocytosis was also found to be significantly impaired just 4 hours after inducing hyperammonemia in patients with stable cirrhosis given an amino acid solution but not in those given a placebo solution and it is possible that ammonia may, in part, account for the increased susceptibility to infection found in patients with liver disease [41]. Hyponatremia was also shown to impair phagocytosis and, when combined with ammonia, these effects were additive supporting the clinical observation in patients with cirrhosis, that hyponatremia is associated with an increased risk of infection [42].

Muscle/metabolic

Muscle plays an important role as an ammonia removing organ and in a hyperammonemic state, muscle detoxifies ammonia through conversion to glutamine [43]. Therefore, malnourished cachectic patients with low muscle mass have less capacity to detoxify ammonia putting them at greater risk for the development of hepatic encephalopathy, particularly during episodes of sepsis. Metabolic disarray is often caused by dehydration, diarrhea and over-diuresis. Strict attention needs to be paid to correcting these factors. Renal replacement therapy may be indicated in the absence of renal impairment to correct hyperlactemia, acid-base disturbances, hyperammonemia and hyponatremia with caution not to raise blood sodium levels too quickly.

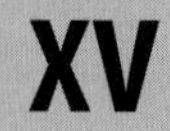

Portal Hypertension/variceal Bleeding

Acute variceal bleeding is now associated with markedly improved survival but it can be extremely challenging to manage patients with bleeding, organ dysfunction and hepatic encephalopathy in a ward environment, and these patients frequently require, and indeed benefit from, augmented levels of care in high dependency and intensive care environments. It is no longer acceptable to battle with agitated, hemodynamically unstable patients with variceal bleeding in the endoscopy suite without the presence of an anesthetist and/or airway protection by way of intubation and performed in an operating room or intensive care facility. Timely endoscopic therapies, including variceal band ligation and histoacryl glue injection, following aggressive resuscitation and correction of clotting abnormalities have been shown to be associated with favorable outcomes in patients with cirrhosis. Patients warrant ICU admission when the bleeding is uncontrolled, the patient is at risk of aspiration, and during periods of hemodynamic instability. Frequently, infection is a precipitant for variceal bleeding and the administration of empirical broad spectrum antibiotics is recommended, particularly when patients are at risk of aspiration pneumonia. The long-acting vasopressin analog, terlipressin, has immediate splanchnic vasoconstrictor action and has been shown in several placebo-controlled trials to reduce failure to control bleeding and to improve survival [44]. Its use is warranted early on during resuscitation before diagnostic endoscopy and administration is recommended every 4 to 6 hours for 2 to 5 days. Measurement of portal pressure is increasingly being used to guide the prescription of secondary prophylactic pharmacotherapy against re-bleeding such as non-specific beta-blockers or nitrates. Rescue therapy for uncontrolled variceal bleeding may warrant TIPS or portocaval shunt surgery. Indeed use of portal pressure measurement may delineate a high-risk group of patients (hepatic venous wedge pressure was > 20 mmHg) who should be considered for early intervention [45]. The most recent evidence-based guidelines for the management of acute variceal bleeding and portal hypertension were published in the consensus proceedings of Baveno IV [46].

Renal

Oligoanuria and renal dysfunction are very common in the critically ill patient with cirrhosis and the development of renal failure confers a poor prognosis particularly in the context of sepsis and the development of multiorgan failure [2–5]. Renal dysfunction is often labeled as 'hepatorenal syndrome' when in actual fact other causes of renal failure (particularly pre-renal) are often the most common culprits. Careful attention should be paid to the administration of nephrotoxic agents and intravenous contrast agents, correction of fluid depletion and over-diuresis, and exclusion of intrinsic renal problems which are common place in patients with alcoholic liver disease, viral hepatitis, and those with diabetes.

Assessing renal function in this cohort is extremely challenging and serum creatinine may not be an accurate representation in patients with poor muscle mass and hyperbilirubinemia. Consequently, a 24 hour creatinine clearance is often more accurate than an estimated glomerular filtration rate. A spot urinary sodium measurement can be invaluable in differentiating acute tubular necrosis (urinary sodium > 40 mmol/l) from pre-renal causes and hepatorenal syndrome (urinary sodium < 10 mmol/l). Renal failure may be the only manifestation of sepsis and patients with spontaneous bacterial peritonitis are particularly vulnerable to developing renal dysfunction. The clinical problem is therefore of distinguishing pre-renal failure due to sepsis, hypovolemia, or hepatorenal syndrome, from acute tubular necrosis and it is interesting to note the significant similarities between pre-renal failure as seen commonly in the critical care setting and hepatorenal syndrome. Regardless of the eventual diagnosis, the initial approach is the same in all patients who will be volume deplete. Fluid resuscitation with 1.5 l of colloid or crystalloid is

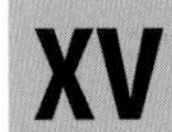

thus the first management step in this cohort. Other causes of renal failure such as virally driven glomerulonephritis, intersitial nephritis, and IgA nephropathy should be considered.

Treatment of hepatorenal syndrome with vasopressin or vasopressin analogs is based on the principle that hepatorenal syndrome results from a reduction in effective arterial blood volume due to arterial vasodilatation and, therefore, that vasoconstrictor drugs may be of benefit. Terlipressin has been evaluated in type 1 hepatorenal syndrome in several studies and has been effective in reversing hepatorenal syndrome in the majority of patients and associated with increased survival, although skeptics have often felt that this may be a reflection on the fact that those given terlipressin (with and without albumin) were more aggressively fluid resuscitated than controls (reviewed in [47]). Data to support the co-administration of albumin and terlipressin have recently been proposed as not only does albumin serve as a volume expander but it has other roles such as an anti-oxidant [48].

Renal replacement therapy is often instituted too late in the course of illness and data is emerging to suggest that it may also dampen down the manifestation of SIRS and reduce arterial ammonia. Studies in the field of renal replacement therapy do not demonstrate any clear benefit of continuous therapies as compared to intermittent ones. Intuitively however, continuous therapy is more likely to be suitable in hemodynamically unstable patients with cirrhosis with metabolic disarray and the risk of cerebral dysfunction [49].

Respiratory

The causes of hypoxia in patients with acute-on-chronic liver failure are diverse and include chest sepsis, acute lung injury (ALI) and acute respiratory distress syndrome (ARDS), splinting of the diaphragms from tense ascites, hepatic hydrothorax, hepatopulmonary syndrome, and pulmonary edema. Some patients may also have intrinsic lung disease, either as part of their liver disease, e.g., alpha-1 antitrypsin deficiency and cystic fibrosis, associated with fibrosing lung disease, or unrelated to their liver disease. Furthermore, the airway is at risk in patients with acute variceal bleeding and severe hepatic encephalopathy. Airway protection is paramount in the latter two populations who have been shown to have good outcomes when managed early and aggressively in a critical care rather than ward environment. It is also important to bear in mind that these patients are immunosuppressed and are at risk of opportunistic fungal infections and cytomegalovirus re-activation.

Bubble echocardiography is a useful tool in the diagnosis of hepatopulmonary syndrome and shunting. This is caused by arteriovenous shunting in the lung leading to a ventilation-perfusion mismatch and hypoxia which improves in the supine position and worsens on sitting/standing.

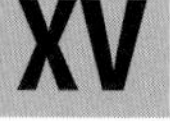

Conclusion

Although consensus has yet to be reached on the precise definition of acute-on-chronic liver failure, it can be viewed simply as the development of one or more organ(s) dysfunction in a patient with cirrhosis. The more organs affected, the bleaker the long-term prognosis in the absence of liver transplantation. It is important not to disregard the impact of hepatic dysfunction on the adrenals, immune system, and gut. The key management principle in the critically ill patient with cirrhosis is to administer early aggressive goal-directed therapies and to remember that admission to a critical care environment is not futile, particularly for those with single organ failure, acute variceal bleeding, and severe hepatic encephalopathy. Management should focus on treating precipitating factors such as infection, metabolic disarray, and hypovolemia. It can be extremely challenging to manage patients with organ dysfunction and hepatic encephalopathy in a ward environment and these patients frequently require, and indeed benefit from, augmented levels of care in high-dependency and intensive care facilities.

References

1. Sen S, Davies NA, Mookerjee RP, et al (2004) Pathophysiological effects of albumin dialysis in acute-on-chronic liver failure: a randomized controlled study. Liver Transpl 10: 1109–1119
2. Gildea TR, Cook WC, Nelson DR, et al (2004) Predictors of long-term mortality in patients with cirrhosis of the liver admitted to a medical ICU. Chest 126: 1598–1603
3. Cholongitas E, Senzolo M, Patch D, et al (2006) Risk factors, sequential organ failure assessment and model for end-stage liver disease scores for predicting short term mortality in cirrhotic patients admitted to intensive care unit. Aliment Pharmacol Ther 23: 883–893
4. Zimmerman JE, Wagner DP, Seneff MG, Becker RB, Sun X, Knaus WA (1996) Intensive care unit admissions with cirrhosis: risk-stratifying patient groups and predicting individual survival. Hepatology 23: 1393–1401
5. Shawcross D, Austin M, Abeles R, et al (2008) Defining the impact of organ dysfunction in cirrhosis: survival at a cost? Gut 57 (Suppl 1):A12-A13 (abst)
6. Levy M, Fink M, Marshall J, et al (2003) 2001 SCCM/ESICM/ACCP/ATS/SIS International Sepsis Definitions Conference. Intensive Care Med 29: 530–538
7. Rivers E, Nguyen B, Havastad S, et al (2001) Early goal-directed therapy in the treatment of severe sepsis and septic shock. N Engl J Med 345: 1368–1377
8. Knaus W, Draper E, Wagner D, Zimmerman J (1985) Prognosis in acute organ-system failure. Ann Surg 202: 685–693
9. Vincent JL, Moreno R, Takala J, et al (1996) The SOFA (Sepsis-related Organ Failure Assessment) score to describe organ dysfunction/failure. Intensive Care Med 22: 707–710
10. Austin M, Shawcross D (2008) Outcome of patients with cirrhosis admitted to intensive care. Curr Opin Crit Care 14: 202–207
11. Pugh R, Murray-Lyon I, Dawson J, Pietroni M, Williams R (1973) Transection of the oesophagus for bleeding oesphageal varices. Br J Surg 60: 646–649
12. Kamath K, Weisner R, Malinchoc M, et al (2001) A model to predict survival in patients with end-stage liver disease. Hepatology 33: 464–470
13. Jenq C, Tsai M, Tain Y, et al (2007) RIFLE classification can predict short-term prognosis in critically ill cirrhotic patients. Intensive Care Med 33: 1921–1930
14. Wasmuth H, Kunz D, Yagmur E, et al (2005) Patients with acute on chronic liver failure display 'sepsis-like' immune paralysis. J Hepatol 42: 195–201
15. Wong F, Bernardi M, Balk R, et al (2005) Sepsis in cirrhosis: report on the 7th meeting of the International Ascites Club. Gut 54: 718–725
16. Antoniades CG, Berry PA, Davies ET, et al (2006) Reduced monocyte HLA-DR expression: a novel biomarker of disease severity and outcome in acetaminophen-induced acute liver failure. Hepatology 44: 34–43
17. Jalan R, Newby DE, Damink SW, Redhead DN, Hayes PC, Lee A (2001) Acute changes in cerebral blood flow and metabolism during portasystemic shunting. Liver Transpl 7: 274–278
18. Van der Linden P, Le Moine O, Ghysels M, Ortinez M, Deviere J (1996) Pulmonary hypertension after transjugular intrahepatic portosystemic shunt: effects on right ventricular function. Hepatology 23: 982–987
19. Harry R, Auzinger G, Wendon J (2002) The clinical importance of adrenal insufficiency in acute hepatic dysfunction. Hepatology 36: 395–402
20. Marik P, Gayowski T, Starzl T (2005) The hepatoadrenal syndrome: a common yet unrecognised clinical condition. Crit Care Med 33: 1254–1259

21. Fernandez J, Escorsell A, Zabalza M, et al (2006) Adrenal insufficiency in patients with cirrhosis and septic shock: Effect of treatment with hydrocortisone on survival. Hepatology 44: 1288–1295
22. Ferenci P, Lockwood A, Mullen K, et al (2002) Hepatic Encephalopathy – Definition, nomenclature, diagnosis and quantification: Final report of the Working Party at the 11th World Congress of Gastroenterology, Vienna, 1998. Hepatology 35: 716–721
23. Cordoba J, Alonso J, Rovira A, et al (2001) The development of low-grade cerebral oedema in cirrhosis is supported by the evolution of 1H-magnetic resonance abnormalities after liver transplantation. J Hepatol 35: 598–604
24. Als-Nielsen B, Gluud L, Gluud C (2004) Non-absorbable disaccharides for hepatic encephalopathy: systematic review of randomised trials. BMJ 328: 1046–1050
25. Cordoba J, Lopez-Hellin J, Planas M, et al (2004) Normal protein diet for episodic hepatic encephalopathy: results of a randomized study. J Hepatol 41: 38–43
26. Rolando N, Wade J, Davalos M, Wendon J, Philpott-Howard J, Williams R (2000) The systemic inflammatory response syndrome in acute liver failure. Hepatology 32: 734–739
27. Shawcross D, Davies N, Williams R, Jalan R (2004) Systemic inflammatory response exacerbates the neuropsychological effects of induced hyperammonemia in cirrhosis. J Hepatol 40: 247–254
28. Liu Q, Duan ZP, Ha dK, Bengmark S, Kurtovic J, Riordan SM (2004) Synbiotic modulation of gut flora: effect on minimal hepatic encephalopathy in patients with cirrhosis. Hepatology 39: 1441–1449
29. Hassanein T, Tofteng F, Brown R, et al (2007) Randomized controlled study of extracorporeal albumin dialysis for hepatic encephalopathy in advanced cirrhosis. Hepatology 46: 1853–1862
30. Bernal W, Auzinger G, Sizer E, Wendon J (2008) Intensive care management for acute liver failure. Semin Liver Dis 28: 188–200
31. Chau T, Chan Y, Patch D, Tokanuga S, Greenslade L, Burroughs A (1998) Thrombelastographic changes and early rebleeding in cirrhotic patients with variceal bleeding. Gut 43: 267–271
32. Papatheodoridis G, Patch D, Webster G, Brooker J, Barnes E, Burroughs A (1999) Infection and hemostasis in decompensated cirrhosis: a prospective study using thrombelastography. Hepatology 29: 1085–1090
33. Fernandez-Seara J, Prieto J, Quiroga J, et al (1989) Systemic and regional haemodynamics in patients with liver cirrhosis and ascites with and without functional renal failure. Gastroenterology 97: 1304–1312
34. Moller S, Henriksen J (2008) Cardiovascular complications of cirrhosis. Gut 57: 268–278
35. Russell J, Walley K, Singer J, et al (2008) Vasopressin versus norepinephrine infusion in patients with septic shock. N Engl J Med 358: 877–887
36. Annane D, Sebille V, Charpentier C, et al (2002) Effect of treatment with low doses of hydrocortisone and fludrocortisone on mortality in patients with septic shock. JAMA 288: 862–871
37. Malbrain M, Chiumello D, Pelosi P, et al (2004) Prevalence of intra-abdominal hypertension in critically ill patients: a multicentre epidemiological study. Intensive Care Med 30: 822–829
38. Rajkovic IA, Williams R (1986) Abnormalities of neutrophil phagocytosis, intracellular killing and metabolic activity in alcoholic cirrhosis and hepatitis. Hepatology 6: 252–262
39. Trevisani F, Castelli E, Foschi FG, et al (2002) Impaired tuftsin activity in cirrhosis: relationship with splenic function and clinical outcome. Gut 50: 707–712
40. Mookerjee R, Stadlbauer V, Lidder S, et al (2007) Neutrophil dysfunction in alcoholic hepatitis superimposed on cirrhosis is reversible and predicts outcome. Hepatology 46: 831–840

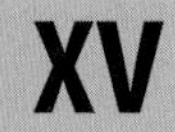

41. Shawcross D, Wright G, Stadlbauer V, et al (2008) Ammonia impairs neutrophil phagocytic function in liver disease. Hepatology 48: 1202–1212
42. Borroni G, Maggi A, Sangiovanni A, Cazzaniga M, Salerno F (2000) Clinical relevance of hyponatraemia for the hospital outcome of cirrhotic patients. Dig Liver Dis 32: 605–610
43. Olde Damink S, Jalan R, Deutz N, et al (2003) The kidney plays a major role in the hyperammonemia seen after a simulated or actual upper gastrointestinal bleeding in patients with cirrhosis. Hepatology 37: 1277–1285
44. Walker S, Stiehl A, Raedsch R, Kommerell B (1986) Terlipressin in bleeding oesphageal varices: a placebo-controlled, double blind study. Hepatology 6: 112–115

45. Monescillo A, Martinez-Lagares F, Ruiz-del-Arbol L, et al (2004) Influence of portal hypertension and its early decompression by TIPS placement on the outcome of variceal bleeding. Hepatology 40: 793–801
46. Laine L, Planas R, Nevens F, Banares R, Patch D, Bosch J (2006) Treatment of the acute bleeding episode. In: De Franchis R (ed) Portal Hypertension IV: Proceedings of the Fourth Baveno International Consensus Workshop. Blackwell Publishing, Boston, pp217–242
47. Salerno F, Gerbes A, Gines P, Wong F, Arroyo V (2007) Diagnosis, prevention and treatment of hepatorenal syndrome in cirrhosis. Gut 56: 1310–1318
48. Ortega R, Gines P, Uriz J, et al (2002) Terlipressin therapy with and without albumin for patients with hepatorenal syndrome: results of a prospective, non randomised study. Hepatology 36: 941–948
49. VA/NIH Acute Renal Failure Trial Network (2008) Intensity of renal support in critically ill patients with acute kidney injury. N Engl J Med 359: 7–20

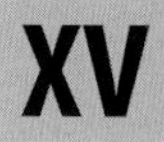

XVI Nutrition

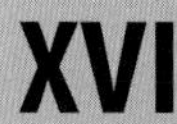

The Curse of Overfeeding and the Blight of Underfeeding

N.-H.W. Loh and R.D. Griffiths

Introduction

Evolution has refined our ability to cope with acute trauma, sepsis and, most importantly, the consequences of short term starvation. Our ancestor when severely ill or injured probably did not eat and either coped with the acute insult and rapidly got better or died. The years of natural selection have not prepared us for modern intensive care management and excess nutrient provision and hyperglycemia. Overfeeding carries a significant metabolic stress and has been associated with prolonged mechanical ventilation, infection risk, and delayed hospital discharge [1]. Difficulties in predicting energy requirements in intensive care further compound the effects of nutrition and overfeeding. In the critically ill, the reality is that enteral nutrition frequently under-delivers the desired calories and micronutrients due to gut intolerance while parenteral nutrition carries a significant risk of overfeeding if used injudiciously. Indeed, historically, particularly in North America dating from 1969, parenteral nutrition took the form of 'hyperalimentation' where excessive carbohydrate calories as the sole non-protein energy source were delivered in the belief that it would reverse the negative nitrogen balance [2]. Not until 1981 was it realized that there were advantages during ventilator support of substituting some of the energy source for lipids [3]. Lipids, however, have featured in European nutrition since their development by Schuberth and Wretlind in 1961 [4].

Energy Requirements in the Critically Ill

Energy requirements in intensive care patients are variable depending on individual activity levels. While sedated and ventilated, a patient's energy requirements approach resting energy expenditure and can double or triple during the recovery, weaning phase. Uehara et al. [5] showed that total energy expenditure rises during the second week after admission to the intensive care unit (ICU). In the first week of admission to intensive care, the ratio of total energy expenditure to resting energy expenditure was 1.0 in septic patients and 1.1 in trauma patients but during the second week rose to 1.7 and 1.8 in patients with sepsis and trauma, respectively. During the first week after admission, total energy expenditure in sepsis and trauma patients, respectively, averaged 25 and 31 kcal/kg of body weight/day, and during the second week for some patients rose to 47 and 59 kcal/kg/day [5]. Resting energy expenditure was still higher than normal (approximately 20 %) when measured 3 weeks after the onset of illness [5].

Increasing energy requirements are often due to diagnosis, severity, duration of illness and even ventilation modes [6]. Predicting energy requirement equations are conceived for resting conditions and defining energy requirements is difficult for ICU patients due to the fluctuating energy consumption. Estimating or measuring requirements in ICU patients frequently leads to errors in excess of 30 % leading to over and under-feeding [7].

Is it Better to Underfeed?

In a Canadian medical critical care study [1] observing the route of feeding and actual caloric intake in 187 patients as compared with American College of Chest Physician (ACCP) recommendations, better outcomes were achieved when patients were moderately underfed. Patients who were given 9–18 kcal/kg/day which was 33–65 % (tertile II) of the ACCP recommendations compared with < 33 % of a target of < 9 kcal/kg/day (tertile I) had a significantly greater likelihood of achieving spontaneous ventilation prior to ICU discharge. Patients who were fed 18–27 kcal/kg/day or more, which was 66 to 100 % of ACCP guidelines (tertile III) had a worse outcome when the SAPS score was greater than 50. Compared with tertile I, tertile II was associated with a significantly higher likelihood of hospital discharge alive, whereas tertile III was associated with a significantly lower likelihood of hospital discharge alive [1].

These data might suggest that a therapeutic window exists when it comes to caloric intake, above which harm and worse outcomes may exist. However, it must be remembered that this was not a randomized controlled trial, merely an observational study and, therefore, open to considerable bias distorted by heterogeneity in patient disease, severity and length of stay that despite best efforts cannot be fully accounted for. In this study, a wide range of caloric intake occurred (from 0 to 227 % of ACCP recommendations) and clearly a proportion of patients were overfed (**Fig. 1**). This may have contributed to the excess mortality in this cohort of medical ICU patients. A target of 66 % of the ACCP guidelines (18 kcal/kg/day) appeared to be more appropriate in this setting and was associated with better ICU outcomes. This is probably not unreasonable since the actual caloric intake values in some patients must have been higher and is masked by the mean value (see the wide variation in **Figure 1**). It should also be realized that length of stay plays a crucial part in this association and cannot be easily corrected for in an observational study. ICU populations are dominated by relatively short stays (less than five to 10 days) where the contribution that any nutrient deprivation could make to influence outcome may be modest. However, the smaller proportion of longer stay ICU patients who have not recovered and have a higher general mortality, are the group that might be more influenced by any nutrient deficiency or excess. As can be seen in **Figure 1**, average intake increases the longer the stay and, as the variation shows, the higher tertile group are also exposed to a greater risk of overfeeding.

Perhaps focusing on calorie intake alone ignores the importance of providing adequate dietary protein. Some commentators suggest that a nutrition support goal of 10–20 kcal/kg of ideal or adjusted weight and 1.5–2 g/kg ideal weight of protein may be more beneficial during the acute stress response [8].

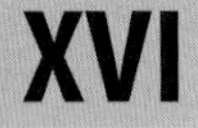

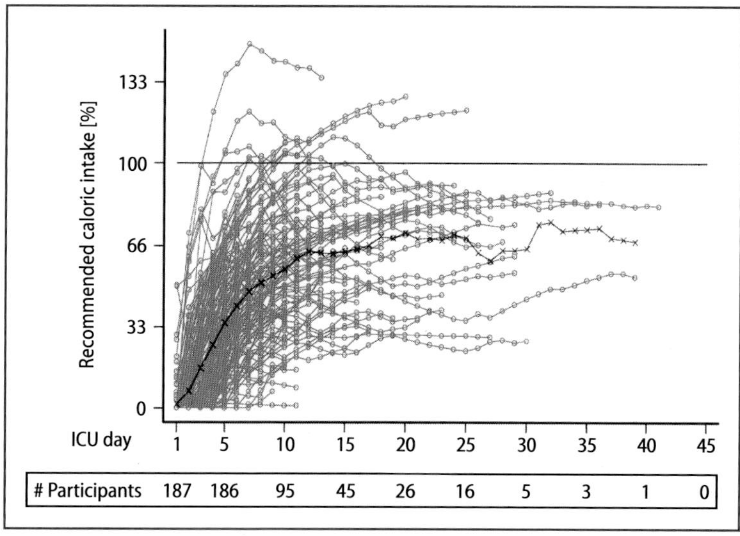

Fig. 1. The cumulative average caloric intake since ICU admission for each of 187 participants. The mean caloric intake for each ICU day for all participants in the ICU is also shown (X). Points above 100 % recommended intake denote patients who were overfed. Note also that much of the data comes from shorter stay patients and "longer-stay" patients dominate the higher feeding tertiles. From [1] with permission.

Underfeeding is also a problem

While taking care to avoid overfeeding acutely, one should not ignore the fact that severe under-feeding and not tailoring energy requirements to patients' requirements may lead to large negative energy balances and septic and non-septic complications in the first week in the ICU [7] and in the longer term [9]. A patient's nutritional requirements should increase with increasing activity when recovering from their critical illness to avoid the metabolic effects of prolonged nutrient deprivation. Resting energy expenditure is usually elevated for several weeks [5] after an acute illness and nutritional demands should be met. Preliminary results from a single center prospective randomized (but not blinded) study of tight caloric control using indirect calorimetry versus conventional 25 kcal/kg feeding suggest outcomes could be improved [10]. Fifty well matched patients were randomized and received both enteral and parenteral nutrition. The tight control group received more parenteral nutrition and had a better cumulative energy daily balance (212 $\pm$ 63 kcal/day vs. –362 $\pm$ 67 kcal/day, $p = 0.001$). Significantly reduced hospital length of stay (29.6 $\pm$ 6.1 days vs. 35.6 $\pm$ 6.4 days, $p < 0.05$) and hospital mortality (26.1 % vs. 52.4 % $p < 0.02$) were seen in the tight control group. This approach avoids both under- and overfeeding and a multicenter study is underway to confirm these striking observations.

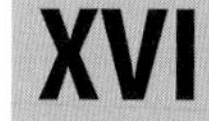

Parenteral versus Enteral Nutrition

Parenteral nutrition is a valuable adjunct in feeding patients on the ICU. However, parenteral nutrition is frequently associated with overfeeding due to the direct delivery of nutrients and the apparent and common failure to account for other routes of calories [11, 12]. Enteral nutrition is usually characterized by underfeeding [11] due to gut intolerance and it is extremely rare to overfeed using enteral nutrition.

In a meta-analysis of 30 randomized controlled trials comparing early enteral and parenteral nutrition, there was no effect of nutrition type on hospital mortality. However, parenteral nutrition was associated with increases in infective complications (7.9 %, $p = 0.001$), catheter-related blood stream infections (3.5 %, $p = 0.003$), non-infectious complications (4.9 %, $p = 0.04$), and hospital length of stay (1.2 days, $p = 0.004$). Enteral nutrition was associated with a significant increase in diarrheal episodes (8.7 %, $p = 0.001$) [13].

Most ICU patients are enterally fed and most are underfed significantly [9, 11]. It is well know that more severely ill ICU patients are more likely to receive parenteral nutrition due to gut dysfunction, where the risk of overfeeding is higher [11] and these patients, therefore, have a higher risk of additional calorie overload.

Why then should there be a Link between Nutritional Excess and Infection?

Glucose and lipids have well defined rates of utilization and storage in humans. When given in normal quantities by either the enteral or parenteral route, they are handled in a range of proportions in the critically ill patient [14] but because of insulin resistance the metabolic consequences are very different as compared with the metabolically unstressed patient [15]. Overfeeding of either fats or glucose stresses the metabolic tolerance and exacerbates the impairment of storage associated with insulin resistance. Obesity and the metabolic syndrome is the equivalent chronic state, intimately linked with inflammation and signaling pathways [16].

Critical to evolutionary survival has been our ability to tolerate starvation and our capacity to mount an inflammatory response and an effective host defense to foreign pathogens [17]. We, therefore, have a signaling system that closely links nutrition monitoring, storage and inflammation and our liver and fat tissues have a cellular tissue organization in which metabolic cells are in immediacy to immune cells (Kupffer cells and macrophages, respectively). This interface and signaling is believed to be behind the development of metabolic disease and chronic inflammation in obesity and diabetes [18]. Evidence suggests that with substrate excess there are metabolically induced increased oxidative processes, increased free radical production, and increased storage challenges carrying consequences for endoplasmic reticulum stress signaling through the major inflammatory pathways [16]. It is, therefore, reasonable to hypothesize that nutritional excess in ICU patients confounds many aspects of immune function and increases the oxidative load in an already critically stressed system.

This metabolic stress has the greatest impact on immune function and inflammatory modulation [16], potentially leading to the infectious and non-infectious complications observed in patients having receiving parenteral nutrition [13].

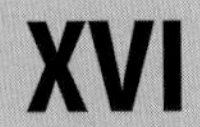

The stress effect of an excessively positive energy balance in humans is only now being explored. Physical inactivity is associated with fat gain and is a complicating factor in the critically ill. Ten normal male volunteers undergoing 35 days of strict bed rest were allowed to adapt their energy intake [19]. The half that gained fat mass ($+2.6 \pm 0.3$ kg $p < 0.001$) were compared with the others who stayed in near neutral balance (1.0 ± 0.5 kg, NS). Markers of inflammation ($p < 0.05$) and muscle atrophy

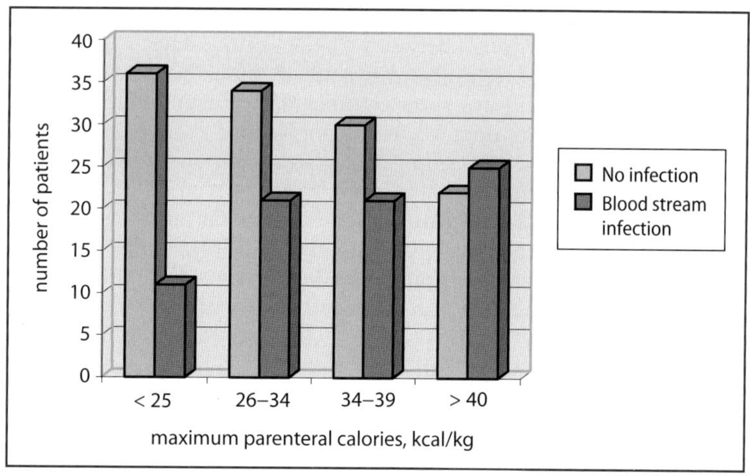

Fig. 2. Occurrence of blood stream infectious according to maximum parenteral caloric intake. Adapted from [12].

($p < 0.01$) were greater in those were had the more positive energy balance, consistent with their overfeeding.

Patients receiving parenteral nutrition have not been shown to have any mortality risk but do have increased infection-related complications. The increase in adverse outcomes was thought to be due to hyperglycemia and insulin resistance due to the large carbohydrate glucose load [12]. However, in an observational study of 200 patients receiving parenteral nutrition where a tight glycemic control protocol was followed in a general ICU, Dissanaike et al. [12] showed that the risk of blood stream infection increased with increased caloric intake unrelated to the level of glucose. Patients receiving > 40 kcal/kg/day had a 4 fold increase in risk for blood stream infection compared to patients receiving < 25 kcal/kg/day [12] (**Fig. 2**). Patients with larger swings of daily caloric intake, and hence greater duration of episodes of overfeeding, also had an increased risk of blood stream infection. Overfeeding episodes were frequently not deliberate, but due to additional calorie load from variable amounts of sedative agents (e.g., propofol) and drugs delivered in dextrose. Obesity was also not an independent risk factor for overfeeding. This study demonstrates the considerable extent of overfeeding that occurs in practice and underlines the misguided belief that tight glycemic control on its own will reduce the infection risk. This is not the case unless the overfeeding is reduced as well. Indeed it may be that a false security is given by a 'normal' glucose level and overfeeding is masked and allowed to persist where in the past the presence of hyperglycemia was an indicator to reduce the rate of parenteral nutrition delivery.

Tight Glycemic Control and Nutrition Delivery are Linked

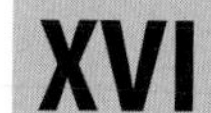

The failure to link nutrition delivery with tight glycemic control protocols may well be a major confounder in the plethora of studies that have tried to emulate the pioneering work of the Leuven Group where attention to consistent nutrient delivery was central in the process [20]. These investigators delivered on average 19 kcal/kg/day (similar to the middle tertile of the Krishnan study [1]) and were neither under- nor overfeeding within a range between 15–25 kcal/kg/day.

A meta-analysis of tight glycemic control studies to date, while showing a reduction in septicemia, did not show significant mortality reduction, but confirmed the increased frequency of documented hypoglycemic events [21]. It is striking that discussion on nutrient delivery and control is absent and perhaps the metabolic stress from under- or overfeeding masks any benefit for glucose control. Instituting such a complex process of care across many centers certainly appears problematic [22] with increased hypoglycemia; but in this study [22] there did not appear to be a detailed nutrition protocol that prescribed a consistent and reasonable glucose or nutrient load to avoid this risk. This contrasts with the careful attention to consistent nutrient delivery that was shown by the Leuven group in a follow-up paper [23]. Studies in septic critically ill patients show that glucose oxidation is not impaired, it is the non-oxidative disposal (e.g., into skeletal muscle) that accounts for reduced total utilization and appearance of hyperglycemia. Therefore, with physiological levels of insulin, an acceptable glucose utilization rate in sepsis is 4 mg/kg fat free mass/min [24] suggesting that not exceeding 16.8 g/h/70 kg or 400 g/day will still be tolerated in the presence of adequate insulin. Under most circumstances, about 150 g/day glucose may be sufficient when other nutrients are present in the feed but it may be important to deliver glucose within a higher but still 'safe' range of between 8–12 g/h initially to avoid hypoglycemia with tight glycemic control protocols. This was done in the original Leuven study while other nutrition was being established; but note also that they avoided overfeeding in the long run.

In another North American study, comparing 20 kcal/kg/day against 30 kcal/kg/day with tight glycemic control, the study showed that with a lower calorie intake, there were fewer and less severe hyperglycemic events and lower insulin requirements as well as greater albumin levels. This study also showed that if the threshold of 4 mg/kg/min of dextrose administered was exceeded, patients were more likely to be hyperglycemic [25]. This is consistent with the recommendations of Carlson [24]. With the 30 kcal/kg/day feeding regimen, significant doses of insulin were required and it was, therefore, highly likely they were masking the signs of overfeeding.

These findings suggest that commonly used rates of parenteral calorie delivery may be higher than optimal in the critically ill. Other complications associated with overfeeding in other studies [26] included increased cardiopulmonary complications, prolonged mechanical ventilation, and increased mortality. The risk of complications may be even higher if tight glycemic control is not used in the management of hyperglycemia in these patients. It is interesting to speculate whether it was hyperglycemia or overfeeding *per se* that resulted in the increased total parenteral nutrition (TPN)-related infections seen in a group of patients who received an average caloric intake of 40 kcal/kg/day in the Veterans Affairs TPN study [27]. When compared with a standard feeding regimen (aiming only for 25 kcal/kg/day) one randomized controlled trial on hypocaloric TPN showed no difference in outcomes [28]. It is highly probable that positive studies that aim for 'hypocaloric' feeding are actually more closely matching individual critically ill patient requirements and avoiding the caloric overfeeding occurring in the control group.

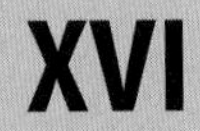

Conclusion

The traditional nutrition support strategy of 'more is always better' may compound the metabolic alterations of the stress response. Benefits of avoiding caloric overfeeding include improved glycemic control, decreased ICU length of stay, and decreased ventilator days and infection rate. Giving the right amount is important since excess feeding may be as harmful as underfeeding and may be even more important than the route of feeding. A clear nutrition protocol and assured consistent calorie delivery is necessary especially with tight glycemic control. Careful attention to less obvious sources of calories from medication and sedatives is essential to avoid overfeeding. Indirect calorimetric measures of energy expenditure remain the gold standard, as most estimations have a large error rate if patient activity is not fully accounted for.

References

1. Krishnan JA, Parce PB, Martinez A, Dietta GB, Brower RG (2003) Caloric intake in medical ICU patients. Consistency of care with guidelines and relationship to clinical outcomes. Chest 124: 297–305
2. Dudrick SJ, Wilmore DW, Vars HM, Rhoades JE (1969) Can intravenous feeding as the sole means of nutrition support growth in the child and restore weight loss in an adult? An affirmative answer. Ann Surg 169: 974–984
3. Askanazi J, Nordenström J, Rosenbaum SH, et al (1981) Nutrition for the patient with respiratory failure: Glucose versus fat. Anesthesiology 54: 373–377
4. Schuberth O, Wretlind A (1961) Intravenous infusion of fat emulsions phosphatides and emulsifying agents. Acta Physiol Scand (Suppl): 278: 1–21
5. Uehara M, Plank LD, Hill GL (1999) Components of energy expenditure in patients with severe sepsis and major trauma: A basis for clinical care. Crit Care Med 27: 1295–1302
6. Hoher JA, Zimermann Teixera PJ, da S Moreira J (2008) Comparison between ventilation modes: How does activity level affect energy expenditure estimates? JPEN J Parenter Enteral Nutr 32: 176–183
7. Berger M, Chiolero R (2007) Hypocaloric feeding: Pros and cons. Curr Opin Crit Care 13: 180–186
8. Boitano M (2006) Hypocaloric feeding of the critically ill. Nutr Clin Pract 21: 617–622
9. Griffiths RD (2007) Too much of a good thing: the curse of overfeeding. Crit Care 11: 176
10. Anbar R, Theilla M, Fisher H, Madar Z, Coehn J, Singer P (2008) Decrease in hospital mortality in tight calorie balance control study: the preliminary results of the TICACOS study. Clin Nutri 3 (Suppl 1): 11 (abst)
11. Griffiths RD (2004) Is parenteral nutrition really that risky in the intensive care unit? Curr Opin Clin Nutr Metab Care 7: 175–181
12. Dissanaike S, Shelton M, Warner K, et al (2007) The risk for bloodstream infections is associated with increased parenteral caloric intake in patients receiving parenteral nutrition. Crit Care 11: R114
13. Peter J, Moran J, Phillips-Hughes J (2005) A metaanalysis of treatment outcomes of early enteral versus early parenteral nutrition in hospitalized patients. Crit Care Med 33: 213–220
14. Tappy L, Schwarz JM, Schneiter P, et al (1998) Effects of isoenergetic glucose-based or lipid-based parenteral nutrition on glucose metabolism, de novo lipogenesis, and respiratory gas exchanges in critically ill patients. Crit Care Med 26: 860–867
15. Tappy L, Berger M, Schwarz JM, et al (1999) Hepatic and peripheral glucose metabolism in intensive care patients receiving continuous high- or low-carbohydrate enteral nutrition. JPEN J Parenter Enteral Nutr 23: 260–267
16. Hotamisligil GS (2006) Inflammation and metabolic disorders. Nature 444: 860–867
17. Levin BR, Lipsitch M, Bonhoeffer S (1999) Population biology, evolution, and infectious disease: convergence and synthesis. Science 283: 806–809

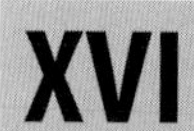

18. Shoelson SE, Lee J, Goldfine AB (2006) Inflammation and insulin resistance. J Clin Invest 116: 1793–1801
19. Antonione R, Agostini F, Guarnieri G, Giolo G (2008) Positive energy balance accelerates muscle atrophy and increases erythrocyte glutathione turnover rate during 35 days bed rest. Clin Nutri 3 (suppl 1): 175 (abst)
20. Van den Berghe G, Wouters P, Weekers F, et al (2001) Intensive insulin therapy in critically ill patients. N Engl J Med 345: 1359–1367
21. Wiener RS, Wiener DC, Larson RJ (2008) Benefits and risks of tight glucose control in critically ill adults: a meta-analysis. JAMA 300: 933–944
22. Brunkhorst FM, Engel C, Bloos F, et al (2008) Intensive insulin therapy and pentastarch resuscitation in severe sepsis. N Engl J Med 358: 125–139
23. Van den Berghe G, Wilmer A, Milants I, et al (2006) Intensive insulin therapy in mixed medical/surgical intensive care unit: Benefits versus harm. Diabetes 55: 3151–3159
24. Carlson G (2004) Insulin resistance in human sepsis: implications for the nutritional and metabolic care of the critically ill surgical patient. Ann R Coll Surg Eng 86: 75–81
25. Ahrens CL, Barletta JF, Kanji S, et al (2005) Effect of low-calorie parenteral nutrition on the incidence and severity of hyperglycaemia in surgical patients: A randomized, controlled trial. Crit Care Med 33: 2507–2512
26. Sandstrom R, Drott C, Hyltander A, et al (1993) The effect of post-operative intravenous feeding (TPN) on outcome following major surgery evaluated in a randomized study. Ann Surg 217: 185–195
27. Veterans Affairs Total Parenteral Nutrition Cooperative Study Group (1991) Perioperative total parenteral nutrition in surgical patients. N Engl J Med; 325:525–532
28. McCowen KC, Friel C, Sternberg J, et al (2000) Hypocaloric total parenteral nutrition: Effectiveness in prevention of hyperglycemia and infectious complications – A randomized clinical trial. Crit Care Med 28: 3606–3611

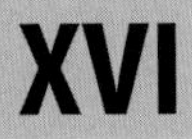

Enteral Feeding during Circulatory Failure: Myths and Reality

M.M. Berger and R.L. Chiolero

Introduction

Cardiovascular disease is a major cause of morbidity and mortality in Western countries, being responsible for a large number of admissions to intensive care units (ICU), after acute myocardial infarction, cardiac surgery, or acute cardiomyopathies. Moreover, the prevalence of cardiovascular diseases is high in patients admitted for primary non-cardiac conditions, since a growing proportion of patients is over 65 years, and chronic cardiac heart failure has a prevalence of 30–130 individuals per 1000 in this age category [1].

The vast majority of patients undergoing cardiac surgery or with acute myocardial infarction do not require nutritional therapy, as they are able to resume oral feeding within 1–2 days. But some patients suffer a more complicated clinical course requiring pharmacological and/or mechanical cardiac support, as well as mechanical ventilation. Such patients are frequently hyper-catabolic, and dependent on artificial nutritional support for many days [2]. Enteral nutrition is considered necessary in acutely ill patients for a variety of metabolic, immune, and practical reasons. Nevertheless, enteral nutrition is commonly considered contraindicated and even hazardous during severe circulatory compromise. The American Society for Parenteral and Enteral Nutrition (ASPEN) 2002 guidelines state that enteral nutrition should be deferred until the patient is hemodynamically stable [2]. Defining stability may be difficult though in patients requiring prolonged inotropic therapy, as well as in patients requiring prolonged mechanical ventricular assistance, such as intra-aortic balloon pump (IABP) [3].

Indeed during cardiogenic shock, the splanchnic circulation is not spared. It may be altered after cardiopulmonary bypass (CPB), exposing the patient to the risk of gastrointestinal complications, particularly bowel ischemia. After cardiac surgery the prevalence of acute mesenteric ischemia varies between 0.5 % [4] and 1.4 % [5], and associated mortality is high ranging between 11 and 27 % [4, 5]. Further, bowel motility is reduced due to a combination of pyloric dysfunction, which is frequent in the critically ill [6], and intestinal atony. But the gut appears functional in many patients, even though bowel sounds are sparse [7], suggesting that enteral nutrition may be possible. This chapter describes under which conditions enteral nutrition is possible, and provides rationale for using specific nutrients and substrates.

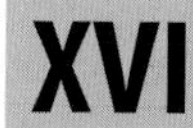

Splanchnic Consequences of Feeding and of Circulatory Failure

The normal cardiovascular response to feeding is complex, including an increase in cardiac output, and vasodilation of mesenteric arteries, and a decrease in peripheral resistance. One of the components of this hemodynamic adaptation to feeding is an increase in local oxygen consumption (VO_2) which may decrease oxygen delivery (DO_2) to vital organs. In healthy subjects, enteral feeding induces increases in flow parameters in the superior mesenteric artery and portal vein in both genders [8]: A study enrolling 44 healthy subjects showed splanchnic postprandial hyperemia in response to intraduodenal feeding using Echo-Doppler technology. Postprandially, diastolic blood pressure fell, and flow in the portal vein increased (ns) and mean velocity in the superior mesenteric artery increased significantly. These changes were paralleled by alterations in systemic hemodynamics.

In acutely ill patients with cardiac failure, this response may be worsened by an already insufficient DO_2 to the tissues and organs. During low cardiac output, splanchnic DO_2 is reduced, while splanchnic VO_2 is maintained; therefore, splanchnic oxygen extraction is high [9]. This is one of the factors explaining the high rate of gastrointestinal complications in this category of patients [4, 5]. In patients with chronic heart failure, continuous enteric feeding set at 1.4–1.5 times resting energy expenditure, compared with intermittent feeding, has been shown to be well tolerated [10]. The authors concluded that enteral nutrition can be provided safely, except in patients with overt cardiac failure [10]. In another metabolic study in cardiac surgery patients with acute cardiac failure requiring inotropic support [11], the introduction of continuous enteral nutrition set at 110 % of resting energy expenditure caused a 10 % increase in cardiac index and splanchnic blood flow, a 10 % decrease in mean arterial pressure (MAP) in parallel with decreased systemic vascular resistance and unchanged heart rate [11]. Metabolic and endocrine responses indicated that nutrients were utilized as energy substrate: On initiation of enteral nutrition, glucose turnover increased, as did plasma glucose concentrations. These data suggest that careful limited continuous enteral feeding can be administered in patients with acute and chronic circulatory failure.

Gastrointestinal complications, and particularly bowel ischemia, are a serious threat after CPB. Indeed, this type of surgery includes periods of aortic cross clamping and of non-pulsatile blood flow, which affect both systemic and regional perfusion patterns. It predisposes the splanchnic region to inadequate perfusion and increases gut permeability. Splanchnic blood flow does not necessarily decrease during CPB nor after surgery as shown by two trials enrolling 10 patients each. In the first study, splanchnic blood flow was measured using infusion of indocyanine green (ICG) dye and low-dose ethanol from induction of anesthesia through hypothermic CPB and until 4 hours after surgery: Splanchnic blood flow and oxygenation parameters did not change significantly [12]. The second trial confirmed the absence of local or global splanchnic ischemia using intestinal laser Doppler flowmetry, gastric tonometry, and measurements of splanchnic lactate extraction [13]. A mismatch between splanchnic oxygen delivery and demand was seen in the latter trial, particularly during rewarming.

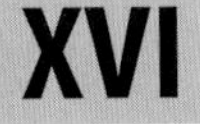

Circulating endotoxin increases during cardiac surgery, and may contribute to cytokine activation, high VO_2, and fever ('postperfusion syndrome') [14]. A trial enrolling 11,202 patients undergoing cardiac surgery requiring CPB with an overall mortality rate of 3 % and a 95 % autopsy rate, showed a 0.49 % incidence of acute mesenteric ischemia [4]. In another trial enrolling 2054 cardiac surgery patients, postoperative gastrointestinal complications were even more frequent at 1.4 % [5]. Mortality associated with intestinal ischemia is high, at 11 % and above [4, 5], and increases with the need for gastrointestinal surgical intervention (44 % versus 0 % in patients not requiring surgery; $p < 0.01$). Risk factors for complications are duration of CPB and cross-clamp time, intra-aortic balloon pump (IABP) support, the development of post-operative renal failure, and operation type and priority [4, 5]. Cardiac surgery for coronary artery bypass grafting (CABG) using the off-pump technique is also associated with hemodynamic alterations, but there are very few data yet. In our experience, this technique is used preferentially in high risk patients and a complicated postoperative course is, therefore, not infrequent.

Bowel ischemia is favored by the abdominal compartment syndrome (ACS) with intra-abdominal pressures (IAP) > 20 mmHg: This complication does occasionally occur after cardiac surgery but is more frequent after descending thoracic and abdominal aortic surgery [15]. Monitoring of IAP belongs to standards of care after major vascular surgery [16].

In addition, the use of vasoactive drugs exerts unpredictable effects on splanchnic perfusion [17]. While dopexamine seems to improve splanchnic perfusion and gastric mucosal perfusion (as reflected by intramucosal pH [pHi]), all the other vasoactive drugs from dopamine to norepinephrine have unpredictable effects. The balance between the effects on systemic and splanchnic hemodynamics is affected by numerous and complex mechanisms, which explain such unpredictable effects.

Gastrointestinal motility is affected by a series of factors in cardiac surgery patients, and gastric emptying is significantly reduced in the postoperative period [18, 19]. Anesthesia, opioids, mechanical ventilation, vasoactive drugs, and sedatives reduce intestinal and gastric motility; these factors may contribute to difficult enteral feeding.

Nutritional Status of the Cardiac Patient

Malnutrition is present in up to 50 % of patients with severe congestive heart failure [2], exposing these patients to the risk of additional rapid malnutrition in absence of adequate support [20]. Cardiac cachexia is observed in patients with severe and prolonged cardiac failure: It has been recognized as an independent predictor of higher mortality in patients with chronic heart failure [21], while moderate obesity appears to be protective. Cardiac cachexia is also associated with poor outcome after cardiac transplantation, with an increase in 30-day mortality (13 versus 7 % in normal weight recipients) and a doubling of 5-year mortality [22]. A trial involving 5168 patients undergoing CABG [23], showed that the operative mortality was highest among those with both low body mass index (BMI < 20 kg/m^2) and albumin level below 25 g/l. The key role played by cardiac failure is illustrated by the progressive improvement in nutritional status after successful heart transplantation [24].

Surgical and medical cardiac patients share many characteristics: Both have chronic metabolic alterations involving mainly energy, carbohydrate, and lipid metabolism, but also may suffer from acute organ dysfunction due to ischemia. A variable degree of systemic inflammatory response syndrome (SIRS) is present in both categories of patients. Malnutrition worsens cardiac function whatever its initial cause: A trial in rats comparing *ad libitum* chow feeding or restriction to 50 % of this amount for 90 days, showed that malnutrition was associated with a reduction in left ventricular systolic function, and with lower contractility and compliance [25].

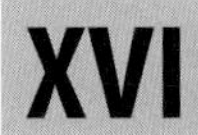

Nutritional assessment is challenging. The frequent presence of edema alters the validity of weight and calculated BMI. In cases where an accurate assessment is required, lean body mass determination by anthropometric measurements (skin fold thickness, arm-muscle circumference), or bioimpedance analysis enables an acceptable estimation of total body water. Practically, the clinician should consider actual weight, i.e., the weight just before the acute condition, recent weight loss, and clinical presentation of the patient. An unintentional weight loss of more than 7.5 % of previous normal weight has been shown to be an independent risk factor for mortality in chronic heart failure [21].

While hypermetabolism is not systematic after myocardial infarction, the majority of surgical patients are hypermetabolic and hypercatabolic as a consequence of the acute phase response triggered by surgery and circulating endotoxins [14]. The acute phase with its endocrine and metabolic consequences [3] contributes to the development of hospital malnutrition.

Energy Target and Substrate Requirements

In patients with cardiac failure, the appetite is poor, which contributes to cachexia [26]. Continuous enteric feeding, compared with intermittent feeding, has been shown to minimize VO_2 and myocardial VO_2: Therefore, enteral nutrition can be provided safely from the cardiac function aspect [27]. The combination of oral food and parenteral nutrition to achieve 20 to 30 kcal/kg per day for 2–3 weeks in patients with cardiac cachexia (severe mitral valve disease and congestive heart failure) is also associated with stable hemodynamics, unchanged whole body VO_2 and CO_2 production [28].

The level of energy requirement in critically ill patients is highly variable: Hypermetabolism is frequent, but in the presence of cachexia, the requirements tend to be below the values calculated with prediction equations. In such patients, determination of resting energy expenditure by indirect calorimetry is the only way to precisely determine their true metabolic rate. In our experience, the energy requirements can be set at 25 kcal/kg/day in most cases [11, 29]; lower requirements may be present in patients with severe persistent cardiogenic shock. Protein requirements do not differ from those of other patients and should be set at 1.3–1.5 g/kg/day.

Enteral Feeding Route

In acute conditions and especially in postoperative states, enteral nutrition is disregarded while parenteral nutrition is believed to be the only possible route of feeding. In circulatory compromise, enteral nutrition is indeed considered to be relatively contraindicated, as it may aggravate gut ischemia (steel); low mesenteric blood flow is a risk factor of bowel necrosis.

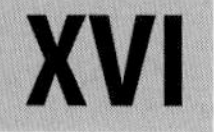

Our team has repeatedly shown that cautious enteral nutrition can be used even during severe cardiac compromise. Paracetamol (acetaminophen) absorption, which is very similar to that of protein absorption, is maintained in postoperative cardiac surgery patients even in low output states [19]: In a series of 23 patients with hemodynamic failure (cardiac index 2–2.5 l/m^2/min), paracetamol jejunal absorption was maintained compared with cardiac surgery controls without cardiac failure (**Fig. 1**).

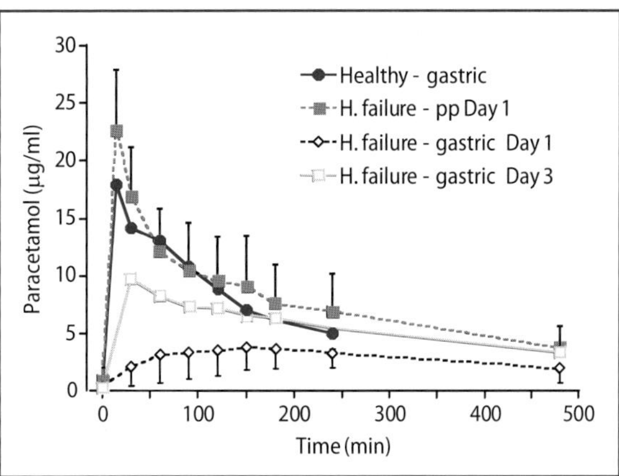

Fig. 1. Paracetamol (acetaminophen) kinetics on days 1 and 3 after cardiac surgery in patients with hemodynamic failure (H. failure) compared to 6 healthy controls having received gastric paracetamol. The figure shows the differences in gastric and postpyloric absorption over time. In the circulatory failure patients, the postpyloric (pp) absorption is already normal on day 1, while gastric absorption is delayed, and recovers slowly by day 3 (data from [19]).

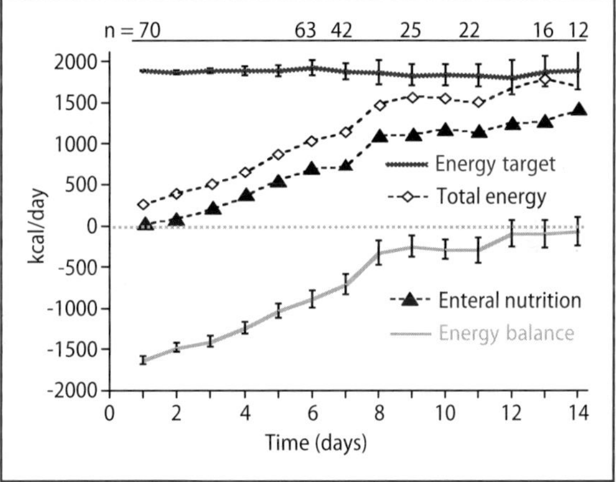

Fig. 2. Evolution of energy delivery and balance in 70 patients with circulatory compromise on pharmacologic and mechanical hemodynamic support [30]. Enteral nutrition, although possible, was not able to cover energy requirements set at 25 kcal/kg.

Such patients can be fed with caution first by the gastric route, or by the jejunal route if the gastric fails, causing large gastric residues. The introduction of enteral nutrition in patients with inotropic support after CPB causes increases in cardiac index and splanchnic blood flow, while metabolic response (endocrine profile) indicates that nutrients are utilized [11]. The data from this trial also suggest that the hemodynamic response to early enteral nutrition is adequate after cardiac surgery. Another recent trial in our ICU, including 70 patients with circulatory compromise, showed that the enteral feeding volume is limited in the presence of severe hemodynamic compromise [30]: As a mean, a maximum of 1000 ml may be delivered by the gastric route, and 1500 ml by the postpyloric route (**Fig. 2**). Among these 70 patients, 17 were dependent on IABP support; analysis of this subset of patients with extremely severe hemodynamic failure showed similar results, enabling the delivery of 15–20 kcal/kg/day by the enteral route. Nevertheless, we have repeatedly observed that although enteral nutrition is possible, the total energy delivery should be monitored as the limited feeding volume tolerance results in energy deficits over prolonged periods of nutritional support if the enteral route is used alone. In our prospective observational study [30], enteral nutrition was started at 20 ml/hour, and

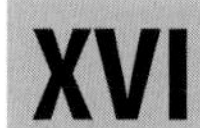

increased stepwise, every 12–24 hours according to tolerance. Clinical criteria used to assess feeding tolerance were the volume of gastric residues (< or > 300 ml), the occurrence of abdominal distension, ileus, vomiting, broncho-aspiration of gastric contents, and impossibility to achieve energy target defined as energy delivery < 50 % of target for more than 3 days [30].

In ACS with an IAP > 20 mmHg, enteral nutrition should not be started, or should be discontinued or reduced to 500 ml/24 hours if already initiated.

Two reviews show that enteral nutrition is well tolerated and probably beneficial in most critically ill patients, as it contributes to restoring splanchnic perfusion and immune function [31, 32]. It should however be used with caution in patients during the shock phase [31].

Enteral Access

Enteral nutrition should be initiated by the gastric route in the absence of any contraindication. Alas, gastric feeding may be difficult in patients with cardiogenic shock, due to pyloric dysfunction [18], and reduced gastrointestinal motility. Gaining postpyloric access may solve this problem: Various techniques can be used, including blind manual placement, endoscopic placement, or fluoroscopic positioning. Endoscopic placement of the feeding tubes is considered a safe method of providing enteral nutrition, as shown by a retrospective study including 15 critically ill cardiothoracic surgery patients [33]; no complications of the procedure were observed. Blind placement in the ICU is worth attempting, and various placement techniques and feeding tubes have been advocated. Self-propelled feeding tubes are an alternative [34] although progression is lowest in those patients on the highest norepinephrine doses: Norepinephrine and morphine doses were the most important determinants of feeding tube progression [34].

Our ICU's enteral feeding protocol specifies a prudent increase in energy delivery to target over 4–5 days, with no enteral feeding during the first hours while in unstable shock, feeding being initiated after 24 to 48 hours.

Timing: Preoperative, Early or Conventional Feeding

Early enteral feeding is now supported by level A evidence [35]. According to international guidelines, cardiac surgery patients do not benefit from early enteral feeding [2], nor are they candidates for use of immunomodulating diets [36]. These guidelines require some discussion though.

Preoperative downregulation of the inflammatory response to surgery by an immunomodulating diet is a promising tool [37], as cardiac surgery typically elicits an inflammatory response [14]. The fish oil ω-3 fatty acids have been shown to have beneficial anti-inflammatory properties which make them candidates for nutritional intervention at the various stages of cardiac disease. Preventing such inflammatory responses may require preoperative intervention. A prospective randomized controlled trial enrolling 50 patients aged 70 years or older with poor ventricular function before cardiac surgery, investigated the effect of an oral supplement containing a mixture of immune-enhancing nutrients (arginine, ω-3 fatty acids and nucleotides) [37]. This trial showed that ≥ 5 days of supplementation improved the general immune response (stronger delayed-type hypersensitivity response), and was associ-

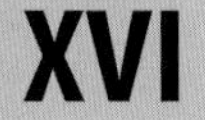

ated with a lower infection rate (4/23 vs 12/22, p = 0.013), a reduction in inotropic drug requirements, lower interleukin (IL)-6 concentrations, and a better preservation of renal function. These data suggest that routine preoperative nutritional intervention should be considered in elective cardiac surgery.

The early postoperative period should also be considered accessible to nutritional therapy. A study of 73 cardiothoracic ICU patients also reported the feasibility and good gastrointestinal tolerance of early enteral nutrition [38]. The only information about daily energy supply was that the energy target could be reached with enteral nutrition only in 9 patients (12 %). In our collective of patients with hemodynamic failure [30], more than 1200 kcal per day could be delivered by the enteral route in all the patients requiring artificial nutrition. The patients included in the study suffered critical circulatory failure as shown by their dependence on norepinephrine and other vasoactive drugs for hemodynamic stability.

Enteral, Intravenous, or Combined Nutrition?

The enteral route is the first choice in the majority of acutely ill patients. On the benefice side, continuous enteric feeding minimizes VO_2 and myocardial VO_2 in patients with congestive heart failure: Enteral nutrition is safe for cardiac function [27].

However, there are a few caveats and contraindications to enteral feeding due to the previously mentioned risk of bowel ischemia [4, 5]. Among these contraindications to enteral nutrition is the development of chylothorax after CABG [39], which favors parenteral nutrition in these patients; however, this complication is not an early complication and is usually diagnosed after several days. This complication may also occur in other types of cardiothoracic procedures in adults and children [40]. Most cases respond successfully to conservative treatment consisting of avoiding enteral nutrition (parenteral nutrition) and pleural drainage: The average duration of the lymph leak is 14 days. In some cases (less than 20 % in literature) a low-fat enteral diet can be used as initial treatment.

Gastrointestinal motility is inversely related to the dose of dopamine and norepinephrine as shown by the reduced migration of feeding tubes in patients on high doses of these drugs [34]. Nevertheless enteral energy delivery, although tending to be lower in patients on high norepinephrine and epinephrine doses [30], is not directly related to the dose as shown in **Figure 3**. Enteral feeding remains possible, although resulting in insufficient energy delivery. Interestingly, in our experience, only a few patients need prokinetic agents confirming the data by Kesek et al. [38], which stressed that gastro-intestinal motility, although impaired in some patients, was not the primary cause of enteral feeding failure. Moreover, in our series of 70 consecutive patients, none experienced any serious gastrointestinal complication.

Nevertheless, the most severely ill patients cannot be fed completely by the enteral route. Combined parenteral feeding is a true option in ICU patients staying longer than 5 days to prevent the installation of an energy deficit and to prevent the build up of energy deficits [20, 30, 41]. The combination of parenteral nutrition with oral food to achieve 20 to 30 kcal/kg/day for 2–3 weeks in patients with cardiac cachexia from severe mitral valve disease and congestive heart failure was associated with stable hemodynamics, unchanged whole body VO_2 and CO_2 production [28].

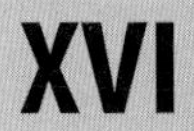

The concept of combined enteral and parenteral nutritional therapy opens new perspectives and questions. Should the supplement be a standard parenteral feed

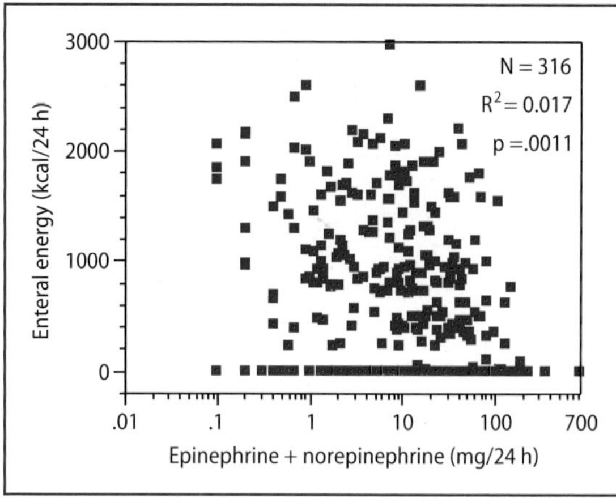

Fig. 3. Scattergram showing the absence of a direct relation between the amount of norepinephrine and epinephrine required for hemodynamic support (log scale) and the energy delivered with enteral feeding. The dose of vasopressor is expressed in mg/24 hours (total amount administered during 24 hours): 100 mg per 24 h is equivalent to 70 μg/min (data from [30]).

aimed at covering energy needs, i.e., provide glucose, amino acids and fat? Should the same types of substrates be delivered by both routes? Should specific nutrients, such as glutamine and antioxidant micronutrients, be delivered intravenously? Should unsaturated fatty acids with anti-inflammatory properties such as ω-3 polyunsaturated fatty acids be delivered intravenously?

Patient Monitoring

The most severe complication after cardiac surgery is splanchnic ischemia with the risk of bowel necrosis, and eventually death [4, 5]. Therefore, the clinical follow up during enteral nutrition includes a careful examination of the abdomen, watching for distension or other signs of sub-ileus. **Table 1** shows commonly encountered problems. Some paraclinical tools can assist the clinician: 1) Monitoring IAP should be the rule after major vascular surgery; any increase in pressure above 20 mmHg puts the gut at risk of ischemia; 2) gastric tonometry and mucosal PCO_2 are helpful; 3) monitoring of arterial blood gases (pH and lactate) can be used to confirm intestinal ischemia; decreasing pH and increasing lactate levels may herald the development of clinically relevant intestinal ischemia, but these are late and non-specific signs.

Daily monitoring of energy delivery should be part of the clinical management. The initial daily energy target should be set at 25 kcal/kg/day: If this target is not reached within 4 days, combination of enteral feeding with intravenous nutrition should be introduced rapidly to avoid the deleterious effects of negative energy balances [20].

The sequential organ failure assessment (SOFA) score [42] which is the most frequently used organ failure score in Europe, does not include any assessment of gastrointestinal function. Recently an additional gastrointestinal failure (GIF) component was proposed for this score [43]. This score will possibly enable detection of patients at the highest risk of intolerance to feeding, who should not be considered for early enteral nutrition.

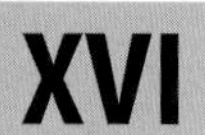

Table 1. Common problems encountered during enteral feeding after cardiac surgery and proposed management (adapted from [19])

Problem	Diagnostic tool	Management	Target
Gastroparesis	Gastric residue > 300 ml	Postpyloric feeding Metoclopramide	Residue < 300 ml
Bowel ischemia	Splanchnic acidosis: ⇓ pHi ⇑ arterial lactate Abdominal distension, ⇑ IAP	Improve hemodynamics Gastric decompression (aspiration) Diuretics	Normal pHi (> 7.2) No distension Normal IAP
Abdominal compartment syndrome	⇑ IAP > 15 mmHg	Reduce fluid loading Diuretics Gastric decompression Reduce enteral nutrition to 500 ml/24 h if IAP > 20 mmHg and initiate combined parenteral feeding	IAP < 20 mmHg
Non occlusive bowel necrosis	Abdominal distension	Surgical resection Parenteral nutrition	No distension Resolution of shock
Gastrointestinal bleeding	Blood in nasogatric tube Endoscopic diagnosis	Prophylaxis: anti-H_2 drugs Treatment: proton pump inhibitors Enteral nutrition (?)	No bleeding
Diarrhea	> 5 liquid stools per day	Fiber	< 3 stools/day
Constipation	No stools for more than 5 days	Fiber Neostigmine (continuous or intermittent)	1 stool every 3 days
Acalculous cholecystitis	Abdominal ultrasound Lab: ⇑ alkaline phosphatase non-specific as in other ICU patients	Postpyloric feeding Interventional radiology Surgery	–

IAP: intra-abdominal pressure

Conclusion

The nutritional management of the patient with acute cardiovascular failure has changed over the recent years. These patients are at higher risk of splanchnic ischemia. Enteral nutrition is possible and safe, though requires close clinical supervision, but will invariably result in insufficient energy delivery prompting combined parenteral and enteral approaches. Based on indirect calorimetry data collected over the last 20 years in our investigation unit, the energy requirements can be set at 25 kcal/kg/day [11, 29], resulting in a mean target of 1900 kcal/day in this type of patient. This target should be reached over a period of 3–4 days, which is not possible by the enteral route alone in most cases. As a mean, 1250 kcal/day can be delivered by the gastric route with large inter-patient variability, and up to1500 kcal by the postpyloric route [30] (**Table 2**), which corresponds to 15–20 kcal/kg/day.

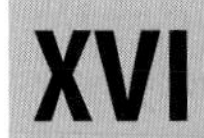

Table 2. Energy delivery according to the enteral feeding route in patients with compromised hemodynamic status (adapted from [30])

Route	Energy delivery (kcal/d)	Calculated energy balance (kcal/d)	Number of days (%)
Gastric	1250 ± 650[1,2]	−210 ± 680	276 (38.6 %)
Jejunal	1545 ± 720[1,2]	−170 ± 770	74 (10.3 %)

[1] Difference gastric versus jejunal energy delivery: ns
[2] Difference intravenous versus jejunal or gastric energy delivery: p = 0.001

In conclusion [30]: 1) Enteral nutrition is possible during the first postoperative week, and even already after 24 hours, in patients with acute severe circulatory failure under careful abdominal monitoring; 2) enteral nutrition generally results in insufficient energy delivery, stressing the importance of careful monitoring of the total daily energy delivery; and 3) combination with parenteral nutrition should be considered to achieve optimal energy delivery.

References

1. Cowie MR, Mosterd DA, Wood DA (1997) The epidemiology of heart failure. Eur Heart J 18: 208–225
2. ASPEN Board of Directors and the Clinical Guidelines Task Force (2002) Guidelines for the use of parenteral and enteral nutrition in adult and pediatric patients. JPEN J Parenter Enteral Nutr 26 (Suppl 1):1SA-138SA
3. Berger MM, Mustafa I (2003) Metabolic and nutritional support in acute cardiac failure. Curr Opin Clin Nutr Metab Care 6: 195–201
4. Venkateswaran RV, Charman SC, Goddard M, Large SR (2002) Lethal mesenteric ischaemia after cardiopulmonary bypass: a common complication? Eur J Cardiothorac Surg 22: 534–538
5. Lazar HL, Hudson H, McCann J, et al (1995) Gastrointestinal complications following cardiac surgery. Cardiovasc Surg 3: 341–344
6. Heyland DK, Tougas G, King D, Cook DJ (1996) Impaired gastric emptying in mechanically ventilated, critically ill patients. Intensive Care Med 22: 1339–1344
7. Payne-James JJ, Rees RG, Silk DBS (1987) Bowel sounds. Anaesthesia 42: 207–220
8. Szinnai C, Mottet C, Gutzwiller JP, Drewe J, Beglinger C, Sieber CC (2001) Role of gender upon basal and postprandial systemic and splanchnic haemodynamics in humans. Scand J Gastroenterol 36: 540–544
9. Jakob SM, Ensinger H, Takala J (2001) Metabolic changes after cardiac surgery. Curr Opin Clin Nutr Metab Care 4: 149–155
10. Heymsfield SB, Bethel RA, Ansely JD, Nixon DW, Rudman D (1979) Enteral hyperalimentation: an alternative to central venous hyperalimentation. Ann Intern Med 90: 63–71
11. Revelly JP, Tappy L, Berger MM, Gersbach P, Cayeux C, Chiolero R (2001) Metabolic, systemic and splanchnic hemodynamic responses to early enteral nutrition in postoperative patients treated for circulatory compromise. Intensive Care Med 27: 540–547
12. Gardeback M, Settergren G, Brodin LA, et al (2002) Splanchnic blood flow and oxygen uptake during cardiopulmonary bypass. J Cardiothorac Vasc Anesth 16: 308–315
13. Thoren A, Elam M, Ricksten SE (2001) Jejunal mucosal perfusion is well maintained during mild hypothermic cardiopulmonary bypass in humans. Anesth Analg 92: 5–11
14. Bouter H, Schippers EF, Luelmo SA, et al (2002) No effect of preoperative selective gut decontamination on endotoxemia and cytokine activation during cardiopulmonary bypass: a randomized, placebo-controlled study. Crit Care Med 30: 38–43
15. Cheatham ML (1999) Intra-abdominal hypertension and abdominal compartment syndrome. New Horiz 7: 96–115
16. Malbrain ML, Cheatham ML, Kirkpatrick A, et al (2006) Results from the International Con-

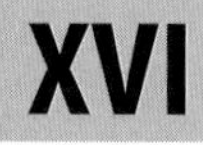

ference of Experts on Intra-abdominal Hypertension and Abdominal Compartment Syndrome. I. Definitions. Intensive Care Med 32: 1722–1732
17. Silva E, DeBacker D, Creteur J, Vincent JL (1998) Effects of vasoactive drugs on gastric intramucosal pH. Crit Care Med 26: 1749–1758
18. Goldhill DR, Whelpton R, Winyard JA, Wilkinson KA (1995) Gastric emptying in patients the day after cardiac surgery. Anaesthesia 50: 122–125
19. Berger MM, Berger-Gryllaki M, Wiesel PH, et al (2000) Gastrointestinal absorption after cardiac surgery. Crit Care Med 28: 2217–2223
20. Villet S, Chioléro RL, Bollmann MD, et al (2005) Negative impact of hypocaloric feeding and energy balance on clinical outcome in ICU patients. Clin Nutr 24: 502–509
21. Anker SD, Ponikowski P, Varney S, et al (1997) Wasting as independent risk factor for mortality in chronic heart failure. Lancet 349: 1050–1053
22. Lietz K, John R, Burke EA, et al (2001) Pretransplant cachexia and morbid obesity are predictors of increased mortality after heart transplantation. Transplantation 72: 277–283
23. Engelman DT, Adams DH, Byrne JG, et al (1999) Impact of body mass index and albumin on morbidity and mortality after cardiac surgery. J Thorac Cardiovasc Surg 118: 866–873
24. Peterson RE, Perens GS, Alejos JC, Wetzel GT, Chang RK (2008) Growth and weight gain of prepubertal children after cardiac transplantation. Pediatr Transplant 12: 436–441
25. Okoshi K, Matsubara LS, Okoshi MP, et al (2002) Food restriction-induced myocardial dysfunction demonstrated by the combination of in vivo and in vitro studies. Nutr Res 22: 1353–1364
26. Heymsfield SB, Smith J, Redd S, Whitworth HB Jr (1981) Nutritional support in cardiac failure. Surg Clin North Am 61: 635–652
27. Heymsfield SB, Casper K (1989) Congestive heart failure: clinical management by use of continuous nasoenteric feeding. Am J Clin Nutr 50: 539–544
28. Paccagnella A, Calò M, Caenaro G, et al (1994) Cardiac cachexia: preoperative and postoperative nutrition management. JPEN J Parenter Enteral Nutr 18: 409–416
29. Revelly JP, Berger MM, Chioléro R (1999) The hemodynamic response to enteral nutrition. In: Vincent JL (ed) Yearbook of Intensive Care and Emergency Medicine. Springer Verlag, Heidelberg, pp:105–114
30. Berger MM, Revelly JP, Cayeux MC, Chiolero RL (2005) Enteral nutrition in critically ill patients with severe hemodynamic failure after cardiopulmonary bypass. Clin Nutr 24: 124–132
31. McClave SA, Chang WK (2003) Feeding the hypotensive patients: does enteral feeding precipitate or protect against ischemic bowel? Nutr Clin Practice 18: 279–284
32. Zaloga GP, Roberts PR, Marik PE (2003) Feeding hemodynamically unstable patient: a critical evaluation of the evidence. Nutr Clin Practice 18: 285–293
33. Vaswani SK, Clarkston WK (1996) Endoscopic nasoenteral feeding tube placement following cardiothoracic surgery. Am Surg 62: 421–413
34. Berger MM, Bollmann MD, Revelly JP, et al (2002) Progression rate of self-propelled feeding tubes in critically ill patients. Intensive Care Med 28: 1768–1774
35. Simpson F, Doig GS (2005) Parenteral vs. enteral nutrition in the critically ill patient: a meta-analysis of trials using the intention to treat principle. Intensive Care Med 31: 12–23
36. Heyland DK, Novak F, Drover JW, Jain M, Su X, Suchner U (2001) Should immunonutrition become routine in critically ill patients? A systematic review of the evidence. JAMA 286: 944–953
37. Tepaske R, Velthuis H, Oudemans-van Straaten HM, et al (2001) Effect of preoperative immune-enhancing nutritional supplement on patients at risk of infection after cardiac surgery: a randomised placebo-controlled trial. Lancet 358: 696–701
38. Kesek DR, Akerlind L, Karlsson T (2002) Early enteral nutrition in the cardiothoracic intensive care unit. Clin Nutr 21: 303–307
39. Brancaccio G, Prifti E, Cricco AM, Totaro M, Antonazzo A, Miraldi F (2001) Chylothorax: a complication after internal thoracic artery harvesting. Ital Heart J 2: 559–562
40. Nguyen DM, Shum-Tim D, Dobell AR, Tchervenkov CI (1995) The management of chylothorax/chylopericardium following pediatric cardiac surgery: a 10-year experience. J Cardiac Surg 10: 302–308
41. Heidegger CP, Romand JA, Treggiari MM, Pichard C (2007) Is it now time to promote mixed enteral and parenteral nutrition for the critically ill patient? Intensive Care Med 33: 963–969

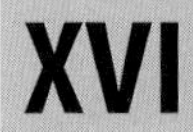

42. Kajdacsy-Balla Amaral AC, Andrade FM, Moreno R, Artigas A, Cantraine F, Vincent JL (2005) Use of the sequential organ failure assessment score as a severity score. Intensive Care Med 31: 243–249
43. Reintam A, Parm P, Kitus R, Starkopf J, Kern H (2008) Gastrointestinal failure score in critically ill patients: a prospective observational study. Crit Care 12:R90

Enteral Nutrition with Anti-inflammatory Lipids in ALI/ARDS

A. Pontes-Arruda and S.J. DeMichele

Introduction

Acute lung injury (ALI) and acute respiratory distress syndrome (ARDS) are two severe forms of respiratory failure characterized by non-cardiogenic pulmonary edema and refractory hypoxemia with massive pulmonary and systemic release of pro-inflammatory mediators. The incidence of these life-threatening pulmonary diseases in the United States is currently estimated at 56–82 cases per 100,000 persons/year [1, 2]. Current strategies adopted to treat patients with ALI and ARDS, including protective ventilation and prone positioning among others, are supportive in nature and have not shown a clear benefit in terms of mortality reduction [3].

Enteral nutrition is gaining in importance as an important adjuvant therapy in a variety of critical illnesses. Among available specialty formulations, the so-called 'immune-enhancing' diets, which are supplemented with arginine as a common pharmaconutrient, have been extensively evaluated in clinical studies over the past two decades. Though a good deal of debate still exists in the clinical community regarding the potential role of such formulas, most authors agree that immune-enhancing diets should not be used routinely in critically ill patients. On the other hand, a new type of enteral formulation enriched with lipids possessing anti-inflammatory properties and with no added arginine, has been used to modulate inflammation in the clinical setting. Moreover, since inflammation, through the release of arachidonic acid and its pro-inflammatory metabolites, is considered the key feature of ARDS [4, 5], the use of lipids, such as eicosapentaenoic acid (EPA, from fish oil) and gamma-linolenic acid (GLA, from borage oil), as a strategy to modulate the inflammatory response is gaining acceptance as an important improvement in the daily management of patients with ALI and ARDS [6–8].

EPA and GLA Mechanisms of Action

Lipid mediators are usually synthesized by three distinct pathways: Cyclooxygenase, 5-lipoxygenase and cytochrome P450 using fatty acids, such as arachidonic acid, EPA and GLA, as substrates. These fatty acids are metabolized to produce several bioactive mediators including prostaglandins, thromboxanes, leukotrienes, lipoxins, hydroxyl and epoxy fatty acids (all considered eicosanoids), as well as other important mediators with relevant biological activities such as platelet-activating factor (PAF) and intercellular signaling molecules. Together, these factors not only have a direct influence on the inflammatory response but also can influence secondary mediators, like reactive oxygen species (ROS) and proteases, regulating the secretion of immune-regulatory cytokines or influencing eutocrine eicosanoid regulation loops [9].

Arachidonic acid (20:4n-6) is a component of immune cell membranes. Following an inflammatory insult, arachidonic acid is mobilized by phospholipase A_2 and metabolized by cyclooxygenase to pro-inflammatory mediators including, but not restricted to, prostaglandin E_2 and thromboxane A_2. These mediators cause inflammation, immune suppression, chemotaxis, and promote platelet aggregation, microvascular thrombosis and the production of pro-inflammatory cytokines. Together, these factors have a pivotal role in the development of ALI and ARDS [10] (**Fig. 1**). Arachidonic acid can also be metabolized by 5-lipoxygenase to produce leukotriene B_4 (LTB_4), a pro-inflammatory prostaglandin which promotes cell adhesion and release of chemoattractive factors (**Fig. 1**). An enteral diet enriched with EPA leads to the incorporation of this fatty acid at the level of the inflammatory cell membranes, replacing arachidonic acid. EPA is metabolized through cyclooxygenase and 5-lipoxygenase producing mediators (e.g., prostaglandin E_3, thromboxane A_3, and LTB_5) with anti-inflammatory activity and inhibiting platelet aggregation. In addition, EPA-derived prostaglandins (e.g., prostaglandin E_3) lack the immunosuppressive activity of prostaglandin E_2.

It is a common misunderstanding that enteral formulas enriched with ω-6 lipids such as linoleic acid (18:2n6; e.g., from corn oil) can produce an upregulation of the inflammatory response and for that reason such formulas may not be used in hyperinflammatory diseases. The formation of arachidonic acid from linoleic acid involves

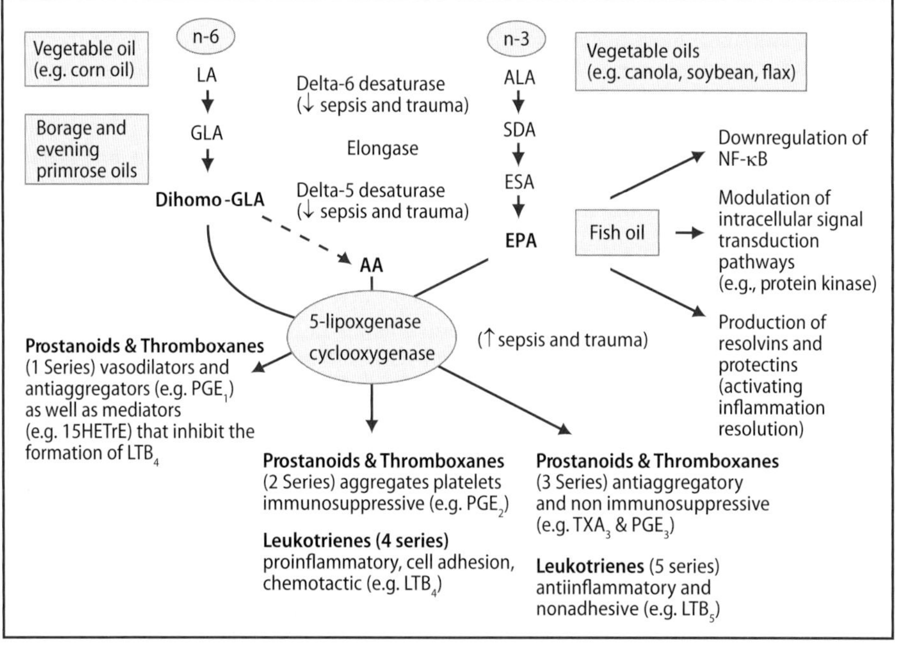

Fig. 1. Eicosapentaenoic acid (EPA) and gamma-linolenic acid (GLA) anti-inflammatory biological pathways. LA: linoleic acid (18:2n-6); ALA: α-linolenic acid (18:3n-3); AA: arachidonic acid (20:4n-6); SDA: stearidonic acid (18:4n-3); ESA: eicosatetraenoic acid (20:4n-3); 15HETrE: 15-hydroxyeicosatrienoic acid; NF-κB: nuclear factor-kappa B. Adapted from [10].

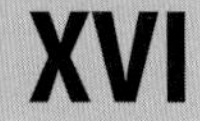

three key enzymatic steps: A delta-6-desaturation to form 18:3n6 (GLA), followed by an elongation to 20:3n6 (di-homo-GLA), and a delta-5-desaturation step to produce 20:4n6. Thus, linoleic acid-enriched formulas cannot worsen inflammation simply because the activity of the enzymes, delta-5-desaturase and delta-6-desaturase, are severely compromised during critical illness by the release of stress and catabolic hormones (e.g., glucocorticoids and catecholamines) [11, 12] limiting the ability to form arachidonic acid despite the provision of linoleic acid [13]. GLA is a metabolite of linoleic acid that can bypass the decreased expression of delta-6-desaturase. Its elongation product, DGLA, is incorporated into the inflammatory cell membranes and the formation of DGLA suppresses leukotriene biosynthesis and can be metabolized to form prostaglandin E_1, a potent pulmonary vasodilator [14, 15]. DGLA is also metabolized by 5-lipoxygenase to form 15-hydroxyeicosatrienoic acid, which inhibits the formation of LTB_4. In fact, an enteral diet enriched with GLA cannot increase arachidonic acid levels in immune cell membranes [16] but, on the other hand, can increase anti-inflammatory activity by incorporating DGLA into the immune cell membranes.

The biological anti-inflammatory activities of EPA go far beyond the simple regulation of eicosanoid production. EPA can affect immune cell responses through the regulation of gene expression and subsequent downstream events by acting as ligands for nuclear receptors [17]. EPA can control transcription factors such as peroxisome proliferator-activated receptors (PPARs) and sterol-regulatory-element binding proteins [18]. PPARs bind to DNA and are involved in the regulation of the inflammatory chain of events, as well as in lipid metabolism and energy utilization by modulating the expression of target genes. EPA can also strongly affect the activity of the pro-inflammatory transcription factor, nuclear factor-κB (NF-κB), which regulates the expression of many pro-inflammatory genes-encoding adhesion molecules, cytokines, chemokines, and other effectors of the innate immune response system [19]. There is enough evidence to say that EPA can affect all three stages of lipopolysaccharide (LPS)-induced NF-κB activity independently (ligand-receptor interaction, IκB phosphorylation leading to the release of NF-κB and its translocation to the cell nucleus, and NF-κB binding to discrete DNA sequences and gene transcription) [19].

Lipids can also modulate intracellular signal transduction pathways since many important pathways are bound or are sensitive to lipid modulation [19]. Phosphatidylinositol-specific phospholipase C can lead to release of intracellular calcium and activation of protein-kinase C through generation of inositol-phosphates and diacylglycerol [20] in a pathway which can be modulated by the phosphatidylinositol lipid composition [21]. It has been described that the lipid composition of diacylglycerol can impact mitogen-activated protein-kinase (MAPK) by a Ras-dependent mechanism [22]. Moreover, ω-3 fatty acids can produce an additional anti-inflammatory impact by downregulating the activity of protein kinase B due to its action upon a phosphatidyl-inositol kinase 3-related signaling pathway [23] (**Fig. 1**).

Finally, it has been recently described that EPA and docosahexaenoic acid (DHA) are substrates of two novel classes of mediators called resolvins and protectins, which are involved in resolution of the inflammatory process. During extensive lung inflammatory diseases, such as ARDS as well as sepsis-induced ARDS, the clearance of inflammatory cells by apoptosis can be delayed, exacerbating the inflammatory damage to the parenchyma [24, 25]. The effective clearance of damaged tissue and microbial infection is an essential part of inflammation resolution and is defined at

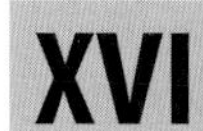

the cellular level by the disappearance of accumulated polymorphonuclear leukocytes (PMNs) [26]; apoptosis of leukocytes is one important route of elimination [27, 28]. Cells that have completed their inflammation roles as phagocytes undergo programmed cell death in response to mediators that regulate the rate of apoptosis [29, 30]. In a subsequent step, the apoptotic neutrophils are phagocytosed by macrophages (efferocytosis) in a non-flogistic process which also stimulates the formation of anti-inflammatory mediators, such as transforming growth factor (TGF)-β, lipoxin (LX) A_4, and interleukin (IL)-10 [31, 32]. Thus, resolvins D and E classes (biosynthesized by DHA and EPA, respectively) can reduce the magnitude of neutrophil infiltrates during inflammation. These important compounds were identified first during the resolution phase of acute inflammation [33, 34] (**Fig. 1**).

From Bench to Bedside: Using EPA and GLA to Modulate Inflammation

Use of the combination of EPA and GLA has been extensively tested during the past two decades in a variety of animal studies [13, 35–41]. Together, these studies demonstrated that this approach can effectively attenuate the severity of inflammation as well as the inflammatory damage to the lungs in sepsis-induced ARDS. In porcine and rodent models of ARDS, an enteral diet enriched with EPA and GLA can promote a decrease in the overall concentration of arachidonic acid in immune cell membrane phospholipids [35, 39, 41]. Several other anti-inflammatory effects were associated with the use of EPA and GLA in animal models of ALI including: A reduction in the production of pro-inflammatory eicosanoids [35–37, 40], an attenuation of endotoxin-induced pulmonary neutrophil recruitment [35], a decrease in microvascular protein permeability [36], an improvement in cardiopulmonary hemodynamics and gas exchange [37] and no impairment of alveolar macrophage function [40]. A summary of the findings from these pre-clinical studies using EPA and GLA to modulate inflammation can be found in **Table 1**.

Table 1. Summary of the results from animal studies of sepsis-induced ARDS using eicosapentaenoic acid (EPA) and gamma-linolenic acid (GLA)

Author	Animal species	Groups, dietary compositions, length of feeding, and challenge	Findings and Implications
Murray et al. [37]	Pigs; endotoxin challenge injury that is similar to the physiological response in humans	1) LA 2) EPA 3) EPA+GLA Diets were fed for 8 days followed by induction of acute lung injury (intravenous endotoxin); measurements were made 2 hours post-challenge	EPA and EPA+GLA • ↓ Proinflammatory TXB_2 levels • ↓ Early phase of cardiopulmonary dysfunction EPA+GLA • ↓ Early and late phase responses to endotoxin-improved gas exchange • ↓ Sustained decrease in pulmonary vascular resistance • ↑ Cardiac output, arterial oxygen saturation and oxygen delivery • EPA+GLA work synergistically versus EPA alone.

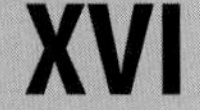

Table 1. *(cont.)*

Author	Animal species	Groups, dietary compositions, length of feeding, and challenge	Findings and Implications
Mancuso et al. [35, 36]	Long-Evans male rats; similarities with respect to dietary fatty acid incorporation into tissues between rats and humans	1) LA 2) EPA 3) EPA+GLA Diets fed for 21 days followed by induction of acute lung injury (intravenous endotoxin); measurements were made 2 hours following challenge	EPA+GLA • ↓ Release of proinflammatory eicosanoids (LTB_4, PGE_2, TXB_2) • ↓ Lung permeability and edema • ↓ Lung myloperoxidase activity • Endotoxin induced hypotension was attenuated with EPA+GLA • EPA+GLA reduced AA in alveolar macrophage phospholipids which reduced inflammatory mediators and lung injury
Palombo et al. [41]	Sprague-Dawley male rats	1) LA 2) EPA 3) EPA+GLA Diets given for 3 and 6 days via feeding tube and assessments made on days 3 and 6	EPA+GLA • ↓ AA concentrations and ↑ EPA and DGLA levels in alveolar and liver macrophage phospholipids by day 3 • Evidence of rapid changes in immune cell phospholipids with continuous enteral feeding
Palombo et al. [39]	Sprague-Dawley male rats	1) LA 2) EPA 3) EPA+GLA Rats were fed for 3 and 6 days either by continuous or cyclical enteral feeding	EPA+GLA • Regardless of either continuous or cyclical enteral feeding – ↓ AA concentrations and ↑ EPA and DGLA levels in alveolar and liver macrophage phospholipids after 3 and 6 days of enteral feeding
Palombo et al. [40]	Pathogen-free Sprague-Dawley male rats	1) LA 2) EPA 3) EPA+GLA Rats were fed LA, EPA, or EPA+GLA to determine if dampening inflammatory responses would compromise immune cell function (alveolar macrophages)	EPA+GLA • ↓ alveolar macrophage levels of AA as well as ↓ ratios of PGE_2/PGE_1, LTB_4/LTB_5 and TXB_2/TXB_3 • Respiratory burst, phagocytosis, and bactericidal activity was not impaired with EPA+GLA diet
Murray et al. [38]	Pigs; endotoxin challenge injury that is similar to physiological response in humans	1) LA 2) EPA 3) EPA+GLA Diets were fed for 8 days followed by induction of acute lung injury (i.v. endotoxin); measurements were made 2 hours post challenge	EPA+GLA • ↑ EPA and DGLA in lung surfactant • Despite changes in fatty acid composition of lung surfactant, there were no adverse affects on either surfactant function or pulmonary compliance.

LA: linoleic acid; AA: arachidonic acid; TXB: thromboxane; PG: prostaglandin; LTB: leukotriene

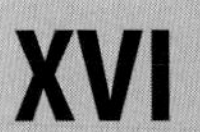

Over the past decade, the effects of an enteral formulation enriched with EPA and GLA have been intensively tested in the clinical setting, resulting in a growing collection of suggested clinical outcome benefits for mechanically ventilated patients with ALI and ARDS (either secondary to sepsis or not) [42–46]. In the first trial, Gadek and colleagues [42] randomized 146 patients with ARDS to receive enteral nutrition with an EPA+GLA formula or an isonitrogenous, isocaloric, high-lipid control diet that differed from the intervention diet only in terms of its lipid composition (although still a well balanced standard n-3/n-6 diet) and levels of antioxidant vitamins. The investigators demonstrated an important improvement in oxygenation status (described as the ratio of partial pressure of arterial oxygen [PaO_2] to percentage of inspired oxygen [FiO_2], or 'P/F' ratio) by study day 4 and maintained until study day 7 in the population of patients fed the EPA+GLA diet, whereas the control group experienced no improvement. This important finding was associated with a reduction in the number of days patients required mechanical ventilation (11 days in the EPA+GLA group versus 16.3 days in the control group, $p = 0.011$) and a decrease in length of intensive care unit (ICU) stay (12.8 days in the EPA+GLA group versus 17.5 days in the control group, $p = 0.016$). Although there was a clear trend towards mortality reduction, this decrease was not statistically significant. Finally, this first study showed an important decrease in the number of new organ failures in the population nourished with the EPA+GLA diet as compared with the control population (8 vs 28 %, $p = 0.015$); this finding is of particular importance since the development of multiple organ system organ failure is the pathway that leads from systemic inflammation to death.

The second study was conducted in Israel by Singer and colleagues [43] in a population of critically ill patients suffering from ALI (with a P/F ratio < 300). This study also demonstrated important improvements in the oxygenation status of the patients nourished with the EPA+GLA diet, as well as an improvement in static pulmonary compliance and resistance. In addition, patients receiving the EPA+GLA diet spent significantly fewer days on mechanical ventilation. But the most relevant finding in this second study was a clear reduction in 28-day all cause mortality; the survival rate was 72 % for the EPA+GLA group versus 43 % for the control group. In an analysis of secondary outcomes in the Singer study, the use of the EPA+GLA diet was also associated with a reduction in the incidence of new pressure ulcers [46].

Shortly after Singer et al. published their findings, Pontes-Arruda and colleagues [44] performed a trial using the same intervention and control diets from the previous studies in a population of 165 patients with ARDS (P/F ratio < 200) secondary to severe sepsis or septic shock. This third trial confirmed the benefits previously described, including an important improvement in the oxygenation status (P/F ratio), significant reduction in the number of days requiring mechanical ventilation, reduction in the number of days in the ICU and in the total number of new organ failures, as well as improvement in the survival rates of patients receiving the EPA+GLA diet (with an absolute reduction in mortality risk of 19.4 %). A summary of the designs and key clinical findings of the three studies can be found in **Table 2**.

Is the Evidence Enough to Change Practice?

Together, the three studies performed in adult patients [42–44] present strong evidence that an enteral diet enriched with EPA and GLA improves outcomes in critically ill patients suffering from ALI/ARDS. The available clinical studies were performed in different patient populations, although sharing a common pathophysiol-

Table 2. Summary of the results from clinical studies using an enteral formula enriched with eicosapentaenoic acid (EPA) and gamma-linolenic acid (GLA) [42–44]

	Gadek et al. [42]	Singer et al. [43]	Pontes-Arruda et al. [44]
Design	Prospective, double-blind RCT	Prospective RCT	Prospective double-blind RCT
Setting	Multicenter – 5 sites, USA	Single center, Israel	Single center, Brazil
Patients	146 ARDS	100 ALI	165 severe sepsis/ septic shock
Interventions	EPA+GLA vs CD	EPA+GLA vs. CD	EPA+GLA vs. CD
Mean Fatty Acid Intake			
EPA (g/day)	6.9	5.4	4.9
DHA (g/day)	2.9	2.5	2.2
GLA (g/day)	5.8	5.1	4.6
Outcomes			
Safety	safe	safe	safe
Improved oxygenation status	+	+	+
Reduced time on ventilator	+	+	+
Reduced ICU length of stay	+	+	+
Reduced new organ failure	+	not assessed	+
Reduced 28-day mortality		+	+

ARDS: acute respiratory distress syndrome; ALI: acute lung injury; CD: Control diet (isocaloric, isolipidic, isonitrogenous); DHA: docosahexaenoic acid; +: statistically significant difference ($p < 0.05$) for EPA+GLA versus control diet.

ogy of respiratory failure due to an increased and persistent systemic inflammation. A recently performed meta-analysis [47] evaluated all the available clinical data on the use of EPA+GLA on clinical outcomes. The three studies in the meta-analysis followed a similar study design comparing the same study diet (enriched with EPA, GLA and antioxidants) with a control diet which is isocaloric, and isonitrogenous with equal amounts of lipids as compared to the study diet. For the patients (n = 296 patients) considered evaluable, the use of an EPA+GLA diet was associated with a 60 % reduction in the risk of 28-day in hospital all-cause mortality (OR = 0.40; 95 % CI 0.24 to 0.68; p = 0.001) with no significant degree of heterogeneity. When evaluating the effects on mortality in an intent-to-treat analysis (n= 411 patients), a 49 % reduction in the risk of 28-day in-hospital all-cause mortality (OR = 0.51; 95 % CI 0.33 to 0.79; p = 0.002) was still evident for use of an EPA+GLA diet. The intent-to-treat analysis remained non-significant in terms of heterogeneity between the included studies. The strong mortality benefit was still present when evaluating the reduction in the mortality risk in terms of relative risk (RR). Using relative risk analysis (n = 296) the risk reduction in the 28-day in-hospital all-cause mortality was 43 % (RR = 0.57, 95 % CI 0.41 to 0.79).

The available clinical data were also consistent in showing a reduction in time on mechanical ventilation; the number of ventilator-free days was 17.0 ± 9.7 days for patients using the EPA+GLA diet versus 12.1 ± 9.9 days for the control population of patients, $p < 0.0001$. This represented a mean increase of 4.9 ventilator-free days within a 28-day observation period for the ALI/ARDS patients randomized to EPA+GLA. In terms of ICU-free days, the use of an enteral diet enriched with EPA and GLA can be associated with a statistically significant improvement in the num-

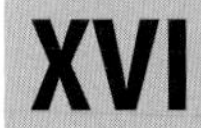

ber of days free of ICU (from 15.1 ± 10.0 ICU-free days when using EPA+GLA to 10.8 ± 9.6 ICU free days when using the control diet; $p < 0.0001$) [47].

Conclusion

Several studies are now underway to evaluate further aspects of the use of anti-inflammatory lipids (EPA and GLA) in a variety of other clinical situations, including their effects in the early stages of sepsis. It is important to consider that the results from all available clinical trials at this point consistently show strong improvements in clinical outcomes of critically ill and mechanically ventilated patients with ALI/ARDS associated or not with severe sepsis/septic shock, in terms of more ICU-free days, more ventilator-free days, improvement in oxygenation status, less development of new organ failures, and reduction in the 28-day all cause mortality. Although some mechanistic aspects regarding the use of enteral diets with EPA+GLA still suggest further basic science investigations, the clinical data available so far and the strong safety profile, clearly point towards a clinical benefit in the use of this approach as an important adjuvant therapy in the treatment of ALI and ARDS.

References

1. Rubenfeld GD, Caldwell E, Peabody E, et al (2005) Incidence and outcomes of acute lung injury. N Engl J Med 353: 1685–1693
2. Mutlu GM, Budinger GR (2006) Incidence and outcomes of acute lung injury. N Engl J Med 354: 416–417
3. Brower RG, Ware LB, Berthiaume Y, Matthay MA (2001) Treatment of ARDS. Chest 120: 1347–1367
4. Bringham KL (1985) Metabolites of arachidonic acid in experimental lung vascular injury. Fed Proc 44: 43–45
5. Henderson WR Jr (1987) Lipid-derivered and other chemical mediators of inflammation in the lung. J Allergy Clin Immunol 79: 543–553
6. Mizock BA (2001) Nutritional support in acute lung injury and acute respiratory distress syndrome. Nutr Clin Pract 16: 319–328
7. Mizock BA, DeMichele SJ (2004) The acute respiratory distress syndrome: role of nutritional modulation of inflammation through dietary lipids. Nutr Clin Pract 19: 563–574
8. Pontes-Arruda A (2007) The use of special lipids in the treatment of inflammatory lung disease. Clin Nutr Insight 33: 1–4
9. Mayer K, Schaefer MB, Seeger W (2006) Fish oil in the critically ill: from experimental to clinical data. Curr Opin Clin Nutr Metab Care 9: 140–148
10. DeMichele SJ, Wood SM, Wennberg AK (2006) A nutritional strategy to improve oxygenation and decrease morbidity in patients who have acute respiratory distress syndrome. Respir Care Clin N Am 12: 547–566
11. de Alaniz MJ, Marra CA (1992) Glucocorticoid and mineralocorticoid hormones depress liver delta 5 desaturase activity through different mechanisms. Lipids 27: 599–604
12. Mills DE, Huang YS, Narce M, Poisson JP (1994) Psychosocial stress, catecholamines, and essential fatty acid metabolism in rats. Proc Soc Exp Biol Med 205: 56–61
13. Palombo JD, DeMichele SJ, Boyce PJ, Noursalehi M, Forse RA, Bistrian BR (1998) Metabolism of dietary alpha-linolenic acid vs eicosapentaenoic acid in rat immune cell phospholipids during endotoxemia. Lipids 33: 1099–1105
14. Fan YY, Chapkin RS (1998) Importance of dietary gamma-linolenic acid in human health and nutrition. J Nutr 128: 1411–1414
15. Karlstad MD, DeMichele SJ, Leathem WD, et al (1993) Effect of intravenous lipid emulsions enriched with gamma-linolenic acid on plasma n-6 fatty acids and prostaglandin biosynthesis after burn and endotoxin injury in rats. Crit Care Med 21: 1740–1749

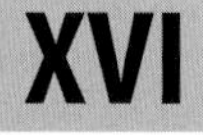

16. Johnson MM, Swan DD, Surette ME, et al (1997) Dietary supplementation with gamma-linolenic acid alters fatty acid content and eicosanoid production in healthty humans. J Nutr 127: 1435–1444
17. Wanten GJA, Calder PC (2007) Immune modulation by parenteral lipid emulsions. Am J Clin Nutr 85: 1171–1184
18. Deckelbaum RJ, Worgall TS, Seo T (2006) n-3 Fatty acids and gene expression. Am J Clin Nutr 83 (Suppl): S1520-S1525
19. Singer P, Shapiro H, Theilla M, Anbar R, Singer J, Cohen J (2008) Anti-inflammatory properties of omega-3 fatty acids and critical illness: novel mechanisms and an integrative perspective. Intensive Care Med 34: 1580–1592
20. Denys A, Hichami A, Khan NA (2005) n-3 PUFAs modulate T-cell activation via protein kinase C-alpha and -epsilon and the NF-kappaB signaling pathway. J Lipid Res 46: 752–758
21. Sperling RI, Benincaso AI, Knoell CT, et al (1993) Dietary omega-3 polyunsaturated fatty acids inhibit phosphoinositide formation and chemotaxis in neutrophils. J Clin Invest 91: 651–660
22. Madani S, Hichami A, Cherkaoui-Malki M, Khan NA (2004) Diacylglycerols containing omega-3 and omega-6 fatty acids bind to RasGRP and modulate MAP kinase activation. J Biol Chem 279: 1176–1183
23. Chen H, Li D, Chen J, et al (2003) EPA and DHA attenuate ox-LDL-induced expression of adhesion molecules in human coronary artery endothelial cells via protein kinase B pathway. J Mol Cell Cardiol 35: 769–775
24. Fialkow L, Fochesatto Filho L, Bozzetti MC, et al (2006) Neutrophil apoptosis: a marker of disease severity in sepsis and sepsis-induced acute respiratory distress syndrome. Crit Care 10: R155
25. Annane D, Bellissant E, Cavaillon JM (2005) Septic shock. Lancet 365: 63–78
26. Willoughby DA, Moore AR, Colville-Nash PR, Gilroy D (2000) Resolution of inflammation. Int J Immunopharmacol 22: 1131–1135
27. Savill JS, Wyllie AH, Henson JE, Walport MJ, Henson PM, Haslett C (1989) Macrophage phagocytosis of aging neutrophils in inflammation. Programmed cell death in the neutrophil leads to its recognition by macrophages. J Clin Invest 83: 865–875
28. Haslett C (1992) Resolution of acute inflammation and the role of apoptosis in the tissue fate of granulocytes. Clin Sci (Lond) 83: 639–648
29. Serhan CN, Savill J (2005) Resolution of inflammation: the beginning programs the end. Nat Immunol 6: 1191–1197
30. Ward C, Walker A, Dransfield I, Haslett C, Rossi AG (2004) Regulation of granulocyte apoptosis by NF-κB. Biochem Soc Trans 32: 465–467
31. Freire-de-Lima CG, Xiao YQ, Gardai SJ, Bratton DL, Schiemann WP, Henson PM (2006) Apoptotic cells, through transforming growth factor-β, coordinately induce anti-inflammatory and suppress pro-inflammatory eicosanoid and NO synthesis in murine macrophages. J Biol Chem 281: 38376–38384
32. Lucas M, Stuart LM, Savill J, Lacy-Hullbert A (2003) Apoptotic cells and innate stimuli combine to regulate macrophage cytokine secretion. J Immunol 171: 2610–2615
33. Serhan CN, Clish CB, Brannon J, Colgan SP, Chiang N, Cronert K (2000) Novel functional sets of lipid-derived mediators with anti-inflammatory actions generated from omega-3 fatty acids via cyclooxygenase 2-nonsteroidal anti-inflammatory drugs and transcellular processing. J Exp Med 192: 1197–1204
34. Serhan CN, Hong S, Gronert K, et al (2002) Resolvins: a family of bioactive products of omega-3 fatty acid transformation circuits initiated by aspirin treatment that counter proinflammation signals. J Exp Med 196: 1025–1037
35. Mancuso P, Whelan J, DeMichele SJ, Snider CC, Guszcza JA, Karlstad MD (1997) Dietary fish oil and fish and borage oil suppress intrapulmonary proinflammatory eicosanoid biosynthesis and attenuate pulmonary neutrophil accumulation in endotoxic rats. Crit Care Med 25: 1198–1206
36. Mancuso P, Whelan J, DeMichele SJ, et al (1997) Effects of eicosapentaenoic and gammalinolenic acid on lung permeability and alveolar macrophage eicosanoid synthesis in endotoxic rats. Crit Care Med 25: 523–532
37. Murray MJ, Kumar M, Gregory TJ, Banks PL, Tazelaar HD, DeMichele SJ (1995) select dietary

fatty acids attenuate cardiopulmonary dysfunction during acute lung injury in pigs. Am J Physiol 269: H2090-H2099

38. Murray MJ, Kanazi G, Moukabary K, Tazelaar HD, DeMichele SJ (2000) Effects of eicosapentaenoic and gamma-linolenic acids (dietary lipids) on pulmonary surfactant composition and function during porcine endotoxemia. Chest 117: 1720–1727
39. Palombo JD, DeMichele SJ, Lydon E, Bistrian BR (1997) Cyclic vs continuous enteral feeding with omega-3 and gamma-linolenic fatty acids: effects on modulation of phospholipid fatty acids in rat lung and liver immune cells. JPEN J Parenter Enteral Nutr 21: 123–132
40. Palombo JD, DeMichele SJ, Boyce PJ, et al (1999) Effect of short-term enteral feeding with eicosapentaenoic and gamma-linolenic acids on alveolar macrophage eicosanoid synthesis and bactericidal function in rats. Crit Care Med 27: 1908–1915
41. Palombo JD, DeMichele SJ, Lyndon EE, et al (1996) Rapid modulation of lung and liver macrophage phospholipid fatty acids in endotoxemic rats by continuous Enteral feeding with n-3 and gamma-linolenic fatty acids. Am J Clin Nutr 63: 208–219
42. Gadek JE, DeMichele SJ, Karlstad MD, et al (1999) Effect of enteral feeding with eicosapentaenoic acid, gamma-linolenic acid, and antioxidants in patients with acute respiratory distress syndrome. Enteral nutrition in ARDS study group. Crit Care Med 27: 1409–1420
43. Singer P, Theilla M, Fisher H, et al (2006) Benefit of an enteral diet enriched with eicosapentaenoic acid and gamma-linolenic acid in ventilated patients with acute lung injury. Crit Care Med 34: 1033–1038
44. Pontes-Arruda A, Aragão AM, Albuquerque JD (2006) The effects of enteral feeding with eicosapentaenoic acid, gamma-linolenic acid and antioxidants in mechanically ventilated patients with severe sepsis and septic shock. Crit Care Med 34: 2325–2333
45. Mayes T, Gottschlich M, Carman B, et al (2005) An evaluation of the safety and efficacy of an anti-inflammatory, pulmonary enteral formula in the treatment of pediatric burn patients with respiratory failure. Nutr Clin Prac 20: 30–31
46. Theilla M, Singer P, Cohen, DeKeyser F (2007) A diet enriched with eicosapentaenoic acid, gamma-linolenic acid and antioxidants in the incidence of new pressure ulcer formation in critically ill patients with acute lung injury: a randomized, prospective, controlled study. Clin Nutr 26: 752–757
47. Pontes-Arruda A, DeMichele SJ, Seth A, Singer P (2008) The use of an inflammation-modulating diet in patients with acute lung injury and acute respiratory distress syndrome: a meta-analysis of outcome data. JPEN J Parenter Enteral Nutr 32: 596–605

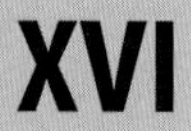

Glutamine Supplementation in ICU Patients

A. Berg, O. Rooyackers, and J. Wernerman

Introduction

Glutamine is a non-essential amino acid with a special role in metabolism and nutrition. The depletion of glutamine is reported to be a predictor of a poor outcome in particular for intensive care unit (ICU) patients [1]. Consequently, supplementation of intravenous nutrition with glutamine improves outcome in terms of mortality and morbidity in ICU patients [2–4]. A number of questions have been raised concerning the handling of glutamine-supplemented nutrition in ICU patients, including the vascular and metabolic tolerance of the dipeptide infusions, the handling of glutamine during renal replacement therapy in ICU patients, and the safety of glutamine administration in head trauma patients. These issues will be dealt with in this short chapter.

Glutamine has a number of key functions in metabolism (**Table 1**). Being a precursor for nucleotide synthesis, glutamine availability is a key factor in cell growth. In the human body, glutamine availability is crucial for intestinal mucosal cells and also for immune-competent cells [5]. When glutamine is used as an energy source, a high metabolic flow rate is present, furthermore a small fraction of that flux will be sufficient to dramatically increase the nucleotide synthesis rate. Therefore, many cells use glutamine as an energy substrate. It has been demonstrated that stressed cells have a particular preference for glutamine as an energy source [6]. The role of glutamine for inter-organ transport is also well established (**Fig. 1**). During metabolic stress there is an increased efflux of glutamine from skeletal muscle and an intracellular depletion of glutamine in muscle. In ICU patients there is essentially no information available about the basal state, but in the fed state the glutamine efflux from skeletal muscle is elevated, although not dramatically [7]. Measurements of glutamine production measured as the rate of appearance of glutamine show unal-

Table 1. Glutamine functions

- Precursor for DNA/RNA
- Constituent for proteins
- Energy substrate for immunocompetent cells and enterocytes
- Substrate for gluconeogenesis
- Precursor for glutamate in the brain – glutamate is an important excitatory neurotransmitter in the brain
- A pathway for glutamate transport out of the brain
- Via glutamate a precursor for glutathione, which is an antioxidant
- A substrate for renal ammoniagenesis and acid-base regulation.

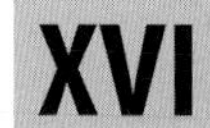

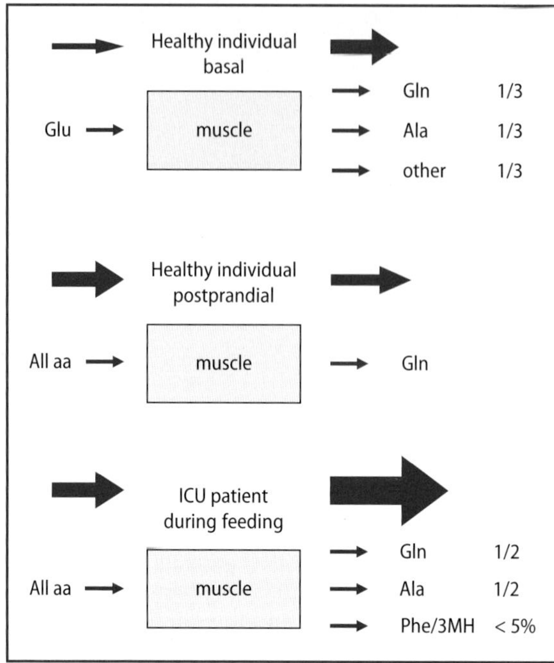

Fig. 1. Muscle amino acid flux in health and disease. The relative quantities of amino acid (aa) influx and efflux occurring in muscle tissue are illustrated by the bold arrows. The small arrows indicate the most important constituents in the different fluxes. Glu: glutamate; Gln: glutamine; Ala: alanine; Phe/3MH: phenylalanine/3-methyl histidine

tered *de novo* production of glutamine in the posttraumatic state of metabolically healthy subjects undergoing elective surgery [8, 9]. Subjects with acute liver failure, however, have extremely high plasma concentrations of glutamine [10]; in contrast, this is not seen in patients with chronic liver failure, even if an acute exacerbation is present. The significance of this finding in acute liver failure is presently not clear.

In ICU patients, several unsuccessful attempts have been made to attenuate the decrease in muscle free glutamine [11, 12]. For plasma free glutamine on the other hand, normalization is always possible, even in ICU patients [12]. However, provision of exogenous glutamine by the intravenous route does not decrease endogenous glutamine production as reflected by the rate of appearance for glutamine, both in healthy volunteers and in trauma patients [8, 13]. Exogenous glutamine, therefore, primarily increases glutamine availability in the splanchnic area.

Background

The clinical effects of glutamine supplementation to ICU patients have been summarized in a meta-analysis [4, 14]. Intravenous glutamine supplementation provides advantages in terms of mortality as well as morbidity [2, 3]. For ICU patients receiving glutamine supplementation by the enteral route, the results are less conclusive [4, 15–17]. For mortality as an end-point, the individual studies of enteral glutamine supplementation are too small in size to be conclusive and no single study has demonstrated a mortality advantage within the ICU. The two studies studying intravenous glutamine supplementation that had a 6-month follow up showed a reduction in mortality at that time point [2, 3]. Other studies involving intravenous gluta-

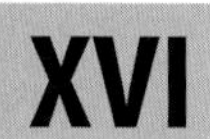

mine supplementation suggest a non-significant tendency towards decreased mortality in the ICU [18–22]. The patients recruited to these studies are multiple organ failure patients with long ICU stays. This is a patient group that carries a very high mortality during ICU stay and during the post-ICU period. In addition, all studies also show beneficial effects in terms of infectious morbidity. Perhaps most importantly so far no studies have reported negative effects attributable to exogenous glutamine supplementation in ICU patients.

From the role of glutamine in physiology, it can be anticipated that glutamine may have beneficial effects on cells that are rapidly turning over. In man, and in particular in diseased states, this is true for immune-competent cells as well as for the gastrointestinal mucosa. This observation has been reported in numerous animal experiments, but there is also good evidence from human studies. Following administration of intravenous glutamine supplementation, the absorption of carbohydrates from the gastrointestinal tract improved in patients with a compromised gut [23, 24]. The histology of the gastrointestinal tract also improved [23]. The effect on immune-competent cells may be the background to the beneficial effect on infectious morbidity reported in a number of patient groups such as intensive care patients [2, 17, 25], hematological patients [26, 27], postoperative patients [28], oncological patients [29], premature children [30], and gastroenterological patients [31].

Metabolic Tolerance

The metabolic tolerance of intravenous glutamine supplementation was studied in a group of ICU patients with only marginal organ failure in the kidney and liver [32]. The protocol used a short infusion period, the rationale being to disclose any tendency for accumulation of the dipeptide, alanyl-glutamine, or the amino acid constituents of the dipeptide. Urinary sampling was also performed to reveal any loss of dipeptide and/or the constituents of amino acids. The treatment group was compared to a control group given saline as placebo. The infusion rate was 0.625 ml/kg/h (corresponding to 0.125 g dipeptide/kg/h or 0.085 g glutamine/kg/h) for 4 h. This infusion rate provides the daily allowance over only four hours. All subjects reached a steady state level in dipeptide concentration during the 4 hours and a rapid elimination phase during the first 2 hours after the infusion was stopped. In addition, there were no losses of dipeptide in the urine. The elimination constants for the dipeptide were slightly longer than what has been reported in healthy subjects [33], but the values seen still indicate complete removal of the dipeptide within 2 hours following the end of infusion.

In addition to the dipeptide, the constituent amino acids, glutamine and alanine, were analyzed together with glutamate. For these amino acids, plasma concentration reached a steady state in some subjects but not in others. The elimination kinetics, as reflected by half-life clearance, demonstrated that the basal plasma concentration was re-established in all subjects within eight hours after termination of the infusion.

When an exogenous supply of glutamine containing dipeptides was given intravenously, the daily dose administered over 24 hours resulted in a mean increase in plasma concentration of approximately 50 % [34, 35]. When a similar dose was infused for 4 hours, a supra-physiological level was achieved in individual subjects [32]. All these levels were cleared back to baseline within 8 hours, but the upper time limit to clear glutamine was needed in some individuals. Approximately 50 % of the subjects included in that study achieved a steady state of plasma glutamine,

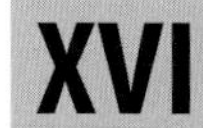

usually within the physiological range or at a slightly elevated level. Some subjects, however, did not attain a steady state in plasma glutamine level during the 4 hours. This indicates that an infusion rate at this level cannot be recommended beyond that time period. In clinical practice in the ICU, a continuous infusion of glutamine containing dipeptide for 24 hours has several advantages. All patients, so far studied attain a steady state within the physiological range, and the plasma concentration is kept within the physiological range, which may have implications for glutamine availability. The mechanisms for glutamine availability to explain the beneficial effects of glutamine supplementation are, however, beyond the scope of this chapter.

Intravenous Glutamine Supplementation during Continuous Renal Replacement Therapy

A question often discussed in the context of ICU nutrition is how to handle patients receiving continuous renal replacement therapy (CRRT). It is well known that any dialysis treatment aimed at the removal of waste products, such as urea and creatinine, will also eliminate free amino acids. In intermittent hemodialysis, the losses are in the magnitude of 10 g amino acids during a 4 hour session [36]. In the ICU setting using continuous hemodialysis often combined with hemofiltration and hemodiafiltration, the flow through the dialysis filter is lower per time unit, but the elimination continues around the clock.

To elucidate the effects of CRRT on glutamine supplementation, a pragmatic design was used [34]. Hence the prescription of renal replacement therapy was entirely left to the attending intensivist. Hence the mode of CRRT and the dialysis dose were not uniform among the patients studied. The pragmatic design also means that the time of dialysis or hemofiltration treatment during each 24 hour period was not standardized. To compensate for this, a design was used where patients were randomized to intravenous glutamine supplementation or placebo on two consecutive days. The randomization was performed by lottery. Each patient therefore served as his/her own control. The necessary prerequisite to attain interpretable results is that the two days were similar in terms of leg circulation, in terms of dialysis dose, and in terms of as many other clinical parameters as possible. If the two days were too far apart in terms of clinical background data, the effects of the studied manipulation, i.e., the infusion of glutamine containing dipeptide or placebo will not be assessable.

The protocol included a 20 hour infusion of alanyl-glutamine 0.5 mg/kg/h [34]. At the end of this infusion, the exchange of glutamine across the leg was studied using the arterio-venous concentration difference combined with a measurement of leg blood flow. Following termination of the infusion, the decay curve over the following hours was studied in order to enable calculation of clearance parameters and the endogenous rate of glutamine appearance. The diafiltrate from the CRRT was sampled, and the glutamine content analyzed.

Plasma concentrations of glutamine increased by 30 % during the infusion. Losses into the ultrafiltrate corresponded to 0.6–6.8 g/24 h. The level of glutamine loss in the ultrafiltrate was related to the blood flow through the dialysis machine and the plasma concentration, with the blood flow through the dialysis machine and filter being the stronger determinant. There were no differences in glutamine exchange across the leg, representing a constant export of glutamine, between treatment and control days.

Glutamate Concentration and Exchange across the Brain in Head Trauma Patients

The role of glutamate as a neurotransmitter is well characterized. There are a number of reports suggesting that severe brain damage, in particular with an unfavorable outcome, is associated with high free glutamate concentration in cerebrospinal fluid and in the interstitial fluid of the brain. Patients with a Glasgow Coma Scale (GCS) score < 8 following head trauma, who were routinely given a microdialysis catheter in the penumbra zone of the injured brain, were studied [35, 37]. The purpose of the study was to provide exogenous intravenous glutamine supplementation and to monitor interstitial brain concentrations of glutamine and glutamate together with the arterio-venous difference of glutamine and glutamate across the brain and the leg. In addition, the endogenous glutamine rate of appearance was calculated. The protocol used was identical to that used in the CRRT patients described above, with the same emphasis upon the need to study two comparable days for the evaluation.

The results showed that interstitial glutamate and glutamine concentrations in the brain were unaffected by glutamine administration. In particular for glutamate, there was considerable inter-individual variation, irrespective of whether exogenous glutamine was provided or not. The subjects studied were too few to make any statement on a possible relation between outcome and the level of glutamate in the micro-dialysate. The overall outcome of the patients included in the study was favorable with 14/15 patients with a Glasgow Outcome Score of 3 or more at hospital discharge and only one death. However, any discussion of the level of glutamate and outcome is beyond the scope of this particular study.

In theory, exogenous glutamine supplementation may hinder the efflux of glutamine from the brain. The background to the importance of glutamine efflux from the brain is that possible elimination pathways of intra-cerebral free glutamate are: 1) re-uptake in the neuron; 2) degradation; 3) uptake into astrocytes and conversion into glutamine, which is then exported out of the brain. Quantitatively, the third alternative is by far the most important. Hence, there is a constant export of glutamine from the brain. Theoretically, an elevation of plasma glutamine concentration may compromise this export. The results from this study indicate that the arterio-venous concentration difference did not decrease during glutamine treatment [37]. As there was no estimate of cerebral blood flow, the assumption is that cerebral blood flow was unaltered and, therefore, the export of glutamine was unaffected. In comparison, the exchange of glutamine across the leg was also studied and there was no difference between the treatment and control days, similar to the results in the patients receiving CRRT [34].

Endogenous Glutamine Rate of Appearance

The advantage of non-compartmental analysis is that it is rather assumption free compared with compartmental models. However, it is assumed that systemic elimination takes place from the measured central compartment and that model parameters are constant over time. All compartmental models are over simplifications, but could still be useful. The simplest model that describes data well should be chosen. This means that the one-compartment model is often the model of choice even if it is known that amino acids are neither produced into nor eliminated directly from

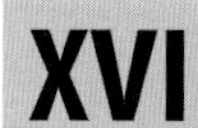

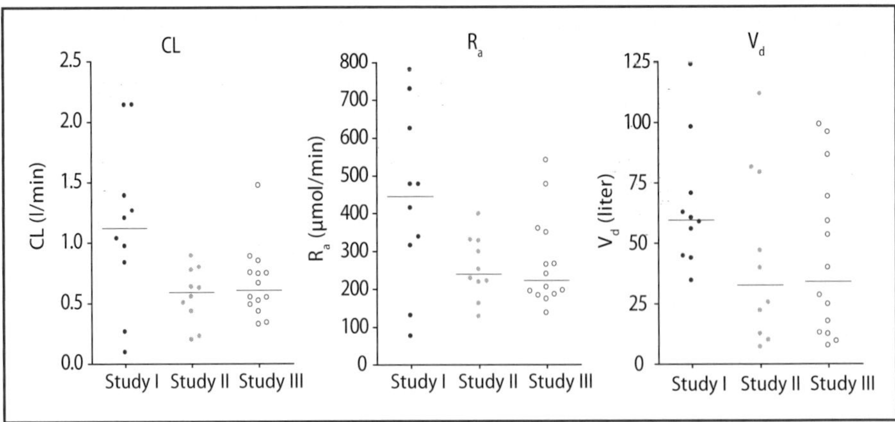

Fig. 2. Clearance (CL), rate of appearance (R_a), and distribution volume (V_d) in three studies [32, 34, 37], illustrated as the individual estimates of the pharmacokinetic model parameters. All data were analyzed by a one-compartment turnover model. Median values are marked.

the central compartment. A too short study time can give falsely high values of the rates of appearance and clearance in both non-compartmental analysis and turnover models and also in isotope tracer studies [9].

In several of our studies, the endogenous rate of appearance for glutamine has been calculated [32, 34, 37] (**Fig. 2**). The hypothesis that exogenous glutamine supplementation may be beneficial for ICU patients rests upon the assumption that the endogenous production is insufficient. So far endogenous glutamine production, usually measured as the endogenous glutamine rate of appearance, has not been quantified. There is literature in healthy individuals or in individuals undergoing elective surgery [8, 38], but measurements among ICU patients, in particular those with multiple organ failure, have so far not been available. The values presented in the studies on metabolic tolerance and in CRRT and head trauma patients show a uniform pattern [35, 37]. The mean and median values are in accord with estimates from healthy individuals: mean values 283±31 umol/kg/min [39] and 280±23 umol/kg/min [40]. The healthy individuals studied are not comparable to ICU patients in terms of age or underlying health status. Nevertheless, the endogenous production of glutamine seems to be on the same level in ICU patients with mean values of 271±120 umol/kg/min in head injury patients and 258±83 umol/kg/min in CRRT patients. It can also be seen that the scatter between individuals is large, but it is not possible to conclude whether the scatter is larger than expected or if it is a reflection of physiology. Again the references to healthy individuals and to elective surgery patients are not sufficiently matched to allow any conclusions regarding the inter-individual scatter.

In several studies, the well defined decay curve after the termination of a constant infusion of glutamine was used to calculate clearance. The accuracy of these calculations are more related to the stability of the basal concentration level, the number of concentration determinations in the decay curve, and to whether or not a steady state plasma concentration was achieved during the period of glutamine supplementation (Cmax). Under the assumption that the rate of appearance of glutamine did not change in relation to glutamine plasma concentration, the rate of appearance was calculated. The rationale for these assumptions was, of course, that there was no change in glutamine export from muscle. Nevertheless, this underlying assumption needs to be validated in future studies. The requisite for a steady state in plasma glutamine concentration during the exogenous infusion was well illustrated during the rapid infusion over a short time period [32], which, for the subjects who did not attain a steady state plasma glutamine, gave erroneously high estimates of their glutamine rate of appearance. The results when the daily infusion was given over 20 hours demonstrated a glutamine rate of appearance on the level of what is seen in the literature [9]. The relation between the glutamine rate of appearance and the factors that may influence the rate of appearance is another fascinating research area that needs to be addressed in future studies.

General Comments

The characteristic decrease in glutamine plasma concentration and the decrease in muscle glutamine concentration are well described among ICU patients [11, 12, 41, 42]. Nevertheless, the mechanisms behind these changes in concentrations have not been satisfactorily explained. Despite the low tissue concentration of glutamine in skeletal muscle, the export of glutamine from leg muscle as well as the rate of appearance as calculated within the framework of current research, are normal or perhaps even slightly elevated [39, 40]. Also, the low plasma concentration does not seem to hinder the export of glutamine from muscle to the splanchnic area keeping it at the same level as when normal plasma glutamine concentrations are present [43]. There is no correlation between plasma concentrations of glutamine in the basal state or during exogenous supplementation, and the efflux of glutamine from the leg or the calculated rate of appearance. The independence of glutamine efflux from the leg in relation to plasma concentration has been demonstrated [7]. This is in contrast to the concentration-dependent uptake of glutamate in skeletal muscle and cardiac muscle [7, 44]. There are data from animal experiments indicative of a concentration-dependent uptake of glutamine within the splanchnic area [45]. This is probably not the case in ICU patients, as export from the leg is independent of plasma concentration, and the reciprocal uptake in the splanchnic area will be of the same magnitude as the export from the leg [13]. Nevertheless, the increase in plasma concentration seen after exogenous supplementation must result in a higher uptake, most likely in the splanchnic area, but without any negative feedback on the export from muscle.

So far the mechanisms behind the regulation of plasma concentration of glutamine remain obscure. Nevertheless, as discussed above, the decrease in plasma and tissue concentration is established quite early during the course of disease [12]. The majority of the patients in the ICU demonstrate plasma concentrations of glutamine below the normal range. This low level is stabile over time and is established quite early in the course of disease. In studies where the initiating event can be controlled, such as the temporal pattern following elective surgical trauma, or the temporal pattern following an endotoxin challenge in healthy volunteers, a decrease in plasma glutamine concentration starting up at 4–6 hours and well established within 12 hours is seen [46, 47]. The decrease in muscle tissue concentration occurs in parallel. The most likely explanation is that the transmembrane transport of glutamine, which maintains the concentration gradients across cell membranes, is somehow set at another level. As a result, dramatic changes in concentrations can be seen, but not in the inter-organ exchange of glutamine. This argues against the concentration being in itself a regulatory mechanism.

When the export of glutamine from muscle tissue is measured quantitatively, no change is seen during an exogenous intravenous glutamine infusion [35, 37]. This lack of change in muscle export has been indirectly demonstrated before [8, 38], but these studies [35, 37] were the first time such measurements had been performed prospectively using the patients as their own controls. As these studies were confined to only one day of glutamine supplementation, it cannot be completely ruled out that the picture may change after several consecutive days of glutamine supplementation; this remains to be studied. However, in earlier studies providing a post-hoc analysis of patients given exogenous glutamine supplementation over a longer time period, no such difference was seen [7].

Conclusion

The purpose of this short chapter is mainly to document the safety of glutamine administration in ICU patients. Beneficial effects have been demonstrated from intravenous glutamine supplementation [2, 3]. The patient groups where a positive effect on mortality has been demonstrated are ICU patients needing total parenteral nutrition. The indications for glutamine supplementation by the enteral or parenteral route in ICU patients on enteral nutrition is less well substantiated. It has been suggested that plasma glutamine concentrations should be used to determine the indication for exogenous glutamine supplementation [48]. However, this suggestion is hypothetical and needs to be verified by prospective studies. The evidence demonstrates that intravenous glutamine is beneficial, but so far it has not been demonstrated that normalization of plasma glutamine levels as a result of the intravenous supplementation is connected to beneficial effects. The reasons for the less convincing results in enterally fed ICU patients may be related to several issues. Enteral supplementation with glutamine is not as effective as parenteral administration in increasing plasma glutamine levels [49]. This observation is related to a relatively high first pass extraction through the splanchnic area and liver when glutamine is provided by the enteral route [50]. The number of studies providing parenteral glutamine to enterally fed patients are so far few, of small size, and, therefore, not conclusive [22]. Studies where enterally fed ICU patients are given enteral supplementation with glutamine contain very different groups of ICU patients. The largest study, comprising more patients than all the other studies of enteral supplementation to ICU patients put together, had a very low mortality rate and a very short mean ICU stay time [16]. The majority of patients included in that particular study [16] were, therefore, different from the patients in whom intravenous glutamine supplementation has been demonstrated to have a beneficial effect on outcome [2, 3].

References

1. Oudemans-van Straaten HM, Bosman RJ, Treskes M, van der Spoel HJ, Zandstra DF (2001) Plasma glutamine depletion and patient outcome in acute ICU admissions. Intensive Care Med 27: 84–90
2. Goeters C, Wenn A, Mertes N, et al (2002) Parenteral L-alanyl-L-glutamine improves 6-month outcome in critically ill patients. Crit Care Med 30: 2032–2037
3. Griffiths RD, Jones C, Palmer TE (1997) Six-month outcome of critically ill patients given glutamine-supplemented parenteral nutrition. Nutrition 13: 295–302
4. Novak F, Heyland DK, Avenell A, Drover JW, Su X (2002) Glutamine supplementation in serious illness: a systematic review of the evidence. Crit Care Med 30: 2022–2029

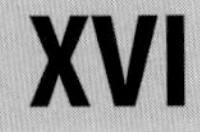

5. Newsholme P, Gordon S, Newsholme EA (1987) Rates of utilization and fates of glucose, glutamine, pyruvate, fatty acids and ketone bodies by mouse macrophages. Biochem J 242: 631–636
6. Ardawi MS, Newsholme EA (1990) Glutamine, the immune system, and the intestine. J Lab Clin Med 115: 654–655
7. Vesali RF, Klaude M, Rooyackers OE, TJäder I, Barle H, Wernerman J (2002) Longitudinal pattern of glutamine/glutamate balance across the leg in long-stay intensive care unit patients. Clin Nutr 21: 505–514
8. van Acker BA, Hulsewe KW, Wagenmakers AJ, von Meyenfeldt MF, Soeters PB (2000) Response of glutamine metabolism to glutamine-supplemented parenteral nutrition. Am J Clin Nutr 72: 790–795
9. Van Acker BA, Hulsewe KW, Wagenmakers AJ, et al (1998) Absence of glutamine isotopic steady state: implications for the assessment of whole-body glutamine production rate. Clin Sci (Lond) 95: 339–346
10. Clemmesen JO, Kondrup J, Ott P (2000) Splanchnic and leg exchange of amino acids and ammonia in acute liver failure. Gastroenterology 118: 1131–1139
11. Gamrin L, Essen P, Forsberg AM, Hultman E, Wernerman J (1996) A descriptive study of skeletal muscle metabolism in critically ill patients: free amino acids, energy-rich phosphates, protein, nucleic acids, fat, water, and electrolytes. Crit Care Med 24: 575–583
12. Tjader I, Rooyackers O, Forsberg AM, Vesali RF, Garlick PJ, Wernerman J (2004). Effects on skeletal muscle of intravenous glutamine supplementation to ICU patients. Intensive Care Med 30: 266–275
13. Boza JJ, Dangin M, Moennoz D, et al (2001) Free and protein-bound glutamine have identical splanchnic extraction in healthy human volunteers. Am J Physiol Gastrointest Liver Physiol 281:G267–274
14. Heyland DK, Dhaliwal R, Drover JW, Gramlich L, Dodek P (2003) Canadian clinical practice guidelines for nutrition support in mechanically ventilated, critically ill adult patients. JPEN J Parenter Enteral Nutr 27: 355–373
15. Garrel D, Patenaude J, Nedelec B, et al (2003) Decreased mortality and infectious morbidity in adult burn patients given enteral glutamine supplements: a prospective, controlled, randomized clinical trial. Crit Care Med 31: 2444–2449
16. Hall JC, Dobb G, Hall J, de Sousa R, Brennan L, McCauley R (2003) A prospective randomized trial of enteral glutamine in critical illness. Intensive Care Med 29: 1710–1716
17. Jones C, Palmer TE, Griffiths RD (1999) Randomized clinical outcome study of critically ill patients given glutamine-supplemented enteral nutrition. Nutrition 15: 108–115
18. Fuentes-Orozco C, Cervantes-Guevara G, Mucino-Hernandez I, et al (2008). L-alanyl-L-glutamine-supplemented parenteral nutrition decreases infectious morbidity rate in patients with severe acute pancreatitis. JPEN J Parenter Enteral Nutr 32: 403–411
19. Estivariz CF, Griffith DP, Luo M, et al (2008) Efficacy of parenteral nutrition supplemented with glutamine dipeptide to decrease hospital infections in critically ill surgical patients. JPEN J Parenter Enteral Nutr 32: 389–402
20. Dechelotte P, Hasselmann M, Cynober L, et al (2006) L-alanyl-L-glutamine dipeptide-supplemented total parenteral nutrition reduces infectious complications and glucose intolerance in critically ill patients: the French controlled, randomized, double-blind, multicenter study. Crit Care Med 34: 598–604
21. Powell-Tuck J, Jamieson CP, Bettany GE, et al (1999) A double blind, randomised, controlled trial of glutamine supplementation in parenteral nutrition. Gut 45: 82–88
22. Wischmeyer PE, Lynch J, Liedel J, et al (2001) Glutamine administration reduces Gram-negative bacteremia in severely burned patients: a prospective, randomized, double-blind trial versus isonitrogenous control. Crit Care Med 29: 2075–2080
23. van der Hulst RR, von Meyenfeldt MF, Deutz NE, Stockbrugger RW, Soeters PB (1996) The effect of glutamine administration on intestinal glutamine content. J Surg Res 61: 30–34
24. Tremel H, Kienle B, Weilemann LS, Stehle P, Furst P (1994) Glutamine dipeptide-supplemented parenteral nutrition maintains intestinal function in the critically ill. Gastroenterology 107: 1595–1601
25. Houdijk AP, Rijnsburger ER, Jansen J, et al (1998) Randomised trial of glutamine-enriched enteral nutrition on infectious morbidity in patients with multiple trauma. Lancet 352: 772–776

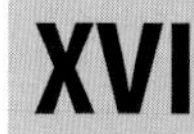

26. Ziegler TR, Young LS, Benfell K, et al (1992) Clinical and metabolic efficacy of glutamine-supplemented parenteral nutrition after bone marrow transplantation. A randomized, double-blind, controlled study. Ann Intern Med 116: 821 – 828
27. Schloerb PR, Amare M (1993) Total parenteral nutrition with glutamine in bone marrow transplantation and other clinical applications (a randomized, double-blind study). JPEN J Parenter Enteral Nutr 17: 407 – 413
28. Mertes N, Schulzki C, Goeters C, et al (2000) Cost containment through L-alanyl-L-glutamine supplemented total parenteral nutrition after major abdominal surgery: a prospective randomized double-blind controlled study. Clin Nutr 19: 395 – 401
29. Cerchietti LC, Navigante AH, Lutteral MA, et al (2006) Double-blinded, placebo-controlled trial on intravenous L-alanyl-L-glutamine in the incidence of oral mucositis following chemoradiotherapy in patients with head-and-neck cancer. Int J Radiat Oncol Biol Phys 65: 1330 – 1337
30. Neu J, Roig JC, Meetze WH, et al (1997) Enteral glutamine supplementation for very low birth weight infants decreases morbidity. J Pediatr 131: 691 – 699
31. van der Hulst RR, von Meyenfeldt MF, Soeters PB (1996) Glutamine: an essential amino acid for the gut. Nutrition 12:S78 – 81
32. Berg A, Rooyackers O, Norberg A, Wernerman J (2005) Elimination kinetics of L-alanyl-L-glutamine in ICU patients. Amino Acids 29: 221 – 228
33. Albers S, Wernerman J, Stehle P, Vinnars E, Furst P (1988) Availability of amino acids supplied intravenously in healthy man as synthetic dipeptides: kinetic evaluation of L-alanyl-L-glutamine and glycyl-L-tyrosine. Clin Sci (Lond) 75: 463 – 468
34. Berg A, Norberg A, Martling CR, Gamrin L, Rooyackers O, Wernerman J (2007) Glutamine kinetics during intravenous glutamine supplementation in ICU patients on continuous renal replacement therapy. Intensive Care Med 33: 660 – 666
35. Berg A, Bellander BM, Wanecek M, et al (2006). Intravenous glutamine supplementation to head trauma patients leaves cerebral glutamate concentration unaffected. Intensive Care Med 32: 1741 – 1746
36. Lofberg E, Essen P, McNurlan M, et al (2000) Effect of hemodialysis on protein synthesis. Clin Nephrol 54: 284 – 294
37. Berg A, Bellander BM, Wanecek M, et al (2008) The pattern of amino acid exchange across the brain is unaffected by intravenous glutamine supplementation in head trauma patients. Clin Nutr 27: 816 – 821
38. Jackson NC, Carroll PV, Russell-Jones DL, et al (2000) Effects of glutamine supplementation, GH, and IGF-I on glutamine metabolism in critically ill patients. Am J Physiol Endocrinol Metab 278:E226 – 233
39. Darmaun D, Matthews DE, Bier DM (1986) Glutamine and glutamate kinetics in humans. Am J Physiol 251:E117 – 126
40. Kreider ME, Stumvoll M, Meyer C, Overkamp D, Welle S, Gerich J (1997) Steady-state and non-steady-state measurements of plasma glutamine turnover in humans. Am J Physiol 272:E621 – 627
41. Biolo G, Zorat F, Antonione R, Ciocchi B (2005) Muscle glutamine depletion in the intensive care unit. Int J Biochem Cell Biol 37: 2169 – 2179
42. Roth E, Funovics J, Muhlbacher F, et al (1982) Metabolic disorders in severe abdominal sepsis: Glutamine deficiency in skeletal muscle. Clin Nutr 1: 25 – 41
43. Boza JJ, Turini M, Moennoz D, et al (2001) Effect of glutamine supplementation of the diet on tissue protein synthesis rate of glucocorticoid-treated rats. Nutrition 17: 35 – 40
44. Svedjeholm R, Svensson S, Ekroth R, et al (1990) Trauma metabolism and the heart: studies of heart and leg amino acid flux after cardiac surgery. Thorac Cardiovasc Surg 38: 1 – 5
45. Bruins MJ, Deutz NE, Soeters PB (2003) Aspects of organ protein, amino acid and glucose metabolism in a porcine model of hypermetabolic sepsis. Clin Sci (Lond) 104: 127 – 141

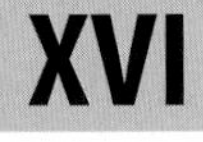

46. Hammarqvist F, Wernerman J, von der Decken A, Vinnars E (1990) Alanyl-glutamine counteracts the depletion of free glutamine and the postoperative decline in protein synthesis in skeletal muscle. Ann Surg 212: 637 – 644
47. Vesali RF, Klaude M, Rooyackers O, Wernerman J (2005) Amino acid metabolism in leg muscle after an endotoxin injection in healthy volunteers. Am J Physiol Endocrinol Metab 288: E360 – 364

48. Wernerman J (2003) Glutamine to intensive care unit patients. JPEN J Parenter Enteral Nutr 27: 302–303
49. Fish J, Sporay G, Beyer K, et al (1997) A prospective randomized study of glutamine-enriched parenteral compared with enteral feeding in postoperative patients. Am J Clin Nutr 65: 977–983
50. Haisch M, Fukagawa NK, Matthews DE (2000) Oxidation of glutamine by the splanchnic bed in humans. Am J Physiol Endocrinol Metab 278: E593–602

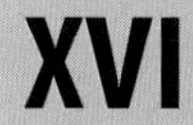

XVII Glucose Control

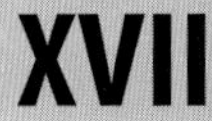

Burn Causes Prolonged Insulin Resistance and Hyperglycemia

G.G. Gauglitz and M.G. Jeschke

Introduction

More than 500,000 burn injuries occur annually in the United States [1]. Although most of these burn injuries are minor, approximately 40,000 to 60,000 burn patients require admission to a hospital or major burn center for appropriate treatment [2]. Advances in therapeutic strategies, based on improved understanding of resuscitation, enhanced wound coverage, improved treatment of inhalation injury, more appropriate infection control, and better support of the hypermetabolic response to injury, have significantly improved the clinical outcome of this unique patient population over the past years [3]. However, severe burns remain a devastating injury affecting nearly every organ system and leading to significant morbidity and mortality [4]. One of the main contributors to adverse outcome of this patient population is the profound metabolic changes associated with insulin resistance and hyperglycemia [4].

Multiple studies have documented insulin resistance and associated hyperglycemia in the acute period following surgery or medical illness [5]. Hyperglycemia is of serious clinical concern as it has been frequently linked to impaired wound healing, increased skin graft loss, increased incidence of infections, increased muscle protein catabolism, and mortality [5, 6]. However, it is currently unknown how long these conditions persist beyond the acute phase post-injury.

This chapter discusses the mechanisms underlying insulin resistance-induced hyperglycemia post-burn and examines the extent and persistence of abnormalities of various clinical parameters commonly utilized to describe insulin resistance.

Metabolic Changes following Severe Burn Injury

Severe burns covering more than 40 % of the total body surface area (TBSA) are typically followed by a period of stress, inflammation, and hypermetabolism, characterized by a hyperdynamic circulatory response with increased body temperature, glycolysis, proteolysis, lipolysis and futile substrate cycling [3]. Marked and sustained increases in catecholamine, glucocorticoid, glucagon, and dopamine secretion are thought to initiate the cascade of events leading to the acute hypermetabolic response with its ensuing catabolic and hyperglycemic state [5]. Interleukin (IL)-1 and IL-6, platelet-activating factor (PAF), tumor necrosis factor (TNF), endotoxin, neutrophil-adherence complexes, reactive oxygen species (ROS), nitric oxide (NO), and coagulation as well as complement cascades have also been implicated in regulating this response to burn injury [7].

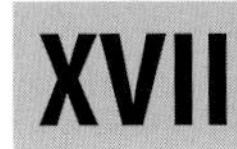

Various studies indicate that these post-burn metabolic phenomena occur in a timely manner, suggesting two distinct patterns of metabolic regulation following injury [8]. The first phase, classically called the 'ebb phase' occurs within the first 48 hours of injury [8, 9], and is characterized by decreased cardiac output, oxygen consumption, and metabolic rates as well as impaired glucose tolerance associated with a hyperglycemic state. These metabolic variables gradually increase within the first five days post-injury to a plateau phase (called the 'flow phase'), characteristically associated with a hyperdynamic circulation and the above mentioned hypermetabolic state. Insulin release during this time period was found to be twice that of controls in response to glucose load [10, 11] and plasma glucose levels are markedly elevated, indicating the development of insulin-resistance [11, 12]. Current understanding has been that these metabolic alterations resolve soon after complete wound closure.

Recent studies have reported that the hypermetabolic response to burn injury may last for more than 12 months after the initial event [13–15] and may thus lead to persistent hyperglycemia and insulin resistance and its associated consequences. Our group, therefore, conducted a prospective study and found that severe burn trauma led to increased hypermetabolism, catabolism, and marked inflammation accompanied by alterations in insulin sensitivity that persisted for up to three years after the initial burn injury. Although the glucose concentrations in our study patients returned to levels of non-burned children after six months post-injury, these children displayed characteristics of impaired insulin sensitivity for up to three years post-burn when compared to normal children.

In healthy subjects, glucose metabolism is tightly regulated: Under physiological conditions, a postprandial increase in blood glucose concentration stimulates the release of insulin from pancreatic β-cells. Insulin mediates peripheral glucose uptake into skeletal muscle and adipose tissue and suppresses hepatic gluconeogenesis, thereby maintaining blood glucose homeostasis [5]. Burn associated metabolic alterations, however, can lead to significant modifications in energy substrate metabolism. In order to provide glucose, a major fuel source to vital organs, release of the above mentioned stress mediators opposes the anabolic actions of insulin [16]. By enhancing adipose tissue lipolysis [17] and skeletal muscle proteolysis [18], these mediators increase gluconeogenic substrates, including glycerol, alanine, and lactate, thus augmenting hepatic glucose production in burned patients [3]. Hyperglycemia fails to suppress hepatic glucose release during this time [19] and the suppressive effect of insulin on hepatic glucose release is attenuated, significantly contributing to post-trauma hyperglycemia [20]. Catecholamine-mediated enhancement of hepatic glycogenolysis, as well as direct sympathetic stimulation of glycogen breakdown, can further aggravate the hyperglycemia in response to stress [21]. Another counter-regulatory hormone of interest during stress of burn victims is glucagon. Glucagon, like epinephrine, leads to increased glucose production through both gluconeogenesis and glycogenolysis. The action of glucagon alone is not maintained over time; however, its action on gluconeogenesis is sustained in an additive manner with the presence of epinephrine, cortisol, and growth hormone [22]. Likewise, epinephrine and glucagon have an additive effect on glycogenolysis [22]. Recent studies reported that pro-inflammatory cytokines contribute indirectly to post-burn hyperglycemia by enhancing the release of the above mentioned stress hormones [23].

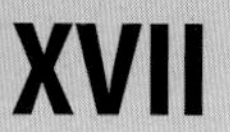

Inflammatory cytokines, such as TNF, as well as the above mentioned metabolic alterations post-burn, have also been implicated in contributing to lean muscle protein breakdown, both during the acute and convalescent phases in response to burn injury [24, 25]. In contrast to starvation, in which lipolysis and ketosis provide energy and protect muscle reserves, burn injury considerably decreases the ability of the human body to utilize fat as an energy source. Skeletal muscle, therefore, serves as a major source of fuel in the burn patient, which leads to marked wasting of lean body mass within days after injury [4]. This muscle breakdown has been demonstrated with whole body and cross leg nitrogen balance studies in which pronounced negative nitrogen balances persisted for 6 and 9 months after injury [26]. Since skeletal muscle has been found to be responsible for 70–80 % of whole body insulin-stimulated glucose uptake, decreases in muscle mass may significantly contribute to this persistent post-burn hyperglycemia. Impaired efficacy of insulin as a muscle protein anabolic agent post-burn, may in turn contribute to this persistent protein catabolism, subsequently leading to the weight loss and growth delay observed in our pediatric patient population for years following thermal injury.

Attenuation of the Hypermetabolic Response and Associated Hyperglycemia Post-burn

In recent years, therapeutic approaches have, therefore, mainly focused on reversing the hypermetabolic response with its ensuing catabolic state post-burn using a large number of different strategies. Besides early excision and closure of the burn wound, which has led to substantially reduced resting energy requirements and subsequent improvement in mortality rates in this patient population, pharmacological strategies, including growth hormone, insulin-like growth factor (IGF)-1, oxandrolone, testosterone, propranolol, and insulin have been successfully utilized in order to attenuate the hypermetabolic response to burn injury [3].

Insulin has, in particular, been extensively studied in this context. In addition to its ability to decrease blood glucose via mediating peripheral glucose uptake into skeletal muscle and adipose tissue and suppressing hepatic gluconeogenesis, insulin is known to increase DNA replication and protein synthesis via control of amino acid uptake, increased fatty acid synthesis and decreased proteinolysis [27]. The latter effect makes insulin particularly attractive for the treatment of hyperglycemia in severely burned patients since insulin given during acute hospitalization has been shown to improve muscle protein synthesis, accelerate donor site healing time, and attenuate lean body mass loss and the acute phase response [5]. In addition to its anabolic actions, insulin was shown to exert unexpected anti-inflammatory effects, potentially neutralizing the pro-inflammatory actions of glucose [28, 29]. In pediatric patients, intensive insulin therapy to maintain glucose levels between 90 and 120 mg/dl was associated with reduced infection rates and improved survival [30]. Other studies have indicated that insulin given to burn children may reduce increases in C-reactive protein (CRP), IL-1β and TNF levels after injury in the absence of normoglycemia [28, 31]. These results suggest a dual benefit of insulin administration: Reduction of the pro-inflammatory effects of glucose by restoration of euglycemia and a proposed additional insulin-mediated anti-inflammatory effect. Van den Berghe and colleagues confirmed the beneficial effects of insulin in a large milestone study [32]. Insulin administered to maintain glucose at levels below 110 mg/dl decreased mortality and the incidence of infections, sepsis and sepsis-associated multi-organ failure in surgically critically ill patients. However, since strict blood glucose control in order to maintain normoglycemia was required to obtain the maximum clinical benefit, the high incidence of hypoglycemic events and difficult

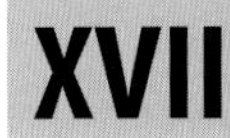

blood glucose titrations have led to the investigation of alternative therapeutic approaches that do not cause hypoglycemia as frequently as insulin, including the use of metformin, a biguanide. By inhibiting gluconeogenesis and augmenting peripheral insulin sensitivity, metformin directly counters the two main metabolic processes that underlie injury-induced hyperglycemia. Indeed, Gore and colleagues showed recently that metformin reduced plasma glucose concentration, decreased endogenous glucose production, and accelerated glucose clearance in severely burned patients [33]. A follow-up study looking at the effects of metformin on muscle protein synthesis, confirmed these observations and demonstrated an increased fractional synthetic rate of muscle protein and improvement in net muscle protein balance in metformin treated patients [34]. Metformin may thus, analogous to insulin, have efficacy in critically injured patients as both an anti-hyperglycemic and a muscle protein anabolic agent. However, the mechanisms by which insulin may improve morbidity and mortality remain unclear. Are these effects due to insulin itself or due to glucose modulation? In order to answer this question, better understanding of the molecular mechanisms underlying the actions of insulin post-burn is needed.

Molecular Mechanisms underlying Insulin Resistance Post-burn

The effects of insulin to maintain normoglycemia occur through the insulin signaling cascade [35]. On binding to the α-subunit on the extracellular portion of its receptor, insulin induces auto-phosphorylation of the β-unit leading to conformational changes and phosphorylation of insulin receptor substrate (IRS)-1 at a critical tyrosine residue, which in turn leads to activation of the phosphatidylinositol-3 kinase (PI3K)/Akt pathway [35]. Several studies have indicated the major role of PI3K in the regulation of metabolic actions of insulin signaling, including stimulation of glucose transport via phosphorylation of Akt and the resultant plasma membrane localization of the GLUT4 glucose transporter within hepatocytes, skeletal muscle, and adipose tissue [36]. Activation of Akt has also been shown to be of major importance for the regulation of hepatic glucose homeostasis via insulin signaling cascades, including inhibition of gluconeogenesis and glycogenolysis pathways and activation of glycolysis pathways via activation or inactivation of several key enzymes [37]. Other effects include activation of glycogen synthesis, lipid synthesis, inhibition of lipolysis, and lipocyte apoptosis [38–41].

Recent work now suggests that stress-induced insulin resistance may be in part due to phosphorylation-based negative-feedback, which may uncouple the insulin receptor or insulin receptor-associated proteins from their downstream signaling pathways, altering insulin action [42]. Epinephrine, for example, seems to exerts its effects on peripheral insulin resistance via this mechanism [43]. Specifically, phosphorylation of IRS-1 at serine residues by various kinases may preclude its tyrosine phosphorylation by the insulin receptor tyrosine kinase, thus inhibiting insulin receptor trafficking [42] (**Fig. 1**). Among these IRS-modifying enzymes, mounting evidence indicates that activation of c-Jun N-terminal kinase (JNK) and inhibitor of nuclear factor-kappa B (NF-κB) kinase-β (IKK) may play a central role in mediating insulin resistance in response to various stressors that occur in obesity and other conditions of insulin resistance (**Fig. 1**) [44]. Both JNK and IKK have been found to inhibit insulin action by serine phosphorylation of IRS-1 [45]; even though the activity of IKK in this regard has not yet been well established under physiological

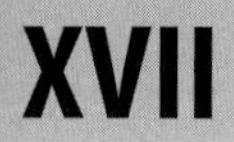

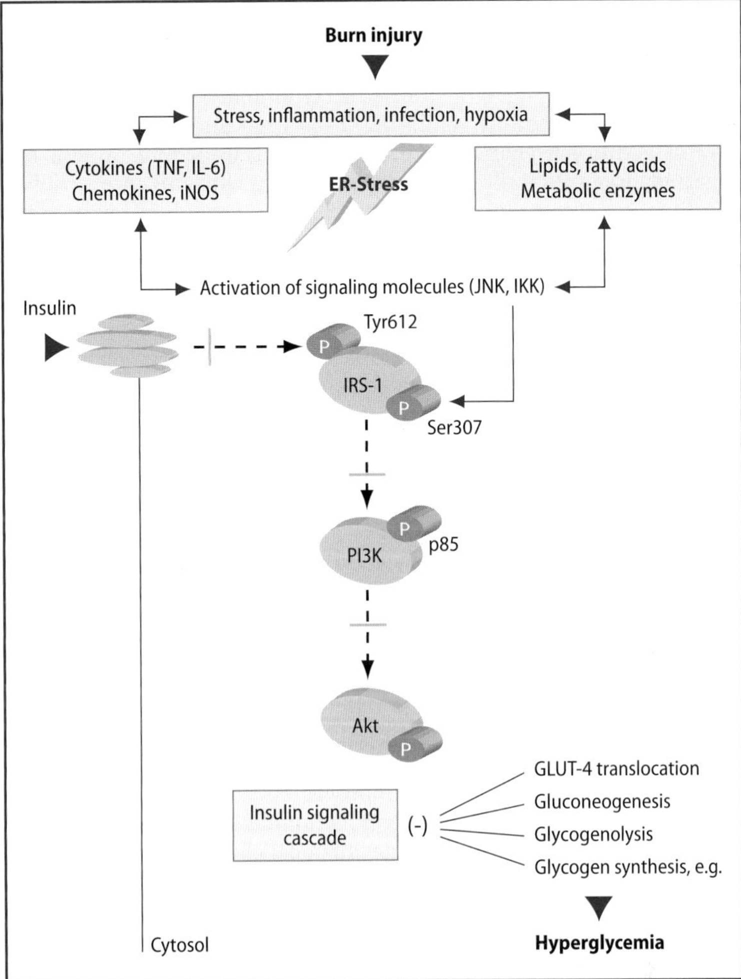

Fig. 1. Molecular mechanisms underlying insulin resistance following thermal injury. Activation of c-Jun N-terminal kinase (JNK) or inhibitor of nuclear factor-κB kinase-β (IKK) by cytokine signaling or lipid products during endoplasmic reticulum (ER) stress may lead to phosphorylation of insulin receptor substrate (IRS)-1 at serine residues which may preclude its tyrosine phosphorylation by the insulin receptor tyrosine kinase, thus resulting in impaired phosphatidylinositol-3 kinase (PI3K)/Akt signaling and insulin resistance with its associated consequences. TNF: tumor necrosis factor; IL: interleukin; iNOS: inducible nitric oxide synthase

conditions. Several studies reported that JNK is activated upon specific stimuli, including the presence of various cytokines, such as IL-6, IL-8, monocyte chemoattractant protein (MCP)-1 and TNF-α, and internal cues, including endoplasmic reticulum stress, all of which are present under conditions leading to hyperglycemia, such as obesity, diabetes mellitus, and stress [46]. It has been well established that a variety of cellular stress signaling and inflammatory pathways are activated as a consequence of burn. A key player in the cellular stress response is the endoplasmic reticulum, a membranous organelle that functions in the synthesis and processing of

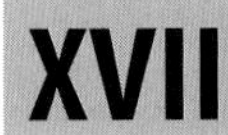

secretory and membrane proteins [45]. Certain pathological stress conditions disrupt the homeostasis of the endoplasmic reticulum and lead to accumulation of unfolded or misfolded proteins in the endoplasmic reticulum lumen [45]. The endoplasmic reticulum stress response limits unfolded protein burden in the endoplasmic reticulum lumen by inhibiting translation and inducing the nuclear transcription of additional chaperone proteins. If the unfolding protein burden cannot be reversed, apoptotic cell death occurs. To cope with this stress, cells activate a signal transduction system linking the endoplasmic reticulum lumen with the cytoplasm and nucleus, called the unfolded protein response (UPR) [45]. Endoplasmic reticulum stress is detected by transmembrane proteins which monitor the load of unfolded proteins in the endoplasmic reticulum lumen, and transmit this signal to the cytosol [46]. Two of these proteins, inositol requiring enzyme-1 (IRE-1) and PKR-like endoplasmic reticulum kinase (PERK), undergo oligomerization and phosphorylation in response to increased endoplasmic reticulum stress [46]. Work in our laboratory has recently demonstrated increased phosphorylation of IRE-1 and PERK in rat livers isolated 24 and 72 hours after burn injury, indicating activation of endoplasmic reticulum stress signaling pathways post-burn. We also found IRE-1 to be activated for up to 60 days after the initial burn injury in muscle samples of pediatric patients (Jeschke and colleagues, unpublished data).

Notably, activity of JNK has been linked to IRE-1 and PERK activity during endoplasmic reticulum stress [5]. Consistent with this phenomenon, we found total JNK activity, indicated by c-Jun phosphorylation, to be markedly elevated upon burn injury, associated with increased glucose and insulin levels for up to 60 days post-burn. The activation status of JNK may thus represent a central and integrating mechanism linking endoplasmic reticulum stress and intracellular glucose homeostasis, since serine phosphorylation of IRS-1 has been shown to impair insulin receptor signaling [46]. Indeed, interventions to block JNK activity in established models of obesity and diabetes improved systemic glucose homeostasis and insulin sensitivity, as well as atherosclerosis. Other novel therapeutic approaches include the use of orally active small-molecule chemical chaperones in order to attenuate endoplasmic reticulum stress by increasing cellular folding capacity. These chaperones have been previously shown to markedly alleviate obesity-induced endoplasmic reticulum stress and JNK activation, as well as treating insulin resistance and type 2 diabetes in mice [47].

Based on the above mentioned pathophysiologic and molecular mechanism underlying post-burn insulin resistance, cytokines and their receptors represent other obvious potential targets in order to attenuate injury-induced insulin resistance. However, even though there have been encouraging results using anti-TNF or anti-CCR2 (chemokine (C-C motif) receptor 2), the benefit of targeting cytokines or signaling receptors is likely to be limited [48, 49]. Thus, tackling a more central locus rather than targeting single molecules may prove more valuable for the development of novel and effective therapeutics to overcome insulin-resistance post-burn.

The insulin sensitizer, metformin, for example, has been recently shown to act via suppression of inducible NO synthase (iNOS), a key mediator of inflammation, in cultured cells as well as in diabetic rodents via activating AMP-activated protein kinase (AMPK), thus leading to improved insulin sensitivity [50]. And peroxisome proliferator-activated receptor (PPAR)-γ agonists, such as fenofibrate, were recently found to significantly decrease plasma glucose concentrations by improving insulin sensitivity and mitochondrial glucose oxidation [20]. Importantly, fenofibrate also

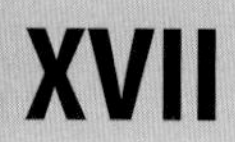

led to significantly increased tyrosine phosphorylation of the insulin receptor and IRS-1 in muscle tissue after hyperinsulinemic-euglycemic clamp when compared to placebo treated patients, indicating improved insulin receptor signaling [20].

These results may place the use of drugs like metformin and fenofibrate in a different light and may help to further elucidate the molecular mechanisms underlying insulin resistance post-burn.

Conclusion

The profound post-burn metabolic alterations associated with persistent changes in glucose metabolism and impaired insulin sensitivity significantly contribute to adverse outcome of this patient population. Recent studies now indicate that these conditions may last for much longer than currently expected. We, therefore, suggest that burned patients should be carefully monitored for the development of diabetes mellitus for a prolonged time after recovery from injury, since medical intervention may be warranted. Given that metabolic alterations and persistent protein catabolism may result in growth delay and may be associated with post-burn insulin resistance thus significantly contributing to adverse outcome of this patient population, therapeutic intervention in order to reverse these post-burn metabolic alterations may significantly improve the clinical outcome of this unique patient population. The weaknesses and potential side effects of currently used drugs reinforce the need for a better understanding of the molecular mechanisms underlying insulin resistance post-burn.

References

1. American Burn Association (2007) Guidelines for the operation of burn centers. J Burn Care Res 28: 134–141
2. Nguyen TT, Gilpin DA, Meyer NA, Herndon DN (1996) Current treatment of severely burned patients. Ann Surg 223: 14–25
3. Herndon DN (2007) Total Burn Care. Saunders Elsevier, New York
4. Herndon DN, Tompkins RG (2004) Support of the metabolic response to burn injury. Lancet 363: 1895–1902
5. Gauglitz GG, Herndon DN, Jeschke MG (2008) Insulin resistance postburn: Underlying mechanisms and current therapeutic strategies. J Burn Care Res 29: 683–694
6. Gore DC, Chinkes D, Heggers J, Herndon DN, Wolf SE, Desai M (2001) Association of hyperglycemia with increased mortality after severe burn injury. J Trauma 51: 540–544
7. Sheridan RL, (2001) A great constitutional disturbance. N Engl J Med 345: 1271–1272
8. Wolfe RR (1981) Review: acute versus chronic response to burn injury. Circ Shock 8: 105–115
9. Cuthbertson DP, Angeles Valero Zanuy MA, Leon Sanz ML (2001) Post-shock metabolic response. Nutr Hosp 16: 175–182
10. Galster AD, Bier DM, Cryer PE, Monafo WW, (1984) Plasma palmitate turnover in subjects with thermal injury. J Trauma 24: 938–945
11. Cree MG, Aarsland A, Herndon DN, Wolfe RR (2007) Role of fat metabolism in burn trauma-induced skeletal muscle insulin resistance. Crit Care Med 35: 476–483
12. Childs C, Heath DF, Little RA, Brotherston M (1990) Glucose metabolism in children during the first day after burn injury. Arch Emerg Med 7: 135–147
13. Hart DW, Wolf SE, Mlcak R, et al (2000) Persistence of muscle catabolism after severe burn. Surgery 128: 312–319
14. Jeschke MG, Mlcak RP, Finnerty CC, et al (2007) Burn size determines the inflammatory and hypermetabolic response. Crit Care 11:90

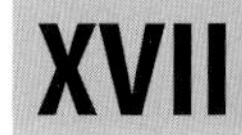

15. Norbury WB, Herndon DN (2007) Modulation of the hypermetabolic response after burn injury. In: Herndon DN (ed) Total Burn Care. Saunders Elsevier, New York, pp 420–433
16. Khani S, Tayek JA (2001) Cortisol increases gluconeogenesis in humans: its role in the metabolic syndrome. Clin Sci (Lond) 101: 739–747
17. Wolfe RR, Herndon DN, Jahoor F, Miyoshi H, Wolfe M (1987) Effect of severe burn injury on substrate cycling by glucose and fatty acids. N Engl J Med 317: 403–408
18. Gore DC, Jahoor F, Wolfe RR, Herndon DN (1993) Acute response of human muscle protein to catabolic hormones. Ann Surg 218: 679–684
19. Wolfe RR, Durkot MJ, Allsop JR, Burke JF (1979) Glucose metabolism in severely burned patients. Metabolism 28: 1031–1039
20. Cree MG, Zwetsloot JJ, Herndon DN, et al (2007) Insulin sensitivity and mitochondrial function are improved in children with burn injury during a randomized controlled trial of fenofibrate. Ann Surg 245: 214–221
21. Robinson LE, van Soeren MH (2004) Insulin resistance and hyperglycemia in critical illness: role of insulin in glycemic control. AACN Clin Issues 15: 45–62
22. Gustavson SM, Chu CA, Nishizawa M, et al (2003) Interaction of glucagon and epinephrine in the control of hepatic glucose production in the conscious dog. Am J Physiol Endocrinol Metab 284: 695–707
23. Lang CH, Dobrescu C, Bagby GJ (1992) Tumor necrosis factor impairs insulin action on peripheral glucose disposal and hepatic glucose output. Endocrinology 130: 43–52
24. Baracos V, Rodemann HP, Dinarello CA, Goldberg AL (1983) Stimulation of muscle protein degradation and prostaglandin E2 release by leukocytic pyrogen (interleukin-1). A mechanism for the increased degradation of muscle proteins during fever. N Engl J Med 308: 553–558
25. Jahoor F, Desai M, Herndon DN, Wolfe RR (1988) Dynamics of the protein metabolic response to burn injury. Metabolism 37: 330–337
26. Hart DW, Wolf SE, Chinkes DL, et al (2000) Determinants of skeletal muscle catabolism after severe burn. Ann Surg 232: 455–465
27. Pidcoke HF, Wade CE, Wolf SE (2007) Insulin and the burned patient. Crit Care Med 35: 524–530
28. Jeschke MG, Klein D, Bolder U, Einspanier R (2004) Insulin attenuates the systemic inflammatory response in endotoxemic rats. Endocrinology 145: 4084–4093
29. Jeschke MG, Klein D, Herndon DN (2004) Insulin treatment improves the systemic inflammatory reaction to severe trauma. Ann Surg 239: 553–560
30. Pham TN, Warren AJ, Phan HH, Molitor F, Greenhalgh DG, Palmieri TL (2005) Impact of tight glycemic control in severely burned children. J Trauma 59: 1148–1154
31. Hansen TK, Thiel S, Wouters PJ, Christiansen JS, Van den Berghe G (2003) Intensive insulin therapy exerts antiinflammatory effects in critically ill patients and counteracts the adverse effect of low mannose-binding lectin levels. J Clin Endocrinol Metab 88: 1082–1088
32. Van den Berghe G, Wouters P, Weekers F, et al (2001) Intensive insulin therapy in the critically ill patients. N Engl J Med 345: 1359–1367
33. Gore DC, Wolf SE, Herndon DN, Wolfe RR (2003) Metformin blunts stress-induced hyperglycemia after thermal injury. J Trauma 54: 555–561
34. Gore DC, Herndon DN, Wolfe RR (2005) Comparison of peripheral metabolic effects of insulin and metformin following severe burn injury. J Trauma 59: 316–323
35. White MF (1997) The insulin signalling system and the IRS proteins. Diabetologia 40 (Suppl 2): 2–17
36. Folli F, Saad MJ, Backer JM, Kahn CR (1992) Insulin stimulation of phosphatidylinositol 3-kinase activity and association with insulin receptor substrate 1 in liver and muscle of the intact rat. J Biol Chem 267: 22171–22177
37. Yu XX, Pandey SK, Booten SL, Murray SF, Monia BP, Bhanot S (2008) Reduced adiposity and improved insulin sensitivity in obese mice with antisense suppression of 4E-BP2 expression. Am J Physiol Endocrinol Metab 294: 530–539
38. Saltiel AR, Pessin JE (2003) Insulin signaling in microdomains of the plasma membrane. Traffic 4: 711–716
39. Ikezu T, Okamoto T, Yonezawa K, Tompkins RG, Martyn JA (1997) Analysis of thermal injury-induced insulin resistance in rodents. Implication of postreceptor mechanisms. J Biol Chem 272: 25289–25295

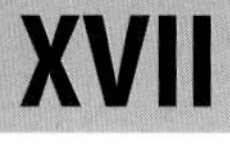

40. Chang L, Chiang SH, Saltiel AR (2004) Insulin signaling and the regulation of glucose transport. Mol Med 10: 65–71
41. Thurmond DC, Pessin JE (2001) Molecular machinery involved in the insulin-regulated fusion of GLUT4-containing vesicles with the plasma membrane. Mol Membr Biol 18: 237–245
42. Le Roith D, Zick Y (2001) Recent advances in our understanding of insulin action and insulin resistance. Diabetes Care 24: 588–597
43. Hunt DG, Ivy JL (2002) Epinephrine inhibits insulin-stimulated muscle glucose transport. J Appl Physiol 93: 1638–1643
44. Hotamisligil GS, Budavari A, Murray D, Spiegelman BM (1994) Reduced tyrosine kinase activity of the insulin receptor in obesity-diabetes. Central role of tumor necrosis factor-alpha. J Clin Invest 94: 1543–1549
45. Ozcan U, Cao Q, Yilmaz E, et al (2004) Endoplasmic reticulum stress links obesity, insulin action, and type 2 diabetes. Science 306: 457–461
46. Ron D, Walter P (2007) Signal integration in the endoplasmic reticulum unfolded protein response. Nat Rev Mol Cell Biol 8: 519–529
47. Ozcan U, Yilmaz E, Ozcan L, et al (2006) Chemical chaperones reduce ER stress and restore glucose homeostasis in a mouse model of type 2 diabetes. Science 313: 1137–1140
48. Wellen KE, Hotamisligil GS (2005) Inflammation, stress, and diabetes. J Clin Invest 115: 1111–1119
49. Shoelson SE, Lee J, Goldfine AB (2006) Inflammation and insulin resistance. J Clin Invest 116: 1793–1801
50. Pilon G, Dallaire P, Marette A (2004) Inhibition of inducible nitric-oxide synthase by activators of AMP-activated protein kinase: a new mechanism of action of insulin-sensitizing drugs. J Biol Chem 279: 20767–20774

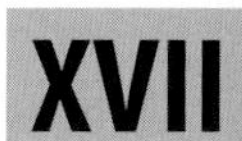

Glucose Variability in Critically Ill Patients

N.A. Ali, J.S. Krinsley, and J.-C. Preiser

Introduction

The presence of stress-induced hyperglycemia in critically ill patients, especially in those without evidence of antecedent diabetes, is a well established marker of poor outcomes [1–4]. Two large single center studies comparing the standard strategy of permissive hyperglycemia to use of intravenous insulin to achieve a blood glucose between 80 and 110 mg/dl (intensive insulin therapy) demonstrated overall clinical benefit with the intensive insulin therapy [5, 6]. However, more recent studies of insulin therapy in critically ill patients have yielded conflicting results [7]. In addition, a growing awareness of the potential risks of hypoglycemia, which can occur more frequently when using intravenous insulin therapy, has raised concerns over the best way to control glucose. Despite this, reverting back to allowing hyperglycemia to continue unchecked is unlikely to be the correct approach either.

It is likely that insulin therapy is not in question, but rather the details of how it should be instituted. In fact, previous reports have suggested that there are wide differences in the insulin treatment algorithms reported in the published literature [8, 9]. Some of these differences could lead to very different recommendations for treatment given similar glucose values and rate of preceding change [9]. In fact many clinical protocols incorporate intentionally vague dose ranges to allow for the experienced bedside practitioner to modify the insulin dose. All of these factors can lead to variation in the amounts of insulin used to treat hyperglycemia in intensive care unit (ICU) patients. Variation in insulin dosing is likely to be one factor that can lead to variation in the rate of glucose reduction. In addition, conditions that necessitate admission to the ICU, like sepsis, major surgery, and trauma, are likely to lead to pulses in endogenous pro-inflammatory cytokines and other counter-regulatory hormones [10, 11]. As these changes are often not clinically apparent at the patient's bedside, clinicians are unlikely to be aware that their patient's insulin sensitivity has changed.

These aspects can lead to a clinical situation where a stable dose of insulin leads to an unpredicted change in plasma glucose. While this situation, similar to the condition in type I diabetes termed 'brittle diabetes', has been interpreted as a risk for unsuspected hypoglycemia, recent studies have suggested that this phenomenon may in and of itself induce harm in critically ill patients. In this chapter, we describe the phenomenon of glucose variability, and explore contributing factors and the basis for its harmful effects. Finally, we speculate on glucose variability as an independent risk factor in critically ill patients and highlight the continued controversies in this area.

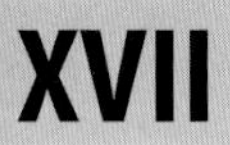

Glucose Elevation versus Variability

Multiple studies in general populations of critically ill patients have suggested that uncontrolled hyperglycemia increases the risk of poor outcomes in terms of mortality [2, 12, 13], prolonged ventilator dependency, and acquired infection [5]. However, closer analysis reveals that the implications of hyperglycemia are exaggerated or mitigated based on other characteristics [14]. For instance, diabetic patients appear to incur less risk if they manifest similar degrees of hyperglycemia compared to non-diabetic patients [15–17].

Despite the consistent observations of adverse effects of hyperglycemia on outcomes, recent studies have given unexpected results when intravenous insulin was used to maintain euglycemia in critically ill patients [6, 7, 18]. Two multicenter randomized controlled trials were stopped early due to evidence that there was no significant benefit of intensive insulin therapy [7, 18]. In these and most previous studies patients receiving aggressive levels of insulin support, had higher rates of hypoglycemia than those whose treatment targeted a higher glucose range [7, 15, 18]. Importantly, at least in patients with severe sepsis, hypoglycemic events were associated with a higher mortality rate [7]. The occurrence of hypoglycemia is very worrying in ICU patients as they are often unable to report premonitory symptoms, leaving active surveillance as the only safety net. Fortunately, because of the similarity of this problem to the diabetic patient with 'hypoglycemia unawareness', glucose trends, which can predict impending hypoglycemia, have been developed. A common element of all of these predictors includes assessment of 'glucose lability'. Several quantitative scores have demonstrated that wide swings in recorded glucose measures in patients with diabetes can predict hypoglycemia [19, 20].

Because of this link and the conflicting results of intensive insulin trials, ICU researchers have analyzed data from several large cohorts to determine the association between glucose variability and outcome. This group of reports has outlined an apparent independent association between variability of glucose and mortality in adult mixed ICU [21, 22], surgical ICU [23], pediatric ICU [24, 25] and adult septic [26] populations. In some studies, it appears that the relationship between variability of glucose and mortality is more direct than that seen with increasing average glucose concentration itself (**Fig. 1**).

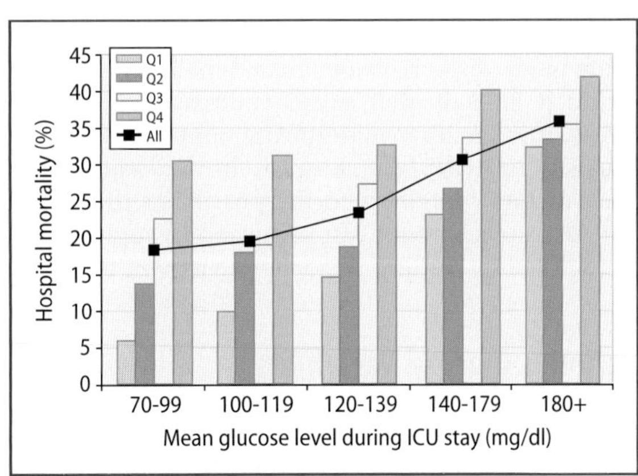

Fig. 1. Observed mortality in critically ill patients by glucose risk category. Each of the increments of mean glucose level is subdivided into four quartiles of glycemic variability. Q1, represents the lowest quartile; Q4, represents the highest quartile. From [22] with permission

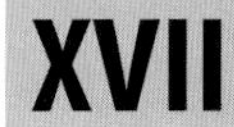

There are several reasons why glucose variability could induce harm in critically ill patients. First, there is evidence that rapid swings in blood glucose concentrations can induce endothelial and other cellular damage [27, 28]. Second, these same swings could result in wide changes in osmolarity that in turn could effect cellular and organ function [29–31]. Finally, because of the special dynamic needs of this vulnerable patient population, the wide swings in blood glucose concentration may mark the occurrence of occult hypoglycemia that could affect neurologic recovery of an already brain-injured patient.

There is ample evidence that cellular injury occurs in the presence of rapidly changing blood glucose concentration. Specifically, endothelial cells appear to undergo rapid apoptosis [27] and cellular signaling in monocytes appears to be deleteriously affected [32]. Previous investigations in diabetic patients have suggested that serum markers of endothelial dysfunction and oxidative stress are increased in those patients who experience glucose fluctuation independent of the average glucose concentration [33]. The specific marker measured in this study, 8-isoprostaglandin-F2α, indicated that oxidative stress was likely to be increased in patients experiencing variable glucose behavior. These authors concluded that this was secondary to endothelial injury [33]. Given the importance of adequate blood flow to the prevention of organ failure, it is reasonable to speculate that harm to the microvasculature accelerated by hyperactive inflammatory cells could lead to poor outcomes. Separately, since glucose is a major contributor to serum osmolarity, it is possible that wide swings in glucose concentration will lead to osmotic shifts. In critically ill patients, serum osmolarity has been shown to be associated with mortality independent of other known conditions [34]. Similar to the effects of hyperglycemia, osmolarity flux has also been shown to result in altered inflammatory response and impaired phagocytic function [29]. The potential reduction in osmolarity and resultant edema shifts have been proposed as a possible mechanism by which insulin therapy improves neurologic recovery in critically ill brain injured patients [30].

Finally, although the most speculative, perhaps the most important reason that variable glucose concentrations may be associated with worsened ICU outcomes is the fact that significant hypoglycemia could occur undetected. There are several factors that can contribute to this including the irregular frequency and accuracy of glucose testing utilized in common practice [9, 35]. Because continuous glucose monitoring has not been widely used in ICU patients, no active surveillance program can eliminate the possibility that significant glucose swings are occurring. Additionally, the well known limitations of measuring blood glucose, especially when point-of-care testing is used [35], make it possible that treatment decisions are being made with erroneous data. Finally, while the frequency of glucose surveillance makes it unlikely that occult mild hypoglycemia could result in neuroglycopenic injury, it is unclear what glucose concentration is required for normal central nervous system (CNS) homeostasis in the hypermetabolic, critically ill patient. All of these factors contribute to the possibility that variability may induce harm, in part due to the occurrence of undetected hypoglycemia or to an excessive correction of hypoglycemia, leading to abrupt swings in blood glucose concentration [36].

Defining Glucose Variability

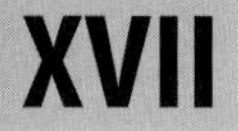

Given the importance of this newly recognized risk factor in critically ill patients, finding an operational definition is essential. However, since research in this area

Table 1. Definitions of variability proposed in critically ill patients.

Expression	Calculation	Population studied	Description
Standard deviation, SD [21, 22]	$\sqrt{\frac{1}{N}\sum_{i=1}^{N}(x_i - \bar{x})^2}$	Diabetics, sepsis, mixed ICU patients	Measure of the range of glucoses measured from the median
Mean amplitude of glycemic excursions, MAGE [26]	$\sum_{i=1}^{N} \lvert Y_i - Y_{i-1} \rvert \cdot N^{-1}$ if (Yi – Yi – 1) ≥ 1 SD of a subject's glucose values	Diabetics, sepsis	In assessing serial glucose values any continuous excursion that exceeds 1 SD of the range of glucose values is averaged.
Glycemic lability index, GLI [19, 26]	$\frac{(\text{mmol/liter})^2}{\text{h}} \cdot \text{week}^{-1}$	Sepsis, diabetes	Quantification of all rates of change between consecutive glucose measures
Maximum glucose change, $BG\Delta_{max}$ [23]	Largest of $\lvert x_{n+1} - x_n \rvert$ for all sequential values in the dataset	Surgical ICU	Maximum glucose change between any 2 consecutive glucose values
Variability Index [25]	$\sum \frac{\lvert x_{n+1} - x_n \rvert}{\lvert t_{n+1} - t_n \rvert} \cdot \text{N}^{-1}$	Pediatric ICU	Average of sequential rates of change between all consecutive glucose values
Glucose variability [24]	Any blood sugar ≥ 150 mg/dl *and* ≤ 60 mg/dl at anytime	Pediatric ICU	Presence of both a hyperglycemic *and* hypoglycemic event during a single hospitalization

ICU: intensive care unit

has only recently begun, there is no current consensus on the definition of glucose variability. Many different expressions of glucose variability have been described in the published literature [19–26] (**Table 1**).

One major discriminator in the methods proposed to assess glucose changes is whether they measure variability which would be observed clinically or not. This essentially can be determined by whether the assessment of variability depends on the assessment of consecutive glucose values or whether the metric is an assessment of the whole population of glucose values that a patient experiences. The maximal glucose change ($BG\Delta_{max}$) [23], Glycemic Lability Index (GLI) [26], and Variability Index [25] all assess the change across sequential glucose values with time being a component of the last two calculations. Glucose variability [24], the Mean Amplitude of Glycemic Excursions (MAGE) [26] and the standard deviation [21, 22] are all generated by an analysis of the entire group of glucose measures available at the time of retrospective analysis. No study has compared the predictive abilities of these measures in a large cohort of critically ill patients; therefore, the 'best' expression of glucose variability is currently unknown.

Contributors to Glucose Variability

The likely factors leading to labile glucose measures can be categorized into those related to clinical treatments including co-interventions, clinical monitoring, or endogenous patient factors. For patients who experience either increased variability

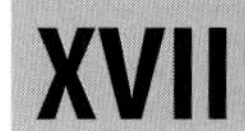

or unexpected hypoglycemia, it is likely that multiple factors are involved; as a result, this categorization is for discussion purposes only. There are several aspects of treatment that could lead to unexpected glucose changes. Insulin therapy itself can be complicated by the route of administration and type of insulin used. Compared to human regular and long acting insulin, the use of rapidly acting short half-life insulin analogs has been shown to reduce glucose variability in diabetic patients [37]. Additionally, problems related to poor circulation can affect drug absorption for insulin administered by the subcutaneous route. As most insulin administered in the ICU is regular insulin this could raise concerns; however, its administration by intravenous infusion likely mitigates the risk. Finally, the unexpected initiation or cessation of nutritional support, when not integrated with coincident insulin therapy can lead to dramatic blood glucose fluctuations [38].

Similarly, clinical monitoring of blood glucose concentration is fraught with imprecision, which can limit the validity of a measured value. The site of blood sample (arterial, venous or capillary) is well known to influence the blood glucose value obtained [26, 35]. Additionally, coincident use of vasopressors is likely to influence the relationship between capillary whole blood and arterial whole blood [35]. Finally, the specific device used to measure glucose, the type of reaction utilized, and the veracity of quality control procedures can all influence measured glucose and, therefore, the treatments recommended [35]. All of these factors can lead to unexpected treatment responses, especially if different samples (capillary or venous) and devices or testing methods are used over time.

Finally, and of most significant concern are the patient factors that can contribute to unpredictable glucose changes. Some obvious non-modifiable factors, like obesity [39], are associated with insulin resistance and, therefore, higher insulin dosing requirements could ultimately lead to higher variability. Other pathologic conditions, like severe sepsis, can lead to unexpected glucose changes likely because the state of counter-regulatory hormone responses and inflammatory cytokines responsible for insulin resistance are dynamic and unpredictable [40]. Finally, unrecognized organ failures, specifically renal and liver failure, can contribute to unexpected glucose changes until their presence is detected and integrated into treatment and drug dosing decisions.

Evidence of Harm in Critically Ill Patients

As alluded to earlier, definitions of glucose variability and the populations studied vary widely in the published literature. However, there has been enough similarity in risk and patient populations to enable some general characteristics to be outlined (**Table 2**). First, subjects at risk of glucose variability have to be in the ICU long enough to have more than two glucose measures in order to calculate any specific measure of variability. This means that patients with very brief ICU stays have been excluded from most of these studies. Second, the cohort studies available to date include a mix of patients who may or may not have been treated with insulin. Additionally, subjects in these studies have been managed with a mix of insulin strategies that vary in terms of routes of administration and glucose target. As a result, there is little known about what the effects of intensive insulin therapy is on glucose variability in these data sets. Finally, whether the variability observed in these studies was clinically apparent is unknown.

In the first report specifically looking at this issue in critically ill patients, Moritoki Egi et al. [21] reported on glucose exposure in a large cohort of adult critically

Table 2. Outcomes of critically ill patients by variability risk factor.

Study population	Variability risk factor	Association with mortality
Sepsis	GLI [26]	OR 4.73 (95 % CI 2.6–8.7) compared to subjects without increased GLI*
Pediatric ICU	Glucose variability [24]	OR 63.6 (95 % CI 7.8–512.2) compared to subjects without glucose variability
	Variability index [25]	> 6-fold increase in observed mortality for those in the highest 2 quintiles of variability
Adult mixed ICU patients	SD [21]	OR 1.28 (95 % CI, 1.14–1.44) per mmol/l increase in SD
	SD [22]	2–5 fold increase in mortality between the highest and lowest variability groups†

GLI: glycemic lability index; SD: standard deviation of glucose; OR: odds ratio; CI: confidence interval; * OR for mortality is the risk adjusted mortality for subjects with higher GLI in the absence of high average glucose; † only in subjects with average glucose < 140 mg/dl.

ill patients admitted to four hospitals in Australia between 2000 and 2004. This retrospective review demonstrated a 28 % (OR 1.28, 95 % CI 1.14–1.44) increase in the odds of hospital mortality for each 1 millimole increase in standard deviation independent of other markers of glucose exposure, severity of illness or admitting reason. This observation was confirmed in a separate cohort of patients in the US studied over a longer period of time between 1999 and 2007 [22]. This study [22] extended this observation by showing the effect of variability in different ranges of glucose exposure. In this analysis, the deleterious effects of increased glucose variability appeared to be greatest in those subjects whose average glucose was near normal. In a third study analyzing a surgical ICU population with the specific goal of assessing a variety of expressions of glucose exposure, a combination of factors that assessed the largest glucose excursion and the dose of insulin was highly associated with hospital mortality [23].

Two subsequent studies using different measures to analyze glucose related outcomes in critically ill pediatric patients have made similar observations [24, 25]. In these two studies, glucose variability, defined as the average of all sequential rates of glucose change [25] or the presence of both a hyper- and hypoglycemic event at any time [24], were both independent predictors of hospital mortality. One important note is that the study that used variability defined as the presence of both hyper- and hypoglycemia excluded patients being treated with insulin [24]. This suggests that the variability observed was more likely to be related to endogenous factors and not to treatments.

In a slightly different cohort analysis of hospitalized patients with severe sepsis, subjects who experienced higher than average variability were found to be at increased risk of hospital mortality, independent of the frequency of blood glucose testing, type of insulin therapy, or other confounding variables [26]. Importantly, in this analysis and the others referenced in this section, there remained a significant risk associated with hyperglycemia that was not completely explained by variability. In other words, it appears that the risk from increased glucose variability is an additional risk, but to get the full picture of glucose-related exposure, hyperglycemia and variability must be assessed and accounted for simultaneously. This is similar to the

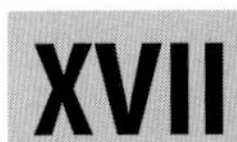

observations made by Krinsley [22], who showed that the risk associated with the standard deviation was attenuated in those subjects who had simultaneous hyperglycemia. Finally, glycemic variability may have different implications for diabetics and non-diabetics. Recent work demonstrated that heightened glycemic variability was strongly associated with increased risk of mortality in a large cohort of non-diabetic medical-surgical ICU patients, but not among diabetics (unpublished data). This finding reinforces other recent data illustrating the different impact of hyperglycemia in critically ill diabetics and non-diabetics. Just as the impact of variability needs to be placed into the context of the acute blood glucose level, it appears it should be placed in the chronic context as well. The long-term glucose dysregulation of diabetes mellitus leads not only to chronic hyperglycemia, but to increased exposure to wide swings in glucose concentration. As a result, it appears that whether a patient has diabetes mellitus may influence the risk observed with highly variable glucose exposure. This is similar to the observations that hyperglycemia appears to be a weaker risk-factor for mortality in critically ill diabetic patients than in non-diabetics [16, 17].

Future Directions

Despite the intriguing hypotheses suggested by the collected work presented in this chapter, there is still much that requires further dissection with respect to the problem of glucose variability. It is possible that untreated, endogenous, 'stress-induced' hyperglycemia may present in two distinct phenotypes: Sustained hyperglycemia or intermittent (or highly variable) hyperglycemia. Are these phenotypes important in the decision to manage blood sugar with insulin therapy? Is glucose variability truly an independent risk factor or simply an epiphenomenon to an as yet unknown process? Should variability be studied as presented here or as an expression of a pathophysiology that is not directly influenced by treatment, like insulin resistance?

Additionally, it remains to be demonstrated what the effect of insulin therapy is on glucose variability. This is an incredibly important question as the replicability of different insulin treatment protocols across different patient populations has been questioned [9]. It is easy to imagine that an overly aggressive protocol or the faulty implementation of a good protocol could in fact contribute to an *increase* in glucose variability. In other cases, patients experiencing spontaneous variability may in fact have their glucose variability reduced by the implementation of intravenous insulin and careful monitoring.

Despite the importance of the questions that remain unanswered, the current controversy that exists in critical care about whom to treat with insulin and to what effect mandates that these newly recognized risk factors be explored. With a better understanding of the effects of glycemic variability, we may gain insight into the inconsistent results of published interventional trials of glycemic control in critically ill patients [41]. It may be of great interest to the critical care community if the authors of the published major interventional trials re-analyzed their outcome data through the prism of these metrics. Finally, this science would be advanced if all future interventional trials explicitly reported indices of glycemic of variability as one of the key outcome parameters.

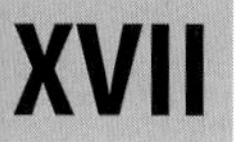

A greater understanding of the risk factors surrounding increased glycemic variability will facilitate the difficult work of designing interventions to control it. Given what we know of the problem at present, it is possible that these interventions could include, in part, protocolized enteral nutrition possibly with pharmacotherapy to slow carbohydrate absorption, variability adjusted insulin therapy, the use of continuous or near-continuous glucose monitors, or even "closed-loop" insulin management systems.

Conclusion

Glucose variability is an emerging risk factor for hospital mortality in critically ill hospitalized patients, as recently demonstrated in several different cohorts of patients from different ICU settings and in those with septic shock. The deleterious effect of increased glucose variability is greatest in patients whose mean glucose values are within or near the euglycemic range, and is much stronger in non-diabetics than in diabetics. Heightened variability may increase the risk of the occurrence of both spontaneous and iatrogenic severe hypoglycemia, a factor linked to increased mortality in these patients. Further clinical investigations are needed to elucidate the contributors to glucose variability and the role insulin therapy plays in its generation. Efforts to minimize glucose variability, including modifications of nutritional therapy, glucose monitoring, and insulin administration, may significantly improve the outcomes of acutely and critically ill patients.

References

1. Ali NA, O'Brien JM Jr, Blum W, et al (2007) Hyperglycemia in patients with acute myeloid leukemia is associated with increased hospital mortality. Cancer 110: 96–102
2. Umpierrez GE, Isaacs SD, Bazargan N, You X, Thaler LM, Kitabchi AE (2002) Hyperglycemia: an independent marker of in-hospital mortality in patients with undiagnosed diabetes. J Clin Endocrinol Metab 87: 978–982
3. Norhammar A, Tenerz A, Nilsson G, et al (2002) Glucose metabolism in patients with acute myocardial infarction and no previous diagnosis of diabetes mellitus: a prospective study. Lancet 359: 2140–2144
4. Silverman RA, Pahk R, Carbone M, et al (2006) The Relationship of Plasma Glucose and HbA1c Levels among Emergency Department Patients with No Prior History of Diabetes Mellitus. Acad Emerg Med 13: 722–726
5. Van den Berghe G, Wouters P, Weekers F, et al (2001) Intensive insulin therapy in the critically ill patients. N Engl J Med 345: 1359–1367
6. Van den Berghe G, Wilmer A, Hermans G, et al (2006) Intensive insulin therapy in the medical ICU. N Engl J Med 354: 449–461
7. Brunkhorst FM, Engel C, Bloos F, et al (2008) Intensive Insulin Therapy and Pentastarch Resuscitation in Severe Sepsis. N Engl J Med 358: 125–139
8. Wilson M, Weinreb J, Hoo GW (2007) Intensive insulin therapy in critical care: A review of 12 protocols. Diabetes Care. 30: 1005–1011
9. Morris AH, Orme JF Jr, Truwit JD, et al (2008) A replicable method for blood glucose control in critically Ill patients. Crit Care Med 36: 1787–1795
10. Marik PE, Raghavan M (2004) Stress-hyperglycemia, insulin and immunomodulation in sepsis. Intensive Care Med 30: 748–756
11. McCowen KC, Malhotra A, Bistrian BR (2001) Stress-induced hyperglycemia. Critical care clinics 17: 107–124
12. Wahl WL, Taddonio M, Maggio PM, Arbabi S, Hemmila MR. (2008) Mean glucose values predict trauma patient mortality. J Trauma 65: 42–48
13. Krinsley JS (2004) Effect of an intensive glucose management protocol on the mortality of critically ill adult patients. Mayo Clin Proc 79: 992–1000
14. Preiser JC, Devos P (2008) Clinical experience with tight glucose control by intensive insulin therapy. Crit Care Med 35:S503-S507

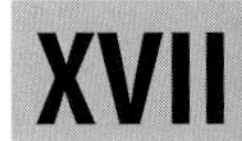

15. Van den Berghe G, Wilmer A, Milants I, et al (2006) Intensive insulin therapy in mixed medical/surgical intensive care units: benefit versus harm. Diabetes 55: 3151 – 3159
16. Egi M, Bellomo R, Stachowski E, et al (2008) Blood glucose concentration and outcome of critical illness: the impact of diabetes. Crit Care Med 36: 2249 – 2255
17. Krinsley JS (2006) Glycemic control, diabetic status, and mortality in a heterogeneous population of critically ill patients before and during the era of intensive glycemic management: six and one-half years experience at a university-affiliated community hospital. Semin Thorac Cardiovasc Surg 18: 317 – 325
18. Devos P, Preiser JC, Melot C (2007) Impact of tight glucose control by intensive insulin therapy on ICU mortality and the rate of hypoglycaemia: final results of the Glucontrol study. Intensive Care Med 33 (Suppl 2): S189 (abst)
19. Ryan EA, Shandro T, Green K, et al (2004) Assessment of the severity of hypoglycemia and glycemic lability in type 1 diabetic subjects undergoing islet transplantation. Diabetes 53: 955 – 962
20. Kovatchev BP, Otto E, Cox D, Gonder-Frederick L, Clarke W (2006) Evaluation of a new measure of blood glucose variability in diabetes. Diabetes Care 29: 2433 – 2438
21. Egi M, Bellomo R, Stachowski E, French CJ, Hart G (2006) Variability of blood glucose concentration and short-term mortality in critically ill patients. Anesthesiology 105: 244 – 252
22. Krinsley JS (2008) Glycemic variability: A strong independent predictor of mortality in critically ill patients. Crit Care Med 36: 3008 – 3013
23. Dossett LA, Cao H, Mowery NT, Dortch MJ, Morris JM Jr, May AK (2008) Blood glucose variability is associated with mortality in the surgical intensive care unit. Am Surg 74: 679 – 685
24. Hirshberg E, Larsen G, Van Duker H (2008) Alterations in glucose homeostasis in the pediatric intensive care unit: Hyperglycemia and glucose variability are associated with increased mortality and morbidity. Pediatr Crit Care Med 9: 361 – 366
25. Wintergerst KA, Buckingham B, Gandrud L, Wong BJ, Kache S, Wilson DM (2006) Association of hypoglycemia, hyperglycemia, and glucose variability with morbidity and death in the pediatric intensive care unit. Pediatrics 118: 173 – 179
26. Ali NA, O'Brien JM Jr, Dungan K, et al (2008) Glucose variability and mortality in patients with sepsis. Crit Care Med 36: 2316 – 2321
27. Risso A, Mercuri F, Quagliaro L, Damante G, Ceriello A (2001) Intermittent high glucose enhances apoptosis in human umbilical vein endothelial cells in culture. Am J Physiol Endocrinol Metab 281: E924-E930
28. Collier B, Dossett LA, May AK, Diaz JJ (2008) Glucose control and the inflammatory Response. Nutr Clin Pract 23: 3 – 15
29. Otto N, Schindler R, Lun A, Boenisch O, Frei U, Oppert M (2008) Hyperosmotic stress enhances cytokine production and decreases phagocytosis in vitro. Crit Care 12:R107
30. Van den Berghe G, Schoonheydt K, Becx P, Bruyninckx F, Wouters PJ (2005) Insulin therapy protects the central and peripheral nervous system of intensive care patients. Neurology 64: 1348 – 1353
31. Capes SE, Hunt D, Malmberg K, Pathak P, Gerstein HC (2001) Stress hyperglycemia and prognosis of stroke in nondiabetic and diabetic patients: A systematic overview. Stroke 32: 2426 – 2432
32. Schiekofer S, Andrassy M, Chen J, et al (2003) Acute hyperglycemia causes intracellular formation of CML and activation of ras, p42/44 MAPK, and nuclear factor {kappa}B in PBMCs. Diabetes 52: 621 – 633
33. Monnier L, Mas E, Ginet C, et al (2006) Activation of oxidative stress by acute glucose fluctuations compared with sustained chronic hyperglycemia in patients with type 2 diabetes. JAMA 295: 1681 – 1687
34. Holtfreter B, Bandt C, Kuhn SO, et al (2006) Serum osmolality and outcome in intensive care unit patients. Acta Anaesthesiol Scand 50: 970 – 977
35. Dungan K, Chapman J, Braithwaite SS, Buse J (2007) Glucose measurement: confounding issues in setting targets for inpatient management. Diabetes Care 30: 403 – 409
36. Suh SW, Gum ET, Hamby AM, Chan PH, Swanson RA (2007) Hypoglycemic neuronal death is triggered by glucose reperfusion and activation of neuronal NADPH oxidase. J Clin Invest 117: 910 – 918
37. Rossetti P, Porcellati F, Fanelli CG, Perriello G, Torlone E, Bolli GB (2008) Superiority of insu-

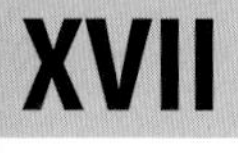

lin analogues versus human insulin in the treatment of diabetes mellitus. Arch Physiol Biochem 114: 3–10
38. Vriesendorp TM, van Santen S, DeVries JH, et al (2006) Predisposing factors for hypoglycemia in the intensive care unit. Crit Care Med 34: 96–101
39. Pieracci F, Hydo L, Eachempati S, Pomp A, Shou J, Barie PS (2008) Higher body mass index predicts need for insulin but not hyperglycemia, nosocomial infection, or death in critically ill surgical patients. Surg Infect (Larchmt) 9: 121–130
40. Rusavy Z, Sramek V, Lacigova S, Novak I, Tesinsky P, Macdonald IA (2004) Influence of insulin on glucose metabolism and energy expenditure in septic patients. Crit Care 8:R213-R220
41. Wiener RS, Wiener DC, Larson RJ (2008) Benefits and risks of tight glucose control in critically ill adults: A meta-analysis. JAMA 300: 933–944

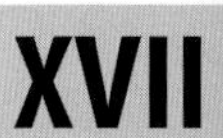

XVIII Adrenal Function

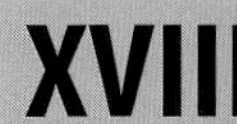

Corticosteroid Biology in Critical Illness: Modulatory Mechanisms and Clinical Implications

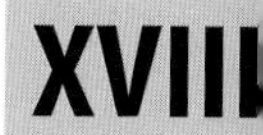

M. Williams and D.K. Menon

Introduction

In recent years there has been renewed interest in the use of steroids in sepsis and septic shock, focusing on lower doses and longer courses with the aim of supplementing a presumed under-activity of the hypothalamic-pituitary-adrenal (HPA) axis due to relative adrenal insufficiency or target tissue glucocorticoid resistance. An international task force of the American College of Critical Care Medicine recently published guidelines for the diagnosis and treatment of what they termed "critical illness-related corticosteroid insufficiency" [1]. This paper makes important recommendations regarding steroid therapy in sepsis and acute respiratory distress syndrome (ARDS). The authors also suggested biochemical definitions of relative adrenal insufficiency. A rational approach would be to use such definitions to make decisions regarding corticosteroid supplementation in critical illness. However, the authors concluded that the available literature provides no evidence to use such biochemical parameters as a basis for treating patients with supplemental steroids. This discordance, in large part, may arise from the fact that classical concepts of the HPA axis ignore many important nuances of glucocorticoid production, bioavailability and cellular action. The purpose of this chapter is to explore these nuances with particular focus on cellular and regional mechanisms of regulation of corticosteroid action, with specific reference to the context of critical illness.

Activation of the HPA Axis

The traditional paradigm of HPA-axis function begins with activation of neuroendocrine cells in the paraventricular nucleus of the hypothalamus, which release corticotropin releasing hormone (CRH) and vasopressin from neurosecretory terminals in the median eminence (**Fig. 1**). These hormones travel to the anterior pituitary, via the portal circulation of the hypophyseal stalk, where they act synergistically to trigger the release of stored adrenocorticotropic hormone (ACTH) from corticotrope cells into the bloodstream. They also induce transcription of pro-opiomelanocortin (POMC) which is cleaved by β-lipotropin to form ACTH. Increased circulating levels of ACTH stimulate ACTH-receptors on the surface of adrenocortical cells in the zona fasciculata of the adrenal glands. These cells respond by increasing the rate of synthesis of glucocorticoids from cholesterol; very little cortisol is stored, such that changes in plasma concentration are closely related to changes in the rate of synthesis.

The release of CRH is influenced by a multitude of factors including the sleep/wake cycle, psychological stress (via neural input from the limbic system), circulat-

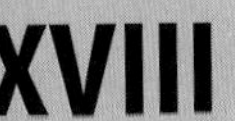

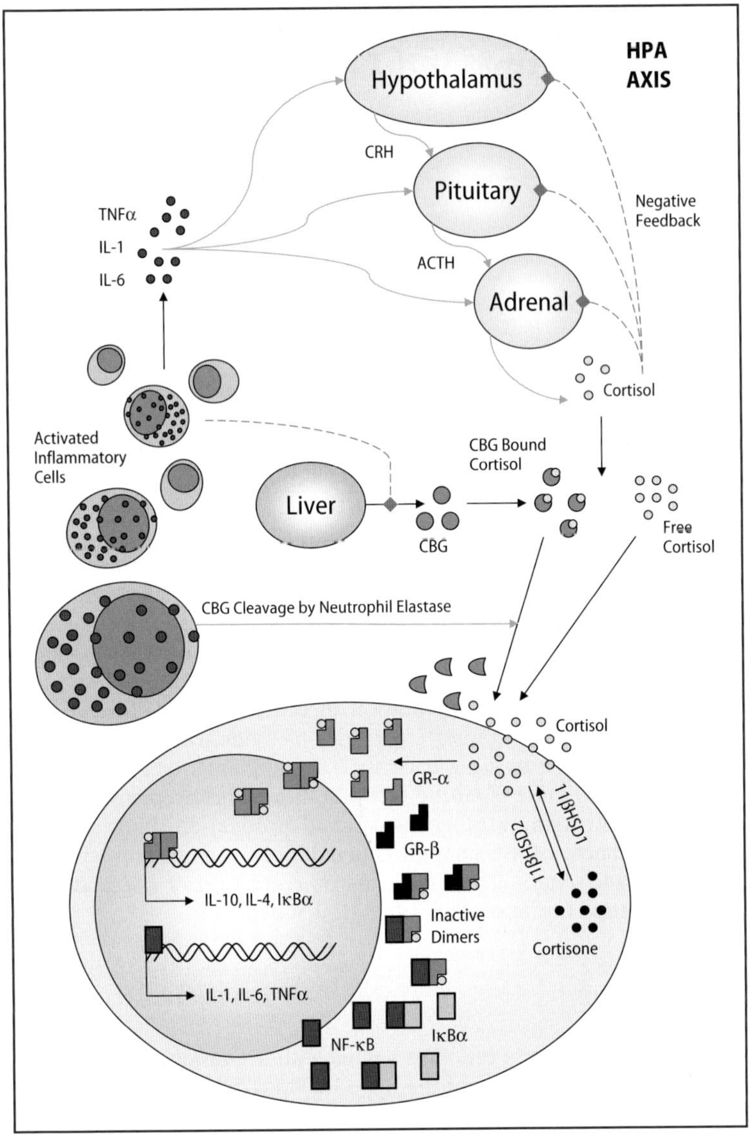

Fig. 1. A schematic representation of the hypothalamic-pituitary-adrenal (HPA) axis and the cellular effects of cortisol. CRH: corticotropin releasing hormone; ACTH: adrenocorticotropic hormone; CBG: cortisol binding globulin; GR: glucocorticoid receptor; 11β-HSD: 11β-hydroxysteroid dehydrogenase; IL: interleukin; TNF: tumor necrosis factor; NF-κB: nuclear factor-kappa B

ing inflammatory cytokines, and plasma levels of cortisol. The latter provides one of several negative feedback loops to regulate plasma glucocorticoid levels. The inflammatory cytokines (tumor necrosis factor [TNF]-α, interleukin [IL]-1, and IL-6) are capable of stimulating CRH release both directly and via afferent vagal fibers. It may seem paradoxical that, in response to inflammation, infection or injury, the body

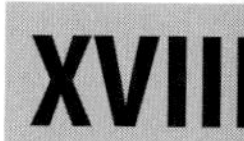

releases an anti-inflammatory agent that causes immunosuppression and delayed wound healing. However, this represents a vital counter-regulatory mechanism that balances positive inflammatory feedback loops.

Under basal conditions, ACTH is secreted in a pulsatile manner with diurnal variation, making individual measurements of ACTH and cortisol difficult to interpret. There is increasing evidence that during critical illness the levels of these two hormones become dissociated, with the chronic phase being characterized by low ACTH levels and high circulating cortisol [2]. There are also a growing number of factors that have been shown to directly stimulate adrenal synthesis of cortisol, independent of ACTH. These include various cytokines (IL-6), endothelial derived factors and direct neural stimulation. These extra-axial stimulatory factors may explain the observation that the hypercortisolemia of sepsis is not suppressible by exogenous dexamethasone [3]. Various stages in the HPA-axis are also subject to additional modulation, with the adrenal response to ACTH being augmented or diminished depending on the stimulus (e.g., physical versus psychological stress). TNF-α may also act to reduce the pituitary response to CRH and the adrenal response to ACTH; this is one of several examples of how the inflammatory cascade acts to antagonize the HPA-axis.

In summary, the changes in critical illness may involve new control mechanisms, as well as alteration of feedback loops that operate in health. These observations may explain some of our difficulties in defining meaningful thresholds for abnormal adrenocortical function in critical illness. A rational approach to corticosteroid supplementation in critical illness depends on a better understanding, not only of the mechanisms affecting cortisol production, but also those affecting its transport, local bioavailability, and intracellular action.

Transport of Cortisol in the Serum by Cortisol Binding Globulin

Approximately 90 % of cortisol in the serum is bound to protein, the majority to cortisol binding globulin (CBG), some to albumin, and a small fraction to sex-hormone-binding globulin. CBG represents a discrete pool of specific, high affinity binding, whereas albumin provides a large reservoir of low affinity, non specific binding sites. It is widely accepted that free cortisol is the biologically active form, as only unbound cortisol is able to cross the cell membrane and bind to the glucocorticoid receptor. CBG is, therefore, ideally placed to facilitate delivery of glucocorticoids to tissues and to control the amount of free cortisol available for utilization by cells.

CBG is a 58 kDa alpha globulin produced by the liver, although low levels of expression have been demonstrated in other tissues. Intriguingly, this protein is structurally unrelated to other steroid-binding proteins, but shares large parts of its sequence with members of the serine protease inhibitor (SERPIN) superfamily [4]. Other family members include α1-antitrypsin and several components of the clotting cascade. These proteins are of particular interest as they undergo radical conformational changes upon interaction with their targets, leaving both proteins irrevocably altered (a suicide interaction). CBG is a non-inhibitory member of this family, its function presumably having diverged and adapted to hormone delivery. It is not the only SERPIN to have done this; thyroxine-binding globulin (TBG) is a SERPIN with similar properties to CBG. These proteins, however, retain their ability to interact with serine proteases. CBG reacts with neutrophil elastase, which cleaves a 5 kDa fragment from CBG, and dramatically reduces its affinity for cortisol.

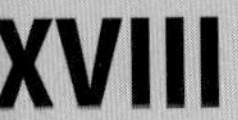

Neutrophil elastase is released by exocytosis from activated neutrophils at sites of inflammation, with a proportion of molecules remaining bound to the cell membrane [5]. Incubation of CBG with activated neutrophils (from septic patients) results in cleavage of CBG and release of cortisol; a phenomenon that has been shown to occur at the cell membrane and not to involve internalization [6]. The presence of a characteristic cleavage product of TBG has been demonstrated in the serum of septic patients [7], although similar studies looking for CBG cleavage in critical illness have yet to be performed. CBG has also been shown to have a reduced affinity for cortisol in the conditions of low pH and high temperature that are seen in inflammation [8]. Thus, the properties of CBG are well suited to allow specific release of cortisol at sites of inflammation.

CBG has been noted to behave as a negative acute phase response protein, its concentration falling in response to a variety of inflammatory stimuli. IL-6 inhibits CBG production in human hepatoblastoma (Hep G2) derived cells, and CBG concentrations in clinical sepsis that do not relate to disease severity or mortality have been shown to be inversely related to IL-6 levels [9]. Glucocorticoids have also been shown to suppress CBG production, glucocorticoid receptor knock out mice display high basal CBG levels that are not suppressed by dexamethasone [10]. However, glucocorticoid receptor-mediated effects of glucocorticoids on CBG levels may be complex and difficult to predict [11].

These mechanisms may represent a two tier system for ensuring the availability of free cortisol to tissues during illness, with local delivery of cortisol being achieved by CBG cleavage at sites of inflammation and central control being exerted through increased cortisol production and decreased CBG concentrations, providing a greater concentration of free cortisol to all tissues during systemic inflammation.

CBG and Biochemical Testing of the HPA-Axis

The occupancy of CBG binding sites at rest is such that increased levels of cortisol following ACTH stimulation result in saturation of CBG and a non-linear rise in the concentration of free cortisol [12]. Coupled with a cortisol-induced decrease in CBG production, this means that the amount of cortisol available to tissues varies more greatly than routine measurements of total serum cortisol might suggest. This difference may be even more pronounced in critical illness, when extra-axial activation of the adrenal glands impairs negative feedback, and CBG concentrations are forced lower still by inflammatory stimuli. It is not surprising that there has been difficulty in the interpretation of short synacthen tests in patients with low CBG levels [13, 14]. A dramatic example is seen in a family affected by a rare null mutation of the CBG gene. Homozygotes have very low basal cortisol levels and a poor response to ACTH testing (as measured by total cortisol), but a normal basal level and response when free cortisol is assayed [15]. It is intriguing that, despite normal free cortisol levels, homozygotes and heterozygotes for the mutation manifest extreme fatigue and hypotension, suggesting that CBG may have independent biological effects beyond cortisol transport.

In response to the challenges of correcting for changes in CBG levels, many groups have tried to calculate or measure directly the concentrations of free cortisol before and after ACTH testing (short synacthen test), as a more accurate measure of cortisol availability during critical illness [16, 17]. However, there remains controversy as to whether these tests are predictive of the need for glucocorticoid therapy

[18]. Although validated in healthy volunteers, there is some doubt as to whether these methods are reliable in critical illness. For example, the Coolens method [19] assumes normal albumin concentrations, and both the free cortisol index (FCI) and the Coolens method use CBG concentration to derive free cortisol levels [19]. This assumes that all of the CBG present participates uniformly in cortisol binding, which would not be the case if a significant proportion of circulating CBG was cleaved.

Cellular Activation and Inactivation of Cortisol by 11βHSD-1 and -2

Once free cortisol enters the cell it is subject to metabolism by two related enzymes: 11β-hydroxysteroid dehydrogenase type 1 (11β-HSD1) and 11β-hydroxysteroid dehydrogenase type 2 (11β-HSD2). These catalyze the interconversion of cortisol to cortisone, which has greatly reduced activity at the glucocorticoid receptor and decreased binding affinity with CBG. Whilst cortisone is generally regarded as an inactive metabolite, it does represent a pool of cortisol precursor that can be rapidly activated if required.

11β-HSD1 is a member of the short chain reductase/dehydrogenase family which catalyzes the reduction of cortisone to form active cortisol. Whilst this enzyme is capable of performing the reverse reaction, the availability of co-factors and the removal of cortisol maintain an equilibrium that favors the forward reaction. Both enzymes are located in the membrane of the endoplasmic reticulum – the catalytic moiety of 11β-HSD1 has been shown to be facing inward and the active site of 11β-HSD2 to be facing outward [20]. The authors of this study [20] propose a system in which hepatocytes reactivate cortisone and load it directly onto CBG prior to excretion, the concentration of 11β-HSD1 within the lumen allowing increased production of cortisol without over stimulation of the cytosolic glucocorticoid receptor.

During early inflammation, IL-1β and TNF-α, produced by T helper 1 (Th1) cells, have been shown to upregulate 11β-HSD1 and to downregulate 11β-HSD2. Later production of IL-2, IL-4 and IL-13 by T helper 2 (Th2) cells seems to upregulate HSD2, possibly preventing prolonged immunosuppression [21]. These findings are supported by the observation that septic patients display a cortisol:cortisone ratio that increases in proportion to the acute phase response. 11β-HSD1 represents another level at which the intracellular availability of cortisol can be regulated during critical illness.

The mineralocorticoid receptor has equal affinity for cortisol, corticosterone, and mineralocorticoids (aldosterone). 11β-HSD2 is present in aldosterone sensitive tissues, where it inactivates cortisol, thus protecting the mineralocorticoid receptor from constant over-stimulation by glucocorticoids, which are present in much higher concentrations than mineralocorticoids. The importance of this function is exemplified by a rare autosomal recessive mutation causing a loss of function of 11β-HSD2; this results in a syndrome of mineralocorticoid excess, characterized by hypertension, salt retention, and metabolic alkalosis. A similar clinical picture can be caused by an excess of licorice and the related drug carbenoloxone, both of which act by inhibiting 11β-HSD2.

An understanding of the function of 11β-HSD2 in providing mineralocorticoid receptor specificity may also offer an explanation for the observed benefit of hydrocortisone over other synthetic glucocorticoids in the treatment of septic shock. Hydrocortisone has a greater affinity for the mineralocorticoid receptor than other

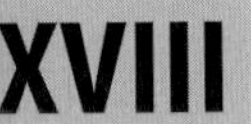

commonly used steroids, and even moderate doses (50 mg three times daily) produce supra-physiological concentrations that are capable of saturating 11β-HSD2 and activating the mineralocorticoid receptor. The hypertension and metabolic alkalosis associated with mineralocorticoids may be useful effects for reversing the hypotension and metabolic acidosis of septic shock [22]. Indeed, the shift toward glucocorticoid and away from mineralocorticoid production during stress may even be a contributing factor in the development of refractory shock. The benefits of hydrocortisone and fludrocortisone (a synthetic mineralocorticoid) in combination have been suggested by clinical studies, in which they were shown to have a beneficial effect on reversing shock but not on survival [23]. Randomized controlled trials comparing hydrocortisone and fludrocortisone with hydrocortisone alone, are currently underway (clinicaltrials.gov identifier NCT00368381).

The Glucocorticoid Receptor

First cloned in 1985, the glucocorticoid receptor was shown to be a member of the nuclear hormone receptor family. The glucocorticoid receptor is a transcription factor which, in its inactive form, is bound to several other proteins, including heat shock proteins 70 and 90 (HSP70, HSP90) and FK506-binding protein 52 (FKBP52). Activation by cortisol binding triggers dissociation from this protein complex, dimerization and translocation to the nucleus. The glucocorticoid receptor exerts many genomic and non-genomic effects, some of which involve binding to specific DNA sequences called glucocorticoid response elements (GREs), with subsequent recruitment of co-activators and increased gene transcription (transactivation). Other actions are DNA independent, and involve direct interactions with other transcription factors, such as nuclear factor-kappa B (NF-κB), which prevents expression of their target genes (transrepression) [24]. This example is of central importance as NF-κB activates the expression of IL-1, IL-6 and TNF-α, key components of the inflammatory response which interact with the HPA-axis at many levels. Glucocorticoid receptors and their co-factors exist in various concentrations in different cells leading to tissue specific responses to cortisol.

The observation that increased levels of cortisol in sepsis and ARDS often fail to suppress inflammatory cytokines led to the concept of systemic inflammation-associated glucocorticoid resistance. In various chronic inflammatory diseases (asthma, chronic obstructive airway disease [COPD], ulcerative colitis), tissue resistance to exogenous steroid has been well documented. Glucocorticoid resistance has been shown to be induced in a cytokine concentration dependant manner that is reversible upon removal of the cytokines [25]. A suggested explanation is that an excess of cytokine-induced transcription factors form complexes with glucocorticoid receptors, preventing their binding to GREs. These transcription factors antagonize each other at several levels. Glucocorticoid receptors form complexes with NF-κB and activator protein-1 (AP-1) preventing their binding to DNA. Glucocorticoid receptors also upregulate anti-inflammatory mediators; and increase levels of IκBα, which sequesters NF-κB in the cytoplasm. Conversely, NF-κB upregulates various pro-inflammatory mediators that exert positive feedback effects upon the inflammatory cascade and interfere with glucocorticoid receptor function: IL-1 may prevent translocation of glucocorticoid receptors to the nucleus and TNF-α can prevent glucocorticoid receptor transactivation independent of NF-κB by binding to the nuclear receptor binding domain of glucocorticoid receptor interacting protein 1 [26]. The

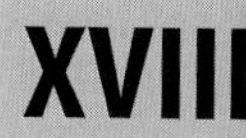

balance of glucocorticoid receptor and NF-κB may underpin the struggle between inflammation and HPA-axis in sepsis and systemic inflammatory response syndrome (SIRS).

The clinical relevance of this concept is demonstrated by the finding that peripheral blood lymphocytes from normal subjects, incubated with the serum from patients with ARDS, express glucocorticoid receptor and NF-κB in ways that correlate with the clinical progress of the patient. Serum from patients who were clinically improving increased glucocorticoid receptor expression and decreased NF-κB expression, whereas sera from patients who remained clinically unwell caused a modest increase in glucocorticoid receptor and a large increase in NF-κB expression. This difference was especially pronounced in non-survivors [27]. Increased glucocorticoid receptor sensitivity and reduced NF-κB were also seen with sera from patients that had been treated with a prolonged course of methylprednisolone. The treated patients showed reductions in levels of IL-1, IL-6, TNF-α, ACTH, and cortisol, that paralleled improvement in organ dysfunction scores [28]. An increase in both NF-κB and glucocorticoid receptor expression in neutrophils has also been demonstrated in SIRS [29]. The simultaneous increase in the expression of two antagonistic transcription factors may seem paradoxical. However, they must remain closely coupled if the immune response is to be balanced and not descend into uncontrolled inflammation or immunosuppression.

The glucocorticoid receptor gene can be alternatively spliced to form an isoform called glucocorticoid receptor-β (GR-β). Unlike the regular form (GR-α), GR-β is not capable of binding cortisol and antagonizes the transactivation of GREs by binding to various co-activators and forming inactive dimers. Studies have suggested that GR-β may account for steroid resistance seen in chronic inflammatory conditions [30]; its significance in acute illness remains to be seen.

There are many other factors that may also contribute to the development of glucocorticoid resistance, including reduced affinity of the glucocorticoid receptor, reduced DNA binding, decreased histone acetylation, altered concentrations of co-activators, and increased conversion of cortisol to cortisone.

Effects of Glucocorticoid Receptor Ligation

Overall, glucocorticoids affect the transcription of thousands of genes, some estimate that up to 20 % of the genome of mononuclear leukocytes is affected by the glucocorticoid receptor. Whilst mice lacking glucocorticoid receptors are not viable, transgenic mice with mutations in the dimerization domain of the glucocorticoid receptor are not only capable of survival but also retain the function of many homeostatic mechanisms that are known to require glucocorticoids. This suggests that many glucocorticoid receptor actions are independent of dimerization and DNA binding.

The traditional model of glucocorticoid receptor function has been that the anti-inflammatory effects are mediated predominantly by transrepression that is independent of DNA binding and dimerization. One example may be the binding of glucocorticoid receptors to NF-κB to form an inert complex that is no longer capable of gene activation. This paradigm has led to the development of dissociating ligands which bind to the glucocorticoid receptor producing allosteric changes that are similar, but not identical, to those induced by cortisol. The resulting conformation may be capable of translocation but not DNA binding, or may only recruit certain co-fac-

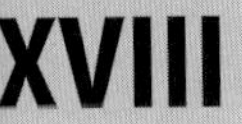

tors, thus dissociating the various glucocorticoid receptor actions. Compound A is a plant derived glucocorticoid receptor agonist whose ligand-receptor complexes are capable of transrepression but not GRE activation, the result being an anti-inflammatory agent with a reduced side effect profile [31].

Recent findings have challenged this traditional view, and re-emphasized the importance of the increased expression of anti-inflammatory genes. Mitogen activated protein kinases (MAPKs) are a group of serine/threonine-specific protein kinases which form intracellular signaling pathways that are triggered by a variety of cell surface stimuli. The JNK, ERK and p38 pathways are of particular relevance to inflammation, and are activated by cellular stress, lipopolysaccharide (LPS), IL-1 and TNF-α. These pathways result in the production and post-transcriptional modification of many pro-inflammatory mediators. Persistent activation of p38 and JNK has been described in glucocorticoid resistant patients [32]. Dual specificity phosphatases (DUSPs – also known as MAPK phosphatases) are enzymes that catalyze the dephosphorylation of MAPKs, thus serving to inactivate the components of these pathways and restrict the inflammatory response. DUSP-1 is activated by pro-inflammatory stimuli, forming a negative feedback loop, the importance of which is seen in DUSP-1 knockout mice which show exaggerated and lethal responses in models of sepsis and autoimmune inflammation. Glucocorticoids also act synergistically with IL-1 and LPS to increase the expression of DUSP-1, thus modulating the amplitude of the negative feedback [33]. The downregulation of many inflammatory products by glucocorticoids is partially impaired in DUSP-1 knockouts, suggesting a wider involvement of this protein.

Importance of Steroid Responsiveness in the Etiology of Sepsis and SIRS

The role of excessive immune activation in conditions such as sepsis and SIRS has been shown by numerous animal models. The importance of the HPA-axis in moderating this response has also been widely demonstrated. Doses of LPS, TNF-α and IL-1 that were tolerated in wild-type animals proved fatal in adrenalectomized or hypophysectomized rats; these fatal effects were blocked by pre-administration of dexamethasone [34].

Increased expression of the glucocorticoid receptor in transgenic mice leads to an increased resistance to the effects of LPS, with a dramatic improvement in survival [35]. Interestingly these shock resistant animals displayed lower levels of CRH, ACTH, POMC and cortisol, with normal responses to exogenous ACTH (synacthen). The negative feedback of cortisol on the hypothalamus is known to be glucocorticoid receptor dependent; greater sensitivity to glucocorticoids and enhancement of this feedback may explain these findings. This also reminds us that low cortisol measurements alone do not necessarily reflect the steroid status of an organism, as changes in the tissue responsiveness can more than compensate for variations in cortisol availability. Arguably, over activity of glucocorticoid receptor in models of true bacterial sepsis may result in worse outcomes by promoting an inappropriate anti-inflammatory response; however there are no studies that address this issue.

Blockade of the glucocorticoid receptor by RU 486 (mifepristone) caused increased mortality to LPS, which was attenuated by pre-treatment with corticosteroids. Concentrations of IL-6 and TNF-α also increased with blockade and decreased with corticosteroid pre-treatment [36]. A potential clinical correlate of

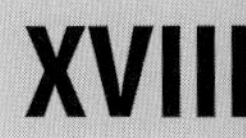

this finding is the report of several cases of rapidly fatal septic shock following medical abortions performed using oral mifepristone and vaginal misoprostol. In each case, the organism *Clostridium sordellii* was identified, but shown to be restricted to the endometrium, suggesting toxic shock as the cause of death [37]. Interestingly these patients presented prior to the onset of infection and shock with symptoms that were consistent with adrenal insufficiency: Abdominal pain, hypotension and fatigue. It has been suggested that blockade of the glucocorticoid receptor resulted in an exaggerated systemic response to this organism as seen in animal models [38, 39]. There remains debate as to the strength of this correlation, given the numbers of uneventful abortions carried out using these agents and reports of several cases of septic shock associated with the use of drugs that do not block the glucocorticoid receptor [40].

In many animal models of septic shock, the administration of exogenous glucocorticoids has dramatic effects, suppressing inflammatory mediators and reducing mortality. However, this finding is not consistently duplicated in clinical practice, where large doses of steroids may even be detrimental. The most obvious difference between these studies and the management of septic patients is the timing of treatment, with most animal models being given glucocorticoids prior to LPS injection, as opposed to the treatment of patients, where the agent is given only when shock is established. A potential molecular explanation for the importance of timing may be found in the actions of nitric oxide (NO) during inflammation [41]. Inducible NO synthase (iNOS) is activated by the inflammatory cascade and suppressed by cortisol, and is thought to contribute to the development of shock through the vasodilatory actions of NO. Dexamethasone given prior to the administration of LPS completely blocked the induction of iNOS and prevented increases in serum nitrate and nitrite concentration. However, administration of dexamethasone as early as four hours post-LPS failed to suppress iNOS, or alter serum nitrite and nitrate levels. Indeed, NO may reduce glucocorticoid effects at the glucocorticoid receptor. Giving an NO donor (S-nitroso-N-acetylpenicillamine, SNAP) prior to glucocorticoids reduced glucocorticoid receptor binding and abolished their suppressive effects, whilst NOS inhibitors prevented the reduction in glucocorticoid receptor binding that is often induced by LPS. These finding suggest a role for NO in mediating inflammatory induced glucocorticoid insensitivity and provide an explanation for the discrepancies between animal models and the clinical effects of steroid therapy.

Notwithstanding the discussion above, it must be recognized that the interaction between NO and glucocorticoids in sepsis is complex. Cortisol has been shown to both upregulate and downregulate iNOS, while NO has been shown to both decrease glucocorticoid receptor sensitivity and to increase its expression. A recent study suggested a synergistic benefit of inhaled NO with intravenous glucocorticoids in models of ARDS. Co-administration of NO was associated with an increased expression of the glucocorticoid receptor and preservation of normal tissue histology following LPS-induced lung injury in pigs [42]; this was prevented by pre-treatment with mifepristone. The opposite effects of NO seen in these two studies [41, 42] may be explained by tissue specific responses to cortisol, but clearly much more work needs to be done to clarify the involvement of NO in the interaction of the HPA-axis and inflammatory processes in critical illness.

It is clear that experimental defects at many levels of the steroid response predispose to the development of uncontrolled inflammation, but what factors influence the susceptibility of normal individuals? Social disruption stress has been shown to decrease glucocorticoid receptor expression in mice, resulting in a greater rise in

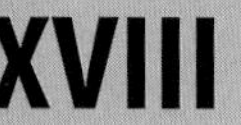

inflammatory markers (TNF-α and IL-1) and increased mortality in response to LPS injection [43]. The rise in serum glucocorticoid concentrations was not significantly different from control animals and glucocorticoid resistance was demonstrated in cultured splenocytes from these animals. Interestingly this effect was specific to social disruption stress, and animals exposed to restraint stress displayed similar increases in cortisol in response to LPS, but without increases in mortality or tissue resistance. Major depression in humans is associated with increased levels of cortisol without any of the features of glucocorticoid excess; it is possible that glucocorticoid resistance accounts for this. Whether this translates into a greater likelihood to develop sepsis or SIRS following infection or injury remains to be seen. It is likely that a myriad of behavioral and physiological differences contribute to whether an individual displays a dominant inflammatory or anti-inflammatory response during critical illness.

Conclusion

It is clear that the function of the HPA-axis, the delivery of cortisol to cells, and their responsiveness are vital processes in the modulation of inflammation during critical illness. Disturbances of function at any level can have profound effects on the balance between inflammatory processes and the suppressive effects of glucocorticoids. It is, therefore, not surprising that testing the integrity of the axis by measurement of cortisol levels alone does not provide accurate information for decisions-to-treat or prognostication. Our attempts to meaningfully define terms such as "relative adrenal insufficiency" and "inflammation-acquired glucocorticoid insensitivity" will continue to be hampered until our understanding of what constitutes an appropriate response of the HPA-axis to critical illness is improved. However, there remains great potential in the design of therapeutic regimens that influence the balance between inflammation and immunosuppression to the benefit of patient outcomes.

Acknowledgements: David Menon is part of the NIHR Biomedical Research Centre at Cambridge, and is supported by grants from the Medical Research Council (UK), Royal College of Anaesthetists, Wellcome Trust, the Evelyn Trust, and Queens' College Cambridge.

References

1. Marik PE, Pastores SM, Annane D, et al (2008) Recommendations for the diagnosis and management of corticosteroid insufficiency in critically ill adult patients: consensus statements from an international task force by the American College of Critical Care Medicine. Crit Care Med 36: 1937–1949
2. Bornstein SR, Engeland WC, Ehrhart-Bornstein M, Herman JP (2008) Dissociation of ACTH and glucocorticoids. Trends Endocrinol Metab 19: 175–180
3. Perrot D, Bonneton A, Dechaud H, Motin J, Pugeat M (1993) Hypercortisolism in septic shock is not suppressible by dexamethasone infusion. Crit Care Med 21: 396–401
4. Pemberton PA, Stein PE, Pepys MB, Potter JM, Carrell RW (1988) Hormone binding globulins undergo serpin conformational change in inflammation. Nature 336: 257–258
5. Owen CA, Campbell MA, Sannes PL, Boukedes SS, Campbell EJ (1995) Cell surface-bound elastase and cathepsin G on human neutrophils: a novel, non-oxidative mechanism by which neutrophils focus and preserve catalytic activity of serine proteinases. J Cell Biol 131: 775–789
6. Hammond GL, Smith CL, Underhill CM, Nguyen VT (1990) Interaction between corticosteroid binding globulin and activated leukocytes in vitro. Biochem Biophys Res Commun 172: 172–177

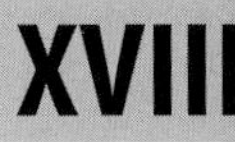

7. Jirasakuldech B, Schussler GC, Yap MG, Drew H, Josephson A, Michl J (2000) A characteristic serpin cleavage product of thyroxine-binding globulin appears in sepsis sera. J Clin Endocrinol Metab 85: 3996-3999
8. Vogeser M, Briegel J (2007) Effect of temperature on protein binding of cortisol. Clin Biochem 40: 724-727
9. Beishuizen A, Thijs LG, Vermes I (2001) Patterns of corticosteroid-binding globulin and the free cortisol index during septic shock and multitrauma. Intensive Care Med 27: 1584-1591
10. Cole TJ, Harris HJ, Hoong I, et al (1999) The glucocorticoid receptor is essential for maintaining basal and dexamethasone-induced repression of the murine corticosteroid-binding globulin gene. Mol Cell Endocrinol 154: 29-36
11. Marti O, Martin M, Gavalda A, et al (1997) Inhibition of corticosteroid-binding globulin caused by a severe stressor is apparently mediated by the adrenal but not by glucocorticoid receptors. Endocrine 6: 159-164
12. Vogeser M, Briegel J, Zachoval R (2002) Dialyzable free cortisol after stimulation with Synacthen. Clin Biochem 35: 539-543
13. Moisey R, Wright D, Aye M, Murphy E, Peacey SR (2006) Interpretation of the short Synacthen test in the presence of low cortisol-binding globulin: two case reports. Ann Clin Biochem 43: 416-419
14. Davidson JS, Bolland MJ, Croxson MS, Chiu W, Lewis JG (2006) A case of low cortisol-binding globulin: use of plasma free cortisol in interpretation of hypothalamic-pituitary-adrenal axis tests. Ann Clin Biochem 43: 237-239
15. Torpy DJ, Bachmann AW, Grice JE, et al (2001) Familial corticosteroid-binding globulin deficiency due to a novel null mutation: association with fatigue and relative hypotension. J Clin Endocrinol Metab 86: 3692-3700
16. Hamrahian AH, Oseni TS, Arafah BM (2004) Measurements of serum free cortisol in critically ill patients. N Engl J Med 350: 1629-1638
17. Ho JT, Al-Musalhi H, Chapman MJ, et al (2006) Septic shock and sepsis: a comparison of total and free plasma cortisol levels. J Clin Endocrinol Metab 91: 105-114
18. Dubey A, Boujoukos AJ (2005) Free cortisol levels should not be used to determine adrenal responsiveness. Crit Care 9: E2
19. Coolens JL, Van Baelen H, Heyns W (1987) Clinical use of unbound plasma cortisol as calculated from total cortisol and corticosteroid-binding globulin. J Steroid Biochem 26: 197-202
20. Odermatt A, Atanasov AG, Balazs Z, et al (2006) Why is 11beta-hydroxysteroid dehydrogenase type 1 facing the endoplasmic reticulum lumen? Physiological relevance of the membrane topology of 11beta-HSD1. Mol Cell Endocrinol 248: 15-23
21. Prigent H, Maxime V, Annane D (2004) Science review: mechanisms of impaired adrenal function in sepsis and molecular actions of glucocorticoids. Crit Care 8: 243-252
22. Druce LA, Thorpe CM, Wilton A (2008) Mineralocorticoid effects due to cortisol inactivation overload explain the beneficial use of hydrocortisone in septic shock. Med Hypotheses 70: 56-60
23. Annane D, Sebille V, Charpentier C, et al (2002) Effect of treatment with low doses of hydrocortisone and fludrocortisone on mortality in patients with septic shock. JAMA 288: 862-871
24. Scheinman RI, Gualberto A, Jewell CM, Cidlowski JA, Baldwin AS Jr (1995) Characterization of mechanisms involved in transrepression of NF-kappa B by activated glucocorticoid receptors. Mol Cell Biol 15: 943-953
25. Meduri GU (1999) New rationale for glucocorticoid treatment in septic shock. J Chemother 11: 541-550
26. Kino T, Chrousos GP (2003) Tumor necrosis factor alpha receptor- and Fas-associated FLASH inhibit transcriptional activity of the glucocorticoid receptor by binding to and interfering with its interaction with p160 type nuclear receptor coactivators. J Biol Chem 278: 3023-3029
27. Meduri GU, Muthiah MP, Carratu P, Eltorky M, Chrousos GP (2005) Nuclear factor-kappaB- and glucocorticoid receptor alpha-mediated mechanisms in the regulation of systemic and pulmonary inflammation during sepsis and acute respiratory distress syndrome. Evidence for inflammation-induced target tissue resistance to glucocorticoids. Neuroimmunomodulation 12: 321-338
28. Meduri GU, Tolley EA, Chrousos GP, Stentz F (2002) Prolonged methylprednisolone treatment suppresses systemic inflammation in patients with unresolving acute respiratory dis-

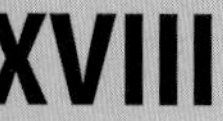

tress syndrome: evidence for inadequate endogenous glucocorticoid secretion and inflammation-induced immune cell resistance to glucocorticoids. Am J Respir Crit Care Med 165: 983–991

29. Nakamori Y, Ogura H, Koh T, et al (2005) The balance between expression of intranuclear NF-kappaB and glucocorticoid receptor in polymorphonuclear leukocytes in SIRS patients. J Trauma 59: 308–314
30. Leung DY, Hamid Q, Vottero A, et al (1997) Association of glucocorticoid insensitivity with increased expression of glucocorticoid receptor beta. J Exp Med 186: 1567–1574
31. van der Laan S, Meijer OC (2008) Pharmacology of glucocorticoids: beyond receptors. Eur J Pharmacol 585: 483–491
32. Sousa AR, Lane SJ, Soh C, Lee TH (1999) In vivo resistance to corticosteroids in bronchial asthma is associated with enhanced phosyphorylation of JUN N-terminal kinase and failure of prednisolone to inhibit JUN N-terminal kinase phosphorylation. J Allergy Clin Immunol 104: 565–574
33. Clark AR, Martins JR, Tchen CR (2008) Role of dual specificity phosphatases in biological responses to glucocorticoids. J Biol Chem 283: 25765–25769
34. Bertini R, Bianchi M, Ghezzi P (1988) Adrenalectomy sensitizes mice to the lethal effects of interleukin 1 and tumor necrosis factor. J Exp Med 167: 1708–1712
35. Reichardt HM, Umland T, Bauer A, Kretz O, Schutz G (2000) Mice with an increased glucocorticoid receptor gene dosage show enhanced resistance to stress and endotoxic shock. Mol Cell Biol 20: 9009–9017
36. Hawes AS, Rock CS, Keogh CV, Lowry SF, Calvano SE (1992) In vivo effects of the antiglucocorticoid RU 486 on glucocorticoid and cytokine responses to Escherichia coli endotoxin. Infect Immun 60: 2641–2647
37. Fischer M, Bhatnagar J, Guarner J, et al (2005) Fatal toxic shock syndrome associated with Clostridium sordellii after medical abortion. N Engl J Med 353: 2352–2360
38. Miech RP (2005) Pathophysiology of mifepristone-induced septic shock due to Clostridium sordellii. Ann Pharmacother 39: 1483–1488
39. Sicard D, Chauvelot-Moachon L (2005) Comment: pathophysiology of mifepristone-induced septic shock due to Clostridium sordellii. Ann Pharmacother 39: 2142–2143
40. Cohen AL, Bhatnagar J, Reagan S, et al (2007) Toxic shock associated with Clostridium sordellii and Clostridium perfringens after medical and spontaneous abortion. Obstet Gynecol 110: 1027–1033
41. Duma D, Silva-Santos JE, Assreuy J (2004) Inhibition of glucocorticoid receptor binding by nitric oxide in endotoxemic rats. Crit Care Med 32: 2304–2310
42. Da J, Chen L, Hedenstierna G (2007) Nitric oxide up-regulates the glucocorticoid receptor and blunts the inflammatory reaction in porcine endotoxin sepsis. Crit Care Med 35: 26–32
43. Quan N, Avitsur R, Stark JL, et al (2001) Social stress increases the susceptibility to endotoxic shock. J Neuroimmunol 115: 36–45

Corticosteroid Treatment of Patients in Septic Shock

C.L. Sprung, S. Goodman, and Y.G. Weiss

Introduction

The use of steroids in septic shock patients has been controversial for decades [1, 2]. High-dose corticosteroids were standard therapy in the 1970s and 1980s [1–4]. During the late 1980s and 1990s, however, the consensus was that corticosteroids should not be used in sepsis and septic shock after studies did not show an improved survival for patients treated with steroids [5–9]. Over the last decade, the recognition of inadequate adrenal corticosteroid production became more important as many critically ill patients were found to have relative adrenal insufficiency [10]. Studies in the late 1990s and early 2000s demonstrated hemodynamic benefits with lower doses of steroids for longer periods of time [11–16]. Unfortunately, steroid use in critically ill patients has been associated with adverse affects [2] especially superinfections [2] and, more recently, critical illness polyneuromyopathy [17, 18]. In view of the ongoing controversy concerning the use of steroids in septic patients and recent studies on the subject, the current chapter attempts to review the topic, weighing the advantages and disadvantages of steroid treatment.

High-dose Steroid Studies

The beneficial effects of corticosteroids were believed to be due to their anti-inflammatory properties which would interrupt the inflammatory cascade in sepsis [19]. Between the late 1950s and mid-1980s, physicians treated patients with short courses of high-dose or pharmacologic doses of corticosteroids (methylprednisolone 30 mg/kg or dexamethasone 3–6 mg/kg in 2–4 intravenous doses). This practice was largely due to the study by Schumer [3], which showed a decrease in mortality from 38 % to 10 % in patients who received steroids. A study by Sprung et al. [4] demonstrated that steroids reversed septic shock and improved survival for a short time and suggested that more prolonged treatment might be beneficial. The use of steroids, however, was questioned by two large prospective randomized trials which noted that corticosteroids did not decrease mortality [5, 6]. In 1995, two meta-analyses [7, 8] concluded that high-dose corticosteroids in patients with severe sepsis and septic shock were ineffective [7] or harmful [8]. Patients treated with steroids had worse outcomes in the trials with the highest quality [8]. High-dose steroids were associated with an increased risk of secondary infections, higher mortality [8], and an increased incidence of renal and hepatic dysfunction [9]. Subsequent to these latter reports [7, 8], doctors stopped using high-dose corticosteroids in septic patients (**Fig. 1**).

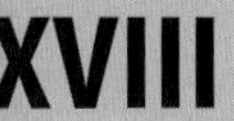

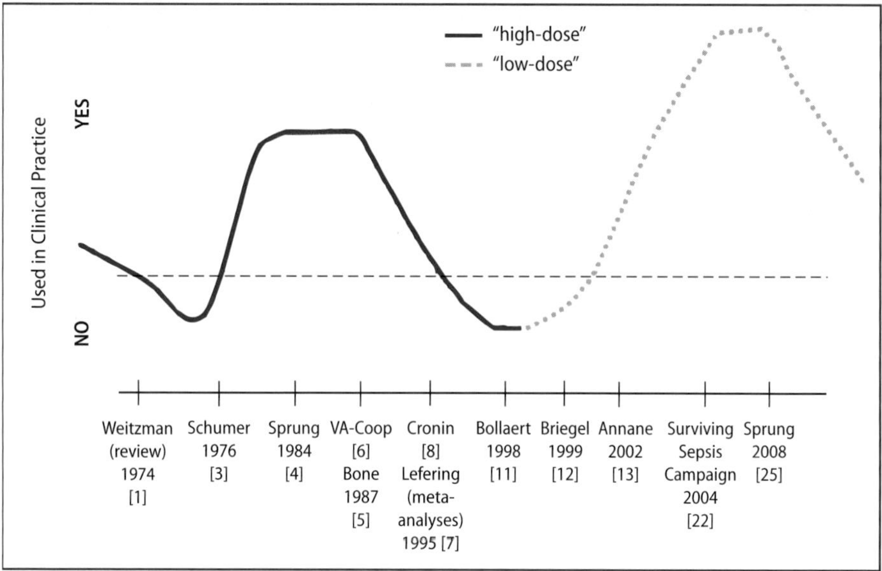

Fig. 1. The use of corticosteroids for patients in septic shock over the years.

Low-dose Steroid Studies

Although the use of high-dose steroids decreased after the above-mentioned studies, doctors began administering low-dose steroids (usually 200–300 mg of intravenous hydrocortisone three times a day) for a new reason – relative adrenal insufficiency. Many septic shock patients have decreased vasopressor sensitivity to catecholamines [20] and do not respond appropriately to corticotropin stimulation [21]. Mortality in septic shock patients was demonstrated to be greatest in patients whose baseline cortisol levels were > 34 μg/dl (938 mmol/l) and did not increase after corticotropin stimulation > 9 μg/dl (248 nmol/l) [21].

Studies have demonstrated improved hemodynamics with corticosteroid treatment [11, 12, 14–16]. Bollaert et al. [11] evaluated the ability of hydrocortisone (100 mg intravenously every 8 hours for at least 5 days) to improve hemodynamics in late septic shock patients. Patients treated with steroids had more reversal of shock at 7 and 28 days [11]. Briegel et al. [12] treated hyperdynamic septic shock patients with hydrocortisone (100 mg followed by 0.18 mg/kg/h intravenously for 6 days) with later tapering. Time to stopping vasopressor therapy was decreased and there was a trend to earlier resolution of sepsis-induced organ dysfunction in patients treated with steroids [12]. Overall reversal of shock and mortality were not affected [12]. Keh et al. performed a crossover study in which patients treated with norepinephrine received hydrocortisone (100 mg followed by 10 mg/h intravenously for 3 days) or a placebo in a random fashion [14]. Patients treated with steroids experienced a significant improvement in blood pressure despite a rapid decrease in the dose and duration of norepinephrine therapy [14]. Oppert et al. [15] treated early hyperdynamic septic shock patients with hydrocortisone (50 mg followed by 0.18 mg/kg/h intravenously until shock reversal) and subsequent tapering. The duration of vasopressor therapy was shorter in the steroid-treated patients [15]. Cicarelli et al. stud-

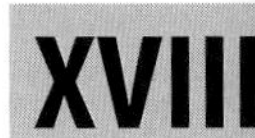

ied septic shock patients evaluating dexamethasone (0.2 mg/kg intravenously every 36 hours for five days) versus placebo [16]. Dexamethasone-treated patients had a shorter duration of vasopressor requirements, a significant reduction in 7-day mortality, and a trend to lower 28-day mortality [16].

Annane et al. [13] evaluated low-dose hydrocortisone in patients with early, severe septic shock in a multicenter, randomized, placebo-controlled, double-blind study. Randomization of patients occurred within 8 hours of shock and patients received intravenous hydrocortisone (50 mg) every 6 hours plus enteral fludrocortisone (50 μg/d) for 7 days. Response to a 250 μg corticotropin stimulation test defined whether patients were "non-responders" or "responders" with non-responders defined by a cortisol increase ≤ 9 μg/dl (248 nmol/l). A total of 299 patients were analyzed. The lungs were the primary source of infection. Shock reversal was more common (57 %) in steroid-treated patients than in patients receiving placebo (40 %) and more rapid. Mortality (28-day) was decreased by steroid therapy in all patients (61 vs. 55 %) and in the non-responders (63 vs. 53 %) [13]. Rates of adverse events were similar in both study groups (22 vs. 21 %).

For many physicians, the above studies suggested that patients with septic shock had impaired adrenal reserve and that steroid replacement would reverse shock and even improve survival. Based primarily on the Annane study [13], the Surviving Sepsis Campaign [22] and two meta-analyses [23, 24] recommended the use of low dose hydrocortisone for patients with septic shock. Once again the use of steroids for septic shock patients became extremely common (**Fig. 1**).

The Corticus Study

Hydrocortisone use and corticotropin testing in septic shock patients was evaluated in a subsequent multicenter, randomized, placebo-controlled, double-blind study – The Corticosteroid Therapy of Septic Shock (Corticus) study [25]. It should be emphasized that the Corticus study was initiated because most of the previous studies had small numbers of patients and the Annane study [13] with large numbers represented a very small percentage of septic shock patients as the entry criteria required that patients not increase their systolic blood pressure > 90 mmHg for one hour despite aggressive fluid resuscitation and/or vasopressor therapy. Patients in the Corticus study could be septic and in shock for up to 72 hours. A total of 499 patients were analyzed. The gastrointestinal tract was the primary source of infection. At enrollment, 99 % of patients received vasopressors and study drug commenced within 12 hours of drug therapy in 77 % of patients. The results of Corticus were that no differences were found in 28-day mortality for patients receiving hydrocortisone or placebo respectively in non-responders to a corticotrophin test (39 vs. 36 %), responders (29 vs. 29 %) or all patients (34 vs. 32 %) [25]. In patients reversing their shock, shock reversal was faster in patients receiving hydrocortisone compared to placebo in all the three groups; in all patients shock reversal occurred in a median time of 3.3 days in the steroid-treated patients and 5.8 days in the placebo patients [25]. Hydrocortisone, however, did not increase the percentage of patients with shock reversal in the three groups [25]. In addition, hydrocortisone treated patients had more episodes of superinfection including new sepsis or septic shock but there was no evidence of increased neuromuscular weakness [25].

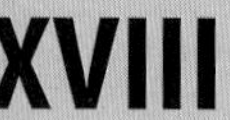

Adverse Effects of Steroids

Unfortunately, the use of steroids in the critically ill is not without adverse effects. Acute complications include superinfection, hyperglycemia, upper gastrointestinal bleeding, hypernatremia, arrhythmias, psychosis, muscular weakness, and delayed wound healing [2]. It has been suggested that the earlier corticosteroid studies using high-dose steroids showed superinfections whereas the more recent studies using low-dose steroids did not. Although recent studies did not find evidence of superinfections [11, 13] or do not report this information [12, 16], the Corticus study, using low-dose steroids, did demonstrate an increased incidence of superinfection including new sepsis or septic shock [25]. Critically ill patients are not only susceptible to bacterial infections but also to viral infections. Heininger et al. [26] showed that critically ill septic patients are more likely to develop cytomegalovirus infections. Jaber et al. [27] noted that cytomegalovirus infection was linked to steroid use in intensive care unit (ICU) non-immunosuppressed patients with fever > 72 hours and that patients with cytomegalovirus infections had a higher mortality, longer mechanical ventilation and longer ICU length of stay.

Studies have shown an association between steroid therapy in critically ill patients and the incidence of critical illness polyneuromyopathy [17, 18]. This may be related to higher doses of steroids, because the Corticus study [25] was unable to demonstrate evidence of muscular weakness in patients receiving steroids.

Some physicians believe that steroids given for septic shock may prevent the development of acute respiratory distress syndrome (ARDS). A recent meta-analysis [28] suggested just the opposite, an association between steroid therapy and the subsequent development of ARDS (ARDS developed in 95/258 [37 %] steroid-treated patients and 68/396 [17 %] placebo patients; odds ratio 1.55 [95 % CI 0.58–4.05]). In fact, the probability suggested a weakly increased risk of death associated with steroid therapy in patients who developed ARDS (mortality in 46/88 [52 %] steroid-treated patients and 26/66 [39 %] placebo patients; odds ratio 1.52 [95 % CI 0.30–5.94]) [28].

The Ongoing Controversy

Despite two recent, large, well performed studies [13, 25], steroid use in septic shock patients continues to be controversial. This may be related to the fact that the studies came to opposite conclusions after studying different patient populations. It cannot be sufficiently emphasized that the two largest studies of low-dose steroids in patients with septic shock evaluated totally different patient groups and this is probably the reason for the differences in study outcomes. Differences between the two studies [13, 25] include: An entry window for patient inclusion in the study that was much shorter in the Annane study (8 vs. 72 hours); systolic blood pressure < 90 mmHg for at least one hour despite fluid resuscitation and vasopressor treatment in the Annane study which represents the minority of septic shock patients (> 1 hour vs. < 1 hour); additional treatment with enteral fludrocortisone in the Annane study which was not given in the Corticus study; shorter duration of treatment in the Annane study (7 vs. 11 days) with no weaning as opposed to Corticus where because of a weaning schedule patients were treated for longer; higher SAPS II severity scores (59 vs. 49) and more non-responders to corticotropin in the Annane study (77 vs. 47 %); differences in steroid effects for non-responders to corticotropin in

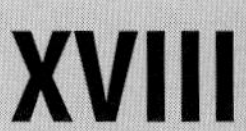

the Annane study whereas there were no differences based on response to corticotropin in the Corticus study; and an increased risk of superinfection in the Corticus but not in the Annane study. Finally, the Annane study was conducted before the publication of practice guidelines recommending steroids which was not the case for the Corticus study, leading to the enrollment of less sick patients in Corticus. Therefore, patients in the study by Annane et al. [13] were treated earlier, were in more severe shock with greater disease severity and received fludrocortisone in addition to a shorter course of hydrocortisone without weaning. Corticus patients [25] were treated later, were in less severe shock with less disease severity, did not receive fludrocortisone and had a longer course of hydrocortisone with weaning.

There are some physicians who believe so strongly in the use of corticosteroids for patients in septic shock that the controversy appears to be based no longer on facts and published literature but rather on faith, similar to strong religious beliefs. In attempting to understand the different points of view in the controversy, the fact that most patients show an immediate effect in reversing their shock after receiving steroids but that patients developing superinfections do so at a later time point and not so evidently caused by steroids may help elucidate the different points of view. It is important to remember, however, that although in the Corticus study 80 % of steroid-treated patients reversed their shock, 74 % of placebo patients also reversed their shock [25]. When deciding on whether to use corticosteroids or not in a septic shock patient, a physician must look at the individual patient, assess his/her severity of shock and response to therapy, and carefully weigh the advantages and disadvantages of steroid use noted in the literature. Only by using objective facts in making decisions can patients receive the "right" treatment from their doctors.

Mechanism of Corticosteroid Action in Reversing Shock

As noted, Corticus showed no difference in mortality or reversal of shock in patients who were responders or non-responders to a corticotropin stimulation test [25]. It may be that many critically ill patients do not respond to corticotropin stimulation but that does not necessarily mean they have relative adrenal insufficiency requiring treatment with steroids. Critically ill patients may have "critical illness-related corticosteroid insufficiency" which may occur as a result of a decrease in adrenal steroid production or tissue resistance to corticosteroids [29]. Although there are probably many mechanisms for the effects of steroids in septic shock, the Corticus findings suggest that the steroid effects in hastening the reversal of septic shock may be unrelated to adrenal insufficiency but might instead be secondary to a direct interaction with mechanisms producing vascular hyporeactivity [30, 31]. The effects of glucocorticoids on vascular tone have been known for decades even before steroids were known to have anti-inflammatory properties [32]. Support for the importance of the steroid effect on vasomotor tone is found by the reversal of the decreased vasopressor sensitivity to catecholamines found in septic shock patients treated with steroids [20].

Recommendations

Corticosteroids are life-saving medications when given for the appropriate indication. Unfortunately, serious harm can ensue with their use, especially in patients who do not have a clear indication for their application. The controversy regarding

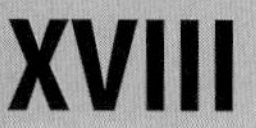

the use of corticosteroids is in those patients who may have critical illness related corticosteroid insufficiency solely because of their septic shock [29]. There is consensus that patients who have previously received steroids for various medical disorders and develop septic shock should receive steroid supplementation [33].

The updated Surviving Sepsis campaign gave the following recommendation for the use of steroids in septic shock patients: "We suggest intravenous hydrocortisone be given only to adult septic shock patients after blood pressure is identified to be poorly responsive to fluid resuscitation and vasopressor therapy [33]." Other recommendations include fludrocortisone therapy as optional therapy when hydrocortisone is used and that corticosteroid therapy should not be guided by the results of corticotropin stimulation tests [33]. The American College of Critical Care Medicine international task force came up with similar recommendations: "Hydrocortisone should be considered in the management strategy of patients with septic shock, particularly those patients who have responded poorly to fluid resuscitation and vasopressor agents [29]."

In trying to develop consensus, the international groups were too general in their recommendations. It is not clear exactly what "poorly responsive to fluid resuscitation and vasopressor therapy" actually means when one has to decide whether to treat a patient with steroids or not. As the recommendations to use corticosteroids come primarily from the Annane study [13], we believe that steroids should be used only in patients who meet the Annane entry criteria. This means that only patients who do not increase their systolic blood pressure to > 90 mmHg with aggressive fluid resuscitation and/or vasopressor therapy after more than one hour should receive steroids. As this scenario is present in only a very small percentage of septic shock patients, most patients in septic shock who can have their systolic blood pressure increased to > 90 mmHg with aggressive fluid resuscitation and/or vasopressor therapy within one hour should *not* receive steroids. The potential benefit of an earlier reversal of shock is not worth the complications of superinfection, new sepsis or new septic shock [25]. An additional two and a half days receiving norepinephrine to maintain blood pressure and perfusion is far better than receiving steroids to reverse shock [25]. In fact, one could argue that similar results could be achieved by using low dose vasopressin which may also increase the vascular responsiveness to norepinephrine [34]. Therefore, based on Corticus [25], the largest study of steroids in septic shock and representing the majority of septic patients, most patients in septic shock should not receive steroids. The importance of the Corticus study is in its evaluation and the findings related to the risk and benefit analysis that must be undertaken every time steroids are prescribed to a patient with septic shock.

Conclusion

The use of corticosteroids in septic shock patients has been controversial for decades. Although high-dose steroid therapy for septic shock patients has not been shown to be beneficial, it was believed that low-dose steroid therapy would be helpful. Steroids appear to be useful only in adult septic shock patients after blood pressure is identified to be poorly responsive to fluid resuscitation and vasopressor therapy. For the majority of septic shock patients, however, steroids cannot be recommended as the benefit of reversing shock is not worth the danger of superinfection, new sepsis and septic shock.

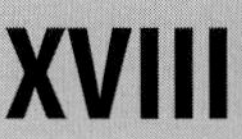

References

1. Weitzman S, Berger S (1974) Clinical trial design in studies of corticosteroids for bacterial infections. Ann Intern Med 81: 36–42
2. Schein RMH, Sprung CL (1986) The use of corticosteroids in the sepsis syndrome. In: Shoemaker W (ed) Critical Care – State of the Art. The Society of Critical Care Medicine, Fullerton, pp 131–149
3. Schumer W (1976) Steroids in the treatment of clinical septic shock. Ann Surg 184: 333–341.
4. Sprung CL, Caralis PV, Marcial EH, et al (1984) The effects of high-dose corticosteroids in patients with septic shock. A prospective, controlled study. N Engl J Med 311: 1137–1143
5. Bone RC, Fisher CJ Jr, Clemmer TP, et al (1987) A controlled clinical trial of high-dose methylprednisolone in the treatment of severe sepsis and septic shock. N Engl J Med 317: 653–658
6. The Veterans Administration Systemic Sepsis Cooperative Study Group (1987) Effect of high-dose glucocorticoid therapy on mortality in patients with clinical signs of systemic sepsis. N Engl J Med 317: 659–665
7. Lefering R, Neugebauer EAM (1995) Steroid controversy in sepsis and septic shock: a meta-analysis. Crit Care Med 23: 1294–1303
8. Cronin L, Cook DJ, Carlet J, et al (1995) Corticosteroid treatment for sepsis: A critical appraisal and meta-analysis of the literature. Crit Care Med 24: 1430–1439
9. Slotman GJ, Fisher CJ Jr, Bone RC, Clemmer TP, Metz CA (1993) Detrimental effects of high-dose methylprednisolone sodium succinate on serum concentrations of hepatic and renal function indicators in severe sepsis and septic shock. The Methylprednisolone Severe Sepsis Study Group. Crit Care Med 21: 191–195
10. Lamberts SWJ, Bruining HA, de Jong FH (1997) Corticosteroid therapy in severe illness. N Engl J Med 337: 1285–1292
11. Bollaert PE, Charpentier C, Levy S, et al (1998) Reversal of late septic shock with supraphysiologic doses of hydrocortisone. Crit Care Med 26: 645–650
12. Briegel J, Frost H, Haller M, et al (1999) Stress doses of hydrocortisone reverse hyperdynamic septic shock: A prospective, randomized, double-blind, single center study. Crit Care Med 27: 723–732
13. Annane D, Sebille V, Charpentier C, et al (2002) Effect of treatment with low doses of hydrocortisone and fludrocortisone on mortality in patients with septic shock. JAMA 288: 862–870
14. Keh D, Boehnke T, Weber-Cartens S, et al (2003) Immunologic and hemodynamic effects of "low-dose" hydrocortisone in septic shock: a double-blind, randomized, placebo-controlled, crossover study. Am J Respir Crit Care Med.167: 512–520
15. Oppert M, Schindler R, Husung C, et al (2005) Low dose hydrocortisone improves shock reversal and reduces cytokine levels in early hyperdynamic septic shock. Crit Care Med 33: 2457–2464
16. Cicarelli DD, Viera JE, Martin Besenor FE (2007) Early dexamethasone treatment for septic shock patients: a prospective randomized clinical trial. Sao Paulo Med J 125: 237–241
17. De Jonghe B, Sharshar T, Lefaucheur JP, et al (2002) Paresis acquired in the intensive care unit: a prospective multicenter study. JAMA 288: 2859–2867
18. Herridge MS, Cheung AM, Tansey CM, et al (2003) One-year outcomes in survivors of the acute respiratory distress syndrome. N Engl J Med 348: 683–693
19. Bone RC (1991) The pathogenesis of sepsis. Ann Intern Med 115: 457–469.
20. Annane D, Bellissant E, Sebille V, et al (1998) Impaired pressor sensitivity to noradrenaline in septic shock patients with and without impaired adrenal reserve. Br J Clin Pharmacol 46: 589–597
21. Annane D, Sebille V, Trocke G, Raphael J-C, Gajdos P, Bellissant EA (2000) 3-level prognostic classification of septic shock based on cortisol level and cortisol response to corticotropin. JAMA 283: 1038–1045
22. Dellinger P, Carlet JM, Masur H, et al (2004) Surviving Sepsis Campaign guidelines for the management of severe sepsis and septic shock. Crit Care Med 32: 858–873
23. Annane D, Bellissant E, Bollaert PE, et al (2004) Corticosteroids for severe sepsis and septic shock: a systematic review and meta-analysis. BMJ 329: 480–488
24. Minneci PC, Deans KJ, Banks SM, et al (2004) Meta-analysis: The effects of steroids on survival and shock during sepsis depend on the dose. Ann Intern Med 141: 47–56

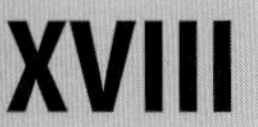

25. Sprung CL, Annane D, Keh D, et al (2008) The CORTICUS randomized, double-blind, placebo-controlled study of hydrocortisone therapy in patients with septic shock. N Engl J Med 358: 111–124
26. Heininger A, Jahn J, Engel C, Notheisen T, Unertl K, Hamprecht K (2001) Human cytomegalovirus infections in nonimmunosuppressed critically ill patients. Crit Care Med 29: 541–547
27. Jaber S, Chanques , Borry J, et al (2005) Cytomegalovirus infection in critically ill patients. Chest 127: 233–241
28. Peter JV, John P, Graham PL, Moran JL, George IA, Bersten A (2008) Corticosteroids in the prevention and treatment of acute respiratory distress syndrome (ARDS) in adults: meta-analysis. BMJ 336: 1006–1009
29. Marik PE, Pastores SM, Annane D, et al (2008) Clinical practice guidelines for the diagnosis and management of corticosteroid insufficiency in critical illness: Recommendations of an international task force. Crit Care Med 36: 1937–1949
30. Silverman HJ, Penaranda R, Orens JB, et al (1993) Impaired beta-adrenergic receptor stimulation of cyclic adenosine monophosphate in human septic shock: Association with myocardial hyporesponsiveness to catecholamines. Crit Care Med 21: 31–39
31. Saito T, Takanashi M, Gallagher E, et al (1995) Corticosteroid effect on early beta-adrenergic down-regulation during circulatory shock: Hemodynamic study and beta-adrenergic receptor assay. Intensive Care Med 21: 204–210
32. Perla D, Marmorston J (1940) Suprarenal cortical hormone and salt in the treatment of pneumonia and other severe infections. Endocrinology 27: 367–374
33. Dellinger RP, Levy MM, Carlet JM, et al (2008) Surviving Sepsis Campaign: International guidelines for management of severe sepsis and septic shock. Crit Care Med 36: 296–327
34. Russell JA, Walley KR, Singer J, et al (2008) Vasopressin versus norepinephrine infusion in patients with septic shock. N Engl J Med 358: 877–887

XIX Coagulation

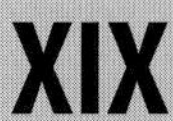

New Anticoagulants: Anti-IIa or Anti-Xa Agents?

C.M. SAMAMA

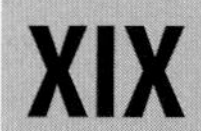

Introduction

The iatrogenicity of vitamin K antagonists is well established. Each year in France, vitamin K antagonists account for more than 17,000 hospital admissions and nearly 4000 deaths. Alternative treatment would be more than welcome. It is hard to imagine a drug that would induce more complications than a vitamin K antagonist.

Low-molecular weight heparins (LMWH), which have been available in France for more than 20 years, are effective as both prophylaxis and cure, but they are non-synthetic (animal-extracted) and induce adverse effects including the much dreaded thrombocytopenia. Thrombocytopenia occurs in about 1 patient in every 1000 receiving LMWH and 1 in every 100 receiving unfractionated heparin (UFH).

There is thus a real need for new anticoagulants whether for injection or oral use. Currently, the pharmaceutical industry has over 20 products in its pipelines. A summary of five of the newer agents is provided in **Table 1**.

Factor Xa Inhibitors

Many products already on the market or in advanced stages of development target activated factor X (factor Xa), either directly or indirectly, and have been designed with the demonstrated efficacy of LMWH in mind.

Table 1. Comparison of new injectable and oral antithrombotic agents [12, 17, 22]

	Fondaparinux	Biotinylated idraparinux	Rivaroxaban	Apixaban	Dabigatran etexilate
Target	Factor Xa	Factor Xa	Factor Xa	Factor Xa	Thrombin
Brand name	Arixtra®	–	Xarelto®	–	Pradaxa®
Route of administration	Subcutaneous	Subcutaneous	Oral	Oral	Oral
Bioavailability	100 %	100 %	80 %	51–85 %	6–8 %
Tmax	1.7 h	2 h	2–4 h	3 h	2 h
Half-Life	17–25 h	90–135 h	9–13 h	9–14 h	14–17 h
Frequency of administration	Once-daily	Once-daily	Once-daily	Twice-daily	Once or twice-daily
Renal excretion	100 %	100 %	66 %	25 %	80 %
Antidote	No	Avidin	No	No	No

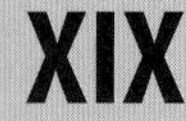

Injectable Indirect Factor Xa Inhibitors

a) Fondaparinux (Arixtra®)

Fondaparinux was the first injected, synthetic, indirect factor Xa inhibitor to be launched and has been on the market for more than 5 years [1]. It is a pentasaccharide that interacts with antithrombin, modifies the binding site for Factor Xa, and, by inhibiting Factor Xa, affects coagulation. Once released, fondaparinux can interact again (2 or 3 times) with antithrombin. This recycling accounts for the drug's high potency.

The pharmacokinetics of fondaparinux has been thoroughly investigated. Its bioavailability after injection is 100 %, peak plasma concentrations are reached within 1.7 hours (Tmax), its half-life is 17 hours in the healthy volunteer but can exceed 30 hours in the elderly. Clearance is by the renal route only. In the Pentathlon dose-ranging study (0.75 mg, 1.5 mg, 3 mg, 6 mg, 8 mg) in patients undergoing total hip replacement surgery, even low doses of fondaparinux gave good results in terms of prevention of thromboembolic events when compared to the LMWH, enoxaparin, injected at the standard North American dose (30 mg twice daily) [2]. The path of the curve describing reduction in thromboembolic events crossed the path of the curve for incidence of major bleeding at a dose of about 3 mg. A dose of 2.5 mg was selected for Phase III trials, even though the antithrombotic activity of fondaparinux was equivalent to that of enoxaparin – or even better – than for a dose 1.5 mg, safety was better.

Outcomes with fondaparinux in four large-scale pivotal studies in major orthopedic surgery (hip replacement, knee, and femoral neck fracture surgery) were good and have been confirmed in a meta-analysis [3]. However, the results of studies in general surgery and medicine have not totally met expectations, because superiority over the standard of care was not fully demonstrated. Bleeding complications were seldom observed during prophylaxis with fondaparinux, no doubt because of its high anticoagulant potency.

The efficacy of fondaparinux has proved greatest in the treatment of deep vein thrombosis (DVT) and pulmonary embolism. It has been compared with continuous intravenous infusion of an adjusted dose of UFH in the treatment of pulmonary embolism [4] and with subcutaneous injection of enoxaparin (1 mg/kg twice daily) in the treatment of DVT [5], in each case followed by a vitamin K antagonist. In both situations, fondaparinux was as effective, if not even a little more effective than standard treatment. Safety was similar. Thus, a once-daily subcutaneous injection of fondaparinux without monitoring is at least as effective and as safe as an adjusted UFH dose in the initial treatment of hemodynamically stable patients with pulmonary embolism.

A rather unexpected but welcome result was observed in the OASIS-5 trial comparing a low dose of fondaparinux (2.5 mg) with enoxaparin (1 mg/kg twice daily) in over 20000 patients with acute coronary syndrome [6]. Fondaparinux had similar efficacy but better safety. It is thus probably the most potent injectable anticoagulant currently available.

Potent anticoagulant activity implies an enhanced risk of bleeding. In 2007, the French Health Products Safety Agency (AFSSAPS) issued a warning after feedback on the administration of fondaparinux to over 250000 patients during the period January 1, 2005, to January 31, 2007. A total of 122 bleeding incidents had been reported. Most had been caused by improper use (overprescription) in patients who were elderly, had a low body weight, or suffered from renal insufficiency, and who

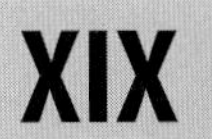

should, therefore, have received other treatment. It has been proposed that such bleeding incidents, if severe, could benefit from the injection of recombinant activated factor VII (Novoseven®). However, data are scant and the thromboembolic risk should not be underestimated. Thrombocytopenia, as induced by heparin, is disputable with fondaparinux; it has been reported only once, in 2007 [7]. It is, therefore, not necessary to monitor coagulation (platelet count) although the administration of fondaparinux to a patient with a history of heparin-induced thrombocytopenia is not recommended.

In conclusion to this brief summary, fondaparinux has been widely studied. It is a highly potent injectable anticoagulant, with proven efficacy in the treatment of DVT and pulmonary embolism. However, attention should be paid to its safety in patients who are frail, who have impaired renal function, are over 75 years old, or weigh less than 50 kg. Thrombocytopenia is unlikely with fondaparinux. The years to come may see its development for surgical procedures carrying a low risk of bleeding (e.g., cancer surgery) or in non-surgical situations such as immobilization of a lower limb after trauma.

b) Idraparinux

Like fondaparinux, idraparinux is a pentasaccharide but with a longer half-life (135 hours). It is administered only once weekly by subcutaneous injection. Its clearance is exclusively renal. Safety in Phase II studies was good at low doses with no bleeding episodes. The indications for Phase III studies have been DVT, pulmonary embolism, and atrial fibrillation. A once-weekly dose of 2.5 mg of idraparinux was as effective as standard therapy (heparin followed by vitamin K antagonist) in the treatment of DVT [8]. However, in the treatment of pulmonary embolism, the 92-day recurrence rate was 3.4 % for idraparinux versus 1.6 % for standard treatment [8]. A possible explanation for recurrence may be the decline in drug concentration during the week. The incidence of clinically relevant bleeding was slightly lower with idraparinux than with standard therapy at 92 days but there was no difference at 6 months.

A companion study to the above compared once-weekly injection of 2.5 mg of idraparinux with placebo in 1215 patients who had undergone 6 months of either idraparinux or standard therapy [9]. Major bleeding was observed in 11 patients on idraparinux but in no patient on placebo. Of these 11 bleeding episodes, 3 were fatal intracranial hemorrhages possibly indicative of drug accumulation. Despite the efficacy of idraparinux, the risk of bleeding was too high to be acceptable.

A randomized controlled trial of idraparinux versus vitamin K antagonists in patents with atrial fibrillation had to be discontinued after randomization of 4576 patients (2283 patients on idraparinux, 2293 on vitamin K antagonist) and a mean follow-up of 10.7 months because of excess bleeding [10]. Clinically relevant bleeding occurred in 346 patients on idraparinux versus 226 patients on vitamin K antagonist; 21 instances of intracranial hemorrhage occurred with idraparinux versus 9 with vitamin K antagonist. Elderly patients and patients with renal impairment were at the highest risk of bleeding.

A new original form of idraparinux coupled to biotin has been developed. Biotinylated idraparinux is immediately neutralized by avidin. The concept is still very interesting but calls for caution as, in theory, avidin carries the risk of an allergic reaction. Studies are ongoing.

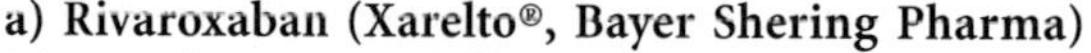

Oral Direct Factor Xa Inhibitors

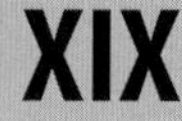

XIX

a) Rivaroxaban (Xarelto®, Bayer Shering Pharma)
Rivaroxaban is an orally active oxazolidone derivative. Its bioavailability is 80 %. It inhibits factor Xa with a Ki of 0.4 nM. It binds to free and clot-bound factor Xa [11, 12]. Its Tmax is 2–4 hours, its half-life is 9–13 hours, two-thirds of the product are eliminated by the kidney. It is a potent anticoagulant with a very wide therapeutic window. In total hip replacement surgery, rivaroxaban efficacy showed no significant dose-relationship but the incidence of bleeding was dose dependent [13]. A low dose was selected for Phase III studies. A randomized double-blind study in 2531 patients (The Regulation of Coagulation in Orthopedic Surgery to Prevent Deep Venous Thrombosis and Pulmonary Embolism, RECORD 3 study) compared 10 mg of rivaroxaban once daily with 40 mg of enoxaparin [14]. Overall incidence of thromboembolic events was 49 % lower with rivaroxaban than with enoxaparin (9.6 vs 18.9 %). For the first time in the history of antithrombotics, the rate of symptomatic events fell from 2.7 to 1 % with no increase in bleeding incidence. The first results for long-term prophylaxis (35 days) with rivaroxaban after hip surgery are promising (RECORD 1 study) [15]. The primary efficacy outcome occurred in 18 of 1595 patients (1.1 %) in the rivaroxaban group and in 58 of 1558 patients (3.7 %) in the enoxaparin group (absolute risk reduction, 2.6; $p < 0.001$). Major venous thromboembolism occurred in 4 of 1686 patients (0.2 %) in the rivaroxaban group and in 33 of 1678 patients (2.0 %) in the enoxaparin group ($p < 0.001$). Major bleeding occurred in 6 of 2209 patients (0.3 %) in the rivaroxaban group and in 2 of 2224 patients (0.1 %) in the enoxaparin group ($p = 0.18$).

The development of rivaroxaban is being pursued in many other indications and users are impatiently awaiting its availability in the market.

b) Apixaban (Bristol Myers Squibb)
Apixaban is an oral, reversible, direct factor Xa inhibitor related to rivaroxaban [16]. Its bioavailability ranges from 51 to 85 %, its Ki (0.08 nM) is better than that of nivaroxaban, its half-life is between 10 and 15 hours. Its elimination is original, only 25 % by the renal route and 75 % by hepatic and biliary metabolism and intestinal excretion. Phase III studies of fairly low doses twice daily are ongoing.

Oral Inhibitors of Activated Thrombin (Factor IIa)

Anesthetists are very familiar with antithrombins. They have used lepirudin (Refludan®) or desirudin (Revasc®), and in particular the first oral thrombin inhibitor, ximegalatran (Exanta®), which had to be withdrawn after 2 years on the market because of hepatotoxicity. Dabigatran etexilate (Pradaxa® - Boehringer-Ingelheim) is the only oral antithrombin to be marketed; others are in much earlier stages of development [17].

The bioavailability of dabigatran etexilate (6–8 %) is not quite as good as that of factor Xa inhibitors. Its Tmax is 2 hours, its terminal half-life is 14–17 hours. There is no interaction with foods; it is eliminated by the kidney [17]. A dose-ranging study (Boehringer Ingleheim Study in Thrombosis, BISTRO II) in 1973 patients undergoing total hip replacement or knee surgery suggested that the effective dose was between 100 and 300 mg but that bleeding episodes increased with dose [18].

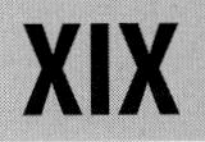

Three pivotal studies have been carried out with dabigatran etexilate in orthopedic surgery (two in knee surgery, one in total hip replacement). In one of the knee surgery studies and the hip study, two once-daily oral doses of dabigatran were used (150 mg and 220 mg starting with a half-dose 1–4 hours after surgery) and compared with daily subcutaneous enoxaparin started the evening before surgery at the 40 mg European dose [19, 20]. The efficacy of dabigatran was not inferior to that of enoxaparin. Venography on Day 10 showed strictly equivalent results in terms of efficacy. Safety was similar and there were no signs of hepatotoxicity. In the total hip replacement study, after 4-weeks of dabigatran results in terms of proximal and symptomatic thromboses were very good. However, unlike rivaroxaban, dabigatran was not superior to enoxaparin. Safety was satisfactory.

The second study on knee surgery compared identical doses of dabigatran and enoxaparin (North American dose – 30 mg twice daily) but could not demonstrate non-inferiority because of the greater number of distal thromboses with dabigatran. However, reassuringly, the rates of proximal thromboses, major bleeding, and symptomatic events did not differ between the two groups [21].

Dabigatran etexilate was granted a European Marketing Authorization on January 24, 2008, and will probably be available for orthopedic surgery in the whole of Europe by the end of the year. Its development in other indications (venous thromboembolism and atrial fibrillation) is ongoing.

Conclusion

The new oral factor Xa and factor IIa inhibitors will probably become available in our hospitals over the next two years. It is not yet possible to say whether one type of inhibitor will have a clear advantage over the other [16]. Whilst awaiting further data and longer follow-ups, clinicians should exert caution, as the long-term effects of these products are still unknown. It is necessary to take account of the products' half-lives, clearance, and specific indications. Only idraparinux has an antidote. The results of ongoing studies in patients with atrial fibrillation receiving high doses for long periods will be decisive. In the meantime, clinicians can only wait and see.

References

1. Bauer KA (2001) Fondaparinux sodium: a selective inhibitor of factor Xa. Am J Health Syst Pharm 58 (Suppl 2):S14–17
2. Turpie AG, Gallus AS, Hoek JA (2001) A synthetic pentasaccharide for the prevention of deep-vein thrombosis after total hip replacement. N Engl J Med 344: 619–625
3. Turpie AG, Bauer KA, Eriksson BI, Lassen MR (2002) Fondaparinux vs enoxaparin for the prevention of venous thromboembolism in major orthopedic surgery: a meta-analysis of 4 randomized double-blind studies. Arch Intern Med 162: 1833–1840
4. Büller HR, Davidson BL, Decousus H, et al (2003) Subcutaneous fondaparinux versus intravenous unfractionated heparin in the initial treatment of pulmonary embolism. N Engl J Med 349: 1695–1702
5. Büller HR, Davidson BL, Decousus H, et al (2004) Fondaparinux or enoxaparin for the initial treatment of symptomatic deep venous thrombosis: a randomized trial. Ann Intern Med 140: 867–873
6. Mehta SR, Granger CB, Eikelboom JW, et al (2007) Efficacy and safety of fondaparinux versus enoxaparin in patients with acute coronary syndromes undergoing percutaneous coronary intervention: results from the OASIS-5 trial. J Am Coll Cardiol 50: 1742–1751

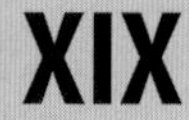

7. Warkentin TE, Maurer BT, Aster RH (2007) Heparin-induced thrombocytopenia associated with fondaparinux. N Engl J Med 356: 2653–2655
8. Buller HR, Cohen AT, Davidson B, et al (2007) Idraparinux versus standard therapy for venous thromboembolic disease. N Engl J Med 357: 1094–1104
9. Buller HR, Cohen AT, Davidson B, et al (2007) Extended prophylaxis of venous thromboembolism with idraparinux. N Engl J Med 357: 1105–1112
10. Bousser MG, Bouthier J, Buller HR, et al (2008) Comparison of idraparinux with vitamin K antagonists for prevention of thromboembolism in patients with atrial fibrillation: a randomised, open-label, non-inferiority trial. Lancet 371: 315–321
11. Weitz JI, Hirsh J, Samama MM (2004) New anticoagulant drugs: the Seventh ACCP Conference on Antithrombotic and Thrombolytic Therapy. Chest 126:265S-286S
12. Weitz JI, Bates SM. New anticoagulants. J Thromb Haemost 2005;3: 1843–53
13. Eriksson BI, Borris LC, Dahl OE, et al (2006) A once-daily, oral, direct Factor Xa inhibitor, rivaroxaban (BAY 59–7939), for thromboprophylaxis after total hip replacement. Circulation 114: 2374–2381
14. Lassen MR, Ageno W, Borris LC, et al (2008) Rivaroxaban versus enoxaparin for thromboprophylaxis after total knee arthroplasty. N Engl J Med 358: 2776–2786
15. Eriksson BI, Borris LC, Friedman RJ, et al (2008) Rivaroxaban versus enoxaparin for thromboprophylaxis after hip arthroplasty. N Engl J Med 358: 2765–2775
16. Lassen MR, Davidson BL, Gallus A, Pineo G, Ansell J, Deitchman D (2007) The efficacy and safety of apixaban, an oral, direct factor Xa inhibitor, as thromboprophylaxis in patients following total knee replacement. J Thromb Haemost 5: 2368–2375
17. Weitz JI (2007) Factor Xa or thrombin: is thrombin a better target? J Thromb Haemost 5 (Suppl 1): 65–67
18. Eriksson BI, Dahl OE, Buller HR, Hettiarachchi R (2005) A new oral direct thrombin inhibitor, dabigatran etexilate, compared with enoxaparin for prevention of thromboembolic events following total hip or knee replacement: the BISTRO II randomized trial. J Thromb Haemost 3: 103–111
19. Eriksson B, Dahl O, Rosencher N, et al (2007) Oral dabigatran etexilate vs. subcutaneous enoxaparin for the prevention of venous thromboembolism after total knee replacement: the RE-MODEL randomized study. J Thromb Haemost 5: 2178–2185
20. Eriksson BI, Dahl OE, Rosencher N, Kurth AA (2007) Dabigatran etexilate versus enoxaparin for prevention of venous thromboembolism after total hip replacement: a randomised, double-blind, non-inferiority trial. Lancet 370: 949–956
21. The RE-MOBILIZE Writing Committee (2009) Oral thrombin inhibitor dabigatran etexilate vs the North American enoxaparin regimen for prevention of venous thromboembolism after knee arthroplasty surgery. J Arthroplasty 24: 1–9
22. Gross PL, Weitz JI (2008) New anticoagulants for treatment of venous thromboembolism. Arterioscler Thromb Vasc Biol 28: 380–386

Emergency Reversal of Anticoagulants

M. Levi

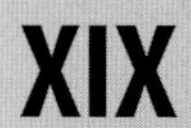

Introduction

Anticoagulant agents are often used for the prevention and treatment of a wide range of cardiovascular diseases. The most frequently used anticoagulants are heparin or its derivatives, vitamin K antagonists (such as warfarin or coumadin) and antiplatelet agents, including aspirin and thienopyridine derivatives, such as clopidogrel. A myriad of clinical studies have demonstrated that these agents (alone or in combination) can prevent or treat acute or chronic thromboembolic complications, such as in patients with atrial fibrillation or prosthetic heart valves, after myocardial infarction or ischemic stroke, and in patients with venous thrombosis or pulmonary embolism [1]. The most important complication of treatment with anticoagulants is hemorrhage, which may be serious, may cause long-term debilitating disease, or may even be life-threatening [2]. In well-controlled patients in clinical trials, treatment with vitamin K antagonists increases the risk of major bleeding by 0.5 %/year and the risk of intracranial hemorrhage by about 0.2 %/year [3]. In a very large series of 34146 patients with acute ischemic coronary syndromes, anticoagulant-associated bleeding was associated with a 5-fold increased risk of death during the first 30 days and a 1.5-fold higher mortality between 30 days and 6 months [4]. Major bleeding was an independent predictor of mortality across all subgroups that were analyzed. In some clinical situations, the incidence of serious bleeding complications may annihilate or even overwhelm the efficacy of antithrombotic agents, as has been shown in the secondary prevention of patients with ischemic stroke by vitamin K antagonists [5]. Nevertheless, in many situations clinical studies show a favorable balance between efficacy and safety in favor of anticoagulant treatment. However, if severe bleeding occurs or if a patient needs to undergo an urgent invasive procedure, such as emergency surgery, it may be necessary to reverse the anticoagulant effect of the various agents [6]. Depending on the clinical situation, i.e., the severity of the bleeding or the urgency and estimated risk of the invasive procedure, this reversal may take place over a few hours, but in some cases immediate reversal is necessary (**Table 1**). Generally, each (immediate) reversal of anticoagulant treatment needs also to take into consideration the indication for the antithrombotic agents. For example, the interruption of combined aspirin and clopidogrel treatment in a patient in whom an intracoronary stent has recently been inserted will markedly increase the risk of acute stent thrombosis with consequent downstream cardiac ischemia or infarction. Likewise, in a patient with a prosthetic mitral valve and atrial fibrillation, interruption of vitamin K antagonists may increase the risk of valve thrombosis and cerebral or systemic embolism. Each of these specific clinical situations requires a careful and balanced assessment of the benefits and risks of

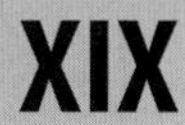

Table 1. Strategies to reverse anticoagulant effect

	Time until restoration of hemostasis after cessation of therapeutic dose	Antidote	Remark
Heparin	3–4 h	Protamine sulfate 25–30 mg	1 mg of protamine per 100 anti-Xa units given in the previous 2–3 h
LMWH	12–24 h	(Partially) protamine sulfate 25–50 mg	1 mg of protamine per 100 anti-Xa units given in the previous 8 h
Pentasaccharides	Fondaparinux: 24–30 h Idraparinux: 5–15 days	Recombinant factor VIIa 90 ug/kg (?)	Based on laboratory end-points, no systematic experience in bleeding patients
Vitamin K antagonists	Acenocoumarol: 18–24 h Warfarin: 60–80 h Phenprocoumon: 8–10 days	Vitamin K i.v: reversal in 12–16 h Vitamin K orally: reversal in 24 h PCCs: immediate reversal	Dose of vitamin K or PCCs dependend on INR and body weight
Oral thrombin and factor Xa inhibitors	Dependent on compound, usually within 12 hrs	Recombinant factor Xa for Xa inhibitors, unsure for IIa inhibitors	Based on laboratory end-points, no systematic experience in bleeding patients
Aspirin	5–10 days (time to produce unaffected platelets)	DDAVP (0.3–0.4 ug/kg) and/or platelet concentrate	Cessation not always required, also dependent on clinical situation and indication
Clopidogrel	1–2 days	Platelet concentrate, possibly in combination with DDAVP (0.3–0.4 ug/kg)	Cessation not always desirable, also dependent on clinical situation and indication
IIb/IIIa inhibitors	Dependent on preparation, usually within 24 h	Platelet concentrate, possibly in combination with DDAVP (0.3–0.4 ug/kg)	

LMWH: low molecular weight heparin; PCC: prothrombin complex concentrate; DDAVP: desamino d-arginine vasopressin or desmopressin

reversing anticoagulants (and potential strategies to keep the period of reversal as short as possible) and will often necessitate consultation with a relevant expert in cardiovascular disease. In this chapter, we will describe the various strategies to reverse the anticoagulant effect of the most widely used antithrombotic agents and some new anticoagulants.

Heparin and Low Molecular Weight Heparin (LMWH)

Herparin and heparin derivatives act by binding to antithrombin and thereby potentiating about 1000-fold the anticoagulant effect of this endogenous inhibitor towards thrombin and factor Xa (and some other coagulation factors). Heparin has a relatively short half-life of about 60–90 minutes and therefore the anticoagulant effect of therapeutic doses of heparin will be mostly eliminated at 3–4 hours after termi-

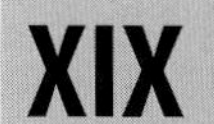

nation of continuous intravenous administration [7]. The anticoagulant effect of high dose subcutaneous heparin, however, will take a longer time to abolish. If a more immediate neutralization of heparin is required, intravenous protamine sulfate is the antidote of choice. Protamine, derived from fish sperm, binds to heparin to from a stable biologically inactive complex. Each mg of protamine will neutralize approximately 100 units of heparin. Hence, the protamine dose in a patient on a stable therapeutic heparin dose of 1000–1250 U/hr should be about 25–30 mg (sufficient to block the amount of heparin given in the previous 2–3 hours). The maximum dose of protamine is 50 mg. Since the half-life of protamine is only about 10 minutes, the reversal of subcutaneous heparin requires a prolonged infusion of protamine sulfate. The effect of protamine can be monitored by measuring the activated partial thromboplastin time (aPTT), which should normalize after its administration.

The reversal of LMWH is more complex, as protamine sulfate will only neutralize the anti-factor IIa activity and has no or only partial effect on the smaller heparin fragments causing the anti-factor Xa activity of the compound [8]. The net effect of protamine reversal of LMWH is not completely clear. There are no clinical studies that have systematically studied this and small case-series and experimental animal studies show contradictory results [9]. As the aPTT is not useful as a monitoring assay when using LMWH, it can also not be used for the monitoring of the neutralizing effect of protamine. Given the relatively long half-life of LMWH, the lack of an adequate strategy to reverse its anticoagulant action may sometimes cause a problem in clinical situations. A practical approach is to give 1 mg of protamine per 100 anti-factor Xa units of LMWH given in the previous 8 hours (where 1 mg of enoxaparin equals 100 anti-factor Xa units). If bleeding continues, a second dose of 0.5 mg per 100 anti-factor Xa units can be given.

The most important adverse effect of protamine is an allergic response, including hemodynamic and respiratory problems [10]. Most adverse reactions can be prevented or minimized by slowing the rate of administration of the drug or by pretreatment with steroids and antihistamines. Risk factors for an adverse reaction are sensitivity to fish (as may occur in traditional fishermen that are often exposed to fish proteins when cutting themselves), a history of vasectomy (which may demolish the blood-testis barrier with consequent formation of anti-semen antibodies), and a history of receiving protamine sulfate-containing insulin. Initial reports that the use of protamine sulfate could lead to an increased risk of rebound thrombosis, in particular ischemic stroke, were not confirmed in a recent randomized controlled study [11].

There are some other strategies to reverse (mostly unfractionated) heparin, such as platelet factor-4, heparanase, or extracorporeal heparin-removal devices, but none of these approaches has been properly evaluated and they are not currently approved for clinical use.

Pentasaccharides

Pentasaccharides are recently developed synthetic compounds that effectively bind and potentiate antithrombin to block factor Xa. Since they lack the additional glycosaminoglycan saccharide residues to bind to thrombin, they have an effect on factor Xa exclusively. The prototype pentasaccharide (and the only one approved for clinical use so far) is fondaparinux. Another pentasaccharide that is currently under study is idraparinux. The main difference between these two agents is the elimination half-life, which is 15–20 hours for fondaparinux and 5½ days for idraparinux. This means that idraparinux can be administered once weekly, which renders the subcutaneous route of administration less cumbersome. Pentasaccharides were shown to be effective in the prophylaxis and treatment of venous thromboembolism and are currently being evaluated in other types of thrombosis. The (very) long half-life of pentasaccharides necessitates the availability of a suitable antidote if major bleeding complicates the treatment, which may especially occur in patients who are treated with therapeutic doses of this type of anticoagulation. So far, no antidote for pentasaccharides has been studied in controlled clinical studies. The only agent that has been systematically evaluated to reverse the anticoagulant effect of pentasaccharides is recombinant factor VIIa (rVIIa). Two randomized placebo-controlled studies in healthy volunteers have tested the hypothesis that rVIIa may be useful as a suitable antidote for pentasaccharide anticoagulation [12, 13]. In the first study, 16 subjects were treated with therapeutic doses of the pentasaccharide, fondaparinux, and after two hours (at the time of maximal anticoagulation) challenged with rVIIa or placebo. Injection of rVIIa (90 μg/kg) after fondaparinux normalized the prolonged aPTT and prothrombin (PT) times and reversed the decrease in prothrombin activation fragments 1+2 (F_{1+2}), as observed with fondaparinux alone. Thrombin-generation time and endogenous thrombin potential, which were inhibited by fondaparinux, normalized up to 6 hours after rVIIa injection [12]. In the second study, 12 subjects received a single subcutaneous dose of 7.5 mg idraparinux (which is 3-fold higher than the currently recommended dose) [13]. The inhibition of thrombin generation by idraparinux, as reflected by an increased thrombin generation time and decreased level of prothrombin F_{1+2}, was partially reversed by injection of rVIIa 3 hours after idraparinux administration. The administration of rVIIa one week after treatment with idraparinux (when much lower, though still therapeutic, doses of the pentasaccharide were present) resulted in a nearly complete reversal of anticoagulation, reflected by normalization of thrombin generation time and other markers of thrombin generation. As mentioned, there are no controlled trials in patients who present with pentasaccharide-induced bleeding but there is some anecdotal experience suggesting that rVIIa may indeed be able to stop bleeding in patients anticoagulated with fondaparinux.

Vitamin K Antagonists

Vitamin K antagonists interfere with the γ-carboxylation of glutamate residues on vitamin K- dependent proteins, which therefore are not capable of a calcium-dependent conformational change by which they can bind to phospholipid surfaces, resulting in a strongly reduced coagulant activity [14]. There are several vitamin K antagonists available, of which warfarin is most widely used, but the coumadin derivatives, acenocoumarol and phenprocoumon, are also frequently prescribed. The most important difference between these three agents is their half-life, which is 9 hours for acenocoumarol, 36–42 hours for warfarin, and 90 hours for phenprocoumon. This variation in half-lives may have important consequences for the optimal strategy to reverse each of these agents. The time to reversal of anticoagulation with vitamin K antagonists will not only be affected by their half-life after cessation of treatment but also by the time it takes to produce properly carboxylated coagulation factors that have not been affected by vitamin K antagonists.

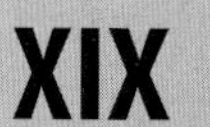

The most straightforward intervention to counteract the effect of vitamin K antagonists is the administration of vitamin K [15, 16]. Although there is some debate on the use of vitamin K in patients with too high an intensity of anticoagulation (i.e., an international normalized ratio [INR] that is too high) but no signs of bleeding, in patients with clinically significant bleeding administration of vitamin K is crucial to reverse the anticoagulant effect of warfarin or coumadin derivatives. Vitamin K can be given orally and intravenously; despite a reasonably quick and good systemic bioavailability of oral vitamin K, the parenteral route has the advantage of a more rapid onset of the treatment effect [17, 18]. After the administration of intravenous vitamin K, the INR will start to decrease within 2 hours and will be completely normalized within 12–16 hours [19]; following oral administration it will take up to 24 hours to normalize the INR [15]. Intramuscular injections of vitamin K should be avoided in patients who are anticoagulated (since they may cause muscle bleeding) and subcutaneous administration of vitamin K results in a less predictable bioavailability [18]. When the INR is less than 7, a dose range of 2.5–5 mg vitamin K has been advocated to completely counteract the anticoagulant effect, whereas with higher INRs a dose of 5 to 10 mg is required. Higher doses of vitamin K are equally effective but may lead to warfarin or coumadin resistance for more than a week, which may hamper the long-term management of these patients [20]. Of note, when reversal of anticoagulation has to be sustained for a longer period, repeated administration of vitamin K may be required, especially in patients treated with vitamin K antagonists with a long half-life, such as phenprocoumon. A potential concern with the use of parenteral vitamin K is the occurrence of anaphylactic reactions, although the incidence of this complication is very low, in particular with the more modern micelle preparations. To avoid this effect, a low infusion rate has been advocated [15].

In very serious or life-threatening bleeding, immediate correction of the INR is mandatory and can be achieved by the administration of vitamin K-dependent coagulation factors. Theoretically, these factors are present in fresh frozen plasma (FFP), however, the amount of plasma that is required to correct the INR is very large, carries the risk of fluid overload, and will probably take hours to administer [21]. Therefore, prothrombin complex concentrates (PCCs), containing all vitamin K-dependent coagulation factors, are more useful. In a small study in patients using vitamin K antagonists who needed urgent reversal of anticoagulation because of major bleeding or emergency invasive procedures, administration of PCCs at a fixed dose of 500 U was sufficient to correct INR values < 5.0. However, at INR values > 5 higher doses were required. Although PCCs can indeed be given using fixed dose schemes, it has been shown that individualized dosing regimens based on the INR at presentation and the body weight are more effective [22]. In a prospective cohort study of patients who presented with major bleeding associated with the use of vitamin K antagonists, patients were treated with PCCs at a relatively high dose of 25–50 U/kg (exact dose per patient was "based on the INR and severity of bleeding"), which was effective in reducing the INR to below 2 in 56 out of 58 patients [23]. Another prospective study in patients being treated with a vitamin K antagonist and presenting with bleeding or the need for an urgent invasive procedure necessitating normalization of the INR also reported that similar doses of PCCs were effective in reducing the INR to below 1.3 in 93 % of patients and resulted in satisfactory and sustained hemostasis in 98 % [24]. In this study, the dose of PCC was tailored at the INR at presentation (INR 2–4: 25 U/kg; INR 4–6: 35 U/kg; and INR > 6: 50 U/kg).

PCCs can be given over a short time frame, have an immediate effect, and the efficacy of the reversal of anticoagulation can be monitored by measuring the INR. PCCs were shown to be safe in a series of 14 retrospective and prospective cohort studies encompassing 460 patients [25]. Thromboembolic complications occurred in 7 patients although in most cases this could also have been explained by the underlying clinical situation and co-morbidity. In recent years, the safety of PCCs, in particular regarding the transmission of blood-borne infectious diseases, has markedly improved by several techniques, such as pasteurization, nanofiltration, and addition of solvent detergent. The often stated risk of disseminated intravascular coagulation (DIC) due to traces of activated coagulation factors in PCCs comes from older literature and modern PCCs seem not to be associated with eliciting or aggravating DIC [26].

Another option for immediate correction of the INR in patients using vitamin K antagonists is the administration of rVIIa, although this treatment is not officially approved for this indication. In healthy volunteers who were given the vitamin K antagonist, acenocoumarol, prolongation of the INR above 2.0 was normalized with the administration of rVIIa at doses between 5 and 320 μg/kg [27]. The duration of the INR correction was dependent on the dose of rVIIa, whereby doses of rVIIa larger than 120 μg/kg resulted in an INR normalization that lasted longer than 24 hours. Correction of the INR after administration of rVIIa may be a 'cosmetic' effect since the PT is very sensitive towards traces of VIIa in plasma; however, a small clinical study found that rVIIa at a dose of 16 μg/kg resulted in satisfactory hemostasis in 14 out of 16 patients who presented with major bleeding while using vitamin K antagonists [28]. Another study demonstrated that reversal of warfarin anticoagulation in a series of 13 patients undergoing invasive procedures resulted in a normalization of the prothrombin time and prevented bleeding in all subjects [29], and a series of 6 patients with central nervous system (CNS) bleeding due to treatment with vitamin K antagonists showed successful reversal of anticoagulation, arrest of bleeding, and uncomplicated drainage of the CNS hematoma in all patients after administration of rVIIa [30].

New Anticoagulants

In recent years a large number of new antithrombotic agents has been developed and tested in clinical trials and many of these new agents will become available for clinical practice in the very near future [31]. The need for new anticoagulant agents is quite obvious: First, current agents are insufficiently effective. For example, 10–15 % of patients undergoing major orthopedic surgery develop venous thromboembolism, despite prophylaxis with LMWH. Furthermore, the available anticoagulants are relatively unsafe, mostly due to the occurrence of bleeding as discussed above. Finally, current anticoagulant agents are often cumbersome with regards to their clinical use, requiring repeated laboratory control and frequent dose adjustments. Increasing knowledge of the function of the hemostatic system *in vivo* has resulted in a new generation of anticoagulant agents. Despite the fact that most of these agents indeed have a somewhat more advantageous benefit-risk profile and are much easier to use with no need for monitoring or dose adjustments, bleeding remains the most important adverse effect of any type of anticoagulant treatment.

An important group of new anticoagulants is the class of direct thrombin inhibitors. Thrombin is the central enzyme in the coagulation process, not only mediating

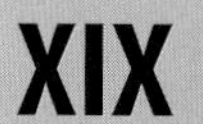

the conversion of fibrinogen to fibrin, but also being the most important physiological activator of platelets and various other coagulation factors. Inhibition of thrombin can be achieved by administration of heparin, but in view of the limited ability of the heparin-antithrombin complex to inhibit surface-bound thrombin, new antithrombin-independent anticoagulants have been developed [32]. The prototype of these thrombin inhibitors is hirudin, originally derived from the saliva of leeches (*hirudo medicinalis*) and now produced by recombinant technology. Melagatran is a synthetic thrombin inhibitor, which has predictable pharmacokinetic properties and can thus be used in a fixed dose [33]. Moreover, the pro-drug ximelagatran is relatively quickly absorbed after oral ingestion and results in sufficient systemic availability, rendering this agent suitable for long-term use as an oral anticoagulant. Clinical trials on the prevention and treatment of venous thromboembolism and in patients with atrial fibrillation showed promising efficacy of (xi)melagatran; however due to the occurrence of enhanced liver enzymes in 6–7 % of patients using melagatran, the compound has been withdrawn by the manufacturer. Nevertheless, there are many similar compounds under evaluation in clinical trials at this moment [34]. For each of these compounds, no established antidote is available in case of serious bleeding complicating the anticoagulant treatment. In a controlled clinical study in healthy subjects, the melagatran-induced effects on aPTT, thrombin generation and platelet activation were not affected by the administration of rVIIa [35]. Based on these results, it seems that rVIIa is not effective in reversing direct thrombin inhibition. Since, however, rVIIa was able to correct the melagatran-induced prolongation of the PT and increased thrombin precursor protein concentrations, it may be that higher doses of rVIIa will have some effect in this situation, but this needs to be studied in future experiments.

Another class of new anticoagulants is directed at factor Xa. The prototypes of these agents are rivaroxaban and apixaban, which have shown promising results in initial experimental and clinical studies [36, 37] There is no evidence so far of any antidote for the anticoagulant effect of any of these orally available factor Xa inhibitors. Based on the experience with rVIIa in the reversal of the anticoagulant effect of fondaparinux, one can postulate that rVIIa may be an effective antidote for these agents, however, direct proof has not been demonstrated.

In view of the central role of the tissue factor-factor VIIa pathway in the initiation of blood coagulation, novel therapeutic strategies aimed at inhibiting this catalytic complex are currently being evaluated. One of these inhibitors is recombinant nematode anticoagulant protein c2 (rNAPc2), a potent and selective inhibitor of the tissue factor-factor VIIa complex in the presence of factor Xa [38]. This compound showed promising antithrombotic properties in clinical trials of prevention and treatment of venous thromboembolism and percutaneous coronary interventions [39]. Recent reports from *in vitro* studies indicate that therapeutic doses of rVIIa may be able to induce activation of coagulation resulting in subsequent thrombin generation possibly independent of tissue factor activity [40]. In a double-blind, randomized, placebo-controlled crossover study administration of rNAPc2 caused a prolongation of the PT, which was immediately and completely corrected by the subsequent injection of rVIIa [41]. Administration of rVIIa in the presence of NAPc2 resulted in a marked generation of thrombin, as reflected by plasma levels of prothrombin fragment F1+2 and thrombin-antithrombin levels.

Aspirin

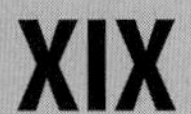

Aspirin is effective in the secondary prevention of atherothrombotic disease, in particular coronary artery disease, cerebrovascular thromboembolism and peripheral arterial disease [42]. As a consequence, aspirin is one of the most widely used agents in the Western world. Aspirin increases the risk of bleeding, in particular gastrointestinal bleeding, and has been associated with a small but consistent increase in intracerebral hemorrhage. In addition, it has been shown that the use of aspirin is associated with increased perioperative blood loss in major procedures, although this does not necessarily translate into clinically relevant endpoints, such as the requirement for transfusion or re-operation [43]. Over the last few years, the approach to the patient who uses aspirin and who presents with bleeding or needs to undergo an invasive procedure has changed considerably. In fact, in current clinical practice, bleeding can almost always be managed with local hemostatic procedures or conservative strategies without interruption of aspirin. In addition, most invasive procedures do not require cessation of aspirin when adequate attention is given to local hemostasis. In contrast, interruption of aspirin has been associated with an increased risk of thromboembolic complications, potentially due to a rebound hypercoagulability [44]. Obviously, in special clinical circumstances, such as intracranial bleeding or the need to undergo a neurosurgical procedure, the antihemostatic effect of aspirin needs to be reversed immediately. The most rigorous measure to achieve this is the administration of platelet concentrate after cessation of aspirin. Another approach is the administration of desamino d-arginine vasopressin (DDAVP, desmopressin). DDAVP is a vasopressin analog that, despite minor molecular differences, has retained its antidiuretic properties but has fewer vasoactive effects [45]. DDAVP induces release of the contents of the endothelial cell-associated Weibel Palade bodies, including von Willebrand factor. Hence, the administration of DDAVP results in a marked increase in the plasma concentration of von Willebrand factor (and associated coagulation factor VIII) and (by yet unexplained additional mechanisms) a remarkable augmentation of primary hemostasis as a consequence. DDAVP is effective in patients with mild hemophilia A or von Willebrand's disease and in patients with qualitative platelet defects, such as in uremia or liver cirrhosis. DDAVP seems also capable of correcting aspirin-induced platelet dysfunction, although large clinical studies employing relevant outcome parameters are lacking [46]. The combined effect of platelet concentrate and subsequent administration of DDAVP has also been advocated to correct the effect of aspirin on platelets. The standard dose of DDAVP is 0.3–0.4 μg/kg in 100 ml saline over 30 minutes and its effect is immediate.

Thienopyridine Derivatives and Other Antiplatelet Agents

Clopidogrel belongs to the class of thienopyridine derivatives, which act by blocking the ADP receptor on the platelet. Clinical studies have shown that clopidogrel is as good as aspirin in the secondary prevention of atherothrombotic events [47]. However, the combination of aspirin and clopidogrel is superior over aspirin alone in patients who have received intracoronary stents or in other patients with high-risk coronary artery disease. The increased efficacy of the combined use of aspirin and clopidogrel is also associated with a higher bleeding risk. The decision whether or not to interrupt or even reverse antithrombotic treatment with clopidogrel and aspi-

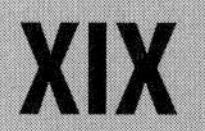

rin in case of serious bleeding or when performing an invasive procedure will depend on the specific clinical situation but also on the indication for the antithrombotic treatment (see above). Especially in patients with recent implantation of an intracoronary stent, the cardiologist will often not, or only reluctantly, agree to cessation of treatment. If, however, the decision is made to stop and even reverse this treatment, administration of platelet concentrate is probably the best way to correct the hemostatic defect [48]. In addition, DDAVP has been shown to correct the defect in platelet aggregation caused by clopidogrel, so this may be another option [49].

Other antiplatelet agents, which are predominantly used in interventional cardiology, include IIb-IIIa receptor antagonists, such as abciximab or eptifibatide. These agents have a very potent antiplatelet effect and – although rare – may carry the risk of thrombocytopenia. If in these situations serious bleeding occurs, administration of platelet concentrate, possibly in combination with DDAVP, will correct the hemostatic defect [50].

Conclusion

Conventional anticoagulant treatment can be reversed by specific interventions when the clinical situation requires immediate correction of hemostasis. For the new generation of anticoagulants, no specific antidotes are available, although some interventions are promising but need further evaluation. Antiplatelet therapy with aspirin can be reversed but this is often not required. More potent antiplatelet strategies can be counteracted with correcting strategies as well; however, in some cases this may not be desirable in view of the indication for this treatment.

References

1. Hirsh J, Guyatt G, Albers GW, Harrington R, Schunemann HJ (2008) Antithrombotic and thrombolytic therapy: American College of Chest Physicians Evidence-Based Clinical Practice Guidelines (8th Edition). Chest 133:110S-112S
2. Mannucci PM, Levi M (2007) Prevention and treatment of major blood loss. N Engl J Med 356: 2301–2311
3. Schulman S, Beyth RJ, Kearon C, Levine MN (2008) Hemorrhagic complications of anticoagulant and thrombolytic treatment: American College of Chest Physicians Evidence-Based Clinical Practice Guidelines (8th Edition). Chest 133 (suppl 6):257S-298S
4. Eikelboom JW, Mehta SR, Anand SS, Xie C, Fox KA, Yusuf S (2006) Adverse impact of bleeding on prognosis in patients with acute coronary syndromes. Circulation 114: 774–782
5. Algra A (2007) Medium intensity oral anticoagulants versus aspirin after cerebral ischaemia of arterial origin (ESPRIT): a randomised controlled trial. Lancet Neurol. 6: 115–124
6. Levi M (2008) Emergency reversal of antithrombotic treatment. Intern Emerg Med (in press)
7. Hirsh J, Bauer KA, Donati MB, Gould M, Samama MM, Weitz JI (2008) Parenteral anticoagulants: American College of Chest Physicians Evidence-Based Clinical Practice Guidelines (8th Edition). Chest 133 (suppl 6):141S-159S
8. Lindblad B, Borgstrom A, Wakefield TW, Whitehouse WM Jr, Stanley JC (1987). Protamine reversal of anticoagulation achieved with a low molecular weight heparin. The effects on eicosanoids, clotting and complement factors. Thromb Res 48: 31–40
9. Van Ryn-McKenna J, Cai L, Ofosu FA, Hirsh J, Buchanan MR (1990) Neutralization of enoxaparine-induced bleeding by protamine sulfate. Thromb Haemost 63: 271–274
10. Caplan SN, Berkman EM (1976) Protamine sulfate and fish allergy. N Engl J Med 295:172
11. Dellagrammaticas D, Lewis SC, Gough MJ (2008) Is heparin reversal with protamine after carotid endarterectomy dangerous? Eur J Vasc Endovasc Surg 36: 41–44

12. Bijsterveld NR, Moons AH, Boekholdt SM, et al (2002). Ability of recombinant factor VIIa to reverse the anticoagulant effect of the pentasaccharide fondaparinux in healthy volunteers. Circulation 106: 2550–2554
13. Bijsterveld NR, Vink R, van Aken BE, et al (2004). Recombinant factor VIIa reverses the anticoagulant effect of the long-acting pentasaccharide idraparinux in healthy volunteers. Br J Haematol 124: 653–658
14. Ansell J, Hirsh J, Hylek E, Jacobson A, Crowther M, Palareti G (2008) Pharmacology and management of the vitamin K antagonists: American College of Chest Physicians Evidence-Based Clinical Practice Guidelines (8th Edition). Chest 133 (suppl 6):160S-198S
15. Dentali F, Ageno W, Crowther M (2006) Treatment of coumarin-associated coagulopathy: a systematic review and proposed treatment algorithms. J Thromb Haemost 4: 1853–1863
16. Baglin T (1998) Management of warfarin (coumarin) overdose. Blood Rev 12: 91–98
17. Whitling AM, Bussey HI, Lyons RM (1998) Comparing different routes and doses of phytonadione for reversing excessive anticoagulation. Arch Intern Med 158: 2136–2140
18. Crowther MA, Douketis JD, Schnurr T, et al (2002) Oral vitamin K lowers the international normalized ratio more rapidly than subcutaneous vitamin K in the treatment of warfarin-associated coagulopathy. A randomized, controlled trial. Ann Intern Med 137: 251–254
19. Lubetsky A, Yonath H, Olchovsky D, Loebstein R, Halkin H, Ezra D (2003). Comparison of oral vs intravenous phytonadione (vitamin K1) in patients with excessive anticoagulation: a prospective randomized controlled study. Arch Intern Med 163: 2469–2473
20. van Geest-Daalderop JH, Hutten BA, Pequeriaux NC, de Vries-Goldschmeding HJ, Rakers E, Levi M (2007) Invasive procedures in the outpatient setting: Managing the short-acting acenocoumarol and the long-acting phenprocoumon. Thromb Haemost 98: 747–755
21. Aguilar MI, Hart RG, Kase CS, et al (2007) Treatment of warfarin-associated intracerebral hemorrhage: literature review and expert opinion. Mayo Clin Proc 82: 82–92
22. van Aart L, Eijkhout HW, Kamphuis JS, et al (2006) Individualized dosing regimen for prothrombin complex concentrate more effective than standard treatment in the reversal of oral anticoagulant therapy: an open, prospective randomized controlled trial. Thromb Res 118: 313–320
23. Lankiewicz MW, Hays J, Friedman KD, Tinkoff G, Blatt PM (2006) Urgent reversal of warfarin with prothrombin complex concentrate. J Thromb Haemost 4: 967–970
24. Pabinger I, Brenner B, Kalina U, Knaub S, Nagy A, Ostermann H (2008) Prothrombin complex concentrate (Beriplex P/N) for emergency anticoagulation reversal: a prospective multinational clinical trial. J Thromb Haemost 6: 622–631
25. Leissinger CA, Blatt PM, Hoots WK, Ewenstein B (2008) Role of prothrombin complex concentrates in reversing warfarin anticoagulation: a review of the literature. Am J Hematol 83: 137–143
26. Levi M (2007) Disseminated intravascular coagulation. Crit Care Med 35: 2191–2195
27. Erhardtsen E, Nony P, Dechavanne M, Ffrench P, Boissel JP, Hedner U (1998) The effect of recombinant factor VIIa (NovoSeven) in healthy volunteers receiving acenocoumarol to an International Normalized Ratio above 2.0. Blood Coagul Fibrinolysis 9: 741–748
28. Dager WE, King JH, Regalia RC, et al (2006) Reversal of elevated international normalized ratios and bleeding with low-dose recombinant activated factor VII in patients receiving warfarin. Pharmacotherapy 26: 1091–1098
29. Deveras RA, Kessler CM (2002) Reversal of warfarin-induced excessive anticoagulation with recombinant human factor VIIa concentrate. Ann Intern Med 137: 884–888
30. Sorensen B, Johansen P, Nielsen GL, Sorensen JC, Ingerslev J (2003) Reversal of the International Normalized Ratio with recombinant activated factor VII in central nervous system bleeding during warfarin thromboprophylaxis: clinical and biochemical aspects. Blood Coagul Fibrinolysis 14: 469–477
31. Levi M (2005) New antithrombotics in the treatment of thromboembolic disease. Eur J Intern Med 16: 230–237
32. Weitz JI, Buller HR (2002) Direct thrombin inhibitors in acute coronary syndromes: present and future. Circulation 105: 1004–1011
33. Wahlander K, Lapidus L, Olsson CG, et al (2002) Pharmacokinetics, pharmacodynamics and clinical effects of the oral direct thrombin inhibitor ximelagatran in acute treatment of patients with pulmonary embolism and deep vein thrombosis. Thromb Res 107: 93–99

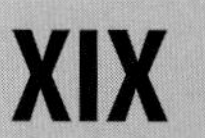

34. Eriksson BI, Dahl OE, Rosencher N, et al (2007) Dabigatran etexilate versus enoxaparin for prevention of venous thromboembolism after total hip replacement: a randomised, double-blind, non-inferiority trial. Lancet 370: 949–956
35. Wolzt M, Levi M, Sarich TC, et al (2004) Effect of recombinant factor VIIa on melagatran-induced inhibition of thrombin generation and platelet activation in healthy volunteers. Thromb Haemost 91: 1090–1096
36. Agnelli G, Gallus A, Goldhaber SZ, et al (2007) Treatment of proximal deep-vein thrombosis with the oral direct factor Xa inhibitor rivaroxaban (BAY 59–7939): the ODIXa-DVT (Oral Direct Factor Xa Inhibitor BAY 59–7939 in Patients With Acute Symptomatic Deep-Vein Thrombosis) study. Circulation 116: 180–187
37. Shantsila E, Lip GY (2008) Apixaban, an oral, direct inhibitor of activated Factor Xa. Curr Opin Investig Drugs 9: 1020–1033
38. Stassens P, Bergum PW, Gansemans Y, et al (1996) Anticoagulant repertoire of the hookworm Ancylostoma caninum. Proc Natl Acad Sci USA 93: 2149–2154
39. Moons AH, Peters RJ, Bijsterveld NR, et al (2003) Recombinant nematode anticoagulant protein c2, an inhibitor of the tissue factor/factor VIIa complex, in patients undergoing elective coronary angioplasty. J Am Coll Cardiol 41: 2147–2153
40. Allen GA, Hoffman M, Roberts HR, Monroe DM III (2002) Recombinant activated factor VII: its mechanism of action and role in the control of hemorrhage. Can J Anaesth 49:S7–14
41. Friederich PW, Levi M, Bauer KA, et al (2001) Ability of recombinant factor VIIa to generate thrombin during inhibition of tissue factor in human subjects. Circulation 103: 2555–2559
42. Patrono C, Baigent C, Hirsh J, Roth G (2008). Antiplatelet drugs: American College of Chest Physicians Evidence-Based Clinical Practice Guidelines (8th Edition). Chest 133 (Suppl 6): 199S-233S
43. Merritt JC, Bhatt DL (2004) The efficacy and safety of perioperative antiplatelet therapy. J Thromb Thrombolysis 17: 21–27
44. Ferrari E, Benhamou M, Cerboni P, Marcel B (2005) Coronary syndromes following aspirin withdrawal: a special risk for late stent thrombosis. J Am Coll Cardiol 45: 456–459
45. Richardson DW, Robinson AG (1985) Desmopressin. Ann Intern Med 103: 228–239
46. Reiter RA, Mayr F, Blazicek H, et al (2003) Desmopressin antagonizes the in vitro platelet dysfunction induced by GPIIb/IIIa inhibitors and aspirin. Blood 102: 4594–4599
47. CAPRIE Steering Committee (1996) A randomised, blinded, trial of clopidogrel versus aspirin in patients at risk of ischaemic events (CAPRIE). Lancet 348: 1329–1339
48. Vilahur G, Choi BG, Zafar MU, et al (2007) Normalization of platelet reactivity in clopidogrel-treated subjects. J Thromb Haemost 5: 82–90
49. Leithauser B, Zielske D, Seyfert UT, Jung F (2008) Effects of desmopressin on platelet membrane glycoproteins and platelet aggregation in volunteers on clopidogrel. Clin Hemorheol Microcirc 39: 293–302
50. Reiter R, Jilma-Stohlawetz P, Horvath M, Jilma B (2005) Additive effects between platelet concentrates and desmopressin in antagonizing the platelet glycoprotein IIb/IIIa inhibitor eptifibatide. Transfusion 45: 420–426

XX Neurological Aspects

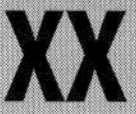

The Role of Imaging in Acute Brain Injury

R.D. Stevens, A. Pustavoitau, and P. van Zijl

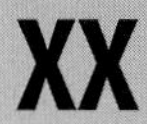

Introduction

There is increasing awareness of the preponderance and complexity of neurological dysfunction in the intensive care unit (ICU). The critical care physician has a central role in the evaluation and treatment not only of patients admitted with complex traumatic and non-traumatic brain injuries, but also of patients who develop secondary neurological dysfunction as a result of a systemic insult such as cardiac arrest, liver failure, or sepsis.

Imaging is a cornerstone of neurologically directed intensive care, identifying critical changes in cerebral structure and function and also yielding valuable insight into the causative mechanisms and natural history of acute brain dysfunction. We review existing and emerging imaging methods for the study of acute brain injury, then we discuss the role of brain imaging in the management of patients with traumatic brain injury (TBI), anuerysmal subarachnoid hemorrhage (SAH), and several common types of encephalopathy. The imaging of acute ischemic stroke and primary intracerebral hemorrhage has been reviewed elsewhere [1, 2].

Brain Imaging Modalities

Brain imaging modalities are centered on the description of anatomy and structure, the determination of brain perfusion and metabolism, and the identification of neural substrates of cognition with functional brain imaging.

Structural Imaging

Computed tomography
Computed tomography (CT) detects acute intracranial hemorrhage, changes in the morphology of the ventricular and subarachnoid systems, moderate to severe degrees of brain edema, and fractures of the skull. Coupled with iodinated intravenous contrast, the head CT becomes more sensitive to regional differences in blood flow or volume (e.g., neovascularization, vasodilatation or hyperemia) or to disruptions in the blood brain barrier (e.g., inflammatory, infectious or neoplastic lesions). These characteristics, along with wide availability, make head CT the imaging modality of choice in the initial or emergent management of a broad range of patients with neurological dysfunction including TBI, ischemic stroke, intracerebral hemorrhage (ICH), and SAH. Limitations of CT include beam-hardening artifact which distorts structures in proximity to bone, an effect typically seen in the poste-

rior fossa and in the temporal and parietal regions; other CT artifacts include partial volume averaging, motion artifact, and streaking from out-of-field objects.

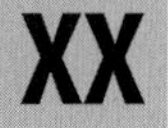

Magnetic resonance imaging

Magnetic resonance imaging (MRI) has greater spatial resolution and is significantly more valuable than CT in evaluating the brainstem, the posterior fossa, and the cerebral cortex. T1 and T2 weighted sequences are routinely complemented with fluid attenuated inversion recovery (FLAIR), which has T2 weighting but suppresses the cerebrospinal fluid (CSF) signal, increasing the visibility of the cortex, subarachnoid space, and periventricular regions. Comprehensive brain MRI often includes gradient recalled echo, an approach that is both T2 weighted and sensitive to field inhomogeneities arising from paramagnetic blood breakdown products such as hemosiderin. Gradient recalled echo identifies areas of intraparenchymal hemorrhage in the subacute to chronic phase when hemorrhagic lesions may not be detectable with CT or other MRI sequences. Recent data have shown that MRI may be as accurate as CT for the detection of acute hemorrhage in patients presenting with acute focal stroke symptoms [3]. Collectively these properties have made MRI routine in the evaluation of patients with ischemic stroke, TBI, and encephalopathy.

Susceptibility weighted imaging

Derived from gradient recalled echo, susceptibility-weighted imaging uses phase post-processing to accentuate the difference in susceptibility (i.e., the degree of magnetization in response to an applied magnetic field) between tissues. Susceptibility-weighted imaging provides excellent contrast for gray-white matter differentiation, detection of hemoglobin breakdown products, and venous blood vessels. Susceptibility-weighted imaging has greater sensitivity than conventional gradient recalled echo in the detection of hemorrhagic lesions associated with trauma (in particular diffuse axonal injury), and is a promising modality in the characterization of non-traumatic intracerebral hemorrhage, vascular malformations, and cerebral venous thrombosis.

Diffusion tensor imaging

Another novel structural imaging modality is diffusion tensor imaging, which is sensitive to the regional diffusion properties of brain water molecules (see below, 'diffusion weighted imaging'). Diffusion tensor imaging contains information on the magnitude and direction of water diffusion and can be used to generate 3-dimensional reconstructions of white matter tracts. In healthy white matter, water diffusion is highly restricted to an axis that is parallel to axons, a property referred to as anisotropy. The diffusion constants in the diffusion tensor (i.e., the 3 x 3 matrix characterizing the directional dependence of diffusion) that are due to anisotropy can be expressed collectively as a 'fractional anisotropy', with decrements in fractional anisotropy indicating white matter disease [4]. Diffusion tensor imaging has been used to identify numerous tracts, such as the commissural fibers of the corpus callosum, the superior and inferior longitudinal fascicules, superior and inferior fronto-occipital fascicules, uncinate fasciculus, and the cingulum; smaller fiber bundles, such as corticothalamic fibers and the corticospinal tract can also be visualized. The information generated by diffusion tensor imaging has been validated in gross anatomical and in histological studies, and evidence indicates that diffusion tensor imaging is a very powerful tool to assess changes in white matter tracts that occur in the setting of ischemic stroke and TBI.

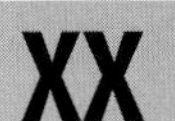

Hemodynamic and Metabolic Imaging

Physiological brain imaging modalities assess cerebral blood flow (CBF), cerebral blood volume (CBV), cerebral oxygen consumption ($CMRO_2$), and brain neurochemistry, and allow inferences regarding cerebral ischemia. Available methods include positron emission tomography (PET), single photon emission CT, xenon-enhanced CT, perfusion CT, perfusion- and diffusion-weighted MRI, arterial spin labeling MRI, and magnetic resonance spectroscopy.

Positron emission tomography

PET is an imaging method that uses positron-emitting radioisotopes to estimate CBF, CBV, $CMRO_2$ and oxygen extraction fraction. Radiotracers derived from ^{15}O are administered intravenously ($H_2{}^{15}O$) or by inhalation ($C^{15}O_2$ and $^{15}O_2$) and CBF, CBV and $CMRO_2$ are estimated using the Kety-Schmidt model which is based on Fick's principle relating tissue uptake, flow, and arteriovenous difference [4, 5]. PET can also be performed with 18-fluorodeoxyglucose (^{18}FDG) to assess regional glucose consumption. Studies indicate that brain tissue in which the oxygen extraction fraction is increased to > 40 % is ischemic or at risk for ischemia. PET is costly, requires an anatomical reference, and is difficult to obtain in emergency settings; its current clinical applications are in the evaluation of selected patients with chronic cerebrovascular disease, encephalopathy and epilepsy. In the context of research, PET has helped delineate abnormal cerebral hemodynamic patterns associated with ischemic stroke, intracerebral hemorrhage, SAH, TBI, and various encephalopathies.

Single photon emission CT

In single photon emission CT (SPECT), gamma-emitting radioisotopes (^{133}xenon, ^{99m}tecnetium-hexamethylpropylenamine oxime, ^{99m}tecnetium-ethyl cysteine dimer, or ^{123}I inosine-5'-monophosphate) are used in conjunction with multiple detector cameras to provide CBF maps which can be quantitative in the case of ^{133}xenon, but which are relative (compared to regions of interest in normal brain or in normal controls) when the other radiopharmaceuticals are used. Advantages of SPECT are that it is rapid and requires comparatively simple and inexpensive hardware; drawbacks are that it is non-anatomic and must be co-registered with either a CT or MRI, has low spatial resolution, and allows only semiquantitative estimates of CBF. In spite of these shortcomings, SPECT is employed in the assessment of patients with acute ischemic stroke, TBI, SAH, encephalopathy, and epilepsy.

Xenon-enhanced CT

In xenon-enhanced CT, the inert radio-opaque inert gas, ^{131}Xe, is inhaled and rapidly distributes to the bloodstream and into the tissues; CBF is estimated using the Kety-Schmidt equation integrating the time course of brain and arterial xenon concentrations and the xenon blood-brain partition coefficient (it is assumed that alveolar and arterial xenon tensions are equivalent). Regional CBF is superimposed on an anatomical scan and resolution is in the order of 4 mm; xenon-enhanced CT does not provide information on $CMRO_2$. Xenon-enhanced CT is rapid, reliable, and has been used to identify changes in CBF and alterations in cerebral autoregulation associated with ischemic stroke, intracerebral hemorrhage, SAH, and TBI. The advantages of xenon-enhanced CT are that it is based on CT which is widely available, that it uses hardware which is relatively simple and inexpensive when compared with other imaging techniques, and that it is quantitative. Drawbacks include the sedative properties of xenon, transient xenon-induced increases in CBF and intracranial pressure (ICP), and reduced accuracy in the presence of pulmonary disease affecting alveolar-arterial diffusion properties.

Perfusion CT

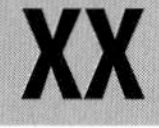

In perfusion CT, high speed helical scanning devices are used to acquire axial images following a rapidly administered bolus of intravenous iodinated contrast. Relative mean transit time (MTT), CBV, and CBF are obtained using the Meier-Zierler model of indicator dilution [6], while absolute quantification requires mathematical processing (deconvolution of the arterial input function) of arterial and tissue enhancement curves [7]. Perfusion maps can be obtained in combination with 3-dimensional CT angiography when an associated vascular lesion is suspected. Perfusion CT is obtained rapidly and spatial resolution is excellent (1–2 mm). however currently available scanners only allow the acquisition of 2–4 axial images.

The accuracy and reliability of perfusion CT estimates of CBF has not been fully validated; quantitative CBF measurements do not consistently correlate with 'standard' methods such as xenon-enhanced CT or PET. On the other hand, in patients with ischemic stroke, perfusion CT estimates of infarct core and ischemic penumbra volumes correlate with diffusion and perfusion MRI measurements, and are predictive of final infarct volume. Advantages of perfusion CT include the fact that it is rapid, uses helical or spiral CT scanners which are widely available, and can be combined with other CT studies such as axial CT or CT angiography; disadvantages are that it entails exposure to radiation and to intravenous contrast, the number of axial images is limited, poor visualization of the posterior fossa, and accuracy of CBF quantification is uncertain. Notwithstanding, perfusion CT is increasingly seen as a valuable tool in the evaluation of patients with acute ischemic stroke, and in the characterization of CBF in patients with TBI, and SAH.

Perfusion-weighted and diffusion-weighted MRI

Dynamic susceptibility contrast brain MRI (often referred to as 'perfusion-weighted imaging' or 'perfusion MRI') assesses changes in brain magnetic susceptibility following the intravenous injection of a gadolinium-based contrast. The passage of contrast through the microvasculature is associated with a loss of signal intensity on T2 or T2* images, and information can be obtained on MTT, time to peak, CBF and CBV using the Meier-Zierler model [6]. In clinical practice, the regional distribution of flow variables is mapped and relative values are inferred by comparison with regions of interest in the contralateral healthy brain. Absolute quantification of cerebral perfusion parameters with perfusion weighted MRI is feasible, however this requires the deconvolution of signal intensity-time curves by an arterial input function; these computations are different than in perfusion CT because of the non-linear relationship between gadolinium concentration changes and magnetic resonance signal intensity. Thus perfusion MRI overestimates CBV and CBF when compared to standard methods such as PET.

Diffusion-weighted imaging is an MRI modality that is sensitive to diffusion of water molecules within tissues. The intracellular accumulation of water that occurs in cytotoxic edema is expressed as a decrease in the apparent diffusion coefficient or as a hyperintense signal on diffusion-weighted imaging. Although diffusion-weighted imaging-hyperintense lesions may be appreciated in brain tumors, abscesses, diffuse and focal TBI, SAH, and intracebrebral hemorrhage, the most frequent cause of increased diffusion-weighted imaging signal is acute ischemic stroke

[8]. Areas of restricted diffusion can be appreciated within minutes after symptom onset, and provide critical information on the site, size, and age of acute ischemic stroke. Comparison of perfusion weighted and diffusion-weighted imaging maps or volumes yields clinically useful inferences on CBF and tissue viability. In the presence of a mismatch (perfusion weighted image larger than diffusion-weighted image), the brain tissue identified after subtracting the diffusion-weighted image from the perfusion-weighted image is postulated to represent a radiological ischemic penumbra, i.e., tissue whose viability is threatened by reduced perfusion, and which might be salvaged with therapeutic intervention. Perfusion/diffusion MRI has many advantages over other imaging modes including the lack of ionizing radiation, the possibility of assessing both perfusion and tissue ischemia, and the ability to image the entire brain; disadvantages include the exposure to gadolinium, inability to accurately quantify CBF, and concerns about the physiological and clinical significance of the mismatch hypothesis.

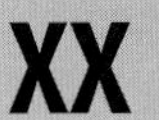

Arterial spin labeling

Arterial spin labeling is a magnetic resonance-based method of assessing cerebral perfusion which uses a radiofrequency pulse to magnetically invert (label) the spin of blood water protons as they enter the brain [9]. Images obtained before and after spin labeling are subtracted, yielding a difference in signal which is proportional to tissue perfusion. Arterial spin labeling provides quantitative estimates of CBF which are reasonably accurate when compared with 'standard' methods such as PET. Existing studies indicate that arterial spin labeling correctly estimates CBF in the gray matter, but tends to underestimate white matter CBF. Quantitative arterial spin labeling CBF measurements change by less than 10 % when the same subject is re-imaged. Arterial spin labeling is an attractive method since no exogenous contrast is needed and spatial resolution is relatively good (1 – 2 mm). While use of this method remains largely confined to research, potential applications of arterial spin labeling include acute ischemic stroke, epilepsy, and TBI.

Magnetic resonance spectroscopy

Brain magnetic resonance spectroscopy (MRS) is a non-invasive method to measure concentrations of biochemical compounds in MRI-specified areas of cerebral tissue. The basis for MRS is that nuclei have a resonance frequency that depends on both the external magnetic field strength and on a nuclear constant, the gyromagnetic radius. Nuclei used in MRS biomedical research are proton (^{1}H), phosphorus (^{31}P), and carbon (^{13}C), with most *in vivo* studies employing ^{1}H due to its natural abundance and greater sensitivity (a consequence of the greater gyromagnetic ratio). Unlike MRI, which is based exclusively on the signal generated by the protons of water molecules, ^{1}H-MRS is dependent on the signal of protons in a number of metabolites. The frequency of the protons in these molecules depends on their magnetic environment and is characterized by the so-called chemical shift that is quantified in parts per million (ppm). For instance, CH_3 protons in N-acetyl aspartate (NAA), a marker of neuronal integrity, resonate at 2.02 ppm. The resolution between resonant frequencies increases with the strength of the magnetic field (frequency in Hz increases but in ppm remains constant), while sensitivity increases with the square of the field.

In humans, ^{1}H-MRS is used to determine concentrations of a number of biologically relevant compounds including: NAA, a marker of neuronal integrity; creatine compounds (creatine and phosphocreatine), which reflect high energy phosphate turnover; choline (Cho), a product of membrane phospholipid metabolism; lactate, an indicator of anaerobic metabolism and ischemia; myo-inositol, a second messenger; and the neurotransmitters, glumatate, glutamine (often expressed together as [Glx]), gamma-amino butyric acid (GABA), and glycine. A broader range of metabolites is detectable with high field MRI scanners. Applications of MRS include the study of brain tumors, encephalopathies, epilepsy, and TBI.

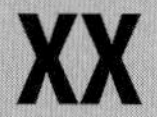

Functional Brain Imaging

The goal of functional brain imaging is to understand the neural basis of cognitive processes. Since there is no validated method to directly image brain function, the latter must be inferred from a surrogate physiological marker, usually a change in cerebral perfusion, working from the hypothesis that neuronal activation is linked temporally and spatially to local changes in blood flow. This can be accomplished with functional PET or functional MRI (fMRI), but much recent research has relied on fMRI because it does not require ionizing radiation and has greater spatial and temporal resolution. The most frequently used fMRI contrast is 'blood oxygenation level-dependent' (BOLD), which reflects inhomogenities in the magnetic field caused by changes in the oxygenation state of hemoglobin in the local vessels of activated regions as well as in draining veins [10]. Neural activation is associated with a local increase in CBF that is of greater magnitude than the increase in $CMRO_2$, leading to a net reduction in the parenchymal concentration of deoxyhemoglobin which is paramagnetic as opposed to oxyhemoglobin which is diamagnetic. It is generally accepted that the BOLD signal is a composite parameter, which depends on the combined effects of changes in CBF, CBV, $CMRO_2$.

Cognitive neuroscience is highly dependent on fMRI, with classic experimental paradigms evaluating BOLD signal changes in response to a specific task or stimulus. An alternative approach evaluates BOLD responses in the absence of any deliberate task, yielding maps of 'resting-state' brain activity. Analysis of fluctuations in the BOLD signal reveals temporal coherence within anatomically distinct areas of the brain, suggesting patterns of functional connectivity [10, 11]. Functional and effective connectivity maps can be corroborated with assessments of structural connectivity obtained with diffusion tensor imaging [12].

Currently the principal clinical application of fMRI is presurgical mapping to localize language and motor areas, and epileptic seizure foci. Recent fMRI studies have characterized brain reorganization patterns following acute injury, as evidenced by an emerging body of work on ischemic stroke and TBI. In survivors of severe brain injury, fMRI has helped generate new insight on the neural substrates of consciousness disorders such as the vegetative or minimally conscious state [13].

Applications of Imaging in Acute Brain Injury (Table 1)

Traumatic Brain Injury

Non-contrast head CT is generally accepted as the initial radiological screen in patients with moderate or severe TBI. CT allows rapid identification of extra-axial hematomas requiring evacuation, intraparenchymal hematomas and contusions, traumatic SAH, and skull fractures. The value of head CT is less clear in patients with milder forms of TBI, and concerns about the efficient use of CT resources have led to the prospective development and validation of specific criteria for obtaining

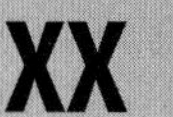

Table 1. Computed tomography (CT) and magnetic resonance imaging (MRI) findings in common causes of acute brain injury

Etiology	CT findings*	MRI findings
Vascular		
Acute ischemic stroke	• Acute: often normal. • Loss of grey-white matter distinction, gyral swelling/sulcal effacement, hyperdense vessel (MCA) • Subacute: parenchymal hypodensity, edema/mass effect, hemorrhagic transformation	• DWI hyperintensity with corresponding low signal on ADC. • PWI: hypoperfusion which may be >, =, or < than DWI volume. • MRA: vessel occlusion/stenosis • GRE may show hypointense lesions (hemorrhage)
Spontaneous intracerebral hemorrhage	• Elliptical hyperdensity; location: basal ganglia > thalamus > lobar > brainstem/ cerebellum. • Often with associated IVH, hydrocephalus	• GRE: multifocal hypointense lesions • DWI: may show restricted diffusion in perihematoma area
Subarachnoid hemorrhage	• Acute (24–48 h): hyperdense CSF, brain edema, IVH, hydrocephalus • Subacute: focal hypodensities	• T2 and FLAIR: hyperintense CSF • DWI in subacute phase: focal areas of restricted diffusion
Cerebral venous thrombosis	• Hyperdense dural sinus (cord sign), venous infarct, petechial hemorrhages, diffuse edema • Contrast CT may show „empty delta sign" (enhancing dura, nonenhancing thrombus).	MRV: absence of flow in occluded sinus
Vasculitis	Often normal. Focal ischemia or hemorrhage.	• FLAIR: Multifocal deep grey/subcortical hyperintensities • GRE: petechial hemorrhages
Posterior reversible encephalopathy syndrome	Patchy bilateral cortical and subcortical hypodensities in parieto-occipital region	• T2 and FLAIR: hyperintense signal in parieto-occipital region • DWI: usually normal • ADC: increased signal (bright)
Trauma		
Cerebral contusions	• Often normal in acute setting (< 24 h). • Patchy hypodensities blossoming at 24–48 h, often with petechial hemorrhage, edema • Typical location: temporal, frontal, parasagittal	• FLAIR: hyperintense cortical edema and CSF • GRE: hypointense foci indicating hemorrhage
Extra-axial hematomas	• EDH: hyperdense, biconcave, not crossing suture lines, often compressing underlying brain • Acute SDH (< 72 h): crescent shaped hyperdensity, may cross suture lines; subacute SDH (3d-3 weeks): iso- to hypodense; chronic SDH (> 3 weeks): hypodense	Not specific Vertex EDH may only be seen on coronal MRI
Diffuse axonal injury	• Often normal initially. • Multifocal small hypodense and/or hyperdense lesions (punctate hemorrhages) in corticomedullary junction, corpus callosum, upper brainstem (dorsolateral midbrain and upper pons), basal ganglia	• FLAIR: multiple hyperintensities • GRE: multiple hypointense lesions (more lesions detected on SWI). • DWI: multiple hyperintense lesions with corresponding ADC hyposignal

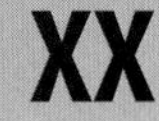

Table 1. (*cont.*)

Etiology	CT findings*	MRI findings
Organ failure		
Hypotensive cerebral infarction	Hypodensity in watershed zone (ACA-MCA, MCA-PCA)	• DWI: hyperintense signal in watershed zone with corresponding ADC hyposignal. • MRA may show vessel stenosis which increases risk of this type of injury
Anoxic-ischemic encephalopathy	• Often normal initially. • After 48 h: diffuse cortical edema, loss of gray white matter distinction, relative hypodensity of basal ganglia	• FLAIR and DWI: hyperintense signal predominantly in the cortex, thalamus and basal ganglia
Hepatic encephalopathy	• Chronic: cerebral atrophy • Acute: diffuse cerebral edema	• T1: increased signal intensity in bilateral basal ganglia, hypothalamus, midbrain • T2: diffusely increased intensity in acute HE • DWI: hyperintense cortical signal in acute HE
Metabolic		
Hypoglycemia	Hypodensity in occipital and parietal lobes	DWI: hyperintense in parietal and occipital lobes with corresponding decrease in ADC signal
Wernicke's encephalopathy	• Often normal or cerebral atrophy • Hypodensity in periaqueductal gray matter, mamillary bodies, thalamus	• T2 hyperintense signal in medial thalamus, mamillary bodies, hypothalamus, midbrain • T1 gadolinium enhancement of mamillary bodies, periaqueductal grey, medial thalamus • DWI: hyperintense around third ventricle, midbrain
Central nervous system infection		
Meningitis (bacterial)	• Noncontrast CT Usually normal. May show hydrocephalus, brain edema • Contrast CT: exudate appears as enhancement in sulci and cisterns	FLAIR: exudate hyperintense in sulci, cisterns
Encephalitis	• Usually normal • Focal hemorrhagic lesions (HSV)	T2: hyperintense gray matter signal (bilateral medial temporal and inferior frontal lobes in HSV) DWI: focal areas of restricted diffusion
Systemic infection		
Septic encephalopathy	• Usually normal	• T2 and FLAIR: hyperintense lesions in white matter (centrum semi-ovale) • DWI: focal areas of restricted diffusion

* Non contrast enhanced unless specified. DWI: diffusion-weighted imaging; PWI: perfusion-weighted imaging; MRA: magnetic resonance angiography; GRE: gradient recalled echo; IVH: intraventricular hemorrhage; CSF: cerebrospinal fluid; FLAIR: fluid attenuated inversion recovery; MRV: magnetic resonance venography; ADC: apparent diffusion coefficient; EDH: epidural hematoma; SDH: subdural hematoma; ACA: anterior cerebral artery; MCA: middle cerebral artery; PCA: posterior cerebral artery; HSV: herpes simplex virus

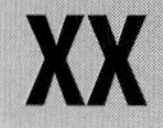

a head CT, including the Canadian CT Head Rule [14], the New Orleans Criteria [15], and the National Institute for Health and Clinical Excellence (NICE) criteria [16], which all specify clinical risk factors in which head CT is recommended.

Numerous studies indicate that MRI has greater sensitivity than CT in the detection of diffuse axonal injury, non-hemorrhagic contusions, brainstem and other posterior fossa lesions, and small extra-axial hematomas. Much interest has centered on the detection of diffuse axonal injury given that it is prevalent, has been linked to poor outcomes, and is not fully appreciated by commonly used neuroimaging modes including CT and MRI. Diffuse axonal injury is seen in up to 50 % of patients with TBI and is characterized histologically by axonal swelling and Wallerian degeneration, microglial clusters, and variable degrees of microvascular damage and focal hemorrhage; the density of lesions is greatest in the gray-white matter junctions of the cerebral cortex, corpus callosum, internal capsule and brainstem.

Diffuse axonal injury is frequently not visible or poorly characterized on CT scan and if suspected should be sought with MRI. Non-hemorrhagic diffuse axonal injury appears as multifocal hyperintense lesions on FLAIR, while hemorrhagic diffuse axonal injury can be identified as hypointense lesions with gradient recalled echo, however even these modalities underestimate the burden of damage. Susceptibility weighted imaging is reported to have a greater sensitivity for hemorrhagic diffuse axonal injury than conventional gradient recalled echo sequences, revealing more lesions and lesions of greater size than gradient recalled echo [17], while diffusion-weighted imaging detects non-hemorrhagic diffuse axonal injury lesions which are occult on FLAIR [18]. Diffusion tensor imaging is emerging as a powerful method to evaluate the integrity of white matter tracts in TBI patients with a broad range of clinical severity. Like diffusion-weighted imaging, diffusion tensor imaging can identify damage in tissue that appears normal on conventional MRI, and the degree of white matter disruption can be quantified with the help of parameters such as fractional anisotropy. Temporal change in fractional anisotropy is emerging as a versatile biomarker in survivors of TBI, potentially indicating ongoing white matter degeneration (decreasing fractional anisotropy) or even regenerative processes (increasing fractional anisotropy) [19].

Physiological brain imaging modalities for TBI patients have included xenon-enhanced CT, SPECT, PET, and perfusion CT. In addition to characterizing the changes in cerebral hemodynamic status that are associated with TBI, these methods can assist in understanding the impact of brain-resuscitative interventions such as hyperventilation, hyperoxia, and cerebral perfusion pressure therapy. Xenon-enhanced CT studies demonstrate both regional and global patterns of cerebral hypoperfusion in patients following TBI, often most pronounced in the pericontusional brain tissue [20]. Xenon-enhanced CT data also indicate a time course of perfusion abnormalities with improved long-term outcomes linked to a normalization of CBF at 3 weeks post-injury [21]. Similar decreases in CBF have been observed with SPECT, even in patients with mild TBI whose CT and MRI showed no structural injury [22]. PET studies of head injured patients demonstrate decreases in CBF and $CMRO_2$ that are often associated with an increased oxygen extraction fraction, underscoring the role of ischemia as a fundamental pathophysiological process in TBI [23]. PET studies also show a regional heterogeneity in CBF, $CMRO_2$, and oxygen extraction fraction, with marked decreases in CBF and $CMRO_2$ and increases in oxygen extraction fraction observed in the tissues surrounding contusions, which some investigators have compared to the ischemic core/penumbra model described in patients with ischemic stroke. The regional heterogeneity of brain injuries has

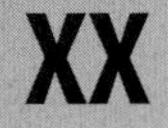

been observed long after the acute phase: In a ^{18}FDG-PET study of patients who remained unconscious months after brain injury, 'islands' of brain tissue with preserved metabolic function were identified and found to correlate with 'fragments' of conscious behavior [24].

Perfusion CT of patients with TBI reveals heterogeneous patterns of regional CBF and may assist in differentiating patients with preserved or abnormal cerebral autoregulatory function. Perfusion CT demonstrates reduced CBF and CBV and increased MTT in proximity to cerebral contusions [25]. In one recent report, perfusion CT derived measurements of MTT correlated inversely with intraparenchymal brain tissue oxygen tension [26].

MRS in patients with TBI reveals an array of neurochemical abnormalities typically identified in tissue which appears normal with other brain imaging modalities, and thus underscoring the complementary nature of the information provided by spectroscopic methods. Abnormalities which have been reported include lactate indicating ischemia, reductions in NAA and glutamate suggestive of neuronal loss or of metabolic depression, and increased choline reflecting membrane lipid turnover [27].

fMRI studies of patients with TBI have centered on the post-acute and chronic phase, revealing patterns of brain activation in patients with consciousness disorders such as the vegetative or minimally conscious state [13], or identifying neural substrates for the cognitive impairments observed in conscious TBI survivors [28]. The value of fMRI in the setting of acute TBI is unknown; research has been hindered by practical and theoretical issues, including the heterogeneity of TBI, limited knowledge of how pathological alterations in cerebral hemodynamics affect the BOLD signal, and the definitions of appropriate control groups.

Aneurysmal Subarachnoid Hemorrhage

The imaging of patients with brain aneurysmal rupture can be considered in three distinct phases: The diagnosis of SAH, the identification of the bleeding source, and the diagnosis of delayed cerebral ischemia. The diagnosis of SAH is based on a careful consideration of history and physical findings and is confirmed by the head CT and/or lumbar puncture. The sensitivity of head CT declines with time, from 98–100 % when obtained within 12 hours of symptom onset [29] to 93 % at 24 hours, decreasing to 50 % at 5–7 days [30]. Head CT can also demonstrate intraparenchymal hematomas, hydrocephalus, and cerebral edema, and may suggest the site of aneurysm rupture. There has been some interest in MRI (in particular FLAIR) as an alternative diagnostic method in subacute SAH in cases where CT findings are inconclusive; however, available studies are not in agreement regarding the accuracy of MRI in this indication.

Digital subtraction angiography is the diagnostic standard for identifying the bleeding source in SAH and for characterizing aneurysm morphology; however, there has been interest in other methods in particular multidetector CT angiography. CT angiography is an appealing alternative since it is not associated with many of the risks and costs of selective cerebral arterial catheterization. Recent prospective data indicate that CT angiography has a very high sensitivity and specificity for aneurysm identification when compared to digital subtraction angiography or surgical findings, and inter-observer reliability is excellent. Nevertheless, there remains considerable debate and controversy regarding the generalization of these findings especially in light of the potentially catastrophic consequences of false negative studies [31].

The detection of delayed cerebral ischemia (often discussed as 'vasospasm') is a diagnostic challenge and requires integration of clinical and radiological data. Although delayed ischemic deficits are observed in about 30 % of patients following SAH, digital subtraction angiography reveals focal or diffuse spasm in the circle of Willis or its branches in up to 80 % of cases. The degree of concordance between clinical signs, angiographic findings and cerebral infarction is low, suggesting that alternative and complementary diagnostic methodologies are needed. SPECT shows global and/or regional hypoperfusion in a high proportion of patients following SAH [32], while PET reveals decreased $CMRO_2$ on days 1–4 after SAH, followed by regional increases in oxygen extraction fraction in patients with delayed ischemic deficits [33]. Recent studies indicate that CT angiography has considerable value in detecting SAH-associated vasospasm, and in addition it may be coupled with perfusion CT thus allowing characterization of both vascular anatomy and associated cerebral perfusion abnormalities [34]. There are also data on diffusion-weighted MRI as a promising diagnostic technique in the assessment of delayed cerebral ischemia [35].

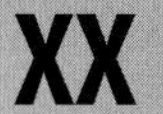

Few studies have investigated MRS in patients with SAH. In a primate model of SAH-induced vasospasm, MRS revealed significant focal reductions in NAA on days 7 and 14 without any associated structural changes on MRI [36]. An early study in humans using ^{31}P-MRS found focal areas of tissue acidosis which correlated with ischemic neurological deficits [37]. In another study combining MRI, perfusion MRI, and MRS, lactate was increased and NAA decreased in the patients with Hunt and Hess grade III and IV SAH, and regions of increased lactate co-localized with focal edema and increased CBV [38].

Anoxic-ischemic Encephalopathy

There are several types of anoxic-ischemic brain injury, the most common being anoxic-ischemic encephalopathy seen in survivors of cardiac arrest. CT findings of anoxic-ischemic encephalopathy include diffuse brain swelling, attenuation of gray white matter differentiation, and relative hypodensity of basal ganglia, however these changes usually become apparent 24–48 hours after the insult, and the initial head CT is often unremarkable.

Brain MRI, in particular diffusion-weighted imaging, has helped to clarify the early changes and also the time course of brain injury in patients with anoxic-ischemic encephalopathy [39]. Characteristic phases in anoxic-ischemic encephalopathy include: An acute phase (< 24 hours) characterized by diffuse edema and a diffusion-weighted hyperintense signal predominantly in the cortex, thalamus and basal ganglia, followed by a subacute phase (14–20 days) with progressive resolution of brain edema, disappearance of diffusion-weighted hyperintensities and occasionally diffuse white matter T2 hyperintense changes, and finally a chronic phase (> 21 days) with the development of diffuse cerebral atrophy. The cortical diffusion-weighted hyperintensity in patients with anoxic-ischemic encephalopathy is believed to be the radiological expression of 'cortical laminar necrosis' a histological pattern of cell death involving the third and fifth layers of the cortical mantle and seen in a variety of global cerebral insults.

Studies investigating physiological imaging in anoxic-ischemic encephalopathy are limited in number. Unconscious survivors of cardiac arrest are reported to have globally decreased CBF and $CMRO_2$ on $^{15}O_2$-PET[40], decreased cerebral metabolism on ^{18}FDG-PET [24], and decreased CBF on SPECT [41]. Studies of anoxic-ischemic encephalopathy patients with xenon-enhanced CT have had mixed results with some showing global hypoperfusion and others suggesting global hyperemia. A recent report using arterial spin labeling found global hyperemia in all anoxic-ischemic encephalopathy patients evaluated a mean of 4.6 days after anoxic injury [42]. MRS in adult patients with anoxic-ischemic encephalopathy showed a significant decrease in the NAA peak in both cerebral cortex and cerebellum consistent with neuronal loss, and diffusely increased lactate [43]. These findings are similar to MRS investigations of perinatal hypoxic-ischemic injury which demonstrate elevated lactate/creatine or lactate/NAA and are predictive of poor prognosis. In neonates, MRS is reported to be one of the most sensitive methods to evaluate cerebral injury within 24 hours of a hypoxic-ischemic insult; however, there are no comparable data in adults.

Hepatic Encephalopathy

Hepatic encephalopathy refers to a spectrum of neuropsychiatric abnormalities associated with chronic and acute liver dysfunction. Liver failure is associated with a profound metabolic brain disturbance which leads to varying degrees of edema. Brain edema is found in 80 % of patients with acute hepatic encephalopathy and is the result of both cytotoxic (intracellular) and vasogenic (extracellular, resulting from blood brain barrier dysfunction) mechanisms. Neuroimaging methods, including MRI, diffusion tensor imaging, MRS, SPECT, PET and fMRI, have provided significant insight into the pathophysiology of hepatic encephalopathy.

Brain MRI in patients with cirrhosis typically reveals varying degrees of cortical and cerebellar atrophy and bilateral T1-hyperintensities (believed to reflect manganese accumulation) involving the basal ganglia, hypothalamus and midbrain; however, the relationship between these findings and clinical manifestations of hepatic encephalopathy is unclear. In chronic non-alcoholic liver failure, FLAIR shows bilateral signal hyperintensities in the corticospinal tract, changes which are believed to reflect cellular (astrocytic) edema, and which resolve after liver transplantation [44]. Diffusion-weighted imaging in patients with chronic liver failure indicates significantly increased apparent diffusion coefficient values in both white and gray matter, suggesting widespread vasogenic edema [45]. Similarly, diffusion tensor imaging in chronic liver failure shows significantly increased mean diffusivity with no change in fractional anisotropy, again signifying vasogenic edema; mean diffusivity values from the corpus callosum and internal capsule are associated with low neuropsychological test scores and these scores and mean diffusivity values improve significantly after treatment with lactulose [46]. In acute, and in particular in fulminant liver failure, the head CT typically discloses diffuse cerebral edema, however CT findings are not strongly predictive of intracranial hypertension [47]. In acute exacerbations of hepatic encephalopathy, cortical T2-weighted and diffusion-weighted hyperintensities may be appreciated, often with sparing of the perirolandic and occipital regions, while the apparent diffusion coefficient tends to decrease diffusely, indicating a predominantly cytotoxic edema mechanism [48]. A recent diffusion tensor imaging investigation of patients with fulminant hepatic failure found decreased fractional anisotropy in all studied brain regions, again suggesting cytotoxic edema [49].

^{18}FDG-PET in patients with chronic liver failure and hepatic encephalopathy show reduced cerebral glucose usage in the inferior and anterior cingulate gyrus, findings which might account for some of the attention deficits observed in many hepatic encephalopathy patients; in addition, overall glucose metabolism is redistributed from cortical to subcortical structures [50]. Consistent with these results, ^{15}O-H_2O PET studies demonstrate significantly increased CBF in the thalamus, basal ganglia, and cerebellum [51]. PET using a $^{13}NH_3$ tracer suggests increases in blood-brain barrier permeability for ammonia as well as increased cerebral ammonia metabolism [52]. PET with ^{11}C-ligand tracers has been used to show increased expression of peripheral benzodiazepine binding sites in the mitochondria of astroglial cells [53]; these sites are involved in the synthesis of neurosteroids and may contribute to the neurological dysfunction of hepatic encephalopathy. Similar to PET studies, SPECT shows redistribution of CBF from cortex to subcortical structures [54].

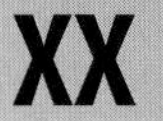

Physiologic probes that have been used for MRS evaluations of hepatic encephalopathy include ^{1}H, ^{13}C, ^{15}N, and ^{31}P. ^{1}H-MRS in chronic liver failure commonly shows a pattern of increased glutamate/glutamine signal attributed to increased glutamine expression, as well as decreased signal intensity of choline and myo-inositol compounds; following liver transplantation these abnormalities tend to normalize in parallel with the resolution of hepatic encephalopathy [55]. ^{15}N-MRS studies have demonstrated that hyperammonemia is associated with increased glutamine fluxes between neurons and astrocytes [56].

Available fMRI studies of patients with hepatic encephalopathy suggest significant abnormalities in activation patterns associated with visual judgment and cognitive control mechanisms. In an intriguing recent study, the task-induced deactivation of the so-called 'default network' normally observed during resting state fMRI was absent in cirrhotic patients [57].

Sepsis-associated Encephalopathy

The term septic encephalopathy describes a subset of patients with severe infections who develop an alteration in mental status associated with diffuse slowing on the electroencephalogram (EEG) and a normal CSF profile. Septic encephalopathy has been reported in up to two thirds of patients with sepsis, and is associated with an increased risk of death.

There are few published reports of neuroimaging in patients with sepsis. In a retrospective analysis of 12 patients with septic encephalopathy, head CT scans were found to be unremarkable [58]. Studies with MRI have been more informative but are based on very small numbers of patients [59, 60]. In a patient who became comatose in the setting of urosepsis, MRI revealed FLAIR-hyperintense, gadolinium non-enhancing changes in bilateral basal ganglia, cerebellum, brainstem, and temporal lobes, associated with diffusion-weighted imaging hyperintense lesions in the basal ganglia [59]; postmortem histology indicated basal ganglia infarctions associated with a profound inflammatory, but non-infectious, infiltrate. Sharshar et al. used MRI to prospectively evaluate nine patients with septic shock who presented with an acute change in neurological exam [60]. They reported diffuse, bilateral FLAIR-hyperintense white matter lesions in five patients and multiple diffusion-weighted imaging hyperintense lesions in two patients; the MRI was normal in the remaining two patients. The lesions of the white matter were associated with increasing duration of shock and with worse Glasgow Outcome Scale at 90 days. Finally, in a recent retrospective report on posterior reversible encephalopathy syndrome, infection or sepsis were identified as potentially causative mechanisms in nearly one quarter of patients [61].

Data are scarce on physiological brain imaging in sepsis, and there are no published studies using PET, SPECT, xenon-enhanced CT, perfusion CT or MR-based assessments of perfusion. In a ^{31}P-MRS investigation conducted in rat models of sepsis, Hotchkiss et al. found no significant change in cellular energy stores nor any significant decrease in pH that would suggest ischemia [62].

Outcome Prediction

Given the increasing sophistication of neuroimaging, there is legitimate interest in deriving prognostic information from specific radiological findings. Most of the published studies concern TBI and anoxic-ischemic encephalopathy.

Traumatic Brain Injury

A number of groups have used MRI in an attempt to predict neurological or functional outcome months to years after the TBI. Features which have been associated with poor outcomes (vegetative state or severe disability) include the presence of brainstem injury, in particular pontine and midbrain lesions that are bilateral and dorsal; lesions in corpus callosum, hippocampus or basal ganglia; the total burden of injury as detected by FLAIR; and the presence of widely distributed lesions, in particular diffuse axonal injury [63, 64].

MRS changes which have been associated with poor neurological or functional outcomes include a low NAA/creatine ratio and an increased choline/creatine ratio [27, 65]. In a recent report, the combination of brainstem abnormalities on FLAIR and MRS obtained 2–3 weeks after injury were highly predictive of low Glasgow Outcome Scores at 18 months [66]. SPECT may also assist in outcome prediction after TBI: poor functional status was noted in patients with a global reduction in CBF [67] and with decrements in regional perfusion affecting the temporal lobes, frontal lobes, and basal ganglia [68]. The time course of perfusion abnormalities may also be important: in one report, patients with total CBF values which remained low 2–6 weeks after injury had significantly worse neurological outcomes [69]. In an intriguing xenon-enhanced CT study of severe TBI patients, unfavorable outcome at 12 months was related to pupillary responsiveness and to low brainstem CBF, leading the authors to speculate that pupillary changes may reflect ischemia of the brainstem rather than its compression from transtentorial herniation [70].

Anoxic-ischemic Encephalopathy

The prognostic value of brain MRI in survivors of cardiac arrest is uncertain. An early study found that MRI findings did not predict functional outcome at 1 year [71]. More recently, the presence of diffuse cortical diffusion-weighted imaging or FLAIR hyperintensities has been associated with poor long term neurological outcome [72]. Data are mixed regarding the prognostic value of PET, SPECT, or xenon-enhanced CT following anoxic-ischemic encephaolopathy, with some studies indicating poor outcome in patients with globally decreased CBF or $CMRO_2$ [73] and other reports suggesting poor outcome in patients with globally increased CBF [74] (part of the variance between these studies reflects the different time points at which patients were imaged). Of the available reports in which adult patients with anoxic-ischemic encephaolopathy were evaluated with MRS, one found that low NAA and elevated lactate predicted poor neurological outcomes 4 weeks after arrest [75]. Based on these data, the American Academy of Neurology in a recent practice parameter concluded that there was insufficient evidence regarding the value of imaging methods to predict outcomes following cardiac arrest [76].

Conclusion

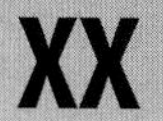

The care of patients with severe brain injury requires a comprehensive approach in which imaging has become an indispensable complement to the clinical information obtained at the bedside. An array of imaging modalities has become available, providing clinicians with powerful tools to probe brain structure and physiology. Brain imaging is routinely used in the diagnosis of patients with a broad range of acute neurological dysfunction, and may assist in the prediction of outcome. With the benefit of theoretical and technological refinements, imaging is also helping to unravel fundamental questions regarding the etiology, pathophysiology, and neuroplasticity associated with critical neurological injury, and it is anticipated that this knowledge will contribute to new and effective therapeutic interventions.

References

1. Moustafa RR, Baron JC (2007) Clinical review: Imaging in ischaemic stroke – implications for acute management. Crit Care 11: 227
2. Kidwell CS, Wintermark M (2008) Imaging of intracranial haemorrhage. Lancet Neurol 7: 256–267
3. Chalela JA, Kidwell CS, Nentwich LM, et al (2007) Magnetic resonance imaging and computed tomography in emergency assessment of patients with suspected acute stroke: a prospective comparison. Lancet 369: 293–298
4. Pierpaoli C, Basser PJ (1996) Toward a quantitative assessment of diffusion anisotropy. Magn Reson Med 36: 893–906
5. Kety SS, Schmidt CF (1948) The nitrous oxide method for the quantitative determination of cerebral blood flow in man: Theory, procedure and normal values. J Clin Invest 27: 476–483
6. Meier P, Zierler KL (1954) On the theory of the indicator-dilution method for measurement of blood flow and volume. J Appl Physiol 6: 731–744
7. Wintermark M, Fischbein NJ, Smith WS, Ko NU, Quist M, Dillon WP (2005) Accuracy of dynamic perfusion CT with deconvolution in detecting acute hemispheric stroke. AJNR Am J Neuroradiol 26: 104–112
8. Warach S, Gaa J, Siewert B, Wielopolski P, Edelman RR (1995) Acute human stroke studied by whole brain echo planar diffusion-weighted magnetic resonance imaging. Ann Neurol 37: 231–241
9. Williams DS, Detre JA, Leigh JS, Koretsky AP (1992) Magnetic resonance imaging of perfusion using spin inversion of arterial water. Proc Natl Acad Sci USA 89: 212–216
10. Ogawa S, Menon RS, Tank DW, et al (1993) Functional brain mapping by blood oxygenation level-dependent contrast magnetic resonance imaging. A comparison of signal characteristics with a biophysical model. Biophys J 64: 803–812
11. Fox MD, Raichle ME (2007) Spontaneous fluctuations in brain activity observed with functional magnetic resonance imaging. Nat Rev Neurosci 8: 700–711
12. Greicius MD, Supekar K, Menon V, Dougherty RF (2009) Resting-state functional connectivity reflects structural connectivity in the default mode network. Cereb Cortex 19: 72–78
13. Coleman MR, Rodd JM, Davis MH, et al (2007) Do vegetative patients retain aspects of language comprehension? Evidence from fMRI. Brain 130: 2494–2507
14. Stiell IG, Lesiuk H, Wells GA, et al (2001) The Canadian CT Head Rule Study for patients with minor head injury: rationale, objectives, and methodology for phase I (derivation). Ann Emerg Med 38: 160–169
15. Haydel MJ, Preston CA, Mills TJ, Luber S, Blaudeau E, DeBlieux PM (2000) Indications for computed tomography in patients with minor head injury. N Engl J Med 343: 100–105

16. Yates D, Aktar R, Hill J (2007) Assessment, investigation, and early management of head injury: summary of NICE guidance. BMJ 335: 719–720
17. Tong KA, Ashwal S, Holshouser BA, et al (2004) Diffuse axonal injury in children: clinical correlation with hemorrhagic lesions. Ann Neurol 56: 36–50
18. Liu AY, Maldjian JA, Bagley LJ, Sinson GP, Grossman RI (1999) Traumatic brain injury: diffusion-weighted MR imaging findings. AJNR Am J Neuroradiol 20: 1636–1641
19. Sidaros A, Engberg AW, Sidaros K, et al (2008) Diffusion tensor imaging during recovery from severe traumatic brain injury and relation to clinical outcome: a longitudinal study. Brain 131: 559–572
20. Schroder ML, Muizelaar JP, Bullock MR, Salvant JB, Povlishock JT (1995) Focal ischemia due to traumatic contusions documented by stable xenon-CT and ultrastructural studies. J Neurosurg 82: 966–971
21. Inoue Y, Shiozaki T, Tasaki O, et al (2005) Changes in cerebral blood flow from the acute to the chronic phase of severe head injury. J Neurotrauma 22: 1411–1418
22. Lewine JD, Davis JT, Bigler ED, et al (2007) Objective documentation of traumatic brain injury subsequent to mild head trauma: multimodal brain imaging with MEG, SPECT, and MRI. J Head Trauma Rehabil 22: 141–155
23. Coles JP, Fryer TD, Smielewski P, et al (2004) Incidence and mechanisms of cerebral ischemia in early clinical head injury. J Cereb Blood Flow Metab 24: 202–211
24. Schiff ND, Ribary U, Moreno DR, et al (2002) Residual cerebral activity and behavioural fragments can remain in the persistently vegetative brain. Brain 125: 1210–1234
25. Soustiel JF, Mahamid E, Goldsher D, Zaaroor M (2008) Perfusion CT for early assessment of traumatic cerebral contusions. Neuroradiology 50: 189–196
26. Hemphill JC 3rd, Smith WS, Sonne DC, Morabito D, Manley GT (2005) Relationship between brain tissue oxygen tension and CT perfusion: feasibility and initial results. AJNR Am J Neuroradiol 26: 1095–1100
27. Friedman SD, Brooks WM, Jung RE, et al (1999) Quantitative proton MRS predicts outcome after traumatic brain injury. Neurology 52: 1384–1391
28. Newsome MR, Scheibel RS, Steinberg JL, et al (2007) Working memory brain activation following severe traumatic brain injury. Cortex 43: 95–111
29. Morgenstern LB, Luna-Gonzales H, Huber JC Jr, et al (1998) Worst headache and subarachnoid hemorrhage: prospective, modern computed tomography and spinal fluid analysis. Ann Emerg Med 32: 297–304
30. Kassell NF, Torner JC (1984) The International Cooperative Study on Timing of Aneurysm Surgery – an update. Stroke 15: 566–570
31. Kallmes DF, Layton K, Marx WF, Tong F (2007) Death by nondiagnosis: why emergent CT angiography should not be done for patients with subarachnoid hemorrhage. AJNR Am J Neuroradiol 28: 1837–1838
32. Leclerc X, Fichten A, Gauvrit JY, et al (2002) Symptomatic vasospasm after subarachnoid haemorrhage: assessment of brain damage by diffusion and perfusion-weighted MRI and single-photon emission computed tomography. Neuroradiology 44: 610–616
33. Carpenter DA, Grubb RL Jr, Tempel LW, Powers WJ (1991) Cerebral oxygen metabolism after aneurysmal subarachnoid hemorrhage. J Cereb Blood Flow Metab 11: 837–844
34. Wintermark M, Ko NU, Smith WS, Liu S, Higashida RT, Dillon WP (2006) Vasospasm after subarachnoid hemorrhage: utility of perfusion CT and CT angiography on diagnosis and management. AJNR Am J Neuroradiol 27: 26–34
35. Condette-Auliac S, Bracard S, Anxionnat R, et al (2001) Vasospasm after subarachnoid hemorrhage: interest in diffusion-weighted MR imaging. Stroke 32: 1818–1824
36. Handa Y, Kaneko M, Matuda T, Kobayashi H, Kubota T (1997) In vivo proton magnetic resonance spectroscopy for metabolic changes in brain during chronic cerebral vasospasm in primates. Neurosurgery 40: 773–780
37. Brooke NS, Ouwerkerk R, Adams CB, Radda GK, Ledingham JG, Rajagopalan B (1994) Phosphorus-31 magnetic resonance spectra reveal prolonged intracellular acidosis in the brain following subarachnoid hemorrhage. Proc Natl Acad Sci USA 91: 1903–1907
38. Rowe J, Blamire AM, Domingo Z, et al (1998) Discrepancies between cerebral perfusion and metabolism after subarachnoid haemorrhage: a magnetic resonance approach. J Neurol Neurosurg Psychiatry 64: 98–103

39. Weiss N, Galanaud D, Carpentier A, Naccache L, Puybasset L (2007) Clinical review: Prognostic value of magnetic resonance imaging in acute brain injury and coma. Crit Care 11: 230
40. Edgren E, Enblad P, Grenvik A, et al (2003) Cerebral blood flow and metabolism after cardiopulmonary resuscitation. A pathophysiologic and prognostic positron emission tomography pilot study. Resuscitation 57: 161–170
41. Rupright J, Woods EA, Singh A (1996) Hypoxic brain injury: evaluation by single photon emission computed tomography. Arch Phys Med Rehabil 77: 1205–1208
42. Pollock JM, Whitlow CT, Deibler AR, et al (2008) Anoxic injury-associated cerebral hyperperfusion identified with arterial spin-labeled MR imaging. AJNR Am J Neuroradiol 29: 1302–1307
43. Wartenberg KE, Patsalides A, Yepes MS (2004) Is magnetic resonance spectroscopy superior to conventional diagnostic tools in hypoxic-ischemic encephalopathy? J Neuroimaging 14: 180–186
44. Rovira A, Cordoba J, Sanpedro F, Grive E, Rovira-Gols A, Alonso J (2002) Normalization of T2 signal abnormalities in hemispheric white matter with liver transplant. Neurology 59: 335–341
45. Lodi R, Tonon C, Stracciari A, et al (2004) Diffusion MRI shows increased water apparent diffusion coefficient in the brains of cirrhotics. Neurology 62: 762–766
46. Kale RA, Gupta RK, Saraswat VA, et al (2006) Demonstration of interstitial cerebral edema with diffusion tensor MR imaging in type C hepatic encephalopathy. Hepatology 43: 698–706
47. Munoz SJ, Robinson M, Northrup B, et al (1991) Elevated intracranial pressure and computed tomography of the brain in fulminant hepatocellular failure. Hepatology 13: 209–212
48. Ranjan P, Mishra AM, Kale R, Saraswat VA, Gupta RK (2005) Cytotoxic edema is responsible for raised intracranial pressure in fulminant hepatic failure: in vivo demonstration using diffusion-weighted MRI in human subjects. Metab Brain Dis 20: 181–192
49. Saraswat VA, Saksena S, Nath K, et al (2008) Evaluation of mannitol effect in patients with acute hepatic failure and acute-on-chronic liver failure using conventional MRI, diffusion tensor imaging and in-vivo proton MR spectroscopy. World J Gastroenterol 14: 4168–4178
50. Lockwood AH (2002) Positron emission tomography in the study of hepatic encephalopathy. Metab Brain Dis 17: 431–435
51. Lockwood AH, Yap EW, Rhoades HM, Wong WH (1991) Altered cerebral blood flow and glucose metabolism in patients with liver disease and minimal encephalopathy. J Cereb Blood Flow Metab 11: 331–336
52. Lockwood AH, McDonald JM, Reiman RE, et al (1979) The dynamics of ammonia metabolism in man. Effects of liver disease and hyperammonemia. J Clin Invest 63: 449–460
53. Cagnin A, Taylor-Robinson SD, Forton DM, Banati RB (2006) In vivo imaging of cerebral „peripheral benzodiazepine binding sites“ in patients with hepatic encephalopathy. Gut 55: 547–553
54. Catafau AM, Kulisevsky J, Berna L, et al (2000) Relationship between cerebral perfusion in frontal-limbic-basal ganglia circuits and neuropsychologic impairment in patients with subclinical hepatic encephalopathy. J Nucl Med 41: 405–410
55. Naegele T, Grodd W, Viebahn R, et al (2000) MR imaging and (1)H spectroscopy of brain metabolites in hepatic encephalopathy: time-course of renormalization after liver transplantation. Radiology 216: 683–691
56. Kanamori K, Ross BD (2006) Kinetics of glial glutamine efflux and the mechanism of neuronal uptake studied in vivo in mildly hyperammonemic rat brain. J Neurochem 99: 1103–1113
57. Zhang LJ, Yang G, Yin J, Liu Y, Qi J (2007) Abnormal default-mode network activation in cirrhotic patients: a functional magnetic resonance imaging study. Acta Radiol 48: 781–787
58. Jackson AC, Gilbert JJ, Young GB, Bolton CF (1985) The encephalopathy of sepsis. Can J Neurol Sci 12: 303–307
59. Finelli PF, Uphoff DF (2004) Magnetic resonance imaging abnormalities with septic encephalopathy. J Neurol Neurosurg Psychiatry 75: 1189–1191
60. Sharshar T, Carlier R, Bernard F, et al (2007) Brain lesions in septic shock: a magnetic resonance imaging study. Intensive Care Med 33: 798–806
61. Bartynski WS, Boardman JF, Zeigler ZR, Shadduck RK, Lister J (2006) Posterior reversible encephalopathy syndrome in infection, sepsis, and shock. AJNR Am J Neuroradiol 27: 2179–2190

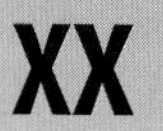

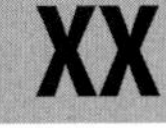

62. Hotchkiss RS, Long RC, Hall JR, et al (1989) An in vivo examination of rat brain during sepsis with 31P-NMR spectroscopy. Am J Physiol 257:C1055–1061
63. Kampfl A, Franz G, Aichner F, et al (1998) The persistent vegetative state after closed head injury: clinical and magnetic resonance imaging findings in 42 patients. J Neurosurg 88: 809–816
64. Paterakis K, Karantanas AH, Komnos A, Volikas Z (2000) Outcome of patients with diffuse axonal injury: the significance and prognostic value of MRI in the acute phase. J Trauma 49: 1071–1075
65. Garnett MR, Blamire AM, Corkill RG, Cadoux-Hudson TA, Rajagopalan B, Styles P (2000) Early proton magnetic resonance spectroscopy in normal-appearing brain correlates with outcome in patients following traumatic brain injury. Brain 123: 2046–2054
66. Weiss N, Galanaud D, Carpentier A, et al (2008) A combined clinical and MRI approach for outcome assessment of traumatic head injured comatose patients. J Neurol 255: 217–223
67. Oder W, Goldenberg G, Podreka I, Deecke L (1991) HM-PAO-SPECT in persistent vegetative state after head injury: prognostic indicator of the likelihood of recovery? Intensive Care Med 17: 149–153
68. Bavetta S, Nimmon CC, White J, et al (1994) A prospective study comparing SPET with MRI and CT as prognostic indicators following severe closed head injury. Nucl Med Commun 15: 961–968
69. Shiina G, Onuma T, Kameyama M, et al (1998) Sequential assessment of cerebral blood flow in diffuse brain injury by 123I-iodoamphetamine single-photon emission CT. AJNR Am J Neuroradiol 19: 297–302
70. Ritter AM, Muizelaar JP, Barnes T, et al (1999) Brain stem blood flow, pupillary response, and outcome in patients with severe head injuries. Neurosurgery 44: 941–948
71. Roine RO, Raininko R, Erkinjuntti T, Ylikoski A, Kaste M (1993) Magnetic resonance imaging findings associated with cardiac arrest. Stroke 24: 1005–1014
72. Wijdicks EF, Campeau NG, Miller GM (2001) MR imaging in comatose survivors of cardiac resuscitation. AJNR Am J Neuroradiol 22: 1561–1565
73. Nogami K, Fujii M, Kashiwagi S, Sadamitsu D, Maekawa T (2000) Cerebral circulation and prognosis of the patients with hypoxic encephalopathy. Keio J Med 49 (Suppl 1): A109–111
74. Cohan SL, Mun SK, Petite J, et al (1989) Cerebral blood flow in humans following resuscitation from cardiac arrest. Stroke 20: 761–765
75. Berek K, Lechleitner P, Luef G, et al (1995) Early determination of neurological outcome after prehospital cardiopulmonary resuscitation. Stroke 26: 543–549
76. Wijdicks EF, Hijdra A, Young GB, Bassetti CL, Wiebe S (2006) Practice parameter: prediction of outcome in comatose survivors after cardiopulmonary resuscitation (an evidence-based review): report of the Quality Standards Subcommittee of the American Academy of Neurology. Neurology 67: 203–210

Monitoring and Managing Raised Intracranial Pressure after Traumatic Brain Injury

M. Smith

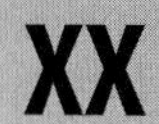

Introduction

The primary aim of the intensive care management of traumatic brain injury (TBI) is to prevent and treat secondary brain injury using a multi-faceted neuroprotective strategy to maintain cerebral perfusion in order to meet the brain's metabolic demands. Raised intracranial pressure (ICP) is an important cause of secondary brain injury and associated with adverse outcome after TBI. It can be related to intracranial mass lesions, contusional injuries, vascular engorgement, and brain edema. The prevention and control of raised ICP, and maintenance of cerebral perfusion pressure (CPP), are fundamental therapeutic goals after TBI. Despite the absence of class-1 studies, ICP monitoring has developed a prominent role in the management of severe TBI and is recommended by international consensus guidance. It is generally accepted as a relatively low-risk, high-yield, and value for money intervention, although there are wide variations in its application.

ICP Monitoring

ICP is a complex variable. ICP monitoring not only quantifies ICP and CPP, but also provides additional information via identification and analysis of pathologic ICP waveforms and can be augmented by measurement of indices describing cerebrovascular pressure reactivity and pressure-volume compensatory reserve [1].

Techniques

ICP cannot be reliably estimated from any specific clinical feature or computed tomography (CT) finding and must actually be measured [1]. Different methods of monitoring ICP have been described (**Table 1**) but two methods are commonly used in clinical practice – intraventricular catheters and intraparenchymal catheter-tip micro-transducer systems. An intraventricular catheter, connected to a standard pressure transducer via a fluid filled catheter, is the 'gold standard' method for monitoring ICP. Ventricular catheters measure global ICP and have the additional advantages of allowing periodic external calibration, therapeutic drainage of cerebrospinal fluid (CSF) and administration of drugs (e.g., antibiotics). However, placement of ventricular catheters may be difficult and their use is complicated by infection in up to 11 % of cases. Microtransducer tipped ICP monitors can be sited in the brain parenchyma or subdural space, either via a cranial access device (skull bolt) or during a neurosurgical procedure. They are almost as accurate as ventricular catheters

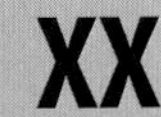

Table 1. Intracranial pressure monitoring devices

Method	Advantages	Disadvantages
Intraventricular catheter	• Gold standard • Measures global pressure • Allows therapeutic drainage of cerebrospinal fluid • *In-vivo* calibration possible	• Insertion may be difficult • Most invasive method • Risk of hematoma • Risk of cerebrospinal fluid infection
Microtransducer system	• Intraparenchymal/subdural placement • Low complication rate • Low infection risk	• Small zero drift over time • No *in-vivo* calibration • Measures local pressure
Epidural catheter	• Easy to insert • No penetration of dura • Low infection rate	• Limited accuracy • Rarely used

and are reliable and easy to use in the clinical setting [1]. They have minimal infection and other complication rates but measured pressure may not be representative of true CSF pressure because of the intraparenchymal pressure gradients that may exist after TBI. *In vivo* calibration is not possible with microtransducer tipped devices but zero drift during long term monitoring lies within a clinically acceptable range and is usually as low as 1 mmHg after 5 days continuous use.

Indications

Although there are no class-1 studies, there is some clinical evidence supporting the use of ICP monitoring to guide therapeutic interventions, detect intracranial mass lesions early and assess prognosis after severe TBI [1]. The Brain Trauma Foundation recommends that ICP should be monitored in all patients with a severe TBI (Glasgow Coma scale score 3–8) and *either* an abnormal CT scan *or* a normal scan *and* the presence of two or more of the following three risk factors at admission: Age > 40 years; unilateral or bilateral motor posturing; systolic blood pressure < 90 mmHg [2]. There is around a 60 % chance of raised ICP in patients with these risk factors. ICP monitoring is accepted as a relatively low-risk, high-yield and value for money intervention during head injury management.

Variations in Practice

Despite the availability of international guidance, there is no general consensus on the benefits of ICP monitoring and considerable variability in its application, and in ICP-directed treatment modalities, between centers [3, 4]. In a study of practice in the USA, ICP monitors were placed in only 58 % of patients who fulfilled established criteria for monitoring, and therapies to reduce raised ICP were routinely applied in those patients in whom ICP was not monitored [3]. In a survey carried out on behalf of the European Brain Injury Consortium, ICP monitoring was undertaken in only 37 % of eligible patients [4] and, in a Canadian study of severe TBI, only 20 % of neurosurgeons believed that outcome was affected by ICP monitoring [5].

Treatment of Intracranial Hypertension

High ICP and low CPP may result in cerebral ischemia after TBI and are associated with increased mortality and worse outcome in survivors [6]. Protocol-driven strategies for head injury management, including treatment of intracranial hypertension, are effective in reducing mortality and improving outcome [7] and usually incorporate step-wise introduction of higher intensity treatment, moving from one step to the next if ICP and CPP targets remain unachieved [8]. Consensus guidance recommends that ICP above 20–25 mmHg should be treated aggressively using a multimodal approach [2].

Sedation and Analgesia

Sedation and analgesia are crucial components of head injury management [9]. They minimize pain, anxiety and agitation, reduce cerebral metabolic rate and facilitate mechanical ventilation. Propofol is a widely used sedative agent because it reduces ICP, has profound cerebral metabolic suppressive effects and a pharmacological profile that allows easy control of sedation levels and ICP and rapid wake-up [8].

Hyperventilation

$PaCO_2$ is a major determinant of cerebral vessel caliber, with a reduction in $PaCO_2$ causing cerebral vasoconstriction and a reduction in cerebral blood volume and ICP. Although hyperventilation has been widely used in the management of raised ICP, it is now appreciated that it can worsen regional ischemia, particularly in the first 24 hours after TBI [10]. The routine application of hyperventilation is discouraged and a $PaCO_2$ target of 4.5–5.0 kPa should be used in the first instance [2]. Hyperventilation to $PaCO_2$ 4.0–4.5 kPa is reserved for those with ICP > 20 mmHg and should be carried out in association with cerebral oxygenation monitoring to detect hyperventilation-induced cerebral ischemia [11]. Acute hyperventilation is relatively safe for short term use (< 30 min) and is effective in controlling severely raised ICP and threatened or actual brain herniation.

Hyperosmolar Therapy

Mannitol (0.5 g/kg) effectively treats elevated ICP and may improve neurological outcome, although it has never been subject to a randomized controlled clinical trial against placebo [12]. Mannitol has two mechanisms of action. Its plasma expanding effect causes an increase in cerebral microcirculatory flow and is responsible for the rapid onset of action whereas its osmotic effect reduces cerebral edema by drawing water across the blood-brain barrier into the vascular space. Treatment directed towards monitored rises in ICP is more beneficial than treatment directed by neurological signs or other physiological indicators [12]. Repeated administration of mannitol may result in unacceptably high serum osmolality (> 320 mOsm/l) and neurological and renal complications [8].

Hypertonic saline is an effective alternative to mannitol and its beneficial effects are likely to be related not only to its osmotic action but also to hemodynamic, vasoregulatory, immunological and neurochemical effects [13]. Hypertonic saline has proven efficacy in controlling ICP resistant to mannitol and is associated with fewer side effects. In particular, the large intravascular volume shifts seen with mannitol are absent and renal complications occur less frequently. However, there are no large, randomized comparisons of hypertonic saline against conventional osmotic agents, or long-term functional outcome studies. Furthermore, there are many different concentrations of hypertonic saline available (1.7 % to 29.2 %) and the optimal osmolar load to lower elevated ICP has not been defined [14].

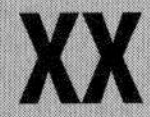

Moderate Hypothermia

Moderate hypothermia (33–35°C) is neuroprotective in animal studies but human trials have been disappointing. A prospective, randomized study of moderate hypothermia (33°C) in TBI was terminated early because of increased morbidity in patients over 45 years of age in the treatment group [15]. There was possible benefit to those who were hypothermic at presentation but older patients had such high rates of medical complications, including the development of pneumonia, that hypothermia was detrimental regardless of admission temperature. It has been suggested that it might be possible to achieve improvements in outcome using hypothermia if its side-effects are proactively managed [16]. Moderate hypothermia is an effective method of reducing raised ICP and is often included in protocols for head injury management [8]. High temperature is associated with worse outcome after TBI and core temperature should be monitored continuously and pyrexia prevented or treated [16].

Barbiturates

Barbiturates lower ICP by many mechanisms and, although there is no good evidence that they improve outcome after TBI [17], there has been a resurgence of interest in the use of high dose barbiturate therapy for the treatment of refractory intracranial hypertension [8]. Hypotension is a frequent complication of treatment and drug accumulation leads to delayed recovery and difficulty with early clinical assessment when the drug is discontinued. Continuous electroencephalogram monitoring (EEG) can be used to titrate barbiturate infusion and minimize side-effects.

Neurosurgical Interventions

The removal of an expanding intracranial mass lesion is the primary goal of neurosurgical treatment after TBI. An external ventricular drain allows drainage of CSF and, because intracranial compliance is reduced when ICP is raised, drainage of even small volumes of CSF can result in dramatic reductions in ICP. Decompressive craniectomy is an extensive neurosurgical procedure where a large area of the skull vault is removed and the dura opened to allow brain expansion with a consequent reduction in ICP. There is divided opinion on the relative benefits and risks of this operation [18] and this issue is currently being addressed by a multicenter, randomized controlled outcome trial – the Rescue-ICP study [http://rescueicp.com/].

Controversies

What is the Target ICP?

Although it is well recognized that elevated ICP correlates with higher risk of mortality and morbidity, not all patients with intracranial hypertension have poor outcome [19]. There is therefore a fundamental dilemma about which patients should be treated and at what levels of ICP. Furthermore, recent evidence suggests that the duration of intracranial hypertension and its response to treatment could be better predictors of neurological outcome than absolute ICP values [20]. It has also recently been demonstrated that brain resuscitation after TBI based on control of ICP and CPP alone does not prevent cerebral hypoxia in more than 20 % of patients [21]. This is unsurprising because monitoring of ICP and CPP does not tell the whole story. It is impossible to know in an individual patient whether the targeted ICP or CPP is sufficient to allow the brain's metabolic demands to be met at a particular moment in time. There is preliminary evidence that therapy directed towards maintenance of brain tissue oxygenation as well as ICP and CPP is associated with reduced mortality after severe TBI [22].

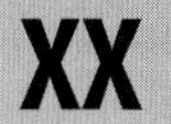

Does ICP Monitoring and Management Improve Outcome?

In a retrospective study, an 'aggressive' management protocol, including the monitoring and management of ICP, was associated with decreased risk of mortality after TBI and shorter length of hospital stay, although there was no difference in functional status in survivors at discharge [3]. Another large retrospective study also concluded that ICP monitoring was associated with significantly decreased mortality [23], but two surveys [4, 5] and one prospective study [24] have not shown benefits from ICP monitoring. The lack of consistency in the approach to ICP monitoring and management is likely to reflect the conflicting evidence available to clinicians and two recent European studies have attempted to clarify this evidence. Cremer and colleagues investigated the use of ICP monitoring and ICP/CPP-targeted therapy in an observational study of 333 patients with severe TBI [24]. This study compared patients managed in two centers but admission to each was determined only by the geographical location in which the original trauma occurred and patient characteristics were well balanced between the two. In center A, ICP was not monitored, but supportive intensive care was provided to maintain mean arterial pressure (MAP) > 90 mmHg and other therapeutic interventions were directed by clinical observations and CT findings. In center B, ICP was monitored and treatment provided to maintain ICP < 20 mmHg and CPP > 70 mmHg, according to standard guidelines. In-hospital mortality was similar in both centers (34 % vs. 33 %, $p = 0.87$) and the odds ratio for a more favorable outcome following ICP/CPP-targeted therapy was 0.95 (95 % confidence interval, 0.62 – 1.44). Intensity of treatment, measured by use of sedatives, vasopressors, mannitol, and barbiturates, was greater in center B and the median time on mechanical ventilation was also greater in center B (12 days vs. 5 days, $p < 0.001$). The second study, of 1856 patients with severe TBI in 32 Austrian ICUs, found that patients who received ICP monitoring had lower raw and risk-adjusted mortality rates than those who were not monitored, although this difference was not statistically significant [25]. Furthermore, the use of ICP monitoring did not show a significant association with neurological outcome at discharge from hospital. Patients admitted to larger centers had the lowest mortality even though ICP was monitored less frequently in these centers than in medium sized centers.

ICP monitoring was also associated with a statistically significant increased use of vasoactive drugs. Both these studies demonstrated increased intensity of treatment following ICP monitoring and management without clear evidence of improvements in outcome.

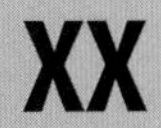

Complications of Treatment

Conventional approaches to the management of TBI have concentrated on a reduction in ICP to prevent secondary cerebral ischemic injury but there has been a shift of emphasis from primary control of ICP to a multi-faceted approach of maintenance of CPP and brain protection. This occurred following evidence that induced hypertension using fluid resuscitation and vasoactive agents to maintain CPP > 70 mmHg is associated with improved outcome [27]. However, therapies to maintain high CPP are controversial because of the high incidence of complications. In one study, there was a five-fold increase in the occurrence of acute lung injury (ALI) in a group of head injured patients managed with a CPP threshold of 70 mmHg vs. 50 mmHg [26]. Furthermore, the successful response of systemic variables to ICP/CPP-directed therapy does not always result in improvement of cerebral microcirculatory or cellular function. For example, CPP augmentation is relatively ineffective in reversing hypoperfusion in pericontusional ischemic areas [28] and only variably effective in improving ICP, cerebral autoregulation and brain tissue oxygenation [29]. The Brain Trauma Foundation now recommends that the CPP target after severe TBI should lie between 50–70 mmHg and that aggressive attempts to maintain CPP > 70 mmHg should be avoided because of the risk of ALI [2].

Multimodal Monitoring

In addition to the evidence that therapy directed towards maintenance of brain tissue oxygenation as well as ICP and CPP may improve outcome after severe TBI [22], it is also possible that targeting treatment only towards changes in ICP and CPP might be inappropriate because, when changes do occur in these variables, irreversible ischemic brain damage may already have occurred [30]. Measurement of ICP and CPP in association with monitors of the adequacy of cerebral perfusion, such as measurement of cerebral oxygenation (e.g., jugular venous oximetry, brain tissue oxygen tension) and metabolic status (e.g., cerebral microdialysis), provide a more complete picture of the injured brain and its response to treatment [11]. Monitoring of several variables simultaneously, multimodal monitoring, allows cross validation between monitors, artifact rejection and greater confidence to make treatment decisions. Developments in multimodal monitoring have allowed a movement away from rigid physiological target setting after TBI toward an individually tailored, patient specific approach that provides early warning of impending brain ischemia and guides targeted therapy [11].

Conclusion

ICP cannot be reliably estimated from any specific clinical feature or CT finding and must actually be measured. ICP monitoring has, therefore, become an established component of brain monitoring after TBI. Different methods of monitoring ICP have been described but intraventricular catheters and microtransducer systems are most widely used in current clinical practice. Although there is considerable variability in the use of ICP monitoring and treatment modalities between head injury centers, there is a body of clinical evidence supporting the use of ICP monitoring to detect intracranial mass lesions early, guide therapeutic interventions and assess prognosis. Prevention and control of raised ICP are fundamental therapeutic goals after TBI but the optimum treatment of raised ICP remains to be established. Management practices have undergone extensive revision as it has become clear that long-standing and established practices are not as efficacious or innocuous as previously believed. Whilst international consensus guidelines are available to assist clinicians, there has been a move away from rigid physiological target setting toward an individually tailored, patient specific approach using multimodality monitoring to guide treatment.

References

1. Smith M (2008) Monitoring intracranial pressure in traumatic brain injury. Anesth Analg 106: 240–248
2. The Brain Trauma Foundation, The American Association of Neurological Surgeons, The Joint Section on Neurotrauma and Critical Care (2007) J Neurotrauma 24:S1-S106
3. Bulger EM, Nathens AB, Rivara FP, Moore M, MacKenzie EJ, Jurkovich GJ (2002) Management of severe head injury: institutional variations in care and effect on outcome. Crit Care Med 30: 1870–1876
4. Stocchetti N, Penny KI, Dearden M, et al (2001) Intensive care management of head-injured patients in Europe: a survey from the European brain injury consortium. Intensive Care Med 27: 400–406
5. Sahjpaul R, Girotti M (2000) Intracranial pressure monitoring in severe traumatic brain injury – results of a Canadian survey. Can J Neurol Sci 27: 143–147
6. Balestreri M, Czosnyka M, Hutchinson P, et al (2006) Impact of intracranial pressure and cerebral perfusion pressure on severe disability and mortality after head injury. Neurocrit Care 4: 8–13
7. Smith M (2004) Neurocritical care: has it come of age? Br J Anaesth 93: 753–755
8. Helmy A, Vizcaychipi M, Gupta AK (2007) Traumatic brain injury: intensive care management. Br J Anaesth 99: 32–42
9. Citerio G, Cormio M (2003) Sedation in neurointensive care: advances in understanding and practice. Curr Opin Crit Care 9: 120–126
10. Coles JP, Fryer TD, Coleman MR, et al (2007) Hyperventilation following head injury: effect on ischemic burden and cerebral oxidative metabolism. Crit Care Med 35: 568–578
11. Tisdall MM, Smith M (2007) Multimodal monitoring in traumatic brain injury: current status and future directions. Br J Anaesth 99: 61–67
12. Wakai A, Roberts I, Schierhout G (2007) Mannitol for acute traumatic brain injury. Cochrane Database Syst Rev CD001049
13. Himmelseher S (2007) Hypertonic saline solutions for treatment of intracranial hypertension. Curr Opin Anaesthesiol 20: 414–426
14. White H, Cook D, Venkatesh B (2006) The use of hypertonic saline for treating intracranial hypertension after traumatic brain injury. Anesth Analg 102: 1836–1846
15. Clifton GL, Miller ER, Choi SC, et al (2001) Lack of effect of induction of hypothermia after acute brain injury. N Engl J Med 344: 556–563
16. Polderman KH, Ely EW, Badr AE, Girbes AR (2004) Induced hypothermia in traumatic brain injury: considering the conflicting results of meta-analyses and moving forward. Intensive Care Med 30: 1860–1864
17. Roberts I (2000) Barbiturates for acute traumatic brain injury. Cochrane Database Syst Rev CD000033
18. Hutchinson PJ, Kirkpatrick PJ (2004) Decompressive craniectomy in head injury. Curr Opin Crit Care 10: 101–104

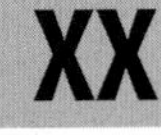

19. Resnick DK, Marion DW, Carlier P (1997) Outcome analysis of patients with severe head injuries and prolonged intracranial hypertension. J Trauma 42: 1108–1111
20. Treggiari MM, Schutz N, Yanez ND, Romand JA (2007) Role of intracranial pressure values and patterns in predicting outcome in traumatic brain injury: a systematic review. Neurocrit Care 6: 104–112
21. Stiefel MF, Udoetuk JD, Spiotta AM, et al (2006) Conventional neurocritical care and cerebral oxygenation after traumatic brain injury. J Neurosurg 105: 568–575
22. Stiefel MF, Spiotta A, Gracias VH, et al (2005) Reduced mortality rate in patients with severe traumatic brain injury treated with brain tissue oxygen monitoring. J Neurosurg 103: 805–811
23. Lane PL, Skoretz TG, Doig G, Girotti MJ (2000) Intracranial pressure monitoring and outcomes after traumatic brain injury. Can J Surg 43: 442–448
24. Cremer OL, van Dijk GW, van Wensen E, et al (2005) Effect of intracranial pressure monitoring and targeted intensive care on functional outcome after severe head injury. Crit Care Med 33: 2207–2213
25. Mauritz W, Steltzer H, Bauer P, Dolanski-Aghamanoukjan L, Metnitz P (2008) Monitoring of intracranial pressure in patients with severe traumatic brain injury: an Austrian prospective multicenter study. Intensive Care Med 34: 1208–1215
26. Robertson CS, Valadka AB, Hannay HJ, et al (1999) Prevention of secondary ischemic insults after severe head injury. Crit Care Med 27: 2086–2095
27. Rosner MJ, Rosner SD, Johnson AH (1995) Cerebral perfusion pressure: management protocol and clinical results. J Neurosurg 83: 949–962
28. Steiner LA, Coles JP, Johnston AJ, et al (2003) Responses of posttraumatic pericontusional cerebral blood flow and blood volume to an increase in cerebral perfusion pressure. J Cereb Blood Flow Metab 23: 1371–1377
29. Cremer OL, van Dijk GW, Amelink GJ, de Smet AM, Moons KG, Kalkman CJ (2004) Cerebral hemodynamic responses to blood pressure manipulation in severely head-injured patients in the presence or absence of intracranial hypertension. Anesth Analg 99: 1211–1217
30. Belli A, Sen J, Petzold A, Russo S, Kitchen N, Smith M (2008) Metabolic failure precedes intracranial pressure rises in traumatic brain injury: a microdialysis study. Acta Neurochir (Wien) 150: 461–469

Sepsis-associated Encephalopathy

S. Siami, A. Polito, and T. Sharshar

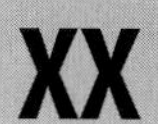

Introduction: Incidence and Diagnosis

Encephalopathy is a frequent but also a severe neurological manifestation of sepsis. It is clinically characterized by changes in mental status and motor activity ranging from delirium to coma and from agitation to hypoactivity [1]. Agitation and somnolence can occur alternately. Paratonic rigidity, asterixis, tremor, and multifocal myoclonus are other but less frequent motor symptoms. Encephalopathy is associated with altered electroencephalographic (EEG) activity that, depending on severity, ranges from excessive theta to burst suppression [1, 2]. Encephalopathy can be accompanied by elevated plasma levels of, for example, neuron-specific enolase (NSE) and S-100 β-protein [1, 2], which are however not correlated with clinical or EEG severity [1, 2]. Brain magnetic resonance imaging (MRI) can reveal cerebral infarcts or posterior reversible encephalopathy syndrome (PRESS) but also localized to diffuse leukoencephalopathy [3, 4]. It has to be noted that brain MRI may fail to detect some brain lesions observed in neuropathological studies, such as hemorrhages related to disseminated intravascular coagulopathy (DIC), microabscesses or multifocal necrotizing leukoencephalopathy [5].

It is clearly established that sepsis is a cause of agitation and delirium [2]. About a third of septic patients have a Glasgow Coma Scale less than 12 [6]. Alteration of alertness and consciousness is an independent prognosis factor, with the mortality rate increasing up to 63 % when Glasgow Coma Scale drops below 8 [6]. It has also been shown that mortality increases with severity of electrophysiological abnormalities and with plasma levels of biomarkers [2].

The incidence and severity of encephalopathy in septic patients should prompt physicians to detect brain dysfunction, diagnose its causes, and, whenever possible, treat them. The diagnostic approach to sepsis-associated encephalopathy has been covered elsewhere [1, 2]. Briefly, changes in mental status can be detected by various validated scores for delirium [1, 2]. Once delirium is identified, neurological examination should look for focal neurological signs, seizures, and meningitis, which are undisputable criteria for performing neuroimaging, EEG, and lumbar puncture, respectively. Encephalopathy should not be simply ascribed to sepsis and drug toxicity, and metabolic disturbance should be systematically sought. Indeed, sepsis-associated encephalopathy is often multi-factorial. However, physicians are well aware that reappearance or persistence of encephalopathy indicates that sepsis is not controlled. Encephalopathy, therefore, becomes a warning sign. This clinical meaning of encephalopathy relates to the fundamental issue of the behavioral response to stress. The behavioral response is mainly controlled by the amygdala and hippocampus which are liable to hemodynamic and metabolic (i.e., hypoxemia and hypoglycemia) insults. It ranges from aggressiveness, anxiety or hyper-alertness to lethargy, and is mainly controlled. Therefore, clinical interpretation of changes in behavior is challenging as they can be adaptive or maladaptive, physiological, or pathophysiological. The crucial role of psychoneuroimmunological interactions in maintaining homeostasis should prompt research into how to evaluate, qualify and modulate behavioral responses during stressful conditions, such as sepsis.

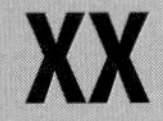

There is no specific treatment for sepsis-associated encephalopathy. Control of sepsis, management of organ failure and metabolic disturbances, and avoidance of neurotoxic drugs constitute the therapeutic approach. However, various treatments have been experimentally tested. These suggested treatments are important to the understanding of pathophysiological mechanisms of sepsis-associated encephalopathy and may also open new therapeutic perspectives for our patients.

Pathophysiology

Brain Signaling in Sepsis

Neuroendocrine, neurovegetative, and behavioral structures involved in the response to stress are physiologically triggered by an activating signal, which encompasses anatomical, cellular, and molecular sequences, as detailed in previous reviews [1, 2]. This brain signaling is mediated by two pathways: The vagus nerve and the circumventricular organs. The former is a sensor of visceral inflammation through its axonal cytokine receptors and its afferents terminate in the nucleus tractus solitarius, which integrates the baroreflex and is connected to other autonomic structures but also to the paraventricular nuclei that control the adrenal axis and vasopressin secretion. The circumventricular organs are deprived of a blood-brain barrier, express components of innate and adaptive immune systems, and are strategically located in the vicinity of the neuroendocrine and neurovegetative nuclei. Once systemic inflammation is detected, the activating signal will spread to the deeper areas involved in controlling the behavioral, neuroendocrine and autonomic response. This activating signal will involve various mediators, including pro-inflammatory and anti-inflammatory cytokines, nitric oxide (NO), and prostaglandins, but also chemokines and carbon monoxide. The signal will directly or indirectly affect migroglial cells, astrocytes, and neurons and finally modulate neurosecretion and neurotransmission. The endothelial cell is another major player as it is, with astrocytes, a major constituent of the blood-brain barrier. Endothelial cells are activated during sepsis, resulting in the release of various mediators into the brain. Because of its deep effects on brain cell functions, this brain activating signal can become, if too intense, pathogenic, altering neurotransmission and leading to encephalopathy.

Alteration of Neurotransmission

Neurotransmitter imbalance is implicated in the pathophysiology of delirium in the intensive care unit (ICU) [7]. Experimental sepsis has been shown to be associated with impairment of the cholinergic [8], brain beta-adrenergic, gamma-aminobutyric acid (GABA), and serotoninergic systems, due to alteration in neurotransmitter release or in the expression of their receptors [9, 10]. These phenomena seem to predominate in the cortex and the hippocampus, which is involved in behavior and emotion. It has been shown that prolonged exposure to lipopolysaccharide (LPS) impaired synaptic transmission and neuronal excitability of pyramid neurons in the hippocampus [11]. There is a body of evidence that NO, cytokines, and prostaglandins modulate beta-adrenergic, GABAergic and cholinergic neurotransmission [10, 12]. The expression of inflammatory mediators and decreased cortical activity have been shown to be associated phenomena in septic rats [13]. Neurotransmitter synthesis is also altered by ammonium and tyrosine, tryptophan, and phenylalanine [14]. Liver dysfunction increases plasma levels of ammonium and, in combination with muscle proteolysis, levels of these amino-acids [14]. A decrease in the ratio of branched-chain to aromatic amino acids may be associated with septic associated encephalopathy [14].

Mitochondrial Dysfunction, Oxidative Stress and Apoptosis

Early but transitory oxidative stress occurs in various brain areas of septic rats, especially in the hippocampus and cortex [15, 16]. It is well established that NO induces oxidative stress, leading to formation of peroxynitrite. For instance, hypotension is preceded by the expression of inducible NO synthase (iNOS), dysfunction of mitochondrial complexes I and IV, and formation of superoxide anions within the medullar autonomic center of septic rats [17]. Other causal factors include a decrease in anti-oxidant factors (heat-shock protein [HSP], ascorbate) [18], imbalance between superoxide dismutase and catalase activity [15], and mitochondrial dysfunction [16]. Oxidative stress may also be induced by hyperglycemia and hypoxemia. However, it is interesting to note that previous studies have shown that brain energy is preserved during sepsis [19].

One major consequence of oxidative stress is apoptosis. Mitochondrial-mediated apoptosis has been demonstrated in septic rats' brains [20] as well as a decrease in intracellular pro-aptoptic (bcl-2) and an increase in anti-apoptotic (bax) factors [20, 21]. In patients who had died from septic shock, neuronal and microglial apoptosis was detected in brain areas involved in the neurovegetative, neuroendocrine and behavioral response to stress [22]. The intensity of apoptosis and endothelial iNOS expression were also correlated. In addition to NO, glutamate, tumor necrosis factor (TNF)-α and glucose have been also incriminated. The role of glutamate-related excito-neurotoxicity has been extensively investigated in various neurological disorders, ranging from acute stroke to chronic neurodegeneration [23]. Briefly, glutamate-induced neuronal death can be mediated by: (1) activation of the N-methyl-D-aspartate (NMDA) subtype of glutamate receptor, resulting in Ca^{2+} and/or Na^{+} overload of the neuron; (2) activation of alpha-amino-3-hydroxy-5-methyl-4-isoxazole-propionic acid (AMPA) receptors, resulting in Ca^{2+} and/or NA^{+} overload of the neuron; and (3) glutamate inhibition of cysteine uptake, resulting in oxidative stress [24]. It has been shown that sepsis inhibits recycling and glutamate export of ascorbate by astrocytes [25, 26] and that plasma and cerebrospinal fluid (CSF) ascorbate levels are lower in patients with sepsis-associated encephalopathy [27]. The activated microglia, which is a consistent phenomenon in sepsis, releases large amounts of glutamate [28].

Although no correlation has been found between TNF-α expression and neuronal or microglial apoptosis [22], its pro-apoptotic role, along with that of other pro-inflammatory cytokines, is supported by the finding of multifocal necrotizing leukoencephalopathy, which is characterized by apoptotic and marked inflammatory lesions of the pons and an excessive systemic inflammatory response, in a patient who had died of septic shock [5]. Interestingly, it has been shown that hyperglycemia increases microglial vulnerability to LPS-mediated toxicity [29].

It must be remembered that brain cell survival depends also on complex interactions between neurons and glial cells, such that activated microglial cells can become neuroprotective or neurotoxic. Moreover, apoptosis must not always be considered a deleterious phenomenon and it has been demonstrated to facilitate plasticity.

Endothelial Activation and Blood-brain Barrier Breakdown

LPS and pro-inflammatory cytokines activate cerebral endothelial cells. They trigger expression of CD40, E-selectin, vascular adhesion molecule-1 and intercellular adhesion molecule-1, activate synthesis of cyclooxygenase 2 and stimulate the IκB-α/nuclear factor-κB (NF-κB) pathway. LPS also induces expression of interleukin (IL)-1 and TNF-α receptors and the production of IL-1β, TNF-α, IL-6, endothelial and inducible NOS [1, 2]. These pro-inflammatory cytokines and NO are able to interact with surrounding brain cells, relaying into the brain's inflammatory response.

The consequences of endothelial activation are: 1) Altered vascular tone, microcirculatory dysfunction, and coagulopathy, which will favor ischemic or hemorrhagic lesions; 2) impairment of oxygen, nutrient, and metabolite movement; 3) blood-brain barrier breakdown, which will facilitate the passage of neurotoxic factors. With regard to the first consequence, changes in cerebral blood flow (CBF) and its autoregulation during sepsis are controversial. Thus, human sepsis studies found an unchanged or a reduced CBF, while experimental studies have reported increased or decreased CBF [1]. Autoregulation of CBF has been also reported as being preserved or altered in human or experimental sepsis [1]. It has recently been shown that in septic patients, delirium was not associated with altered CBF or tissue oxygenation but with disturbed autoregulation [30]. If present, these alterations of cerebral hemodynamics could result in ischemia, which is consistently observed in brain areas susceptible to low CBF [5]. Neuropathological examination reveals hemorrhages in about 9 % of septic shock patients. Clotting tests, platelet count, and incidence of DIC were not significantly different in septic shock patients with and without hemorrhages [5].

Breakdown of the blood-brain barrier has been demonstrated in an experimental model of sepsis [31]. Recently, Handa et al. [32], showed that stimulation of cerebrovascular endothelial cells with septic plasma induced dissociation of the tight junction protein, occludin, from the cytoskeletal network and subsequent increase in size-selective trans-endothelial solute flux. This has also been documented in septic patients, with the help of brain MRI. According to these neuroradiological studies [3, 4], breakdown of the blood-brain barrier can be localized around the Wirchow-Robin spaces, diffuse to the whole white matter, or be localized in posterior lobes, then corresponding to a posterior reversible encephalopathy syndrome. Interestingly, glutamate, which is also involved in brain oxidative stress and cell death, plays an important role in blood-brain barrier permeability [24].

Experimental Therapeutic Approach

Among treatments currently used in septic patients, intensive insulin therapy, activated protein C, and steroids may have some effects on endothelial activation, blood-brain barrier breakdown, neuroinflammation, and oxidative stress or apoptosis, which are the main and entwined pathophysiological mechanisms of sepsis-associated encephalopathy (**Fig. 1**).

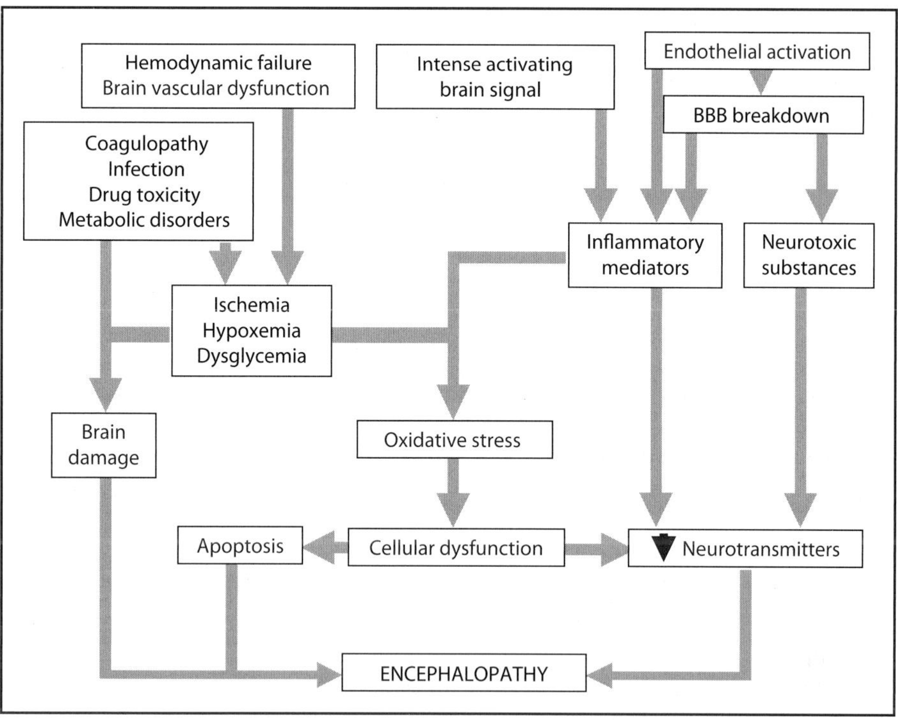

Fig. 1. Mechanisms of sepsis-associated encephalopathy (adapted from [2]). BBB: blood brain barrier

Insulin as a neuroprotective therapy is supported by experimental evidence that hyperglycemia induces oxidative stress and apoptosis. Although insulin therapy may improve the outcome of brain-injured patients [33], it has been recently shown not to be beneficial in acute stroke [34]. However, it is impossible to anticipate its effect on the incidence and severity of sepsis-associated encephalopathy as cerebral glucose metabolism is highly complex and its disturbances in sepsis have been insufficiently elucidated. For instance, it is unknown how sepsis alters the brain cell expression of glucose transporters (GLUT), notably of GLUT4 which is modulated by insulin [35]. Therefore, neuronal sensitivity to hypoglycemia and hyperglycemia may be considerably altered in sepsis, making the effect of insulin on neuronal metabolism unpredictable. Moreover, LPS increased the permeability of the blood-brain barrier to insulin, potentiating its central effects [36]. One must remember that hypoglycemia is harmful for the brain, notably for the hippocampus.

Steroids may act on all these mechanisms. It has experimentally been shown that steroids decrease systemic inflammation, reduce brain edema [37], improve blood-brain barrier function [38], and also modulate microglia functions [39]. The expression of steroid receptors in hippocampus, reduction of NMDA receptor expression in the hippocampus [40], and prevention by hydrocortisone of post-traumatic stress syndrome [41] are supportive arguments for the role of steroids in behavioral response to stress.

The anti-inflammatory and endothelial effects of activated protein C in sepsis and experimental brain ischemia are also appealing. However, there is no evidence from

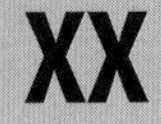

clinical trials that insulin therapy, activated protein C, or steroids reduce the incidence or severity of sepsis-associated encephalopathy.

Among experimental treatments, inhibition of iNOS was one of the first to be tested because of the pathogenic role of iNOS. iNOS inhibition did not improve consciousness but reduced LPS-induced neuronal apoptosis in septic rats [42], aggravated brain ischemia [43] and increased cardiovascular deaths [44]. Serum amyloid P or magnesium [45, 46] have also been proposed and have been shown to reduce blood-brain barrier permeability in septic animals. Antioxidant molecules have also been tested. For instance, Riluzole, a glutamate release inhibitor, diminished brain edema, blood-brain barrier permeability, oxidative damage, and brain injury in septic rats; the two latter being also reduced by Silymarin [24, 47]. While infusion of branched-chain amino acids can reduce aromatic amino acids in the brain by competing with their transport, its effect on septic encephalopathy has not been demonstrated [48]. Calcium channel blockers and removal of circulating cytokines, notably by coupled plasma filtration adsorption, have also been proposed for reducing blood-brain barrier permeability [49]. Modulation of brain signaling is another option; it has recently been demonstrated that pharmacological inhibition of the cholinergic pathway improves sickness behavior [50].

Conclusion

The diagnosis of encephalopathy in septic patients is crucial as it is a frequent and severe complication. Diagnosis relies essentially on neurological examination. Mechanisms of sepsis-associated encephalopathy are highly complex, resulting from both inflammatory and non-inflammatory processes that affect all brain cells and induce blood-brain barrier breakdown, dysfunction of intracellular metabolism, brain cell death, and brain injury. Currently, treatment of sepsis-associated encephalopathy consists mainly of control of sepsis. The effects of insulin therapy, activated protein C, and steroids on sepsis-associated encephalopathy need to be assessed. Benefits from experimental treatments of sepsis-induced blood-brain barrier dysfunction, brain oxidative stress and inflammation, and also brain signaling, are interesting but need to be confirmed.

References

1. Ebersoldt M, Sharshar T, Annane D (2007) Sepsis-associated delirium. Intensive Care Med 33: 941–950
2. Siami S, Annane D, Sharshar T (2008) The encephalopathy in sepsis. Crit Care Clin 24: 67–82
3. Sharshar T, Carlier R, Bernard F, et al. (2007) Brain lesions in septic shock: a magnetic resonance imaging study. Intensive Care Med 33: 798–806
4. Bartynski WS, Boardman JF, Zeigler ZR, Shadduck RK, Lister J (2006) Posterior reversible encephalopathy syndrome in infection, sepsis, and shock. AJNR Am J Neuroradiol 27: 2179–2190
5. Sharshar T, Annane D, de la Grandmaison G, et al. (2004) The neuropathology of septic shock. Brain Pathol 14: 21–33
6. Eidelman LA, Putterman D, Putterman C, Sprung CL (1996) The spectrum of septic encephalopathy. Definitions, etiologies, and mortalities. JAMA 275: 470–473
7. Girard TD, Pandharipande PP, Ely EW (2008) Delirium in the intensive care unit. Crit Care 12 (Suppl 3):S3
8. Semmler A, Frisch C, Debeir T, et al (2007) Long-term cognitive impairment, neuronal loss and reduced cortical cholinergic innervation after recovery from sepsis in a rodent model. Exp Neurol 204: 733–740

9. Kadoi Y, Saito S (1996) An alteration in the gamma-aminobutyric acid receptor system in experimentally induced septic shock in rats. Crit Care Med 24: 298–305
10. Kadoi Y, Saito S, Kunimoto F, Imai T, Fujita T (1996) Impairment of the brain beta-adrenergic system during experimental endotoxemia. J Surg Res 61: 496–502
11. Hellstrom IC, Danik M, Luheshi GN, Williams S (2005) Chronic LPS exposure produces changes in intrinsic membrane properties and a sustained IL-beta-dependent increase in GABAergic inhibition in hippocampal CA1 pyramidal neurons. Hippocampus 15: 656–664
12. Pavlov VA, Ochani M, Gallowitsch-Puerta M, et al (2006) Central muscarinic cholinergic regulation of the systemic inflammatory response during endotoxemia. Proc Natl Acad Sci USA 103: 5219–5223
13. Semmler A, Hermann S, Mormann F, et al (2008) Sepsis causes neuroinflammation and concomitant decrease of cerebral metabolism. J Neuroinflammation 5:38
14. Basler T, Meier-Hellmann A, Bredle D, Reinhart K (2002) Amino acid imbalance early in septic encephalopathy. Intensive Care Med 28: 293–298
15. Barichello T, Fortunato JJ, Vitali AM, et al (2006) Oxidative variables in the rat brain after sepsis induced by cecal ligation and perforation. Crit Care Med 34: 886–889
16. d'Avila JC, Santiago AP, Amancio RT, et al (2008) Sepsis induces brain mitochondrial dysfunction. Crit Care Med 36: 1925–1932.
17. Chan JY, Chang AY, Wang LL, Ou CC, Chan SH (2007) Protein kinase C-dependent mitochondrial translocation of proapoptotic protein Bax on activation of inducible nitric-oxide synthase in rostral ventrolateral medulla mediates cardiovascular depression during experimental endotoxemia. Mol Pharmacol 71: 1129–1139
18. Christians ES, Yan LJ, Benjamin IJ (2002) Heat shock factor 1 and heat shock proteins: critical partners in protection against acute cell injury. Crit Care Med 30: S43–50
19. Hotchkiss RS, Karl IE (1992) Reevaluation of the role of cellular hypoxia and bioenergetic failure in sepsis. JAMA 267: 1503–1510.
20. Messaris E, Memos N, Chatzigianni E, et al (2004) Time-dependent mitochondrial-mediated programmed neuronal cell death survival in sepsis. Crit Care Med 32: 1764–1770
21. Semmler A, Okulla T, Sastre M, Dumitrescu-Ozimek L, Heneka MT (2005) Systemic inflammation induces apoptosis with variable vulnerability of different brain regions. J Chem Neuroanat 30: 144–157
22. Sharshar T, Gray F, Lorin de la Grandmaison G, et al (2003) Apoptosis of neurons in cardiovascular autonomic centres triggered by inducible nitric oxide synthase after death from septic shock. Lancet 362: 1799–1805
23. Villmann C, Becker CM (2007) On the hypes and falls in neuroprotection: targeting the NMDA receptor. Neuroscientist 13: 594–615
24. Toklu HZ, Uysal MK, Kabasakal L, et al (2009) The effects of riluzole on neurological, brain biochemical, and histological changes in early and late term of sepsis in rats. J Surg Res (in press)
25. Wilson JX, Dragan M (2005) Sepsis inhibits recycling and glutamate-stimulated export of ascorbate by astrocytes. Free Radic Biol Med 39: 990–998
26. Korcok J, Wu F, Tyml K, Hammond RR, Wilson JX (2002) Sepsis inhibits reduction of dehydroascorbic acid and accumulation of ascorbate in astroglial cultures: intracellular ascorbate depletion increases nitric oxide synthase induction and glutamate uptake inhibition. J Neurochem 81: 185–193
27. Voigt K, Kontush A, Stuerenburg HJ, et al (2002) Decreased plasma and cerebrospinal fluid ascorbate levels in patients with septic encephalopathy. Free Radic Res 36: 735–739
28. Brown GC, Bal-Price A (2003) Inflammatory neurodegeneration mediated by nitric oxide, glutamate, and mitochondria. Mol Neurobiol 27: 325–355
29. Wang JY, Yang JM, Tao PL, Yang SN (2001) Synergistic apoptosis induced by bacterial endotoxin lipopolysaccharide and high glucose in rat microglia. Neurosci Lett 304: 177–180
30. Pfister D, Siegemund M, Dell-Kuster S, et al (2008) Cerebral perfusion in sepsis-associated delirium. Crit Care 12:R63
31. Papadopoulos MC, Lamb FJ, Moss RF, et al (1999) Faecal peritonitis causes oedema and neuronal injury in pig cerebral cortex. Clin Sci (Lond) 96: 461–466
32. Handa O, Stephen J, Cepinskas G (2008) Role of eNOS-derived nitric oxide (NO) in activation and dysfunction of cerebrovascular endothelial cells during early onsets of sepsis. Am J Physiol Heart Circ Physiol 1712–1719

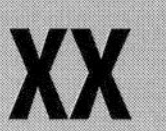

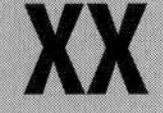

33. Van den Berghe G, Schoonheydt K, Becx P, Bruyninckx F, Wouters PJ (2005) Insulin therapy protects the central and peripheral nervous system of intensive care patients. Neurology 64: 1348–1353
34. Bruno A, Kent TA, Coull BM, et al (2008) Treatment of hyperglycemia in ischemic stroke (THIS): a randomized pilot trial. Stroke 39: 384–389
35. Maher F, Vannucci SJ, Simpson IA (1994) Glucose transporter proteins in brain. FASEB J 8: 1003–1011.
36. Xaio H, Banks WA, Niehoff ML, Morley JE (2001) Effect of LPS on the permeability of the blood-brain barrier to insulin. Brain Res 896: 36–42
37. Kaal EC, Vecht CJ (2004) The management of brain edema in brain tumors. Curr Opin Oncol 16: 593–600
38. Bauer B, Hartz AM, Fricker G, Miller DS (2005) Modulation of p-glycoprotein transport function at the blood-brain barrier. Exp Biol Med (Maywood) 230: 118–127
39. Sierra A, Gottfried-Blackmore A, Milner TA, McEwen BS, Bulloch K (2008) Steroid hormone receptor expression and function in microglia. Glia 56: 659–674
40. Weiland NG, Orchinik M, Tanapat P (1997) Chronic corticosterone treatment induces parallel changes in N-methyl-D-aspartate receptor subunit messenger RNA levels and antagonist binding sites in the hippocampus. Neuroscience 78: 653–662
41. Schelling G, Roozendaal B, Krauseneck T, et al (2006) Efficacy of hydrocortisone in preventing posttraumatic stress disorder following critical illness and major surgery. Ann NY Acad Sci 1071: 46–53
42. Kadoi Y, Goto F (2004) Selective inducible nitric oxide inhibition can restore hemodynamics, but does not improve neurological dysfunction in experimentally-induced septic shock in rats. Anesth Analg 99: 212–220
43. Li H, Forstermann U (2000) Nitric oxide in the pathogenesis of vascular disease. J Pathol 190: 244–254
44. Lopez A, Lorente JA, Steingrub J, et al (2004) Multiple-center, randomized, placebo-controlled, double-blind study of the nitric oxide synthase inhibitor 546C88: effect on survival in patients with septic shock. Crit Care Med 32: 21–30
45. Veszelka S, Urbanyi Z, Pazmany T, et al (2003) Human serum amyloid P component attenuates the bacterial lipopolysaccharide-induced increase in blood-brain barrier permeability in mice. Neurosci Lett 352: 57–60
46. Esen F, Erdem T, Aktan D, et al (2005) Effect of magnesium sulfate administration on blood-brain barrier in a rat model of intraperitoneal sepsis: a randomized controlled experimental study. Crit Care 9:R18–23
47. Toklu HZ, Tunali Akbay T, Velioglu-Ogunc A, et al (2008) Silymarin, the antioxidant component of Silybum marianum, prevents sepsis-induced acute lung and brain injury. J Surg Res 145: 214–222
48. Hasselgren PO, Fischer JE (1986) Septic encephalopathy. Etiology and management. Intensive Care Med 12: 13–16
49. Wratten ML (2008) Therapeutic approaches to reduce systemic inflammation in septic-associated neurologic complications. Eur J Anaesthesiol Suppl 42: 1–7
50. Johnson DR, O'Connor JC, Dantzer R, Freund GG (2005) Inhibition of vagally mediated immune-to-brain signaling by vanadyl sulfate speeds recovery from sickness. Proc Natl Acad Sci USA 102: 15184–15189

XXI Malignancies

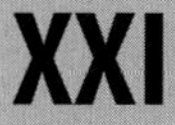

Acute Tumor Lysis Syndrome: Diagnosis and Management

M. Darmon, M. Roumier, and E. Azoulay

Introduction

Tumor lysis syndrome is a potentially life-threatening complication of cancer treatment in patients with extensive, rapidly growing, chemosensitive malignancies. Tumor lysis syndrome results from the rapid destruction of malignant cells, which abruptly release intracellular ions, proteins, and metabolites into the extracellular space [1]. Potassium, calcium, phosphates, and uric acid, which are present in high concentrations within malignant cells, pour into the extracellular space. The result is a constellation of metabolic disturbances that can cause acute kidney injury (AKI), of which the most common mechanism is uric-acid crystal formation in the renal tubules. Another cause of AKI is calcium-phosphate deposition related to hyperphosphatemia. AKI may, in itself, cause substantial morbidity and mortality [2]. In addition, AKI leads to further increases in the above-listed metabolites, most notably potassium and phosphate, which may lead to cardiac arrhythmia or sudden death [3, 4].

Although tumor lysis syndrome typically occurs in patients with high-grade hematological malignancies, cases have been reported in a variety of other hematological malignancies, including low-grade non-Hodgkin's lymphoma and Hodgkin's disease, as well as in fast-growing solid tumors such as testicular cancer [1, 5]. Early recognition of patients at high risk for acute tumor lysis syndrome may allow the initiation of prophylactic measures.

The objectives of this chapter are to describe the diagnostic criteria of tumor lysis syndrome, to review the clinical and biological consequences of this syndrome, and to provide up-to-date guidelines for the prevention and prompt management of tumor lysis syndrome.

Pathophysiology

Massive cell destruction leads to the rapid release of intracellular anions, cations, and metabolic products of proteins and nucleic acids into the bloodstream (**Fig. 1**) [1]. Although tumor lysis syndrome usually develops shortly after the initiation of cytotoxic chemotherapy, up to one-third of cases may occur before treatment [6–8].

Malignant cells carry a large burden of nucleic-acid products, which reflects their high cellular activity and turnover. The release into the extracellular space of purine nucleic acids and their subsequent transformation into uric acid causes hyperuricemia [9–11]. Uric acid is poorly soluble in water, and hyperuricemia may therefore lead to the deposition of uric-acid crystals. A low urinary flow and an acidic pH may

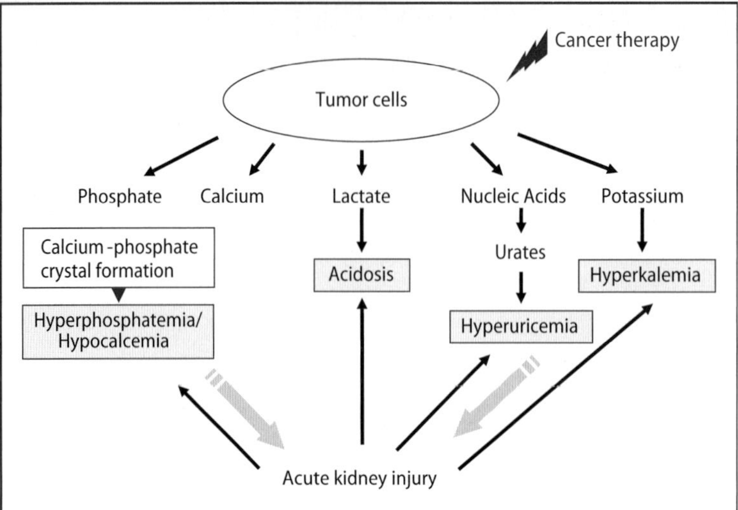

Fig. 1. Pathophysiology of tumor lysis syndrome

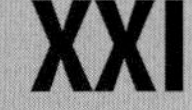

decrease the threshold at which uric acid precipitates into crystals, thereby increasing the risk of tubular obstruction [12].

The potassium released by destroyed cells may overwhelm renal excretion capabilities, causing hyperkalemia. In addition, an early peak in serum potassium concentration may occur as a result of mitochondrial dysfunction induced by cancer therapy [1]. Thus, leakage of potassium out of the tumor cells may antedate complete tumor lysis or the development of AKI.

Nucleotides and phosphate are among the compounds contained in the degenerated nuclear material released by destroyed cells. Malignant cells may contain as much as four times the amount of phosphate contained in mature lymphocytes [13]. Hyperphosphatemia may lead to precipitation of calcium-phosphate crystals, which may cause nephrocalcinosis, urinary obstruction, and tissue deposits. Furthermore, hyperphosphatemia and the precipitation of calcium-phosphate crystals may cause hypocalcemia, which, however, is usually asymptomatic. No validated methods for predicting the threshold at which deposition of calcium-phosphate crystal occurs are available [14]. Hypocalcemia (reflecting calcium-phosphate crystal deposition) and persistent hyperphosphatemia despite hydration are the only reliable warning signs of impending symptomatic calcium-phosphate crystal deposition.

Lactate dehydrogenase (LDH) is a surrogate of tumor burden and predicts tumor lysis syndrome. However, tumor lysis may further increase LDH levels.

As many as one-third of patients with tumor lysis syndrome experience clinical manifestations [8]. AKI is the most common and may lead to fluid overload and pulmonary edema. Cardiac arrhythmia or sudden death may result from hyperkalemia or hyperphosphatemia. Finally, calcium and phosphate abnormalities may lead to muscle cramps or seizures. In addition to these life-threatening clinical consequences, symptomatic tumor lysis syndrome may jeopardize the chances for achieving a complete remission by causing chemotherapy-limiting AKI [15].

Diagnosis, Classification, and Risk Factors

The diagnosis of tumor lysis syndrome usually rests on the occurrence of suggestive laboratory test abnormalities in a patient who has a fast-growing malignancy. However, none of the signs is specific, and careful attention should, therefore, be paid to the course of the symptoms and metabolic disturbances over time. AKI related to any cause may lead to hyperkalemia, hyperphosphatemia, and hyperuricemia, thus mimicking tumor lysis syndrome. Differentiating tumor lysis syndrome with secondary AKI from AKI without tumor lysis syndrome may be challenging.

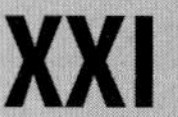

Until very recently there was no diagnostic criterion for tumor lysis syndrome. The first diagnostic classification was developed by Hande and Garrow in 1993 then modified by Cairo and Bishop (**Table 1**) [3]. According to this classification, a constellation of metabolic disturbances (hyperkalemia, hyperphosphatemia, hyperuricemia, and hyperkalemia) defines laboratory tumor lysis syndrome in high-risk patients, whereas clinical manifestations (cardiac, renal, or neurological manifestations of tumor lysis syndrome) in a patient with laboratory tumor lysis syndrome defines clinical tumor lysis syndrome. Guidelines developed in 2008 rest on this classification [16].

Early recognition of high-risk patients may allow a risk-based strategy for preventing both tumor lysis syndrome and AKI. Tumor lysis syndrome typically occurs in patients with high-grade hematological malignancies (acute leukemia, Burkitt's lymphoma, or other high-grade non-Hodgkin lymphomas) [6, 13, 17–20]. Despite routine urate oxidase therapy, tumor lysis syndrome develops in 10 to 50 % of patients with these high-grade malignancies [8, 21–23] and AKI in up to one-third [8, 22, 23]. In addition to the type of tumor and to its sensitivity to chemotherapeutic agents, features related to the tumor burden (large tumor burden, LDH > 1500 IU, and extensive bone marrow involvement) influence the risk of tumor lysis syndrome [18]. Finally, patient characteristics may affect the risk of tumor lysis syndrome. For example, pre-existing renal failure is associated with an increased risk of laboratory and clinical tumor lysis syndrome.

The spectrum of patients at risk for tumor lysis syndrome is changing. Tumor lysis syndrome was known to occur in several fast-growing solid tumors, such as testicular cancer [1, 5]. Tumor lysis syndrome was recently described in patients with low-grade hematological malignancies, including chronic lymphoid lymphoma, solid tumors, and myeloma [24–28]. The increasing effectiveness of new anticancer therapies (e.g., rituximab, bortezumib, thalidomide, tamoxifen, and interferon-α) may partly explain this phenomenon [26–31]. In addition, recent studies suggest that spontaneous tumor lysis syndrome may be more common than previously thought [6–8]. As many as one-third of cases of tumor lysis syndrome predate the ini-

Table 1. Definitions of laboratory and clinical tumor lysis syndrome in adults, according to Cairo and Bishop [3]

Laboratory tumor lysis syndrome = at least two of the following, in serum	
Non-ionized calcium	< 1.75 mmol/l or -25 % from baseline
Potassium	> 6 mmol/l or +25 % from baseline
Uric acid	> 476 μmol/l or +25 % from baseline
Phosphate	> 1.45 mmol/l or +25 % from baseline
Clinical tumor lysis syndrome = laboratory tumor lysis syndrome (above) plus one of the following	
Renal involvement	Acute kidney injury
Cardiovascular involvement	Cardiac arrhythmia or sudden death
Neurological involvement	Seizure

tiation of cancer chemotherapy [6–8]. Some of these cases may be related to diagnostic procedures (e.g., biopsies) or corticosteroid administration (e.g., before contrast-agent administration). However, high-grade hematological malignancies, especially with heavy tumor burdens, may be associated with spontaneous tumor lysis syndrome. In our experience, spontaneous tumor lysis syndrome is usually more severe and more often associated with clinical tumor lysis syndrome, compared to tumor lysis syndrome induced by cancer chemotherapy. Spontaneous tumor lysis syndrome should probably be looked for routinely in patients with high-grade malignancies.

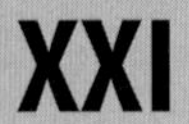

Treatment

Three steps must be distinguished: a) Prevention of tumor lysis syndrome; b) prevention of clinical manifestations in patients with laboratory tumor lysis syndrome; and c) prevention of further organ dysfunction in clinical tumor lysis syndrome. The goal of these measures is to prevent AKI, which severely exacerbates the laboratory and clinical manifestations of tumor lysis syndrome. In addition, this strategy may help to avoid not only excess mortality, but also residual organ dysfunction.

Therefore, control of hyperuricemia and prevention of nephrocalcinosis are key treatment goals. Renal replacement therapy should be started if the metabolic disorders are not controlled within 6 hours of treatment initiation. If AKI develops despite prevention, extra-renal therapy should be initiated quickly to clear the excess uric acid and phosphates, thus limiting further kidney impairment [32]. Patients with highly aggressive tumors may have hypophosphatemia and hypokalemia before cancer chemotherapy initiation. These abnormalities indicate a high risk of tumor lysis syndrome; therefore, they should not be corrected. Preventive and curative measures are summarized in **Table 2**.

Table 2. Prevention and treatment of tumor lysis syndrome

General Measures
Avoid correction of hypokalemia or hypophosphatemia before induction
Avoid urine alkalinization
Avoid correcting hypocalcemia, unless symptomatic
Prevention of Tumor Lysis Syndrome
Volume expansion
Urate oxidase if high risk for tumor lysis syndrome, allopurinol otherwise
No phosphate, potassium, or calcium in the intravenous fluids
Prevention of Clinical Tumor Lysis Syndrome
Volume expansion
Urate oxidase
No phosphate, potassium, or calcium in the intravenous fluids
Initiate renal replacement therapy if phosphatemia remains high after 6 hours of management
Treatment of Clinical Tumor Lysis Syndrome
Volume expansion
Urate oxidase
No phosphate, potassium, or calcium in the intravenous fluids
Initiate renal replacement therapy:
After 6 hours in patients with persistent hyperphosphatemia or renal function impairment
Immediately in patients with cardiac or neurological manifestations

Although no scientific proof exists to support this statement, intensive care unit (ICU) admission should be discussed routinely for high-risk patients and patients with overt tumor lysis syndrome, especially spontaneous tumor lysis syndrome. In addition, close metabolic monitoring should be performed, including measurement of serum potassium, calcium, phosphate, urea, creatinine, and uric acid at least every 8 hours.

Fluid Expansion

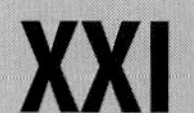

The mainstay for prophylaxis or treatment of tumor lysis syndrome is aggressive hydration with saline solution to maintain a high urinary output capable of flushing out uric acid and phosphate [3, 12, 32]. In patients whose urinary output decreases despite adequate fluid intake, diuretic therapy with or without mannitol has been suggested [3, 16]. In our experience, the effectiveness of diuretics is limited. In addition, the development of oliguria usually indicates AKI, which requires renal replacement therapy as opposed to diuretics, especially when oliguria develops despite adequate prevention. As a general rule, caution is required when using diuretics in critically ill patients [33].

Urine Alkalinization

Urine alkalinization has long been used to promote the elimination of uric acid. However, the introduction of fast-acting urate oxidase has considerably reduced the risk of urate nephropathy [20, 34]. In addition, urine alkalinization may promote calcium-phosphate deposition [35, 36]. Furthermore, the efficacy of urine alkalinization remains unclear. High tubular fluid flow is the key to protecting against acute uric-acid nephropathy, and urine alkalinization may play only a minor preventive role, at least in animal models of hyperuricemia [12]. Given the limited effectiveness and potential adverse effects of urine alkalinization, this method is no longer recommended routinely when urate oxidase is available (level of evidence V; grade D recommendation) [16]. However, the role for urine alkalinization in patients treated with allopurinol remains unclear [16].

Hypouricemic Agents

Several agents are available for decreasing uric acid levels. Recombinant urate oxidase converts uric acid to allantoin, which is 5 to 10 times more soluble in urine [3]. Recombinant urate oxidase (rasburicase) decreases the median uric acid concentration from 577 to 60 μmol/l within 4 hours [19]. Moreover, recombinant urate oxidase significantly decreases the uric-acid exposure time compared to allopurinol in children at high risk for tumor lysis syndrome [20]. Recombinant urate oxidase ensures the control of plasma uric acid within 4 hours [19, 34, 37]. Last, urate oxidase has long been known to decrease the risk of AKI during tumor lysis syndrome [38]. Although very effective, recombinant urate oxidase is costly. In 2003, the cost of rasburicase treatment of a 70-kg adult for 4 days was estimated at 2200€ in Europe [39]. Whereas rasburicase treatment of established tumor lysis syndrome in adults was highly cost-effective, the cost-effectiveness of tumor lysis syndrome prevention with rasburicase varied widely, being extremely sensitive to tumor lysis syndrome risk [39]. Therefore, rasburicase should be restricted to the prevention of tumor lysis syndrome in high-risk patients, the treatment of established tumor lysis syndrome, and the prevention of tumor lysis syndrome in low- or intermediate-risk patients who have pre-existing hyperuricemia or who develop hyperuricemia despite allopurinol [16, 39]. Rasburicase is contraindicated in patients with glucose-6-phosphate dehydrogenase (G6PD) deficiency, as uric acid breakdown leads to excessive hydrogen peroxide production with a risk of hemolysis [40].

In patients at low or intermediate risk for tumor lysis syndrome, allopurinol can be used as a hypouricemic agent. Allopurinol is a xanthine analog that decreases the conversion of xanthine to uric acid [37]. However, although allopurinol may decrease the risk of uric acid nephropathy in some patients, it also increases serum xanthine and hypoxanthine concentrations. Both compounds are less soluble in water than uric acid, so that xanthine nephropathy may develop [36]. This complication is uncommon, however, and allopurinol is still recommended provided the treatment is started 24 to 48 hours before cancer chemotherapy and continued for 3 to 7 days after the cancer chemotherapy initiation (level of evidence: II; grade B recommendation) [16]. In addition, since allopurinol prevents the formation of uric acid but does not decrease the amount of uric acid present before treatment initiation, rasburicase should be preferred in patients with baseline hyperuricemia (> 450 μmol/l) (level of evidence: II; grade B recommendation) [16].

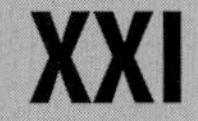

Prevention of Nephrocalcinosis

Nephrocalcinosis prevention requires the correction of hyperphosphatemia. Calcium should not be administered. Apart from hydration, few methods are available for preventing or treating hyperphosphatemia. Oral phosphate binders are not effective. The persistence of hyperphosphatemia 4 to 6 hours after the initiation of a saline infusion should lead to renal replacement therapy. Although hyperphosphatemia remains a good marker for the response to hydration, the occurrence of hypocalcemia with persistent hyperphosphatemia usually indicates calcium-phosphate crystal deposition.

Indication and Timing of Renal Replacement Therapy

Although the indications for renal replacement therapy in tumor lysis syndrome have not been the focus of specific studies, emergency renal replacement therapy is probably appropriate when hydration fails to promptly improve the metabolic disturbances or when AKI develops. AKI carries a poor prognosis in patients with tumor lysis syndrome [8]. Renal replacement therapy may prove effective in controlling the metabolic disturbances and preventing AKI. A few case-reports and case-series suggest that phosphate clearance may be higher with sequential dialysis than with hemofiltration. However, phosphate rebound is common 30 to 60 minutes after the end of hemodialysis [4]. Extended daily dialysis or isolated sequential dialysis followed by continuous hemofiltration may, therefore, be helpful in patients with tumor lysis syndrome requiring renal replacement therapy.

Management of Cancer Chemotherapy in Patients with Tumor Lysis Syndrome

In patients at high risk for tumor lysis syndrome or with spontaneous tumor lysis syndrome, the appropriateness of delaying cancer chemotherapy until preventive measures are initiated should be discussed based on patient status and on the nature of the underlying malignancy (level of evidence II; grade A recommendation) [16].

In addition, increasing the time over which cancer chemotherapy is administered may deserve consideration, especially in patients with overt tumor lysis syndrome. However, in our experience, the full chemotherapy dose can be given to most patients. Dose reduction should be avoided whenever possible in order to minimize the risk of failed induction treatment [15].

Future Research

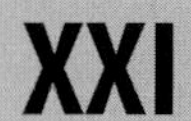

Recommendations have been issued recently regarding the diagnosis and treatment of tumor lysis syndrome [16]. However, few studies focusing on patients with tumor lysis syndrome are available. Therefore, most recommendations are grade D, that is, based on little or no systematic empirical evidence. Further studies are needed.

Studies should seek to clarify the mechanisms of renal toxicity during tumor lysis syndrome, to develop better means of evaluating the risk for tumor lysis syndrome and of AKI complicating tumor lysis syndrome, and to validate preventive and curative treatments. Ideas for future studies are listed below.

- The mechanisms of calcium-phosphate precipitation need to be elucidated. Methods for predicting the threshold at which precipitation occurs must be developed. Both *in vitro* studies and *in vivo* animal studies may help to achieve these objectives.
- The risk of tumor lysis syndrome has been the focus of a few small retrospective cohort studies. At present, no methods are available for assessing the risk of laboratory or clinical tumor lysis syndrome in the individual patient. Large prospective studies are required to evaluate the risk for laboratory and clinical tumor lysis syndrome associated with various malignancies.
- Currently used aggressive strategies for limiting the adverse clinical effects of tumor lysis syndrome have not been validated. These strategies are widely accepted for patients with overt tumor lysis syndrome, most notably overt clinical tumor lysis syndrome. In contrast, potential benefits from early ICU admission of patients at high risk for tumor lysis syndrome and from preventive renal replacement therapy (started before AKI develops) need to be evaluated.
- The optimal timing and modalities of preventive renal replacement therapy need to be evaluated. The best method for phosphate removal must be determined. The pharmacokinetics of cancer chemotherapy in critically ill patients and in patients receiving renal replacement therapy should be investigated.

Conclusion

Tumor lysis syndrome is a common and life-threatening complication of newly diagnosed malignancies. The development of AKI or metabolic derangements may prompt ICU admission. Identifying patients at risk for tumor lysis syndrome and prevention of tumor lysis syndrome (or of its clinical manifestations in patients with laboratory tumor lysis syndrome) are crucial to limit the mortality and morbidity associated with this syndrome.

In high-risk patients and in patients with overt tumor lysis syndrome, aggressive management including hydration and urate oxidase should be started on an emergency basis to limit the metabolic disturbances and to decrease the risk of AKI. ICU admission and renal replacement therapy are required if these symptomatic measures fail to control the metabolic abnormalities within 4 to 6 hours. The main treatment objective is to avoid excess mortality and residual organ dysfunction in these patients.

Objective data on tumor lysis syndrome are scarce. Studies are needed to better delineate the spectrum of patients at risk for tumor lysis syndrome and to determine the optimal modalities and timing for tumor lysis syndrome prevention and treatment.

References

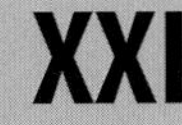

1. Yarpuzlu AA (2003) A review of clinical and laboratory findings and treatment of tumor lysis syndrome. Clin Chim Acta 333: 13–18
2. Metnitz PG, Krenn CG, Steltzer, et al (2002) Effect of acute renal failure requiring renal replacement therapy on outcome in critically ill patients. Crit Care Med 30: 2051–2058
3. Cairo MS, Bishop M (2004) Tumour lysis syndrome: new therapeutic strategies and classification. Br J Haematol 127: 3–11
4. Davidson MB, Thakkar S, Hix JK, et al (2004) Pathophysiology, clinical consequences, and treatment of tumor lysis syndrome. Am J Med 116: 546–554
5. Kalemkerian GP, Darwish B, Varterasian ML (1997) Tumor lysis syndrome in small cell carcinoma and other solid tumors. Am J Med 103: 363–367
6. Altman A (2001) Acute tumor lysis syndrome. Semin Oncol 28:S3–8
7. Darmon M, Thiery G, Ciroldi M, et al (2005) Intensive care in patients with newly diagnosed malignancies and a need for cancer chemotherapy. Crit Care Med 33: 2488–2493
8. Montesinos P, Lorenzo I, Martin G, et al (2008) Tumor lysis syndrome in patients with acute myeloid leukemia: identification of risk factors and development of a predictive model. Haematologica 93: 67–74
9. Seegmiller JE, Laster L, Howell RR (1963) Biochemistry of uric acid and its relation to gout. N Engl J Med 268: 821–827
10. Seegmiller JE, Laster L, Howell RR (1963) Biochemistry of uric acid and its relation to gout. N Engl J Med 268: 764–773
11. Seegmiller JE, Laster L, Howell RR (1963) Biochemistry of uric acid and its relation to gout. N Engl J Med 268: 712–716
12. Conger JD, Falk SA (1977) Intrarenal dynamics in the pathogenesis and prevention of acute urate nephropathy. J Clin Invest 59: 786–793
13. Flombaum CD (2000) Metabolic emergencies in the cancer patient. Semin Oncol 27: 322–334
14. Hebert LA, Lemann J Jr, Petersen JR (1966) Studies of the mechanism by which phosphate infusion lowers serum calcium concentration. J Clin Invest 45: 1886–1894
15. Munker R, Hill U, Jehn U, et al (1998) Renal complications in acute leukemias. Haematologica 83: 416–421
16. Coiffier B, Altman A, Pui CH, et al (2008) Guidelines for the management of pediatric and adult tumor lysis syndrome: an evidence-based review. J Clin Oncol 26: 2767–2778
17. Jeha S (2001) Tumor lysis syndrome. Semin Hematol 38:S4–8
18. Cohen LF, Balow JE, Magrath IT, et al (1980) Acute tumor lysis syndrome. A review of 37 patients with Burkitt's lymphoma. Am J Med 68: 486–491
19. Pui CH (2001) Urate oxidase in the prophylaxis or treatment of hyperuricemia: the United States experience. Semin Hematol 38:S13–21
20. Goldman SC, Holcenberg JS, Finklestein JZ, et al (2001) A randomized comparison between rasburicase and allopurinol in children with lymphoma or leukemia at high risk for tumor lysis. Blood 97: 2998–3003
21. Annemans L, Moeremans K, Lamotte M, et al (2003) Incidence, medical resource utilisation and costs of hyperuricemia and tumour lysis syndrome in patients with acute leukaemia and non-Hodgkin's lymphoma in four European countries. Leuk Lymphoma 44: 77–83
22. Mato AR, Riccio BE, Qin L, et al (2006) A predictive model for the detection of tumor lysis syndrome during AML induction therapy. Leuk Lymphoma 47: 877–883
23. Razis E, Arlin ZA, Ahmed T, et al (1994) Incidence and treatment of tumor lysis syndrome in patients with acute leukemia. Acta Haematol 91: 171–174

24. Hussain K, Mazza JJ, Clouse LH (2003) Tumor lysis syndrome (TLS) following fludarabine therapy for chronic lymphocytic leukemia (CLL): case report and review of the literature. Am J Hematol 72: 212–215
25. Fassas AB, Desikan KR, Siegel D, et al (1999) Tumour lysis syndrome complicating high-dose treatment in patients with multiple myeloma. Br J Haematol 105: 938–941
26. Terpos E, Politou M, Rahemtulla A (2004) Tumour lysis syndrome in multiple myeloma after bortezomib (VELCADE) administration. J Cancer Res Clin Oncol 130: 623–625
27. Yang H, Rosove MH, Figlin RA (1999) Tumor lysis syndrome occurring after the administration of rituximab in lymphoproliferative disorders: high-grade non-Hodgkin's lymphoma and chronic lymphocytic leukemia. Am J Hematol 62: 247–250
28. Cany L, Fitoussi O, Boiron JM, et al (2002) Tumor lysis syndrome at the beginning of thalidomide therapy for multiple myeloma. J Clin Oncol 20:2212
29. Lee CC, Wu YH, Chung SH, et al (2006) Acute tumor lysis syndrome after thalidomide therapy in advanced hepatocellular carcinoma. Oncologist 11: 87–88
30. Cech P, Block JB, Cone LA, et al (1986) Tumor lysis syndrome after tamoxifen flare. N Engl J Med 315: 263–264
31. Stoves J, Richardson D, Patel H (2001) Tumour lysis syndrome in a patient with metastatic melanoma treated with biochemotherapy. Nephrol Dial Transplant 16: 188–189
32. Humphreys BD, Soiffer RJ, Magee CC (2005) Renal failure associated with cancer and its treatment: an update. J Am Soc Nephrol 16: 151–161
33. Mehta RL, Pascual MT, Soroko S, et al (2002) Diuretics, mortality, and nonrecovery of renal function in acute renal failure. JAMA 288: 2547–2553
34. Coiffier B, Mounier N, Bologna S, et al (2003) Efficacy and safety of rasburicase (recombinant urate oxidase) for the prevention and treatment of hyperuricemia during induction chemotherapy of aggressive non-Hodgkin's lymphoma: results of the GRAAL1 (Groupe d'Etude des Lymphomes de l'Adulte Trial on Rasburicase Activity in Adult Lymphoma) study. J Clin Oncol 21: 4402–4406
35. Baeksgaard L, Sorensen JB (2003) Acute tumor lysis syndrome in solid tumors--a case report and review of the literature. Cancer Chemother Pharmacol 51: 187–192
36. Haas M, Ohler L, Watzke H, et al (1999) The spectrum of acute renal failure in tumour lysis syndrome. Nephrol Dial Transplant 14: 776–779
37. Goldman SC (2003) Rasburicase: potential role in managing tumor lysis in patients with hematological malignancies. Expert Rev Anticancer Ther 3: 429–433
38. Patte C, Sakiroglu C, Ansoborlo S, et al (2002) Urate-oxidase in the prevention and treatment of metabolic complications in patients with B-cell lymphoma and leukemia, treated in the Societe Francaise d'Oncologie Pediatrique LMB89 protocol. Ann Oncol 13: 789–795
39. Annemans L, Moeremans K, Lamotte M, et al (2003) Pan-European multicentre economic evaluation of recombinant urate oxidase (rasburicase) in prevention and treatment of hyperuricaemia and tumour lysis syndrome in haematological cancer patients. Support Care Cancer 11: 249–257
40. Browning LA, Kruse JA (2005) Hemolysis and methemoglobinemia secondary to rasburicase administration. Ann Pharmacother 39: 1932–1935

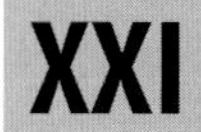

Life-threatening Neurological Complications in Patients with Malignancies

S. Legriel and E. Azoulay

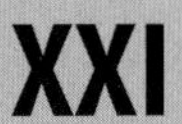

Introduction

A growing number of patients with malignancies experience infectious and toxic complications related to their disease or to its treatment. The population of patients likely to require medical attention for malignant disease is expanding for three reasons: 1) The incidence of cancer is rising [1, 2], survival of patients with malignancies is improving as a result of new treatments and management strategies [2], and 3) life expectancy has increased in older individuals, patients infected with human immunodeficiency virus (HIV), and patients treated with anticancer medications or immunosuppressants [3, 4].

Acute respiratory, cardiovascular, and renal events in patients with malignancies have been the focus of many epidemiological, diagnostic, and outcome studies [5–11]. Neurological failure, in contrast, although present in 10 % to 20 % of cancer patients admitted to the intensive care unit (ICU), has received little attention. Outside the critical care setting, a few descriptive studies have provided information on the features of, and reasons for, neurological events [12–15], but little is known about patient outcomes [16].

The objective of this chapter is to provide clinicians with guidance for managing cancer patients with acute neurological disorders. We describe an empirical classification system based on the relationship of the neurological disease with the malignancy (direct or indirect) and on its causes. A management algorithm is suggested.

Direct Involvement of the Nervous System by the Malignancy

Infiltration of the Brain Parenchyma

Primary parenchymatous brain tumors constitute a heterogeneous group of lesions composed chiefly of solid tumors. Their classification has been recently updated in the fourth edition of the World Health Organization (WHO) Classification of Tumors of the Central Nervous System [17]. The clinical manifestations of these tumors vary, in particular with the site of the tumor. The presenting symptom may be a seizure, which is often focal. Headaches are reported by more than 50 % of patients. Behavioral disorders or hemicorporal motor deficits are present in 5 to 50 % of patients [18]. In nearly 3 % of patients, the presenting picture suggests a cerebrovascular accident [19]. Cerebral computed tomography (CT) with or without contrast injection or, preferably, magnetic resonance imaging (MRI) with gadolinium injection may suggest the diagnosis, which must be confirmed histologically. Stereotactic biopsy may fail to consistently provide the diagnosis. Primary surgical excision may deserve consideration in patients with suspected solid primary malignancies of the central nervous system (CNS) [20].

Hematological malignancies may cause primary lesions of the brain parenchyma. Nearly 25 % of patients with non-Hodgkin's lymphoma have brain involvement, with diffuse large B cell lymphomas accounting for most of these cases [21]. Multifocal lesions are the rule, with preferential involvement of the periventricular region. Cognitive dysfunction and behavioral disorders are the most common presenting symptoms. Hemiparesis, aphasia, and visual disorders are often present also. The onset may be insidious, and routinely testing for chin numbness (which suggests skull base infiltration at the trigeminal nerve exit) may help to make the diagnosis. Seizures occur in 15 % of patients [18]. MRI may visualize suggestive lesions. In 25 % of patients, the lumbar puncture shows lymphoma cells. Stereotactic biopsy is often necessary and provides the definitive diagnosis [18]. Leptomeningeal or cerebral infiltration by a known lymphoma may be suspected on clinical grounds when the manifestations are typical. In contrast, cerebral biopsy is indispensable in patients with primary lymphoma of the brain.

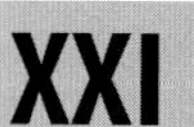

Cerebral and Epidural Metastases

Metastases to the central nervous system occur in 20 to 25 % of patients with cancer [22]. In an autopsy study, brain metastases were found in 572 of 3219 patients who died with cancer [23]. Although no cancer type was exempt, brain metastases were chiefly associated with lung cancer, breast cancer, and melanoma but were rare in other types such as prostate cancer [23]. Common presenting symptoms include cognitive dysfunction (34 %) and/or incapacitating headaches (31 %). Typical headaches that start in the morning and fade as the day wears on are rare. Seizures occur at presentation in 19 % of cases and indicate a poor prognosis [22]. The diagnosis rests on brain imaging studies -- chiefly MRI with gadolinium injection -- and on the response to chemotherapy [22]. Importantly, a suspicious brain mass is ten times more likely to be a metastasis than a primary cerebral tumor. The primary is unknown in 5 to 10 % of patients diagnosed with brain metastases. In this situation, investigations are needed to confirm the malignant nature of the lesion and to identify the primary. CT of the chest and abdomen should be performed. When no tumor is found, a mammogram and/or colonoscopy may be in order, depending on the circumstances. Positron emission tomography (PET) shows the primary in about 45 % of patients [25] but is of limited availability. When the primary is not found and there are no metastases elsewhere, a stereotactic or open biopsy should be performed unless this procedure is expected to be life-threatening [26]. The presence of brain metastases is of adverse prognostic significance. The outcome depends chiefly on treatment intensity: median survival is 1 month without treatment, 2 to 3 months with corticosteroid therapy and anticonvulsants, 4 to 6 months with radiation therapy alone, and 6 to 12 months with surgery, which also provides the definitive diagnosis [27].

Epidural metastases may develop, causing spinal cord compression. The most common causes of epidural spread are solid tumors, including lung cancer (26 %), prostate cancer (19 %), breast cancer (13 %), genitourinary cancer (11 %), gastrointestinal cancer (6 %), and melanoma (6 %). Only 10 % of cases are related to myeloma and 5 % to lymphoma. Several months usually elapse between symptom onset and MRI visualization of a mass putting pressure on the spinal cord [8]. A lumbar puncture should be performed, as concomitant meningeal involvement is common.

Complete suprajacent spinal cord compression should be ruled out before the procedure [13, 15].

Carcinomatous Meningitis

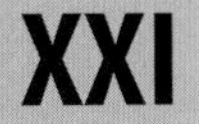

Carcinomatous meningitis occurs in 5 to 8 % of all patients with malignant disease [29]. Fewer than 10 % of cases of carcinomatous meningitis are diagnosed in patients who have no known history of cancer [30]. The rate of carcinomatous meningitis is 6 % in small-cell lung cancer, 3 % in breast cancer, 1.5 % in melanoma, 1 % in non-small-cell lung cancer, and 3 % in malignant disease with an unknown primary. Carcinomatous meningitis affects 1 % to 10 % of patients with primary solid malignancies of the CNS. A number of hematological malignancies may involve the meninges. Thus, carcinomatous meningitis occurs in 5 to 15 % of patients with non-Hodgkin's lymphoma (Burkitt lymphoma or lymphoblastic lymphoma). Meningeal involvement is noted at the diagnosis of acute lymphoblastic leukemia in 6 % of patients [31]. Meningitis is a feature in only 1 % of patients with myeloma [32].

The clinical manifestations of carcinomatous meningitis vary, their main determinant being the site of involvement. Headache is present in 66 % of patients, behavioral disorders in 45 %, ataxia in 50 %, cranial nerve involvement in 75 %, and spinal cord involvement in 60 %. A meningeal syndrome is found in only 21 % of patients [29]. The diagnosis relies on examination of the cerebrospinal fluid (CSF). The typical pattern includes high pressure (> 200 mmHg), high protein (> 0.5 g/dl), low glucose (< 0.6 g/dl), and numerous malignant cells [31]. None of these findings is consistently present, however, and the first lumbar puncture provides the diagnosis in only 50 % of patients with carcinomatous meningitis. The second lumbar puncture is diagnostic in an additional 25 % of patients. Subsequent lumbar punctures, in contrast, supply the diagnosis in only 2 % of additional patients [31]. Isolated protein elevation strongly suggests the diagnosis and requires a repeat lumbar puncture, particularly if the patient has a known history of cancer. Collecting at least 10 ml of CSF increases the likelihood of establishing the diagnosis.

Brain imaging studies provide valuable diagnostic orientation. MRI is 70 % sensitive, compared to only 30 % for CT, and should visualize the entire CNS including the spinal cord [29, 33]. Gadolinium injection is typically followed by signal enhancement in the leptomeningeal spaces [31].

Rarely, a meningeal biopsy must be performed to establish the diagnosis. However, both sensitivity and specificity are low. Meningeal biopsy is appropriate only when the imaging study findings are highly suggestive, CSF examination fails to establish the diagnosis, and potentially life-extending treatment is available should the diagnosis of carcinomatous meningitis be confirmed [33].

Tumors of the Peripheral Nervous System

Primary tumors of the peripheral nervous system are rare. Direct peripheral involvement with malignancies is usually due to infiltration by local or metastatic tumor spread, chiefly from carcinomas and non-Hodgkin lymphomas [34]. When a plexus is involved, the site of the involvement suggests the site of the underlying malignancy: Solid tumors of the head and neck and malignant lymphomas may lead to involvement of the cervical plexus; lung and breast cancer and malignant lymphoma to involvement of the brachial plexus; and solid tumors of the prostate, female reproductive organs, colon, and rectum, as well as malignant lymphoma, to involvement of the lumbosacral plexus. Monoradicular involvement suggests a schwannoma (or neurilemoma) associated with neurofibromatosis or a metastasis from a solid tumor or malignant lymphoma. Finally, polyneuropathy should suggest primary neurolymphomatosis [35]. The definitive diagnosis depends on obtaining a nerve biopsy [35].

Indirect Involvement of the Nervous System by the Malignancy

Autologous and Allogeneic Bone Marrow Transplant Recipients

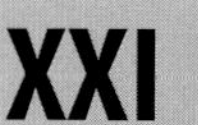

Recipients of autologous and, even more so, allogeneic bone marrow transplants are at high risk for indirect neurological involvement. In a recent retrospective study, 57 (16 %) of 361 patients had neurological complications, in the following categories: Infections (4 % of the total population), metabolic encephalopathy (3 %), tumor recurrence (4 %), cerebrovascular events (2 %), and peripheral nerve involvement (3 %). The inhospital mortality rate was 32 % among patients with neurological complications. Four-year survival was significantly lower in patients with than without neurological complications (12 vs 58 %) [16].

Infections

The diagnostic strategy in cancer patients with suspected CNS infection is complex and differs in many ways from the approach to immunocompetent patients [36]. The diversity of the underlying immune dysfunctions translates into a broad spectrum of causes (**Table 1**). The presenting symptoms are often limited, as immune deficiencies lead to impairments in the local inflammatory response (**Table 1**). In a recent retrospective study [37], the typical triad of fever, nuchal rigidity, and altered mental status was found in only 5 % of patients with cancer and positive CSF cultures, compared to 44 % in the general population [38]. Many microorganisms may be involved (**Table 2**), with the most common being *Listeria monocytogenes, Nocardia*

Table 1. Diagnostic orientation in patients with central nervous system infection, based on the type of immune deficiency

	Defective phagocytosis (granulocytes)	Defective humoral immunity (B cells – immunoglobulins)	Defective cell-mediated immunity (T cells – macrophages)	Blood-brain barrier damage
Hematological diagnosis	Acute leukemia Lymphoma Solid tumor Chemotherapy Radiation therapy Allogeneic or autologous bone marrow transplant	Chronic lymphoid leukemia Multiple myeloma Allogeneic bone marrow transplant Splenectomy	Hodgkin's disease Long-term steroid therapy Immunosuppressants Allogeneic bone marrow transplantation	Neurosurgery Internal or external ventricular shunt
Causative organisms	Bacteria Yeasts Viruses	Bacteria Viruses	Bacteria Yeasts Viruses Parasites	Bacteria Yeasts

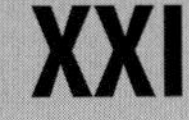

Table 2. Microorganisms often found in cancer patients with central nervous system infection

Bacteria	**Yeasts**
Gram-positive cocci	*Cryptococcus neoformans*
Coagulase-negative *Staphylococcus*	*Candida albicans*
Staphylococcus aureus	*Aspergillus fumigatus*
Streptococcus pneumoniae	Mucormycoses
	Histoplasma capsulatum
Gram-positive rods	*Pseudallescheria boydii*
Listeria monocytogenes	
Corynebacterium spp	**Viruses**
Propionibacterium spp	Cytomegalovirus
Nocardia asteroides	Herpes simplex virus
Gram-negative rods	Other human herpes viruses
Enterobacteria	Varicella-zona virus
Escherichia coli	Adenovirus
Klebsiella pneumoniae	Epstein-Barr virus
Serratia marcescens	JC virus
Proteus mirabilis	Enterovirus
Pseudomonas aeruginosa and related organisms	Measles or Paramyxoviridae virus
Acinetobacter baumanii	
Haemophilus influenzae	**Parasites**
Mycobacteria	*Toxoplasma gondii*
Mycobacterium tuberculosis	*Strongyloides stercoralis*

asteroides, Aspergillus fumigatus, Mucoraceae, *Candida* spp., *Cryptococcus neoformans*, JC virus, and *Toxoplasma gondii* [39]. Therefore, a rational diagnostic approach based on the type of the immune deficiency (**Table 1**), course, and type of syndrome (**Table 3**) is crucial to ensure early initiation of probabilistic antiinfectious drugs [40].

In addition, a vast array of microbiological tests selected according to the suspected causative pathogens should be performed. The CSF should be analyzed in detail (pressure, glucose, protein, cell counts, smear, standard bacteriological cultures, cultures for slow-growing microorganisms, India ink, mycological cultures, *Cryptococcus* antigens, viral polymerase chain reaction (PCR) and cultures, acid-fast bacilli test, and PCR and cultures for the tubercle bacillus). Blood specimens are usually taken for further tests to identify the suspected microorganisms (blood cultures, *Aspergillus* antigen, *Cryptococcus* antigen, viral PCR and cultures, HIV serology, and p24 antigen). Other investigations may include tests for slow-growing organisms in respiratory tract specimens, sputum tests for the tubercle bacillus, urinary cytology and cultures, and *Legionella* antigenuria [40]. Imaging studies of the brain often contribute to the diagnosis. Cerebral CT with contrast injection should be performed routinely, if possible together with cerebral MRI [41]. When the diagnosis remains in doubt, a brain biopsy should be performed promptly, most notably when an abscess is suspected [41].

Cerebrovascular Disease

Cerebrovascular disease is common in cancer patients and can affect any level of the CNS [42]. In an autopsy study published in 1985, 500 (14.6 %) of 3424 cancer patients had cerebrovascular disease. Ischemia and hemorrhage each contributed

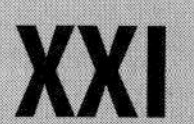

Table 3. Diagnostic orientation in patients with central nervous system infection, based on the clinical features

	Focal deficit	Meningitis	Meningoencephalitis	Rhombencephalitis
Bacteria	*S. aureus* *Listeria monocytogenes* *Nocardia asteroides* Gram-negative rods *Streptococcus pneumoniae* Enterobacter	*Listeria monocytogenes* *Haemophilus influenzae* *Streptococcus pneumoniae* Gram-negative rods	*Listeria monocytogenes* *Legionella pneumophila* Gram-negative rods	*Mycobacterium tuberculosis* *Listeria monocytogenes*
Yeasts	*Aspergillus fumigatus* *Cryptococcus neoformans* Mucoraceae Candida spp.	*Cryptococcus neoformans* Candida spp. *Coccidioides immitis* *Histoplasma capsulatum*	*Aspergillus fumigatus* *Cryptococcus neoformans* Mucoraceae	*Aspergillus fumigatus* *Cryptococcus neoformans* Mucoraceae
Viruses	JC virus Varicella-zona virus Papovavirus	Herpes simplex viruses 1 and 2 Other herpes viruses Cytomegalovirus Varicella-zona virus Epstein-Barr virus	Herpes simplex viruses 1 and 2 Other herpes viruses Cytomegalovirus Varicella-zona virus Coxsackie virus Papovavirus Epstein-Barr virus	Cytomegalovirus
Parasites	*Toxoplasma gondii*	*Toxoplasma gondii* *Strongyloides stercoralis*	*Toxoplasma gondii* *Strongyloides stercoralis*	

about half the cases. Only half the patients had clinical symptoms suggesting cerebrovascular disease [43]. The risk of cerebrovascular disease may be particularly high in some cancer types, such as lung cancer (30 % of patients with cancer and stroke [44]); other cancers were found in 6 to 9 % of patients: Primary CNS tumors, prostate cancer, breast cancer, lymphoma, leukemia, cancer of the female reproductive tract, urinary bladder cancer, and gastroesophageal cancer [44].

The many causes of cerebrovascular disease in cancer patients fall into four main categories: Coagulopathies, iatrogenic events, infections, and the underlying malignancy. Few data are available on the incidences of these complications in the overall population of cancer patients. A retrospective study of 125 autologous or allogeneic bone marrow transplant recipients found that 36 patients (2.9 %) experienced stroke [45]. Intracranial bleeding related to thrombocytopenia accounted for 38.9 % of cases and ischemia or bleeding due to fungal infections for 30.6 % of cases. The stroke was fatal in 69.4 % of patients [45].

Coagulation disorders occur in many malignant diseases and can cause ischemia or bleeding. Disseminated intravascular coagulation (DIC) is associated with acute promyelocytic leukemia or breast cancer. At the stage of terminal disease, however, DIC may occur in patients with any form of cancer. Bleeding may occur in the CNS parenchyma and/or meninges. Arterial occlusion may lead to brain infarction.

Acute leukemia is often responsible for thrombocytopenia, which is frequently severe, even in the absence of ongoing chemotherapy. Thrombocytopenia may cause bleeding in the CNS parenchyma or meninges. Myeloma and Waldenström's macroglobulinemia are associated with increased blood viscosity, which can cause ischemic events. Finally, all forms of cancer increase the risk not only of deep vein thrombosis, but also of cerebral thrombophlebitis originating in venous thrombosis of the sagittal sinus or of a cortical vein. This complication is most common in patients with leukemia, lymphoma, or solid tumors.

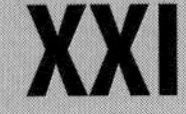

Chemotherapy is often associated with bleeding. Various pathophysiological mechanisms may be involved. Nitrosourea compounds may induce thrombocytopenia after 4 to 6 weeks. Gemcitabine and mitomycin may cause thrombotic microangiopathy. L-asparaginase is associated with clotting disorders (decreased prothrombin time, increased thromboplastin time, and decreases in fibrinogen, antithrombin III, and plasminogen). Finally, nitrosoureas, anthracyclines, and busulfan induce bone marrow hypoplasia, which is most marked after 6 to 15 days. L-asparaginase, cisplatin, and hormone therapy can cause ischemic events.

The following anticancer medications have been reported to be associated with ischemic or hemorrhagic stroke: L-asparaginase, bleomycin, carboplatin, cisplatin, doxorubicin, erythropoietin, estramustine, gemtuzumab, imatinib, methotrexate, tamoxifen, and toremifene [12]. Radiation therapy can lead to ischemic stroke due to stenosis of the carotid artery (see below). Intracerebral hematoma may develop after surgery. Furthermore, all cerebral infections, most notably those caused by fungi, can cause septic embolism, vasculitis, and aneurysms, which in turn may lead to ischemia or bleeding.

Primary or secondary cerebral involvement by solid tumors or hematological malignancies can cause cerebrovascular lesions. Compression and/or infiltration of the sagittal sinus occur chiefly in patients with lung cancer, breast cancer, neuroblastoma, or lymphoma. Leptomeningeal metastases from gliomas or solid tumors may cause arterial thrombosis responsible for cerebral infarction. Another cause of cerebral infarction is compression by a parasellar meningioma. Lung cancer and cardiac tumors may cause embolism with ischemic stroke.

Intraparenchymatous bleeding can be caused by primary gliomas or by metastases from melanoma, choriocarcinoma, or skin carcinoma. A metastasis within the brain parenchyma may result in an aneurysmal lesion, which may rupture; this complication has been reported in patients with bronchial carcinoma or choriocarcinoma. Tumor spread to the bone or dura mater may lead to subdural or epidural bleeding, most notably in patients with skin carcinoma, leukemia, lymphoma, or hepatocellular carcinoma.

Neurological Paraneoplastic Syndromes

Paraneoplastic syndromes involving the nervous system are defined as neurological manifestations that occur at a distance from a malignancy and have no relation to the primary, metastases, or other complications such as infections or vascular damage [46]. Recent advances have shed light on the underlying pathophysiological mechanisms. Neurological paraneoplastic syndromes are caused by antibodies to a tumor antigen that share similarities with antigens expressed by the central or peripheral nervous system [47].

The CNS can be affected indirectly by paraneoplastic syndromes. Examples include Cushing's syndrome and paraneoplastic hypercalcemia with encephalopathy [48]. These types of syndromes are not discussed here. Neurological paraneoplastic syndromes constitute a highly complex set of conditions that can affect the entire nervous system [47–50]. Rather than listing their many causes, a syndromic

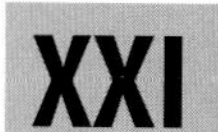

Table 4. Diagnostic orientation in patients with suspected paraneoplastic syndromes involving the central nervous system

Site involved	Clinical features	Antibodies incriminated in the manifestations		
Cerebral hemispheres	Limbic encephalitis	Anti-Hu (ANNA-1) Anti-Ma2 (Ta) Anti-amphiphysin	Anti-CRMP3–4 Anti-GluRε2 Anti-CV2 (CRMP5) Anti-NR1/NR2 of NMDA receptors	ANNA-3 Anti-GAD Anti-VGKC
	Opsoclonus myoclonus syndrome	Anti-Ri (ANNA-2) Anti-Zic2	Anti-genomic APC (Adenomatous Polyposis Coli)	
Cerebellum	Cerebellar degeneration	Anti-Hu (ANNA-1) Anti-Yo (PCA-1) Anti-Ri (ANNA-2) Anti-CV2 (CRMP5) Anti-Ma2 (Ta)	Anti-Tr Anti-Zic 4 mGluR1 Anti-VGCC Anti-CARP VIII	Anti-Zic1, Zic4 Anti-PKCγ Anti-proteasome ANNA-3
	Cerebellar ataxia	Anti-GAD		
Brainstem	Brainstem encephalitis	Anti-Hu (ANNA-1)	Anti-Ri (ANNA-2)	Anti-Ma2 (Ta)
Spinal cord	Myelitis	Anti-Hu (ANNA-1)	Anti-amphiphysin	
	Motor neuron disease	Unknown		
	Necrotizing myelopathy	Unknown		
	Stiff-person syndrome	Anti-amphiphysin	Anti-GAD	
Cerebral hemi-spheres/cerebellum/brainstem/spinal cord	Encephalomyelitis	Anti-Hu (ANNA-1) Anti-CV2 (CRMP5)	Anti-amphiphysin	Anti-Ma2 (Ta)
Retina	Optic neuritis	Anti-CV2 (CRMP5)		
	Retinopathy	Anti-Recoverin		
	Uveitis	Anti-CV2 (CRMP5)		
Peripheral nerves	Sensory neuropathy	Anti-Hu (ANNA-1)	Anti-amphiphysin	Anti-CV2 (CRMP5)
	Chronic intestinal pseudoobstruction	Anti-Hu (ANNA-1)	Anti-CV2 (CRMP5)	
	Sensory motor neuropathy	Anti-CV2 (CRMP5)		
	Dysautonomia	Anti-Hu (ANNA-1)	Anti-nAChR	
Neuromuscular junction	Myasthenia	Anti-AChR		
	Lambert-Eaton myasthenic syndrome	Anti-VGCC		
	Acquired neuromyopathy	Anti-VGKC		
Muscle	Dermatopolymyositis	Anti-Mi2		
	Acute necrotizing myopathy	Unknown		
	Chorea	Anti-CV2 (CRMP5)		

approach is more relevant to everyday clinical practice. Antibody assays in blood and CSF specimens can be selected based on the clinical features (**Table 4**). However, antibody assays have low sensitivity (0.9 to 25 % depending on the study [47, 49], **Table 5**). Targeted investigations for the underlying malignancy consist of CT with

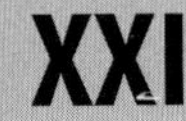

Table 5. Etiological orientation based on the type of antibody identified in patients with suspected paraneoplastic syndromes involving the central nervous system

Antibody	Malignancy	Specificity
Anti-Hu (ANNA-1)	Small-cell lung cancer Neuroblastoma Prostate cancer	high specificity
Anti-Yo (PCA-1)	Ovarian and uterine cancer Breast cancer Non-small-cell lung cancer	high specificity
Anti-Ri (ANNA-2)	Uterine cancer Breast cancer Small-cell lung cancer Cancer of the urinary bladder	high specificity
Anti-CV2 (CRMP5)	Small-cell lung cancer Thymoma	high specificity
Anti-Ma2 (Ta)	Germ-cell testicular tumors Non-small-cell lung cancer Other solid tumors	high specificity
Anti-amphiphysin	Small-cell lung cancer Breast cancer Leukemias Lymphomas	high specificity
Anti-Recoverin (Antiretinal)	Small-cell lung cancer Melanoma Ovarian and uterine cancer	high specificity
Anti-Zic 1, Anti-Zic 4	Small-cell lung cancer	low specificity
Anti-proteasome	Ovarian cancer	low specificity
Anti-Tr	Hodgkin's lymphoma	low specificity
Anti-mGluR1	Hodgkin's lymphoma	low specificity
ANNA-3	Small-cell lung cancer	low specificity
PCA2	Small-cell lung cancer	low specificity
Anti-NR1/NR2 of NMDA receptors	Ovarian teratoma	low specificity
Anti-VGKC	Thymoma Small-cell lung cancer	nonspecific
Anti-VGCC	Small-cell lung cancer	nonspecific
Anti-AChR	Thymoma	nonspecific
Anti-nAChR	Small-cell lung cancer	nonspecific
Anti-GAD	Thymoma	nonspecific
Anti-CARP VIII	Melanoma	nonspecific
Anti-PKCγ	Non-small-cell lung cancer	nonspecific
Anti-genomic APC (adenomatous polyposis coli)	Small-cell lung cancer	nonspecific
Anti-Zic2	Small-cell lung cancer	nonspecific
Anti-CRMP3 – 4	Thymoma	nonspecific
Anti-GluRε2	Ovarian teratoma	nonspecific

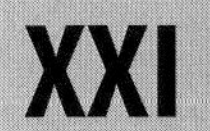

Table 6. Diagnostic criteria for paraneoplastic syndromes involving the central nervous system

Criteria for a definitive diagnosis of neurological paraneoplastic syndrome
• syndrome typically associated with a malignancy diagnosed within 5 years before the onset of the neurological manifestations
• syndrome not typically associated with the malignancy but complete resolution or substantial improvement with anticancer treatment, in the absence of immunomodulating treatment
• syndrome not typically associated with a malignancy diagnosed within 5 years before the onset of the neurological manifestations, but positive assays for antibodies typically associated with the syndrome
• typical or atypical syndrome, without known cancer, with highly specific anti-neuron antibodies (Anti-HU, Yo, Ri, CRMP5, Ma2, or amphiphysin)
Criteria for a possible diagnosis of neurological paraneoplastic syndrome
• typical syndrome and risk factors for malignant disease, without anti-neuron antibodies
• typical or atypical syndrome, without known cancer, with anti-neuron antibodies characterized by low specificity
• atypical syndrome and malignancy diagnosed within 2 years before the onset of the neurological manifestations, without anti-neuron antibodies

contrast injection combined, if needed, with PET. When no tumor is found, the investigations should be repeated every 4 to 6 months. However, some antibodies are nonspecific, so that tests for a malignancy may remain negative [51]. Criteria have been suggested to assist in the diagnosis of paraneoplastic syndromes (**Table 6**) [49].

Iatrogenic Events

Adverse neurological effects of chemotherapy are common. The broad diversity of their clinical manifestations reflects the multiplicity of sites vulnerable to neurotoxicity. Patients may present with a variable combination of coma, acute encephalopathy, mood and behavioral disturbances, headaches, seizures, dementia-like episodes, visual disorders, cortical blindness, myelopathy, extrapyramidal syndrome, cerebellar syndrome, meningeal syndrome, and peripheral neuropathy.

Peripheral neuropathies are the most common chemotherapy-induced neurological events. They may be related to either direct axonal damage or demyelination. Sensory, motor, and autonomic fibers may be involved. Risk factors include alcohol abuse, diabetes, liver function disturbances, and a history of treatment with neurotoxic anticancer agents [52]. Central involvement is less common, perhaps because many anticancer agents are high-molecular-weight molecules that cannot cross the blood-brain barrier. The dosages and administration modalities explain the toxicity mechanisms. For instance, intrathecal or intracerebral administration leads to aseptic meningitis in 10 to 50 % of patients, with a febrile meningeal reaction in 60 % of patients that resolves within 72 hours [14]. Posterior reversible encephalopathy syndrome, another common neurotoxic event, is characterized by the sudden onset of neurological manifestations (confusion, seizure or status epilepticus [53], headaches, visual disorders, nausea, and vomiting) with imaging study abnormalities that are best visualized by MRI [54]. MRI typically shows bilateral symmetric signal abnormalities from the posterior parieto-occipital white matter [55]. Cortical areas are involved occasionally. The frontal or temporal lobes or the posterior fossa are less often affected. T2-weighted and FLAIR sequences show high signal intensity, whereas diffusion sequences are normal. The apparent diffusion coefficient is high when the lesions are reversible and low when they are infracted [55]. Many cytotoxic agents have been incriminated in the occurrence of posterior reversible encephalopathy syndrome [56] (**Table 7** lists the central and peripheral neurological events reported with widely used anticancer agents [12, 14]).

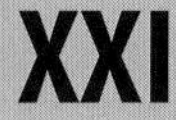

Table 7. Neurotoxicity of anticancer medications

Class	Agent	Adverse neurological effects
Alkylating agents	Cisplatin	Peripheral neuropathy, dysautonomic neuropathy, Lhermitte's sign, encephalopathy, optic neuritis, cortical blindness, PRES, headaches, myelopathy
	Carboplatin	Peripheral neuropathy, optic neuritis, PRES, encephalopathy, seizures, cortical blindness
	Oxaliplatin	Peripheral neuropathy, visual field alterations, PRES
	Ifosphamide	Encephalopathy, seizures, coma, peripheral neuropathy, extrapyramidal syndrome, cerebellar syndrome
	Cytarabine	Cerebellar syndrome, seizures, encephalopathy, peripheral neuropathy, dementia, aseptic meningitis
	Carmustine	Encephalopathy
	Busulfan	Seizures
	Chlorambucil	Seizures, encephalopathy
	Cyclophosphamide	Encephalopathy, visual disorders, seizures
	Temozolomide	Headaches
	Thiotepa	Aseptic meningitis, myelopathy, encephalopathy
Antimetabolites	Methotrexate	Aseptic meningitis, encephalopathy, myelopathy after intrathecal injection, seizures, dementia, PRES, headaches, cortical blindness
	5 Fluorouracil	Cerebellar syndrome, encephalopathy, seizures, extrapyramidal syndrome
	Capecitabine	Confusion
	Hydroxyurea	Headaches, encephalopathy, seizures
	Cladribine	Confusion, headaches, peripheral neuropathy, tetraparesis
	Fludarabine	Headaches, confusion, paresthesia, dementia , cortical blindness, seizures, coma, encephalopathy
	Gemcitabine	Somnolence, paresthesia, PRES
	Cytarabine	Encephalopathy, myelopathy, seizures, headaches, cerebellar syndrome
Topo-isomerase inhibitors	Topotecan	Headaches, paresthesia
	Irinotecan hydrochloride	Encephalopathy, PRES
	Etoposide	Sensory-motor axonal neuropathy, guillain-barre syndrome, encephalopathy, headaches, seizures
Plant alkaloids	Paclitaxel	Peripheral neuropathy, encephalopathy
	Docetaxel	Peripheral neuropathy, myelopathy, Lhermitte's sign
	Vincristine	Peripheral neuropathy, dysautonomic neuropathy, ataxia, headaches, Seizures, cortical blindness, PRES, extrapyramidal syndrome
	Vinblastine	Peripheral neuropathy, ataxia, diplopia
	L asparaginase	Encephalopathy, seizures, headaches
	Thalidomide	Drowsiness, peripheral neuropathy, headaches, tremor, encephalopathy, seizures, cerebellar syndrome
	Corticosteroids	Tremor, visual disorders
	Tamoxifen	

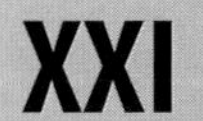

Table 7. (*cont.*)

Class	Agent	Adverse neurological effects
DNA polymerase inhibitor	Suramin	Sensory-motor axonal neuropathy, Guillain-Barré syndrome, encephalopathy, headaches
Monoclonal anti-CD20 Ab	Rituximab	Headaches, paresthesia, PRES
Monoclonal anti-ErbB2 Ab	Trastuzumab	Headaches, paresthesia
Monoclonal anti-CD33 Ab	Gentuzumab	Headaches
Tyrosine kinase inhibitor	Imatinib	Headaches, confusion
Immunomodulating cytokines	Interferon-alfa	Encephalopathy, PRES, headaches, seizures, dementia, myelopathy, extrapyramidal syndrome
	Interleukin-2	Encephalopathy, PRES, headaches, seizures, dementia, cortical blindness, cerebellar syndrome
Anti-angiogenic agents	Bevacizumab	Encephalopathy, PRES,
	Sunitinib	Encephalopathy, PRES,
	RAF kinase inhibitor BAY 43–9006	Encephalopathy, PRES,
Intravenous immunoglobulins		Encephalopathy, PRES,
Anti-lymphocyte globulins		Encephalopathy, PRES,
Immuno-suppressants	Cyclosporine A	Encephalopathy, PRES,
	Tacrolimus (FK 506)	Encephalopathy, PRES,
	Sirolomus	Encephalopathy, PRES,
	High-dose corticosteroids	Encephalopathy, PRES, headaches, myelopathy,
Hematopoietic growth factors		Encephalopathy, PRES, seizures, Cortical blindness
Antitumor antibiotics	Mitomycin C	Encephalopathy
	Doxorubicin	Encephalopathy, myelopathy, aseptic meningitis
Erythropoietin		Seizures, PRES, cortical blindness

PRES: Posterior reversible encephalopathy syndrome

Radiation therapy plays a major role in the management of malignant disease. Radiation exposure is associated with specific and potentially life-threatening lesions of the brain. Damage to the spinal cord and peripheral nerves may occur also. Radiation-induced brain damage moves through three main phases [57, 58]. The acute phase, which lasts a few weeks after radiation exposure, is characterized by acute reversible manifestations ascribed to exacerbation of cerebral edema (e.g., headaches, nausea, vomiting, drowsiness, and exacerbation of preexisting neurological symptoms). At the subacute phase, which extends roughly from the second to the sixth postradiation month, encephalopathy develops, seemingly as a result of diffuse demyelination. The manifestations may include headaches, drowsiness, fatigability, and exacerbation of preexisting deficits. Finally, the late phase, which starts 6

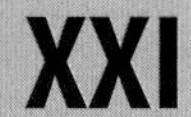

months after radiation exposure, is characterized by variable clinical manifestations usually related to demyelination and/or to vascular damage that may be so severe as to cause brain tissue necrosis. The symptoms depend on the site of the lesions. Focal necrosis usually leads to symptoms of intracranial hypertension or to seizures. White-matter involvement manifests as memory loss and dementia, which may be severe. Leukoencephalopathy may cause ataxia, confusion, dysarthria, seizures and, at the worst, dementia of variable severity. Risk factors for these serious radiation-induced events are age older than 60 years and cerebral lymphoma. Hypertension, diabetes, and hyperlipidemia may be additional risk factors [57, 58]. Maximum doses of 50 Gy for total irradiation and 60 Gy for focal irradiation are associated with a 5-year risk of necrosis of less than 5 %, provided the dose per session is less than 2 Gy [58, 59]. Irradiation of the brain can cause vascular lesions such as intracranial arterial stenosis, thrombosis of the internal carotid artery, lacunar syndrome, rupture of the internal carotid artery, intracranial arterial aneurysms, cavernous angiomas, and cryptic vascular malformations [58].

The main differential diagnosis of radiation-induced brain damage is tumor progression. The diagnosis may prove extremely challenging. PET or magnetic resonance spectroscopy (MRS) may be helpful. Radiolabeled metabolic markers are taken up by tumor tissue but not by foci of radiation-induced necrosis. However, the definitive diagnosis rests on a stereotactic brain biopsy [58].

Spinal cord irradiation can cause motor neuropathy, usually in the lumbosacral region, with weakness, muscle wasting, loss of the deep tendon reflexes, and sphincter dysfunction. The lesions develop within 2 to 8 months after radiation exposure [60]. The brachial and lumbar plexuses are the main sites of peripheral radiation-induced damage, with symptoms occurring within 5 months to 5 years of exposure [60].

The psychotropic and analgesic medications usually administered to patients undergoing anticancer treatment are associated with many adverse events [60, 61]. In the absence of contraindications, the injection of antidotes such as naloxone or flumazenil can provide the diagnosis.

Metabolic Complications

Failure to recognize metabolic complications usually leads to exacerbation of the clinical manifestations, often with the emergence of highly suggestive neurological symptoms. In most cases, encephalopathy is combined with alterations in consciousness of variable severity, ranging from confusion to a coma. The main causes of metabolic neurological complications are hypoglycemia, hypercalcemia, hypo- and hypernatremia, hyperuremia related to acute renal failure, hyperammonemia, lactic acidosis, and adrenal insufficiency. The clinical features suggest the underlying metabolic disturbance. They are easy to recognize and should be looked for routinely in cancer patients with new neurological manifestations. Causes of metabolic disturbances include organ failure related to tumor progression, treatment toxicity (most notably with anticancer medications), and paraneoplastic syndromes [62].

Diagnostic Strategy in Cancer Patients with New Neurological Manifestations

The diagnostic strategy is fairly well standardized. After a careful history and thorough physical examination, investigations should be performed as appropriate, starting with the simplest and moving to the more sophisticated (**Fig. 1**). CT, electroencephalography (EEG), and a lumbar puncture are easy to perform. MRI should be obtained almost routinely, as the large amount of information provided is valuable in sifting through the long list of possible causes.

When the diagnosis remains in doubt despite these investigations, a stereotactic brain biopsy, meningeal biopsy, or nerve biopsy is required. Nevertheless, the diagnosis remains unknown in nearly 15 % of patients [16].

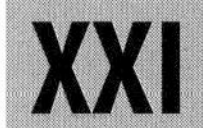

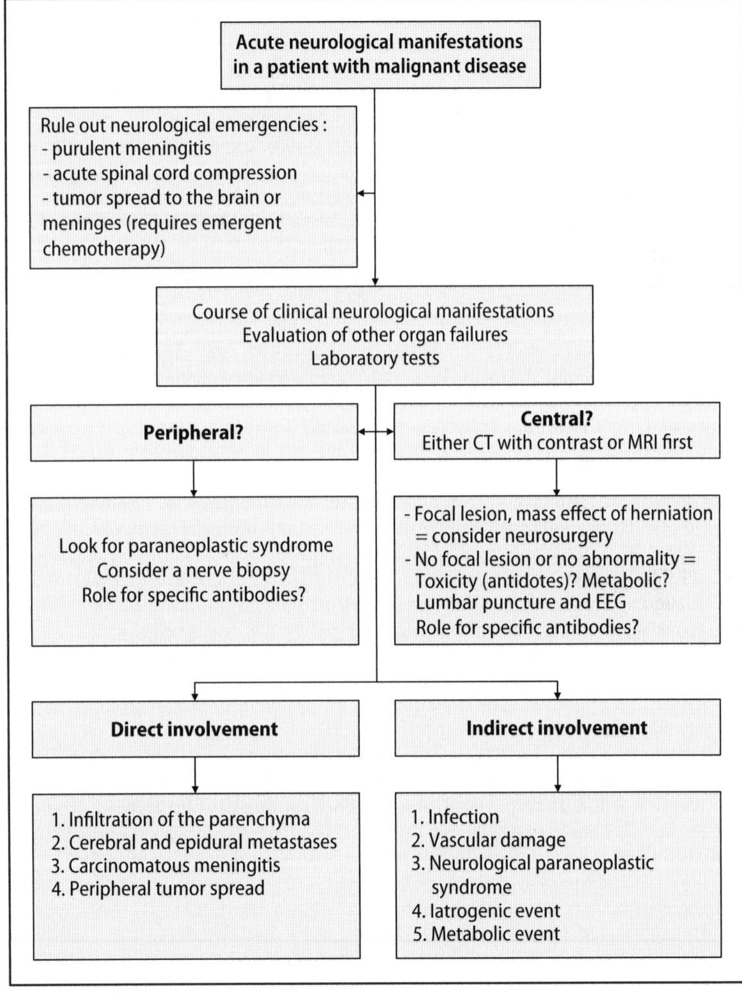

Fig. 1. Diagnostic strategy in cancer patients with acute neurological manifestations. CT: computed tomography; MRI: magnetic resonance imaging; EEG: electroencephalogram

Conclusion

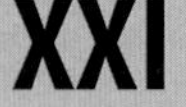

This chapter supplies objective data on acute neurological complications in patients with malignancies. An empirical classification is used to discuss data from the literature. Further studies are needed to accurately delineate the incidence of neurological complications, their causes, and the outcomes associated with each diagnosis. Their results should enable clinicians to identify those patients who are most likely to benefit from aggressive diagnostic and therapeutic management. Furthermore, neurosurgical biopsy is a major diagnostic tool. The current practice of reserving neurosurgical biopsy for patients whose diagnosis remains in doubt despite multiple investigations may deserve reappraisal should studies establish that failure to make the diagnosis adversely affects patient outcomes.

References

1. Ferlay J, Autier P, Boniol M, Heanue M, Colombet M, Boyle P (2007) Estimates of the cancer incidence and mortality in Europe in 2006. Ann Oncol 18: 581–592
2. Brenner H (2002) Long-term survival rates of cancer patients achieved by the end of the 20th century: a period analysis. Lancet 360: 1131–1135
3. Patel P, Hanson DL, Sullivan PS, et al (2008) Incidence of types of cancer among HIV-infected persons compared with the general population in the United States, 1992–2003. Ann Intern Med 148: 728–736
4. Yabroff KR, Lamont EB, Mariotto A, et al (2008) Cost of care for elderly cancer patients in the United States. J Natl Cancer Inst 100: 630–641
5. Azoulay E, Schlemmer B (2006) Diagnostic strategy in cancer patients with acute respiratory failure. Intensive Care Med 32: 808–822
6. Azoulay E, Thiery G, Chevret S, et al (2004) The prognosis of acute respiratory failure in critically ill cancer patients. Medicine (Baltimore) 83: 360–370
7. Larche J, Azoulay E, Fieux F, et al (2003) Improved survival of critically ill cancer patients with septic shock. Intensive Care Med 29: 1688–1695
8. Pene F, Percheron S, Lemiale V, et al (2008) Temporal changes in management and outcome of septic shock in patients with malignancies in the intensive care unit. Crit Care Med 36: 690–696
9. Darmon M, Thiery G, Ciroldi M, Porcher R, Schlemmer B, Azoulay E (2007) Should dialysis be offered to cancer patients with acute kidney injury? Intensive Care Med 33: 765–772
10. Soares M, Salluh JI, Carvalho MS, Darmon M, Rocco JR, Spector N (2006) Prognosis of critically ill patients with cancer and acute renal dysfunction. J Clin Oncol 24: 4003–4010
11. Darmon M, Ciroldi M, Thiery G, Schlemmer B, Azoulay E (2006) Clinical review: specific aspects of acute renal failure in cancer patients. Crit Care 10: 211
12. Plotkin SR, Wen PY (2003) Neurologic complications of cancer therapy. Neurol Clin 21: 279–318
13. Recht L, Mrugala M (2003) Neurologic complications of hematologic neoplasms. Neurol Clin 21: 87–105
14. Sul JK, Deangelis LM (2006) Neurologic complications of cancer chemotherapy. Semin Oncol 33: 324–332
15. Wen PY, Schiff D (2003) Neurologic complications of solid tumors. Neurol Clin 21: 107–140
16. Denier C, Bourhis JH, Lacroix C, et al (2006) Spectrum and prognosis of neurologic complications after hematopoietic transplantation. Neurology 67: 1990–1997
17. Louis DN, Ohgaki H, Wiestler OD, et al (2007) The 2007 WHO Classification of Tumours of the Central Nervous System. Acta Neuropathol (Berl) 114: 97–109
18. DeAngelis LM (2001) Brain tumors. N Engl J Med 344: 114–123
19. Morgenstern LB, Frankowski RF (1999) Brain tumor masquerading as stroke. J Neurooncol 44: 47–52
20. Metcalfe SE, Grant R (2001) Biopsy versus resection for malignant glioma. Cochrane Database Syst Rev CD002034

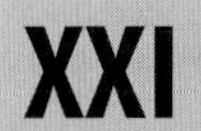

21. Bataille B, Delwail V, Menet E, et al (2000) Primary intracerebral malignant lymphoma: report of 248 cases. J Neurosurg 92: 261–266
22. Lassman AB, DeAngelis LM (2003) Brain metastases. Neurol Clin 21: 1–23
23. Posner JB, Chernik NL (1978) Intracranial metastases from systemic cancer. Adv Neurol 19: 579–592
24. Demir H, Berk F, Raderer M, et al (2004) The role of nuclear medicine in the diagnosis of cancer of unknown origin. Q J Nucl Med Mol Imaging 48: 164–173
25. Lassen U, Daugaard G, Eigtved A, Damgaard K, Friberg L (1999) 18F-FDG whole body positron emission tomography (PET) in patients with unknown primary tumours (UPT). Eur J Cancer 35: 1076–1082
26. Fédération Nationale Des Centres De Lutte Contre Le Cancer (2002) Standards, Options et Recommandations 2002 pour la prise en charge des patients atteints de carcinome de site prise en charge des patients atteints de carcinome de site primitif inconnu (rapport intégral). Available at: http://www.sor-cancer.fr/index.php?tg=fileman&idx=get&inl = 1&id = 2&gr=Y&path=Tumeurs+d+origine+inconnue%2Fcarcinome+de+site+primitif+inconnu&file=APC_DIV_CAPI_int.pdf Accessed Nov 2008
27. Andrews DW (2008) Current neurosurgical management of brain metastases. Semin Oncol 35: 100–107
28. Byrne TN, Borges LF, Loeffler JS (2006) Metastatic epidural spinal cord compression: update on management. Semin Oncol 33: 307–311
29. Pavlidis N (2004) The diagnostic and therapeutic management of leptomeningeal carcinomatosis. Ann Oncol 15 (Suppl 4): iv285–291
30. Chamberlain MC (2005) Neoplastic meningitis. J Clin Oncol 23: 3605–3613
31. Gleissner B, Chamberlain MC (2006) Neoplastic meningitis. Lancet Neurol 5: 443–452
32. Nieuwenhuizen L, Biesma DH (2008) Central nervous system myelomatosis: review of the literature. Eur J Haematol 80: 1–9
33. Jaeckle KA (2006) Neoplastic meningitis from systemic malignancies: diagnosis, prognosis and treatment. Semin Oncol 33: 312–323
34. Ramchandren S, Dalmau J (2005) Metastases to the peripheral nervous system. J Neurooncol 75: 101–110
35. Antoine JC, Camdessanche JP (2007) [Paraneoplastic neurological syndromes]. Presse Med 36: 1418–1426
36. Pruitt AA (2004) Central nervous system infections in cancer patients. Semin Neurol 24: 435–452
37. Safdieh JE, Mead PA, Sepkowitz KA, Kiehn TE, Abrey LE (2008) Bacterial and fungal meningitis in patients with cancer. Neurology 70: 943–947
38. van de Beek D, de Gans J, Spanjaard L, Weisfelt M, Reitsma JB, Vermeulen M (2004) Clinical features and prognostic factors in adults with bacterial meningitis. N Engl J Med 351: 1849–1859
39. Klastersky J, Aoun M (2004) Opportunistic infections in patients with cancer. Ann Oncol 15 (Suppl 4): iv329–335
40. Dougan C, Ormerod I (2004) A neurologist's approach to the immunosuppressed patient. J Neurol Neurosurg Psychiatry 75 (Suppl 1): i43–49
41. Segal BH, Freifeld AG, Baden LR, et al (2008) Prevention and treatment of cancer-related infections. J Natl Compr Canc Netw 6: 122–174
42. Rogers LR (2003) Cerebrovascular complications in cancer patients. Neurol Clin 21: 167–192
43. Graus F, Rogers LR, Posner JB (1985) Cerebrovascular complications in patients with cancer. Medicine (Baltimore) 64: 16–35
44. Cestari DM, Weine DM, Panageas KS, Segal AZ, DeAngelis LM (2004) Stroke in patients with cancer: incidence and etiology. Neurology 62: 2025–2030
45. Coplin WM, Cochran MS, Levine SR, Crawford SW (2001) Stroke after bone marrow transplantation: frequency, aetiology and outcome. Brain 124: 1043–1051
46. Darnell RB, Posner JB (2003) Paraneoplastic syndromes involving the nervous system. N Engl J Med 349: 1543–1554
47. Dalmau J, Rosenfeld MR (2008) Paraneoplastic syndromes of the CNS. Lancet Neurol 7: 327–340
48. Darnell RB, Posner JB (2006) Paraneoplastic syndromes affecting the nervous system. Semin Oncol 33: 270–298

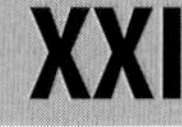

49. Honnorat J, Antoine JC (2007) Paraneoplastic neurological syndromes. Orphanet J Rare Dis 2: 22
50. de Beukelaar JW, Sillevis Smitt PA (2006) Managing paraneoplastic neurological disorders. Oncologist 11: 292–305
51. Vedeler CA, Antoine JC, Giometto B, et al (2006) Management of paraneoplastic neurological syndromes: report of an EFNS Task Force. Eur J Neurol 13: 682–690
52. Verstappen CC, Heimans JJ, Hoekman K, Postma TJ (2003) Neurotoxic complications of chemotherapy in patients with cancer: clinical signs and optimal management. Drugs 63: 1549–1563
53. Kozak OS, Wijdicks EF, Manno EM, Miley JT, Rabinstein AA (2007) Status epilepticus as initial manifestation of posterior reversible encephalopathy syndrome. Neurology 69: 894–897
54. Hinchey J, Chaves C, Appignani B, et al (1996) A reversible posterior leukoencephalopathy syndrome. N Engl J Med 334: 494–500
55. Lamy C, Oppenheim C, Meder JF, Mas JL (2004) Neuroimaging in posterior reversible encephalopathy syndrome. J Neuroimaging 14: 89–96
56. Legriel S, Bruneel F, Spreux-Varoquaux O, et al (2008) Lysergic acid amide-induced posterior reversible encephalopathy syndrome with status epilepticus. Neurocrit Care 9: 247–252
57. Laack NN, Brown PD (2004) Cognitive sequelae of brain radiation in adults. Semin Oncol 31: 702–713
58. Cross NE, Glantz MJ (2003) Neurologic complications of radiation therapy. Neurol Clin 21: 249–277
59. Soffietti R, Cornu P, Delattre JY, et al (2006) EFNS Guidelines on diagnosis and treatment of brain metastases: report of an EFNS Task Force. Eur J Neurol 13: 674–681
60. Delaney A, Fleetwood-Walker SM, Colvin LA, Fallon M (2008) Translational medicine: cancer pain mechanisms and management. Br J Anaesth 101: 87–94
61. Miovic M, Block S (2007) Psychiatric disorders in advanced cancer. Cancer 110: 1665–1676
62. Spinazze S, Schrijvers D (2006) Metabolic emergencies. Crit Rev Oncol Hematol 58: 79–89

Should We Admit Critically Ill Cancer Patients to the ICU?

D.D. Benoit, P.O. Depuydt, and J.M. Decruyenaere

Introduction

The long-term survival of patients with hematological malignancies has substantially improved over the past two decades. Nowadays, approximately 40 % of patients with acute myelogeneous leukemia or non-Hodgkin lymphoma survive for more than 5 years and it is estimated that nearly 30 % of these patients can be cured [1]. Although diseases such as multiple myeloma, low grade non-Hodgkin lymphoma and chronic lymphocytic leukemia remain incurable, half of the patients will survive for more than 4 years and survival for more than 8 to 10 years is no longer exceptional today. Similar figures can be drawn for patients with solid tumors. While the prognosis of, for instance, lung cancer and cancer of the upper gastrointestinal tract remains very grim if not detected early, substantial advances have been made in chemo-sensitive tumors such as tumors of the breast, prostate, head-and-neck region and, to a lesser extent, lower gastrointestinal tract, even in rather advanced stages of disease [1]. These improvements have been mainly achieved through the use of new and/or intensive chemotherapeutic regimens coupled with a better risk stratification of patients due to advances in radiology, immuno-histology and cytogenetics, and through advances in supportive care. Unfortunately, the therapeutic intensification coupled with longer survival time has led to an increased occurrence of potential life-threatening complications requiring intensive care unit (ICU) admission in these immunosuppressed patients [2, 3].

The substantial improvements in long-term outcome of cancer patients over the past two decades have not really influenced ICU triage decision in daily practice [2, 3]. In contrast with other patient populations with severe co-morbidities and similar long-term survival rates, such as for instance patients with chronic heart [4] or renal [5] failure, critical care physicians in general still tend to be reluctant to admit cancer patients to the ICU in case of life-threatening complications [2, 3]. The high mortality reported in older series, of more than 80 % in patients requiring mechanical ventilation [6–13], towering to 90–95 % in patients developing multiple organ failure or requiring renal replacement therapy during the ICU stay [9,13–15], particularly in the bone marrow or peripheral stem cell transplant setting [16], probably still contributes to feed this reluctance together with the severe emotional and physical burden endured by these patients and their relatives, and the considerable costs of advanced and prolonged life-supporting therapy [11].

The aim of the current chapter is: 1) To describe the improvement in outcome that has been observed over the past two decades in general and more particularly in the severely ill subgroups of cancer patients admitted to the ICU; 2) to discuss the reasons for these improvements, including the use of non-invasive ventilation (NIV);

3) to focus on prognostic indicators and to identify the subgroups of patients who should, in our opinion, be considered for ICU admission; and finally, 4) to focus on the decision making in an individual patient and on the importance of good communication in this population.

Outcome in Critically Ill Cancer Patients Requiring Advanced Life Supporting Therapy

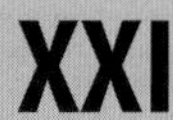

Over the past few years, several centers throughout the world have reported improved survival in critically ill patients with hematological malignancies and solid tumors [17–29], approaching the survival rates reported in critically ill non-cancer patients [30]. In a case-historical study from a large cancer center, Azoulay et al. reported a decrease in hospital mortality in ventilated cancer patients from 82 % in the period 1990–1995 to 61 % in the period 1996–1998 ($p < 0.001$) despite a significant increase in severity of illness between these periods, resulting in a four-fold lower odds of death after adjustment for confounders [17]. In a subsequent study, the same group reported 30 day mortality lowering from 79 % to 55.5 % ($p = 0.01$) between the period 1995–1997 and 1998–2000 in septic shock cancer patients resulting in a five-fold lower odds of death in the multivariate analysis [18]. This finding was recently confirmed in another case-historical study by Pène et al. [19] who observed a decrease in hospital mortality in cancer patients with septic shock from 78.9 % in the period 1998–2001 to 63.5 % in the period 2002–2005 ($p < 0.01$). The most obvious improvement was observed in patients who did not require renal replacement therapy; mortality was 78.6 % in the first period versus 35.0 % in the latter period ($p < 0.001$). The decrease in crude mortality rates reported in the literature over the past two decades in general cancer patients [20–23] and in more severely ill subgroups [24–29] further supports the finding of these case-historical studies. While most centers reported a mortality of 85–90 % in ventilated cancer patients until the end of the previous century, most arrive at a mortality of 65–70 % today (**Table 1**). In a recent large prospective study including 463 cancer patients who were ventilated > 24 hours, Soares et al. [26] described a 64 % hospital mortality. The survival of ventilated allogeneic bone marrow or peripheral stem cell transplantation recipients, however, remains particularly poor [16], although here also some improvement has been achieved [31, 32]. Encouraging results have also been obtained in cancer patients requiring renal replacement therapy for acute renal failure, even in case of multiple organ failure or in combination with ventilatory support [27–29]. While renal replacement therapy was unequivocally associated with a 90–95 % ICU mortality in case of multiple organ failure two decades ago [9,15], Soares et al. [29] recently reported 65 % 6-month mortality in patients with one or two associated organ failures and a 93 % 6-month mortality in case of three associated organ failures [30]. Moreover, Benoit et al. found no difference in 6-month survival in critically ill patients with and without hematological malignancies who received renal replacement therapy after accounting for the severity of illness upon ICU admission or the duration of hospitalization prior to admission [27]. This finding was recently confirmed by Darmon et al. [28] in critically ill patients with acute kidney injury (AKI). Cancer and non-cancer patients had similar hospital (51.1 % vs 42.9 %, $p = 0.3$) and 6-month (65 % vs 63.1 % ($p = 0.99$) mortality rates, and the presence of cancer was again not associated with a higher risk of death after adjusting for confounders [28]. Although these latter two studies probably suffered a lack

Table 1. Hospital mortality in ventilated cancer patients; evolution over the past two decades[a]

Author [ref], year	n	Solid tumors, n	Hematologic malignancies, n	Mortality rate(s) (%)
Schuster [6], 1983	52	0	52	92
Ewer [7], 1986	46	46	0	91
Peters [8], 1988	116	0	116	82
Brunet [9], 1990	111	0	111	85
Sculier [10], 1991	64	37	27	80/70
Schapira [11], 1993	54	24	30	75/76
Epner [12], 1996	86	0	86	75
Groeger [13], 1999	782	305	477	63/84
Kress [20], 1999	153	95	58	67[b]
Azoulay [17], 2001	237	68	169	76/71[c]
Massion [22], 2002	48	0	48	75
Benoit [23], 2003	88	0	88	68
Depuydt [24], 2004	166	0	166	71
Azoulay [25], 2004	203	23	180	75[b]
Soares [26], 2005	463	359	104	65/68

[a] Limited to the most important studies which did not focus exclusively on bone marrow or peripheral stem cell transplant recipients.
[b] Subgroup mortality rates are not reported.
[c] 30-day mortality rates

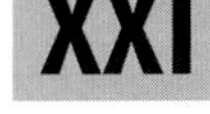

of power, both clearly indicate that the difference in mortality between cancer and non-cancer patients was not as large as commonly perceived and that the presence of underlying cancer alone is not enough to withhold renal replacement therapy.

Recently, improvement in a rather unexpected subgroup of critically ill patients was reported. Two large centers, independently from each other, reported the survival rates of cancer patients who required chemotherapy while being critically ill [33, 34]. Although clearly these patients were highly selected, meaningful long-term survival was observed despite the need for advanced life-supporting therapy during ICU stay in patients with hematological malignancies or chemo-sensitive solid tumors at first presentation of their disease, a finding that no one would have thought possible a few years ago. Finally, changes over the past two decades in recommendations regarding the duration of advanced life-supporting therapy in cancer patients further reflect the results of the case-historical studies and the improvement in crude survival rates over time. Until the end of 1980, most authors recommended that cancer patients receive mechanical ventilation for no longer than 5–7 days because of 100 % mortality [6, 7]. However, the duration of mechanical ventilation is no longer reported to be of prognostic importance [17, 24–26]. For instance, of the 112 patients with hematological malignancies who received mechanical ventilation in our center for > 7 days between 1997 and 2007, 26 % survived to hospital discharge and 20 % were still alive at 6 months (unpublished data). Recently Soares et al. [35] found no difference in hospital and 6 month mortality rates in cancer patients with a length of ICU stay ≥ 21 days compared to patients with an ICU length of stay of < 21 days, which again confirms that the duration of ICU support alone cannot be used as a reason to withhold supportive care, at least in patients who are admitted to the ICU with stable disease or in complete remission and in whom subsequent revalidation and recovery will not be compromised by the need of chemotherapy.

Reasons for Improvement in Outcomes and the Role of Non-invasive Ventilation

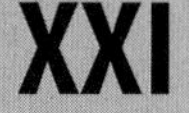

Several factors may have contributed to the improvement in outcome of critically ill cancer patients over the past decades. Better patient selection with regard their underlying malignancy and subsequent expected long-term prognosis has undeniably contributed to these improvements [17–19, 23, 25]. More rapid engraftments thanks to the increasing use of peripheral blood stem cells instead of bone marrow may have been responsible for the encouraging results in transplant recipients [31]. Congruently, a shorter duration of neutropenia, with the generalized use of granulocyte colony stimulating factors (G-CSF) in hematological malignancies since the early 2000s, may also be partially responsible for the positive evolution outside the transplant setting. While neutropenia has been found to be associated with an increased risk of death in several older series [6, 14], particularly in ventilated adult patients with hematological malignancies who experienced prolonged neutropenia, this is no longer the case today [17, 18, 24–29]. For instance, mortality rates in neutropenic and non-neutropenic patients with hematological malignancies admitted to Ghent University Hospital medical ICU between 1997 and 2000 were 43.3 % (15/57) versus 26.3 % (29/67), $p = 0.06$ [23], compared with 25.6 % (46/167) and 27.5 % (43/168), $p = 0.71$ between 2001 and 2007 [36]. Although neutropenic patients are certainly more susceptible to infection, there is no longer convincing evidence that such patients do worse once admitted to the ICU. Another, underestimated factor that may have contributed to this improvement is the more rapid referral of unstable patients to the ICU over the years thanks to better communication and collaboration between critical care physicians and hemato-oncologists [19, 34, 36, 37]. This may be of upmost importance in septic patients refractory to an initial fluid challenge [36, 37] and for the early initiation of NIV in patients with respiratory failure (see below) [24, 25, 38].

Last but not least, advances have been made over the past decade in the treatment of sepsis and in ICU support in general [17, 18, 19, 36–38, 42]. One of these advances, the use of NIV, has been claimed by several authors to be one of the major contributors to the improvement in outcome over the past decade [17, 38]. The evidence supporting the use of NIV in patients with hematological malignancies stems from two controlled trials and from several observational studies. Antonelli et al. [39] and Hilbert et al. [38] randomized immunosuppressed hypoxemic patients to NIV or standard oxygen delivery, thus testing a concept where ventilatory support was provided in relatively stable patients at an early phase of their respiratory failure. The study by Antonelli et al. [39] recruited solid organ transplant patients, whereas Hilbert et al. [38] also included a small number of hematological and/or neutropenic patients. In both studies, patients assigned to oxygen therapy more often required endotracheal intubation, which was associated with a very high rate of complications. Both studies were single center and had a heterogeneous case mix, and complications in the invasive mechanical ventilation arms were associated with a higher fatality rate (almost 100 %) than seen in most other reports. The observational studies examining the association between NIV and outcome in patients with hematological malignancies present conflicting results [17, 24–26]. In a multivariable regression analysis on predictors of ICU mortality in 237 mechanically ventilated cancer patients, and in an accompanying matched cohort analysis, Azoulay et al. observed a protective effect of NIV [17]. In contrast, in a similarly designed study on 166 ventilated patients with hematological malignancies [24], NIV was not associated with improved outcome. The severity of hypoxemia was similar in both studies; however, a different timing of initiation of ventilatory support or, alternatively, a different case-mix in terms of the underlying cause of respiratory failure could be responsible for these discordant results. When evaluating the merits of NIV, it is important to mention that in non-cancer ICU patients, NIV has been shown to be especially beneficial in patients with predominantly hypercapnic, i.e., respiratory pump failure, such as patients with exacerbations of chronic obstructive pulmonary disease (COPD), and in patients with rapidly reversible hypoxemic failure, such as cardiogenic pulmonary edema. In hypoxemic respiratory failure other than that caused by cardiogenic edema, the data are more ambiguous [40]. Moreover, it still remains unclear what proportion of hypoxemic cancer patients may be candidates for NIV outside a trial setting, as both Depuydt et al. [24] and Soares et al. [26] observed that only a small minority of cancer patients, 15 % (26/166) and 9 % (40/463), respectively, was offered NIV. Summarizing the evidence, it can be concluded that a judicious trial of NIV may be appropriate in selected cancer patients with hypercapnic, or early-onset hypoxemic respiratory failure, in order to postpone or avoid intubation with its frequently associated complications. The overall framework of general indications and contra-indications should be respected and patients should be monitored closely to avoid the adverse effects of unduly delayed intubation [24, 25]. A trial of NIV will only be successful if the underlying cause of respiratory failure is identified and reversed. Hypoxemic respiratory failure may be due to infectious pneumonia, invasion by the underlying malignancy, chemotherapy-related acute lung injury (ALI), cardiogenic and non-cardiogenic pulmonary edema or diffuse alveolar bleeding, whereas hypercapnic respiratory failure may result from comorbidity such as COPD. Mortality from acute hypoxemic respiratory failure in patients with hematological malignancies relates not only to the choice of mechanical ventilation, but also to the underlying diagnosis [22, 24–27, 36–38, 41–43]. In the aforementioned study by Hilbert et al. [38], more patients in the NIV arm had a diagnosis of infectious bacterial pneumonia, a potentially more rapidly reversible condition compared to many other non-bacterial and non-infectious complications in patients with hematological malignancies [22–25, 36–38, 41–43], and this may in part have biased towards the good outcome in the NIV patients. As a final remark, NIV may be applied as the upper limit of ventilatory support in patients with a limited prognosis [44]. The success rate of this approach will again depend on the underlying cause, with best results in hypercapnic failure. However, in a highly selected subset of cancer patients with irreversible respiratory failure, a limited trial of non-invasive respiratory support, with appropriate palliation and attention to good communication between the patient and his or her relatives, may add a short but emotionally meaningful time to the patient's life [44].

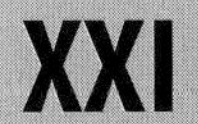

Prognostic Indicators: Subgroups with a Better and Worse Outcome

From the previous data it must be clear that the presence of an underlying cancer alone can no longer be considered to be a contraindication to refer or admit patients to the ICU, even for advanced life-supporting therapy. Of course, the type of cancer and its available treatments, the cancer status, and the remaining therapeutic options in case of relapse or active disease are important aspects to take into account on admission, although cancer characteristics *per* se, with the exception of extensive metastatic disease in solid tumor patients [26, 43], has only a minor impact on the 6-month survival [21, 22, 26, 29, 35, 45]. Age also has only a minimal impact on 6-month survival in critically cancer patients [45] whereas performance status and comorbidity are much more important [26, 29, 43, 45]. Short term survival, however, will essentially depend upon the number and severity of organ failures and the subsequent need for advanced life-supporting measures such as mechanical ventilation, vasopressor use, and/or renal replacement therapy on the one hand [13–29], and the reversibility of the organ failure on the other [14,18, 19]. This latter factor will in turn depend on the availability of an effective treatment and the time until response to such treatment. An effective treatment can, however, only be started after having made a final diagnosis, which is unfortunately not always so easy to obtain in immunosuppressed patients [42]. Several authors have claimed that critically cancer patients in whom a final diagnosis can be made have a better outcome [25, 38, 41]. For instance, in bone marrow transplant recipients presenting to the ICU with respiratory failure, Gruson et al. [41] reported a mortality of 56 % in patients with a final diagnosis made by bronchoalveolar lavage (BAL) as compared to 91 % (p = 0.03) in those without a diagnosis. In immunosuppressed patients who were randomly assigned to NIV versus invasive mechanical ventilation, the same group [38] reported a mortality of 38 % versus 76 % (p = 0.007), respectively, a factor which may have biased the results in favor of NIV as discussed above. Congruently, Azoulay et al. reported a nearly four fold higher odds of death in cancer patients with an unclear diagnosis [25].

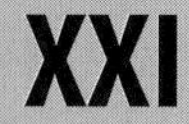

However, in our opinion, having a final diagnosis may not be enough [42]. Preferably, it should be a final diagnosis of a disease for which an effective treatment is available and which is relatively rapidly reversible; a relatively quick recovery is essential for patients who still require subsequent intravenous chemotherapy. Paradoxically, bacterial infection has been found to be associated with a better outcome regardless of the degree of advanced life-supporting therapeutic requirements in several studies [22–24, 27, 37, 38, 41], particularly in patients with hematological malignancies. In the previously mentioned studies by Gruson et al. [41] and by Hilbert et al. [38], the mortality rates in patients with versus without microbiologically documented bacterial infection diagnosed by BAL were 36 % versus 89 % (p < 0.001) and 25 % versus 65 % (p = 0.01) respectively, indicating that the beneficial effect of a final diagnosis was essentially attributable to bacterial infection. In a study by Massion et al., patients with bacterial infection had a hospital mortality of 52 % as compared to 70 % in patients with viral infection, and 90 % in those with fungal infection [22]. In a study by Benoit et al. [23], patients with hematological malignancies had a hospital mortality of 37 % when bacteremia had precipitated ICU admission compared with 59 % when other ICU admission diagnosis were present (p = 0.052). After adjusting for severity of illness, bacteremia was associated with a five-fold lower odds of death (p = 0.005). This finding was confirmed by the same authors in a subsequent new cohort of patients with hematological malignancies, regardless of the diagnostic certainty of bacterial infection [42]. In this prospective study, 172 critically ill patients with hematological malignancies admitted over a 4-year period were categorized by an independent panel of physicians blinded to the patient's outcome and C-reactive protein (CRP). The authors found no difference in mortality rates between patients with a microbiologically confirmed and those with a clinically suspected bacterial infection: Both were associated with a five-fold lower odds of death compared to other complications after adjusting for confounders (odds ratio 0.20, 95 % CI 0.06–0.62, p = 0.006 and odds ratio 0.18, 95 % CI 0.06–0.52, p = 0.002, respectively). Since the authors did not routinely use BAL in their center, this finding indicates that

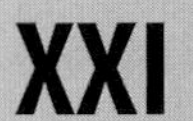

it is possible to identify patients with a high likelihood of bacterial infection precipitating ICU admission in daily practice without using potentially harmful invasive techniques. Moreover, bacterial infection was associated with a better outcome within the most severely ill subgroups of patients such as those with high grade malignancies, those hospitalized > 2 days, with an APACHE II > 25 upon admission, and those requiring mechanical ventilation or vasopressor therapy [42]. It is important to note that the mortality rates reported in the most severely subgroups were similar to those of general ICU patients with sepsis [30]. This finding was also observed in patients with hematologic malignancies requiring renal replacement therapy [27]. Of course, bacterial infection precipitating ICU admission is a serious complication in these immunosuppressed patients, which is associated with an average mortality of 30 % in patients without pulmonary infiltrates [37, 42], increasing to 65 % in patients with pulmonary infiltrates [24, 37, 42] or who require ventilatory support [18, 19, 23, 24, 37, 42], and up to 75 % in those with multiple organ failure [19, 27, 37, 42]. However, it is at least a treatable and potentially more rapidly reversible complication [23, 24, 27, 37, 42] compared to many other complications in cancer patients, such as major organ involvement by solid tumor [26, 43] or hematological malignancy [24, 26, 33, 34], invasive pulmonary aspergillosis [22–25, 37, 41, 42], post-transplant related complications [16, 31, 32, 41, 42], viral pneumonia [22–24, 37, 41], or an uncertain diagnosis [23–25, 37, 38, 41, 42]. Notable exceptions are, of course, uncomplicated pulmonary edema [25] and COPD exacerbations, and, to a lesser extent, *Pneumocystis jiroveci* pneumonia [24, 37, 42]. Of course the beneficial effect of bacterial infection on outcome is a relative one and will essentially depend upon the incidence of severe non-bacterial and non-infectious complications in the population. This is probably the reason why this finding has essentially been documented in patients with hematological malignancies who are much more susceptible to such severe complications than solid tumor patients. Although neutropenia is no longer associated with higher mortality rates [36], until recently it remained unclear whether recently administrated chemotherapy had an impact on mortality as developing sepsis and septic shock in this setting is often considered the worst case scenario in daily practice. Moreover, chemotherapy may influence mortality by other ways than neutropenia, such as by inducing major bleeding in critically ill patients because of thrombocytopenia. In a 2008 paper, Vandijck et al. studied outcome in 186 severe sepsis and septic shock patients with hematological malignancies who were admitted to the ICU over a 6-year period, and made a comparison between patients who had received and those who had not received recent chemotherapy [37]. Crude 28-day mortality rates were 40.7 % in patients who had received recent chemotherapy versus 57.4 % in those who had not ($p = 0.027$). The lower crude mortality in patients who received chemotherapy could be attributed to a lower incidence of pulmonary infiltrates (49.5 % vs. 69.5 %, $p = 0.007$) and a subsequent lower need for ventilator support (57.1 % vs. 72.6 %, $p = 0.041$). While the 28-day mortality in patients with pulmonary infiltrates was about 60 % regardless of the recent administration of chemotherapy, in patients without pulmonary infiltrates these figures were 21.7 % in those who had received versus 48.3 % in those who had not received recent chemotherapy ($p = 0.023$). The authors explained their finding by the fact that sepsis induced by bacterial translocation from the gut, which is supposed to be the major portal of entry during and after chemotherapy treatment, is more readily contained by early appropriate antibiotic therapy compared to pneumonia or any other site of infection, with the potential exception of catheter-related infection, in patients not treated with chemotherapy. This is probably related to a rapid achievement of source control in bacterial translocation as less local tissue inflammation and destruction is present [37]. Only after adjustment for the probability of having received chemotherapy by a propensity score, was recent chemotherapy no longer associated with outcome (odds ratio 0.50, 95 % CI 0.23–1.08, p = 0.07) in multivariate analysis. Whereas selection bias still could not fully be excluded given the observational nature of the study, the complete absence of a detrimental effect of chemotherapy on outcome after adjustment for confounders and a propensity score presents a strong argument against this bias.

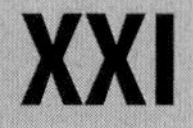

From the previous data, it is clear that cancer patients with microbiologically documented or clinically suspected bacterial infections should benefit from ICU admission since the mortality rates are similar to the general non-cancer ICU population with sepsis [30] regardless of the severity of illness and the previous recent administration of chemotherapy. Moreover, the majority of these patients will survive for more than 6 months after ICU admission [18, 19, 22–24, 37, 42]. However, this does not mean that patients with other severe complications such as for instance fungal or viral infections, or major organ failure caused by infiltration by the underlying malignancy should be denied ICU admission. With the development of new fungostatics, management of fungal infection may improve in the near future and two recently published studies have already indicated that it is feasible and justifiable to administer chemotherapy in the ICU to critically ill patients with chemo-sensitive tumors, at least at first presentation of the disease [33, 34]. However, given the higher mortality rates in these patients, good and honest communication with the relatives and if possible with the patient will be of utmost importance before proposing an ICU trial.

Triage Decisions in an Individual Patient and the Importance of Good Communication

The relatively good results achieved over the past decades in cancer patients should not be used to justify therapeutic perseverance or to withhold palliative care in patients who are in a desperate situation. As in every patient who is referred to the ICU, the degree and duration of advanced life-supporting therapy should be in proportion with the expected long-term survival and quality of life. Systematically providing advanced life-supporting therapy to patients with a dismal chance of successful recovery, regardless of whether it is related to an underlying cancer or other severe co-morbidities, is associated with a huge emotional burden for patients and relatives, and may induce emotional distress and burn-out in caregivers as well, which in turn will have an impact on the quality of care in general. Moreover, this approach is associated with considerable cost for society since the majority of ICU-generated costs are accounted for by the non-survivors [11]. However, the decision to provide or withhold advanced life-supporting therapy remains difficult in an individual patient in daily practice and is even more challenging in cancer patients. Even ICU physicians who often deal with such patients fail to discriminate well between survivors and non-survivors [46]. In a study by Thiéry et al., 26 % of the cancer patients who were considered "too sick" to benefit from ICU admission by both the hemato-oncologist and critical care physicians survived to day 30, while 16.7 % were still alive at 6 months. Importantly, among the patients considered "too well" to benefit from ICU admission in this study, the 30-day survival was a worrisome 78.7 % [46]. Although is it clear that such a decision cannot simply be replaced by a number of prognostic indicators, by a rule of thumb or even by a more complex scoring systems, it certainly can assist physicians in their decision-making [23, 47]. Beside these prognostic indicators, the quality of life and above all the preferences of the patient and/or the relatives should also be taken into account. However, preferences are only known in a minority of the patients upon referral to the ICU. Moreover, critical care physicians are often confronted in daily practice with overoptimistic referring physicians, patients and/or relatives. Although, for instance, oncologists are able to predict long-term outcome relatively accurately, 70.2 % of them communicate overoptimistic survival estimates to their patients [48]. Similarly, according to a recent French survey, only 17.8 % and 65.9 % of the oncologists admitted to systematically informing their patient about the diagnosis and therapy, respectively [49]. Differences in expectations between the parties involved may be a source of important conflicts, which may in turn fuel the reluctance of the ICU team to admit future critically ill cancer patients. Providing appropriate care to these complex patients is only possible after honest communication of the most probable case scenario(s) with the relatives, and preferably, if allowed by her or his acute illness at that moment, with the patient. The effect of prolonged ICU support as a potential interference with subsequent cancer treatment should also be taken into account, particularly in patients with active or unstable disease. In case of doubt, an ICU trial for a couple of days can be considered [50].

Conclusion

Reluctance to admit cancer patients to the ICU for advance life supporting therapy is no longer justified. Over the past decade, several centers across the world have shown that is possible to achieve meaningful outcomes in certain subgroups of patients. For instance, patients with severe sepsis and septic shock, particularly resulting from bacterial infection, have short-term and long-term survival rates that are similar to the general ICU population, regardless of the degree of advanced life-supporting therapeutic requirements. However, these relatively good results should not be used to justify therapeutic perseverance or to postpone palliative care in patients who are in a desperate situation. Similarly to any other critically ill patient, the degree and duration of advanced life-supporting therapy provided should be in proportion to the patient's expected long-term survival and quality of life. Honest communication regarding these issues between the caregivers, the patient, and the relatives before and upon referral to the ICU as well as during the ICU stay is therefore essential.

References

1. Brenner H (2002) Long-term survival rates of cancer patients achieved by the end of the 20th century: a period analysis. Lancet 360: 1131–1135
2. Azoulay E, Afessa B (2006) The intensive care support for patients with malignancy. Do everything that can be done. Intensive Care Med 32: 3–5
3. Pène F, Soares M (2008) Can we still refuse ICU admission of patients with hematological malignancies? Intensive Care Med 34: 847–855
4. Gustafsson I, Brendorp B, Seibaek M, et al (2004) Influence of diabetes and diabetes-gender interaction on the risk of death in patients hospitalized with congestive heart failure. J Am Coll Cardiol 43: 771–777
5. Mc Alister FA, Ezekowitz J, Tonelli M, et al (2004) Renal insufficiency and heart failure. Circulation 109: 1004–1009

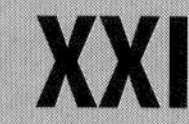

6. Schuster DP, Marion JM (1982) Precedents for meaningful recovery during treatment in a medical intensive care unit. Outcome in patients with hematologic malignancy. Am J Med 75: 402–408
7. Ewer MS, Ali MK, Atta MS, Morice RC, Balakrishna PV (1986) Outcome in lung cancer patients requiring mechanical ventilation for pulmonary failure. JAMA 256: 3364–3366
8. Peters SG, Meadows JA, Gracey DR (1988) Outcome of respiratory failure in hematologic malignancy. Chest 94: 99–102
9. Brunet F, Lanore JJ, Dhainaut JF, et al (1990) Is intensive care justified for patients with haematological malignancies ? Intensive Care Med 16: 291–297
10. Sculier JP, Markiewicz E (1991) Medical cancer patients and intensive care. Anticancer Res 11: 2171–2174
11. Schapira DV, Studnicki J, Bradham DD, et al (1993) Intensive care, survival, and expense of treating critically ill cancer patients. JAMA 269: 783–786
12. Epner DE, White P, Krasnoff M, et al (1996) Outcome of mechanical ventilation for adults with hematologic malignancy. J Invest Med 44: 254–260
13. Groeger JS, White Jr P, Nierman DM, et al (1999) Outcome for cancer patients requiring mechanical ventilation. J Clin Oncol 17: 991–997
14. Guiguet M, Blot F, Escudier B, et al (1998) Severity-of-illness scores for neutropenic cancer patients in an intensive care unit: which is the best predictor? Do multiple assessment times improve the predictive value? Crit Care Med 26: 488–493
15. Lanore JJ, Brunet F, Pochard F, et al (1991) Hemodialysis for acute renal failure in patients with hematologic malignancies. Crit Care Med 19: 346–351
16. Bach PB, Schrag D, Nieman DM, et al (2001) Identification of poor prognostic features among patients requiring mechanical ventilation after hematopoietic stem cell transplantation. Blood 98: 3234–3240
17. Azoulay E, Albertti C, Bornstain C, et al (2001) Improved survival in cancer patients requiring mechanical ventilatory support: impact of noninvasive mechanical ventilatory support. Crit Care Med 29: 519–525
18. Larché J, Azoulay E, Fieux F, et al (2003) Improved survival of critically ill cancer patients with septic shock. Intensive Care Med 29: 1688–1695
19. Pène F, Percheron S, Lemiale V, et al (2008) Temporal changes in management and outcome of septic shock in patients with malignancies in the intensive care unit. Crit Care Med 36: 690–696
20. Kress J, Christenson J, Pohlman A, et al (1999) Outcomes of critically ill cancer patients in an university hospital setting. Am J Respir Crit Care Med 160: 1957–1961
21. Staudinger T, Stoiser B, Müllner M, et al (2000) Outcome and prognostic factors in critically ill cancer patients admitted to the intensive care unit. Crit Care Med 28: 1322–1328
22. Massion PB, Dive AL, Doyen C, et al (2002) Prognosis of hematologic malignancies does not predict intensive care unit mortality. Crit care Med 30: 2260–2270
23. Benoit DD, Vandewoude KH, Decruyenaere JM, Hoste EA, Colardyn FA (2003) Outcome and early prognostic indicators in patients with a hematologic malignancy admitted to the intensive care unit for a life-threatening complication. Crit Care Med 31: 104–112
24. Depuydt PO, Benoit DD, Vandewoude K, Decruyenaere J, Colardyn F (2004) Outcome in noninvasively and invasively ventilated hematologic patients with acute respiratory failure. Chest 126: 1299–1306
25. Azoulay E, Thiery G, Chevret S, et al (2004) The prognosis of acute respiratory failure in critically ill cancer patients. Medicine 83: 360–370
26. Soares M, Salluh JI, Spector N, Rocco JR (2005) Characteristics and outcome of cancer patients requiring mechanical ventilatory support > 24 hrs. Crit Care Med 33: 520–526
27. Benoit DD, Hoste EA, Depuydt PO, et al (2005) Outcome in critically ill medical patients treated with renal replacement therapy for acute renal failure: comparison between patients with and those without haematological malignancies. Nephrol Dial Transplant 20: 552–558
28. Darmon M, Thiery G, Ciroldi M, Porcher R, Sclemmer B, Azoulay E (2007) Should dialysis be offered to cancer patients with acute kidney injury ? Intensive Care Med 33: 765–772
29. Soares M, Salluh JI, Carvalho MS, Darmon M, Rocco JR, Spector N (2006) Prognosis of critically ill patients with cancer and acute renal dysfunction. J Clin Oncol 24: 4003–4010
30. Alberti C, Brun-Buisson C, Buchardi H, et al (2002) Epidemiology of sepsis and infection in ICU patients from an international multicenter cohort study. Intensive Care Med 28: 108–121

31. Price KJ, Thall PF, Kish SK, et al (1998) Prognostic indicators for blood and marrow transplant patients admitted to an intensive care unit. Am J Respir Crit Care Med 158: 876–884
32. Pène F, Aubron C, Azoulay E, et al (2006) Outcome of critically ill allogeneic hematopoetic stem cell transplantation recipients: a reappraisal for indications of organ failure support. J Clin Oncol 24: 643–649
33. Darmon M, Thiery G, Ciroldi M, et al (2005) Intensive care in patients with newly diagnosed malignancies and a need for cancer chemotherapy. Crit Care Med 33: 2488–2493
34. Benoit DD, Depuydt PO, Vandewoude KH, et al (2006) Outcome in severely ill patients with hematological malignancies who received intravenous chemotherapy in the intensive care unit. Intensive Care Med 32: 93–99
35. Soares M, Salluh JI, Torres VB, Leal JV, Spector N (2008) Short- and long-term outcomes of critically ill patients with cancer and prolonged ICU length of stay. Chest 134: 520–526
36. Vandijck DM, Benoit DD (2008) Impact of recent intravenous chemotherapy on outcome in severe sepsis and septic shock patients with haematological malignancies. Intensive Care Med 34: 1930–1931
37. Vandijck DM, Benoit DD, Depuydt PO, et al (2008) Impact of recent intravenous chemotherapy on outcome in severe sepsis and septic shock patients with hematological malignancies. Intensive Care Med 34: 847–855
38. Hilbert G, Gruson D, Vargas F, et al (2001) Noninvasive ventilation in immunosupressed patients with pulmonary infiltrates, fever, and acute respiratory failure. N Engl J Med 344: 481–487
39. Antonelli M, Conti G, Bufi M, et al (2000) Nonivasive ventilation for treatment of acute respiratory failure in patients undergoing solid organ transplantation. JAMA 283: 235–241
40. Keenan S, Sinuff T, Cook D, Hill NS (2004) Does noninvasive positive pressure ventilation improve outcome in acute hypoxemic failure? A systematic review. Crit Care Med 32: 2516–2523
41. Gruson D, Hilbert G, Portel L, et al (1999) Severe respiratory failure requiring ICU admission in bone marrow transplant recipients. Eur Respir J 13: 883–887
42. Benoit DD, Depuydt PO, Peleman RA, et al (2005) Documented and clinically suspected bacterial infection precipitating Intensive Care Unit admission in severely ill patients with hematological malignancies: impact on outcome. Intensive Care Med 31: 934–942
43. Soares M, Darmon M, Salluh JI, et al (2007) Prognosis of lung cancer patients with life-threatening complications. Chest 131: 840–846
44. Schettino G, Altobelli N, Kacmarek RM (2008) Non-invasive positive-pressure ventilation in acute respiratory failure outside clinical trials: experience at the Massachusetts General Hospital. Crit Care Med 36: 441–447
45. Soares M, Carvalho MS, Salluh JI, et al (2006) Effect of age on survival in critically ill patients with cancer. Crit Care Med 34: 715–721
46. Thiery G, Azoulay E, Darmon M, et al (2005) Outcome of cancer patients considered for intensive care unit admission: a hospital-wide prospective study. J Clin Oncol 23: 4406–4413
47. Soares M, Fontes F, Dantas J, et al (2004) Performance of six severity-of-illness scores in cancer patients requiring admission to the intensive care unit: a prospective observational study. Crit Care 8:R194–203
48. Lamont EB, Christakis NA (2001) Prognostic disclosure to patients with cancer near the end of life. Ann Intern Med 134: 1096–1105
49. Peritti-Watel P, Bendiane MK, Pegliasco H, et al (2003) Doctor's opinion on euthanasia, end of life care and doctor-patient communication: telephone survey in France. BMJ 327: 595–596
50. Lecuyer L, Chevret S, Thiery G, Darmon M, Schlemmer B, Azoulay E (2007) The ICU trial: a new admission policy for cancer patients requiring mechanical ventilation. Crit Care Med 35: 808–814

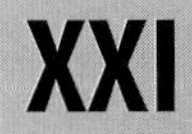

XXII Drug Dosing

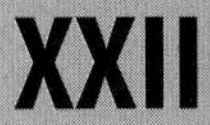

Optimizing Drug Dosing in the ICU

X. Liu, P. Kruger, and M.S. Roberts

Introduction

Patients admitted to the intensive care unit (ICU) may exhibit multiple organ dysfunctions and usually require treatment with a wide range of drugs such as sedatives, analgesics, neuromuscular blockers, and antimicrobials [1]. Recommendations for the dosing regimens in ICU patients are often extrapolated from clinical trials in healthy volunteers or non-ICU patients. This extrapolation assumes similar drug behavior (pharmacokinetics and pharmacodynamics) among ICU and other patients or healthy volunteers. However, it is well described that many drugs used in critically ill patients may have alterations of the pharmacokinetic and pharmacodynamic properties due to pathophysiological changes or drug interactions [1–4]. These changes may occur even within a single patient at varying stages of their illness and, therefore, critically ill patients offer unique challenges in drug dosing.

The ultimate goal of drug administration in the critically ill patient is to achieve a desired clinical effect and limit the drug toxicity. This relies on the delivery of a safe and effective concentration of the drug to the target tissue which then results in an appropriate physiological effect. The action of a given drug normally shows a better relationship with its concentration in blood or at its site of effect than with the dose of the drug. Linking the blood concentration (pharmacokinetic) and effects (pharmacodynamic) seeks to improve our understanding of the dose-concentration and concentration-effect relationships. In recent years, more research has been done to define pharmacokinetic/pharmacodynamic models for common drugs in the ICU [5–8]. These models provide a description of drug concentrations and subsequent response in a variety of ICU patients, thus offering the potential to develop more appropriate dosing regimens and improve patient outcome and drug safety. In general, the most common examples relate to improving dosing for antimicrobial therapy [9, 10].

Pharmacokinetic and Pharmacodynamic Alterations in Critically Ill Patients

Pharmacokinetic Alterations

Patients in the ICU may display a range of organ dysfunctions related to severe acute illness. These pathophysiological changes, together with drug interactions and other therapeutic interventions (e.g., renal replacement therapy, vasopressor support, fluid loading) [1], can have a great impact on the pharmacokinetic properties of absorption, distribution, metabolism, and excretion. **Figure 1** shows an overview of the key

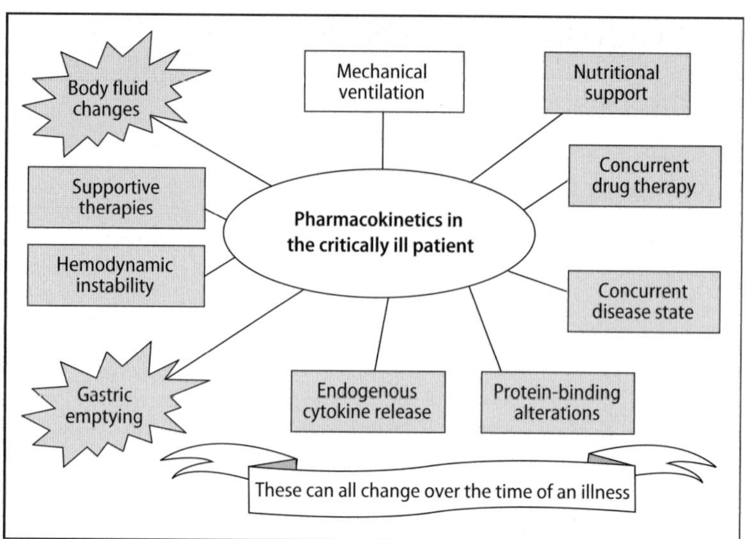

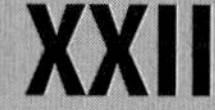

Fig. 1. An overview of the key pathophysiological changes and therapeutic interventions that can impact on pharmacokinetics and pharmacodynamics in ICU patients (adapted from [11])

pathophysiological changes that can be seen in an ICU patient. The impact of each of these aspects on pharmacokinetics and pharmacodynamics is considered in more detail below.

Alterations in distribution

The extent of drug distribution in the body is normally expressed in terms of a volume of distribution for the drug, a pharmacokinetic parameter defined by the ratio of the amount of drug in the body to the concentration in the blood or plasma. Multiple factors such as pH of the environment, protein binding in plasma and tissue, cardiac output, blood flow and permeability of tissue could substantially affect this distribution, as discussed below. These factors may change greatly during the process of illness in critically ill patients, thereby altering the volume of distribution of drug.

pH changes: Most drugs are weak acids or bases and their ionization state is affected by the pH of the environment. The unionized drug is more lipophilic than its ionized form and penetrates the lipid-based cellular membrane more easily (these principles are sometimes utilized to our advantage such as pH-adjusted solutions to optimize delivery and onset or urine pH manipulation for enhanced excretion). The pH of body fluid may change in critically ill patients as a result of respiratory failure, shock states, renal failure, or exocrine pancreatic dysfunction. These alterations in pH may cause a change in drug ionization and increase or decrease drug absorption and distribution. Weak basic drugs are also more concentrated in acidic organelles such as lysosomes and mitochondria and this can be a significant component in the distribution volume for these drugs [12].

Protein binding: Many drugs demonstrate non-specific protein binding in plasma and tissues to constituent proteins, which principally include albumin (acidic drugs) and α_1-acid glycoprotein (basic drugs) [13]. The bound drug is in equilibrium with the free (unbound) drug and the amount bound is dependent on both the affinity of the drug for the protein and the binding capacity of each protein. It is generally assumed that only unbound drug is free to cross the cell membrane and be subject to distribution, metabolism, and excretion process, and subsequently interact with its corresponding receptor to show pharmacological or toxicological effect [14]. ICU patients may have substantial protein extravasation as a result of increased endothelial permeability and tissue perfusion. As a consequence, bound drug will be carried across into tissues and the area under the unbound concentration – time profiles in the tissue space are often greater than in the plasma for drugs with significant protein binding (Dalley A et al., personal communication).

Albumin concentrations frequently decrease and α_1-acid glycoprotein synthesis often increases in critically ill patients during and after traumatic or physiologic stress [15, 16]. These changes will result in the increase of unbound fraction of acidic drugs primarily bound to albumin (e.g., diazepam) but decrease in the unbound fraction of basic drugs primarily bound to α_1-acid glycoprotein (e.g., meperidine). In a review by Benet and Hoener [17], the authors listed 25 drugs for which protein binding may affect the drug exposure. Among those listed are drugs frequently administered to critically ill patients such as fentanyl, propofol, midazolam, diltiazem, and haloperidol. On occasions, critically ill patients are exposed to huge doses of drug, either deliberately or inadvertently, and this can saturate protein binding sites and lead to greater than expected free drug levels.

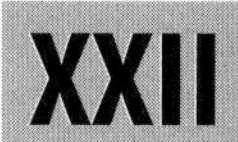

Fluid shifts: After a drug enters the body, it must be distributed via the systemic circulation and subsequently penetrate through tissue to its site of effect. This involves the endothelium, interstitial fluid and cell membranes. Variations in these compartments caused by fluid shift have been implicated as a major pathophysiological mechanism possibly affecting drug distribution (the volume of distribution) and/or elimination processes. Both increased capillary permeability and reduction of oncotic pressure due to severe hypoalbuminemia may cause fluid shifts responsible for the leakage of large volumes into the interstitium. This is often referred to as the 'third spacing' phenomenon. Edema [18], pleural effusion [19], ascites [20], peritoneal exudate [21], abundant intravenous therapies [22], and total parenteral nutrition [23] may lead to a significant increase in the volume of distribution of hydrophilic drugs. Increased volume of distribution will result in a lower plasma concentration for any given dose and this may be clinically relevant especially for drugs, such as antibiotics, that display concentration-dependent antimicrobial activity. Clinical failure of antimicrobial therapy in sepsis and trauma has been documented due to increasing volume of distribution and lowing antimicrobial concentrations [24].

The impact of organ dysfunction: Alterations in cardiac output and peripheral blood flow will alter the distribution of many drugs. Those drugs whose distribution is restricted to the extracellular fluid space are likely to be most affected. A common event associated with trauma is a reduction in distribution volume as a consequence of tissue hypoperfusion. For instance, the higher plasma level for amoxicillin in trauma is due more to the subsequent decrease in distribution volume than in clearance [25].Vasopressor use and changes in endothelial permeability may further alter the redistribution of many agents, although the details are poorly understood.

Alterations in metabolism

The liver is the major organ responsible for drug metabolism. Hepatic dysfunction is present in up to 54 % critically ill patients and may cause changes in drug clearance via effects on hepatic blood or bile flow or cytochrome P450 (CYP450) enzyme activity [1]. The predominant metabolism reactions in humans are oxidation by the various isoforms of CYP450 (phase I metabolism) and conjugation with glucuronide, sulphate or glutathione (phase II metabolism) [26]. Pro-inflammatory cytokines (interleukin [IL]-1β, IL-6, tumor necrosis factor [TNF]-α) and possibly even catecholamines, may impact on CYP450 enzyme activity [27, 28]. The metabolism of certain drugs (phenytoin, pentobarbital, lorazepam) has been demonstrated to increase in trauma patients, especially those with severe head injury [2, 29].

Hepatic blood flow can vary widely in critically ill patients. In addition to the underlying disease process, a variety of interventions may also cause changes of blood flow. Alpha-adrenoceptor agonists (e.g., phenylephrine, norepinephrine) [30] and vasopressin [31] have been reported to decrease total hepatic blood flow. In contrast, nitroglycerin may increase blood flow. De Backer et al. [32] demonstrated variations in splanchnic perfusion with individual vasoactive agents even in the setting of preserved or increased cardiac output. Mechanical ventilation also has well described effects on organ blood flow. Hemorrhage, hypovolemia from other causes, and acute heart failure in critically ill patients may all result in a reduction of hepatic blood flow and, thus, decreased drug clearance. The opposite situation may be seen during the hyperdynamic stage of sepsis where cardiac output typically increases and blood flow distribution changes to shunt blood flow to vital organs.

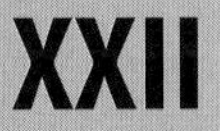

These alterations in hepatic or splanchnic blood flow will impact on the first pass metabolism of enterally administered medication and also effect metabolism following intravenous administration of drugs highly extracted by the liver (extraction ratio > 0.7) (e.g., lidocaine, beta-blockers, morphine, and midazolam).

Alterations in Excretion

The kidneys are responsible for the excretion of many small drugs and their metabolites. Larger polar molecules (> 500 Da) are often excreted in the bile. Whilst glomerular filtration is the major mechanism responsible for renal excretion, some organic anions and cations do have an active secretion component. Water soluble drugs and metabolites are removed by glomerular filtration and eliminated through the urine. The renal clearance of drugs can be severely impaired in patients with acute renal failure or pre-existing chronic renal failure, which results in the accumulation of both parent drug and metabolites.

An increase in creatinine clearance may be seen in some critically ill patients and is often underappreciated. This may result from increases in cardiac output and renal blood flow, although the exact magnitude of these changes is not known. Typically seen in patients with extensive burns [33], sepsis [34], or traumatic brain injuries [35] it can result in the renal clearance of hydrophilic drugs being increased significantly.

Pharmacodynamic Alterations

Pharmacodynamics describes the relationship between drug concentrations at the site of action (receptor) and the pharmacologic response, including physiologic effects that influence the interaction of drug with the receptor. Although not as extensively studied as pharmacokinetics, the changes of drug effect resulting from pharmacodynamic changes have been documented in critically ill patients [4, 36]. For example, tolerance to neuromuscular blockers in sepsis or major burns has been previously reported [37].

Pharmacodynamic changes are probably due to changes in the affinity of the receptor for the drug or alterations in the intrinsic activity of the receptor under pathophysiological conditions. Genetic differences in ICU patients could be another important factor responsible for the inter-individual variability in drug pharmacodynamics. Numerous polymorphisms have been described in genes encoding drug-metabolizing enzymes, transporters, and receptors. A recent study by Link et al. [38] identified common genetic variants in SLCO1B1 (encoding the transporter-OATA1B1) strongly associated with alterations in risk of simvastatin-induced myopathy.

Most drugs exert their action in the tissue rather than in the blood. Therefore, the local tissue concentration of drug can be more relevant than drug plasma concentrations to determine a concentration-effect profile. Microdialysis is a technique increasingly used in pharmacodynamic studies to allow direct assessment of drug levels in the interstitial fluid of a target tissue. In addition, microdialysis also allows the continuous measurement of endogenous substances (e.g., neurotransmitter, hormone) which may serve as a biological marker for drug response. By using microdialysis to determine the concentration of levofloxacin in the interstitial fluid space of skeletal muscle in patients with sepsis, Zeitlinger et al. [39] found that the drug concentration in tissue was inadequate for efficacy even though effective concentrations were attained in plasma. As a consequence, dosing regimens based on plasma concentration may lead to therapy failure. Further research to understand the factors altering tissue drug concentration in critically ill patients is likely to lead to more effective dosing regimens.

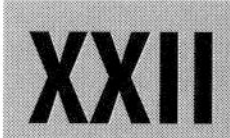

Pharmacokinetic and Pharmacodynamic Modeling

For drugs with rapid onset, short duration, and easily assessable end-points of action (such as vasoactive agents), the dosing regimen is often titrated to an effect rather than to a specific dose. As a consequence of this, changes in drug behavior during a patient's illness are not of great concern as they can easily be adjusted for during the patient's clinical management. However, for drugs that have less readily assessable effects and effects that are directly related to the plasma, or subsequent effect site, concentration, getting the optimal dose can be difficult. Drugs for which distribution is restricted to the extracellular fluid space are potentially the most affected by the changes in pathophysiology and body fluid spaces seen in critically ill patients.

Back to Basics

Traditional approaches assess plasma levels and make assumptions about the movement of drug to the effect site. They treat the body as a series of potential compartments and use measured plasma levels to generate pharmacokinetic data and a separate study of pharmacodynamics to link in drug effects

Bayesian Forecasting

Bayesian forecasting provides a method to predict steady-state plasma drug concentration and individual pharmacokinetic parameters. It has been used to individualize aminoglycoside therapy in critically ill patients since the 1980s [40]. The use of this method has been reported to allow the safe use of large doses of aminoglycosides in the first few critical days in sepsis [40]. However, it is desirable to have some clinical feel for approximately what answers you might expect from such predictions as significant errors are possible. Initial forecasts are based on population assumptions which may in some cases not accurately reflect an individual patient's circumstances.

Population Pharmacokinetics/pharmacodynamics

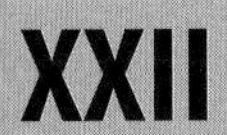

Population pharmacokinetics/pharmacodynamics provides a full description of a drug's pharmacokinetic/pharmacodynamic behavior in the population in terms of typical parameter estimates (mean with a statistical distribution) as well as variability between patients. It studies the covariants (factors that alter behavior) and correlates the variability in drug concentrations and effect among individuals in the population of interest [40]. Some pharmacokinetic/pharmacodynamic variations can be explained by certain patient demographic, pathophysiological, and therapeutic features, such as gender, body weight, age, hepatic and renal impairment, and the presence of other therapies. Population pharmacokinetics/pharmacodynamics facilitates investigation of the measurable factors that may cause changes in the dose-concentration or concentration-effect relationship. It assesses the extent of these changes and may lead to a better prediction of dose and/or response in individuals receiving the drug in the future.

Over the past two decades, population pharmacokinetics/pharmacodynamics have been widely applied in drug development programmes in the pharmaceutical industry and are described in the Food and Drug Administration (FDA)'s guidance document [42]. Population pharmacokinetics/pharmacodynamics may also play an important role in the selection of the optimal dose for an individual patient by identifying patient characteristics previously related to drug exposure or treatment outcome.

The problem in applying this technique for critically ill patients is the very heterogeneous nature of the ICU population. Critically ill patients have wide and varied pathology and every patient is also likely to have differing pathophysiology at varying stages of their illness. To make these techniques more applicable to the ICU, perhaps we need to consider specific sub-population pharmacokinetic/pharmacodynamic modeling, which appropriately recognizes the time dependency of pharmacokinetics/pharmacodynamics in an ICU setting. We have recently completed a pharmacokinetics/pharmacodynamics study of the neuromuscular blocking drug, cisatracurium (unpublished data). We specifically selected a subpopulation of ICU patients, those with severe sepsis in the early phase of their illness. This study confirmed that these patients exhibited resistance to cisatracurium. Interestingly, this was not due to changes in pharmacokinetics, as the clearance and volume of distribution parameters obtained from these ICU patients were comparable to those previously published for healthy volunteers and other patient groups. The increased median effective concentration (EC50) in these patients suggested a pharmacodynamic reason for the altered drug dose response.

Methods of population modeling

Population pharmacokinetic/pharmacodynamic modeling provides a statistical model for the estimation of both intra-subject and inter-subject variability. Most population analyses aim at estimating the population pharmacokinetic/pharmacodynamic parameters and the variability. They identify potential covariates that explain some of the variability in the dose-concentration or concentration-effect relationship.

There are three common methods for the analysis of population pharmacokinetic/pharmacodynamic data: 1) Naïve pooled approach; 2) standard two-stage approach; and 3) non-linear mixed-effects modeling approach. Only the last two approaches enable an accurate estimation of intersubject variability.

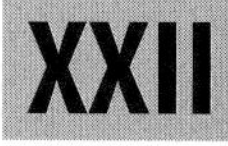

- Naïve pooled approach: The naïve pooled approach is, in fact, a method to analyze population data, but not a population approach. With this method, all the observations from the population are pooled together and are treated as if they represent a single subject or patient. Overall population mean pharmacokinetic/pharmacodynamic parameters can then be estimated. However, no information can be obtained on different sources of variability. In addition, it does not allow incorporation of potential influential factors (e.g., patient characteristics). This approach is seldom used but may be helpful to obtain the initial estimates of parameters for a more appropriate method.
- Standard two-stage approach: This traditional method involves controlled experimental investigations with a relatively small number of subjects (healthy volunteers or selected homogeneous patients) and relatively large numbers of data points per subject (e.g., 8–16 blood samples). The first stage of this approach is to estimate the pharmacokinetic parameters through non-linear regression using individual concentration-time data. In the second stage, individual parameter estimates obtained from the first stage serve as input data for a simple statistical description of the population distribution (mean values, standard deviation) of each parameter of interest. Analysis of the relationship between parameters and covariates (e.g., patient characteristics) using classic statistical analysis (stepwise regression, covariance analysis, cluster analysis) can be performed in the second stage. The method generally provides unbiased mean estimates but systematically overestimates variance and covariance [43]. Refinements have been proposed (e.g., iterative two-stage Bayesian approach) to improve the standard two-stage approach through bias correction for the random effects covariance.
- Non-linear mixed effect modeling: This method of population modeling, first introduced in the late seventies by Sheiner et al. [44], was the first true population modeling method. It considers the population study sample, rather than the individual, as a unit of analysis and estimates the distribution of parameters and their relationships with covariates within the population. The method can function with sparse, unbalanced data as well as the dense data situation. It can allow one to combine heterogeneous types of data from varying sources (e.g., pooled data from several clinical trials or study centers).

The most common statistical models used in population pharmacokinetics/pharmacodynamics are mixed-effects models, which simultaneously estimate fixed and random effects (therefore, mixed-effects). The fixed effects representing the typical population parameters (e.g., clearance, volume of distribution), are related to covariates (body weight, age, gender, creatinine clearance) by the defined 'structure' of the model. The random effects quantify the variability among individuals, within-individuals, or among occasions (e.g., due to disease progress), along with the residual 'unexplained' variability. In the mixed-effects context, population parameters are reported by a population typical value, generally the mean, and a population-variability value, generally the variance. The individual parameters are assumed to be normally distributed and to vary around the population mean.

Non-linear mixed effect modeling is particularly useful in application to clinically relevant situations where only sparse data are available from each individual. This situation often happens in pharmacokinetics studies of certain groups of patients such as critically ill, children, elderly, and outpatients. The collected data are insufficient for the estimation of individual pharmacokinetic parameters using the standard two-stage approach. The population approach is also able to accommodate unstructured and unbalanced study designs, which often occur in clinical situations. An unstructured study is depicted as one where the purpose of blood sampling is not related to the current study, e.g., retrospective collection of data arising from routine therapeutic drug monitoring measurements. An unbalanced study refers to datasets with different number of samples for each individual and different times of sampling. The number of subjects required in non-linear mixed effect modeling analysis can range from 50 to several hundred depending on the variability and the range of population characteristics possibly to be encountered.

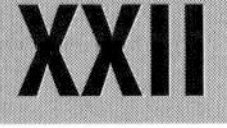

Population pharmacokinetic/pharmacodynamic modeling involves sophisticated statistical analysis to estimate the model parameters and their variability. Although several computer programs are available to perform such analyses, the most widely used program is non-linear mixed effect modeling. For non-linear mixed effect modeling to perform the analysis, the data has to be collected and organized and then a model describing underlining pharmacokinetics must be stated. Population pharmacokinetic/pharmacodynamic modeling involves complex statistical analysis and a certain expertise is required for the analyses.

Application to Critically Ill Patients

The application of population pharmacokinetics/pharmacodynamics may provide a better rationale for the proper selection of an optimal dose, type, and duration of administration for a drug to an individual patient. Increasing interest has been seen with population pharmacokinetics/pharmacodynamics studies evaluating ICU patients, particularly for antibiotic therapy [10]. Most of these studies aim to better estimate appropriate dosing regimens in ICU patients by applying population pharmacokinetics/pharmacodynamics models. The importance of antibiotic dosing relates not only to efficacy but could potentially impact on antimicrobial resistance [45].

A recent example of population pharmacokinetic/pharmacodynamic analysis is a study of vancomycin in ICU patients [46]. The purpose of this study was first to identify the variables responsible for vancomycin pharmacokinetic changes in medical ICU patients, and then to evaluate the potential efficacy of a dosage regimen applied to this group of patients. A retrospective pharmacokinetic analysis was performed using sparse serum data collected during routine clinical care. Patient information, such as age, total body weight, albumin and serum creatinine levels, and APACHE II score, was also collected. Population pharmacokinetic analysis was performed and clearance was found to be highly correlated to renal function, APACHE II score, age, and serum albumin. The pharmacodynamic effect (probability of achieving the recommended value of the 24 hour area under the concentration-time curve/minimum inhibitory concentration [AUC_{24h}/MIC ratio]) was estimated by the Monte Carlo simulation technique. This technique allows the prediction of the potential efficacy of different dosage regimens using population pharmacokinetics when therapeutic drug monitoring is not possible. Therefore, the best therapeutic option could be selected to achieve the highest probability of clinical success in ICU patients. The results from this study provide some insight into individualization of vancomycin dosing in critically ill patients.

Conclusion

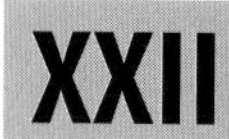

Drug dosing in ICU patients is challenging for clinicians due to the complex pathophysiological conditions of these patients. Pharmacokinetic/pharmacodynamic principles could be applied to maximize the clinical response, improve efficacy, minimize side effects of drug therapy and improve cost efficiency. Population pharmacokinetic/pharmacodynamic modeling is a powerful tool to investigate the influence of demographic parameters and pathophysiological conditions on the dose-concentration or concentration-response relationship. While it is increasingly being applied for selected drugs in ICU patients, it is likely these techniques could gain wider clinical application by considering the 'sub-population' pharmacokinetic/pharmacodynamic approach. A vital tool missing from current practice is the ability to teach a 'clinical feel' for approximate pharmacokinetic/pharmacodynamic relationships and how they change over time or between patients. We need to develop techniques that will allow clinicians to use pharmacokinetic/pharmacodynamic information in routine clinical care and so optimize drug use in the ICU and potentially improve patient outcomes.

Acknowledgements: We recognize the support of the Australian National Health & Medical Research Council.

References

1. Power BM, Forbes AM, van Heerden PV, Ilett KF (1998) Pharmacokinetics of drugs used in critically ill adults. Clin Pharmacokinet 34: 25–56
2. Boucher BA, Wood GC, Swanson JM (2006) Pharmacokinetic changes in critical illness. Crit Care Clin 22: 255–271
3. Lipman J (2000) Towards better ICU antibiotic dosing. Crit Care Resusc 2: 282–289
4. Wagnerand BK, O'Hara DA (1997) Pharmacokinetics and pharmacodynamics of sedatives and analgesics in the treatment of agitated critically ill patients. Clin Pharmacokinet 33: 426–453
5. Benko R, Matuz M, Doro P, et al (2007) Pharmacokinetics and pharmacodynamics of levofloxacin in critically ill patients with ventilator-associated pneumonia. Int J Antimicrob Agents 30: 162–168
6. Fish DN, Teitelbaum I, Abraham E (2005) Pharmacokinetics and pharmacodynamics of imipenem during continuous renal replacement therapy in critically ill patients. Antimicrob Agents Chemother 49: 2421–2428
7. Johnston AJ, Steiner LA, O'Connell M, Chatfield DA, Gupta AK, Menon DK (2004) Pharmacokinetics and pharmacodynamics of dopamine and norepinephrine in critically ill head-injured patients. Intensive Care Med 30: 45–50
8. Vincent JL, Spapen HD, Creteur J, et al (2006) Pharmacokinetics and pharmacodynamics of once-weekly subcutaneous epoetin alfa in critically ill patients: results of a randomized, double-blind, placebo-controlled trial. Crit Care Med 34: 1661–1667
9. Mohr JF, Wanger A, Rex JH (2004) Pharmacokinetic/pharmacodynamic modeling can help guide targeted antimicrobial therapy for nosocomial gram-negative infections in critically ill patients. Diagn Microbiol Infect Dis 48: 125–130

10. de Wildt SN, de Hoog M, Vinks AA, van der Giesen E, van den Anker JN (2003) Population pharmacokinetics and metabolism of midazolam in pediatric intensive care patients. Crit Care Med 31: 1952–1958
11. Herfindaland ET, Gourley DR (2000) Textbook of Therapeutics: Drug and Disease Management. Lippincott Williams and Wilkins, Philadelphia
12. Siebert GA, Hung DY, Chang P, Roberts MS (2004) Ion-trapping, microsomal binding, and unbound drug distribution in the hepatic retention of basic drugs. J Pharmacol Exp Ther 308: 228–235
13. Laznicekand M, Laznickova A (1995) The effect of lipophilicity on the protein binding and blood cell uptake of some acidic drugs. J Pharm Biomed Anal 13: 823–828
14. Herve F, Urien S, Albengres E, Duche JC, Tillement JP (1994) Drug binding in plasma. A summary of recent trends in the study of drug and hormone binding. Clin Pharmacokinet 26: 44–58
15. Martyn JA, Abernethy DR, Greenblatt DJ (1984) Plasma protein binding of drugs after severe burn injury. Clin Pharmacol Ther 35: 535–539
16. Hammons KB, Edwards RF, Rice WY (2006) Golf-inhibiting gynecomastia associated with atorvastatin therapy. Pharmacotherapy 26: 1165–1168
17. Benet LZ, Hoener BA (2002) Changes in plasma protein binding have little clinical relevance. Clin Pharmacol Ther 71: 115–121
18. Vrhovac B, Sarapa N, Bakran I, et al (1995) Pharmacokinetic changes in patients with oedema. Clin Pharmacokinet 28: 405–418
19. Barlage S, Frohlich D, Bottcher A, et al (2001) ApoE-containing high density lipoproteins and phospholipid transfer protein activity increase in patients with a systemic inflammatory response. J Lipid Res 42: 281–290
20. Sampliner R, Perrier D, Powell R, Finley P (1984) Influence of ascites on tobramycin pharmacokinetics. J Clin Pharmacol 24: 43–46
21. Buijk SL, Gyssens IC, Mouton JW, Van Vliet A, Verbrugh HA, Bruining HA (2002) Pharmacokinetics of ceftazidime in serum and peritoneal exudate during continuous versus intermittent administration to patients with severe intra-abdominal infections. J Antimicrob Chemother 49: 121–128
22. Botha FJ, van der Bijl P, Seifart HI, Parkin DP (1996) Fluctuation of the volume of distribution of amikacin and its effect on once-daily dosage and clearance in a seriously ill patient. Intensive Care Med 22: 443–446
23. Ronchera-Oms CL, Tormo C, Ordovas JP, Abad J, Jimenez NV (1995) Expanded gentamicin volume of distribution in critically ill adult patients receiving total parenteral nutrition. J Clin Pharm Ther 20: 253–258
24. Reaand RS, Capitano B (2007) Optimizing use of aminoglycosides in the critically ill. Semin Respir Crit Care Med 28: 596–603
25. Mimoz O, Schaeffer V, Incagnoli P, et al (2001) Co-amoxiclav pharmacokinetics during posttraumatic hemorrhagic shock. Crit Care Med 29: 1350–1355
26. Park GR (1996) Molecular mechanisms of drug metabolism in the critically ill. Br J Anaesth 77: 32–49
27. McKindley DS, Hanes S, Boucher BA (1998) Hepatic drug metabolism in critical illness. Pharmacotherapy 18: 759–778
28. Aninat C, Seguin P, Descheemaeker PN, Morel F, Malledant Y, Guillouzo A (2008) Catecholamines induce an inflammatory response in human hepatocytes. Crit Care Med 36: 848–854
29. Boucher BA, Kuhl DA, Fabian TC, Robertson JT (1991) Effect of neurotrauma on hepatic drug clearance. Clin Pharmacol Ther 50: 487–497
30. Meier-Hellmann A, Reinhart K, Bredle DL, Specht M, Spies CD, Hannemann L (1997) Epinephrine impairs splanchnic perfusion in septic shock. Crit Care Med 25: 399–404
31. Obritsch MD, Bestul DJ, Jung R, Fish DN, MacLaren R (2004) The role of vasopressin in vasodilatory septic shock. Pharmacotherapy 24: 1050–1063
32. De Backer D, Creteur J, Silva E, Vincent JL (2003) Effects of dopamine, norepinephrine, and epinephrine on the splanchnic circulation in septic shock: which is best? Crit Care Med 31: 1659–1667
33. Weinbren MJ (1999) Pharmacokinetics of antibiotics in burn patients. J Antimicrob Chemother 44: 319–327

34. Kumar A, Roberts D, Wood KE, et al (2006) Duration of hypotension before initiation of effective antimicrobial therapy is the critical determinant of survival in human septic shock. Crit Care Med 34: 1589–1596
35. Lipman J, Wallis SC, Boots RJ (2003) Cefepime versus cefpirome: the importance of creatinine clearance. Anesth Analg 97: 1149–1154
36. Han TH, Lee JH, Kwak IS, Kil HY, Han KW, Kim KM (2005) The relationship between bispectral index and targeted propofol concentration is biphasic in patients with major burns. Acta Anaesthesiol Scand 49: 85–91
37. Tschida SJ, Hoey LL, Nahum A, Vance-Bryan K (1995) Atracurium resistance in a critically Ill patient. Pharmacotherapy 15: 533–539
38. Link E, Parish S, Bowman L, et al (2008) SLCOBI Variants and statin-induced myopathy – a genomewide study. N Engl J Med 359: 789–799
39. Zeitlinger MA, Dehghanyar P, Mayer BX, et al (2003) Relevance of soft-tissue penetration by levofloxacin for target site bacterial killing in patients with sepsis. Antimicrob Agents Chemother 47: 3548–3553
40. Denaroand CP, Ravenscroft PJ (1989) Comparison of Sawchuk-Zaske and Bayesian forecasting for aminoglycosides in seriously ill patients. Br J Clin Pharmacol 28: 37–44
41. Aarons L (1991) Population pharmacokinetics: theory and practice. Br J Clin Pharmacol 32: 669–670
42. U.S. Department of Health and Human Services, FDA, CDER, CBER (1999) Guidance for industry: population pharmacokinetics. Available at: http://www.fda.gov/cber/gdlns/popharm.pdf Accessed Nov 2008
43. Steimer JL, Mallet A, Golmard JL, Boisvieux JF (1984) Alternative approaches to estimation of population pharmacokinetic parameters: comparison with the nonlinear mixed-effect model. Drug Metab Rev 15: 265–292
44. Sheiner LB, Beal S, Rosenberg B, Marathe VV (1979) Forecasting individual pharmacokinetics. Clin Pharmacol Ther 26: 294–305
45. Roberts JA, Kruger P, Paterson DL, Lipman J (2008) Antibiotic resistance--what's dosing got to do with it? Crit Care Med 36: 2433–2440
46. del Mar Fernandez de Gatta Garcia M, Revilla N, Calvo MV, Dominguez-Gil A, Sanchez Navarro A (2007) Pharmacokinetic/pharmacodynamic analysis of vancomycin in ICU patients. Intensive Care Med 33: 279–285

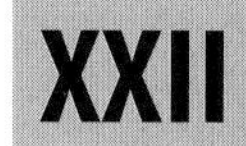

Relevant CYP450-mediated Drug Interactions in the ICU

I. Spriet and W. Meersseman

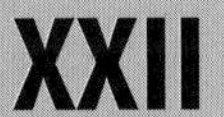

Introduction

As multiple drug therapies are often used at the same time, the potential for clinically significant drug interactions in intensive care unit (ICU) patients is large [1]. Moreover, disease-related factors, such as altered drug distribution, renal insufficiency, and hepatic disease or altered protein binding, typically occurring in the critically ill will contribute to the wide interindividual variability in drug exposure and response and to the high risk of drug interactions [2]. The majority of drugs used in the ICU are metabolized by the iso-enzymes of the cytochrome P450 (CYP450) system [3]. This chapter provides a practical overview of CYP450-mediated drug interactions with high relevance to ICU patients.

The Role of CYP450 in Drug Metabolism

Drug interactions can be pharmacokinetic or pharmacodynamic in nature. Pharmacokinetic interactions will result in altered concentrations of a drug or its metabolites while pharmacodynamic interactions will change the response to a drug. Pharmacokinetic interactions can occur during the absorption, distribution, or excretion phase; however, the most dangerous and most prevalent pharmacokinetic interactions will involve drug metabolism [4].

The liver is the major organ handling drug metabolism, and two phases can be distinguished as shown in **Figure 1**. During phase I, a parent compound will be converted into a more water-soluble metabolite, which can be either pharmacologically

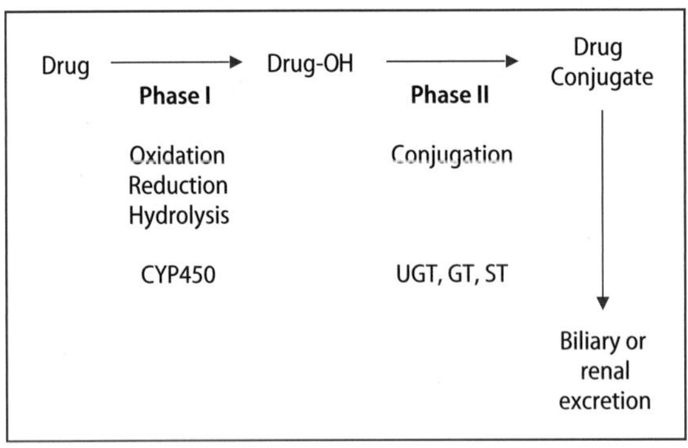

Fig. 1. Drug metabolism in the liver. CYP450: cytochrome P450 enzyme system; UGT: uridine glucuronosyl transferase; GT: glutathione transferase; ST: sulfotransferase

active or inactive [4]. The majority of these phase I reactions are handled by the CYP450-isoenzymes. Phase II reactions are not mediated by CYP450 and will result in the conjugation of the parent drug or the phase I metabolite with endogenous molecules such as glucuronic acid or glutathione. During phase II, the compound will be rendered even more water soluble, so that excretion is facilitated [4].

CYP450 is a family of enzymes that catalyzes the metabolism of many endogenous substances such as steroids, fatty acids, and bile acids. In addition, it also handles the metabolism of xenobiotics [5]. The enzymes are located in the smooth endoplasmic reticulum of the hepatocytes, and to a lesser extent in the epithelium of the small intestine, lungs, kidney, and brain. Fifty-seven enzymes have been identified in humans; each of them is encoded by a separate gene. Based on similarity in amino-acid sequence, the enzymes are grouped into families and subfamilies [5]. In that way, enzymes in the same family, e.g., CYP3A, are homologous for about 50 % of amino-acid sequences, and enzymes within the same subfamily, e.g., CYP3A4, are homologous for more than 55 %. In humans, six enzymes are responsible for the bulk of drug metabolism: CYP1A2, 2C9, 2C19, 2D6, 2E1, and 3A4 [5].

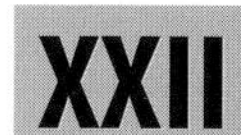

Inhibition and Induction

CYP450-mediated metabolism can be inhibited or induced. Enzyme induction occurs when an inducer enhances the synthesis or slows down the breakdown of a CYP450 enzyme. This will lead to an increase in enzyme activity and will result in lower plasma concentrations of the substrate [4, 6]. In the case of an active parent compound, this will result in a decreased effect. However, in the case of a prodrug requiring metabolism to its active metabolite, enzyme induction will lead to an increased effect. The maximal effect will develop over several days or weeks, as new protein synthesis is usually required. Similarly, after withdrawal of the inducing agent, the effect will generally persist for a similar period, depending on both the half-life of the inducer and the induced enzyme [4, 6].

In contrast, enzyme inhibition will lead to higher plasma concentration and an increased effect of the inhibited substrate, except in the case of prodrugs. The onset of enzyme inhibition is usually rapid, the effect takes place as soon as sufficient concentrations of the inhibitor reach the CYP450 enzyme. The effect will be maximal if steady state concentrations of the inhibitor are reached. In general, enzyme inhibition can occur based on two mechanisms: Competitive inhibition, in which the substrate and inhibitor compete for the same site on the enzyme, and mechanism-based inhibition, in which the inhibitor is metabolized to an active intermediate which binds covalently to the CYP450 enzyme so that the enzyme is no longer functional. Competitive inhibition is also called reversible, as it is transient: The enzyme will act normally once the inhibitor has been excreted. Mechanism-based inhibition is irreversible as the intermediate-enzyme complex cannot be reversed, and new protein synthesis is required to restore enzyme activity [4, 6].

Interindividual Variability in CYP450-mediated Metabolism

Among the population, it is shown that people can have either an extensive or a poor ability to metabolize drugs dependent on CYP450-activity; the distribution of the activity of certain CYP450-isoenzymes is polymodal [7]. This distribution is determined by genetic polymorphisms, which refer to a mutation in CYP450-genes determining enzyme activity. Genetic polymorphism has been described for CYP1A2, 2C9, 2C19, 2D6 and 2E1. Variant alleles can lead to increased, decreased, or no activity of the CYP450 enzyme, according to three phenotypes: Poor, extensive and ultrarapid metabolizers [7]. The last group exhibits increased metabolic activity due to duplicated alleles. If the elimination of a drug is primarily determined by metabolism, and a single CYP450 enzyme is responsible, a functional polymorphism may have important clinical consequences. The administration of a standard dose will result in distinct clinical effect. The frequency of variant alleles en enzyme activity varies among populations according to race and ethnic background [7].

In addition to genetic polymorphism, it has been shown in *in vitro* studies that CYP450 metabolism is inhibited by the release of the pro-inflammatory cytokines, interleukin (IL)-6 and tumor necrosis factor (TNF)-α. Many ICU patients are, therefore, more prone to adverse drug interactions [8].

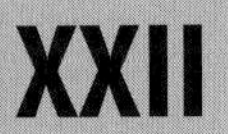

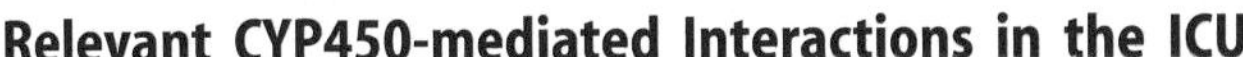

Relevant CYP450-mediated Interactions in the ICU

Drugs metabolized by CYP3A4, 2C9, 2C19 and 2D6 are discussed in this chapter, as these are most relevant for ICU practice. We based the evaluation of reviews on the azoles, rifampicin, proton pump inhibitors, glucocorticoids, anti-epileptics, antibiotics, and immunosuppressants [9–15].

Drug Interactions Involving CYP3A4

CYP3A4 is probably the most important of all drug metabolizing enzymes as it accounts for nearly 50 % of the CYP450 enzymes, and because it handles the oxidative biotransformation of more than half of the drugs that undergo metabolism by oxidation [4]. The activity of CYP3A4 can vary among the population, but its distribution is unimodal. This suggests that several genes regulate the protein but that individual genetic factors, such as genetic polymorphism, do not play a role [4].

CYP3A4 is expressed both in the liver and in the epithelium of the small intestine, so inhibition or induction can occur at both sites [4, 16]. As a result, CYP3A4-mediated drug interactions are likely to be more relevant after oral than intravenous drug administration. In the small bowel, CYP3A4 forms a barrier against drug absorption together with the transporter protein, P-glycoprotein (P-gp). P-gp works as an efflux pump which limits and regulates access to CYP3A4. As an orally administered substrate is repeatedly transported out by P-gp towards the gut lumen and then passively reabsorbed, this continuous repeated exposure leads to more efficient metabolism. Thus, after oral administration of a drug, CYP3A4/P-gp located in the intestine together with CYP3A4 in the liver may reduce the portion of the dose that reaches the systemic circulation leading to a lower bio-availability, a phenomenon called the first-pass effect [4, 16].

Many drugs inhibit CYP3A4. Potent inhibitors include the azoles, calcium antagonists and macrolide antibiotics such as erythromycin and clarithromycin [4, 9, 14]. On the contrary, rifampicin, phenytoin, phenobarbital, and carbamazepine will all lead to a reduction in plasma concentrations of compounds metabolized by CYP3A4. These drugs are potent CYP3A4 inducers [4, 10, 13].

Substrates of CYP3A4: Midazolam, tacrolimus, cyclosporine, (su)fentanyl and methylprednisolone

Midazolam, which is widely used as a sedative in ICU because of its predictable effect and easy titration is primarily metabolized by CYP3A4, and thus, particularly prone to drug interactions. Excessive sedation is reported when combined with potent inhibitors such as itraconazole, voriconazole, and the macrolides [9, 14, 17]. Only one study has investigated the combination of midazolam as a continuous infusion and fluconazole in ICU patients [18]. Plasma levels rose variably with increases from minimal up to 300 %. The authors recommended reducing midazolam infusion rate when fluconazole is initiated and when the degree of sedation is increasing [18]. Sedative effects should be carefully monitored if azoles or macrolides are associated [9, 14]. To prevent weaning problems, daily interruption of midazolam until patients are awake or alternative regimens with propofol or lorazepam can be considered [19].

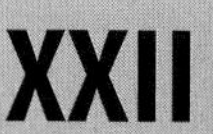

In contrast, although not studied for intravenous midazolam pharmacokinetics, the effect of midazolam will be completely lost if it is combined with potent inducers such as phenytoin or rifampicin [10, 13].

Tacrolimus and cyclosporine, both frequently used immunosuppressants, are for the most part metabolized by CYP3A4 in the liver and the small bowel and, therefore, often victims of CYP3A4 inhibition and induction [20]. Moreover, both drugs are regularly administered by mouth and, as a result, CYP3A4 interactions will be more pronounced after oral administration [16]. Both drugs have a narrow therapeutic window and increased concentrations can lead to important toxicity [20]. The list of drugs interacting with tacrolimus and cyclosporine plasma levels contains nearly all known CYP3A4 inhibitors and inducers [20]. Daily monitoring of plasma levels of both drugs is necessary to avoid toxicity and warrant efficacy, if combined with interacting drugs. Plasma levels of both can be markedly increased by clarithromycin and erythromycin; for cyclosporine this is reported to be often complicated by acute renal failure [20]. When macrolides are used to treat *Mycoplasma* or *Legionella* pneumonia, azithromycin, which is not believed to inhibit CYP3A4, or quinolones are the best choice. The azoles also inhibit metabolism of both drugs [15]. Dosages of tacrolimus and cyclosporine should be reduced if combined with voriconazole, respectively by 66 and 50 % [15, 20]. Inadequate levels caused by induction of rifampicin may lead to graft rejection. Interestingly, the potent inducers phenytoin and phenobarbital, have been used as treatment for acute tacrolimus overdose [21, 22].

Fentanyl and sufentanil are strong opioids that are also both metabolized by CYP3A4. However, these drugs are known to have a high hepatic extraction ratio. This makes these drugs less sensitive to CYP450-mediated drug interactions, as hepatic clearance is less likely to be affected by changes in metabolic activity. For example, if itraconazole is associated, the pharmacokinetics of fentanyl will not change [23]. Even so, in patients on long term carbamazepine or phenytoin, higher doses of fentanyl will be required [24]. Remifentanil can be used as alternative if important CYP3A4 inhibitors or inducers cannot be avoided. It is metabolized by aspecific esterases in plasma and no pharmacokinetic interactions have been reported. But the drug is significantly more expensive than other opioids [25].

Methylprednisolone is partially metabolized by CYP3A4 and the potent CYP3A4 inhibitors voriconazole, itraconazole and macrolides can, therefore, increase its plasma levels [12]. This may lead to enhanced adrenal suppression, or, more important, to an increased immunosuppressive effect, which is undesirable in patients at risk for infections. As expected, it is also sensitive to enzyme induction by phenobarbital, carbamazepine, phenytoin and rifampicin [12].

Little is known about the interactive properties of hydrocortisone, although this drug is frequently used in patients with septic shock and inadequate adrenal response .

Drug Interactions involving CYP2C9 and CYP2C19: Phenytoin and Warfarin

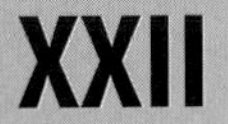

CYP2C9 and CYP2C19 appear to play a major role in the complex metabolism of phenytoin. Genetic polymorphism is described for both iso-enzymes, so higher phenytoin levels can be observed, especially in CYP2C9 poor metabolizers. If phenytoin plasma levels rise above 25 mg/dl, toxicity presenting with confusion, respiratory depression and coma can occur. It is prudent to regularly monitor plasma levels in order to prevent adverse effects [26]. When phenytoin is associated with azole therapy, especially fluconazole, complex interactions take place. On the one hand, plasma levels of phenytoin will increase rapidly as fluconazole strongly inhibits both CYP2C9 and 2C19. However, phenytoin itself is a potent inducer, leading to a marked reduction in fluconazole levels [9].

Warfarin is worth mentioning; it is still commonly used and potentially involved in many drug interactions sometimes leading to life-threatening bleeding. Warfarin has complex pharmacokinetics, as it is a racemic mixture with two active isomers having separate metabolism [27]. The S-warfarin is the more active isomer and is inactivated by CYP2C9; consequently potent CYP2C9 inhibitors, such as fluconazole, may potentiate the effect of warfarin. CYP2C9 inducers, such as rifampicin, will do the converse. The R-isomer is metabolized by different hepatic enzymes, and as it has less activity, drug interactions are generally of less clinical relevance [27]. It is well known that the warfarin dose to obtain therapeutic International Normalized Ratio (INR) values varies widely among patients. Recently this has been explained, as genetic polymorphisms are discovered both in the CYP2C9 gene coding for the isoenzyme that is responsible for its metabolism, but also in the gene (VKORC) coding for the vitamin K epoxide reductase enzyme (which is the hepatic target protein for the mechanism of action of warfarin) [28]. Patients with certain common genetic variants of CYP2C9 will metabolize warfarin more slowly, and are more likely to have higher INR values during warfarin initiation. Moreover, patients with a VKORC polymorphism will typically require lower warfarin doses [28]. Based on this information, clinicians may consider using pharmacogenetic information before warfarin therapy is initiated [29].

Drug Interactions Involving CYP2D6

CYP2D6 plays a major role in the metabolism of drugs frequently used in the ambulatory setting, such as opioids, selective serotonin reuptake inhibitors (SSRIs) and beta-blocking agents. Quinidine, haloperidol, and some of the SSRIs, such as paroxetine and fluoxetin, are known to be inhibitors. Induction has not been described [4].

In the superfamily of CYP450-enzymes, CYP2D6 was the first example of genetic polymorphism identified. Ultrarapid metabolizers, generally rare (1–3 %) in Caucasians, have higher enzyme activity leading to accelerated metabolism of the parent compound. In poor metabolizers (5–10 % of Caucasians), plasma levels of the parent drug will rise even with usual doses [30]. CYP2D6 is responsible for the conversion of codeine to morphine, an active metabolite, so clinical pain relief is more difficult to achieve in persons with poor metabolism. In contrast, several cases have been reported in which morphine-induced side effects are related to ultrarapid metabolism of codeine [31, 32].

Future Perspectives

Individual variation in response to drugs is a problem that physicians routinely face in clinical practice. The clinical consequences of drug interactions involving CYP450-mediated metabolism are well known for some drugs outside the ICU setting and has led to removal from the market of some agents (e.g., terfenadine, astemizole, and mibefradil). As drug interactions involving the inhibition and induction of CYP450, especially CYP3A4, will undoubtedly continue to be of scientific interest, a lot of effort is now being put into *in vitro* tests using recombinant CYP450 to predict drug interactions during drug development. Using recombinant CYP450, it is possible to determine a particular substance's metabolic pathways, genetic polymorphisms, and its ability to inhibit or induce drug metabolism.

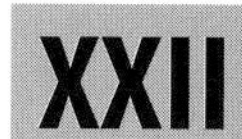

Interestingly, recent screening programs for new drugs try to filter out chemical substances that display high affinities for CYP450, so that CYP450-mediated drug interactions can be avoided. However, as a consequence, it has been demonstrated that hepatic drug interactions frequently extend beyond the classical involvement of CYP450 metabolism. It has also been shown that drug interactions can also be expected at the level of drug transport handled by transport proteins over the apical and basolateral membrane of the hepatocyte. As a result, it is expected that a substantial number of drug-drug interactions occurring at the hepatic uptake phase will be reported within the next few years.

For many years, there has been strong evidence that the presence of variant CYP450 alleles has important clinical consequences; however, a patient's particular genotype is rarely determined in clinical practice. Recently, the US Food and Drug Administration approved the first genotype test designed to guide the selection of medications metabolized by CYP450-enzymes with polymorphisms. The Amplichip CYP450 test is a DNA micro-array test that can detect 29 polymorphisms of CYP2D6 and two polymorphisms of CYP2C19. Large, prospective studies are now needed to determine whether use of genotyping in clinical practice increases drug efficacy, prevents or reduces adverse drug reactions, or lowers the overall costs of therapy [33].

Conclusion

The complex environment of the ICU makes the potential for clinically relevant drug interactions very high. The majority of drugs used in the ICU are metabolized by CYP3A4. As a result of this enzyme's critical role in drug metabolism, inhibition or induction of drugs metabolized by this enzyme will lead to marked changes in plasma concentrations. Knowledge of CYP3A4's most important substrates, inhibitors, and inducers is fundamental to achieve therapeutic efficacy and avoid drug-related toxicity.

References

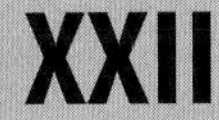

1. Kopp BJ, Erstad BL, Allen ME, Theodorou AA, Priestley G (2006) Medication errors and adverse drug events in an intensive care unit: direct observation approach for detection. Crit Care Med 34: 415–425
2. Krishnan V, Murray P (2003) Pharmacologic issues in the critically ill. Clin Chest Med 24: 671–688
3. Mann HJ(2006) Drug-associated disease: cytochrome P450 interactions. Crit Care Clin 22: 329–345
4. Wilkinson GR (2005) Drug metabolism and variability among patients in drug response. N Engl J Med 352: 2211–2221
5. Lewis DF (2004) 57 varieties: the human cytochromes P450. Pharmacogenomics 5: 305–318
6. Lin JH, Lu AYH (1998) Inhibition and induction of cytochrome P450 and the clinical implications. Clin Pharmacokinet 35: 361–390
7. Pirmohamed M, Park BK (2003) Cytochrome P450 enzyme polymorphisms and adverse drug reactions. Toxicol 192: 23–32
8. Renton KW (2004) Cytochrome P450 regulation and drug biotransformation during inflammation and infection. Curr Drug Metab 5: 235–243
9. Venkatakrishnan K, von Moltke LL, Greenblatt DJ (2000) Effects of the antifungal agents on oxidative drug metabolism. Clin Pharmacokinet 38: 111–180
10. Finch CK, Chrisman CR, Baciewicz AM, Self TH (2002) Rifampin and rifabutin drug interactions. An update. Arch Intern Med 162: 985–992
11. Gerson LB, Triadafilopoulos G (2001) Proton pump inhibitors and their drug interactions: an evidence-based approach. Eur J Gastroenterol Hepatol 13: 611–616
12. Czock D, Keller F, Rasche FM, Häussler U (2005) Pharmacokinetics and pharmacodynamics of systemically administered glucocorticoids. Clin Pharmacokinet 44: 61–98
13. Perucca E (2005) Clinically relevant drug interactions with antiepileptic drugs. Br J Clin Pharmacol 61: 246–255
14. Pai MP, Momary KM, Rodvold KA (2006) Antibiotic drug interactions. Med Clin N Am 90: 1223–1255
15. Saad AH, DePestel D, Carver P (2006) Factors influencing the magnitude and clinical significance of drug interactions between azole antifungals and select immunosuppressants. Pharmacotherapy 26: 1730–1744
16. Doherty MM, Charman WH (2002) The mucosa of the small intestine: how clinically relevant as an organ of drug metabolism. Clin Pharmacokinet 41: 235–253
17. Gorski JC, Jones DR, Haehner-Daniels BD, Hamman MA, O'Mara EM, Hall SD (1998) The contribution of intestinal and hepatic CYP3A to the interaction between midazolam and clarithromycin. Clin Pharmacol Ther 64: 133–143
18. Ahonen J, Olkkola KT, Takala A, Neuvonen PJ (1999) Interaction between fluconazole and midazolam in intensive care patients. Acta Anaesthesiol Scand 43: 509–514
19. Kress JP, Pohlman AS, O'Connor MF, Hall JB (2000) Daily interruption of sedative infusions in critically ill patients undergoing mechanical ventilation. N Engl J Med 342: 1471–1477
20. Leather HL (2004) Drug interactions in the hematopoetic stem cell transplant (HSCT) recipient: what every transplanter needs to know. Bone Marrow Transplant 33: 137–152
21. Karasu Z, Gurakar A, Carlson J, et al (2001) Acute tacrolimus overdose and treatment with phenytoin in liver transplant recipients. J Okla State Med Assoc 94: 121–123
22. McLaughlin GE, Gonzalez-Rossique M, Gelman B, Kato T (2000) Use of phenobarbital in the management of acute tacrolimus toxicity: a case report. Transplant Proc 32: 665–668
23. Palkama VJ, Neuvonen PJ, Olkolla KT (1998) The CYP3A4 inhibitor itraconazole has no effect on the pharmacokinetics and pharmacodynamics of i.v. fentanyl. Br J Anaesth 81: 598–600
24. Tempelhoff R, Modica P, Spitznagel E (1988) Increased fentanyl requirement in patients receiving long-term anticonvulsant therapy. Anesthesiology 69: A594 (abst)
25. Beers R, Camporesi E (2004) Remifentanil update: clinical science and utility. CNS Drugs 18: 1085–1104
26. Anderson GD (2008) Pharmacokinetic, pharmacodynamic, and pharmacogenetic targeted therapy of antiepileptic drugs. Ther Drug Monit 30: 173–180

27. Holbrook AM, Pereira JA, Labiris R, et al (2005) Systematic overview of warfarin and its drug and food interactions. Arch Intern Med 165: 1095–1106
28. Schwarz UI, Ritchie MD, Bradford Y, et al (2008) Genetic determinants of response to warfarin during initial anticoagulation. N Engl J Med 358: 999–1008
29. Limdi NA, Veenstra DL (2008) Warfarin pharmacogenetics. Pharmacother 28: 1084–1087
30. Ozawa S, Soyama A, Saeki M, et al (2004) Ethnic differences in genetic polymorphisms of CYP2D6, CYP2C19, CYP3As and MDR1/ABCB1. Drug Metab Pharmacokinet 19: 83–95
31. Stamer UM, Stüber F, Muders T, Musshoff F (2008) Respiratory depression with tramadol in a patient with renal impairment and CYP2D6 gene duplication. Anesth Analg 107: 926–929
32. Gashe Y, Daaili Y, Fathi M, et al (2004) Codeine intoxication associated with ultrarapid CYP2D6 metabolism. N Engl J Med 351: 2827–2837
33. U.S. Food and Drug Administration. Center for Devices and Radiological Health consumer information. New device clearance. Roche Amplichip cytochrome P450 genotyping test and Affymetrix GeneChip Microarray Instrumentation System – K042259. Available from: http://www.fda.gov/cdrh/mda/docs/k042259.html Accessed, Nov 2008

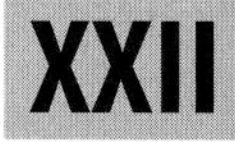

XXIII Sedation and Analgesia

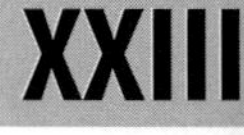

Sedation and Pain Management in the ICU

M.A. Mirski and J.J. Lewin III

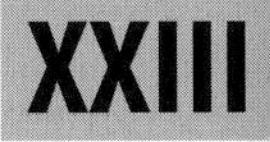

Introduction

During the past decade, critical care physicians have recognized that routinely maintaining patients in a pharmacological deep stupor or unconsciousness as a consequence of sedation is not beneficial. Data has since emerged to support the concept that more optimal, lower dosing of sedatives with preservation of the wakeful state is important in reducing mortality and shortening the duration of mechanical ventilation and overall intensive care unit (ICU) length of stay (LOS) [1–4]. Such emphasis also aids in supporting patient autonomy and in the prevention of and early intervention for evolving neurological deterioration [5–7]. Such tenets are in keeping with the guidelines from the Society of Critical Care Medicine (SCCM) for patient sedation [8]. More interactive patients require that regular assessments be made to ensure adequacy of comfort and analgesia. Along parallel lines, the US Joint Commission on Accreditation of Healthcare Organizations (JCAHO) introduced in 2000 their mandate for the implementation of standards for pain assessment and treatment in hospitalized patients [9].

This renaissance of encouraging a more interactive state for ICU patients has required adaptation on the part of the medical and surgical intensivists in their approach to sedation. It has also forced a pharmacological reappraisal of the medications selected, dosing algorithms, routes and modes of administration, and sedation scales appropriate for titration. Both the depths and duration of sedation have come under critical review, with the emphasis now clearly towards low-dose continuous regimens or intermittent periods of arousal incorporating a titration scheme to use the least medication necessary to achieve a comfortable and controlled behavioral state.

The Need for Sedation or Analgesia in the ICU

The pharmacological therapy for sedation commonly embraces provision for analgesia, anxiolysis, antipsychosis, or a combination thereof. Correct diagnosis of a single or overlapping disturbance thus becomes the starting point, as there are medications with broad therapeutic effects as well as those directed towards a specific pathology. To minimize toxicity and side effects, it is best to select agents appropriate for the indication.

Management of Pain

The prerequisite for analgesic therapy is discomfort. Unfortunately, the ICU is replete with reasons for patients to complain of pain (**Table 1**). Most are due to primary physiological discomfort associated with focal disease or injury (e.g., broken bones, surgical incisional pain), and other forms of superficial or visceral discomfort that may have poorly localizable foci. Pain may also occur as a primary consequence of neurophysiological dysfunction as in the case of neuropathic pain, headache, intracranial pressure (ICP) elevation, etc. Unfortunately, critical care therapies themselves often lend themselves to discomfort in the form of ICU procedures and management processes such as mechanical ventilation, therapeutic suctioning, patient turning and positioning.

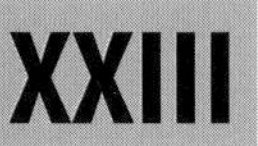

Not all pain should be suppressed in its entirety, particularly discomfort that provides a clinical guide to the evolution of a pathological process such as an acute abdomen or compartment syndrome. Nevertheless, studies have demonstrated that patients cared for in an ICU are apt to be in considerable discomfort during some portions of their stay, and overall management of pain during critical care has remained sub-optimal. In a recent large series of mechanically ventilated patients, procedural discomfort was specifically managed in less than 25 % of the population, and the use of guidelines for analgesia and sedation promoted less, not more therapy for pain management [10]. Specific to procedure, a nursing report documented that patients commonly expressed great differences between pre- and post-procedural levels of discomfort with interventions of drain removal, deep breathing and coughing exercises, suctioning, and line removal [11]. In that series, less than 50 % of patients received pre-procedural analgesia. The authors also noted that routine monitoring of hemodynamic parameters, such as heart rate and blood pressure, often failed to serve as indicators of patient discomfort.

To quantify patient discomfort, a considerable number of pain measures are employed in the ICU setting. Some are used primarily in awake, responsive patients, such as the commonly used Numerical Rating Scale (1 to 10) and the Visual Analog Scale (VAS, 1 to 100) [12]. Other quantitative measures have been adopted to assess discomfort in patients unable to self-rate their level of pain as in the case of a sedated, mechanically ventilated patient. Such examples include the Behavioral Pain Rating Scale (BPRS) [13], Behavioral Pain Scale (BPS) [14], Critical-Care Pain Observational Tool (CPOT) [15], Nonverbal Pain Scale (NVPS) [16], and the Pain Assessment and Intervention Notation (PAIN) Algorithm [17]. All of the latter scor-

Table 1. Examples of ICU pain syndromes

Localized pain	Diffuse visceral	Neurologic	Complex
Surgical wound	Acute abdomen	Intracranial hemorrhage	Mechanical ventilation
Bone fracture	Myocardial ischemia	Headache-migraine	Diffuse joint pain – arthralgia
Ulceration	Pneumonia	Elevated intracranial pressure	Sickle cell
Pleurodynia	Myocarditis	Compressive neuropathy	Metabolic disorders
Invasive procedure	Pulmonary embolus	Subarachnoid hemorrhage	Febrile – sepsis
Local burn injury	Vascular ischemia	Cranial neuritis	
Compartment syndromes	Gastritis	Diabetic neuropathy	
Uretheral stone	Pancreatitis	Reflex dystrophy	
Appendicitis	Bowel obstruction	Meningismus	

ing devices include measures of a variety of behavioral dimensions to provide a comprehensive assessment in the non-verbal patient. Both the BPRS and the BPS have undergone complete content, criterion, and construct validity testing, and the BPS has further documented inter-rater reliability testing [14]. Many studies assessing quantification of pain in ICU patients have demonstrated that self-reporting of discomfort indeed has the greatest correlation with multi-domain behavioral ratings compared with single item scoring [18].

Unfortunately, ICU pain management regimens do risk diminishing the overall level of arousal when administered in a fashion to eliminate all of the patient's perception of pain or stigmata of discomfort. In lieu of such hazard, especially in the neurologically compromised patient, analgesia should be titrated to effect with preservation of responsiveness, typically to reduce the pain to less than a 3 on a 0–10 ordinal scale. Medications utilized include non-steroidal anti-inflammatory drugs (aspirin, acetaminophen, ibuprofen, ketorolac), narcotics (both pure and mixed mu-opioid receptor agonists), α_2-agonists (clonidine and dexmedetomidine), steroids, ketamine, and local anesthetics.

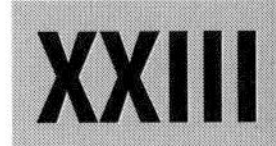

Anxiolysis

Anxiolysis represents the therapy most sought after when delivering 'sedation'. It is the provision of pharmacotherapy to lessen feelings of apprehension, anxiety, diminish general nervous tension or 'stress', and to treat the most severe form of excited disequilibrium – agitation. Psychologically demanding circumstances in critical care are numerous, with common general ICU stressors being the psychological responses to a life-threatening illness, unfamiliar surroundings, near constant noise and activity, disturbed sleep-wake cycles, and overall sense of lack of control. Specific ICU treatments and conditions that add to this mix include endotracheal intubation and mechanical ventilation, need for restraints, traumatic head injury, sepsis, febrile state, medication effects, and other etiologies of encephalopathy.

Since both pain and anxiety are commonly combined, it is important to discern whether pain is paramount, leading to agitation, or if anxiety/agitation are separate signs or symptoms of the patient. Several agents are very effective in anxiolysis, such as the benzodiazepines or the sedative/hypnotic agents, like the barbiturates and propofol. Some provide both analgesia and anxiolysis, e.g., α_2-agonists, ketamine, and some narcotics in low doses.

Delirium

Delirium is a dysfunctional cognitive state that has gained great interest as a predictor of poor outcome in hospitalized patients, particularly in the ICU [19, 20]. It is not easily diagnosed unless the diagnosis is specifically entertained, and even then the clinical features of delirium may be confounded by coincident neurological disturbances. Specific scoring batteries have been designed for diagnostic purpose (the most popular is the Confusion Assessment Method for the Intensive Care Unit [CAM-ICU]) [19], and their introduction has led to data supporting that delirium is an independent predictor of longer hospital stay, greater mortality, and ICU costs [20]. It remains unclear, however, whether all forms of delirium are equally hazardous. Especially in the ICU setting, there is a breadth of conditions that incite the encephalopathic state and delirium in a transient or persistent manner, and each with likely different effect on the patient's physiological state. Several examples include metabolic dysfunction, electrolyte abnormalities, relative hypoxia, acid-base disturbances, drug-induced cognitive dysfunction, and loss of adequate sleep and sleep-wake cycling. It still remains to be seen whether effective treatment of delirium improves these indices.

Choice of Agent

Once a decision is made to treat an individual with sedative medication, the choice of pharmacotherapy is expansive. There exist many classes of drugs, including the narcotics, benzodiazepines, barbiturates, propofol, neuroleptics, α_2-adrenergic agents, ketamine, and several other lesser classes of chemical agents. Each has advantages and disadvantages in the ICU patient, and between and within each class are agents with varied pharmacokinetics, routes of administration, titratability, adverse reactions, and hemodynamic profiles. It is generally recommended that shorter-acting agents be used in the critical care setting when serial neurological examinations are important [7]. Where relevant, the reversibility, drug-drug interactions, and cost-effectiveness will also be discussed. We present a summary of the main characteristics of preferred sedatives and analgesics in ICU patients in **Tables 2** and **3**.

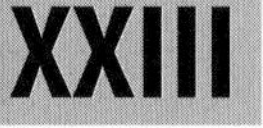

Table 2. Pharmacological profile of common ICU sedative/analgesic agents

Drug	Type of medication	Sedation	Analgesia	Mechanism of action	Advantages	Adverse effects
Fentanyl	Opioid	+	+++	Mu receptor agonist	Potent, reversible, rapid onset, short duration	Respiratory depression, chest wall rigidity, gastric dysmotility, hypotension
Remifentanil	Opioid	+	+++	Mu receptor agonist	Potent, reversible, rapid onset, short duration	Respiratory depression, chest wall rigidity, gastric dysmotility, hypotension
Morphine sulfate	Opioid	+	+++	Mu receptor agonist	Reversible, promotes sleep	Respiratory depression, gastric dysmotility, hypotension, hallucinations
Hydromorphone	Opioid	+	+++	Mu receptor agonist	Reversible, longer duration	Respiratory depression, gastric dysmotility,
Ketamine	Non-barbiturate anesthetic/analgesic agent	+++	+++	NMDA agonist	Preserves ventilatory drive, pharyngeal-laryngeal reflexes, & cardiovascular stability	Dissociative state, hallucinations, delirium, tachyarrythmia
Diazepam	Benzodiazepine	+++	+	$GABA_a$ receptor agonist	Reversible, short duration	Respiratory depression, hypotension, confusion, long-acting active metabolite

Table 2. (*cont.*)

Drug	Type of medication	Sedation	Analgesia	Mechanism of action	Advantages	Adverse effects
Lorazepam	Benzodiazepine	+++	–	$GABA_a$ receptor agonist	Reversible, longer duration	Respiratory depression, hypotension, confusion
Midazolam	Benzodiazepine	+++	–	$GABA_a$ receptor agonist	Reversible, short duration, titratable, water soluble	Respiratory depression, hypotension, confusion
Haloperidol	Neuroleptic (butyrophenone)	+++	–	Blocks dopamine, adrenergic, serotonin, acetylcholine, and histamine receptors	Preserves level of arousal, airway reflexes	Extrapyramidal signs; may lower seizure threshold
Droperidol	Neuroleptic (butyrophenone)	+++	+	Blocks dopamine, adrenergic, serotonin, acetylcholine, and histamine receptors	Combined sedation, antipsychotic. anti-emetic, analgesia in headache syndromes	Extrapyramidal signs; may lower seizure threshold; QT prolongation
Clonidine	Alpha-2 agonist	++	++	Alpha-2 receptor agonist (pre- and post-synaptic	Useful in setting of alcohol or drug withdrawal	Dry mouth, bradycardia, hypotension, rebound hypertension
Dexmedetomidine	Alpha-2 agonist	++	++	Alpha-2 receptor agonist (pre- and post-synaptic	Short acting, Little effect on consciousness & blood pressure	Dry mouth, bradycardia, hypotension, adrenal suppression, atrial fibrillation
Propofol		+++	–	Unclear	Very short duration, titratable	Hypotension, respiratory depression, metabolic acidosis, rhabdomyolysis, anaphylaxis, sepsis, pain at venous site

+ mild; ++ moderate; +++ high; GABA: gamma-amino-butyric acid; NMDA: N-methyl-D-aspartate

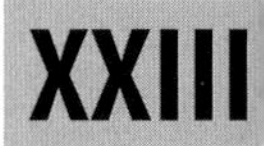

Table 3. Pharmacokinetics and dosing of common ICU sedatives

Drug	Half-life	Starting dose	Titration	Protein binding	Metabolism	Active metabolite
Fentanyl	30–60 min (single i.v. dose). Repeated is hours	12.5–50 μg i.v. q 20–30 min	Infusion 0.01–0.03 μg/kg/min and titrate q 15–30 min, up to 50–100 μg/h	80–86 %	Hepatic	–
Remifentanil	3–10 min after single dose	Bolus not necessary	Infusion 0.05–0.2 μg/kg/min	92 %	Plasma esterases	–

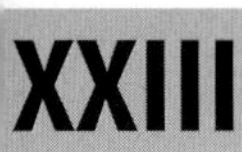

Table 3. *(cont.)*

Drug	Half-life	Starting dose	Titration	Protein binding	Metabolism	Active metabolite
Morphine sulfate	1.5–4.5 hours i.v., i.m., s.c.	5–20 mg i.m. q 4 hours 2–10 mg i.v. q 4 hours	Caution: metabolites may accumulate For post-operative pain (PCAP): 0.2–3.0 mg and 5–20 min lockout intervals	20–30 %	Hepatic	Morphine-3-glucuronide Morphine-6-glucuronide
Diazepam	30–60 hours	2 mg i.v. q 30–60 min	–	99 %	Hepatic	Desmethyldiazepam, oxazepam, hydroxydiazepam
Lorazepam	10–20 hours	0.25–0.5 mg i.v. q 1–2 hours	–	91–93 %	Hepatic	–
Midazolam	1–2.5 hours	0.5–1 mg i.v. q 5–30 min	0.02 to 0.1 mg/kg/hour (1 to 7 mg/hour),	97 %	Hepatic	1-Hydroxymethylmidazolam
Haloperidol	12–36 hours	0.5–5 mg i.v.	–	92 %	Hepatic	–
Droperidol	4–12 hours	0.625–2.5 mg i.v.	–	92 %	Hepatic	–
Clonidine	12–16 hours	0.1 mg PO q 8–24 hours. Increase 0.1 mg/d q 1–2 d up to 0.6 mg/d	–	20–40 %	Hepatic (50 %) and urine (unchanged, 50 %)	–
Dexmedetomidine	2 hours	1 μg/kg i.v. over 10 min	Infusion 0.2–0.7 μg/kg/h	94 %	Hepatic	–
Propofol	4–10 min	1–2.5 mg/kg i.v. (anesthesia induction) 5 μg/kg/min for 5 min i.v. (sedation)	Increase infusion by 5–10 μg/kg/min q 5–10 min to maintenance 25–100 μg/kg/min up to 100–300 μg/kg/min	Not found	Hepatic and extra hepatic	–

i.v.: intravenous; i.m.: intramuscular; s.c.: subcutaneous; PCAP: patient-controlled analgesia pump.

It is of course necessary to eliminate all alternative explanations for agitation, confusion, or sympathetic hyperactivity prior to actively suppressing these potential symptoms and signs of a serious underlying condition. Hypoxemia or hypercarbia related to decreased respiratory drive or poor airway protection must be detected and treated appropriately. Metabolic disturbances, including acidosis, hyponatremia, hypoglycemia, hypercalcemia, hyperamylasemia, hyperammonemia, or hepatic or renal insufficiency may contribute to behavioral changes in critically ill patients. Cardiac ischemia, infection, and hypotension, which may often be associated with cerebral hypoperfusion, contribute to mental status changes, and must be ruled out as a cause of delirium in the critically ill. Psychoactive medications such as antidepressants, anticonvulsants, and other commonly used medications may promote cognitive dysfunction and agitation.

Monitoring of Sedation

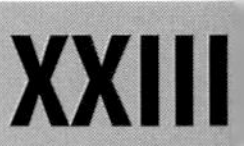

In order to monitor the administration of sedatives, particularly in the ICU where frequent dosing and titrations are necessary, numerous sedation scoring systems have been crafted. The first scale popularized was the Ramsay Scale introduced in 1974, and representative of the sedation goals that were popular at that time. Focused primarily on the post-cardiac surgery patient, the Ramsay Scale places great emphasis on deep levels of sedation, with the clinical target arousal level being the semi- or fully unconscious state [21]. Three of the six stages of sedation are within the asleep or unconscious state, one describes a sedated but awake phase, and one corresponds to an anxious/agitated condition. Subsequently, in an effort to focus on less obtunded states of sedation and to delineate exaggerated levels of arousal – restlessness and agitation – evaluation tools were devised placing greater descriptive weight on specific motor behaviors and hemodynamic parameters. Recent scoring tools include the Riker Sedation-Agitation Scale (SAS, 1999) [22], Motor Activity Assessment Scale (MAAS, 1999) [23], the Richmond Agitation-Sedation Scale (2002) [24], and recently the Adaptation to Intensive Care Environment (ATICE, measuring sedation and tolerance) [25] and Avripas Scale (four components: Agitation, alertness, heart rate, and respiration) [26]. Of those listed, only the RASS has been validated for its ability to detect changes in sedation status over consecutive days. Some intensivists have argued that representation of several domains of level of arousal – including cognitive state and degrees of anxiety or agitation – into a single numerical value diminishes the potential utility of an assessment tool. Two-domain instruments have, therefore, been developed and validated, and include the Vancouver Interaction and Calmness Scale (VICS) and the Minnesota Sedation Assessment Tool (MSAT) scale [27, 28].

One criticism of sedation scales to date is that for the most part, they are nursing tools for recording or charting levels of sedation, rather than a tool to easily and rapidly communicate the patient's clinical status. To that end, we have recently developed and introduced a symmetrical 7-level scale (+3 "dangerously agitated" to -3 "deeply sedated") that is both intuitive and easy to use, the Nursing Instrument for the Communication of Sedation (NICS) [29]. In addition to excellent criteria, construct and face validity, NICS was highly rated by nurses as easy to score, intuitive, and a clinically relevant measure of sedation and agitation. NICS performed better than RASS when asked which scale is easiest to communicate, and when asked which was preferred overall (83 % NICS, 17 % RASS, 6 % Other). NICS also demonstrated a high degree of inter-rater reliability (ICC = 0.945).

All such scales have utility in monitoring sedation, and a tool should be routinely used in all sedated ICU patients in order to provide an objective target for the depth of sedation, minimize the amount of drug required to obtain the sedation goal, and facilitate communication among providers. Selection depends primarily on the particular needs of an ICU, in particular their efficiency in transfer of well-categorized patient status from one caregiver to another, and in charting a patient's arousal state over time in the medical record.

Cognitive Function Evaluation

In keeping with recent trends of maintaining a more awake and alert patient during ICU sedation, it becomes desirable to afford pharmacotherapy that limits the common adverse effects on cognitive function. Unfortunately, few intensivists routinely assess awake critically ill patients with detailed neurological examinations or tests of intellect. Yet at least 30 % of ICU patients are known to suffer neurological sequelae from ICU management, the most common diagnosis being encephalopathy [7]. Despite technological advances in radiographic and physiological imaging, the bedside neurological exam remains the most sensitive evaluation of neurological function. Hence, it is appropriate to have tools to assess cognition that can be easily incorporated into the management of ICU patients. The Mini-Mental Status Examination (MMSE) is often used, but is not suited for intubated patients. Recently, a specific tool for critically ill patients has been developed, the Adapted Cognitive Exam (ACE) [30]. The ACE is a 10 minute, 100-point scale assessing cognition through orientation, language, registration, attention/calculation, and recall. It has been validated in ICU patients, and has been shown to be easier to use and more sensitive than the MMSE. The ACE also demonstrated excellent inter-rater reliability (ICC = 0.998).

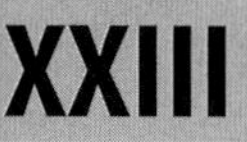

Physiological and Brain Functional Monitors

There have been attempts to effectively titrate sedative agents in an ICU using both a patient's hemodynamic response to pharmacological intervention and changes in cerebral electrical function. Although logical and often presumed, neither heart rate nor blood pressure changes have been supported in studies as useful parameters for guidance. In fact, published guidelines for sedation specifically discourage their use as markers of sedation [8]. The neurological monitors have their origin in the raw electroencephalogram (EEG), and typically have been variants of signal-processed EEG and more recently the bispectral index (BIS) monitor. These evolved devices take EEG data from the frontal cortex site via a dual electrode patch and generalize the electrical phenomena to a global state. The BIS is by far the most tested proprietary algorithm, and compares the patient's frontal EEG to processed data from over 5,000 volunteer EEG samples to scale the output of the measured EEG to between 0 and 100. The 'fully awake state' is scored 100, whereas 0 is an isoelectric EEG reading. The score of 60 is the fundamental threshold established by the proprietary analysis that places the patient at high probability of unconsciousness with a reading below 60. For general anesthetic purposes, a range of 40–60 is commonly used, whereas sedation targets are typified by ranges of 60–75.

Although some ICUs enjoy the benefits of a simple numerical scale to assist physician/nursing titration of sedation, particularly when continuous infusions of medication are used, the BIS monitor suffers from several shortcomings. From a pharmacological perspective, the BIS is best used when administering a short acting barbiturate anesthetic (thiopental) or barbiturate-like drug (propofol) which the processed EEG algorithm is based on. These agents induce a very stereotypic alteration in the EEG as a patient transitions from the completely awake to the sedated and finally unconscious/comatose state. Agents such as the benzodiazepines, narcotics, or other classes of sedatives differentially influence the EEG, and the BIS is not programmed to interpret such changes as well [31]. For example, benzodiazepines cause a rise in EEG frequency following modest to moderate doses, not slowing as does propofol. Narcotics on the other hand, can have a profound effect on a patient's state of anxiety without untoward disturbance on the underlying cortical EEG. Combination pharmacotherapy also makes it difficult to readily translate a BIS 'score' to a clinical state of arousal as different agents have such varying actions on the EEG as they contribute to the sedation scheme. Another major limitation of using the BIS as an ICU sedation monitor stems from the inability of the device to fully eliminate the electromyographic (EMG) signal artifact that originates from the frontalis muscle underneath the electrode patch, contaminating the EEG signal input and rendering the numerical output unreliable under conditions of a pharmacologically non-paralyzed state.

Classes of Sedative Agents

Narcotics (Opioids)

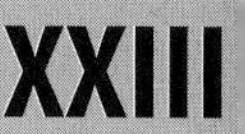

A large number of natural opioids (e.g., morphine sulfate, codeine), semi-synthetic opioids (e.g., fentanyl, hydromorphone, oxycodone), and completely synthetic (e.g., meperidine) opioid-like compounds are available. These compounds act primarily as analgesics, but also serve as sedative-hypnotics at low dosages. Their major disadvantage is their coincident action of suppressing ventilatory drive and gastrointestinal motility. Advantages include easy titratability, provision of patient comfort, and reversibility. Three opioids in particular are common sedative-analgesics used in the critical care setting – morphine, fentanyl, and remifentanil.

Mechanism of action

All opioids act by binding to mu opioid receptors in the central and peripheral nervous systems as agonists, partial agonists, or agonist-antagonists [32]. These receptor interactions are the basis for the pharmacological effects of opioids (analgesia, decreased level of consciousness, respiratory depression, miosis, gastrointestinal hypomotility, antitussive effects, euphoria or dysphoria, and vasodilatation), and vary by the specific opioid receptor subtypes bound by each drug.

Of particular interest to clinicians using narcotics for sedation and analgesia is the recent evidence that the mu opioid receptor (MOR-1) is constructed via translation of a combination of exon fragments of the MOR-1 gene. Certain exon fragments, such as 1, 2, and 3, define the receptor complex at the cell surface for all variants of the MOR-1 construct, thus supporting the observation that all mu receptor opioid agonists have similar high affinity for the receptor. However, the interior cell receptor component is composed of a variety of potential constructs owing to the possible mix of splice variants from at least 5 potential exon fragments. Thus, although all opioids bind to MOR-1, the physiological response may vary from individual to individual, owing to the receptor differences located inside the cell. This phenomenon may help explain the subtle distinctions between drugs as well as support the concept that opioid administration – both type and dose – needs to be tailored to each patient [33].

Pharmacokinetics and dynamics

Opioids are readily absorbed through mucosal surfaces, from the gastrointestinal tract, or through subcutaneous, intramuscular, intrathecal, epidural, and intravenous routes of administration. Fentanyl is also easily absorbed via transdermal application. Morphine and other opioids are rapidly distributed to the brain, with the more lipophilic compounds (e.g., fentanyl, remifentanil) having the shortest time of onset. Peak effect following intravenous administration of morphine is approximately 15 minutes; that for fentanyl is 5 minutes, and remifentanil is 1–2 minutes.

After enteral administration, the bioavailability of morphine sulfate is only approximately 20–40 % due to first pass hepatic metabolism. Intramuscular and intravenous morphine sulfate is rapidly and readily available. Morphine is 20–36 % protein bound in plasma, and has a volume of distribution of 1–6 l/kg, depending on the route of administration. However, the majority of systemically administered morphine does not cross the blood-brain barrier.

Morphine is eliminated in the liver by *N*-demethylation, *N*-dealkylation, *O*-dealkylation, conjugation and hydrolysis. The majority of clearance is by glucuronidation to the active metabolites, morphine-3-glucuronide (~ 50 %) and morphine-6-glucuronide (5–15 %), which are renally excreted; the latter is a more potent analgesic than the parent compound, and may accumulate in patients with renal insufficiency. The half-life of morphine varies greatly by route of administration, ranging from 1.5–4.5 hours for intravenous, intramuscular, and subcutaneous injection, to 15 hours or more for sustained-release oral preparations.

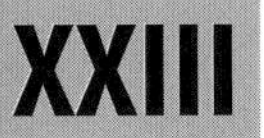

Time to onset following buccal administration of fentanyl is 5–15 minutes, with a peak response at 20–30 minutes. For intramuscular injection of fentanyl, onset is at 7–8 minutes, and effects last 1–2 hours. Transdermal fentanyl has a much slower onset of action, 12–24 hours, although rate of absorption increases with higher skin temperature (e.g., febrile patients). Steady state is reached at 36–48 hours, and duration of action is up to 72 hours after removal of transdermal fentanyl. Following intravenous administration, the onset of action of fentanyl is immediate, although peak effects take several minutes to manifest. Duration of action after a single intravenous dose of fentanyl is 30–60 minutes, which increases after repeated or prolonged dosing due to accumulation in fat and skeletal muscle.

Fentanyl is extensively plasma protein bound (80–86 %), with a volume of distribution of 3–6 l/kg in adults. Fentanyl is metabolized via *N*-dealkylation by the hepatic cytochrome P450 system, producing norfentanyl and other inactive metabolites, which are renally excreted. The half-life of fentanyl is ~200 minutes following intravenous injection, and up to 17 hours for transdermal administration. As up to 10 % of fentanyl is excreted unchanged in the urine, its duration of action may be prolonged following high cumulative doses in patients with renal insufficiency. Fentanyl does not appear to be removed from the plasma compartment by hemodialysis.

Remifentanil is typically given by intravenous infusion, with a time to peak onset of action of 1 to 3 minutes. Duration of action is only 3–10 minutes after a single dose, increased slightly after prolonged infusions. Remifentanil is 92 % plasma protein bound, with a volume of distribution of 25–60 l and a distribution half-life of one minute. Remifentanil is rapidly metabolized by plasma esterases to an inactive carboxylic acid, which is 90 % renally excreted. Metabolism is independent of the cumulative remifentanil dose, and unaffected by hepatic or renal function.

Due to its rapid onset and short duration of action, which is independent of hepatic and renal clearance, remifentanil is the most easily titratable of the opioids. Preliminary use of continuous remifentanil infusion for sedation of intubated patients in an ICU setting has shown promising results, with blunting of hemodynamic instability and intracranial hypertension associated with agitation, coughing, and tracheal suctioning. It is expensive relative to fentanyl or morphine, but when the need to have a true on-off drug is manifested, remifentanil possesses ideal pharmacokinetic properties to facilitate this. The downside of the ultra-short half-life of remifentanil manifests itself upon abrupt discontinuation of the infusion (this is analogous to rapid reversal with naloxone), which can precipitate acute exacerbations of pain, or possibly withdrawal in patients receiving long-standing opioid therapy. For this reason, it is imperative that a plan for transition to a longer-acting opioid and strategy for pain management be implemented prior to discontinuation.

Fentanyl is more readily accessible than remifentanil in many medical centers, and many physicians are more familiar with this intravenous opioid. Fentanyl may be given by either bolus dosing or continuous intravenous infusion. By its lipophilic nature and longer clearance time, however, fentanyl may be less easily titrated than remifentanil and may require greater periods of drug interruption to permit frequent neurologic assessment. However, doses of 1–2 μg/kg/h are typically well tolerated, and continuous uninterrupted infusion for several days can provide analgesia/sedation with minimal neurological or respiratory compromise. Morphine is the most difficult of these opioids to titrate, again due to its longer duration of action, dependence on hepatic and renal clearance, and prolonged clearance of active metabolites. For these reasons, infusions of morphine are not recommended for ICU patients requiring short-term sedation, although intermittent administration may facilitate patient comfort and hemodynamic stability.

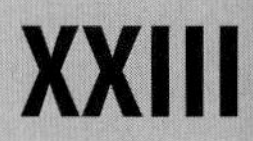

Comparing remifentanil and fentanyl, a recent randomized, double-blind trial of ICU sedation found that analgesia-based sedation with each of the two agents provided effective sedation and rapid extubation without the need for propofol in most patients. Fentanyl was similar to remifentanil with respect to achievement of appropriate level of sedation and its context-sensitive half life as measured to time to extubation once the medications was discontinued following 12–72 hrs of continuous sedation (1–2 μg/kg/h) [34]. Sedation with remifentanil incurred the risk of higher degrees and longer duration of pain upon discontinuation than fentanyl. These results emphasize the need for proactive pain management when discontinuing remifentanil, transitioning to longer acting analgesics during the weaning period.

One of the advantages of sedation with opioid narcotics is their rapid reversibility with the antagonist naloxone. Although the recommended dosage for reversal of narcotic overdose is generally 0.4 mg or above, in ICU patients the starting dosage should be lower (e.g., 0.04 to 0.08 mg by intravenous push) to avoid 'overshoot' phenomena such as hypertension, tachycardia, and emergence agitation, all of which may precipitate or worsen myocardial ischemia, ventilatory mismatch, or intracranial hypertension. Dosage may be titrated to the desired level of arousal and reversal of respiratory depression, with effects seen within 1–2 minutes of each subsequent administration.

Rationale for ICU use and adverse reactions

The narcotics as a class of drug present as a highly useful pharmacological tool in an ICU setting. Analgesia is commonly required, and the opioids are typically well-tolerated with minimal adverse physiological effects. Although modest bradycardia can occur with high-dose narcotic administration, typically these agents have little or no effect on chronotropy or systemic pressure. Caution has been issued regarding administration of morphine to patients with traumatic brain injury (TBI) due to increases in ICP, although the mechanism is unclear. In general, opioids *per se* have no effects on ICP or cerebral blood flow (CBF), but any hypercarbia related to respiratory depression by opiates may lead to cerebral vasodilatation and its sequelae.

Very high doses of both morphine and fentanyl have been shown to induce seizure-like activity in patients undergoing general anesthesia [35]. As none of these cases had documented electrographic seizure activity, others have suggested that the reported 'seizures' were actually manifestations of narcotic-induced rigidity or myoclonus. Indeed, non-epileptic myoclonus has been reported in numerous cases when very high doses of intravenous or intrathecal morphine were given. Meperidine has a renally eliminated active metabolite, normeperidine, which has been associated with an excitatory syndrome that includes seizures. Patients with underlying renal dysfunction are particularly susceptible to this.

Common adverse responses of narcotics include pruritus, excessive somnolence, respiratory depression, chest wall and other muscular rigidity (primarily fentanyl and other high potent opioids), dysphoria or hallucinations (primarily morphine), nausea and vomiting, gastrointestinal dysmotility, hypotension, histamine release causing urticaria and flushing (primarily meperidine and morphine), anaphylaxis (rare), and immune suppression after repeated dosing [32]. Although morphine may induce hypotension even at low therapeutic doses (partly due to promotion of histamine release), fentanyl and remifentanil tend to have little effect on blood pressure at sedative doses. Fentanyl also tends to reduce heart rate, which is favorable in the setting of cardiovascular disease. Because of their potential to suppress respiratory drive, it is recommended that all patients receiving narcotic sedation have frequent (preferably continuous) monitoring of pulse oximetry and respiratory rate. Additional frequent hemodynamic assessments including blood pressure and heart rate are prudent due to the potential for hypotension, bradycardia, and tachycardia with selective narcotic agonists.

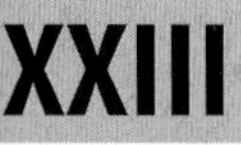

Drug-drug interactions

Combined use of morphine and neuroleptics may produce greater than expected decreases in blood pressure. Additionally, the depressant effects of narcotics on respiration and level of consciousness may be potentiated by concurrent administration of phenothiazine neuroleptics, tricyclic antidepressants, and monoamine oxidase inhibitors [32].

Dosage recommendations

Dosage recommendations are for narcotic-naïve patients. As a general guideline, fentanyl and remifentanil are approximately 100 times more potent than morphine.

Fentanyl: Although fentanyl may also be given by buccal, transdermal, intramuscular, intrathecal, and epidural routes, intravenous administration is recommended for ICU patients. For mild sedation and analgesia, recommended starting dosage is 25–50 μg intravenously every 5–10 minutes until comfort is achieved, recognizing that time-to-peak is approximately 3 min following each dose. Thus the next dose occurs as the previous effect begins to wane. A cumulative effect gradually occurs. Alternatively, for more durable effect, a continuous infusion of 0.5–2.5 μg/kg/h may be used, titrating to effect every 15–30 minutes. Continuous infusions above 2 μg/kg/h are not recommended in narcotic-naïve patients unless they are endotracheally intubated or otherwise have a protected airway, and mechanical ventilation is possible. For deeper sedation, as an adjunct to general anesthesia, or in narcotic-tolerant patients, continuous infusions greater than those above may be advocated.

Remifentanil: Being extremely short acting, remifentanil can be effectively and quickly titrated by continuous infusion. Dosing range for sedation begins at approximately 0.02–0.05 μg/kg/min, and upwards as needed to a typical maximum of

0.1 μg/kg/min. Larger doses rapidly lead to apnea and subsequently general anesthetic doses. No adjustment is needed for renal or hepatic insufficiency, although decreasing the dose by 50 % is recommended for patients older than 65 years of age.

Morphine sulfate: The time-to-peak of this longer acting narcotic is 20–30 min. with duration of approximately 4 hours. Thus, intermittent bolus delivery constitutes a sensible dosing regimen. For analgesic dosing, titration doses of 5–20 mg intramuscularly every 4 hours or 2–10 mg intravenously over 4–5 minutes every 2–4 hours is recommended. Preference should be given to intravenous dosing in an ICU setting to minimize patient discomfort. For oral dosing when appropriate, 15–30 mg of the immediate release formula every 4 hours is reasonable.

These dosages are for narcotic naïve individuals, and may be increased substantially (with appropriate monitoring) in patients tolerant to opioids. It is quite common to admit patients to an ICU with preconditions requiring large doses of oral opioids at baseline. These patients are best served by initial bedside titration of intravenous fentanyl until immediate discomfort is relieved. This minimizes the time to comfort. It is not unusual in some circumstances to titrate upwards of 1000 μg of fentanyl over a 30 minute time span in a highly narcotic tolerant patient. Thereafter, logical dose substitution for a longer acting agent such as morphine is warranted. Due to hepatic metabolism and renal clearance, dosages should be reduced in patients with hepatic or renal insufficiency or those at the extremes of age.

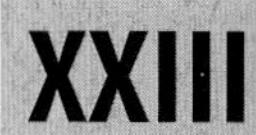

Benzodiazepines

Benzodiazepines rank as the most common agent used for ICU sedation. Three principal agents are found within this category that are commonly used in the ICU – diazepam, lorazepam, and midazolam. These medications are sedatives by virtue of predominant anxiolytic action. Some analgesic effect has been suggested for diazepam via GABAergic receptor function [36].

Mechanism of action

The majority, if not all, of the effects of benzodiazepines are through potentiation of the central nervous system (CNS) actions of the inhibitory neurotransmitter, gamma aminobutyric acid (GABA). Benzodiazepines experimentally increase the frequency of opening of the $GABA_a$ chloride channel in response to binding of GABA [36]. Subsequent effects include anxiolysis, sedation, muscle relaxation, anterograde amnesia, respiratory depression (especially in children, patients with chronic pulmonary disease, hepatic insufficiency, or when combined with other sedatives), anticonvulsant activity (not all benzodiazepines), and analgesia (only intravenous diazepam). Very high doses of several benzodiazepines will also lead to coronary vasodilatation and neuromuscular blockade through interaction with peripheral sites [36].

Pharmacokinetics and dynamics

Time to onset and offset of single intravenous doses of a benzodiazepine is largely determined by the agent's relative lipophilicity. Upon a single intravenous injection, benzodiazepines are rapidly distributed to the brain, followed by redistribution to muscle and fat. Of the three, diazepam is the most rapid in onset, and likewise the most rapidly redistributed due to its higher lipophilicity, followed by midazolam and lorazepam. With multiple doses or continuous infusions, the time to offset is more dependent on the agent's half-life, and presence or absence of active metabolites. Thus, diazepam has a very short onset time and initial duration of effect following a single bolus (due to redistribution), but has the longest half-life of > 50 h. In addition, a primary metabolite, dimethyl-diazepam, retains considerable potency as a sedative, and with its elimination half-life of > 90 h, may prolong recovery from the effects of repeated dosing or lengthy infusion of the agent. Midazolam is the most easily titratable as an intravenous drug owing to its shorter duration of action and shortest half-life (1–4 h), and is most appropriate for use as a continuous infusion. Midazolam does possess an active metabolite (alpha-hydroxy-midazolam) which is renally eliminated. Accumulation of this metabolite in the renally impaired may contribute to prolonged sedation. Lorazepam is the most water soluble with the smallest redistribution effect, which enhances its duration of action following a single bolus. Thus, duration of 4–6 hours may be expected following a single dose, as compared with 5–20 min following either midazolam or diazepam. Lorazepam does not possess any active metabolites. All benzodiazepines are highly bound to plasma proteins, and all are hepatically metabolized.

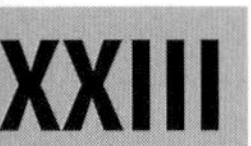

Benzodiazepines are reversible with the selective antagonist, flumazenil. Caution must be exerted with flumazenil, however, as this agent may precipitate rapid rises in ICP, systemic hypertension, and lowering of seizure threshold, particularly in TBI and neurosurgical patients. Additionally, because of its short duration of action, patients may become re-sedated from longer-acting benzodiazepines after flumazenil has been metabolized.

Rationale for ICU use and adverse reactions

As anxiolytics and amnestics, benzodiazepines provide often-needed relief from the stressful ICU environment. Small, titrated doses can usually be given to effect without overt compromise of cognitive function. Anterograde amnesia is a profoundly useful attribute when performing discomforting procedures, although analgesia should also be offered. Similar to the opioids, benzodiazepines provide their positive effects without undue alteration in either blood pressure or heart rate, and respiratory drive is well preserved unless high doses are entertained. Low (oral hypnotic) doses of benzodiazepines have little effect on blood pressure, but higher intravenous (sedative or anesthetic) doses may cause hypotension and increased heart rate. Alone, benzodiazepines have little or no effect on ICP. However, decreases in mean arterial pressure associated with midazolam administration may impair cerebral perfusion. As with opioids, high doses of benzodiazepines may induce respiratory dysfunction and apnea, and the hypercarbia associated with these respiratory-depressant effects may stimulate an increase in ICP.

With that stated, the most common unintended action from use of the benzodiazepines is over sedation, but it is dose-dependent and usually avoidable. Another unintended consequence of benzodiazepine administration is inducing frank delirium. Although a tranquil state coupled with anterograde amnesia are principal reasons for their use, these agents also precipitate altered cognition that defines in part the delirious state. Delirium is diagnosed if features of acute onset of mental status change or fluctuating level of consciousness occur along with inattention and either feature disorganized thinking or altered level of consciousness are present. Measures have been recently developed for the screening of delirium such as the CAM-ICU [19] or the Intensive Care Delirium Screening Checklist [20]. Clearly, benzodiazepine use has been attributed to the etiology of delirium, and this likely adverse event must be considered when administration of this drug class is initiated [37].

With nearly all sedative agents, additive or synergistic effects may occur with benzodiazepines and any other medication that may alter level of consciousness, suppress respiratory drive, or decrease systemic blood pressure. In particular, apnea can commonly be precipitated when used in conjunction with opioids, and caution must be used when this combination therapy is pursued. As with opioid narcotics, the potential for respiratory depression and hypotension with high-dose benzodiazepines necessitates careful monitoring of pulse oximetry and blood pressure. This is especially prudent in patients maintained on continuous infusions, and those who are not mechanically-ventilated.

An adjunctive benefit to the neurological population is the anticonvulsant property of the benzodiazepines, and data support them as primary therapy for treatment of acute seizures, including convulsive status epilepticus. In this regard, lorazepam is the drug advocated in this life threatening condition. Animal studies demonstrate that benzodiazepines inhibit many types of experimentally induced seizure activity, but not all. When seizures are provoked by mechanisms other than antagonism of the GABA receptor, such as theophylline-induced seizures, benzodiazepine therapy is typically unsuccessful. In treating seizure disorders, however, tolerance develops rapidly and diminishes their efficacy with time.

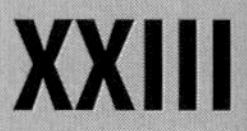

Propylene glycol is the solvent used for intravenous lorazepam and diazepam, and in high doses has been implicated in the development of hyperosmolar states, lactic acidosis, and reversible acute tubular necrosis. An absolute dosing threshold in which the development of this complication is likely has not been identified, but it is more commonly reported in patients receiving higher doses (lorazepam infusion > 18 mg/h) for prolonged periods of time. Calculation of the osmolar gap can be used as a surrogate for serum propylene glycol concentrations. This should be monitored closely in patients receiving high doses, with an osmolar gap > 10 suggestive of potentially toxic propylene glycol concentrations.

Other side effects of these agents include headache, nausea or vomiting, vertigo, confusion, excessive somnolence to obtundation, respiratory depression, hypotension, hypotonia/loss of reflexes, or muscular weakness.

Drug-drug interactions

Both diazepam and midazolam are susceptible to numerous drug interactions, as they are metabolized by the cytochrome P450 family of enzymes. Inducers of the P450 system (e.g., rifampin, carbamazepine, phenytoin, and phenobarbital) may enhance clearance of these agents, while inhibitors (e.g., macrolides, azole antifungals, and non-dihydropyridine calcium channel blockers) may inhibit clearance. In contrast, lorazepam is prone to very few drug interactions, as it is metabolized by glucuronidation.

Dosage recommendations

Diazepam: For sedation, initial doses of 1–2 mg intravenously every 10–20 min is recommended, incrementally increasing up to 5 mg per dose. The short duration limits this drug to brief sedation (for invasive procedures, etc.) or as an attempt to induce sleep. If multiple high dosing or continuous intravenous infusion is considered, the possibility of prolonged sedation must be considered owing to its previously stated pharmacokinetic properties.

Lorazepam: For sedation, 0.25–0.5 mg intravenously every 2–4 h is usually sufficient, and a 1–2 mg intravenous bolus will often provide moderately deep sedation for 4–8 h. In acute withdrawal syndromes, higher dosing is often required, but provisions for respiratory support must be made available, especially if other sedatives are being used in conjunction.

Midazolam: Administer 0.5–2 mg intravenously every 5–10 minutes as needed. This drug can also be administered intramuscularly (0.07 mg/kg) in contrast to diazepam where the propylene glycol based mixture may cause myonecrosis. Maintenance infusions may be started at 0.02 to 0.1 mg/kg/hour (1 to 7 mg/hour), and titrated to the target sedation score.

Alpha$_2$ Agonists

The two agents now in use in the ICU setting for the management of anxiety and agitation are clonidine and dexmedetomidine. Clonidine has long been used as an adjunct to general, neuraxial, and regional anesthesia due to its sedative and analgesic properties, but its cardiovascular depressant effects limit its utility when combined with most other agents. Dexmedetomidine has been recently approved in the United States for post-operative and ICU settings, and shows promise as an alternative to traditional sedatives, as it reduces the discomfort of mechanical ventilation while permitting rapid patient arousability for neurologic examination. Neither clonidine nor dexmedetomidine alone are capable of inducing general anesthesia, but both agents markedly enhance the efficacy of inhalational anesthetics as well as opioids, decreasing the requirements for these other substances.

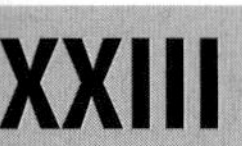

Mechanism of action
Both clonidine and dexmedetomidine are selective α_2-adrenergic receptor agonists. Dexmedetomidine, however, is considered a 'super' selective α_2-agonist with 8–10x more avid binding to α_2 receptors than clonidine. The sedative and analgesic properties of these compounds result from presynaptic inhibition of descending noradrenergic activation of spinal neurons, as well as activation of post-synaptic α_2-adrenergic receptors coupled to potassium-channel activating G-proteins [38]. The summation of these effects is a decrease in sympathetic outflow from the locus coeruleus, a decrease in tonic activity in spinal motor neurons and spinothalamic pain pathways, and subsequent decreases in heart rate and blood pressure. At recommended doses, respiratory drive is not compromised.

Pharmacokinetics and dynamics
Clonidine is available in oral and transdermal formulations in the United States. As with the other lipophilic sedatives described previously, clonidine is rapidly distributed to the brain and spinal cord following administration. Decreases in blood pressure and heart rate may be noted within 30–60 minutes following oral dosing, although peak effects are not seen for 2–4 hours. The half-life varies between 12–16 hours in healthy individuals, but may be prolonged to 41 hours in patients with impaired renal function. Only about 5 % of plasma clonidine is removed by hemodialysis. Approximately 50 % of plasma clonidine is cleared by hepatic metabolism, with the remainder of the drug eliminated unchanged in urine. Clonidine is moderately bound to serum proteins (20–40 %), and may compete with other substances for these binding sites.

Although the initial action of oral doses of clonidine may be relatively rapid, there may remain undesirable effects on heart rate and blood pressure for several days after initiation of drug therapy. As the time of onset for transdermal clonidine is 24–72 hours, this system is not useful as a sedative agent. However, transdermal clonidine may be useful in the setting of alcohol or drug withdrawal in ICU patients, or as an adjunct for reduction of sympathetic hyperactivity in severe TBI patients.

Dexmedetomidine is only given as an intravenous infusion, and is rapidly distributed to the brain with an equilibrium half-life of 6–9 minutes. The elimination half-life is 2 hours in healthy volunteers, but due to extensive metabolism by the liver this may increase to 7.5 hours in individuals with hepatic insufficiency. Due to its relatively short half-life, dexmedetomidine is easily titrated. Excretion of dexmedetomidine is primarily through the kidney as inactive methyl- and glucuronide- conjugates.

Rationale for ICU use and adverse reactions

A potential advantage of clonidine and dexmedetomidine as sedative agents compared to current popular classes of drugs, particularly propofol, benzodiazepines, and narcotics, is the nominal effect on reduction of level of arousal. Experience suggests that these agents may induce effective degrees of sedation without concomitant loss of attentive behavior and cognition following low levels of auditory or tactile stimulation. In the ICU, this agent has recently been demonstrated to possess advantageous characteristics for sedation in the critically ill [39]. We recently completed a prospective, randomized, double-blinded cross-over comparing sedation between dexmedetomidine and propofol which demonstrated that the selective α_2-adrenergic agonist improved cognition while sedating patients to a calm, awake state [40]. Higher cognitive test results with dexmedetomidine may be a consequence of the intellect-sparing yet calming effect of this drug, permitting improved patient concentration.

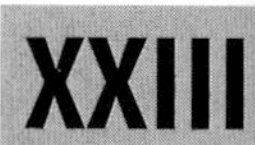

Using dexmedetomidine, neurological assessment may be preserved while achieving the goal of a non-agitated or anxious patient. Additionally, the combination of both sedative/anxiolytic and analgesic action of clonidine and dexmedetomidine may permit single drug use for both sedation and modest pain control during the post-operative and medical ICU period in select patients.

From an intraoperative perspective, dexmedetomidine has been effectively used as a sedative for both awake craniotomy and sedation cases. Some evidence suggests prolonged cognitive deficits may persist beyond the sedative action of the drug. As in the operating arena, the ability to easily arouse patients appears to be a distinctive quality.

The most common undesirable effects of clonidine include dry mouth, bradycardia, hypotension, lightheadedness, and anxiety. Acute withdrawal of chronic clonidine administration may lead to rebound hypertension, and possible subsequent stroke or cerebral hemorrhage; dosage should thus be tapered off after prolonged use. Like clonidine, dexmedetomidine has been reported to cause hypotension and bradycardia, but to a lesser degree, and this is more commonly associated with the initial bolus dose. Treatment is supportive, with decrease or discontinuation of the infusion, intravenous fluids, and rarely pressors or vagolytics. In the management of TBI patients, clonidine had no significant effects on ICP but did impair cerebral perfusion pressure (CPP) via a reduction in systemic arterial pressure. Similar data now exists for dexmedetomidine [41]. In a study of 39 neurosurgical patients, the mean CPP increased while ICP decreased during sedation. Agitation was the predominant adverse reaction while hypotension occurred in 10 of the 39 patients. This class of drug appears suitable for sedation in the cerebrally-injured patient.

Paradoxical transient hypertension may also be observed in association with a loading dose of dexmedetomidine, and thus infusions are often begun without a bolus. Other reported adverse reactions with dexmedetomidine include nausea, vomiting, fever, dry mouth, anxiety, and atrial fibrillation, although the incidence of these side effects did not differ significantly from placebo. Rare elevation of hepatic enzymes has also been reported.

Drug-drug interactions
Due to their sedating properties, both clonidine and dexmedetomidine may exacerbate the effects of other centrally acting depressants. Additionally, hypotension and bradycardia may be worsened by concomitant administration of antihypertensive and antidysrhythmic medications. Conversely, tricyclic antidepressants combined with clonidine may produce a paradoxical increase in blood pressure. As with all of the aforementioned sedatives, caution must be exercised when combining α_2-agonists with multiple medications, particularly in hypovolemic or otherwise hemodynamically unstable patients. *In vitro* studies suggest inhibition of the cytochrome P450 microsomal system by dexmedetomidine, however this does not appear to have clinically significant effects on the metabolism of other substances utilizing this metabolic pathway.

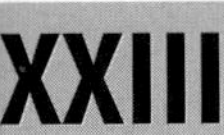

Dosage recommendations
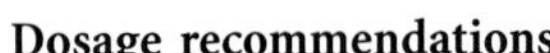
Frequent monitoring of blood pressure and heart rate is recommended with initiation of clonidine or dexmedetomidine therapy.

Clonidine: Initial oral dosing may be started at 0.1 mg orally every 8–24 hours, increasing by 0.1 mg/day every 1–2 days to a maximum of 1.2 mg/day. Transdermal clonidine is started with the 0.1 mg/day patch, applied to hairless skin and changed every 7 days; dosage may be incrementally-increased to the 0.2 and 0.3 mg/day patches each week.

Dexmedetomidine: Use of dexmedetomidine infusions for greater than 24 hours has not been approved by the Food and Drug Administration (FDA). A loading dose may be given as 1 μg/kg over 10 minutes, although this is not mandatory. For sedation in the ICU, maintenance infusions are titrated from 0.2–0.7 μg/kg/h per the product labeling. More recent data suggest doses of up to 1.4 μg/kg/h, and durations up to 30 days have been invoked. Dosage adjustment may be necessary in individuals with hepatic insufficiency.

Neuroleptics/'antipsychotics'

Neuroleptics are considered the drug of choice for patients diagnosed with delirium. In addition, the lack of respiratory depression makes them potentially attractive alternatives to more conventional sedatives for non-intubated patients with pulmonary compromise. Discussion shall be limited to the two agents used most commonly in the ICU and anesthesia realms, the butyrophenones, haloperidol and droperidol.

Mechanism of action
Neuroleptics produce both therapeutic and adverse effects by blocking cerebral and peripheral (but not spinal) dopamine, adrenergic, serotonin, acetylcholine, and histamine receptors, with variable selectivity depending on the agent. These effects include sedation (tolerance develops with repeated dosing), anxiolysis, restlessness, suppression of emotional and aggressive outbursts, reduction of delusions, hallucinations, and disorganized thoughts (over repeated dosing), antiemetic properties, hypotension (varies by agent), and extrapyramidal side effects. Haloperidol and dro-

peridol have limited anticholinergic properties compared with other neuroleptics, reducing the occurrence of blurred vision, urinary retention, and gastrointestinal hypomotility [42].

Pharmacokinetics and dynamics

Haloperidol is highly lipophilic and plasma-protein bound. Sedative effects may be seen within minutes of intravenous administration. Although plasma half-life varies from 12–36 hours (depending on hepatic microsomal and conjugation activities), the effective half-life may be much longer (a week or more) due to accumulation in brain and other tissues with a high blood supply. The very young and very old have a reduced capacity to metabolize haloperidol and related agents. When administered intravenously, droperidol has a rapid onset of action (1–3 minutes), although peak effects may not be noted for 30 minutes. Duration of action varies from 2–12 hours, and elimination appears to follow more linear (first-order) kinetics even at high doses. Systemic elimination mirrors hepatic blood flow, and thus metabolism is presumably similar to that of haloperidol.

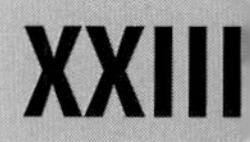

Haloperidol is available for oral, intramuscular, and intravenous administration. Droperidol is given intramuscularly or intravenously. Because of their onset within minutes of intravenous administration, both haloperidol and droperidol are readily titratable with initial bolus dosing. However, as metabolism and elimination may be highly variable, repeated dosing should be done with caution due to potential systemic accumulation.

Rationale for ICU use and adverse reactions

The major utility of the phenothiazines or butyrophenones is in the treatment of acute agitation secondary to psychosis or delirium. Their adverse effects negate the use of these agents for mild sedation. However, where appropriate, the effects can be dramatic and provide the necessary conditions to greatly enhance ICU management. Recent studies have illustrated the adverse effect of ICU delirium on patient ICU length-of-stay and mortality [37].

Unfortunately, the use of these agents is replete with potential physiological and neurological complications, thereby limiting their utility in the ICU. Extrapyramidal side effects (Parkinsonism, acute and tardive dystonias, tardive dyskinesia, akathesia, and perioral tremor) may be expressed. Although less common with butyrophenones than with phenothiazine antipsychotics, such motor disturbances may still occur with both haloperidol and droperidol. Regarding possible other CNS effects, droperidol had little effect on ICP, although CPP was decreased by moderate systemic hypotension.

Lowering of the seizure threshold has been a longstanding concern with the phenothiazines. Neuroleptics do induce slowing and synchronization (with associated increased voltage) of the EEG. However, effects on the seizure threshold are highly variable, depending on the agent. Haloperidol and related butyrophenones (including droperidol) have unpredictable effects on seizure threshold, and although most studies suggest a low risk, these drugs should be used with caution in patients with known seizure disorders.

Other potential side effects including increased prolactin secretion, orthostatic hypotension (rare with haloperidol and droperidol), neuroleptic malignant syndrome, and jaundice (rare with butyrophenones) have all been reported for neuroleptics in general [42]. Both haloperidol and droperidol can induce QT prolongation and torsades-de-pointes, and warnings have been issued regarding this adverse effect with even low doses of droperidol, greatly limiting the use of this agent for its perioperative sedation and antiemetic properties [43]. As such, droperidol is contraindicated in patients with pre-existing QT prolongation, and should be used with extreme caution in those at risk for cardiac dysrhythmias. Although chlorpromazine and other typical phenothiazine antipsychotics have been associated with hypotension, negative inotropy, and nonspecific ST and T-wave changes (including QT prolongation), significant hemodynamic side effects are rare with haloperidol and droperidol [42]. Both droperidol and haloperidol may cause systemic hypotension via peripheral vasodilatation when given intravenously.

Prior to treatment with droperidol, a 12-lead electrocardiogram (EKG) should be performed to evaluate for pre-existent QT prolongation that would preclude use of this medication. Continuous EKG monitoring must be performed for several hours following administration of droperidol, and appropriate treatments for hypotension, QT prolongation, and ventricular dysrhythmias must be readily available. Because of potential hypotension from intravenous haloperidol or droperidol, frequent blood pressure measurement should also be performed with use of these medications.

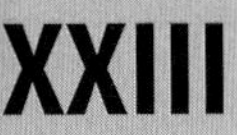

Because of the risk of ventricular dysrhythmias, droperidol should not be concurrently administered with any medications that may prolong the QT interval [43]. These include, but are not limited to, antihistamines, several antibiotics, class I or III antiarrhythmics, and many antidepressants. Hypomagnesemia and hypokalemia should be avoided or treated.

Drug-drug interactions

Because of their sedative and potential autonomic effects, haloperidol and droperidol may enhance the effects of other sedative agents (including anticonvulsants). Additionally, any medications that induce the hepatic microsomal enzyme system may increase the rate at which neuroleptics are metabolized. Selective serotonin reuptake inhibitors (SSRIs) compete with neuroleptics for hepatic oxidative enzymes and may, therefore, increase circulating levels of haloperidol and droperidol [42]. In addition, co-administration with any agent which can prolong the QT interval may increase the likelihood of torsades-de-pointes, and routine EKG monitoring is necessary. As with all medications, non-specific adverse effects, including anaphylaxis, laryngospasm, and bronchospasm, have been reported.

Dosage recommendations

Haloperidol: For sedation, initial intravenous doses of 0.5–5 mg may be used. Dosage should be low in the elderly and in those with hemodynamic instability or high risk of seizures. The half-life is 12–36 hours, but active metabolites may remain for a much longer period.

Droperidol: For sedation in the setting of agitation, a starting dosage of 0.625 mg to a maximum of 2.5 mg intravenously is recommended. Additional dosages should not exceed 0.625–1.25 mg every 2–4 hours.

Propofol

Propofol, an ultra-short acting alkylphenol, is an agent that has been extensively used both as a sedative agent in critically ill patients as well as a general anesthetic. Although structurally distinct, its clinical action and effects on cerebral activity and intracranial dynamics are very similar to the short-acting barbiturates, such as thiopental. However, its extreme high rate of clearance results in even shorter duration of action, especially noted following prolonged infusions as compared to barbiturates [7]. This novel compound has other advantages over the older class of drugs, including less emetic properties than barbiturates as well as being a mood enhancer rather than frank depressant. However, reports of fatal metabolic acidosis and myocardial failure following long-term administration of propofol (especially in children) has tempered these beneficial properties to a degree and in some cases has led to disfavor and a return to alternative methods of sedation [44]·

Mechanism of action

A GABA-ergic mechanism of action has been suggested for propofol based on both *in vivo* and *in vitro* binding studies [45], with evidence that propofol may directly bind to $GABA_a$ receptors and activate inhibitory chloride channels in the absence of GABA. Other studies suggest a nonspecific but structurally-dependent effect on neuronal plasma membrane fluidity [46]. The specific mechanism(s) of action of propofol thus remain unclear.

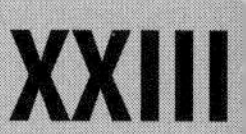

Pharmacokinetics and dynamics

Similar to thiopental in its lipophilicity, propofol is rapidly distributed to the brain following intravenous administration. It has a distribution half-life of 1–8 min, substantially shorter in time than most sedative agents with an equally rapid recovery following redistribution to other less perfused tissues [7]. Repeated or continuous dosing of propofol is cleared far more rapidly than thiopental. This is the result of a high degree of clearance, calculated to approach or exceed 1.5–2 l/min, which is greater than that of hepatic blood flow. Such kinetics suggests extra-hepatic sites of metabolism. This brief elimination time allows for more rapid recovery following cessation of sedative infusions. Propofol is also highly plasma protein bound, with free circulating levels increased in hypoalbuminic states.

Propofol is administered intravenously at a premixed concentration of 10 mg/ml (1 %). For the purposes of ICU sedation it is given as a continuous infusion, however, it may also be given as boluses for other indications. Due to its insolubility in water, propofol is suspended as an emulsion in a mixture of soybean oil, glycerol, and egg phospholipids, leaving it susceptible to bacterial contamination. Despite the presence of ethylenediaminetetraacetate (EDTA) as a bacteriostatic agent, propofol must be handled in an aseptic manner, and unused solutions discarded within 6–12 hours after a sterile seal is broken.

For continuous sedation in the ICU the dose ranges from 5–80 μg/kg/min. For other ICU indications (burst suppression EEG for refractory status epilepticus or refractory intracranial hypertension) general anesthesia doses such as 100–300 μg/kg/min may be required.

Rationale for ICU use and adverse reactions

The major utility of propofol in an ICU setting is its ultra-short duration of action, making it thus readily titratable and rapidly eliminated. It produces a stereotypic suppression of EEG activity similar to the barbiturates, from increasing theta and delta to a flat EEG pattern during deep general anesthesia. Thus, this drug can also be used to suppress seizure activity at high doses. As a sedative-hypnotic, propofol provides sedation devoid of any analgesia. Owing to a dose-dependent effect on cerebral metabolism, propofol also has a niche in the control of intracranial hypertension.

Propofol is by no means an ideal drug, especially in the ICU. As mentioned, no analgesic action is provided, so this sedative should not be used alone during sedation for painful maneuvers. Propofol may cause hypotension due to both vasodilation and a negative inotropic effect, and impairs the cardio-accelerator response to decreased blood pressure. This hypotension may be especially pronounced in patients with reduced cardiac output, hypovolemia, on other cardio-depressant medications, or the elderly. When used as a sedative for severe TBI patients, propofol may impair cerebral perfusion even as it induces a fall in ICP. Dose-dependent respiratory depression is a predictable result of the drug, and propofol should be used only in the setting of a controlled airway or in the continuous presence of experienced critical care or anesthesia personnel. During bolus or continuous infusions of propofol, frequent or continuous monitoring of pulse-oximetry, respiratory rate and depth of respiration, and blood pressure is recommended. Invasive monitoring of blood pressure and cardiac output may be necessary for high-dose propofol (e.g., burst suppression EEG).

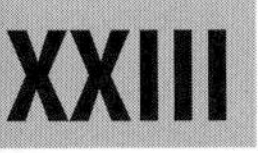

Pain on injection, which is common and due to the carrier solution, may be lessened by administration through central or larger veins, or pretreatment of peripheral injection sites with intravenous lidocaine (0.5 to 1 mg/kg). Far less common are potential anaphylactoid reactions with propofol. Usually, an immunological reaction is due not to the parent compound but to the emulsion which contains egg and soy product. Thus, administration of propofol is contraindicated in individuals who have had a severe allergic reaction to these food substances. Given the lipid vehicle of propofol, hypertriglyceridemia may occur, particularly at higher doses or prolonged duration.

Although the side effect profile for propofol is far more favorable than that for barbiturates, a syndrome of metabolic acidosis, hyperkalemia, rhabdomyolysis, and hypoxia has been described in children [44], and more recently in adults [46], receiving prolonged infusions of propofol. The etiology of this syndrome is unclear, and in the majority of reported cases the affected individuals were critically ill and on multiple other medications that may have initiated the metabolic disarray. Nonetheless, careful monitoring of electrolytes, lactic acid, creatine kinase, and triglycerides is highly recommended in patients receiving doses greater than 80 μg/kg/min for prolonged periods of time.

Drug-drug interactions

As with nearly all of the preceding sedatives, propofol may potentiate the sedative and cardiovascular effects of alcohol, opioids, benzodiazepines, barbiturates, other general anesthetics, antihypertensives, and antiarrhythmics. Propofol does not appear to alter the metabolism, elimination, or plasma protein binding of other drugs. Because of the scattered reports of rhabdomyolysis, metabolic acidosis, and myocardial failure following prolonged infusions of propofol, this agent should be used with caution when combined with other medications with similar potential. In addition, the high lipid content of propofol should be kept in mind when prescribing nutrition regimens, as the lipid vehicle constitutes a significant source of calories (1.1 kcal/ml) from fat.

Conclusion

Sedation of critically ill patients is common and provided as part of an optimal care plan. Neurological patients represent a particularly challenging subset given the need to balance comfort with maintenance of the neurologic exam. A detailed knowledge of the available agents, and patient-specific variables is necessary to strike this balance, necessitating the need for an interdisciplinary approach. Careful selection from the classes of available sedative agents is important to reduce toxicity and relieve patient anxiety, agitation or delirium. The incorporation of appropriate sedation scales is a valuable adjunct to define depth of sedation and to assure optimal drug titration and seamless communication of the goals of therapy. Due to the individualized nature of drug response, careful selection and dosing must be carried out in each patient to meet the intended sedation goal while preserving patient safety.

References

1. Kress JP, Pohlman AS, O'Connor MF, Hall JB (2000) Daily interruption of sedative infusions in critically ill patients undergoing mechanical ventilation. N Engl J Med 342: 1471–1477
2. Hogarth DK, Hall J (2004) Management of sedation in mechanically ventilated patients. Curr Opin Crit Care 10: 40–46
3. Hsiang JK, Chesnut RM, Crisp CB, Klauber MR, Blunt BA, Marshall LF (1994) Early, routine paralysis for intracranial pressure control in severe head injury: is it necessary? Crit Care Med 22: 1471–1476
4. Robinson BR, Mueller EW, Henson K, Branson RD, Barsoum S, Tsuei BJ (2008) An analgesia-delirium-sedation protocol for critically ill trauma patients reduces ventilator days and hospital length of stay. J Trauma 65: 517–526
5. Stocchetti N, Pagan F, Calappi E, et al (2004) Inaccurate early assessment of neurological severity in head injury. J Neurotrauma 21: 1131–1140
6. Servadei F, Nasi MT, Cremonini AM, Giuliani G, Cenni P, Nanni A (1998) Importance of a reliable admission Glasgow Coma Scale score for determining the need for evacuation of posttraumatic subdural hematomas: a prospective study of 65 patients. J Trauma 44: 868–873
7. Mirski MA, Muffelman B, Ulatowski JA, Hanley DF (1995) Sedation for the critically ill neurologic patient. Crit Care Med 23: 2038–2053
8. Jacobi J, Fraser GL, Coursin DB, et al (2002) Clinical practice guidelines for the sustained use of sedatives and analgesics in the critically ill adult. Crit Care Med 30: 119–141
9. Phillips DM (2000) JCAHO pain management standards are unveiled. Joint Commission on Accreditation of Healthcare Organizations. JAMA 284: 428–429
10. Payen JF, Chanques G, Mantz J, et al (2007) Current practices in sedation and analgesia for mechanically ventilated critically ill patients: a prospective multicenter patient-based study. Anesthesiology 106: 687–695
11. Siffleet J, Young J, Nikoletti S, Shaw T (2007) Patients' self-report of procedural pain in the intensive care unit. J Clin Nurs 16: 2142–2148
12. Li D, Puntillo K, Miaskowski C (2008) A review of objective pain measures for use with critical care adult patients unable to self-report. J Pain 9: 2–10
13. Mateo O, Krenzischek D (1992) A pilot study to assess the relationship between behavioral manifestations and self-report of pain in postanesthesia care unit patients, J Post Anesth Nurs 7: 15–21
14. Payen J, Bru O, Bosson J, et al (2001) Assessing pain in critically ill sedated patients by using a behavioral pain scale. Crit Care Med 29: 2258–2263
15. Gelinas C, Fillion L, Puntillo K, Viens C, Fortier M (2006) Validation of the Critical-Care Pain Observation Tool in adult patients. Am J Crit Care 15: 420–427
16. Odhner M, Wegman D, Freeland N, Steinmetz A, Ingersoll G (2003) Assessing pain control in nonverbal critically ill adults. Dimens Crit Care Nurs 22: 260–267
17. Puntillo K, Miaskowski C, Kehrle K, Stannard D, Gleeson S, Nye P (1997) Relationship between behavioral and physiological indicators of pain, critical care patients' self-reports of pain, and opioid administration, Crit Care Med 25: 1159–1166
18. Labus J, Keefe F, Jensen M (2003) Self-reports of pain intensity and direct observations of pain behavior: When are they correlated? J Pain 102: 109–124
19. Ely EW, Siegel MD, Inouye S (2001) Delirium in the intensive care unit: an under-recognized syndrome of organ dysfunction. Semin Respir Crit Care Med 22: 115–126

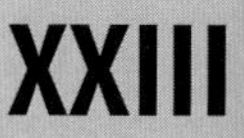

20. Thomason JWW, Shintani A, Peterson JF, et al (2005) Intensive Care Delirium is an independent predictor of longer hospital stay: a prospective analysis of 261 non-ventilated patients. Crit Care Med 9: R375–381
21. Ramsay MA, Savege TM, Simpson BR, Goodwin R (1974) Controlled sedation with alphaxalone-alphadolone. BMJ 2: 656–659
22. Riker RR, Picard JT, Fraser GL (1999) Prospective evaluation of the Sedation-Agitation Scale for adult critically ill patients. Crit Care Med 27: 1325–1329
23. Devlin JW, Boleski G, Mlynarek M, et al (1999) Motor Activity Assessment Scale: A valid and reasonable sedation scale for use with mechanically ventilated patients in an adult surgical intensive care unit. Crit Care Med 27: 1271–1275
24. Sessler CN, Gosnell MS, Grapp MJ, et al (2002) The Richmond Agitation-Sedation Scale. Validity and reliability in adult intensive care unit patients. Am J Respir Crit Care Med 166: 1338–1344
25. DeJonghe B, Cook D, Griffith L, et al (2003) Adaptation to the Intensive Care Environment (ATICE): development and validation of a new sedation assessment instrument. Crit Care Med 31: 2344–2354
26. Avripas MB, Smythe MA, Carr A, Begle RL, Johnson MH, Erb DR (2001) Development of an intensive care unit bedside sedation scale. Ann Pharmacother 35: 262–263
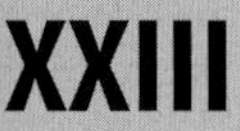
27. de Lemos, J, Tweeddale, M, Chittock, D (2000) Measuring quality of sedation in adult mechanically ventilated critically ill patients: the Vancouver Interaction and Calmness Scale. J Clin Epidemiol 53: 908–919
28. Weinert C, McFarland L (2004) The state of intubated ICU patients. Development of a two-dimensional sedation rating scale for critically ill adults. *Chest* 126: 1883–1890
29. Mirski M, Lewin JJ, Thompson C, LeDroux S, Zink EK, Mirski KT (2008) Validity and reliability of the Johns Hopkins nursing instrument for the communication of sedation (NICS). Crit Care Med 36 (suppl): A126 (abst)
30. Mirski M, Lewin JJ, LeDroux S, Bishop J, Griswold M, Thompson C (2008) Measurement of cognition in intubated & non-intubated critically ill patients: validity and reliability of the Johns Hopkins Adapted Cognitive Exam (ACE). Crit Care Med 36 (suppl): A125 (abst)
31. Park KS, Hur EJ, Han KW, Kil HY, Han TH (2006) Bispectral index does not correlate with observer assessment of alertness and sedation scores during 0.5 % bupivacaine epidural anesthesia with nitrous oxide sedation. Anesth Analg 103: 385–389
32. Gutstein HB, Akil H (2001) Opioid Analgesics. In: Hardman JG, Limbird LE (eds) Goodman and Gilman's The Pharmacological Basis of Therapeutics, 10th ed. McGraw-Hill, New York, pp 569–619
33. Pan YX, Xu J, Bolan E, Moskowitz HS, Xu M, Pasternak GW (2005) Identification of four novel exon 5 splice variants of the mouse mu-opioid receptor gene: functional consequences of C-terminal splicing. Mol Pharmacol 68: 866–875
34. Muellejans B, López A, Cross MH, Bonome C, Morrison L, Kirkham AJ (2004) Remifentanil versus fentanyl for analgesia based sedation to provide patient comfort in the intensive care unit: a randomized, double-blind controlled trial. Crit Care Med 8: 13–14
35. Rao TLK, Mummaneni N, El-Etr AA (1982) Convulsions: an unusual response to intravenous fentanyl administration. Anesth Analg 61: 1020–1021
36. Charney DS, Mihic SJ, Harris RA (2001) Hypnotics and Sedatives. In: Hardman JG, Limbird LE (eds) Goodman and Gilman's The Pharmacological Basis of Therapeutics, 10th ed. McGraw-Hill, New York, pp 399–427
37. Pandharipande P, Jackson J, Ely EW (2005) Delirium: acute cognitive dysfunction in the critically ill. Curr Opin Crit Care 11: 360–368
38. Khan ZP, Munday IT, Jones RM, Thornton C, Mant TG, Amin D (1999) Effects of dexmedetomidine on isoflurane requirements in healthy volunteers. 1: Pharmacodynamic and pharmacokinetic interactions. Br J Anaesth 83: 372–380
39. Szumita PM, Baroletti SA, Anger KE, Wechsler ME (2007) Sedation and analgesia in the intensive care unit: evaluating the role of dexmedetomidine. Am J Health Syst Pharm 64: 37–44
40. Mirski MA, LeDroux, S, Thompson, C, Zink EK, Griswold M, Lewin JJ (2008) Preservation of cognition during ICU sedation – The Johns Hopkins Acute Neurological ICU Sedation Trial (ANIST). Crit Care Med 36 (suppl): A10 (abst)

41. Aryan HE, Box KW, Ibrahim D, Desiraju U, Ames CP (2006) Safety and efficacy of dexmedetomidine in neurosurgical patients. Brain Inj 20: 791–798
42. Baldessarini RJ, Tarazi FI (2001) Drugs and the Treatment of Psychiatric Disorders: Psychosis and Mania. In: Hardman JG, Limbird LE (eds) Goodman and Gilman's The Pharmacological Basis of Therapeutics, 10th ed. McGraw-Hill, New York, pp 485–520
43. Lischke V, Behne M, Doelken P, Schledt U, Probst S, Vettermann J (1994) Droperidol causes a dose-dependent prolongation of the QT interval. Anesth Analg 79: 983–986
44. Vasile B, Rasulo F, Candiani A, Latronico N (2003) The pathophysiology of propofol infusion syndrome: a simple name for a complex syndrome. Intensive Care Med 29: 1417–1425
45. Alkire MT, Haier RJ (2001) Correlating in vivo anaesthetic effects with ex vivo receptor density data supports a GABAergic mechanism of action for propofol, but not for isoflurane. Br J Anaesth 86: 618–626
46. Perrier ND, Baerga-Varela Y, Murray MJ (2000) Death related to propofol use in an adult patient. Crit Care Med 28: 3071–3074

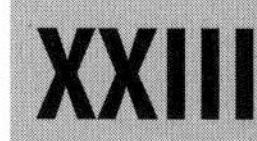

The Role of Dexmedetomidine in Intensive Care

R. Rahman West, A. Rhodes, and R.M. Grounds

Introduction

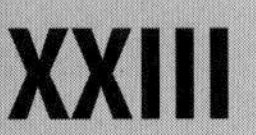

The US Food and Drug Administration (FDA) first approved dexmedetomidine in December 1999 for use as a continuous infusion in post-operative ventilated patients for up to 24 hours in the intensive care unit (ICU). It is not yet approved in the European Union. Its use is currently being evaluated in a number of different situations: Longer-term use, perioperative care, anesthesia, and postoperative analgesia. This chapter will focus on its potential for intensive care patients.

Mechanism of Action

Dexmedetomidine is an imidazole compound and is also a potent centrally acting α_2-receptor agonist [1]. It is highly selective for α_2-receptors compared to α_1-receptors, with a binding affinity ratio of 1620:1 [2]. As a sedative, its mechanism of action is similar to clonidine, however dexmedetomidine has eight times more affinity for the α_2-receptor [1]. Dexmedetomidine is the dextro-enantiomer of medetomidine, an agent that has been used for many years for sedation and analgesia in veterinary medicine [2, 3].

Three sub-types of α_2-adrenoceptor (α_{2a}, α_{2b} and α_{2c}) have been identified. Data from animal work suggests that these three receptors have different functional roles, α_{2a} mediating sedative/hypnotic, analgesic and anesthesia sparing effects whereas the α_{2c} sites are responsible for hypothermic effects. The sedative/hypnotic effects of

Table 1. Key properties of dexmedetomidine

Empirical formula	$C_{13}H_{16}N_2.HCL$
Molecular weight	236.7
pH as solution	4.5–7
pKa	7.1
Partition coefficient in octanol:water	2.89 at pH 7.4
Indication	Up to 24 hours for sedation of initially mechanically ventilated ICU patients
Main action site	Alpha$_{2a}$ receptor, locus coeruleus
Main effects	'Arousable sedation', moderate analgesia, no respiratory effect
Dosage	Slow loading 1 μg/kg over 10 minutes, followed by 0.2–0.7 μg/kg/h infusion
Common adverse effects	Hypotension, bradycardia
Caution	Hepatic impairment, heart block, severe ventricular dysfunction

dexmedetomidine are mediated through pertussis-sensitive inhibitory G proteins in the locus coeruleus. This consists of small bilateral nuclei in the upper brain stem containing a large number of adrenergic receptors [4]. The α_{2a} receptor subtype has been reported to be the predominant subtype in the brain, and is involved in a variety of physiological functions including antinoiciceptive, sedative, sympatholytic, hypothermic, and behavioral actions [5]. The dorsal horn of the spinal cord is also thought to be an important site of the analgesic action although spinal and supraspinal sites are also evident [4].

Pharmacokinetics

In the dosage range of 0.2 to 0.7 µg/kg/h, dexmedetomidine exhibits a linear relationship between dose and plasma concentration when administered by intravenous infusion, for up to 24 hours. Dexmedetomidine has a rapid onset of action with a distribution half life of 6 minutes and a terminal elimination half life of approximately 2 hours [6]. It has a relatively large volume of distribution of about 1.33 l/kg and a total body clearance of 0.495 l/h/kg. Ninety-four percent of dexmedetomidine is bound to plasma protein [1].

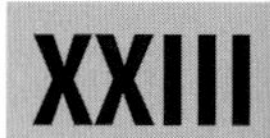

Dexmedetomidine undergoes extensive metabolism in the liver by direct glucuronidation and oxidative metabolism by the cytochrome P450 enzyme system. Hence the metabolism of the drug is heavily affected by severe liver disease. Ninety-five percent of the inactive metabolites are excreted in the urine and 5 % in the feces [7].

General Pharmacodynamics

Cardiorespiratory Effects

The cardiorespiratory effects of dexmedetomidine have been extensively studied in a variety of animal models and different species and states of consciousness. Intravenous infusion of dexmedetomidine can produce transient hypertension and coronary vasoconstriction (peripheral post-synaptic effects) and these are dependent on the dose and rate of delivery. This is followed by hypotension and bradycardia (central and peripheral pre-synaptic sympatholytic effects and increased vagal tone). In general no adverse events are seen on cardiac function as myocardial oxygen demand is reduced in response to the reduction in heart rate.

Respiratory Effects

Respiratory depression is noted with dexmedetomidine but it does not potentiate the respiratory depression associated with fentanyl.

Central Nervous System Effects

Tolerance or desensitization of effect is noted with high doses in some species. Dexmedetomidine has shown no convulsant or anticonvulsant effects. It is reported to be neuroprotective in a variety of ischemic injury models and may reduce neuronal damage induced by ethanol intoxication. Intracranial pressure (ICP) is slightly reduced or unaffected by use of doses up to 320 µg/kg in rabbits but doses of up to 10 µg/kg in dogs produced profound reduction in cerebral blood flow.

Gastrointestinal and Other Effects

Dexmedetomidine may reduce the transit time of food and may increase urinary volume and electrolytes. Dexmedetomidine increases prolactin and growth hormone levels and decreases thyroid stimulating hormone (TSH) levels. Sedative doses of dexmedetomidine elevate plasma glucose levels and higher doses inhibit insulin release.

Interactions

Dexmedetomidine acts synergistically when given in combination with midazolam, diazepam and fentanyl. There is a synergistic analgesic effect between μ, but not δ, opioid agonists and dexmedetomidine.

Dosage and Duration of Administration

Dosage for use of dexmedetomidine for sedation in the ICU has been recommended as a slow loading infusion of 1 μg/kg over 10 minutes followed by a continuous infusion of 0.2 to 0.7 μg/kg/h for up to 24 hours [8]. The dosage should be titrated according to the level of sedation required. However, there have been several clinical trials that have shown that the maximum dosage allowed is inadequate to produce the desired clinical effect. Between 10 to 20 % of patients receiving the maximum dosage of 0.7 μg/kg/h need additional sedative agents [9–15, 21–24, 27]. Dosages used have been increased up to 2.5 μg/kg/h and studies have found that above 0.7 μg/kg/h patients needed much less or no supplement of other sedative agents at all to be sufficiently sedated [6, 9, 16]. On the other hand, in a phase II study evaluating the efficacy of dexmedetomidine in a medical ICU, the authors suggested that dosages higher than 1.5 μg/kg/h add little value to the quality of sedation but merely increased the number of complications; but the drug was only tested on 8 patients in this study [9].

The licensed maximum duration of infusion has been approved to be not more than 24 hours, however several studies have investigated its use for a longer duration [13, 14, 17]. Two of these studies continued dexmedetomidine infusion for up to 7 days. When comparing adverse events, one of the randomized controlled studies found that the incidence of bradycardia and hypotension were similar in the dexmedetomidine group compared to a midazolam group after 24 hours of infusion [13]. In another open-label, uncontrolled study, the authors reported an approximately 20 % decrease in mean heart rate from baseline over the first 12 hours of dexmedetomidine infusion. After 12 hours, the rest of the infusion time only caused minimal changes in heart rate [14]. In a 30 patient randomized controlled trial comparing dexmedetomidine to placebo with rescue therapy of morphine and propofol, infusion duration continued for up to 72 hours [17]. The results showed that the incidence of adverse events including bradycardia and hypotension were similar in the two groups. In another report where patients were treated with dexmedetomidine for up to 124 hours, the frequency of adverse events was not higher when treatment was prolonged for more than 24 hours [18].

Loading and maximizing dosage will have implications on the safety profile and adverse events. To date the optimum dosage in view of risk and benefit is still unclear. In terms of increasing the duration of infusion for more than the recommended time, even though it seems that dexmedetomidine is quite well tolerated, more evidence is still needed to provide guidance for its use.

Sedative and Analgesia Profile

At certain dosages, dexmedetomidine induces a state of 'arousable sedation' where patients are well sedated but can be woken up when stimulated allowing communication and cooperation [19]. Once left alone, they return to sleep in a very short time period. The literature has also described dexmedetomidine's other properties, which include possible anxiolysis, moderate analgesia, and only very mild respiratory depression.

Post-surgical Patients

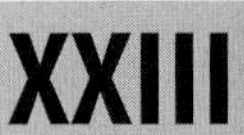

Most clinical trials have evaluated the use of dexmedetomidine as a short-term sedative agent (< 24 hours) in patients admitted to the ICU following surgery. Several studies have established the ability of dexmedetomidine to provide sufficient sedation and analgesia in mechanically ventilated patients following cardiac surgery [9, 10, 17, 20–24]. In a prospective trial of 401 intubated patients following major surgery, significantly less propofol rescue ($p < 0.001$) and morphine requirements ($p < 0.001$) were needed in patients sedated with dexmedetomidine when compared to placebo groups [10], suggesting that dexmedetomidine not only had sedative properties but had mild analgesic properties as well. However, a significantly higher incidence of hypotension and bradycardia were also observed in the dexmedetomidine groups ($p < 0.001$ and $p = 0.003$, respectively) whereas significantly more hypertension was observed in control group ($p = 0.005$) [10]. In another trial involving 119 postoperative general and cardiothoracic ICU patients and comparing dexmedetomidine groups with placebo, there was a significant reduction in the mean amount of midazolam and morphine rescue requirements observed in the dexmedetomidine group during mechanical ventilation ($p = 0.0001$ and $p = 0.0006$, respectively) [20]. Overall adverse events for dexmedetomidine group were more than placebo (53 versus 39 events) although this was not significant statistically. Conversely in a trial examining the bispectral index in 30 post-cardiac surgical patients where dexmedetomidine was compared to placebo treatment for up to 72 hours, efficacy was assessed using the need for additional propofol and morphine [17]. Although additional propofol requirements were significantly lower in the dexmedetomidine group before and during weaning from mechanical ventilation ($p = 0.006$ and $p < 0.001$, respectively), there were no significant differences in morphine dose requirement or mean bispectral index before, during and post-extubation and mean time to extubation. The overall incidence of adverse events was also similar in the two groups (15 vs 13 events, $p = 0.483$). The results from these studies suggest that dexmedetomidine is similarly efficacious to the comparator sedatives (propofol and midazolam) and that it is able to provide adequate short-term sedation but that more evidence than merely a reduction in opioid use was required to demonstrate that it had powerful analgesic effects.

A number of other clinical studies have been published comparing dexmedetomidine with propofol in post-surgical patients [16, 21, 24, 25]. The sedative profile of dexmedetomidine measured using the Ramsay Sedation Score was found to be similar to propofol [16, 21, 25]. These trials also demonstrated that opioid requirements were significantly less in post-operative patients receiving dexmedetomidine. However, in a study of 89 patients undergoing elective coronary artery bypass graft (CABG) surgery, the authors found that the median Ramsay Sedation Score was significantly lower in patients receiving dexmedetomidine than in those receiving propofol, and there were no differences in patient-reported responses between the two groups when dosages were titrated to achieve the same level of sedation. Other findings included similar needs for rescue treatment with midazolam and morphine in both groups of patients [24]. MacLaren and colleagues showed that analgesic requirements were not different in patients who were already receiving either propofol or lorazepam and fentanyl and who received additional dexmedetomidine [26]. Thus, these two studies question the suggestion that dexmedetomidine has no additional benefit in reducing analgesia requirement.

The mean time to extubation was found to be similar with dexmedetomidine and propofol [16, 21, 24, 25]. Patients receiving dexmedetomidine appeared to have more recall of their stay in the ICU, but described it as being overall pleasant [16, 17]. All of these clinical trials also demonstrate that the incidence of decrease in blood pressure was similar in both groups of patients but heart rates were reported to be significantly lower in the dexmedetomidine group, although the lowest values were still more than 60 beats per minute.

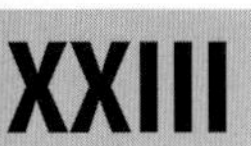

Medical Patients

In the medical population, fewer data are available regarding the clinical application of dexmedetomidine. In a phase II trial, Venn and colleagues evaluated the efficacy of dexmedetomidine for sedation in critically ill medical patients [9]. Twelve patients were recruited within 12 hours of sedation and mechanical ventilation, with a minimum requirement for mechanical ventilation of greater than six hours. The primary outcome of this study was the dosage of dexmedetomidine needed to reach a Ramsay Sedation Score of > 2. The regime was a loading infusion of 1 µg/kg of dexmedetomidine over 10 minutes, followed by 0.2–0.7 µg/kg/h with rescue boluses of propofol. After the first four patients, the protocol had to be changed, allowing an increase in the maximum dosage of up to 2.5 µg/kg/h, which is higher than the recommended dose [8]. The durations of dexmedetomidine infusion were up to 72 hours with a mean of 33 hours. The mean dosage received by the first four patients was 0.7 µg/kg/h. The other eight patients received a mean dosage of 1.0 ± 0.7 µg/kg/h after the protocol was amended. During the loading infusion, four patients developed hypotension that responded to intravenous fluid administration. Dexmedetomidine was stopped prematurely in one patient due to persistent hypotension despite intravenous fluid administration; another patient developed bradycardia down to 45 beats per minute [9]. The mean heart rate decreased from 90 to 80 beats per minute. The sedative use of dexmedetomidine in non-surgical patients will inevitably require a longer duration of use than the current license allows for and the optimal dose regimen for these patients will need to be further evaluated in order to better define the role of dexmedetomidine as a sedative.

Respiratory Profile

The ability of dexmedetomidine to provide sedation together with an opioid sparing effect leads it to produce less respiratory depression and have fewer other adverse effects of opioids. The reduction in respiratory depression may lead to easier or faster weaning from mechanical ventilation and ultimately reduce the length of stay in the ICU. In several clinical studies, dexmedetomidine has demonstrated its ability to reduced opiate requirements in mechanically ventilated patients [17, 20, 21, 23, 27]. In one study, morphine consumption was significantly less in patients receiving dexmedetomidine than patients receiving morphine alone [27]. In another study, the respiratory effects of dexmedetomidine were retrospectively examined in 33 post-surgical patients involved in a randomized placebo-controlled study after extubation in the ICU [23]. Morphine requirements decreased by 50 % when dexmedetomidine was administered; nevertheless, there were no significant differences in respiratory rate, pH, oxygen saturation, or arterial carbon dioxide between the two groups. The respiratory effects of dexmedetomidine have also been compared to remifentanil in a study of six healthy volunteers. Remifentanil induced respiratory depression by reducing respiratory rate and minute ventilation, the respiratory acidosis and apnoeic episodes resulting in arterial oxygen desaturations. On the contrary, dexmedetomidine allowed the respiratory rate to increase whilst simultaneously decreasing the apnea/hypopnea index. Furthermore during a 5 % carbon dioxide challenge, the hypercapnic arousal response was preserved during sedation with dexmedetomidine [28].

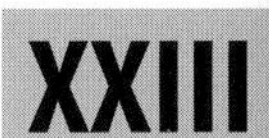

Non-sedative Use in the ICU

Delirium is now thought to be a common complication of ICU stay and is linked with an increase in morbidity and mortality [29]. When comparing dexmedetomidine infusion with propofol and midazolam, a single center study showed that the incidence of delirium was 1/30 with dexmedetomidine, as opposed to 15/30 with propofol and with midazolam ($p = 0.01$) [30]. In a clinical trial involving 106 patients from two centers, ventilated for up to 120 hours, which compared dexmedetomidine with lorazepam for sedation, there was a reduction in duration of delirium and coma while providing adequate sedation [31]. Patients were monitored twice daily for delirium using the Confusion Assessment Method for the ICU (CAM-ICU). The outcome of the study demonstrated that sedation with dexmedetomidine resulted in more patient days alive without delirium or coma (median days, 7.0 vs 3.0; $p = 0.01$) and a lower prevalence of coma (63 vs 92 %; $p < 0.001$); however, since the "delirium free days" alone were not found to be statistically significant ($p = 0.09$) this suggests that the reduction in delirium might be due to beneficial use of dexmedetomidine in avoiding oversedation. Dexmedetomidine may have a role in reducing sedation-related delirium but more evidence is needed to better define this.

Dexmedetomidine may also be used to facilitate weaning from mechanical ventilation and to reduce dosages of other sedatives and opiates [18]. Some case series have reported the success of introducing dexmedetomidine in weaning agitated patients off mechanical ventilator when they had previously failed [32]. Also from case studies, treatment of drug or alcohol withdrawal syndromes has been described with dexmedetomidine [33–35]. Another reported non-sedative use includes a reduction in the threshold for shivering [36].

Safety Profile/adverse Events

Dexmedetomidine is associated with a number of adverse reactions. The most commonly described adverse events are associated with its sympatholytic activity leading to dose-related bradycardia and hypotension which are usually reversed if the dosage is reduced or discontinued [19]. Results from a phase III trial involving 401 patients showed that the most common adverse events were hypotension (30 %), hypertension (12 %), nausea (11 %), bradycardia (9 %), and dry mouth (3 %) [1]. These findings, except for hypertension, were more frequent in patients treated with dexmedetomidine than in control groups. In another phase III trial involving 353 patients, hypertensive episodes were more predominant in the dexmedetomidine groups (22 %) compared to control (12 %) [1]. In a study by Ebert and colleagues, the effects of increasing plasma concentrations of dexmedetomidine were evaluated in ten healthy men. These authors showed that with increasing concentration the heart rate and cardiac output decreased progressively. The mean arterial pressure, however, decreased at low plasma concentrations of the drug but progressively increased at higher concentrations [37]. Several studies have also implied that bradycardia and especially hypotension can be linked to loading dose administration [9, 10, 13, 21]. Transient hypertension on the other hand has been associated with very rapid loading dose administration. As with higher dosage, the transient hypertension is thought to be the effect of direct peripheral α_{2b} receptor stimulation leading to vasoconstriction, counteracting the hypotensive effects of the α_{2a} receptor subtype [38]. This effect can be avoided by slowing down the loading dose administration rate [20]. Severe bradycardia leading to cardiac arrest has also been reported in one case report but multiple other issues might have been contributing factors [39]. Other very rare adverse events that have been reported include fever, vomiting, hypoxia, xerostomia, paradoxical agitation, oliguria, and anemia [8].

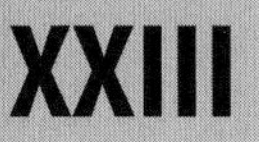

Conclusion

Dexmetetomidine has a broad range of potential applications, both within the ICU and beyond. Probably the most appealing feature is its ability to produce cooperative sedation, a quality not as well pronounced in other sedative agents. It may also produce less delirium than equivalent agents. It has adverse effects mainly related to its sympatholytic action though concomitant patient factors contribute to this. Although a large body of work has already been done on dexmedetomidine, fundamental questions remain unanswered, such as its suitability over other currently available sedative agents, optimal dosing ranges, whether it has analgesic effects, the true nature of its lack of respiratory depression, its potential to reduce the number of cases of delirium, maximum length of infusion, and adverse events. To date, the maximum recommended infusion rate has been found inadequate to produce satisfactory sedation by a number of authors.

There is much further research and development to be done before dexmedetomidine is ready for widespread routine use.

References

1. Bhana N, Goa KL, McClellan KJ (2000) Dexmedetomidine. Drugs 59: 263–268
2. Savola J-M, Virtanen R (1991) Central alpha2-adrenoceptors are highly stereoselective for dexmedetomidine, the dextro enantiomer of medetomidine. Eur J Pharmacol 195: 193–199
3. Szumita PM, Baroletti SA, Anger KE, Wechsler ME (2007) Sedation and analgesia in the intensive care unit: evaluating the role of dexmedetomidine. Am J Health Syst Pharm 64: 37–44
4. Kamibayashi T, Maze M (2000) Clinical uses of alpha2-adrenergic agonists. Anesthesiology 93: 1345–1349
5. MacMillan LB, Hein L, Smith MS, et al (1996) Central hypotensive effects of the alpha2a-adrenergic receptor subtype. Science 273: 801–803
6. Venn RM. Karol MD. Grounds RM (2002) Pharmacokinetics of dexmedetomidine infusions for sedation of postoperative patients requiring intensive care. Br J Anaesth 88: 669–675
7. Maze M, Scarfini C, Cavaliere F (2001) New agents for sedation in the intensive care unit. Crit Care Clin 17: 881–897
8. Product information Precedex® (dexmedetomidine). Available at: http://precedex.hospira.com/_docs/PrecedexPI.pdf Accessed Nov 2008
9. Venn RM, Newmann PJ, Grounds RM (2003) A phase II study to evaluate the efficacy of dexmedetomidine for sedation in the medical intensive care unit. Intensive Care Med 29: 201–207
10. Martin E, Ramsay G, Mantz J, Sum-Ping ST (2003) The role of the alpha2-adrenoceptor agonist dexmedetomidine in postsurgical sedation in the intensive care unit. J Intensive Care Med 18: 29–41
11. Bachand R, Scholz J, Pinaud M, et al (1999) The effects of dexmedetomidine in patients in the intensive care setting. Intensive Care Med 25 (Suppl 1): S160 (abst)
12. Martin E, Lehott JJ, Manikis P Torres L, Cote D, Mooi B (1999) Dexmedetomidine: a novel agent for patients in the intensive care setting. Intensive Care Med 25 (Suppl 1): S160 (abst)
13. Riker RR, Ramsay MAE, Prielipp RA, Jorden VSB (2001) Dexmedetomidine provides effective long-term sedation for intubated ICU patients compared to midazolam: a randomized open-label pilot study. Chest 120: 260s (abst)
14. Shehabi Y, Ruettimann U, Adamson H, Innes R, Ickeringill M (2004) Dexmedetomidine infusion for more than 24 hours in critically ill patients: sedative and cardiovascular effects. Intensive Care Med 30: 2188–2196
15. Richard R. Riker RR, Fraser GL (2005) Adverse events associated with sedatives, analgesics and other drugs that provide patient comfort in the intensive care unit. Pharmacotherapy 25: 8S-18S
16. Venn RM, Grounds RM (2001) Comparison between dexmedetomidine and propofol for sedation in the intensive care unit: patient and clinician perceptions. Br J Anaesth 87: 684–690
17. Triltsch AE, Welte M, Von Homeyer P, et al (2002) Bispectral index-guided sedation with dexmedetomidine in intensive care: a prospective, randomized, double blind, placebo-controlled phase II study. Crit Care Med 30: 1007–1014
18. Dasta JF, Kane-Gill SL, Durtschi AJ (2004) Comparing dexmedetomidineprescribing patterns and safety in the naturalistic setting versus published data. Ann Pharmacother 38: 1130–1135
19. Chrysostomou C, Schmitt C (2008) Dexmedetimidine: sedation, analgesia and beyond. Expert Opin Drug Metab Toxicol 4: 619–627
20. Venn RM, Bradshaw CJ, Spencer R, et al (1999) Preliminary UK experience of dexmedetomidine, a novel agent for postoperative sedation in the intensive care unit. Anaesthesia 54: 1136–1142
21. Herr DL, Sum-Ping ST, England M (2003) ICU sedation after coronary artery bypass surgery: dexmedetomidine-based versus propofol-based sedation regimens. J Cardiothor Vasc Anesth 17: 576–584
22. Ickeringill M, Shehabi Y, Adamson H, Ruettimann U (2004) Dexmedetomidine infusion without loading dose in surgical patients requiring mechanical ventilation: haemodynamic effects and efficacy. Anaesth Intensive Care 32: 741–745

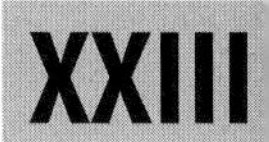

23. Venn RM. Hell J (2004) Grounds RM. Respiratory effects of dexmedetomidine in the surgical patient requiring intensive care. Crit Care 4: 302–308
24. Corbett SM, Rebuck JA, Greene CM, et al (2005) Dexmedetomidine does not improve patient satisfaction when compared to propofol during mechanical ventilation. Crit Care Med 33: 940–945
25. Elbaradie S, El Mahalawy FH, Solyman AH (2004) Dexmedetomidine vs propofol for short-term sedation of postoperative mechanically ventilated patients. J Egyptian Nat Cancer Inst 16: 153–158
26. MacLaren R, Forrest LK, Kiser TH (2007) Adjunctive dexmedetomidine therapy in the intensive care unit: a retrospective assessment of impact on sedative and analgesic requirements, levels of sedation and analgesia, and ventilatory and hemodynamic parameters. Pharmacotherapy 27: 351–359
27. Arain Sr, Ruehlow RM, Uhrich TD, et al (2004) The efficacy of dexmedetomidine versus morphine for postoperative analgesia after major inpatient surgery. Anesth Analg 98: 153–158
28. Hsu YW, Cortinez LI, Robertson KM, et al (2004) Dexmedetomidine pharmacodynamics. Part 1: Crossover comparison of the respiratory effects of dexmedetomidine and remifentanil in healthy volunteers. Anesthesiology 101: 1066–1076

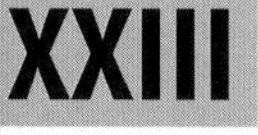

29. Ely EW, Shintani A, Truman B, et al (2004) Delirium as a predictor of mortality in mechanically ventilated patients in the intensive care unit. JAMA 291: 1753–1762
30. Maldonado JR, Wysong A, Van Der Starre PJ, et al (2005) Alpha-2 agonist induced sedation prevents ICU delirium in post-cardiotomy patients. J Psychosom Res 58: 61 (abst)
31. Pandharipande PP, Pun BT, Herr DL, Maze M (2007) Effect of sedation with dexmedetomidine vs lorazepam on acute brain dysfunction in mechanically ventilated patients. JAMA 298: 2644–2653
32. Siobal MS, Kallet RH, Kivett VA, Tang JF (2006) Use of dexmedetomidine to facilitate extubation in surgical intensive-care-unit patients who failed previous weaning attempts following prolonged mechanical ventilation: a pilot study. Respir Care 51: 492–496
33. Baddigam K, Russo P, Russo J, Tobias JD (2005) Dexmedetomidine in the treatment of withdrawal syndromes in cardiothoracic surgery patients. J Intensive Care Med 20: 118–123
34. Maccioli GA (2003) Dexmedetomidine to facilitate drug withdrawal. Anesthesiology 98: 575–577
35. Multz AS (2003) Prolonged dexmedetomidine infusion as an adjunct in treating sedation-induced withdrawal. Anesth Analg 96: 1054–1055
36. Doufas AG, Lin CM, Suleman MI, et al (2003) Dexmedetomidine and meperidine additively reduce the shivering threshold in humans. Stroke 34: 1218–1223
37. Ebert TJ, Hall JE, Barney JA, Uhrich TD, Colinco MD (2000) The effects of increasing plasma concentrations of dexmedetomidine in humans. Anesthesiology 93: 382–394
38. Paris A, Tonner PH (2005) Dexmedetomidine in anaesthesia. Curr Opin Anaesthesiol 18: 412–418
39. Ingersoll-Weng E, Manecke GR Jr, Thistlethwaite PA (2004) Dexmedetomidine and cardiac arrest. Anesthesiology 100: 738–739

Monitoring Delirium in the ICU

M. Seeling, A. Heymann, and C. Spies

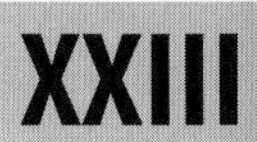

Introduction

For most of us, critical care used to consist of directly applying physiological and pathophysiological knowledge – which we so proudly and diligently acquired during medical school – in the real world. Pulmonary, cardiac, renal, and later metabolic functions were the concerns of the day and their dysfunction comprised the major determinants of disease. Introducing a new dimension, Pronovost et al. [1] showed us that team efforts make a great contribution towards improving critical care outcomes. Since Bedford observed the postoperative long-term confusional state back in 1955 [2], we have come a long way, to understand that the acute impairment of cognitive functions is not only an annoying side issue which is difficult to deal with on the critical care ward, but that it all too often determines the outcome of patients when all other organ functions should have been under control. Defining this 'sixth vital sign' necessitated some evolutionary development in that international terminology had to be agreed on – a process that is still underway. Despite international clarification by means of the International Statistical Classification of Diseases (ICD)-10 and the Diagnostic and Statistical Manual of Mental Disorders (DSM), there is no real gold-standard for diagnosing acute confusional state.

Increasingly, we – the medical community – understand the impact delirium has on our patients. However, the authors believe that it is time to step back and review a few points on the way to internationally implemented intensive care unit delirium screening programs. In this chapter, we will consider the impact that postoperative confusional states have on relevant outcome parameters, what a strategic approach towards prevention and treatment could look like, what the current technology and knowledge base is, and what we as clinicians, researchers, and policy makers have to do in the future in order to accomplish interventions that are worth the resources employed.

Burden of Illness

Concept

Delirium is characterized by an acutely changing or fluctuating mental state, inattention, disorganized thinking, and an altered level of consciousness that may or may not be accompanied by agitation. The term, delirium, as a diagnostic entity did not even appear in the formal nomenclature until 1980 when it achieved recognition in DSM-III as a diagnostic entity. Gary Tucker, a member of the APA Work Group on Organic Disorders of the DSM-IV Task Force wrote, "I feel the diagnostic criteria for

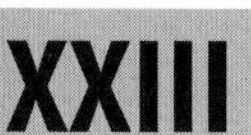

Table 1. DSM-IV-TR criteria for the diagnosis of delirium [66]

a. Disturbances of consciousness (e.g., reduced clarity of awareness of the environment) with reduced ability to focus, sustain or shift attention.

b. A change in cognition (such as memory deficit, disorientation, language disturbance) or the development of a perceptual disturbance that is not better accounted for by a pre-existing, established, or evolving dementia.

c. The disturbance develops over a short period of time (usually hours to days) and tends to fluctuate during the course of the day.

d. Where the delirium is due to a general medical condition – there is evidence from the history, physical examination, or laboratory findings that the disturbance is caused by the direct physiological consequences of a general medical condition.
Where the delirium is due to substance intoxication – there is evidence from the history, physical examination, or laboratory findings of either 1 or 2:
1. The symptoms in criteria (a) and (b) developed during substance intoxication
2. Medication use etiologically related to the disturbance
Where delirium is due to substance withdrawal – there is evidence from the history, physical examination, or laboratory findings that the symptoms in criteria (a) and (b) developed during or shortly after withdrawal syndromes
Where delirium is due to multiple etiologies – there is evidence from the history, physical examination, or laboratory findings that the delirium has more than one etiology (for example, more than one etiological general medical condition, a general medical condition plus substance intoxication, or medication side effects)

e. Delirium not otherwise specified – this category should be used to diagnose a delirium that does not meet criteria for any of the specific types of delirium described. Examples include a clinical presentation of delirium that is suspected to be due to general medical condition or substance use but for which there is insufficient evidence to establish a specific etiology or where delirium is due to causes not listed (for example, sensory deprivation).

delirium are still a work in progress, as are most of the entities of psychiatry, and that we will eventually add laboratory measures to the diagnosis of delirium" [3]. The current diagnostic criteria for delirium according to the DSM-IV are shown in **Table 1.**

"We need to be sure what delirium is. But we are not" Yoanna Skrobik recently remarked in an editorial in *Critical Care Medicine* [4]. Such a comment from a renowned figure in delirium research might be surprising in the face of increasing intervention and outcome studies in which the term delirium seems to be used with comfort and confidence. In the majority of studies delirium is perceived as defined by the DSM. The first edition (DSM-I) was published in 1952 shortly before PD Bedford presented his seminal paper on the phenomenon of postoperative cerebral adverse effects of anesthesia in 1953, published in 1955 [2]. In the subsequent decades, the DSM underwent radical changes but was still based primarily on expert opinion and case reports. This changed only with the development of the 4th edition for which a working group solicited comments from the field (mainly psychiatrists, neurologists, and neuropsychologists) nationally and internationally about their thoughts on the DSM-III-R organic disorders, then undertook an up-to-date comprehensive literature review of each diagnostic category and the diagnostic criteria. Preliminary ideas were formed and examined in light of several large patient databases that had good symptomatic descriptions of delirium (Harvard – Liptzin; University of Pennsylvania – Gottlieb) and dementia (Johns Hopkins – Folstein; University of Rochester – Caine). The results were then resubmitted to the consultants. The aim was to arrive at evidence-based, explicit criteria that could be operationalized [2]. Concern has been raised about the dimension 'attention' being difficult to operationalize as a criterion. Also, the possibility of coding whether the patient is hyperactive or somnolent or whether there are any corroborating laboratory data or subthreshold conditions, was opposed by the majority of task force members.

Research in the area of acute brain dysfunction develops more and more rapidly. However, there are still relevant international differences in terminology. Morandi et al., through expert interviews, reviewed 13 languages utilizing Romanic characters (Italian, Portuguese, Portuguese-Brazil, Spanish-Spain, Spanish-Latin America, French, French-Swiss, Dutch, Norwegian, Danish, Swedish and German) and found coma, delirium, delirio, delirium tremens, de'lire, confusion mentale, delir, delier, Durchgangs-Syndrom, acute verwardheid, intensivpsykose, IVA-psykos, IVA-syndrom, akutt konfusion/forvirring as terms being utulized to describe the acute deterioration of brain function [5]. Coma, describing patients who were unresponsive to verbal and/or physical stimuli, and delirium, defining delirium due to alcohol withdrawal, were the most consistent terms across all languages. Only 54 % of experts used the term delirium according to DSM-IV as an acute change in mental status, inattention, disorganized thinking and altered level of consciousness.

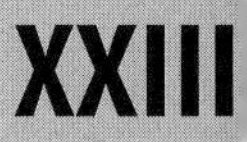

DSM-IV criteria define delirium independent of its etiology. Cheung et al. asked: "How do intensivists diagnose delirium? Does diagnosis affect management?" [6]. These authors were unaware of any literature that examined how delirium was diagnosed in the ICU. They, therefore, surveyed 130 Canadian intensivists registered with the Canadian Critical Care Society and found that when an etiological cognitive dysfunction diagnosis was obvious, 83–85 % responded with the medical diagnosis to explain the cognitive abnormalities; only 43–55 % used the term 'delirium'. In contrast, where an underlying medical problem was lacking, 74 % of respondents diagnosed 'delirium'. This is in contrast with the DSM-IV criteria of delirium which in its latest version includes the etiology in the title (delirium due to a general medical condition, substance intoxication, substance withdrawal, multiple etiologies, or not otherwise specified if the etiology is unknown) but assigns 'delirium' to all disturbances qualifying the criteria irrespective of the cause. Indeed, as Skrobik suggests [4], the construct of delirium to date is less than clear as is its conceptualization.

Currently, research into delirium detection focuses mainly on the validation of screening tools and their implementation into clinical routine. Little is known, however, about how exactly delirium is diagnosed in the 'real' environment. Despite conceptual shortcomings, data collection and analysis mainly focuses on numbers, which cannot provide the rich information that words can.

Occurrence Rate

Delirium has been reported to occur in 20–40 % of non-critically ill and up to 80 % of critically ill hospitalized patients [7–10]. Apart from real differences in patient populations, variations in reader characteristics, such as professional background, choice of instruments used, time frame of testing, and other factors have influenced the reported incidence rates [7, 8]. As mentioned above, all the incidence and prevalence studies are somewhat flawed when a real gold standard is missing. Loney et al. [11] suggested guidelines to appraise studies of occurrence rates for dementia,

Table 2. Guidelines for critically appraising studies of prevalence or incidence of a health problem [11]

A. Are the study methods valid?
1. Are the study design and sampling method appropriate for the research question?
2. Is the sampling frame appropriate?
3. Is the sample size adequate?
4. Are objective, suitable and standard criteria used for measurement of the health outcome?
5. Is the health outcome measured in an unbiased fashion?
6. Is the response rate adequate? Are the refusers described?
B. What is the interpretation of the results?
7. Are the estimates of prevalence or incidence given with confidence intervals and in detail by subgroup, if appropriate?
C. What is the applicability of the results?
8. Are the study subjects and the setting described in detail and similar to those of interest to you?

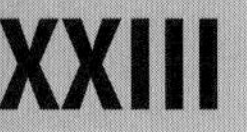

which similarly apply in the context of delirium (**Table 2**). In particular, sampling frame, sampling size, standard criteria used for measurement of the health outcome, measurement bias, and description of refusers, raise concern in quite a few of the available incidence studies of ICU delirium.

Peterson et al. [12] described the motoric subtypes of delirium in critically ill patients and their occurrence rates in a prospective cohort study of 156 patients on a medical intensive care unit (ICU). The authors detected delirium in 72 % of the subjects aged 65 and older and in 57 % of patients younger than 65. Mixed type appeared in 55 %, followed by hypoactive delirium with 44 %. Purely hyperactive delirium occurred in only a few patients (not even 2 %). They noticed hypoactive delirium at a significantly greater rate in patients aged 65 and older (41 % vs 22 %), while in the older group they did not detect hyperactive delirium at all.

Risk Factors

In a prospective cohort study of 304 patients 60 years or older admitted to an ICU, Pisani et al. [13] assessed the occurrence of delirium that developed within 48 hours of ICU admission. Patients were assessed for delirium using the Confusion Assessment Method for the ICU (CAM-ICU) as well as by reviewing medical records. The authors found a striking 70 % incidence and determined that dementia (odds ratio [OR] 6.3; 95 % confidence interval [CI] 2.9 – 13.8], receipt of benzodiazepines before ICU admission (OR 3.4; CI 1.6 – 7.0), elevated creatinine level (OR 2.1; CI 1.1 – 4.0), and low arterial pH (OR 2.1; CI 1.1 – 3.9) were independent risk factors. This study nicely distinguishes admission factors from ICU related factors in the development of delerium in a high risk population [13].

Dubois et al. [14], in a prospective cohort study of 216 patients admitted to a mixed medical/surgical ICU for more than 24 hours, established an incidence of delirium of 19 %; hypertension, smoking history, abnormal bilirubin level, epidural use, and morphine were independent risk factors. Delirium assessment included diagnosis at the discretion of the individual physician, the 8-item Intensive Care Delirium Checklist (ISDSC), and confirmatory diagnosis by a psychiatrist. These authors noted that a third of patients labeled delirious were not agitated indicating hypoactive delirium [14].

Recently Lin et al. [15], assessing early-onset delirium in a prospective cohort study of 143 ventilated patients, found an incidence of 22 % in the first 5 days and identified hypoalbuminemia (OR, 5.94; CI, 1.23–28.77] and sepsis (OR, 3.65; 95 % CI, 1.03–12.9) as independent risk factors. They used the CAM-ICU as screening tool.

Cost and Consequences

Research has also shown that the development of delirium in ICU patients is an independent predictor of longer hospital stay [16, 17], higher hospital costs [18], and, more alarmingly, a threefold increase in death at 6 months [9]. Delirium may be associated with long-term cognitive impairment [18], impaired activities of daily living [19], and decreased quality of life [20] in survivors of critical illness.

The cost of informal care depends on the way health systems are structured and financed [21]. Leslie et al. [22] demonstrated that health care costs per each survival day were 2.77 times greater in people who were delirious during a hospital stay than non-delirious patients (unadjusted data). Interestingly, receipt of a delirium prevention intervention did not significantly affect costs [22]. It should be noted that this study only referred to reimbursed direct costs. The real societal costs of delirium would be much greater.

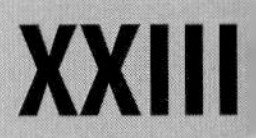

The likelihood of receiving nursing home care could not be reduced by a multi-component targeted intervention for delerium. However, those patients who received a multi-component targeted intervention who went into nursing home care, had 15 % reduced costs [23]. Here again, analysis of costs and consequences focussed on one section of the full costs and consequences accrued by society. It is unclear whether the savings would be offset by extra costs if all patients (including those not receiving nursing home care) were analyzed.

A multi-component targeted intervention significantly reduced non-intervention costs among subjects at intermediate risk for developing delirium, but not among subjects at high risk. When multi-component targeted intervention costs were included, the multi-component targeted intervention had no significant effect on overall health care costs in the intermediate risk cohort, but raised overall costs in the high risk group [24]. It should be noted that these three studies [22–24] all used data from the same trial [25]. Deterioration of health related quality of live (here measured by the 15D instrument) deteriorated slower and was higher during hospital stay after receiving a multi-component targeted intervention. Costs after one year did not differ significantly between groups. Indirect, intangible, as well as important direct costs (social services), were not included in the analysis. Although the 15D instrument carries the potential of being used as a single index as well as a profile measure, the authors failed to use a full cost-utility analysis [26]. The cost analysis was based on a previous randomized study in which there was no significant difference in any hard primary outcome was significantly different between patients managed with or without a multi-component targeted intervention [27].

In the ICU, delirious patients had 1.5-fold higher costs than those without delirium [18]. Costs were calculated at a patient-ledger level and were, therefore, seen from the perspective of the hospital.

Screening

First, we would like to stress the differences between diagnosis and screening. A screening tool does not provide the definite diagnosis defined by the gold standard. Rather it takes a risk stratification approach, making the diagnosis in the positively tested population more efficient thus rendering the otherwise Herculean labor into a feasible diagnostic process. A psychiatric consultation may still be valuable, particularly in situations where a patient's symptoms are atypical or the medical history is unknown.

In a survey of 912 health professionals, Ely et al. [28] found that underdiagnosis was acknowledged by 78 %; only 40 % reported routinely screening for delirium, and only 16 % indicated using a specific tool for delirium assessment. This was despite delirium being considered a significant or very serious problem in the ICU by 92 % of the respondents.

Albeit not in the ICU setting, a more recent Belgian survey among 2256 nurses and 982 physicians (response rate of 26 %) showed that 72 % of the respondents overall considered delirium as a minor problem or no problem at all. However, over half of the respondents working on a palliative care unit (87 %), trauma ward (67 %), cardiothoracic surgery ward (58 %), ICU (55 %), or geriatric ward (55 %) reported that delirium was a serious problem. Delirium was considered as an underdiagnosed (85 %) but preventable (75 %) syndrome, yet repondents stated that patients at risk were rarely (34 %) or never (52 %) screened for delirium. When screening was used (48 %), only 4 % used a specific validated assessment tool. Ninety-seven percent of all respondents were convinced that delirium requires an active and immediate intervention of nurse and physician [29].

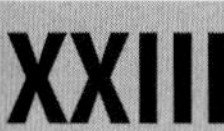

The 2002 guidelines of the Society of Critical Care Medicine (SCCM) and the 2005 guideline of the German Society of Anesthesiology and Intensive Care Medicine (DGAI) for sedation and analgesia recommend that all critically ill patients be simultaneously monitored for level of sedation and for delirium [30, 31]. Other guidelines are more cautious in their recommendations [32].

While delirium is classically described as a hyperactive condition (i.e., patient is agitated and combative), current epidemiological evidence suggests that more patients with delirium in the ICU are hypoactive (i.e., psychomotor slowing) or have a mixed picture [8, 12]. This is why the use of an assessment tool that can identify the hallmark signs of delirium (inattention, disorganized thinking, fluctuating course) is so important. Considering the fluctuating nature of delirium, a single evaluation is usually erratic and has been shown to be a poor strategy to identify delirium in acutely ill patients. A number of characteristics in the critically ill create particular difficulties for screening, such as the inability of intubated patients to give verbal responses, the reduced and often fluctuating level of consciousness inhibiting more complex questions, the instability of many ICU patients, and the lack of expertise among personnel. Essential qualities of delirium assessment instruments that should be used in the ICU setting have been proposed [33, 34]:

- The instrument has to evaluate the primary components of delirium (e.g. consciousness, inattention, disorganized thinking, fluctuating course)
- It has to have proven validity and reliability in ICU populations
- It can be completed quickly and easily, and
- It does not require the presence of psychiatric personnel

Available Tools

Recently, Devlin et al. in a systematic search identified six delirium assessment instruments including the Cognitive Test for Delirium (CTD), abbreviated CTD, CAM-ICU, Intensive Care Delirium Screening Checklist, NEECHAM scale, and the Delirium Detection Score validated for use in the ICU setting [33]. The authors described fundamental differences among the scales in terms of the quality and extent of validation, the specific components of the delirium syndrome that the scores addressed, their ability to identify hypoactive delirium, their use in patients with a compromised level of consciousness, and their ease of use (**Table 3**).

The CAM-ICU [35] and its later versions has been used extensively in practice as well as research settings. In a recent systematic review of current usage, of 239 original articles, 10 were categorized as validation studies, using a reference standard for

Table 3. Available delirium screening tools for the ICU. From [33] with permission

Instrument	Study	Population	Assessments	Validity	Reliability
CTD	Hart et al. 1996 [67]	22 MICU patients with delirium per DSM-III-R, mechanical ventilation (NR)	44 assessments, no. of raters not clear	Versus MMSE r =0.82 (p < 0.001) ROC analysis: sensitivity 100 %, specificity 95 %	r = 0.87 (p < 0.001)
Abbreviated CTD	Hart et al. 1997 [68]	19 medical ward and MICU patients with delirium per DSM-III-R, mechanical ventilation (NR)	38 assessments, no. of raters not clear	Versus CTD r= 0.91 (p < 0.001) ROC analysis: sensitivity 94.7 %, specificity 98.8 %	r =0.79 (p < 0.001)
CAM-ICU	Ely et al. 2001 [69]	38 MICU patients, mechanical ventilation (58 %)	293 assessments, 4 raters	Accuracy vs. delirium expert assessment using DSM-IV criteria: intensivist 96 % (95 % CI 80–100), nurse 1 95 % (95 % CI 86–100), nurse 2 96 % (95 % CI 86–100)	Intensivist vs. nurse 1 κ = 0.84 (95 % CI 0.63–0.99), intensivist vs. nurse 2 κ = 0.79 (95 % CI 0.64–0.95), nurse 1 vs. nurse 2 κ = 0.95 (95 % CI 0.84–1.00)
	Ely et al. 2001 [8]	96 MICU and CCU patients, mechanical ventilation (100 %)	471 paired daily assessments by 2 nurses	Accuracy vs. delirium expert assessment using DSM-IV criteria: nurses 1 and 2 combined 98.4 % (95 % CI 92–100)	Nurse 1 vs. nurse 2 κ = 0.6 (95 % CI 0.92–0.99)
	Lin et al. 2004 [70]	111 MICU and CCU patients, mechanical ventilation (100 %)	204 paired daily assessments by 2 research assistants	Versus psychiatrist evaluation using DSM-IV criteria: sensitivity: assessor 1.91 % (p NR); assessor 2.95 % (p NR); specificity: assessor 1.98 % (p NR); assessor 2.98 % (p NR)	Assessor 1 vs. assessor 2 κ = 0.96 (p NR)

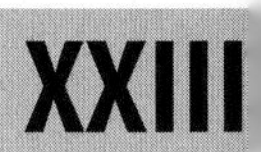

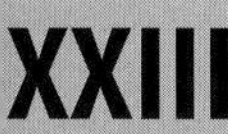

Table 3. (*cont.*)

Instrument	Study	Population	Assessments	Validity	Reliability
	McNicoll et al. 2003 [10]	22 alert elderly MICU patients, mechanical ventilation (0 %)	22 assessments by 2 trained clinician-researchers	Versus CAM: sensitivity: 73 % (95 % CI 60–86), specificity: 100 % (95 % CI 56–100)	Interrater reliability between CAM-ICU and CAM: 82 %, κ = 0.64 (95 % CI 32–94)
	Pun et al. 2005 [51]	377 MICU patients at teaching hospital, mechanical ventilation (57.2 %); 131 MICU patients at community hospital, mechanical ventilation (20.1 %)	Random paired spot checks (n = 508) by the patient nurse and pre-trained expert nursing raters	–	Versus "expert nursing raters": teaching hospital κ = 0.92 (95 % CI 0.90–0.94), community hospital κ = 0.75 (95 % CI 0.68–0.81)
ICDSC	Bergeron et al. 2001 [7]	93 mixed medical/ surgical ICU patients, mechanical ventilation (% NR)	Daily (independent) grouped assess-ments for 93 patients by: patient nurse, research nurse, intensivist, psychiatrist (total no. of assessments NR)	Versus psychiatrist evaluation using ICDSC: Sensitivity 99 %, specificity 64 %	Nurse vs. nurse: r > 0.94 (p NR), nurse vs. intensivist: r > 0.94 (p NR)
NEECHAM	Csokasy 1999 [71]	19 mixed medical/ surgical ICU patients, mechanical ventilation (0 %)	19 subjects; no. raters not clear	Accuracy vs. DSM-III score r = 0.68 (p NR)	Researcher vs. patient nurse 0.81 (p NR)
	Immers et al. 2005 [72]	105 patients in mixed medical/ surgical ICU unknown med/surg ICU, mechanical ventilation (% NR)	253 ratings performed daily by both ICU research and bedside nurses	Vs. DSM-IV $\chi 2$ = 67.52 (p = 0.001), sensitivity 97.2 %, specificity 82.8 %	Research nurse vs. patient nurse κ =0.60 (p NR)
DDS	Otter et al. 2005 [73]	1,073 SICU patients, mechanical ventilation (% NR) at	3,588 paired assessments by patient's physician and nurse least once every shift	Versus SAS (> 5 = delirium) area under the ROC 0.80 (95 % CI 0.72–0.90, p< 0.001), sensitivity 69 %, specificity 75 %	Cronbach's α = 0.667 (p NR)

CTD: Cognitive Test for Delirium; CAM-ICU: Confusion Assessment Method for the Intensive Care Unit; ICDSC: Intensive Care Unit Delirium Screening Checklist; DDS: Delirium Detection Score; CCU: cardiac care unit; MMSE: Mini-Mental State Examination; MICU: medical intensive care unit; CI: confidence interval; NR: not reported; ROC: receiver operator characteristic curve; DSM-III-R: Diagnostic and Statistical Manual of Mental Disorders – revised third edition comparison, 16 as adaptations (e.g. CAM-ICU), 12 as translations, and 222 as applications [36]. Combined results showed an overall sensitivity of 94 % (CI, 91 %-97 %) and specificity of 89 % (CI, 85 %-94 %).

Conditions for Screening Programs

Underlying principles of an effective screening program include the following: The condition screened for is an important health problem; there is an asymptomatic phase of the disease during which screening is the only means to identify affected individuals; tests or examinations are simple, reliable, and acceptable to the population being screened; there is an accepted and effective treatment for the condition; and benefits from treatment outweigh costs of the screening. These principles follow roughly the classic text by Wilson and Jungner [37] and are shown in **Table 4**. Although public health based screening programs aim to detect disease on a population basis and are, therefore, different from clinical in-hospital screening programs, the underlying principles provide a rational framework to analyze whether current evidence is sufficient to support the notion of implementing a comprehensive system-wide screening algorithm.

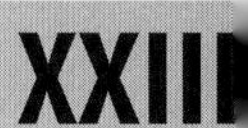

Additional questions regarding screening programs evoked by Cadman et al. include [38]:

- Has the effectiveness of the program been demonstrated in a randomized trial?
- Are efficacious treatments available?
- Does the burden of suffering warrant screening?
- Is there a good screening test?
- Does the program reach those who could benefit?
- Can the health system cope with the program?
- Do persons with positive screenings comply with advice and interventions?

How does delirium screening fare in this light today? As we have seen, among the ICU community, there is little doubt that delirium is an important health problem. This is certainly true from a hospital perspective in general and the ICU perspective in particular. From a national or global burden of disease perspective the importance still seems evident but is not yet iron-clad [39]. As we will see in the next sections, evidence on effective treatment is scare. It is, therefore, not surprising that wide variation exists in the approach to management [6]. Facilities for diagnosis and

Table 4. Criteria for the evaluation of screening programs [37].

1. The condition sought should be an important health problem.
2. There should be an accepted treatment for patients with recognized disease.
3. Facilities for diagnosis and treatment should be available.
4. There should be a recognizable latent or early symptomatic stage.
5. There should be a suitable test or examination.
6. The test should be acceptable to the population.
7. The natural history of the condition, including development from latent to declared disease, should be adequately understood.
8. There should be an agreed policy on whom to treat as patients
9. The cost of case-finding (including diagnosis and treatment of patients diagnosed) should be economically balanced in relation to possible expenditure on medical care as a whole.
10. Case-finding should be a continuing process and not a "once and for all" project.

treatment do not really need to be available since delirium is currently diagnosed and screened for clinically. However, the distribution and application of knowledge and skills should be seen as the facilities applicable in this context. Again looking at current opinion amongst staff and carers, this still seems to be a big problem outside the academic context. Is there a latent or early symptomatic stage? We do know something about the risk factors (see above), and there is rising suspicion about subsyndromal forms of delirium being a prodromal stage of full-blown delirium. Yet it is unclear to date whether early rather than later detection or treatment would make a difference. Regarding the natural history of disease, we are still in the dark. There is some evidence that early postoperative delirium does progress to delirium on the ward from a study by Sharma et al. [40] after hip surgery. Surprisingly, some patients labeled delirious at first were not labeled delirious during the follow-up period in this study. Hence, our knowledge about disease progression is still limited. As noted above, there is to date no proper economic evaluation that compares costs with consequences of delirium screening.

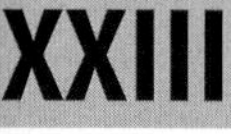

Devlin et al. [41] used two script concordance case scenarios, a slide presentation regarding scale-based delirium assessment, and two further cases in order to teach ICU nursing staff about recognizing delirium. After education, the number of nurses able to evaluate delirium using any scale (12 vs 82 %)] and use it correctly (8 vs 62 %) increased significantly.

Interventions

Prevention and Therapy

Not only young doctors, but also experienced physicians, vary considerably in their approach to the therapeutic management of delirium [42]. Cheung et al. [6] noticed a considerable variation in non-pharmacological and pharmacological management by physician and scenario but independently from whether the term "delirium" was selected. Commonly selected pharmacological agents were antipsychotics and benzodiazepines, followed by narcotics, non-narcotic analgesics, and other sedatives [5]. Therapeutic interventions carry potential side effects and should be used according to an evidence based rational. This is particularly true since anxiolytics and sedatives, often used in the ICU, increase hospital length of stay [43].

Siddiqi et al. [44] in a meta-analysis of interventions for preventing delirium in hospitalized patients identified six studies with a total of 833 participants that fulfilled the inclusion criteria (randomized controlled trial, RCT). All were conducted in surgical settings, five in orthopedic surgery, and one in patients undergoing resection for gastric or colon cancer. Only one study of 126 hip fracture patients comparing proactive geriatric consultation with usual care was sufficiently powered to detect a difference in the primary outcome, incident delirium. The authors did not identify any completed studies in hospitalized medical, care of the elderly, general surgery, cancer or ICU patients. In terms of outcomes, no studies examined for death, use of psychotropic medication, activities of daily living, psychological morbidity, quality of life, carer or staff psychological morbidity, cost of intervention, or cost to health care services. Outcomes were only reported up to discharge, with no studies reporting medium or longer-term effects. In particular there was no randomized controlled intervention study in the ICU setting

More recently, Bourne et al. [45] conducted a meta-analysis of medical treatment for delirium. They described 33 prospective studies including 1880 patients of which only four were randomized, double-blind, placebo-controlled studies. All the RCTs examined drug prevention not treatment of delirium. Almost two-thirds of the prospective studies identified were published within the last 5 years.

Lonergan et al. [46] in a review of antipsychotics for delirium found three studies satisfying the selection criteria. These studies compared haloperidol with risperidone, olanzapine, and placebo in the management of delirium and in the incidence of adverse drug reactions. Decreases in delirium scores were not significantly different comparing low dose haloperidol (< 3.0 mg per day) with the atypical antipsychotics, olanzapine and risperidone (OR 0.63, CI 10.29–1.38). Low dose haloperidol was not associated with a higher incidence of adverse effects than the atypical antipsychotics. High dose haloperidol (> 4.5 mg per day) in one study was associated with an increased incidence of extrapyramidal adverse effects, compared with olanzapine. Low dose haloperidol decreased the severity and duration of delirium in postoperative patients, although not the incidence of delirium compared to placebo controls in one study. There were no controlled trials comparing quetiapine with haloperidol.

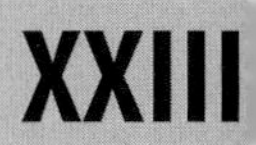

In several RCTs for alcohol withdrawal delirium, Spies et al. [47–49] demonstrated preventative as well as therapeutic efficacy for symptom-orientated adjusted bolus therapy in the ICU using flunitrazepam, clonidine, or haloperidol.

Since many risk factors are already 'at work' before the diagnosis of delirium [13], effective prevention strategies have to start before the commencement of ICU treatment. Therefore, we will briefly mention some prevention strategies. Inouye et al. [25], in a classic risk reduction multicomponent strategy for the prevention of delirium, studied, by means of a prospective matching strategy, 852 patients 70 years of age or older who had been admitted to the general medicine service at a teaching hospital. The intervention consisted of standardized protocols for the management of six risk factors for delirium: Cognitive impairment, sleep deprivation, immobility, visual impairment, hearing impairment, and dehydration. Delirium developed significantly less frequently in the intervention group (9.9 vs. 15.0 %). The total number of days with delirium (105 vs. 161) and the total number of episodes (62 vs. 90) were also significantly reduced. However, the severity of delirium and the recurrence rates were not reduced. The adherence rate to the intervention was 87 % [25]. This prevention program formed the Hospital Elder Life Program (HELP), a model of care to prevent cognitive and functional decline in older hospitalized patients.

In a randomized controlled trial of 227 patients, Cole et al. [50] analyzed the systematic detection and multidisciplinary care of delirium in older medical inpatients. The authors found no significant differences in primary or secondary outcomes within 8 weeks after enrolment.

In another prospective observational cohort study, Pun et al. [51] followed 711 patients admitted to two academic medical ICUs over 4163 days. They implemented a sedation scale (Richmond Agitation-Sedation Scale, RASS) and delirium instrument (CAM-ICU) after a 20-min introductory session for all ICU nurses, followed by graded, staged educational interventions at regular intervals. Compliance with the RASS was over 90 % and with the CAM-ICU over 80 %. The agreement (kappa) with reference raters for the RASS was between 0.89 and 0.77 and for the CAM-ICU between 0.92 and 0.75. Physician buy-in and time were the main barriers to implementation. Currently screening algorithms have to be developed and require strategies to improve outcome quality measures.

Implication for Research and Policy Information

The current gold standard will have to be further developed by field-testing to evaluate results in relation to relevant outcome parameters and to test criteria in different patient populations and settings. False positives would be a significant problem since in studies of the epidemiology, pathophysiology or treatment of delirium it is crucial for the population under study to be as pure as possible [52]. From a screening and secondary prevention point of view, it would be desirable to reliably detect specific subtypes, such as subsyndromal delirium or delirium due to specific etiologies or in different subpopulations (medical, surgical). In terms of treatment, false negatives would prevent patients from being further examined, monitored and treated. All of the above holds true even if we assume a screening tool that is 100 % specific and 100 % sensitive to the gold standard. In fact to date we do not even know if the available screening tools may possess higher accuracy with regard to construct validity than the gold standard against which they have been compared. Experienced psychiatrists do not agree well with one another, a fact that is underestimated in studies where the gold standard comprises a single reference diagnosis by a psychiatrist. Moreover, intensivists familiar with the ICU setting and dedicated to the detection of delirium might at times possess more expertise in accurately diagnosing delirium than the so called 'expert' in the field.

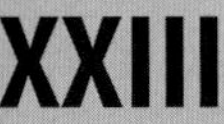

Surveying the status quo of delirium management within but especially outside academic institutions should give us a better picture of what is really happening and how far we still have to go. We should be prepared to expect contradicting opinions and practices [6, 28, 29].

Devlin et al. [33, 41] found important differences among delirium screening tools, including the specific components of the delirium syndrome addressed, the criterion threshold for diagnosing delirium, accuracy, the ability to identify both forms of delirium (i.e., hypoactive and hyperactive), the ability to be used in a patient with a compromised level of consciousness or compromised visual/auditory acuity, and the ease of use. They suggest that clinicians consider these differences before implementing any of these scales in clinical practice [33, 41].

For research purposes, augmenting delirium instruments with multiple sources, such as the medical chart, is a method that might be of some help to better identify this high-risk condition and to intervene outside [53] and more importantly within the ICU [54].

As a role model, we could consider how the approach to ventilator weaning has changed over the past 30 years as a result of research into three areas: Pathophysiology, weaning-predictor testing, and weaning techniques. Research uncovered the reason for weaning failure as well as revealing markers of weaning success. Reliable prediction helps patients to be weaned more rapidly. Tobin [55] suggests the following lessons to be learnt from the weaning story:

- The importance of creativity
- The asking of heretical questions
- Serendipity
- Mental-set psychology
- Cross-fertilization
- The hazards of precocity

He argues that weaning research also illustrates how Kuhnian normal (me-too) science dominates any field [55]. Maybe we are seeing the first signs of this in delirium research with more and more screening tools being 'discovered' before we are sure about the validity of the gold standard in the ICU setting.

Devlin et al. [33] suggest several strategies to improve delirium assessment practices in the ICU. First, a member of the ICU team who is dedicated to and responsible for routine delirium monitoring should be appointed. These authors suggest a bedside nurse because of their ability to detect fluctuations in agitation, the presence of hallucinations, changes in emotional responsiveness, and alterations in sleep [56]. Ultimately Devlin et al. see the need for a 'champion' as the driving force. We pursue a similar but somewhat different approach in our institution, placing the emphasis on a dedicated team (the delirium core team). We feel that a team as the champion is more able to perform this complex task and is less sensitive to frustration and fatigue. This is in accordance with Pandharipande et al. who also feel that a multimodal, multidisciplinary team approach is required [34].

Ubiquitous pocket cards, wall charts, flow sheets and incorporation into the patient data management system (PDMS) improve awareness and use. However, it cannot be overemphasized that effective delirium screening is a team effort and relies for the most part on people-to-people interaction. Education and training is the foremost task of any improvement program and has been shown to have great effect [51, 57].

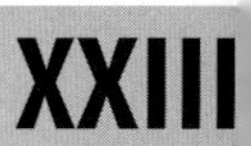

Lately, delirium has jumped onto the policy agenda and is, therefore, more visible for decision makers, researchers, and patients alike, than some other important components of ICU practice. This should not preclude using the potential of synergy that delirium screening has with issues like sedation, respirator therapy, weaning, early ambulation, consent etc. Indeed a delirium screening program without the use of a sedation scale (e.g., RASS) defies any utility. As with all improvement efforts, continuous monitoring of the progress made has to be insured. The necessary systems for this, such as core team meetings, interviews, surveys and data management system reporting, have to be installed. These in themselves sustain awareness and continuous improvement.

Adding a third dimension to our current understanding of how delirium is being monitored clinically, could certainly aid in our quest to devise and implement effective prevention and treatment programs across whole health systems and not just academic institutions. Qualitative research, e.g., by participatory and non-participatory observations into patient-staff interactions, would be one way. We do not know enough about delirium to force our data to converge upon a single proposition or a single score. Triangulation, a research method combining quantitative and different qualitative research methods conveys the potential to give us a richer picture of a complex phenomenon [58].

Other than clinical prediction and screening, increasingly biomarkers emerge which may play a role in the pathophysiology of delirium and which may need to be incorporated into delirium screening algorithms in the future. Some of these markers are serum chemistry, renal function, apolipoprotein E4 allele, A9 allele of the dopamine transporter, serum amino acids (especially tryptophan), cytokines (inflammatory markers), C-reactive protein, hypercortisolism, neuron-specific enolase, S-100 beta, and tau protein [59]. It should be fascinating to watch development in this area with the hope that excitement will not distract from the strict standards in diagnostic accuracy studies that are needed to arrive at valid and valuable results [60].

Once additional trials have been accomplished, they must be reviewed by systematic review and meta analyses; however, these approaches have to be viewed with a certain degree of suspicion [61].

Recent claims not to go ahead with screening before proven treatments are available should be treated with great caution. Awareness of delirium is the key stone for improvement and inherent in any proper carer-patient relationship. The evidence for intraoperative blood pressure monitoring is even scarcer. Nevertheless, blood pressure monitoring has been standard practice for decades [62] without being sure how to define 'good' or 'bad' blood pressure [63]. Likewise delirium, as an organ dysfunction, should not be invisible to the clinical team [64, 65].

Conclusion

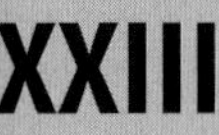

Delirium inside and outside the ICU creates suffering and kills. We know of important risks, some modifiable, some not. We know that detection can be drastically improved and sustained monitoring does work. We are certain that risk reduction strategies most probably make a difference. We do not know for certain whether pharmacological interventions, either preventative or therapeutic, are of definite help and which ones we should use. In order to convince policy makers to shift resources towards delirium screening prevention and screening programs we need to do more. We have to do it fairly quickly in order to avoid investing great efforts to implement strategies that we later find out to be inferior to others. Future tasks will be on two levels: Laboratory science for better therapeutics and people science to improve the team efforts needed to bring our knowledge to the patient.

References

1. Pronovost P, Holzmueller CG, Clattenburg L, et al (2006). Team care: beyond open and closed intensive care units. Curr Opin Crit Care 12: 604–608
2. Bedford PD (1955) Adverse cerebral effects of anaesthesia on old people. Lancet 269: 259–263
3. Tucker GJ (1999) The diagnosis of delirium and DSM-IV. Dement Geriatr Cogn Disord 10: 359–363
4. Skrobik Y (2007) Delirium as destiny: clinical precision and genetic risk. Crit Care Med 35: 304–305
5. Morandi A, Pandharipande, P, Trabucchi, et al (2008) Understanding international differences in terminology for delirium and other types of acute brain dysfunction in critically ill patients. Intensive Care Med 34: 1907–1915
6. Cheung CZ, Alibhai SM, Robinson M, et al (2008) Recognition and labeling of delirium symptoms by intensivists: Does it matter? Intensive Care Med 34: 437–446
7. Bergeron N, Dubois MJ, Dumont M, Dial S, Skrobik Y (2001) Intensive care delirium screening checklist: Evaluation of a new screening tool. Intensive Care Med 27: 859–864
8. Ely EW, Inouye SK, Bernard GR, et al (2001) Delirium in mechanically ventilated patients: validity and reliability of the confusion assessment method for the intensive care unit (CAM-ICU). JAMA 286: 2703–2710
9. Ely EW, Shintani A, Truman B, et al (2004) Delirium as a predictor of mortality in mechanically ventilated patients in the intensive care unit. JAMA 291: 1753–1762
10. McNicoll L, Pisani MA, Zhang Y, Ely EW, Siegel MD, Inouye SK (2003) Delirium in the intensive care unit: occurrence and clinical course in older patients. J Am Geriatr Soc 51: 591–598
11. Loney PL, Chambers LW, Bennett KJ, Roberts JG, Stratford PW (1998) Critical appraisal of the health research literature: prevalence or incidence of a health problem. Chronic Dis Can 19: 170–176
12. Peterson JF, Pun BT, Dittus RS, et al (2006) Delirium and its motoric subtypes: a study of 614 critically ill patients. J Am Geriatr Soc 54: 479–484

13. Pisani MA, Murphy TE, Van Ness PH, Araujo KL, Inouye SK (2007) Characteristics associated with delirium in older patients in a medical intensive care unit. Arch Intern Med 167: 1629–1634
14. Dubois MJ, Bergeron N, Dumont M, Dial S, Skrobik Y (2001) Delirium in an intensive care unit: a study of risk factors. Intensive Care Med 27: 1297–1304
15. Lin SM, Huang CD, Liu CY, et al (2008) Risk factors for the development of early-onset delirium and the subsequent clinical outcome in mechanically ventilated patients. J Crit Care 23: 372–379
16. Ely EW, Gautam S, Margolin R, et al (2001) The impact of delirium in the intensive care unit on hospital length of stay. Intensive Care Med 27: 1892–1900
17. Ouimet S, Kavanagh BP, Gottfried SB, Skrobik Y (2007) Incidence, risk factors and consequences of ICU delirium. Intensive Care Med 33: 66–73
18. Milbrandt EB, Deppen S, Harrison PL, et al (2004) Costs associated with delirium in mechanically ventilated patients. Crit Care Med 32: 955–62
19. Jackson JC, Gordon SM, Hart RP, Hopkins RO, Ely EW (2004) The association between delirium and cognitive decline: a review of the empirical literature. Neuropsychol Rev 14: 87–98
20. Inouye SK, Schlesinger MJ, Lydon TJ (1999) Delirium: a symptom of how hospital care is failing older persons and a window to improve quality of hospital care. Am J Med 106: 565–573
21. Bellelli G, Bianchetti A, Trabucchi M (2008) Delirium and costs of informal home care. Arch Intern Med 168:1717
22. Leslie DL, Marcantonio ER, Zhang Y, Leo-Summers L, Inouye SK (2008) One-year health care costs associated with delirium in the elderly population. Arch Intern Med 168: 27–32
23. Leslie DL, Zhang Y, Bogardus ST, Holford TR, Leo-Summers LS, Inouye SK (2005) Consequences of preventing delirium in hospitalized older adults on nursing home costs. J Am Geriatr Soc 53: 405–409
24. Rizzo JA, Bogardus ST Jr, Leo-Summers L, Williams CS, Acampora D, Inouye SK (2001) Multicomponent targeted intervention to prevent delirium in hospitalized older patients: what is the economic value? Med Care 39: 740–752
25. Inouye SK, Bogardus ST Jr, Charpentier PA, et al (1999) A multicomponent intervention to prevent delirium in hospitalized older patients. N Engl J Med 340: 669–676
26. Rockwood K, Brown M, Merry H, Sketris I, Fisk J (2002) Societal costs of vascular cognitive impairment in older adults. Stroke 33: 1605–1609
27. Pitkala KH, Laurila JV, Strandberg TE, Kautiainen H, Sintonen H, Tilvis RS (2008) Multicomponent geriatric intervention for elderly inpatients with delirium: effects on costs and health-related quality of life. J Gerontol A Biol Sci Med Sci 63: 56–61
28. Ely EW, Stephens RK, Jackson, et al (2004) Current opinions regarding the importance, diagnosis, and management of delirium in the intensive care unit: a survey of 912 healthcare professionals. Crit Care Med 32: 106–112
29. Verstraete L, Joosten, E, Milisen, K (2008) [Opinions of physicians and nurses regarding the prevention, diagnosis and management of delirium]. Tijdschr Gerontol Geriatr 39: 26–34
30. Jacobi J, Fraser, GL, Coursin et al. (2002) Clinical practice guidelines for the sustained use of sedatives and analgesics in the critically ill adult. Crit Care Med 30: 119–141
31. Martin J, Bäsell K, Bürkle H, et al (2005) Analgesie und Sedierung in der Intensivmedizin-S2-Leitlinien der Deutschen Gesellschaft für Anästhesiologie und Intensivmedizin. Anästh Intensivmed 46 (Suppl1/2005): 1–20
32. Mattia C, Savoia G, Paoletti F, et al (2006) SIAARTI Recommendations for analgo-sedation in intensive care unit. Minerva Anestesiol 72: 769–805
33. Devlin JW, Fong JJ, Fraser GL, Riker RR (2007) Delirium assessment in the critically ill. Intensive Care Med 33: 929–940
34. Pandharipande P, Jackson J, Ely EW (2005) Delirium: Acute cognitive dysfunction in the critically ill. Curr Opin Crit Care 11: 360–368
35. Inouye SK, van Dyck CH, Alessi CA, Balkin S, Siegal AP, Horwitz RI (1990) Clarifying confusion: the confusion assessment method. a new method for detection of delirium. Ann Intern Med 113: 941–948
36. Wei LA, Fearing MA, Sternberg EJ, Inouye SK (2008) The confusion assessment method: a systematic review of current usage. J Am Geriatr Soc 56: 823–830
37. Wilson JMG, Jungner G (1968) Principles and Practice of Screening for Disease. WHO, Geneva

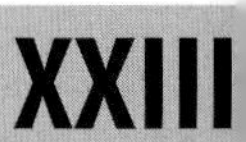

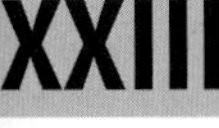

38. Cadman D, Chambers L, Feldman W, Sackett D (1984) Assessing the effectiveness of community screening programs. JAMA 251: 1580–1585
39. Eaton WW, Martins SS, Nestadt G, Bienvenu OJ, Clarke D, Alexandre P (2008) The burden of mental disorders. Epidemiol Rev 30: 1–14
40. Sharma PT, Sieber FE, Zakriya KJ, et al (2005) Recovery room delirium predicts postoperative delirium after hip-fracture repair. Anesth Analg 101: 1215–1220
41. Devlin JW, Marquis F, Riker RR, et al (2008) Combined didactic and scenario-based education improves the ability of intensive care unit staff to recognize delirium at the bedside. Crit Care 12:R19
42. Carnes M, Howell T, Rosenberg M, Francis J, Hildebrand C, Knuppel J (2003) Physicians vary in approaches to the clinical management of delirium. J Am Geriatr Soc 51: 234–239
43. Gardner DM, Baldessarini RJ, Waraich P (2005) Modern antipsychotic drugs: a critical overview. CMAJ 172: 1703–1711
44. Siddiqi N, Stockdale R, Britton AM, Holmes J (2007) Interventions for preventing delirium in hospitalised patients. Cochrane Database Syst Rev: CD005563
45. Bourne RS, Tahir TA, Borthwick M, Sampson EL (2008) Drug treatment of delirium: past, present and future. J Psychosom Res 65: 273–282
46. Lonergan E, Britton AM, Luxenberg J, Wyller T (2007) Antipsychotics for delirium. Cochrane Database Syst Rev: CD005594
47. Spies CD, Dubisz N, Funk W, et al. (1995) Prophylaxis of alcohol withdrawal syndrome in alcohol-dependent patients admitted to the intensive care unit after tumour resection. Br J Anaesth 75: 734 739
48. Spies CD, Dubisz N, Neumann T, et al (1996) Therapy of alcohol withdrawal syndrome in intensive care unit patients following trauma: results of a prospective, randomized trial. Crit Care Med 24: 414–422
49. Spies CD, Otter HE, Huske B, et al (2003) Alcohol withdrawal severity is decreased by symptom-orientated adjusted bolus therapy in the ICU. Intensive Care Med 29: 2230–2238
50. Cole MG, McCusker J, Bellavance F, et al (2002) Systematic detection and multidisciplinary care of delirium in older medical inpatients: a randomized trial. CMAJ 167: 753–759
51. Pun BT, Gordon SM, Peterson JF, et al (2005) Large-scale implementation of sedation and delirium monitoring in the intensive care unit: a report from two medical centers. Crit Care Med 33: 1199–1205
52. Liptzin B (1999) What criteria should be used for the diagnosis of delirium? Dement Geriatr Cogn Disord 10: 364–367
53. Simon SE, Bergmann MA, Jones RN, Murphy KM, Orav EJ, Marcantonio ER (2006) Reliability of a structured assessment for nonclinicians to detect delirium among new admissions to postacute care. J Am Med Dir Assoc 7: 412–415
54. Pisani MA, Araujo KL, Van Ness PH, Zhang Y, Ely EW, Inouye SK (2006) A research algorithm to improve detection of delirium in the intensive care unit. Crit Care 10: R121
55. Tobin MJ (2006) Remembrance of weaning past: the seminal papers. Intensive Care Med 32: 1485–1493
56. Justic M (2000) Does "ICU psychosis" really exist? Crit Care Nurse 20: 28–37
57. Inouye SK, Foreman MD, Mion LC, Katz KH, Cooney LM Jr (2001) Nurses' recognition of delirium and its symptoms: comparison of nurse and researcher ratings. Arch Intern Med 161: 2467–2473
58. Mathison S (1988) Why triangulate? Educational Researcher 17: 13–17
59. Marcantonio ER, Rudolph JL, Culley D, Crosby G, Alsop D, Inouye SK (2006) Serum biomarkers for delirium. J Gerontol A Biol Sci Med Sci 61: 1281–1286
60. Bossuyt PM, Reitsma JB, Bruns DE, et al (2003) The STARD statement for reporting studies of diagnostic accuracy: explanation and elaboration. Ann Intern Med 138:W1–12
61. Tobin MJ, Jubran A (2008) Meta-analysis under the spotlight: focused on a meta-analysis of ventilator weaning. Crit Care Med 36: 1–7
62. Eichhorn JH, Cooper JB, Cullen DJ, Maier WR, Philip JH, Seeman RG (1986) Standards for patient monitoring during anesthesia at harvard medical school. JAMA 256: 1017–1020
63. Bijker JB, van Klei WA, Kappen TH, van Wolfswinkel L, Moons KG, Kalkman CJ (2007) Incidence of intraoperative hypotension as a function of the chosen definition: literature definitions applied to a retrospective cohort using automated data collection. Anesthesiology 107: 213–220

64. Bowton DL (2004) Delirium--the cost of inattention. Crit Care Med 32: 1080–1081
65. Pun BT, Ely EW (2007) The importance of diagnosing and managing ICU delirium. Chest 132: 624–636
66. American Psychiatric Association (2000) Diagnostic and statistical manual of mental disorders, 4th edn. American Psychiatric Association, Washington
67. Hart RP, Levenson JL, Sessler CN, Best AM, Schwartz SM, Rutherford LE (1996) Validation of a cognitive test for delirium in medical ICU patients. Psychosomatics 37: 533–546
68. Hart RP, Best AM, Sessler CN, Levenson JL (1997) Abbreviated cognitive test for delirium. J Psychosom Res 43: 417–423
69. Ely EW, Margolin R, Francis J, et al (2001) Evaluation of delirium in critically ill patients: validation of the Confusion Assessment Method for the Intensive Care Unit (CAM-ICU). Crit Care Med 29: 1370–1379
70. Lin SM, Liu CY, Wang CH, et al (2004) The impact of delirium on the survival of mechanically ventilated patients. Crit Care Med 32: 2254–2259
71. Csokasy J (1999) Assessment of acute confusion: use of the NEECHAM Confusion Scale. Appl Nurs Res 12: 51–55
72. Immers HE, Schuurmans MJ, van de Bijl JJ (2005) Recognition of delirium in ICU patients: a diagnostic study of the NEECHAM confusion scale in ICU patients. BMC Nurs 4:7
73. Otter H, Martin J, Basell K, et al (2005) Validity and reliability of the DDS for severity of delirium in the ICU. Neurocrit Care 2: 150–158

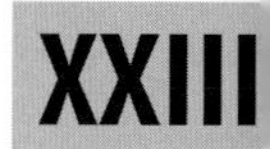

XXIV ICU Management

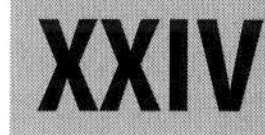

Intensive Care for the Elderly: Current and Future Concerns

H. Wunsch, A.T. Jones, and D.C. Scales

Introduction

Around the world, the elderly population is growing faster than the total population, and this difference in growth rates is increasing [1]. In 1950, 1 in every 20 individuals was aged 65 years or older; by the year 2050, this figure is projected to increase to nearly 1 in 6 (**Fig. 1**) [1]. These population trends represent a looming crisis for healthcare systems around the world, and understanding patterns of care and outcomes for the ageing segment of the population is vital when planning for future healthcare needs in all countries.

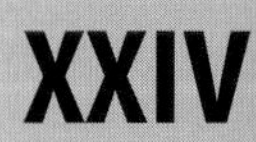

Intensive care is an integral component of healthcare across the developed world [2], and intensive care beds already account for approximately 1–10 % of all inpatient acute care beds in developed countries [3]. The ageing of the world's population may have profound implications on the provision of this expensive component of healthcare [4]. In this chapter, we examine special issues related to intensive care for the elderly, and we consider the impact increasing numbers of older patients will have on the delivery of intensive care in the future.

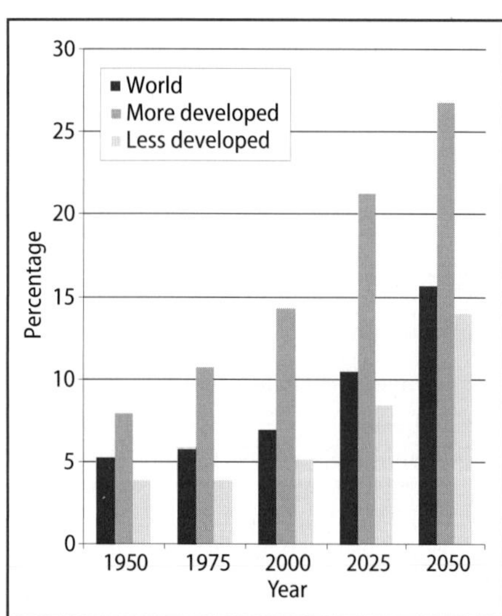

Fig. 1. Percentage of the population aged 65 and over: world and development regions 1950–2050 (data from United Nations [1])

Current Provision of Intensive Care

Definition of Elderly

There is currently no consensus regarding the definition of an 'elderly' patient. Previous research has often used varying cut-offs – anywhere from age 50 to 90 – making comparisons between studies difficult. In the US and Europe, elderly patients are often defined as those who are age 65 years and older, reflecting a common retirement age and, in the US, the age at which most Americans become eligible for health coverage by Medicare, the national health insurance program. However, persons greater than age 65 certainly do not comprise a homogeneous group. Furthermore, attempts to simply subdivide elderly groups according to chronological age can have significant limitations, ignoring differences in baseline functional capacity and pre-existing organ function. Such factors are often considered when describing a person's 'physiological age'. To further complicate matters, the perception of what age constitutes elderly appears to be shifting. In many Western countries, statutory retirement age is increasing: In Italy from 57 to 58, in Germany and the UK from 65 to 67 and 68, respectively. These increases suggest a growing societal recognition of the size of this demographic and also reflect the improved overall health status of many older people [1].

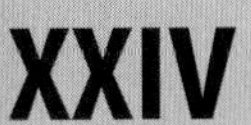

Current Age Distribution of Intensive Care Patients

Regardless of which definition of elderly is used, current data suggest that older patients routinely receive intensive care. For example, in an international cohort of 20,000 intensive care patients from 35 countries, the median age was 63 (interquartile range 49–74) [5]. Large cohort studies in both the US and Canada have reported similar median ages for intensive care patients [6, 7]. In studies where serial measurements have been taken over time, intensive care unit (ICU) patients appear to be getting older; in the Paris area (Collège des Utilisateurs de Bases de données en Réanimation, CUB-REA) database, the mean age has increased by 6 months per year over the past decade in the ICU population compared to only 3 months per year in the general population [8]. Similarly, there was a 16 % increase in the use of intensive care per 1,000 Medicare beneficiaries (age $\geq$ 65 years) from 1994 until 2004, at which time one third of hospitalizations for this group included admission to either an ICU or coronary care unit [9].

Caring for the Elderly

Triage Decisions

A controversial issue regarding intensive care for elderly patients is one of triage – whether age does, or should, factor into decisions about the appropriateness of ICU admission. Specific studies of ICU triage decisions are relatively small in number, but increasing age is often a factor associated with ICU refusal [10]. In one study, advanced age was documented as a contributing reason in over 90 % of cases where admission was refused for perceived lack of benefit [11]. Interestingly, in this study of octogenarians referred for ICU care, mortality was 63 % in those admitted, 71 % in those deemed too sick to benefit, and 18 % in those deemed too well to benefit, highlighting the difficulty in predicting clinical outcomes. Clinical decision-making is not helped by the large body of conflicting literature exploring the role of advanced age on outcomes for patients who *are* admitted to ICU. Some studies conclude that age is not a predictor of survival after adjusting for other co-morbidities [12, 13], while others conclude that increasing age is independently associated with higher ICU and hospital mortality [14, 15]. These different results are likely due to variation in study design, ICU population and type, ability to control for co-morbidities, and, most importantly, the difficulty of studying patients not admitted to ICU, leading to a potential selection bias.

Cook and colleagues studied patients admitted to 15 Canadian ICUs to examine clinical determinants that were associated with the withdrawal of mechanical ventilation [16]. Rather than age or the severity of illness, they found that the strongest determinants of the withdrawal of life support were the physician's perception that the patient preferred not to use life support, the physician's prediction of low survival likelihood, and high likelihood of poor cognitive function. However, there is evidence that differences often exist between physician assessments of patient preferences and quality of life, and the actual preferences and perceptions of patients and their families, and that these assessments are often influenced by cultural and religious factors [17]. In an attempt to aid objectivity and thus improve triage decision making, detailed recommendations for ICU admission and discharge have been developed [18]. However, clinicians do not always employ such guidelines in routine practice [19]. The recently completed ELDICUS study (Triage Decision Making for the Elderly in European ICUs), should help clarify which factors influence the triage decisions made for elderly patients [20].

Co-morbidities

Once admitted to the ICU, elderly patients are a potentially vulnerable population: They often have diagnoses associated with high mortality, suffer from chronic illnesses, have limited physiological reserve to withstand superimposed critical illness, and may often have more limited support systems than do younger patients [21, 22]. Furthermore, clinicians may struggle to recognize and deal with often hidden co-morbidities such as cognitive dysfunction and frailty. In one study of patients aged 65 and older, the prevalence of pre-existing cognitive impairment was 37 %, although ICU physicians were unaware of this in more than half of cases [23]. Factors associated with increased clinician awareness of cognitive impairment included admission from a nursing home or need for assistance with activities of daily living. Delirium is also more common among elderly patients in the ICU [24]. One study that examined risk factors for delirium found an association between older age and risk of developing delirium that was independent of other factors, such as choice of sedative [25]. In a cohort of elderly patients (aged 65 and older) admitted to a medical ICU, 70 % were found to have delirium during their hospitalization [26]. As already discussed, pre-existing cognitive function is more common in the elderly, and is also an independent risk factor for delirium in the ICU, which in turn is associated with higher mortality [24].

Mechanical Ventilation for Elderly Patients

The elderly also make up a large proportion of mechanically ventilated patients in the ICU. An international, 28-day study of mechanical ventilation found that the median age of patients was 63 [27]. Similarly, a Canadian study showed that two-thirds of mechanically ventilated patients are over the age of 60 [7]. Overall, mechanically ventilated patients have much longer ICU and hospital lengths of stay compared with non-ventilated patients [28]. A study of patients in one state (North Carolina) found that patients over age 65 had the highest age-specific incidence of mechanical ventilation, with the peak incidence between age 75–84 (1.14 per 1,000 population in 2002) [29]. Outcomes for elderly mechanically ventilated patients are not clear cut; in older patients with acute lung injury (ALI) and the acute respiratory distress syndrome (ARDS), older age (70 years and over) was associated with a much longer length of mechanical ventilation compared with younger patients (19 days versus 10 days) and a longer length of ICU and hospital stay [30]. However, a study of a cohort of mechanically ventilated patients found a similar duration of mechanical ventilation and ICU length of stay for patients age 75 and older compared with younger patients [31]. Both the recent international 28 day survey of mechanical ventilation, and the study of ALI and ARDS patients reported higher hospital mortality for elderly patients receiving mechanical ventilation [27, 30].

Life after Intensive Care

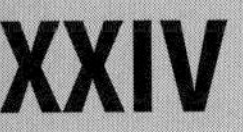

The subsequent healthcare requirements for elderly patients who are discharged from ICU may be much greater than for younger patients due to underlying co-morbidities as well as increased disability and de-conditioning that occur after a critical illness. Over the 1990s, it was noted that there was a decrease in the standardized mortality ratio (SMR) for intensive care patients in the US [32]. This decrease was attributed to the large concomitant increase in the use of skilled nursing facilities on discharge from the hospital. Elderly cardiac surgery patients have also been noted to be discharged to skilled nursing facilities in increasing numbers [33]. One study that tracked discharge transitions after leaving hospital found that many elderly patients required multiple transfers between institutions, and a large percentage of these involved a return to higher intensity care environments [34]. Older age was also associated with an increased hospital readmission rate among patients who received prolonged (> 96 hours) mechanical ventilation [35]. Interventions have been proposed to target elderly patients considered at risk of poor outcomes after hospitalization, such as nurse-led discharge planning and home visits, but such interventions remain difficult to coordinate and are labor and cost intensive [36].

Caregiver Burden

The care needs of elderly people who have survived intensive care may place a large burden on families and caregivers [37]. One study found that three quarters of ICU survivors who received mechanical ventilation required help from a caregiver 2 months after hospital discharge [38]. Another study of patients who needed prolonged mechanical ventilation (> 48 hours) found that more than half still required caregiver assistance one year after discharge from the ICU [39]. A high rate of depression has been described among the informal caregivers of patients who have received mechanical ventilation (> 48 hours), and older patient age was identified as an independent risk factor for caregiver depression [40].

End-of-life Decisions

One in five Americans who die now receive intensive care services before death [41]. Providing care for patients at the end of life now represents a large component of intensive care. A survey of European practice surrounding deaths found great variation in the amount of discussion with patients and families regarding end-of-life decisions [42]. Similarly, the ETHICUS study, which examined end-of-life practices in European ICUs, demonstrated great variation regarding limitation of treatments in the ICU. However, the study observed only a modest association between increasing age and the withholding or withdrawing of life-sustaining treatments (odds ratio 1.02, 95 % CI 1.01 – 1.03) [43]. The correlation between patient preferences for end-of-life care and actual clinical practice has been observed to be poor, suggesting a need to help patients communicate and enact their stated preferences [44]. In the US, the use of do-not-resuscitate (DNR) orders in hospitalized patients may be increasing, and there appears to be an increasing awareness worldwide that quality end-of-life discussions and interventions are needed to improve both patient and family satisfaction [45, 46].

Future of Intensive Care for the Elderly

Estimating the resource requirements needed to care for the elderly in the coming years is complicated and must take into account changes in population demographics, technology, and our approach to care (**Fig. 2**). The largest driving factor affecting the care of the elderly over the next twenty to forty years clearly will be the dramatic anticipated increase in the size of the elderly population worldwide. Intensive care occupancy rates already range from 65 % in the US to 85 % in the UK [47, 48]. Recent projections from Ontario, Canada show that if current trends continue, the demand for mechanical ventilation will only continue to increase between now and 2026 (**Fig. 3**). Although individual countries may have a greater or lesser ability to cope with an increase in the overall demand for intensive care arising from the increased absolute number of elderly patients, no country will be able to handle this increase without either some expansion of intensive care beds or by rationing access [4]. Furthermore, it seems unlikely that future rationing guidelines will incorporate age alone as a restricting factor for ICU admission. Therefore, we need to continue to seek to accurately identify those patients, of all ages, who will benefit most from admission to the ICU.

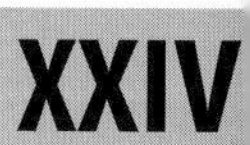

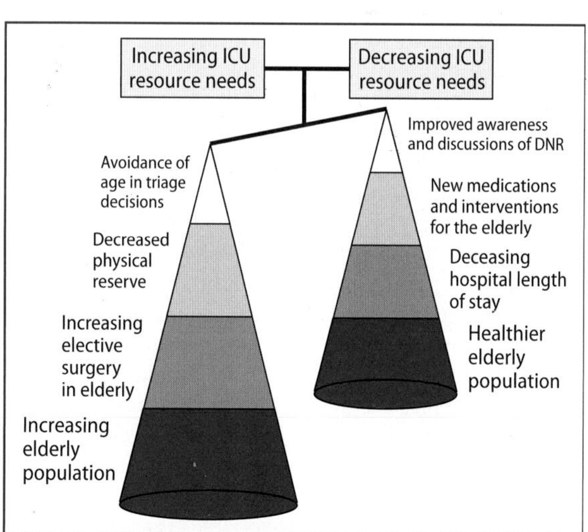

Fig. 2. Factors affecting future delivery of critical care in the elderly. DNR: do-not-resuscitate

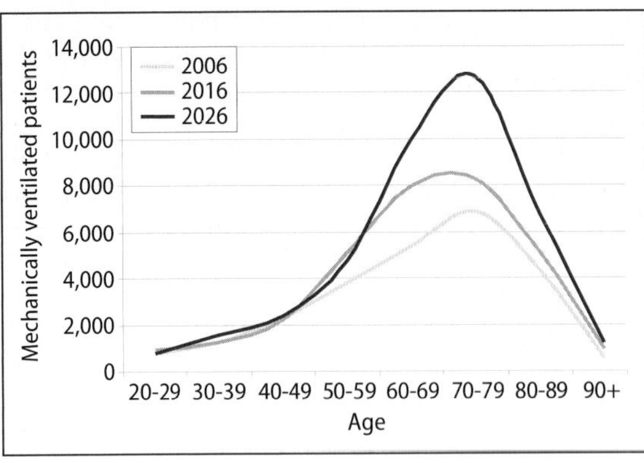

Fig. 3. Projected future requirements for mechanical ventilation in Ontario, Canada (2001 to 2026), by age group [7].

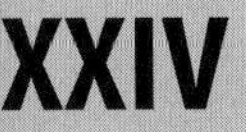

Increases in the overall demand for intensive care by elderly populations could potentially be off-set by improvements in care or efficiency that lead to decreased need for intensive care or shorter lengths of stay in the ICU. However, recent data from the US show no decrease in the average ICU length of stay for Medicare beneficiaries from 1994 to 2004, but a substantial increase in the number and rate of ICU admissions [9]. The incidence of mechanical ventilation was also found to be increasing over time in all age groups, and similar trends were found for patients receiving prolonged (> 96 hours) mechanical ventilation [49]. These observations suggest that improvements in efficiency are unlikely to offset the increasing numbers of patients vying for ICU care [7].

The demand for intensive care may also increase due to advances in technology and treatments that allow for older patients to receive (and survive) more aggressive treatments, such as coronary artery bypass grafting (CABG) and chemotherapeutic regimens. Conversely, the increasing use of other less invasive modalities, such as coronary stents, may help to decrease the need for intensive care. Future changes in case-mix and treatment are extremely difficult to predict due to the complicated interplay between different advances in technology and medical care. Studies are clearly needed to monitor the changes in demand for intensive care that occur within different sub-groups of the population and following the introduction of healthcare innovations. The downstream effects of caring for more elderly patients in the ICU will also need to be considered. The need for skilled nursing facilities and caregivers will only increase as more elderly patients experience the debilitating effects of prolonged hospitalizations.

As the population ages, there will likely be even greater heterogeneity between different 'elderly' patients when considering the combined effect of chronological age and functional status. A recent editorial in the *American Journal of Public Health* lamented the general lack of data reporting that further subdivides people age 85 and older. It observed that US federal agencies always present summary statistics including *everyone* above this age, despite a growing recognition of substantial differences in disease incidence and mortality even within this group [50]. Again, this is an area where further research is needed to elucidate these differences and allow for better prognostication in this large group.

Conclusion

The shift in demographics towards an older population is occurring in many countries worldwide. This change is expected to have wide-spread social and economic impacts. The increasing number of elderly patients needing healthcare poses unique ethical challenges regarding decision-making for ICU triage decisions, appropriateness of complex interventions, and end-of-life planning. In the ICU, elderly patients appear to be at higher risk of delirium, may require increased length of mechanical ventilation and hospital stay, and pose unique challenges for discharge planning and management after hospital discharge. Yet, the data available do not always substantiate common opinions regarding the functional status, preferences, and outcomes for elderly patients. More research into the effects of age on intensive care utilization and outcomes, and on post-ICU care, is urgently needed to allow for appropriate planning of future healthcare delivery to the increasing number of elderly patients in the coming years.

References

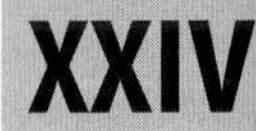

1. Anonymous (2001) World population aging: 1950–2050. United Nations Department of Economic and Social Affairs, New York
2. Fan E, Ferguson ND (2008) One for all, and all for one? The globalization of critical care. Crit Care Med 36: 2942–2943
3. Wunsch H, Angus DC, Harrison DA, et al (2008) Variation in critical care services across North America and Western Europe. Crit Care Med 36: 2787–2793
4. Halpern NA, Pastores SM, Greenstein RJ (2004) Critical care medicine in the United States 1985–2000: an analysis of bed numbers, use, and costs. Crit Care Med 32: 1254–1259
5. Metnitz PG, Moreno RP, Almeida E, et al (2005) SAPS 3--From evaluation of the patient to evaluation of the intensive care unit. Part 1: Objectives, methods and cohort description. Intensive Care Med 31: 1336–1344
6. Kahn JM, Goss CH, Heagerty PJ, et al (2006) Hospital Volume and the Outcomes of Mechanical Ventilation. N Engl J Med 355: 41–50
7. Gomes T and Scales DC (2007) Projected incidence of mechanical ventilation in Ontario to 2026 – Working Report. (Update [2007] of Needham DM, Bronskill SE, Calinawan JR, Sibbald WJ, Pronovost PJ, Laupacis A. Projected incidence of mechanical ventilation in Ontario to 2026: Preparing for the aging baby boomers. Crit Care Med 2005;33: 574–9). Institute for Clinical Evaluative Sciences, Toronto, Ontario, Canada
8. Boumendil A, Somme D, Garrouste-Org M, Guidet B (2007) Should elderly patients be admitted to the intensive care unit? Intensive Care Med 33: 1252–1262
9. Milbrandt EB, Kersten A, Rahim MT, et al (2008) Growth of intensive care unit resource use and its estimated cost in Medicare. Crit Care Med 36: 2504–2510
10. Sinuff T, Kahnamoui K, Cook DJ, Luce JM, Levy MM (2004) Rationing critical care beds: a systematic review. Crit Care Med 32: 1588–1597
11. Garrouste-Org, Timsit JF, Montuclard L, et al (2006) Decision-making process, outcome, and 1-year quality of life of octogenarians referred for intensive care unit admission. Intensive Care Med 32: 1045–1051
12. Somme D, Maillet JM, Gisselbrecht M, et al (2003) Critically ill old and the oldest-old patients in intensive care: short- and long-term outcomes. Intensive Care Med 29: 2137–2143
13. Torres OH, Francia E, Longobardi V, et al (2006) Short- and long-term outcomes of older patients in intermediate care units. Intensive Care Med 32: 1052–1059
14. Boumendil A, Aegerter P, Guidet B (2005) Treatment intensity and outcome of patients aged 80 and older in intensive care units: a multicenter matched-cohort study. J Am Geriatr Soc 53: 88–93
15. de Rooij SE, Govers A, Korevaar JC, et al (2006) Short-term and long-term mortality in very elderly patients admitted to an intensive care unit. Intensive Care Med 32: 1039–1044

16. Cook D, Rocker G, Marshall J, et al (2003) Withdrawal of mechanical ventilation in anticipation of death in the intensive care unit. N Engl J Med 349: 1123–1132
17. The SUPPORT Principal Investigators (1995) A controlled trial to improve care for seriously ill hospitalized patients. The study to understand prognoses and preferences for outcomes and risks of treatments (SUPPORT). JAMA 274: 1591–1598
18. Task Force of the American College of Critical Care Medicine, Society of Critical Care Medicine (1999) Guidelines for intensive care unit admission, discharge, and triage. Crit Care Med 27: 633–638
19. Azoulay E, Pochard F, Chevret S, et al (2001) Compliance with triage to intensive care recommendations. Crit Care Med 29: 2132–2136
20. Levin PD, Sprung CL (2006) Intensive care triage--the hardest rationing decision of them all. Crit Care Med 34: 1250–1251
21. Hennessy D, Juzwishin K, Yergens D, Noseworthy T, Doig C (2005) Outcomes of elderly survivors of intensive care: a review of the literature. Chest 127: 1764–1774
22. de Rooij SE, bu-Hanna A, Levi M, de Jonge E (2005) Factors that predict outcome of intensive care treatment in very elderly patients: a review. Crit Care 9: R307-R314
23. Pisani MA, Redlich C, McNicoll L, Ely EW, Inouye SK (2003) Underrecognition of preexisting cognitive impairment by physicians in older ICU patients. Chest 124: 2267–2274
24. Girard T, Pandharipande P, Ely EW (2008) Delirium in the intensive care unit. Crit Care 12: S3
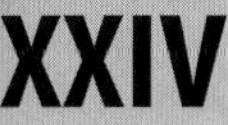
25. Pandharipande P, Ely EW (2006) Sedative and analgesic medications: risk factors for delirium and sleep disturbances in the critically ill. Crit Care Clin 22: 313–327
26. McNicoll L, Pisani MA, Zhang Y, et al (2003) Delirium in the intensive care unit: occurrence and clinical course in older patients. J Am Geriatr Soc 51: 591–598
27. Esteban A, Anzueto A, Frutos F, et al (2002) Characteristics and outcomes in adult patients receiving mechanical ventilation: a 28-day international study. JAMA 287: 345–355
28. Moran JL, Bristow P, Solomon PJ, George C, Hart GK (2008) Mortality and length-of-stay outcomes, 1993–2003, in the binational Australian and New Zealand intensive care adult patient database. Crit Care Med 36: 46–61
29. Carson SS, Cox CE, Holmes GM, Howard A, Carey TS (2006) The changing epidemiology of mechanical ventilation: a population-based study. J Intensive Care Med 21: 173–182
30. Ely EW, Wheeler AP, Thompson BT, et al (2002) Recovery rate and prognosis in older persons who develop acute lung injury and the acute respiratory distress syndrome. Ann Intern Med 136: 25–36
31. Ely EW, Evans GW, Haponik EF (1999) Mechanical ventilation in a cohort of elderly patients admitted to an intensive care unit. Ann Intern Med 131: 96–104
32. Sirio CA, Shepardson LB, Rotondi AJ, et al (1999) Community-wide assessment of intensive care outcomes using a physiologically based prognostic measure: implications for critical care delivery from Cleveland Health Quality Choice. Chest 115: 793–801
33. Lichtman JH, Kapoor R, Wang Y, et al (2007) Temporal trends of outcomes for nonagenarians undergoing coronary artery bypass grafting, 1993 to 1999. Am J Cardiol 100: 1630–1634
34. Coleman EA, Min SJ, Chomiak A, Kramer AM (2004) Posthospital care transitions: patterns, complications, and risk identification. Health Serv Res 39: 1449–1465
35. Douglas SL, Daly BJ, Brennan PF, Gordon NH, Uthis P (2001) Hospital readmission among long-term ventilator patients. Chest 120: 1278–1286
36. Naylor MD, Brooten D, Campbell R, et al (1999) Comprehensive discharge planning and home follow-up of hospitalized elders: a randomized clinical trial. JAMA 281: 613–620
37. Angus DC, Carlet J (2003) Surviving intensive care: a report from the 2002 Brussels Roundtable. Intensive Care Med 29: 368–377
38. Im K, Belle SH, Schulz R, Mendelsohn AB, Chelluri L (2004) Prevalence and outcomes of caregiving after prolonged (> or =48 hours) mechanical ventilation in the ICU. Chest 125: 597–606
39. Chelluri L, Im KA, Belle SH, et al (2004) Long-term mortality and quality of life after prolonged mechanical ventilation. Crit Care Med 32: 61–69
40. Van Pelt DC, Milbrandt EB, Qin L, et al (2007) Informal caregiver burden among survivors of prolonged mechanical ventilation. Am J Respir Crit Care Med 175: 167–173
41. Angus DC, Barnato AE, Linde-Zwirble WT, et al (2004) Use of intensive care at the end of life in the United States: an epidemiologic study. Crit Care Med 32: 638–643

42. van der Heide A, Deliens L, Faisst K, et al (2003) End-of-life decision-making in six European countries: descriptive study. Lancet 362: 345–350
43. Sprung CL, Cohen SL, Sjokvist P, et al (2003) End-of-life practices in European intensive care units: the Ethicus Study. JAMA 290: 790–797
44. Barnato AE, Herndon MB, Anthony DL, et al (2007) Are regional variations in end-of-life care intensity explained by patient preferences?: A Study of the US Medicare Population. Med Care 45: 386–393
45. Lautrette A, Darmon M, Megarbane B, et al (2007) A communication strategy and brochure for relatives of patients dying in the ICU. N Engl J Med 356: 469–478
46. Jackson EA, Yarzebski JL, Goldberg RJ, et al (2004) Do-not-resuscitate orders in patients hospitalized with acute myocardial infarction: the Worcester Heart Attack Study. Arch Intern Med 164: 776–783
47. Halpern NA, Pastores SM, Thaler HT, Greenstein RJ (2006) Changes in critical care beds and occupancy in the United States 1985–2000: Differences attributable to hospital size. Crit Care Med 34: 2105–2112
48. Harrison DA, Lertsithichai P, Brady AR, Carpenter JR, Rowan K (2004) Winter excess mortality in intensive care in the UK: an analysis of outcome adjusted for patient case mix and unit workload. Intensive Care Med 30: 1900–1907
49. Zilberberg MD, de WM, Pirone JR, Shorr AF (2008) Growth in adult prolonged acute mechanical ventilation: implications for healthcare delivery. Crit Care Med 36: 1451–1455
50. Boscoe FP (2008) Subdividing the age group of 85 years and older to improve US disease reporting. Am J Public Health 98: 1167–1170

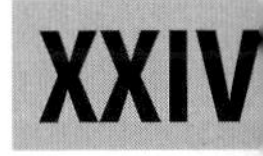

ICU Performance: Managing with Balanced Scorecards

K. Shukri and F.S.M. Ali

Introduction

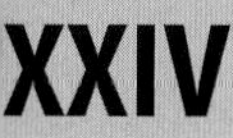

Intensive care units (ICUs) are dynamic organizations with one of the most complex environments of all healthcare facilities. Defining or measuring ICU performance is, therefore, challenging. The meaning, scope, and measurement of performance in health care has evolved and expanded over the past two decades. Some of the most widely used approaches to improving performance in health care have proved inadequate, all the more as, since 2000, healthcare organizations are faced with increasing challenges, including changing demographics, increased customer expectations, increased competition, and intensified governmental pressure, that demand unprecedented levels of change. Meeting these challenges will require healthcare organizations to undergo fundamental changes and to seek new ways to improve performance.

The balanced scorecard represents a technique used in strategic management to translate an organization's mission and strategy into a comprehensive set of performance indicators that provides the framework for implementation of strategic management.

The following are four scenarios of ICU performance which could occur in any ICU:

- ICU 1 has all the resources of supplies, medications and technology but the quality of care is poor with many medical errors and worsening clinical outcomes.
- ICU 2 faces high staff turnover, vacancy rate, and absenteeism, and poor employee satisfaction score. The management is concerned more about patient volume than about quality of care and staff morale is decreasing.
- ICU 3 has a new director who implements evidence based guidelines and a closed system resulting in better clinical outcomes and who sets an international benchmark. Staff and patient satisfaction rates improve dramatically.
- ICU 4's reputation has been affected and the hospital's annual operating is in crisis with ICU loss of revenue. The administration is introducing cutbacks and community complaints are increasing. The ICU staff is working in an information silo.

Looking at the four scenarios, several questions are raised: What is ICU performance? Which factors contribute to high performance? How do we really assess and manage ICU performance? Should we look at performance only in terms of outcomes or using other measures? Does your ICU have a vision, with mission and objectives to achieve? How can we execute the objectives to achieve our goals? How can we select the right indicators?

This chapter provides an ICU framework and model for developing a balanced scorecard and demonstrates the remarkable success of this process, which helps focus leadership decisions about the allocation of resources to improve ICU performance.

What is ICU Performance?

Defining ICU performance is a complicated task, involving medical knowledge, ethics, economics, systems, engineering, sociology, and philosophy. Efforts to measure ICU performance should adhere to the following two essential principles: (1) Evaluate a variety of parameters that span the dimensions of ICU performance; and (2) use performance measures that are primarily relevant or that have a proven relationship to primary measures. Assessing performance requires the quantification of parameters that are relevant to patients, society, and the hospital [1]. Based on the literature, we can divide ICU performance into six categories: Outcomes, patient safety, cost and resource utilization, workforce, leadership, and intensive care environment.

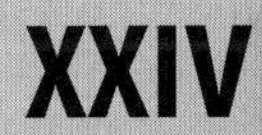

Outcomes

Traditionally ICU performance can be evaluated using the standard mortality ratio (SMR), the ratio between the observed (O) and predicted hospital mortality rates (P), based on a statistical model. If, for 100 consecutive unselected patients, the O/P ratio is less than 1, then the performance is considered good, otherwise bad [2]. However, as Zimmerman [3] suggested that "It would nice if we could measure ICU performance and everyone believed the results". It will be difficult to relate quality of care to a severity model in view of case mix and variations in SMR. Glance and colleagues [4] determined whether the identity of ICU quality outliers depended on the ICU scoring system (APACHE II, SAPS II and MPMII) used to calculate the SMR within a single database of 16000 patients from 32 US Hospitals. The authors concluded that these models were of limited usefulness for benchmarking. Current risk adjustment systems are not able to completely control for case mix in the ICU. A study in Brazilian ICUs reported that there were substantial and significant variations in their SMRs compared to those in US ICUs [5]. Another study in Europe evaluated the performance of SAPS II and MPMII in 16060 patients from 89 ICUs in 12 European countries from the EURICUS database; the result revealed that studies utilizing general outcome prediction systems without previous validation in the target population should be interpreted with caution [6]. In 2000, Metnitz et al. confirmed that caution should be exercised when using risk-adjusted mortality rates to distinguish ICUs with widely divergent case mix [7]. Even though the risk-adjusted hospital mortality is used by the Joint Commission for Accreditation of Healthcare Organizations (JCAHO) [8] and the severity-adjusted mortality by the Solucient Leadership Institute when ranking the best 100 ICUs in the US [9], mortality is the only outcome measure which does not reflect other components, such as efficiency, effectiveness, timeliness of intervention, process indicators, survival from different conditions in ICUs, adverse events, rate of infections, financial cost, resource and technology utilization, and safety in view of the high costs of healthcare globally. Therefore, mortality during hospitalization is a limited measure of the effectiveness of intensive care [10].

Patient Safety

There is a high risk of iatrogenic injury in the ICU because of the patients' underlying severe illnesses. There are, therefore, cumulative data regarding the incidence of diagnostic and therapeutic errors in the ICU, which can reflect poor performance in specific areas of ICU systems. The data reveal that 31 % of all ICU patients suffer iatrogenic complications during their stay and for the ICU as a whole, about 1.7 errors occur per patient day [11]. Twice a day a severe or potentially detrimental error is committed; 60 % of adverse events were errors in medication [11]. In a study assessing medication errors, adverse events occurred in 3.6 % of orders; 81 % were clinically important [12]. In the Critical Care Safety Study, supported in part by the Agency for Healthcare Research and Quality (AHRQ), 120 adverse events were identified in 79 patients (20.2 %); adverse events occurred at a rate of 81 per 1,000 patient days. Forty-five percent of the adverse events in this study were preventable; serious errors occurred at a rate of 150 per 1,000 patient days [13]. Sixty-three to eighty-three percent of all critical incidents can be attributed to human error and one in three errors in the ICU is caused by communication problems [14]. Thirteen to fifty-one percent of all critical incidents pose a major threat for patient safety [15].

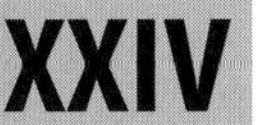

Cost and Resource Utilization

Under ideal circumstances, economic pressures and financial constraints can have a positive impact on healthcare delivery, as processes and structures can be streamlined and waste eliminated without reduction in quality of care [16]. More than 4 million US patients receive care in an ICU each year at an annual cost of more than $180 billion, making the ICU a high volume and high cost environment [17]. One day in an ICU cost $2,000 to $3,000 in America, which is six fold higher than the costs for non-ICU care; ICUs consume 20 % of total in-patient expenditure [18].

Workforce Performance

Of all the controllable factors affecting performance, the human capital or workforce is the most critical underperforming asset in most business organizations. It is the people who improve performance, process, and systems; therefore, upgrading skills and education and promoting a mindset culture are major elements of success for human resource performance management. The needs of ICU patients are often complex, requiring caregivers who work under stressful conditions. Despite a high level of knowledge, dedication and competency of ICU caregivers, mortality rates for critical care patients remain high ranging from 10–20 % in well established ICU facilities [19].

Leadership Performance

Numerous studies of business management models have substantiated the important role of leadership in achieving the desired result. It has been shown that leadership has a strong relationship with business results, more than twice the effect of any other variable [20]. As intensive care medicine is a specialty that is highly interactive and interdisciplinary there are few data on ICU leadership and management skills. Strack van Schijndel and Burchardi described how non-medical management competencies can be applied to ICU leadership, including directing, communication skills, daily rounds, team briefings, staffing, planning, organizing, budgeting, controlling, conflict management, and negotiations [21].

Another challenge for ICU leadership is to reduce staff turnover and burn out and create a positive team culture often amid a lack of supportive resources and good working relationships between staff and disciplines [22]. Therefore, ICU leadership is vital for a successful performance of the ICU. Pronovost and colleagues [23] presented a model to help health care organizations reliably deliver effective interventions. The overall objective of the study was to improve patient safety using a "Safety Score Card". This system was used in over 100 ICUs in Michigan to improve organizational culture and eliminate catheter-related blood stream infections. The model focused on learning from mistakes and system redesign. It targeted three important groups – senior leaders, team leaders, and front line staff – and facilitated change management by a manual of operations – engage, educate, execute, and evaluate – for planned interventions. Use of this model was associated with a significant reduction in catheter-related blood stream infections and improvement in culture. However, this model has limitations as it requires huge resources; in addition, further validation is needed and further studies to measure patient safety.

The ICU environment

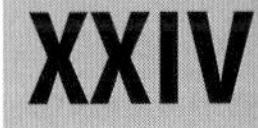

This includes: ICU organization model, staffing, credentialing and privileges, healthy culture, equipment and technology. Using an intensivist and a closed system has improved outcomes and been associated with potential cost savings [24]. Lower ICU nurse:patient ratios have been associated with an increased infection risk for patients [25]; therefore, adequate nursing is highly recommended to ensure quality care for patients. The American Association of Critical Care Nurses (AACN) set six essential standards for a healthy working environment to improve ICU performance: Skilled communication, true collaboration, effective decision making, appropriate staffing, meaningful recognition, and authentic leadership [26]. These six categories have a major impact on ICU performance and all are linked to each other, so how do we integrate the six into one framework?

What is the Balanced Scorecard

In the 1990s, Kaplan and Norton [27] undertook a study to examine how organizations measure their performance. However, their study uncovered a number of reporting practices that many leading organizations were using to measure their performance. Therefore, the Balanced Scorecard Framework has been developed to allow organizations to:

- Develop and deploy a scorecard economically using an existing infrastructure.
- Manage and display the data and knowledge pertinent to balanced scorecards.
- Facilitate analysis of measures so that prompt corrective action can take place.

The framework provides a comprehensive, flexible, cost-effective way to deploy the balanced scorecard and to deliver superior returns on people, processes, customers, and technologies.

Drs. Norton and Kaplan describe the balanced scorecard as follows: "A balanced scorecard is a system of linked objectives, measures, targets, and initiatives, which collectively describe the strategy of an organization and how the strategy can be achieved. It can take something as complicated and frequently nebulous as strategy and translate it into something that is specific and can be understood". Tradition-

Table 1. Classic balanced scorecard in non-healthcare industries

Perspective	Key question	Objectives	Initiatives	Measure/ indicator	Target
Financial	To succeed financially, how should we appear to our stakeholders?				
Customer	To achieve our vision, how should we appear to our customers?				
Process	To satisfy our customers and shareholders, at what business processes must we excel?				
Learning and growth	To achieve our vision, how will we sustain our ability to change and improve?				

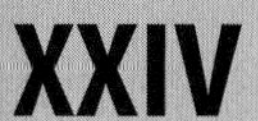

ally, the unbalanced scorecard allocates 70 % of the total to the financial perspective leaving only 30 % for the other three perspectives (internal processes, customers, learning and growth). While this type of allocation may have a short term benefit, it could have a deleterious impact on the organization's financial and non-financial outcomes in the long run. A balanced scorecard approach allocates approximately 30 % each to the financial and internal perspectives and 20 % each to customers and learning and growth.

The classic balanced scorecard describes strategy and performance management from multiple perspectives. The classic balanced scorecard in non-healthcare industries has four perspectives (**Table 1**); each perspective can be explained by a key question with which it is associated. The answers to each key question become the objectives associated with that perspective, and performance is then judged by the progress to achieving these objectives. There is an explicit causal relationship between the perspectives: Good performance in the Learning and Growth objectives generally drives improvements in the Internal Process objectives, which should improve the organization in the eyes of the customer, which ultimately leads to improved financial results.

Objectives are desired outcomes. The progress toward attaining an objective is gauged by one or more measures. As with perspectives, there are causal relationships between objectives. In fact, the causal relationship is defined by dependencies among objectives. So, it is critical to set measurable, strategically relevant, consistent, time-delineated objectives.

Measures are the indicators of how a business is performing relative to its strategic objectives. Measures, or metrics, are quantifiable performance statements. As such, they must be:

1. Relevant to the objective and strategy.
2. Placed in context of a target to be reached in an identified time frame.
3. Capable of being trended.
4. Owned by a designated person or group who has the ability to impact those measures

The balanced scorecard is a key element in such a system and provides an effective tool to move an organization's strategy and vision into action. If used properly, it can enhance strategic feedback and learning.

Balanced Scorecards in Healthcare Organizations

The balanced scorecard has been modified by many healthcare organizations, most commonly by placing the patient/customer at the top of the strategy map. Finance then becomes a means to achieve superior patient outcomes and satisfaction (**Table 2**). The balanced scorecard has been adopted by leading healthcare organizations in the USA, including Duke's Children's Hospital (Durham, NC [28], Mayo Clinic (Rochester, MN) [29] and Saint Mary's Duluth Clinic (Duluth, MN), and in countries like Canada [30] Japan, China, and Korea.

The use of the balanced scorecard in healthcare has been shown to improve the competitive marketing position, financial results, and patient satisfaction. Chen and colleagues described the use of a balanced scorecard to compare hospital performance in China and Japan. The use of the balanced scorecard showed benefits that not only suggested performance improvements in individual hospitals but also revealed effective health factors allowing implementation of valid national health policies [31]. Hong et al. concluded that there was a high degree of validity and reliability of the balanced scorecard when assessing performance measurement of a Korean hospital nursing organization [32]. The balanced scorecard can be used in different departments. For example, performance in the emergency department improved significantly after implementing the balanced scorecard, including hours of continuing education attended by the staff, staff job satisfaction, the rate of incomplete laboratory tests within 30 minutes, the average monthly inappropriate return rate, and hospital profit [33]. The indicators used in this study [33] may also be reasonable for a hospital that has limited resources or as a management business tool for building a new program or center [34].

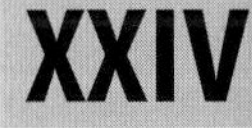

Table 2. Balanced scorecard in healthcare and the intensive care unit (ICU)

Perspective	Key question
Financial	To succeed financially, how should we appear to our stakeholders?
Resource and service utilization	To achieve cost effectiveness, how can we use the resources appropriately?
Customer	To achieve our vision, how should we appear to our patients, families and the community?
Process	To satisfy our patients, families, vendors, and shareholders, at what business processes must we excel?
Learning and growth	To achieve our vision, how will we sustain our ability to change and improve?
Financial	To financially sustain our mission, what must we focus on?

Balanced Scorecard Application in the ICU

An organization that adopts a balanced scorecard approach should also adopt specific metric indicators at a departmental level. The ICU department is one the most dynamic units in the hospital, therefore metrics should be aligned with and support the organization indicators, and ICU leadership must be completely aware of them and must be accountable for their achievement.

As Studer stated, we are not measuring just to measure [35]. We are measuring to align specific leadership and employee behaviors that cascade throughout the organization to drive results [35]. The scorecard can be used at many different levels in an organization. However, departmental scorecards should be linked to divisional, and ultimately to corporate, levels. The development and operation of scorecards requires disciplined communication which can be an incentive for action. A good methodology in the ICU would include the following actions:

1. Develop an executable business/department strategy: Determine the important objectives of the ICU dept and base the strategy on those goals, the strategy should be aligned with hospital vision and mission and objectives. The process entails finding out what key performance indicators contribute the most to the success of the ICU and the hospital.
2. Describe the strategy: ICU leadership should hold meetings with key stakeholders, including nursing and physician personnel, and other hospital staff who support daily work activities in the ICU, i.e., pharmacy, laboratory, radiology, etc. Explanations are given as to why certain indicators were chosen and how these indicators make an impact on ICU and hospital outcomes.
3. Design and develop the scorecard framework with performance metrics: The indicators should closely follow the strategic objectives outlined by the hospital. In this way the ICU scorecard is not just a set of unrelated metrics, but represents the hospital's organizational system for financial and non-financial goals and for monitoring goals to achieve preferred outcomes.

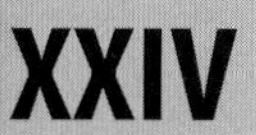

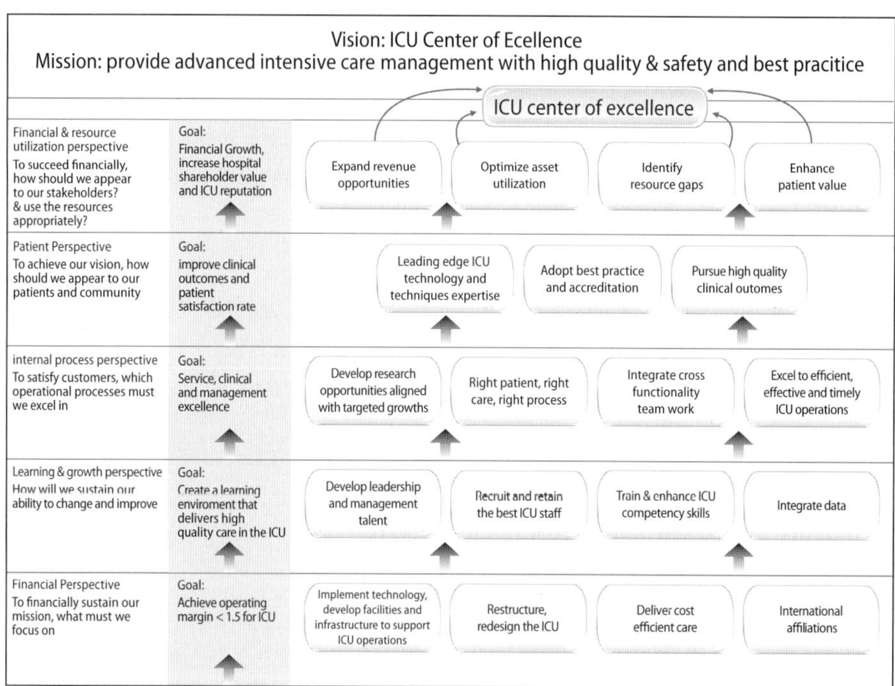

Fig. 1. Intensive care unit strategy map

The ICU-strategic map (**Fig. 1**) consists of series of linked initiatives. Each initiative should have a quantitative measure and a target, some will be cross–departmental, for example ICU and laboratory, radiology or pharmacy. The ICU leadership must be a role model to lead the staff members, physicians and other stakeholders in building a vision and maximizing resources to carry out the job. The leadership must create an environment in which the following occur:

- There is a clear focus on meeting the needs and expectations of patients and other stakeholders
- Learning and innovation are embraced
- The hospital and ICU direction is well defined and communicated, continuously addressing priorities and performance expectation
- Good ethical principles are developed and adhered to.
  An ICU strategy map would describe:
- If there is adequate financial support to provide staff, space, resources, and technology, then the vision, mission, and goals can be accomplished and sustained
- If the ICU staff has the skills, tools, education, and motivation then operations and processes will improve
- If operations and processes run efficiently and effectively then patient outcomes will improve and the ICU's reputation will grow
- If outcomes and operations improve then resource utilization will be adequate and cost-effective
- If resources and services are utilized adequately then financial performance will improve and grow.

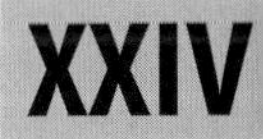

The five perspectives of a balanced scorecard with examples of ICU indicators for each are described as follows (**Table 3**).

ICU Workforce Learning and Growth Perspective

To effectively execute a strategy, the ICU staff must have the necessary tools and resources to succeed. Therefore, investment in this aspect is important. There are three aspects of learning and growth: Employee skills, information technology, and motivation. [36]. ICUs worldwide have a diverse multinational staff. Continuous updating of clinical skills and competency with accreditation standards is vital. Other important skills which should be improved are leadership, communication, quality improvement skills, and teamwork. A progressive culture and motivated employees are clearly competitive, therefore, it is important to monitor ICU staff satisfaction with respect to various factors including involvement with decisions, recognition of doing a job, access to sufficient information to do the job well, and encouraging creativity. Examples of objectives for learning and growth could be: Achieving sepsis management expertise, developing effective multidisciplinary and cross functional teams, deploying computer technology for simulation, and fostering a culture of learning and innovation. Examples of indicators to measure performance from a staff learning and growth perspective include: Turnover, absenteeism, training hours per employee, retention rate, number of simulation classes attended, hours of continuous medical education (CME) gained per year.

Table 3. ICU performance indicators in the balanced scorecard format

Financial perspective	Learning and growth perspective	Internal process/ operating efficiency perspective	Patient outcome focus perspective	Resource utilization perspective
Percent of hospital budget: ICU budget ratio (revenue and expense) Cost per ICU bed Research grant revenue Growth, revenue, expense and profit-product line Growth, revenue, expense and profit-dept Growth, revenue and cost per adjusted patient day Growth, revenue and cost per physician full time equivalent (FTE) Cost of top antibiotic utilization in the ICU Cost of ICU patients who are in clinical pathways/protocols	Vacancy rate Turnover rate Number of ACLS trained nurses/physicians Number of staff with new competency training skills Staff satisfaction rate	Turn-around time for starting sedation, inotropes and vasopressors Turn-around time for urgent radiology reports Timing of antibiotics Turn-around time for stat blood transfusions Operating efficiency timing for protocol guidelines for sepsis, CRRT, HFOV, hypothermia Percent compliance for DVT prevention, early enteral feeding, H_2-blockers Percent compliance to IHI (Institute for Health Improvement) guidelines for VAP, central line infection prevention	Rate of central line infections Rate of VAP Rate of MRSA, VRE Rate of multidrug resistant organisms Survival rate of severe sepsis Survival of ARDS/ALI Number of ICU incident reports ICU-readmission rate within 72 hours Unplanned extubation Medication errors rate Adverse events rate Sentinel events rate Near miss rate Outcome of abdominal catastrophes, such as ACS Outcome of post-CPR treated with hypothermia Patient satisfaction rate Family satisfaction Percent of decubitus ulcers grade 3–4 Outcomes of hemodialysis and CRRT	Nurse: patient ratio ICU bed occupancy Utilization of CRRT Blood utilization Emergency admissions Elective admissions Unplanned surgical cases Length of stay Mechanical ventilation days Compliance with evidence based guidelines Reputation Availability of resources Patient turnover Patient care volume by different category of disease (sepsis, ARDS, acute renal failure) Antibiotic utilization Blood utilization and wastage ICU stock utilization (CRRT filters, arterial lines, isolation gowns, etc)

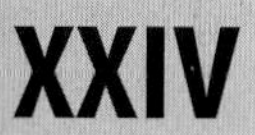

VAP: ventilator-associated pneumonia; MRSA: methicillin-resistant *S aureus*; VRE: vancomycin-resistant enterococcus; ACS: abdominal compartment syndrome; ARDS: acute respiratory distress syndrome; ALI: acute lung injury; ACLS: advanced cardiac life support; CPR: cardiopulmonary resuscitation; CRRT: continuous renal replacement therapy; HFOV: high frequency oscillatory ventilation

ICU Internal Process and Operation Efficiency Perspective

The internal process or operation has three major components: Innovation, ongoing process improvement, and post-discharge service. A well performing and organized ICU will have a purposeful innovation process. The first step in an ICU innovation process is to identify a potential patient segment, then to answer two primary questions: 1) What benefits will customers value in tomorrow's market; and 2) How can the organization innovate to deliver those benefits. Four innovation processes are: Identifying opportunities for new services, managing the research and development portfolio, designing and developing new services, and introducing new services into the healthcare market, for example, adding a neuro-ICU as a new service, remodeling and redecorating the ICU, increasing ICU partnerships or affiliations, creating a cross-functional process with multidisciplinary teams to improve the work flow of patient care efficiently and effectively.

ICU Patient Perspective

In most healthcare organizations, the customer is the patient; therefore it is important to determine the value proposition that will be delivered to each patient and build a reputation for the hospital, taking, for example, a segment of critically ill patients with severe sepsis, acute respiratory distress syndrome (ARDS), or post-cardiac arrest survivors, and determining the indicators for this category of patients. Berenholtz and colleagues [37] evaluated the quality of sepsis care by identifying ten potential measures: Vancomycin administration, time to vancomycin initiation, broad-spectrum antibiotic administration, time to broad-spectrum antibiotic initiation, blood culture collection, steroid administration, corticotrophin stimulation test administration, activated protein C eligibility assessment, activated protein C administration, and vancomycin discontinuation. These measures helped caregivers to focus on evidence-based interventions that improve mortality and to evaluate their current performance [37]. Examples of ICU indicators to measure performance from a patient perspective include: Patient care volumes by different category of illness, turnover of patients, readmission rates, complication rates, compliance with evidenced based guidelines, medical errors, and patient satisfaction.

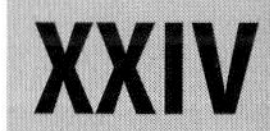

ICU Resource Utilization Perspective

Using appropriate resources with cost-effectiveness and providing high quality care is a major task for the ICU. Examples include bed utilization of non-acute admissions, antibiotic utilization, length of stay, utilization of continuous renal replacement therapy (CRRT) and its filters, blood products transfusion utilization, unused equipment and technology. All these factors may affect cost and future financial revenues. Identifying resource gaps and optimizing asset utilization is a target to be achieved.

ICU Financial Perspective

If the ICU is in growth mode, the focus should be on increasing revenue to accommodate this growth. If it is operating in a relatively stable environment then profitability is emphasized. If it is stable and profitable, the focus can shift to investment in terms of both physical assets and human capital (workforce). Therefore, financial measures are an important component: They ensure that we are achieving our results, but doing so in an efficient manner which minimizes cost. Examples of indicators include revenue, profitability, asset utilization, operating margin, cost per ICU case, research grant revenue, and ICU department growth. Overall, the target is to achieve vision and mission, sustain it with financial strength, develop a reputation and brand image, be cost-effective, and create reduction with productivity.

Successful Implementation of an ICU Balanced Scorecard System

The criteria for successful implementation of a balanced scorecard system in the ICU include:

1. Hospital senior management must be committed to change
2. Leadership commitment and skills (ICU director, nurse manager)
3. Organizational mission and vision
4. Promote a culture of safety, learning, and team building
5. Perspectives (finance, customer, internal business process, learning and growing, resource utilization)
6. Selecting the right and relevant indicators in each perspective
7. Strategy maps/strategy alignment
8. Balanced scorecard framework (**Table 4**)
9. Process for identifying targets, resources, initiatives, and budgets
10. Feedback and strategic learning process

As ICU indicators are linked to each other, the following are examples of key decisions when interpreted using a balanced scorecard framework

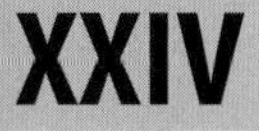

- if the rate of procedure complications is high then competency skills of staff need to be re-evaluated
- if the staff satisfaction loyalty index is below the setting benchmark then the staff workload (nurse:patient ratio, healthy culture) should be re-evaluated
- if the rate of central line infections is above the benchmark then re-assessing compliance to guidelines should be taken seriously
- if the survival rate from severe sepsis is low then the physicians' credentials and training skills in managing sepsis, compliance with protocols, availability and timing of antibiotics should be re-assessed
- if the rates of sentinel events, adverse events, and near-misses are increasing then it suggests a non-punitive culture and policies of cross-functional team building must be re-evaluated and re-structured.
- if the use of CRRT filters is high over 24–48 hours, this may be attributed to poor skills in handling CRRT machines, unavailability of proper guidelines, or lack of training in CRRT.
- if the rate of pressure ulcers is high then this could be linked to poor skills in mobilizing ICU patients
- if there is a high rate of post-cardiac arrest patients admitted to the ICU, then a rapid response team initiative and therapeutic hypothermia should be considered.
- if patient clinical outcomes are very good this suggests that the staff is skillful and competent and the internal process of the unit is efficient leading to a better reputation
- if there is high grant research revenue then this may be attributed to highly qualified staff where your target is to have a high retention rate

Conclusion

The balanced scorecard is a proven performance measurement system. It is a framework for defining, refining, and communicating strategy, for translating strategy to operational terms, and for measuring the effectiveness of strategy implementation.

Table 4. Example of intensive care unit (ICU) balanced scorecard framework

	Objective	Measure	Target	Initiative	Accountability
Financial	Increase reputation Financial growth	Revenue growth	20 %		
Resource utilization ↑	Provide a tertiary level of ICU care	Average length of stay for patients with severe sepsis	2005, > 7 days		ICU multidisciplinary team
		ICU bed utilization for planned surgical case	< 10 %		ICU director/ nurse manager
Patient outcomes ↑	Decrease rate of central line infections	Rate of central line infections	2005, < 5 %	Participate in IHI campaign	ICU doctors Nursing
	Decrease rate of decubitus ulcers	Rate of decubitus ulcer grade 3 – 4	< 2 %	protocol prevention of decubitus ulcers	Multidisciplinary team ICU director and staff
	Improve survival of sepsis patients with APACHE 2	Survival rate of Severe sepsis	75 %	Implement sepsis campaign guidelines	ICU doctors
	High patient and family satisfaction	Patient and family loyalty index	90 %	Survey for patient and family satisfaction	
		ICU-readmission rate within 72 hours	< 5 %		
		Rate of VAP	10 – 15 %		
Internal process ↑	Compliance with IHI guidelines and JCAHO	% compliance	2005, 100 % compliance		ICU staff
		Timing of antibiotics	< 1 hour		
Learning and growth ↑	Provide education/training in infection control and accreditation standards	% ICU staff trained	2005, 100 % compliance		
	ACLS training	Percent of doctors ACLS certified			
	CME education	Percent of ICU staff attending ESICM Congress			
	Effective managerial skills	Percent of nurses attending the managerial course			
	Retain the best staff	Retention rate			
Financial ↑	Budget for ICU staff training	ICU operating margin	> 1.5 %		

IHI: Institute of Healthcare Improvement; JCAHO: Joint Commission on the Accreditation of Healthcare Organizations; CME: continuing medical education; ACLS: advanced cardiac life support

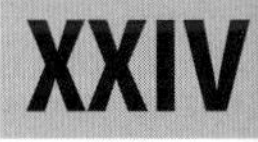

ICUs can use the balanced scorecard approach to achieve high peak performance and identify areas for improvement in outcomes, processes, quality and safety, cost and resource utilization, in a systemic organized way; this requires leadership commitment. There is a need for a consensus for defining ICU performance, high peak performance, and performance excellence in order to benchmark indicators and to be able to identify the leading ICUs in the world.

References

1. Garland A (2005) Improving the ICU: Part 1. Chest 127: 2151–2164
2. Le Gall JR (2007) Performance of adult intensive care units. Thirty years' experience. Bull Acad Natl Med 191: 869–877
3. Zimmerman JE (2002) Measuring intensive care unit performance: a way to move forward. Crit Care Med 30: 2149–2150
4. Glance TG, Osler TM, Dick A (2002) Rating the quality of intensive care units: is it a function of the intensive care unit scoring system? Crit Care Med 30: 1976–1982
5. Bastos PG, Sun X, Wagner DP, Knaus WA, Zimmerman (1996) Application of APACHE III prognostic system in Brazilian intensive care units: a prospective multicenter study. Intensive Care Med 22: 564–570

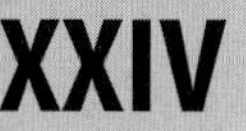

6. Moreno R, Metnitz PG, et al (2005) On behalf of the SAPS 3 investigators. SAPS 3 -from evaluation of the patient to evaluation of the intensive care unit. Part 2: development of a prognostic model for hospital mortality at ICU admission. Intensive Care Med 31: 1345–1355
7. Metnitz PG, Lang T, Vesley H (2000) Ratio of observed to expected mortality is affected by differences in case mix and quality of care. Intensive Care Med 26: 1466–1472
8. Joint Commission on Accreditation of Healthcare Oragniztions (2007) ICU measure overview. Available at: www.jointcommision.org
9. Solucient Leadership Institute (2007) Top 100 hospitals. National benchmarks for success 2006. Available at: www.100tophospitals.com
10. Thibault GE, Mulley AG, Barnett GO (1980) Medical intensive care: indications, interventions and outcomes. N Engl J Med 302: 938–942
11. Donchin Y, Gopher D, Olin M, et al (1995) A look into the nature and causes of human errors in the intensive care unit. the hostile environment of the intensive care unit. Crit Care Med 23: 294–300
12. Buckley MS, Erstad B, Kopp B, Theodorou AA, Priestley G (2007) Direct observation approach for detecting medication errors and adverse drug events in pediatric intensive care unit. Pediatr Crit Care Med 8: 145–152
13. Rothschild JM, Landrigan CP, Cronin JW (2005) The critical care safety study: the incidence and nature of adverse events and serious medical errors in intensive care. Crit Care Med 33: 1694–1700
14. Wright D, Mackenzie SJ, Buchan I (1991) Critical incidents in intensive care therapy unit. Lancet 338: 676–678
15. Giraud T, Dhainaut J, Vaxelaire J (1993) Iatrogenic complications in adult intensive care units, a prospective two center study. Crit Care Med 21: 40–51
16. Chalfin DB, Cohen IL, Lambrinos J (1995) The economics of cost effectiveness of critical care med. Intensive Care Med 21: 952–961
17. Pronovost PJ, Goeschel C (2005) Improving ICU care: it takes a team. Health Exec 20: 15–22
18. Norris C, Jacobs P, Rapport J, et al (1995) ICU and non-ICU cost per day. Can J Anaesth 42: 192–196
19. The leapfrog group (2004) ICU physician staffing fact sheet. Available at: http://www. leapfroggroup.org/media/file/Fact_Sheet_IPS_081104.pdf Accessed Nov 2008
20. Pannirselvam GP, Ferguson LA (2001) A study of the relationships between the Baldrige categories. International Journal of Quality and Reliability Management 18: 14–34
21. Strack van Schijndel RJ, Burchardi H (2007) Bench-to-bedside review: leadership and conflict management in the intensive care unit. Crit Care 11: 234
22. Laporta DP, Burns J, Doig CJ (2005) Bench-to-bedside review: dealing with increased intensive care unit staff turnover: a leadership challenge. Crit Care 9: 454–458

23. Pronovost PJ, Berenholtz SM, Goeschel CA (2006) Creating high reliability in health care organizations. Health Serv Res 41: 1599–1617
24. Pronosvost P, Needham DM, Waters H, et al (2004) Intensive care unit physician staffing ,financial modeling of leapfrog standard. Crit Care Med 32: 1247–1253
25. Hugonnet S, Chevrolet JC, Pittet D (2007) The effect of workload on infection risk in critically ill patients. Crit Care Med 35: 76–81
26. American Association of Critical Care Nurses (2005) AACN standards for establishing and sustaining healthy work environments. Available at: http://classic.aacn.org/aacn/pubpolcy.nsf/Files/HWEStandards/$file/HWEStandards.pdf Accessed Nov 2008
27. Kaplan RS, Norton DP (1992) The balanced scorecard – measures that drive performance. Harv Bus Rev 70: 71–79
28. Meliones J (2000) Saving money, saving lives. Harv Bus Rev 78: 57–62
29. Curtright JW, Stolp-Smith SC, Edell ES (2000) Strategic performance management: development of a performance measurement system at the Mayo Clinic. J Health Manag 45: 58–68
30. Baker GR, Pink GH (1995) A balanced scorecard for Canadian hospitals. Healthc Manage Forum 8: 7–21
31. Chen XY, Yamauchi K, Kato K, Nishimura A, Ito K (2006) Using the balanced scorecard to measure Chinese and Japanese hospital performance. Int J Health Care Qual Assur 19: 339–350
32. Hong Y, Hwang KJ, Kim MJ, Park CG (2008) [Balanced scorecard for performance measurement of a nursing organization in a Korean hospital] Taehan Kanho Hakhoe Chi 38: 45–54
33. Huang SH, Chen PL, Yang MC, Chang WY, Lee HJ (2004) Using a balanced scorecard to improve the performance of an emergency department. Nurs Econ 22: 140–146
34. Wachtel TL, Hartford CE, Hughes JA (1999) Building a balanced scorecard for a burn center. Burns 25: 431–437
35. Studer Q (2003) Hardwiring Excellence. Fire Starter Publishing, Gulf Breeze
36. Kaplan RS, Norton DP (1996) The Balanced Scorecard: Translating Strategy into Action. Harvard Business School Press, Boston
37. Berenholtz SM, Pronovost PJ, Ngo K (2007) Developing quality measures for sepsis care in the ICU. Jt Comm J Qual Patient Saf 33: 559–568

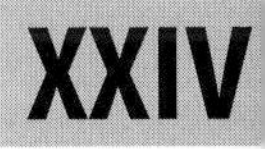

XXV End-of-Life Issues

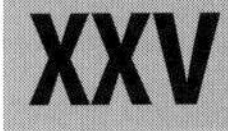

Towards a Neuro-scientific Explanation of Near-death Experiences?

A. Vanhaudenhuyse, M. Thonnard, and S. Laureys

Introduction

Near-death experiences can be defined as "profound psychological events with transcendental and mystical elements, typically occurring to individuals close to death or in situations of intense physical or emotional danger. These elements include ineffability, a sense that the experience transcends personal ego, and an experience of union with a divine or higher principle" [1]. Common elements recurring in near-death experiences are experiencing a panoramic life review, feelings of peace and quiet, seeing a dark tunnel, experiencing a bright light, or out-of-body experiences [1] (**Fig. 1**). During an out-of-body experience, people seem to be awake and see their own body and the world from a location outside their physical body [2] (**Fig. 2**). Some spiritual and psychological theories have been developed in order to explain near-death experiences and out-of-body experiences. Clinical studies have aimed at determining their frequency and assessing precipitating factors. Recent studies have shown the involvement of the temporo-parietal cortex in the generation of out-of-body experiences and offer a neurological account for the phenomenon, rebuffing dualistic, non-physical explanations. In this chapter, we discuss what is and is not known about the neuronal correlates of these extraordinary experiences.

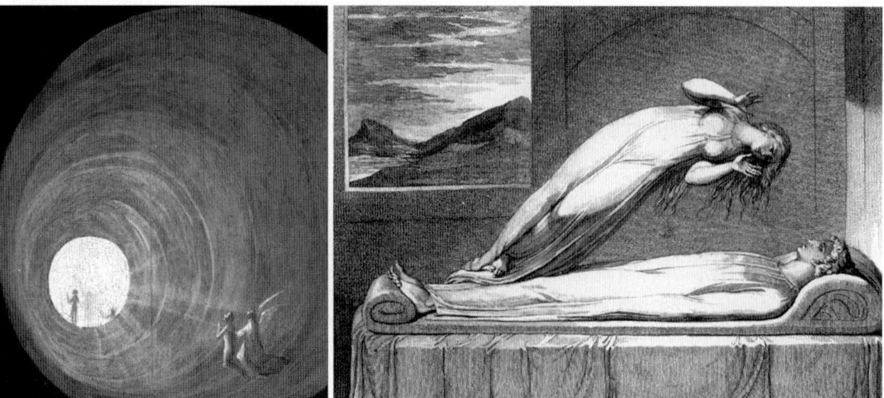

Fig. 1. Common elements recurring in near-death experiences are seeing a dark tunnel, experiencing a bright light, feelings of peace and quiet, experiencing a panoramic life review or out-of-body experience (from Hieronymus Bosch, 1500s "Paradise and the Ascent in the Empyrean" *left*; and Schiavonetti, 1808 "The soul leaves the body at the moment of death" *right*).

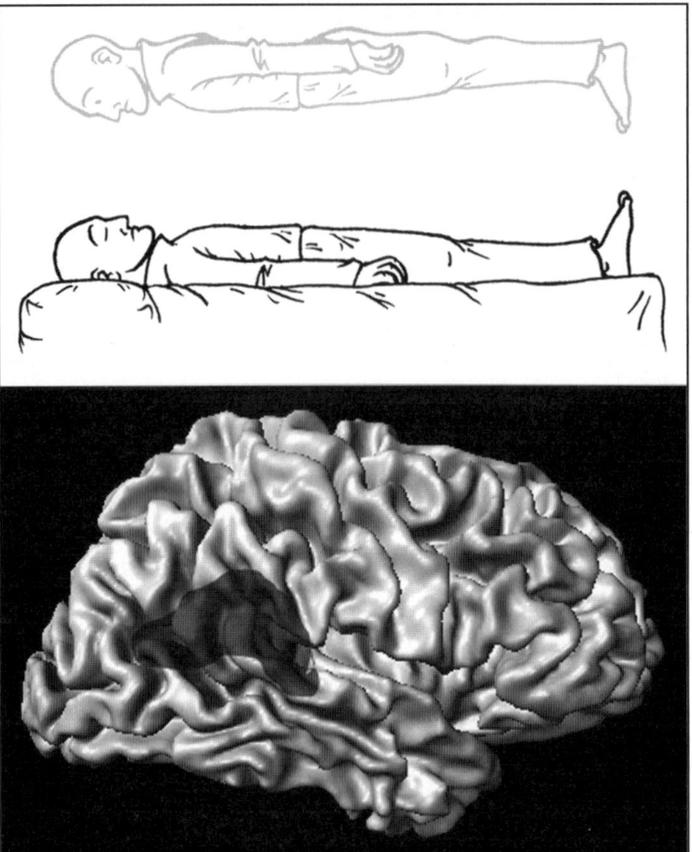

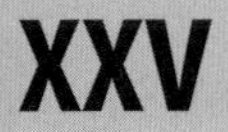

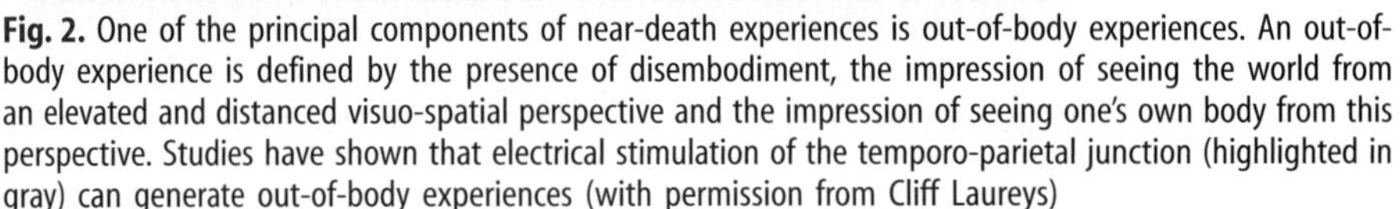

Fig. 2. One of the principal components of near-death experiences is out-of-body experiences. An out-of-body experience is defined by the presence of disembodiment, the impression of seeing the world from an elevated and distanced visuo-spatial perspective and the impression of seeing one's own body from this perspective. Studies have shown that electrical stimulation of the temporo-parietal junction (highlighted in gray) can generate out-of-body experiences (with permission from Cliff Laureys)

Near-death Experiences

Definition

It is important to stress that near-death experiences occur in what is considered 'near-death', i.e., the patient being in transitory and reversible cardiac arrest (clinical death). Under the US Uniform Determination of Death Act [3], a person is dead when physicians determine, by applying prevailing clinical criteria, that cardiorespiratory or brain functions are absent and cannot be retrieved. Clinical death is a term to be avoided, referring in popular media to cessation of blood circulation and breathing. Without resuscitation, recovery of brain function more than 3 minutes after a cardiac arrest is rare. This notion of irreversible is reflected in the 'Pittsburgh Protocol' for non-heart-beating organ donation (now called organ donation after cardiac death). Here, patients who are hopelessly brain-damaged (but not brain dead) can have their life-sustaining therapy (e.g., positive-pressure ventilation) withdrawn. Once their heart stops beating for a period of 3–10 minutes (length varies by protocol), they can be declared dead (and only then can organs be procured) [4, 5].

At present, there are no universally accepted definitions of near-death experiences. Nevertheless, there are many ways of categorizing its phenomenological elements. Moody [6] identified a number of common elements recurring in near-death experiences: Ineffability, hearing oneself pronounced dead, feelings of peace and quiet, hearing unusual noises, seeing a dark tunnel, being 'out of the body', meeting 'spiritual beings', experiencing a bright light or a "being of light", panoramic life review, experiencing a realm in which all knowledge exists, experiencing cities of light, experiencing a realm of bewildered spirits, experiencing a 'supernatural rescue', sensing a border or limit, coming back 'into the body'.

Structured interview of individuals who have had a near-death experience have identified five stages occurring in the following order: (1) A feeling of peace and well-being; (2) separation from the physical body; (3) entering a region of darkness; (4) seeing a brilliant light; (5) going through the light and entering another realm. The two scales most commonly used to quantify the subjective experience of near-death experiences are the Weighted Core Experience Index (WCEI) [7] and the Greyson Near-death Experience Scale [8]. The WCEI includes ten components which are scored for their presence or absence (maximum score is 29) (**Table 1**).

The Greyson Near-death Experience Scale [8] is a revision of the WCEI and has 146 questions (maximum score of 32). In order to consider the subjective report as being a true near-death experience, a minimum score of 7 needs to be recorded (**Table 2**).

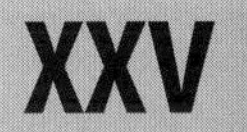

Theoretical Approaches: Spiritual, Psychological and Organic Hypotheses

Spiritual interpretations consider the existence of near-death experiences as strong evidence that the mind (i.e., soul) can be separated from the physical body. Supporters of this theory consider that near-death experiences provide a glimpse of the spiritual realm to which the soul migrates after death. The second category encompasses psychological theories according to which near-death experiences are a type of depersonalization, acting as a protection against the threat of death in situations of intense danger, by allowing an engagement in pleasurable fantasies [9]. Others have proposed a concept of psychological absorption, which may be defined as the tendency to focus attention on imaginative or selected sensory experiences to the exclu-

Table 1. Characteristics of near-death experiences as reported by 62 cardiac arrest survivors, according to the Weighted Core Experience Index (WCEI) [22].

	Number of patients (%)
Awareness of being dead	31 (50 %)
Positive emotions	35 (56 %)
Out-of-body experiences	15 (24 %)
Moving through a tunnel	19 (31 %)
Communication with light	14 (23 %)
Observation of colors	14 (23 %)
Observation of a celestial landscape	18 (29 %)
Meeting with deceased persons	20 (32 %)
Life review	8 (13 %)
Presence of border	5 (8 %)

Table 2. Characteristics of near-death experiences according to the Greyson Near-death Experience Scale.

	Number of cardiac arrest survivors (%)	
	Parnia et al., 2001 [21] (n = 4)	Greyson, 2003 [24] (n = 27)
Cognitive features		
Did time seem to speed up or slow down?	2 (50 %)	18 (66 %)
Were your thoughts speeded up?	0	12 (44 %)
Did scenes from your past come back to you?	0	8 (30 %)
Did you suddenly seem to understand everything?	1 (25 %)	8 (30 %)
Emotional features		
Did you have a feeling of peace or pleasantness?	3 (75 %)	23 (85 %)
Did you see, or feel surrounded by, a brilliant light?	3 (75 %)	19 (70 %)
Did you have a feeling of joy?	3 (75 %)	18 (66 %)
Did you feel a sense of harmony or unity with the universe?	2 (50 %)	14 (52 %)
"Paranormal" features		
Did you feel separated from your body?	2 (50 %)	19 (70 %)
Were your senses more vivid than usual?	2 (50 %)	4 (15 %)
Did you seem to be aware of things going on elsewhere, as if by extrasensory perception?	2 (50 %)	3 (11 %)
Did scenes from the future come to you?	0	2 (7 %)
Transcendental features		
Did you seem to enter some other, unearthly world?	2 (50 %)	17 (63 %)
Did you seem to encounter a mystical being or presence, or hear an unidentifiable voice?	2 (50 %)	14 (52 %)
Did you come to a border or point of no return?	4 (100 %)	11 (41 %)
Did you see deceased or religious spirits?	1 (25 %)	7 (26 %)

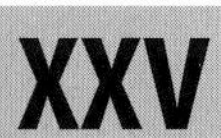

sion of stimuli from the external environment [10]. However, some authors have pointed out that near-death experiences differ from depersonalization in the sense that what is distorted is not one's sense of identity but the association of one's identity with one's bodily sensations. In this view, near-death experiences are considered as a dissociation of self-identity from bodily sensations and emotions [11].

The last category encompasses so-called organic hypotheses. A large number of theories have attempted to account for components of near-death experience in terms of brain dysfunctions. Some authors have considered the possible role of abnormal levels of blood gases. Indeed, anoxia [12] and hypercarbia [13] can produce symptoms including seeing bright lights, having out-of-body experiences, reliving past memories, and inducing mystical experiences. Other authors have suggested that near-death experience can be reported as hallucinatory experiences caused in part by, for example, endorphin [14], serotonin [15], or ketamine [16, 17] release. More recent theories have proposed that temporal lobe dysfunction may explain out-of-body experiences [2] and bodily hallucinations [18]. Finally, it was also shown that individuals who reported having near-death experience had more significant epileptiform electroencephalogram (EEG) activity compared to control patients [19].

An integrative model of these organic theories has proposed that brain stress caused by traumatic events leads to the release of neurotransmitters producing effects such as analgesia, euphoria and detachment. These effects combine with the effect of decreases in oxygen tension to produce epileptiform discharges in the hippocampus and amygdala, possibly leading to hallucinations and life review. After-discharges, propagating through limbic connections to other brain areas, could produce further hallucinations and the sensation of seeing a brilliant light [20]. Finally, there exists no EEG data about brain functions in the critical clinical period that is assumed to be associated with near-death experiences. Indeed, loss of consciousness was diagnosed only by electrocardiogram (EKG) examinations, independent of neurological or EEG records.

Clinical Studies

Parnia et al. [21] prospectively studied cardiac arrest patients over a one year period. Of the 63 survivors interviewed within a week of cardiac arrest, 7 (11 %) reported memories of their period of unconsciousness, 4 of whom (6 %) had near-death experiences according to the Greyson Near-death Experience scale [8]. All patients reported that the near-death experience was pleasant. Due to the small number of patients, it was not possible to draw any clear conclusions regarding possible causative physiological factors such as hypoxia, hypercarbia, electrolyte disturbances, specific cardiac dysrhythmia, carbon dioxide, sodium and potassium obtained from arterial blood gas and peripheral blood, or the administration of drugs around the period of arrest. Only the partial pressure of oxygen was reported to be higher in the near-death experience group as compared to non-near-death experience survivors.

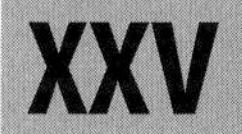

Another prospective study was conducted by Van Lommel et al. [22] and involved 344 cardiac arrest survivors. Sixty-two (18 %) patients reported a near-death experience, 41 (12 %) of whom reported a "core near-death experience experience" (i.e., scoring 6 or more on the WCEI [7]). No patients reported distressing near-death experiences. Duration of cardiac arrest, medication, fear of death before cardiac arrest, and the duration between the near-death experience and the interview were not related to the occurrence of near-death experiences. However, people younger than 60 were more likely to report a near-death experience than older people, as were those suffering their first myocardial infarction. More vivid near-death experience (i.e., higher WCEI scores) were reported by patients surviving cardiac arrest outside the hospital, and were more frequently reported by women and those reporting being afraid of death before the cardiac arrest. Two and eight years after the near-death experience, patients were re-interviewed and compared with a control group (cardiac arrest survivors who did not report a near-death experience). This longitudinal follow-up showed that near-death experiences produce long-lasting effects in terms of increased belief in an afterlife and decreased fear of death, increased interest in the meaning of one's own life, and increased social awareness such as showing love and accepting others.

Schwaninger et al. [23] prospectively studied 174 cardiac arrest patients (of whom 119 [68 %] died). Of the remaining 55 patients, 30 (17 %) were interviewed using the Greyson Near-death Experience scale [8] (25 were excluded due to neurological impairment or intubation until discharge). Seven patients reported a near-death experience (13 % of survivors). A 6-month follow-up confirmed previous findings of long-lasting transformational effects of near-death experiences with regard to personal understanding of life and self, social attitudes, and changes in social customs and religious or spiritual beliefs.

Finally, Greyson [24] prospectively studied 1595 cardiac survivors patients, of whom 27 (2 %) scored 7 or more points on the Greyson Near-death Experience scale

Table 3. Frequency of near-death experiences in cardiac arrest survivors according to the Weighted Core Experience Index (WCEI) or the Greyson Near-death Experience Scale [8].

Authors	Scale	Total number of patients	Number of patients having reported near-death experience (%)
Van Lommel et al. (2001) [22]	WCEI	344	41 (12 %)
Parnia et al. (2001) [21]	Greyson scale	63	4 (6 %)
Schwaninger et al. (2002) [23]	Greyson scale	55	7 (13 %)
Greyson (2003) [24]	Greyson scale	1595	27 (2 %)

[8]. Near-death experiencers, comprising 2 % of the entire sample, included 10 % of patients admitted with cardiac arrest, 1 % of those with myocardial infarction, 1 % of those with unstable angina, and 1 % of those with other cardiac diagnoses. Patients who reported a near-death experience were younger, more likely to have lost consciousness, and more likely to report prior so-called "paranormal experiences" but not extrasensory perceptions. Religious beliefs prior to the near-death experience were not related to the frequency of near-death experiences.

In summary, these studies report incidence rates of near-death experiences in survivors from cardiac arrest ranging from 2 % to 13 % (**Table 3**) and show a higher incidence in younger patients. The reported experiences suggest that features of near-death experiences are similar among patients (**Tables 1** and **2**).

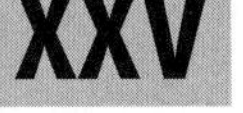

Out-of-body Experiences

Definition

One of the principal components of near-death experiences is the out-of-body experience. Out-of-body experience is defined by the presence of three phenomenological characteristics: Disembodiment (i.e., location of the self outside one's body); the impression of seeing the world from an elevated and distanced visuo-spatial perspective; and the impression of seeing one's own body from this perspective (i.e., autoscopy) [25] (**Fig. 2**, upper part). Understanding how the brain generates the abnormal self during out-of-body experiences is particularly interesting since out-of-body experiences are not only found in clinical populations, but also appear in approximately 10 % of the healthy population [25, 26]. The out-of-body experience can also be present in various situations, such as psychiatric disorders, drug abuse, general anesthesia, and sleep.

Neuroanatomical Correlates

There is increasing evidence showing that out-of-body experiences may result from a deficient multisensory integration at the temporo-parietal junction area [2, 18, 27]. Focal electrical stimulation of this area in a patient who was undergoing evaluation for epilepsy treatment induced repeated out-of-body experiences and illusory transformations of the patient's arm and legs [18]. In a study of six neurological patients (with epilepsy or migraine), Blanke et al. [2] showed that out-of-body experiences were always described from one visuo-spatial perspective, which was localized in a second body outside the physical body (e.g., inverted by 180° with respect to the extra personal visual space and the habitual physical body position). All patients showed immediate self-recognition and their lesion overlap was centered on the temporo-parietal junction, including the anterior part of the angular gyrus and the posterior temporal gyrus. De Ridder et al. [27] induced an out-of-body experience in a 63-year-old man with an implanted electrode over the right temporo-parietal junction. Using a positron emission tomography (PET) scan, these authors also showed that the out-of-body experience was related to increased activity in the right temporo-parietal junction, superior temporal, and right precuneal cortices. They suggested that the induced altered spatial self-recognition was mediated by the temporo-parietal junction, which is involved in vestibular-somatosensory integration of body orientation in space. Similarly, Blanke [28] suggested a model to explain out-of-body experiences proposing that "out-of-body experiences are related to a disintegration within personal space (multisensory dysfunction) and disintegration between personal space (vestibular) and extrapersonal (visual) due to interference with the temporo-parietal junction". In these models, the experience of seeing one's body in a position that does not coincide with the felt position of one's body is assumed to be related to temporo-parietal junction dysfunction (**Fig. 2**, lower part).

Conclusion

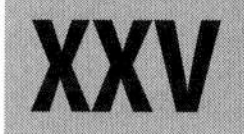

Near-death experiences and out-of-body experiences remain fascinating phenomena which are abundant in popular beliefs, mythology, and spiritual experiences of many ancient and modern societies. Clinical studies suggest that characteristics of near-death experiences are culturally invariant and can be investigated neuroscientifically. The frequency of near-death experiences in cardiac arrest survivors varies from 2 to 13 % and near-death experiences seem to be more common in younger patients. Longitudinal studies have shown profound long-lasting transformational effects of near-death experiences with regard to personal understanding of life and self, social attitudes, and changes in social customs and religious or spiritual beliefs. One of the principal components of near-death experiences is the out-of-body experience that is associated with partial impairments in consciousness and disturbed own body processing. Recent studies employing deep brain stimulation and neuroimaging have demonstrated that out-of-body experiences result from a deficient multisensory integration at the temporo-parietal junction. Ongoing studies aim to further identify the functional neuroanatomy of near-death experiences by means of standardized EEG recordings.

Acknowledgements: This research was funded by the Belgian National Funds for Scientific Research (FNRS), the European Commission, the James McDonnell Foundation, the Mind Science Foundation, the French Speaking Community Concerted Research Action (ARC-06/11 – 340), the Fondation Médicale Reine Elisabeth, and the University of Liège. A.V. was funded by ARC 06/11 – 340 and S.L. is senior research associate at the FNRS.

References

1. Greyson B (2000) Near-death experiences. In: Cardena E, Lynn SJ, Krippner S (eds) Varieties of Anomalous Experiences: Examining the Scientific Evidence. American Psychological Association, Washington, pp 315–352
2. Blanke O, Landis T, Spinelli L, Seeck M (2004) Out-of-body experience and autoscopy of neurological origin. Brain 127: 243–258.
3. Uniform Determination of Death Act (1997) 598 (West 1993 and West Supp. 1997.) Uniforms Laws Annoted (ULA), 12.
4. Bernat JL, D'Alessandro AM, Port FK, et al (2006) Report of a National Conference on Donation after cardiac death. Am J Transplant 6: 281–291
5. Laureys S (2005) Science and society: death, unconsciousness and the brain. Nat Rev Neurosci 6: 899–909
6. Moody RA (1975) Life After Life. Bantam Books, New York
7. Ring K (1980) Life at Death: A Scientific Investigation of the Near-Death Experience. Coward, McCann, and Geoghegan, New York
8. Greyson B (1983) The near-death experience scale. Construction, reliability, and validity. J Nerv Ment Dis 171: 369–375
9. Noyes R, Jr., Kletti R (1976) Depersonalization in the face of life-threatening danger: a description. Psychiatry 39: 19–27
10. Tellegen A, Atkinson G (1974) Openness to absorbing and self-altering experiences ("absorption"), a trait related to hypnotic susceptibility. J Abnorm Psychol 83: 268–277
11. Irwin HJ (1993) The near-death as a dissociative phenomenon: An empirical assessment. J Near Death Stud 12: 95–103
12. Whinnery J (1997) Psychophysiologic correlates of unconsciousness and near-death experiences. J Near Death Stud 15: 231–258
13. Meduna L (1950) Carbon Dioxide Therapy. Charles Thomas, Springfield
14. Carr DB (1982) Pathophysiology of stress-induced limic lobe dysfunction: A hypothesis relevant to near-death experiences. Anabiosis: J Near Death Stud 2: 75–89
15. Morse ML, Venecia D, Milstein J (1989) Near-death experiences: A neurophysiologic explanatory model. J Near Death Stud 8: 45–53
16. Jansen KLR (1989) Near death experience and the NMDA receptor. BMJ 298:1708
17. Jansen KLR (1997) The ketamine model for the near-death experience: A central role for the N-methyl-D-aspartate receptor. J Near Death Stud 16: 79–95
18. Blanke O, Ortigue S, Landis T, Seeck M (2002) Stimulating illusory own-body perceptions. Nature 419: 269–270.
19. Britton WB, Bootzin RR (2004) Near-death experiences and the temporal lobe. Psychol Sci 15: 254–258
20. Saavedra-Aguilar JC, Gómez-Jerias JS (1989) A neurobiological model of near-death experiences. J Near Death Stud 7: 205–222
21. Parnia S, Waller DG, Yeates R, Fenwick P (2001) A qualitative and quantitative study of the incidence, features and aetiology of near death experiences in cardiac arrest survivors. Resuscitation 48: 149–156
22. Van Lommel P, van Wees R, Meyers V, Elfferich I (2001) Near-death experience in survivors of cardiac arrest: a prospective study in the Netherlands. Lancet 358: 2039–2045
23. Schwaninger J, Eisenberg PR, Schectman KB, Weiss AN (2002) A prospective analysis of near death experiences in cardiac arrest patients. J Near Death Stud 20: 215–232
24. Greyson B (2003) Incidence and correlates of near-death experiences in a cardiac care unit. Gen Hosp Psychiatry 25: 269–276
25. Bünning S, Blanke O (2005) The out-of body experience: precipitating factors and neural correlates. Prog Brain Res 150: 331–350
26. Faguet RA (1979) With the eyes of the mind: autoscopic phenomena in the hospital setting. Gen Hosp Psychiatry 1: 311–314
27. De Ridder D, Van Laere K, Dupont P, Menovsky T, Van de Heyning P (2007) Visualizing out-of-body experience in the brain. N Engl J Med 357: 1829–1833
28. Blanke O (2004) Out of body experiences and their neural basis. BMJ 329: 1414–1415

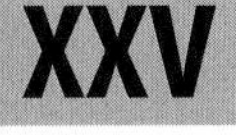

Managing Conflict at the End-of-Life

K. Hillman and J. Chen

Introduction

There are increasing pressures to admit patients to intensive care units (ICUs). The majority of people now die in institutions, rather than at home. Even terminally ill patients in nursing homes sometimes find their way into acute hospitals. Once in the emergency department, they are often assessed and admitted to hospital as the history and prognosis may not initially be clear; and because it is usually easier, in purely practical terms, to admit a terminally ill elderly patient rather than to arrange appropriate support in the community. Once in an acute hospital there are expectations, realistic or not, that there is some hope. The conveyor belt to intensive care is further facilitated by increasingly specialized physicians who often do not understand the way different co-morbidities and multiorgan involvement influences the patient's prognosis.

Conflict can occur as a result of a difference of opinion between an admitting clinician and an intensive care physician or even between intensive care clinicians. These are usually resolved in-house. Conflict can occur between relatives/friends of a patient who is incompetent, where there is a difference of opinion about the appropriateness of further treatment. These are also usually resolved without referral to a third party outside the hospital system. The most challenging conflict occurs when relatives/friends of an incompetent patient, usually in an ICU, do not agree with the caring clinicians.

This chapter covers all these forms of conflict in general terms but concentrates on conflict between clinicians and the relatives or friends of patients, as most decisions of this nature in the ICU involve incompetent patients.

There are many documents and studies around strategies that potentially may decrease conflict, such as policy statements from governments and professional bodies, and large bodies of work on concepts such as communication and mediation. However, there is little in the way of evidence to suggest which approaches may work in practice.

This chapter first addresses strategies which may prevent or minimize conflict and then strategies that may be useful when the conflict becomes seemingly intractable. It soon becomes obvious that in order to address conflict at the end-of-life, the whole journey from the patient's site of transfer to hospital to the inevitability of dying in the ICU needs to be analyzed. Each step in the patient's journey represents a possible opportunity for preventing and managing conflict in an effective way.

Strategies to Prevent Conflict at the End-Of-Life

Community Awareness and Advance Directives

Many countries have a provision for people to make their wishes about the extent and type of care they want at the end-of-life explicitly stated while they are physically and mentally competent – so-called advance directives. A model for the widespread uptake of advance directives has been developed in Oregon in the USA. Here they use a one page Physician Order for Life-Sustaining Treatment (POLST) document (www.ohsu.edu/ethics/polst). Knowledge of a patient's wishes is made electronically available to many potential points of care such as ambulance services and emergency departments ensuring the wishes of the patient are known and respected before the patient is admitted to hospital.

Futility

One of the challenges in resolving conflict around end-of-life issues is the concept of certainty of death inevitably occurring in the near future, despite active measures. Prognosis almost always has certain degrees of certainty attached to it [1]. Prognostic information substantially influences treatment decisions and physicians' prognostic estimates are reasonably accurate [2]. There usually comes a time when the disease process is so advanced that the patient's condition is worsening despite massive amounts of support. The challenge is to predict futility at a time which minimizes the patient's and their carers' suffering.

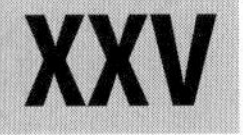

Clinicians are usually conservative in withdrawing and withholding treatment. Part of the reason is a failure to agree on how to define futility. Despite broad agreement around the meaning of the word futility – 'because it offers no reasonable hope of recovery or improvement', or 'because the patient is permanently unable to experience any benefit' – in one of the more comprehensive surveys, 87 % of doctors in intensive care and 95 % of nurses reported that futile care was still provided in the ICU [3].

Strategies to Avoid Conflict in Acute Hospitals Before Admission to the ICU

There is a paucity of scientific references on managing conflict at the end-of-life outside the ICU. Presumably this is related to the fact that patients outside the ICU are usually competent and able to make decisions around how their own end-of-life care should be managed. If a patient being managed on the general wards is incompetent, it is usually as a result of a temporary and reversible disorder or as part of a natural and predictable dying process. Others, who are incompetent as part of their illness and where there is doubt about their prognosis, are often transferred to the ICU.

Although there is little scientific literature on avoiding conflict in patients outside the ICU, usually on the general wards of a hospital, many of the reasons for conflict within the ICU have their origins there.

The reasons are many and include: Failure of doctors to diagnose dying; reluctance to discuss death and dying with patients and relatives; and fear of criticism or litigation. Admitting doctors often do not know what intensive care can offer and may give relatives false hope by the way they communicate with them. For example, they may offer care, which is inappropriate by asking them ... "do you want everything done". Following this, the message passed on to the intensivist is "the relatives want everything done". The seeds of conflict are sewn when the intensivist has to either refuse admission or withdraw/withhold treatment.

Rapid response systems, such as the Medical Emergency Team (MET) concept [4], are becoming increasingly employed to identify and respond to seriously ill patients. The response teams are not only being called to seriously ill patients where there is a large reversible element but also to patients who are dying in an expected fashion [5]. The reasons for this are many, but include a general reluctance to discuss dying amongst clinicians, and sometimes just an inability to diagnose dying. Thus, the response teams, usually as an outreach of intensive care have, in many cases, become the surrogate 'dying team', often having to explain to the relatives and home medical team that there is little more to offer in the way of active management.

In order to institute a more effective plan for management of the dying in acute hospitals, consideration could be given to a standardized and integrated care plan. Perhaps the best know of these is the Liverpool Care Pathway for the Dying Patient (LCP) (www.mcpcil.org.uk). The program recognizes the transition from active to palliative care, encouraging early recognition of patients who may eventually move wholly into end-of-life care.

While palliative care services are traditionally available to patients with cancer, there is little awareness about similar services being offered to seriously ill hospitalized patients. And yet the rate of death from chronic conditions is far higher than deaths from cancer [6]. One of the reasons for this is that accurate prognostication is more difficult for patients with conditions such as chronic heart failure, chronic obstructive pulmonary disease (COPD) and dementia [7–9]. This is sometimes referred to as "prognostic paralysis" [7]. It is suggested that this very uncertainty should be the basis for initiating end-of-life discussions. Some units are documenting a care plan with parallel palliative and active care for patients with COPD [9].

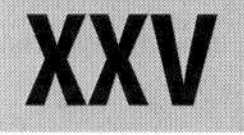

Communication

Communication is one of the more important strategies to avoid conflict at the end-of-life, not only in the ICU, but also throughout the patient's hospital journey. There are specific needs of the family at this time in regard to content, timing, and settings in which bad news can be delivered [10]. There is also some evidence that end-of-life family conferences assist them when difficult decisions need to be made [11]. The use of a brochure on bereavement and using a proactive communication strategy in the ICU were associated with a lower burden of bereavement using three validated scales 90 days after the patient's death [12]. This is the only multicenter, randomized study demonstrating that a proactive communication strategy conducted according to specific guidelines improved relative satisfaction.

Communication skills are generic in managing end-of-life conflict. However, there are some special circumstances which are challenging. Conflict between functional and legal family units can occur. There has often been simmering resentment and disagreement between the two units, sometimes over many years. This then comes to a head when end-of-life issues arise. The same failure of communication exists in pediatric [13, 14] and neonatal ICUs [15].

The concept of improved communication is probably easier to include in documents than to actually ensure there is a comprehensive plan of implementation. Even with senior clinicians who supposedly understand the importance of communication, the actual application of the principles can fall short of what happens in practice. The standardized approach to family conferences and a specifically designed brochure available in the ICU could be part of a comprehensive care plan aimed at patients who may be likely to need end-of-life care, similar to that used in the National Health Service (www.mcpcil.org.uk).

Then, there is the daunting task of improving communication skills around end-of-life issues across all nursing and medical undergraduate and postgraduate educational facilities. The American Medical Association has an education program aimed at improving the communication skills of undergraduates and postgraduates – Education for Physicians in End-of-Life Care (EPEC) (www.ama-assn.org/EPEC).

Clinical Practice Guidelines for End-of-Life Care and Decision Making

There are many excellent guidelines for end-of-life care and decision making [16–19]. The assumption appears to be that if all of these guidelines were applied in a clinically relevant way then it would be unusual to have to resort to conflict resolution. There is probably a lot of truth in this assumption as the recommendations are exhaustive and clinically relevant. Despite these guidelines being freely available many families are dissatisfied with the care they receive at the end-of-life [20].

Another challenge is considering how much of this literature, including well thought out national guidelines, is actually translated into the every day practice in ICUs and other places where end-of-life patients are managed.

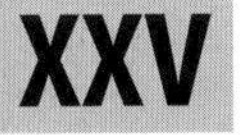

Cultural, Religious and Racial Aspects around End-of-Life Conflicts

In order to minimize any potential conflict, health care workers should have some understanding of different cultural attitudes around end-of-life issues. Recently, summaries of Islamic, Hindu, Jewish, Buddhist, and Christian views of end-of-life issues were published [21–26]. The articles discuss how families can negotiate their rituals within the space of secular health care initiatives.

However, there are dangers in designing end-of-life care specifically around different cultural, religious and racial groups. For example, African Americans prefer more aggressive end-of-life interventions [27]. There would be an inherent injustice in shaping end-of-life decisions around the different wishes of individual groups to demand more aggressive treatment. The right of the individual, as a determinant in conflict resolution, would probably not be as paramount in some parts of the world as it is in the USA.

Specific material could be developed and used as a resource for educating health care deliverers and also made freely available for staff working in acute hospital areas such as emergency departments, ICUs and palliative care units. As communication is crucial around conflict at the end-of-life, the use of interpreters would need to be freely available (**Table 1**).

Direct Interventions Dealing with Conflict at the End-of-Life

The guidelines covering strategies dealing with end-of-life issues listed in the previous section [16–19] cover pre-emptive strategies to prevent conflict. They cover many of the same areas, despite coming from many different countries, organizations, and professional bodies. The issue around prevention of conflict is probably

Table 1. Possible strategies for avoiding conflict at the end-of-life

Strategies	Comments	Possible Action
Advanced care directives	General consensus by community and health industry that these would make end-of-life care easier and would improve care.	Need to provide interdisciplinary and multi-level strategies to improve uptake and include general practitioners/acute hospitals/nursing homes legal services and community in a concerted and coordinated way.
Early identification and involvement of palliative care services for dying patients in hospital	Early response systems are already widely used as a vehicle for early recognition of the dying patients. Palliative care services could interact more formally with early response systems and other parts of the hospital to provide early palliative care interventions for a wide range of dying patients	Need to develop systems for more effective integration of acute and palliative care services in acute hospitals.
Improved communication	Well developed and organized specialties of intensive care and emergency medicine. Large multicultural population. High level of clinical services in acute hospitals.	Standardized care plans for dying which cover patient's hospital journey, including guidelines for withholding and withdrawing care once patient identified. Specific communication courses for clinicians working in acute hospitals. Specifically designed material for both patients from a multicultural background as well as for staff treating them.
Ethics' committees	Seem to be more commonly employed in the USA and is institutionally based.	Could integrate a version of this strategy in combination with communication and mediation strategies.
Mediation adjudication tribunals	Potential to develop specifically designed system using a combination of these strategies.	
Legal solutions	Universal desire to avoid legal intervention if possible in the literature; by individual institutions, by governments and usually by the community as well. Where specific end-of-life laws are in place e.g., Texas and Israel there remain value laden questions which do not lend themselves to simple solutions.	

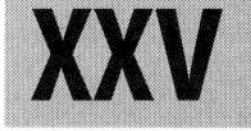

not so much related to the comprehensiveness of the guidelines but more to the effectiveness of the implementation of the guidelines.

Once there is conflict around decisions being contemplated at the end-of-life, there are various strategies to defuse and limit the conflict. These include: Time and repeated discussions; seeking another medical opinion or another opinion from within the health service; transfer to another institution; or referral to ethics' committees. If these measures fail and conflict is either unresolved or escalates, there is the possibility of mediation or referral to a body which is more at arm's length from the health system such as a Tribunal. Finally, if these measures fail the matter can be referred to the legal system.

Recent UK guidelines from the General Medical Council offer a framework for dealing with conflict at the end-of-life. Some of the more relevant principles include [28]:

- A competent patient has the right to refuse treatment and their refusal must be respected, even if it will result in their death.
- Doctors are under no legal or ethical obligation to agree to a patient's request for treatment if they consider the treatment is not in the patient's best interests.
- A decision for, or on the behalf of, a person who lacks capacity must be done, or made, in his best interests.

The guidelines are consistent with laws across the UK.

Striving For Consensus

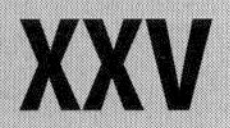

It is important that the transition from pre-emptive conflict resolution to more direct forms of intervention is not abrupt. There is always hope that the conflict will be resolved by continuing pre-emptive strategies. Moreover, it is important that both parties feel that the process has been fair, whatever the ultimate outcome, and that health care deliverers have acted in a professional and sensitive way. Strategies include 'time and repeat discussion', emphasizing that time to come to terms with impending death is important and further discussions are important to resolve outstanding issues. A 'time limited treatment trial' in order to clarify prognostic uncertainty can be useful. Continued use of sound communication principles and end-of-life guidelines outlined in the first section of this chapter is probably also important.

All of these strategies are intuitively sensible but, as with many suggestions around resolving conflict in end-of-life issues, there is little specific evidence apart from that already described under communication.

The Role of Ethical Guidelines in Conflict Resolution

The word ethics used in situations of conflict resolution around end-of-life care in itself implies that a rational and just framework for resolving issues exists. It is probably more common in the USA than in other countries to refer end-of-life conflict situations to an ethics committee. In the case of intractable conflict, an institutional ethics committee can negotiate with clinicians and family, usually around differences on withdrawing treatment when it is thought to be futile by the treating clinicians. However, the ethical committee can merely act as a surrogate judge and jury [29]. In many cases, the committee is made up of mainly 'insiders', employed by the hospital and hospital appointed community representatives.

One of the main challenges with using the word 'ethics' to resolve conflict is that the four main ethical principles governing provision of medical care lack precision and can be contradictory.

The four ethical principles are:

- Beneficence – to do good.
- Non-maleficence – avoid harm.
- Justice – provision of health for all.
- Autonomy – patient orientated decision making.

While these principles are universally accepted, they are difficult to apply in practice and, in many cases, are ambiguous and, even in conflict with one another. For example, patients in intensive care are often not competent and, therefore, autonomy can be a problem; doing harm (prolonging suffering) or good (prolonging life) may depend on the clinical outcome and this is often uncertain; and acting in the patient's interest can be open to different interpretations. Moreover, for a clinician to simultaneously consider whether providing extra resources to sustain the life of one patient is consistent with the fair provision of therapy for all makes the application of these principles even less relevant [30, 31].

Applying ethical theory is also made difficult by factors such as the lack of robustness around the concept of 'futility'. The medico-legal position in some countries is that withdrawal of treatment is not causing death; the disease is causing the death, which would not have been prevented by the provision of therapy. Allowing for problems around defining futility, there may be no moral obligation by clinicians to continue treatment that is futile [32].

While intuitively appealing, referring patients to 'ethical' adjudicators has problems. Ethics in intensive care medicine has many inherent ambiguities and conflicts [33]. It may be useful to employ ethical perspectives in decision making but the 'right' thing to do will vary depending on the ethical perspective adopted and there will never be an ethical system satisfactory to all people, or even to a single person in different circumstances.

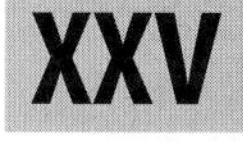

Mediation

Mediation could be considered as an extension of guidelines [34] such as using time and repeated discussions to defuse and limit conflict. There is no evidence to suggest that it should be used in parallel to, or after, efforts by treating clinicians and relatives to resolve conflict. Nor is there any information on the timing of mediation in relation to seeking second opinions, transferring to another institution, referral to Tribunals or recourse to the legal system.

For the purposes of this chapter, the following definitions have been used:

- Mediation or conciliation refers to someone trained in mediation who brokers an agreement between two parties. The expert acts purely as a facilitator and the final decision comes from the two parties. The decision can be legally binding. For example, in the case of divorce and disagreement around property arrangements, mediation can be compulsory in some societies before the matter is referred to the legal system.
- Adjudication (also called expert determination, arbitration or third party decision making) can be used as a process in its own right or after mediation has failed. It is used when two parties, who are having a disagreement over a matter, are referred to an expert who makes a decision based on factors such as written submissions or interviews and in line with the processes of natural justice. The adjudicator can call on other experts in assisting him/her within his/her determination. In some cases the expert determination can be legally binding under specific legislation.
- Tribunals are usually independent bodies developed to deal with specific issues, usually indirectly or directly associated with government and often empowered by government statutes. They can facilitate the mediation and adjudication process.

Examples of mediation and adjudication usually remain subject to appeals to a traditional legal system. The process of mediation and adjudication results in most cases being resolved before recourse to traditional legal systems. Both mediation and adjudication use people specifically trained in the generic aspects of dispute resolution as much as, if not more than in the content area of the particular dispute.

The Legal System

An important general comment on the role of the law in resolving end-of-life conflicts was published in the *New England Journal of Medicine* [35]. Its conclusions included:

- These cases are extremely rare and, as such, the problem should not be overstated.
- Patient's families and friends should be encouraged to be involved in early conversations around end-of-life questions.
- Issues should be solved largely by encouraging communication and reconciliation; avoiding regrets and resentment wherever possible.
- There should be increased use of mediator based methodology such as that used with divorcing couples and estranged business partners.
- Caregivers should be encouraged to 'assert themselves gently'.

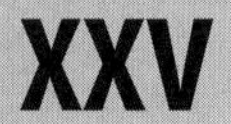

The editorial [35] emphasizes avoiding clear winners and losers involved in legal solutions. It suggests that governments should make legal recourse difficult, encouraging conversation, reconciliation, and accommodation. The editorial also outlines the limits of the law in such matters being restricted to areas such as active killing, clear advance directives being followed, and the assistance of physicians in suicide. But within these boundaries, it is suggested that end-of-life questions need to be almost totally resolved within the private sphere by patients, their physicians, family members, social workers, nurses and others where relevant.

It would appear that there is little satisfactory and consistent legal resolution of the ethical and practical dilemmas surrounding end-of-life care [36]. Legal resolution can be used but it relies on an approach that can be more illusory than real and can even risk becoming a rubber-stamp mechanism [37].

The legal framework is poorly adapted to the special situations and demands of modern medicine. The failure of the legal system to reflect the changing relationships between illnesses which would have been otherwise fatal and the ability of modern medicine to sustain life, has resulted in 'legal liabilities anxieties' amongst ICU doctors [38]. In subtle ways, the failure of the legal system to offer clarity around end-of-life issues, together with the fear, by doctors, of not acting within an ill-defined legal framework has lead to a perverse situation, where the law is often determining the nature of end-of-life medical care. A doctor acting out of fear of prosecution is probably not a positive incentive for appropriate medical treatment. This also has implications in terms of financial cost to our society as well as prolonging suffering of both patients and carers.

While there are many descriptions of different legal systems and reports of cases there is no scientific evidence to suggest what may best decrease conflict around end-of-life issues.

Conclusion

One of the problems with dealing with end-of-life matters in intensive care is related to the way our society approaches dying and death and the way the health system concentrates on active treatment of diseases throughout the patient's journey from their home and increasingly ending in their admission to intensive care. There are many strategies, such as advance care planning, for preventing hospital admission. There are also many opportunities to openly and honestly discuss end-of-life care in a more open and transparent way once patients are admitted to hospital.

Increasingly, intensivists will be involved in the diagnosis of dying as they are in the best position to advise on whether escalation of active treatment will be of benefit to the patient. Early and parallel involvement of palliative care colleagues will improve the dying process. In the rare event of irresolvable conflict between clinicians and patients or their carers, strategies such as mediation facilitated by professionals may be an option. Most people want to avoid recourse to a legal system, as the law usually allows great discretion in withdrawing and withholding treatment. There are, therefore, no specific guidelines under which the law can make hard and fast decisions.

Finally, the profession of intensive care medicine could be leading debates within our society about the reality of dying and death and the often unreal expectations of a society that believes modern medicine has all the answers.

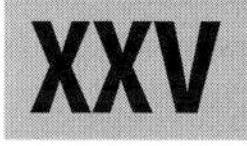

References

1. Miller DW Jnr, Miller CG (2005) On evidence, medical and legal. J Am Phys Surg 10: 70–75
2. Lloyd CB, Nietert PJ, Silvestri GA (2004) Intensive care decision making in the seriously ill and elderly. Crit Care Med 32: 649–654
3. Palda VA, Bowman KW, McLean RF, Chapman MG (2005) "Futile" care: Do we provide it? Why? A semistructured, Canada-wide survey of intensive care unit doctors and nurses. J Crit Care 20: 207–213
4. Lee A, Bishop G, Hillman KM. Daffurn K (1995) The medical emergency team. Anaesth Intensive Care 23: 183–186
5. Jones DA, McIntyre T, Baldwin I, Mercer I, Kattula A, Bellomo R (2007) The medical emergency team and end-of-life care: A pilot study. Crit Care Resus 9: 151–156
6. World Health Organization (2005) Preventing Chronic Diseases: A Vital Investment. WHO, Geneva
7. Murray SA, Boyd K, Sheikh A (2005) Palliative care in chronic illness. BMJ 330: 611–612
8. Coventry PA, Grande GE, Richards DA, Todd CJ (2005) Prediction of appropriate timing of palliative care for older adults with non-malignant life-threatening disease: A systematic review. Age Ageing 34: 218–227
9. Murray, SA, Sheikh A (2008) Making a difference. Palliative care beyond cancer. Care for all at the end of life. BMJ 336: 958–959
10. Ptacek JT, Ederhardt TL (1996) Breaking bad news: A review of the literature. JAMA 276: 496–502
11. Curtis JR, Patrick DL, Shannon SE, Treece PD, Engelberg RA, Rubenfeld GD (2001) The family conference as a focus to improve communication about end-of-life care in the intensive care unit: Opportunities for improvement. Crit Care Med 29 (Suppl): N26-N33
12. Lautrette A, Darmon M, Megarbane B, et al (2007) A communication strategy and brochure for relatives of patients dying in the ICU. N Eng J Med 356: 469–478
13. Committee on Bioethics, American Academy of Pediatrics (1994) Guidelines of foregoing life-sustaining treatment. Pediatrics 3:532–536
14. Committee on Bioethics, American Academy of Pediatrics (1996) Ethics and the care of critically ill infants and children. Pediatrics 98:149–152

15. de Leeuw R, de Beaufort AJ, de Kleine MJK, et al (1996) Forgoing intensive care treatment in newborn infants with extremely poor prognoses. J Pediatr 129: 661–666
16. Truog RD, Cist AF, Brackett SE, et al (2001) Recommendations for end-of-life care in the intensive care unit. The Ethics Committee of the Society of Critical Care Medicine. Crit Care Med 29: 2332–2348
17. Rocker G, Dunbar S (2000) Withholding or withdrawal of life support: The Canadian Critical Care Society Position Paper. J Palliat Care16:S53-S63
18. British Medical Association Ethics Committee (1999) Withholding and Withdrawing Life-prolonging Medical Treatment. Guidance for Decision Making. BMJ Publishing Group, London
19. General Medical Council (2002) Withhold and Withdrawing Life-prolonging Treatments: Good Practice in Decision-Making. General Medical Council, London
20. Rabow MW, Hardy GE, Fair GM, et al (2000) An evaluation of the end-of-life care content in 50 textbooks from multiple specialties. JAMA 283: 771–778
21. Sachedina A (2005) End-of-Life: The Islamic view. Lancet 366: 774–1132
22. Firth S (2005) End of Life: A Hindu view. Lancet 366: 682–686
23. Dorff EN (2005) End of Life: A Jewish perspective. Lancet 366:862–865
24. Keown D (2005) End of Life: The Buddhist view. Lancet 366: 952–955
25. Englehardt HT Jnr, Iltis AS (2005) End of Life: The traditional Christian view. Lancet 366: 1045–1049
26. Markwell H (2005) End of Life: A Catholic view. Lancet 366: 1132–1135
27. Hopp FP, Duffy SA (2000) Racial variations in end of life care. J Am Geriatr Soc 48: 658 663
28. General Medical Council (2008) Consent: patients and doctors making decisions together. Available at: http://www.gmc-uk.org/news/articles/Consent_guidance.pdf. Accessed Nov 208

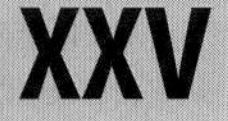

29. Fine RL, Mayo TW (2003) Resolution of futility by due process: early experience with the Texas advance directives. Ann Intern Med 138: 743–746
30. American Lung Association, American Thoracic Society (1997) Official statement on the fair allocation of intensive care unit resources. Am J Respir Crit Care Med 156: 1282–1301
31. The American College of Chest Physicians and Society of Critical Care Medicine. Consensus Panel (1990) Ethical and moral guidelines for the initiation, continuation and withdrawal of intensive care. Chest 97: 949–958
32. McCullough LB (1998) A transcultural, preventive ethics approach to critical-care medicine: restoring critical care physicians power and authority. J Med Philos 23: 628–642
33. Cook D (2001) Patient autonomy versus parentalism. Crit Care Med 29:N24–25
34. NSW Health Department (2005) Guidelines for End-Of-Life Care and Decision-Making. Better Health Centre. Publications Warehouse, Gladesville
35. Bloche MG (2005) Managing conflict at the end of life. N Engl J Med 352: 2371–2373
36. Fisher MM, Raper RF (2005) Courts, doctors and end-of-life care. Intensive Care Med 31: 762–764
37. Carlet J, Thijs LG, Antonelli M, et al (2004) Challenges in end-of-life care in the ICU. Statement of the 5th International Consensus Conference in Critical Care: Brussels, Belgium, April 2003. Intensive Care Med 30: 770–784
38. Faunce T (2005) Emerging roles for law and human rights in ethical conflicts surrounding neuro critical care. Crit Care Resus 7: 221–227

Strengths and Weaknesses of Substitute Decision Making in the ICU

A. Lautrette, E. Azoulay, and B. Souweine

Introduction

The doctor-patient relationship is at the heart of patient management. The trend in recent years has been towards patient autonomy. Frequently, intensive care unit (ICU) patients lack the capacity to make decisions about their health. In this case, surrogacy or substitute decision-making is one means of preserving patient autonomy. The legitimacy of surrogates is now widely recognized by physicians and many countries have passed legislation that offers the possibility of guaranteeing patient autonomy. Substitute decision-making involves three active participants: The patient, the surrogate, and the physician (with caregivers). For each of the three, substitute decision-making has both strengths and weaknesses.

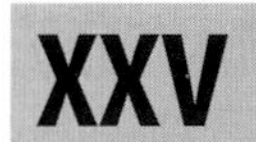

Strengths for the Patient (Table 1)

Substitute Decision-Making Is a Substitute for the Paternalism Model

Physician paternalism and patient autonomy are the two main patient-doctor relationships. In the paternalism model it is the physician who possesses knowledge and takes decisions alone. The physician informs family members but does not include them in the radical decision-making process. There are several drawbacks to this model. The physician's choices are guided by subjective elements such as beliefs, temperament, and personal values to the detriment of the patient's own individual characteristics [1]. The paternalistic model assigns a passive, dependent role to the patient and it is at variance with current principles of medical ethics [2]. In the patient autonomy model, the physician gives advice but takes no decision that might run counter to the patient's wishes. The model stipulates certain requirements for patient decision-making: (i) Patients must be aware that a decision is to be taken; (ii) they must understand the information given by the physician; (iii) they must understand the different therapeutic possibilities and their relative risks and benefits; (iv) they must incorporate the objective medical information into their own set of subjective values; (v) they must be able to make reasoned judgements in order to take the decision that is in their best interests [3]. Many ICU patients lose decisional capacity, either because of encephalopathy resulting from the causal disorder, or because they are sedated. In this case, the medical team can maintain patient autonomy by the process of substitute decision-making. A relative of the patient will be designated as surrogate and, thereafter, be involved in decision-making. A relative who knows the life story, convictions, beliefs, and philosophy of life of the patient is probably the most appropriate person to express his or her wishes.

Table 1. Strengths and weaknesses of substitute decision-making for the patient, surrogate, physician, and community

	Strength	Weakness
Patient	• substitute decision-making replaces paternalistic model • substitute decision-making replaces advance directives • substitute decision-making is the wish of ICU patients • substitute decision-making is a real-time decisional process	• Designation of surrogate is problematic • substitute decision-making is not relevant for all ICU patients (incapacitated patient without relatives)
Surrogate	• family has a legitimacy to protect the patient's interest • substitute decision-making is the wish of the family	• substitute decision-making depends on information from physician and patient • surrogate is not always objective • surrogate sometimes lacks capacity
Physician	• substitute decision-making is the wish of ICU staff member • substitute decision-making induces physician-family communication	• assessment of surrogate or patient capacity is problematic • substitute decision-making is a source of family-physician conflict
Community	• substitute decision-making is the wish of national legislators	• substitute decision-making is not a consensual process

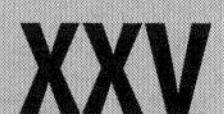

Substitute Decision-Making is a Substitute for Advance Directives

Although advance directives remain a major expression of patients' wishes in many countries, they are rarely available [4, 5]. Despite information campaigns, few patients know they exist and many are averse to formulating plans for a critical situation and to drawing up advance directives. Studies show that physicians are not sufficiently diligent in finding out whether an incapacitated patient has made an advance directive [6]. Some studies suggest that the use of advance directives does not avoid the expense of futile treatment and is of no benefit in patient care [7, 8]. Because of these major limitations, substitute decision making seems to be more readily available for ICU patients than advance directives.

Substitute Decision-making is the Wish of ICU Patients

An ICU patient who has the capacity to make a medical decision, should be the one to take that step. In this case, the patient does not require a substitute decision-maker. When a patient lacks decision-making capacity, the ICU team should turn to a surrogate decision-maker. The majority of ICU patients are too ill or sedated and consequently lack decisional capacity [9]. Studies report that patients express the desire for a relative to be involved in the decision-making process [10]. They want to be represented by a person in whom they have confidence and who would be able to express their convictions, philosophy of life, and beliefs. Generally, this surrogate is a family member or a close friend.

Substitute Decision-making is a Real-time Decisional Process

Another advantage of substitute decision making for the patient lacking decisional capacity is that the decisional process is adapted to medical circumstances. After being informed about diagnosis, prognosis, and therapeutic possibilities, the surrogate can make a decision in real time that will take account of the medical problem and reflect the patients' wishes. If the patient has drawn up advance directives, the physician can refer to them. However, the use of advance directives sometimes leads to problems either because they do not pertain to the situation the patient is faced with [4] or because they were drawn up on the basis of inaccurate or outdated scientific information [5]. For these reasons, a real-time decision taken by a surrogate may have precedence over patient directives formulated before the event [11].

Weaknesses for the Patient (Table 1)

The Designation of a Substitute Decision-maker is Problematic

If ICU patients are sedated, they inevitably lose their decision-making capacity. However, for alert patients, there exist no established criteria in the ICU for defining incapacity. Studies using the Mini Mental Status Examination (MMSE) have shown that more than half of patients who are able to communicate when admitted to the ICU nevertheless have impaired cognitive function [9]. One fundamental problem for the physician is to decide what level of competence is required for the patient to be autonomous and what calls for the intervention of a substitute decision-maker. The level needed to make a decision about medical treatment is high whereas that required to appoint a surrogate is lower. As there is a high risk of losing decisional capacity in the ICU, patient designation of a surrogate must be done swiftly. At present, the physician alone considers whether the patient has the capacity to designate his or her surrogate [12] and it is likely that there are wide variations between physicians in their assessment of what constitutes capacity.

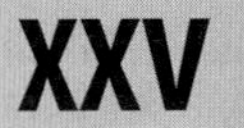

Substitute Decision-making is not Appropriate for all Patients

Some ICU patients lack both decision making capacity and surrogate decision-makers. A study reported that 16 % of patients admitted to an ICU lacked decision-making capacity and a surrogate during their entire ICU stay [13]. For 37 % of these patients, physicians considered withholding or withdrawing treatment. Decisions to limit life support were made by physicians with the opinion of another attending physician in 56 % of the cases, with the input of the court or the hospital ethics committee in 11 % of cases and independently in 33 %. The process of substitute decision-making is not appropriate for at least 10 % of ICU patients. In these cases, physicians fall back on the paternalism model.

Strengths for the Surrogate (Table 1)

Substitute Decision-making is Legitimate

When a patient is unable to make a decision, physicians automatically turn to a close relative. There are several arguments in support of this practice. The ethical argument states that it is appropriate for a close relative to be involved in the decision-making process because a family will naturally tend to protect the patient's interests [2, 14]. The legitimacy of substitute decision-making is now recognized by physicians. The practice also has social acceptability: A survey performed among 8000 French persons showed that 90 % of those taking part were in favor of having a surrogate to represent them and be involved in decision-making if they were incapacitated [15].

Substitute Decision-making is the Wish of the Family

In the sharing model, the substitute decision-maker has a major role, which can be decisional or consultative depending on the law of the country. However, this role is also the choice of surrogate who makes decisions alone or who can share decisions with the medical staff. A multicenter study conducted by Heyland et al. in Canadian ICUs found that about 61 % of family members wanted to share in decisions or to make decisions alone [16]. The majority of respondents (81 %) preferred some form of shared decision-making process. In terms of overall satisfaction with decision-making, 71 % of the respondents were either completely or very satisfied. However, the authors reported that family members who wanted to leave decisions entirely to physicians had significantly higher satisfaction scores. Factors contributing the most to satisfaction with decision-making included complete satisfaction with level of health care the patient received, completeness of information received, and feeling supported during the decision-making process. In France, where the role of surrogate is only consultative, a study reported that a desire to share in decision-making was expressed by 47 % of family members, but that only 15 % of these members actually took part in the process [17]. Interestingly, the relevance of the information provided influenced this desire. The authors concluded that French physicians should ask how much participation in decision-making the family would like to have. In contrast, a Spanish study reported that 71.7 % of family members were involved in the decision to withhold or withdraw life support therapy [18]. On the whole, families wish to be involved in decisions concerning their relative, probably because they want to be sure that any medical action taken will be consistent with the patients' wishes.

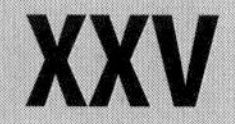

Weaknesses for the Surrogate (Table 1)

Substitute Decision-making is Dependent on Information

At least two conditions have to be fulfilled for the surrogate's role to be carried out. First, the surrogate must be informed of, and fully understand, the diagnosis, prognosis, and treatment of the patient. The information provided by the ICU team should be exact and relevant to the situation. Medical staff should agree on what information will be given. Some studies report that families were unable to take decisions because they did not have the necessary information [19]. Various tools, such as leaflets, can improve the quality of communication [20]. Second, the surrogate must be aware of the patient's wishes and properly understand them. These wishes are often expressed before the patient is admitted to hospital and subsequent changes or clarification depend on how well the physician informs the patient. Hines and colleagues reported that families have little awareness of patients' wishes, including end-of-life issues [21]. Furthermore, conversations between a patient and a surrogate about end-of-life issues did not increase the surrogate's knowledge of the patient's values or preferences [21]. This is a major limitation of substitute decision-making. A surrogate who lacks information, cannot make appropriate decisions in the patient's best interest.

The Substitute Decision-maker is not always Objective

In the process of substitute decision-making, the surrogate must give an objective account of the patient's wishes. Surrogates commonly project their own wishes onto those of the patient [22]. But the surrogate is a substitute decision-maker and not a substitute for the patient. Studies of medical scenarios showed that in only 66 % of cases was the decision of the surrogate in accordance with that of the patient [23]. The agreement rate was not affected by how the surrogate was designated and was not improved by previous discussions between surrogate and patient. Studies on the ability of family members to accurately predict a patient's consent to take part in critical research produced similar results [24]. This inaccuracy can be explained by a lack of information or misinterpretation, voluntary or not. The surrogate's decision-making is based on: (i) Conversations (knowledge of their loved ones' preferences), (ii) documents (advance directives), (iii) shared experience (believing an inner sense would guide decisions because of shared lived experiences), (iv) surrogates' own values and preferences, and (v) surrogates' network (enlisting the help of others) [25].

Surrogates' decisions are often influenced by religious convictions or spiritual values especially in times of crisis [26]. Religious values may differ but they have in common the aim of doing what is best for the patient's welfare. A fuller awareness of the major religions' basic tenets will allow the physician to understand the surrogate's beliefs and avoid conflicts that may arise from requests for inappropriate treatment [27]. Financial concerns may also influence a surrogate's decision. Medical expenses are met either by the state, as in France, or by private insurance, as in the USA. In many cases, the families of end-of-life ICU patients encounter difficulties [28] and the surrogate's decision-making process may be governed by the concern to avoid extra expense.

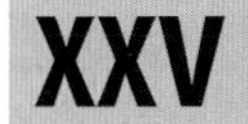

The Substitute Decision-maker can lack Capacity

The problem of capacity also concerns the surrogate. It has been suggested that a surrogate's capacity should be formally assessed but as yet there exists no valid assessment procedure [29]. Chronic or acute mental illness may prevent the surrogate from making informed and rational healthcare decisions. If the physician has serious doubts about the decision-making capacity of the surrogate, the opinion of an outside consultant or an ethics committee should be sought. Disagreement between surrogate and physician should not be considered as proof of incapacity. In the event of conflict, the physician should establish with the surrogate whether the dissension affects the patient's interests [30]. If it does so adversely, then either the physician in charge can be changed for another or the surrogate can be replaced after approval from an independent source.

It is widely documented that symptoms of anxiety, depression, and post-traumatic stress disorder are commonly observed in relatives of ICU patients, and in particular in wives [31, 32]. These psychological problems are proportionate to the extent of the family's involvement in end-of-life decisions. A recent study reported that up to 34 % of substitute decision-makers had features of psychiatric illness following their involvement in decision-making [33]. Preventing the effects of anxiety, depression, and post-traumatic stress disorder should be a priority for the medical team. A proactive communication strategy decreases these symptoms in family members of patients who die in ICU [34]. Studies are needed to assess whether this strategy could be used to decrease similar symptoms in substitute decision-makers.

Strengths for the Medical Team (Table 1)

Substitute Decision-making is the Wish of ICU Staff Members

Nurses and doctors are in favor of families being involved in decision-making. A French study reported that of 2754 ICU staff members, 91 % of physicians and 83 % of non-physicians (nurses and assistant nurses) believed that participation in decision-making should be offered to families [17]. However, only 39 % of physicians had involved family members in decisions. The authors suggest that the gap between intention and practice may indicate that ICU staff members in France are in a transitional period from paternalism to autonomy. These results show that substitute decision-making is the wish of the ICU team, but that practice is dependent on the evolving concept of patient autonomy, which differs between countries.

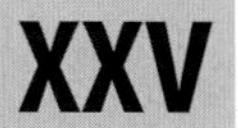

Substitute Decision-making Requires Communication with the Family

The process of substitute decision-making involves close communication between family members and the ICU team. The major communication is about information on diagnosis, prognosis and treatment. The information given by the ICU team physician is an essential element in the involvement of the family in substitute decision-making. A recent questionnaire survey reported that most surrogate decision-makers have good understanding and excellent staff communication [35]. Another study reported that adequate communication, feeling supported, and achieving the appropriate level of care for their family member were key determinants of satisfaction with decision-making in the ICU [16]. The satisfaction of surrogates and their involvement in substitute decision-making require good communication based on clear, relevant information.

Weaknesses for the Medical Team (Table 1)

The Substitute Decision-maker Requires an Assessment of Capacity

The patient's and surrogate's level of capacity is assessed by the physician, which entails several drawbacks. Physicians are not trained to make this assessment and tend to make a subjective judgement. In most cases they compare the patient's decision with that they consider to be in the patient's best interest, whereas they should assess capacity on the basis of objective, concrete facts [29]. Several ICU members could be asked to assess capacity, thereby decreasing subjectivity. Often only one assessment is made of decision-making capacity instead of regular re-assessments as the patient's condition changes.

Substitute Decision-making is an Interpretation also for Physicians

Upadya and colleagues reported substantial differences between patients, physicians, and family members in the understanding of living wills [36]. Misunderstanding of medical vocabulary and of a patient's will, can be confusing for family members. Often, the ICU physician is not the attending patient's physician and so has not had sufficient time to discuss the patient's beliefs or will arrangements. The patient's declarations can be interpreted according to the physician's own wishes and, as a result, the ICU team and the family can differ widely in their interpretation of the patient's intentions.

Strengths for the Community (Table 1)

Substitute Decision-making is the Wish of Legislators

Over the two last decades, many countries have created a legal framework for patients' rights. The legislation of these countries is consistent with the patient autonomy model [29, 37–40]. Although the laws of these countries reflect the same approach, there are several differences in the mode of designation of surrogates and in their decisional authority.

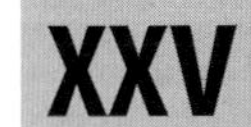

Weaknesses for the Community (Table 1)

Substitute Decision-making is not a Consensual Process

The legal power of surrogates varies between countries. In some countries, surrogates have a decisional role, while in others their role is merely consultative. In North America (US, Canada), patient-designated surrogates have a decisional role. **Figure 1** shows the legal framework of surrogacy in Belgium, Denmark, England, France, Germany, the Netherlands, Spain, and Switzerland. Of these European countries, France confers the weakest power to surrogates in decision-making [37].

The role of patient-designated surrogates is established by the laws of the country. In the absence of a specific designation, some countries appoint a surrogate according to legal hierarchy. In other countries there are no legal provisions when the patient has not designated a surrogate [37, 40]. In some countries, including England, the surrogate can have durable power of attorney. In others countries, including France, the patient is invited to designate a surrogate on each admission to hospital [37, 40].

Conclusion

The process of substitute decision-making allows physician and patient to maintain the latter's autonomy. The surrogate gives expression to the patient's values in making decisions that will be in the best interest of the patient. This represents a major advance in the doctor-patient relationship. Although patient, physician, surrogate, and the community gain a lot from the process, certain difficulties prevent it from being put into general use. Some measures could improve substitute decision-making such as developing tools to assess patients' or surrogates' decision-making capacity, preventing the projection of surrogate's wishes onto those of the patient,

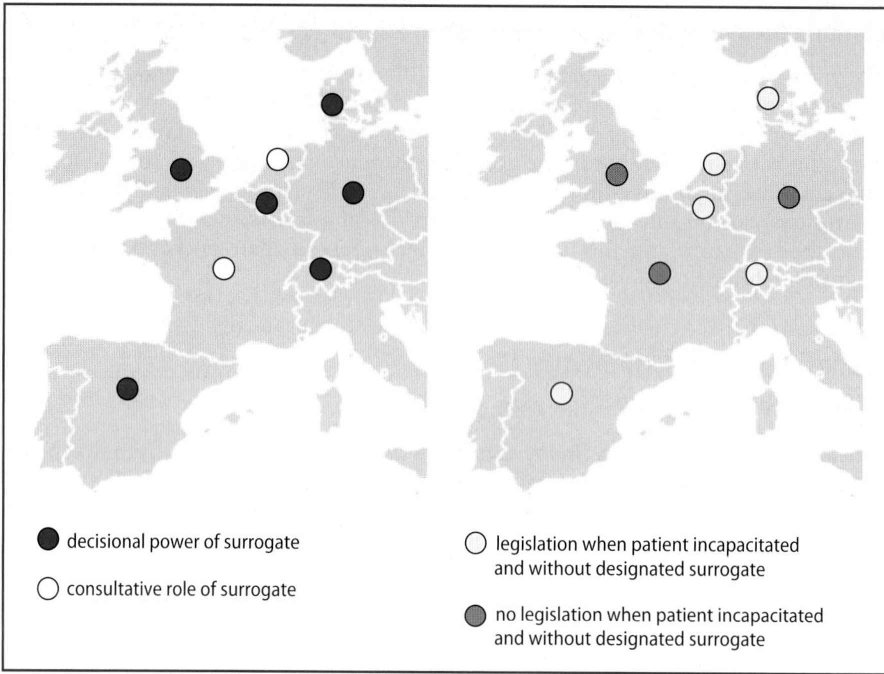

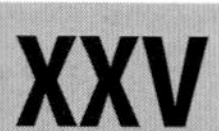

Fig. 1. Legislations in eight western European countries

removing surrogates' guilt feelings, raising the awareness of physicians and the general population, and training physicians. Anticipating the difficulties of substitute decision-making should be a priority in developing a reliable and effective process.

References

1. Schneiderman LJ, Kaplan RM, Pearlman RA, Teetzel H (1993) Do physicians' own preferences for life-sustaining treatment influence their perceptions of patients' preferences? J Clin Ethics 4: 28–33
2. Arnold RM, Kellum J (2003) Moral justifications for surrogate decision making in the intensive care unit: implications and limitations. Crit Care Med 31:S347–353
3. Appelbaum PS (2007) Clinical practice. Assessment of patients' competence to consent to treatment. N Engl J Med 357: 1834–1840.
4. Teno J, Lynn J, Wenger N, Phillips RS, et al (1997) Advance directives for seriously ill hospitalized patients: effectiveness with the patient self-determination act and the SUPPORT intervention. SUPPORT Investigators. Study to Understand Prognoses and Preferences for Outcomes and Risks of Treatment. J Am Geriatr Soc 45: 500–507
5. Collins LG, Parks SM, Winter L (2006) The state of advance care planning: one decade after SUPPORT. Am J Hosp Palliat Care 23: 378–384
6. Morrison RS, Olson E, Mertz KR, Meier DE (1995) The inaccessibility of advance directives on transfer from ambulatory to acute care settings. JAMA 274: 478–482
7. Prendergast TJ (2001) Advance care planning: pitfalls, progress, promise. Crit Care Med 29: N34–39
8. Covinsky KE, Goldman L, Cook EF, et al (1994) The impact of serious illness on patients' families. SUPPORT Investigators. Study to Understand Prognoses and Preferences for Outcomes and Risks of Treatment. JAMA 272: 1839–1844

9. Ferrand E, Bachoud-Levi AC, Rodrigues M, Maggiore S, Brun-Buisson C, Lemaire F (2001) Decision-making capacity and surrogate designation in French ICU patients. Intensive Care Med 27: 1360–1364
10. Puchalski CM, Zhong Z, Jacobs MM, et al (2000) Patients who want their family and physician to make resuscitation decisions for them: observations from SUPPORT and HELP. Study to Understand Prognoses and Preferences for Outcomes and Risks of Treatment. Hospitalized Elderly Longitudinal Project. J Am Geriatr Soc 48:S84–90
11. Sehgal A, Galbraith A, Chesney M, Schoenfeld P, Charles G, Lo B (1992) How strictly do dialysis patients want their advance directives followed? JAMA 267: 59–63
12. Emanuel EJ, Fuchs VR (2008) Who really pays for health care? The myth of "shared responsibility". JAMA 299: 1057–1059
13. White DB, Curtis JR, Lo B, Luce JM (2006) Decisions to limit life-sustaining treatment for critically ill patients who lack both decision-making capacity and surrogate decision-makers. Crit Care Med 34: 2053–2059
14. Emanuel EJ, Emanuel LL (1992) Proxy decision making for incompetent patients. An ethical and empirical analysis. JAMA 267: 2067–2071
15. Azoulay E, Pochard F, Chevret S, et al (2003) Opinions about surrogate designation: a population survey in France. Crit Care Med 31: 1711–1714
16. Heyland DK, Cook DJ, Rocker GM, et al (2003) Decision-making in the ICU: perspectives of the substitute decision-maker. Intensive Care Med 29: 75–82
17. Azoulay E, Pochard F, Chevret S, et al (2004) Half the family members of intensive care unit patients do not want to share in the decision-making process: a study in 78 French intensive care units. Crit Care Med 32: 1832–1838
18. Esteban A, Gordo F, Solsona JF, et al (2001) Withdrawing and withholding life support in the intensive care unit: a Spanish prospective multi-centre observational study. Intensive Care Med 27: 1744–1749
19. Nelson JE, Mercado AF, Camhi SL, et al (2007) Communication about chronic critical illness. Arch Intern Med 167: 2509–2515
20. Azoulay E, Pochard F, Chevret S, et al (2002) Impact of a family information leaflet on effectiveness of information provided to family members of intensive care unit patients: a multicenter, prospective, randomized, controlled trial. Am J Respir Crit Care Med 165: 438–442
21. Hines SC, Glover JJ, Babrow AS, Holley JL, Badzek LA, Moss AH (2001) Improving advance care planning by accommodating family preferences. J Palliat Med 4: 481–489
22. Fagerlin A, Ditto PH, Danks JH, Houts RM, Smucker WD (2001) Projection in surrogate decisions about life-sustaining medical treatments. Health Psychol 20: 166–175
23. Shalowitz DI, Garrett-Mayer E, Wendler D (2006) The accuracy of surrogate decision makers: a systematic review. Arch Intern Med 166: 493–497
24. Ciroldi M, Cariou A, Adrie C, et al (2007) Ability of family members to predict patient's consent to critical care research. Intensive Care Med 33: 807–813
25. Vig EK, Taylor JS, Starks H, Hopley EK, Fryer-Edwards K (2006) Beyond substituted judgment: How surrogates navigate end-of-life decision-making. J Am Geriatr Soc 54: 1688–1693
26. Ankeny RA, Clifford R, Jordens CF, Kerridge IH, Benson R (2005) Religious perspectives on withdrawal of treatment from patients with multiple organ failure. Med J Aust 183: 616–621
27. Orr RD, Genesen LB (1997) Requests for "inappropriate" treatment based on religious beliefs. J Med Ethics 23: 142–147
28. Cuthbertson SJ, Margetts MA, Streat SJ (2000) Bereavement follow-up after critical illness. Crit Care Med 28: 1196–1201
29. Welie SP, Dute J, Nys H, van Wijmen FC (2005) Patient incompetence and substitute decision-making: an analysis of the role of the health care professional in Dutch law. Health Policy 73: 21–40
30. Bramstedt KA (2003) Questioning the decision-making capacity of surrogates. Intern Med J 33: 257–259
31. Pochard F, Azoulay E, Chevret S, et al (2001) Symptoms of anxiety and depression in family members of intensive care unit patients: ethical hypothesis regarding decision-making capacity. Crit Care Med 29: 1893–1897
32. Azoulay E, Pochard F, Kentish-Barnes N, et al (2005) Risk of post-traumatic stress symptoms in family members of intensive care unit patients. Am J Respir Crit Care Med 171: 987–994

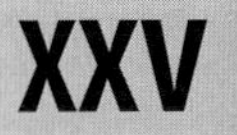

33. Siegel MD, Hayes E, Vanderwerker LC, Loseth DB, Prigerson HG (2008) Psychiatric illness in the next of kin of patients who die in the intensive care unit. Crit Care Med 36: 1722–1728
34. Lautrette A, Darmon M, Megarbane B, et al (2007) A communication strategy and brochure for relatives of patients dying in the ICU. N Engl J Med 356: 469–478
35. Rodriguez RM, Navarrete E, Schwaber J, et al (2008) A prospective study of primary surrogate decision makers' knowledge of intensive care. Crit Care Med 36: 1633–1636
36. Upadya A, Muralidharan V, Thorevska N, Amoateng-Adjepong Y, Manthous CA (2002) Patient, physician, and family member understanding of living wills. Am J Respir Crit Care Med 166: 1430–1435
37. French Senate (2004) Patients rights at the end-of-life in European countries. Comparative Law Study n°139, November 2004. Available at: http://www.senat.fr/lc/lc139/lc1390.html Accessed Nov 2008
38. French Public Health Code, law of 4 March 2002 on Patients Rights, article: L1111. Available at: http://www.legifrance.gouv.fr/affichTexte.do?cidTexte=JORFTEXT000000227015&dateTexte =Accessed Nov 2008
39. Jox RJ, Michalowski S, Lorenz J, Schildmann J (2008) Substitute decision making in medicine: comparative analysis of the ethico-legal discourse in England and Germany. Med Health Care Philos 11: 153–163
40. Truog, RD, Campbell ML, Curtis JR, et al (2008) Recommendations for end-of-life care in the intensive care unit: a consensus statement by the American College of Critical Care Medicine. Crit Care Med 36: 953–963

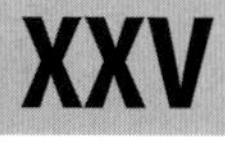

Subject Index

Printing and Binding: Stürtz GmbH, Würzburg